Exotic Animal Hematology and Cytology

FIFTH EDITION

Exotic Animal Hematology and Cytology

■ FIFTH EDITION

TERRY W. CAMPBELL, DVM, PHD

Associate Professor Emeritus of Zoological Medicine
College of Veterinary Medicine and Biomedical Sciences
Colorado State University
Fort Collins, CO, USA

Former Head Veterinarian, Downtown Aquarium, Denver, CO, USA

KRYSTAN R. GRANT, DVM, PHD, CERTAQV

Director of Pet Health, PetSmart Home Office
Phoenix, AZ, USA

WILEY Blackwell

This fifth edition first published 2022

Edition History
Iowa State University Press (1e, 1988); Iowa State University Press (2e, 1992); Blackwell Publishing Professional (3e, 2007); Wiley Blackwell (4e, 2015)

Registered Office
John Wiley & Sons, Inc., 111 River Street, Hoboken, NJ 07030, USA

Editorial Office
111 River Street, Hoboken, NJ 07030, USA

For details of our global editorial offices, customer services, and more information about Wiley products visit us at www.wiley.com.

Wiley also publishes its books in a variety of electronic formats and by print-on-demand. Some content that appears in standard print versions of this book may not be available in other formats.

Library of Congress Cataloging-in-Publication Data

Names: Campbell, Terry W., 1949– author. | Grant, Krystan R., author.
Title: Exotic animal hematology and cytology / Terry W. Campbell, Krystan R. Grant.
Description: Fifth edition. | Hoboken, NJ : Wiley-Blackwell, 2022. | Includes bibliographical references and index.
Identifiers: LCCN 2021045164 (print) | LCCN 2021045165 (ebook) | ISBN 9781119660231 (hardback) | ISBN 9781119660248 (adobe pdf) | ISBN 9781119660262 (epub)
Subjects: MESH: Animal Diseases–diagnosis | Animals, Domestic–physiology | Pets–physiology | Hematologic Tests–veterinary | Cytodiagnosis–veterinary | Case Reports
Classification: LCC SF997.5.E95 (print) | LCC SF997.5.E95 (ebook) | NLM SF 997.5.E95 | DDC 636.089/607561–dc23
LC record available at https://lccn.loc.gov/2021045164
LC ebook record available at https://lccn.loc.gov/2021045165

Cover Design: Wiley
Cover Image: © Krystan R. Grant, Terry W. Campbell

Set in 11/12pt TimesLTStd by Straive, Pondicherry, India
Printed and bound by CPI Group (UK) Ltd, Croydon CR0 4YY

C9781119660231_260124

CONTENTS

PREFACE

This book is the latest edition of a book that was first published in 1988 with the original title, *Avian Hematology and Cytology*. Since then, the book has developed into a more comprehensive reference on exotic animal hematology and cytology with a focus on the most common species of small mammals, birds, reptiles, amphibians, and fish seen in exotic pet practice. This edition has been completely reorganized from the previous edition. The new structure of this book is based upon the suggestions from users of the previous edition and their preferred organization to the book.

The book is divided into four sections that are assembled into the basic animal groupings: Section I Mammals; Section II Avian; Section III Herptile; and Section IV Fish. Each section follows the same pattern of chapter order with the exception of Section IV Fish. Each section begins with chapters dealing with hematology followed by chapters involving cytodiagnosis. The hematology portions begin with blood sample collection for hematology (which include bone marrow sampling); hematologic techniques; evaluation of the peripheral blood; evaluation of hematopoiesis; and hematology clinical case presentations. The cytodiagnosis portions begin with sample collection for cytodiagnosis; cytodiagnosis; and clinical case presentations in cytodiagnosis. Section III Herptile has separate chapters for reptile and amphibian evaluation of the peripheral blood. Section IV Fish includes separate chapters for wet-mount studies beginning with sample collection for wet mounts and followed by wet-mount evaluation and clinical case presentation in piscine wet mounts.

The hematology chapters discuss erythrocyte, leukocyte, and thrombocyte (platelet) morphology and their responses to disease with updated references. Representations of normal and abnormal hemic cytology are provided. Abnormal hemic cytology includes identification and meaning of toxic neutrophils and heterophils, immature cells, and leukemic cells. Commonly seen blood parasites on blood films are also represented.

The cytodiagnosis chapters provide updated information involving the basic cellular responses (normal, inflammatory, hyperplasia, and malignant neoplasia) observed in samples obtained from exotic animal patients as well as the cytology of the various body systems. Along with description and interpretation of the cellular responses, major species differences, the cytology of effusions, and identification of the commonly seen etiologic agents are also provided.

There are also changes and additions to the appendices. Appendix B, comprising hematology and cytochemical staining tables, is updated to include additional studies. Appendix C is new. This section provides color plates of representative hemic cells from the basic animal groupings (mammals, birds, reptiles, amphibians, and fish). This serves as an atlas for those wishing for quick access to examples of hemic cells in exotic animals. Appendix D is new. This section provides an overview of common artifacts observed in blood films and cytologic samples. Although information provided in Appendices C and D are found throughout the text, these appendices compile and present the cells and artifacts and serve as a quick guide.

As with previous editions, this book is designed to provide a reference for those engaged in exotic animal practice, especially when laboratory testing is performed on site. The target audience not only includes veterinarians and veterinary technicians in clinical practice, but also clinical pathologists, laboratory technicians, veterinary students, veterinary pathologists, wildlife rehabilitators, and those engaged in exotic animal research.

A good-quality microscope is one of the most useful diagnostic tools available for veterinarians engaged in clinical practice. This book, positioned beside the microscope, will not only provide a quick reference to the various types of cells observed in blood films and cytological samples from exotic animal patients, but will also be a resource for understanding and interpreting laboratory results and explaining the pathologic diagnosis.

ACKNOWLEDGMENTS

I was once called "a scope jockey," and I suppose I am. I love peering through the lenses of a microscope, especially when searching for the meaning behind the assortment of cells harvested from my animal patients. The author Bill Bryson once wrote, "The basic challenge of any book is you know you're going to be working on it for three or four years or more. So, you want to have a subject that will keep you engaged." For me, that subject is hematology and cytology. However, this edition of my book, *Exotic Animal Hematology and Cytology*, would not have been possible without my coauthor, Dr. Krystan Grant. When I was asked by the publisher to write another edition to this book, I thought about Bill Bryson's words and the time and effort that went into the production of the previous editions. Mentioning this to Dr. Grant, her response was, "you should do it!" I replied, "I'll only do it with you as my coauthor." So, here we are.

I have known Dr. Grant since her senior year at Colorado State University as she was finishing her degree in veterinary medicine from Ross University School of Veterinary Medicine in St. Kitts, West Indies. When we first met, I had just returned from vacationing in St. John, U.S. Virgin Islands, and she was starting her rotation in my service in zoological medicine. At that time, I would tell folks that they should feel sorry for me as I had just returned from the Caribbean. When they laughed, I explained that the reason I deserve their pity was that I knew what I was missing now that I had returned to my normal life. I was half joking, of course; however, my new student from Ross University understood the serious part of my plea for sympathy. Recognition of a mutual Caribbean soul was the beginning of a close kinship.

Although I was trained in clinical pathology, my veterinary career involved clinical exotic animal medicine. When it came to honing cytological skills, I felt a distinct advantage in being involved with each animal patient from the time of presentation in the examination room to sample collection and processing, and finally the microscopic assessment of the material collected with the aid of the clinical workup as well as information obtained from pathology. Along the way, it has been an inspirational experience working with clinical pathologists at Kansas State University and Colorado State University as together, we explored the world of comparative clinical pathology.

This book and its previous editions would not be possible without having animal patients and their varying diseases to teach me along the way. Therefore, I dedicate this book to all the animal patients out there in the world guiding humankind to a better understanding of veterinary medicine.

Terry W. Campbell, DVM, PHD

Nearly 17 years ago, I had finished an intense first week of clinics as a fourth-year veterinary student and was wondering what I had gotten myself into by going back to vet school for a second career. I had no idea what to expect during the next week on the exotics service. I was sitting in the zoo med ward eagerly waiting for the next clinician and in walked Dr. Campbell. I'll never forget his opening statement giving me my first (and lasting) impression of him: "You all should be kind and feel sorry for me as I've recently returned from a vacation in St. John, the U.S. Virgin Islands, and therefore know what I'm missing out on." Little did I know then that I would be fortunate to enjoy a flurry of dad jokes, learn more than I ever knew existed about cells, and gain a trusted Caribbean-soul friend and colleague with whom I would travel, learn, and teach with for decades to come. His passion and enthusiasm for clinical pathology is infectious; therefore, it didn't take me long to understand the value and adopt that passion. Of course, when he asked me to join him on this edition, I was honored and humbly agreed. The year or so of collaboration did not disappoint – I've learned and laughed more – so, thank you, Terry. I appreciate your encouragement, inspiration, and introduction to a world that has enriched my life.

To those whose support granted me the time, focus, and energy to stay on track: Adwyn Lim, Kristi Yee, Greg Costanzo, and Lee Chichester. Adwyn, thank you for cooking dinner for me nearly every day for six months during the home stretch of this project. Kristi, thank you for being a sounding board, keeping things real, and upgrading to Köhler illumination. Greg and Lee, I appreciate your solidarity especially in times for when the sun is getting real low – thank you for everything you have done this past year while I worked on this project.

Finally, our commitment and completion of this project (as well as all of our other projects) are reflections of the commitment and never-ending support from our spouses, Susie Campbell and Paul Grant. Susie, thanks (again and again) for putting up with our shenanigans and sharing in some of the adventure – you are a saint! Paul, first of all, thank you for your willingness to help – for your time spent on Appendix C and for reviewing and editing for continuity! But most importantly, thank you for the love, care, and comfort you provide me and the crew; your ingenuity to get us where we need to go; and your acceptance and partnership with all my ideas, projects, and animals that you helped care for with me. I'm so glad you talked me into taking the plunge to the island! I appreciate and love you more, obviously.

Krystan R. Grant, DVM, PHD, CERTAQV

ABOUT THE COMPANION WEBSITE

This book is accompanied by a companion website:

www.wiley.com/go/campbell/exotic

The website includes:

- Video clips
- Case Studies
- Additional hematologic values tables (Appendix B): Erythrocyte and Leukocyte parameters for selected Elasmobranchs

SCIENTIFIC NAMES

Mammals

African hedgehog (*Atelerix albiventris*)
African lion (*Panthera leo*)
Bengal tiger (*Panthera tigris tigris*)
Chinchilla (*Chinchilla lanigera*)
Cottontail rabbit (*Sylvilagus floridanus*)
Domestic dog (*Canis lupus familiaris*)
Domestic ferret (*Mustela putorius furo*)
Domestic mouse (*Mus musculus*)
Domestic rabbit (*Oryctolagus cuniculus*)
Domestic rat (*Rattus norvegicus*)
Gerbil (*Meriones unguiculatus*)
Goeldi's monkey (*Callimico goeldii*)
Guinea pig (*Cavia porcellus*)
Hamster (*Mesocricetus auratus*)
Horse (*Equus caballus*)
Leopard (*Panthera pardus*)
Macacque (*Macaca arctoides*)
North American river otter (*Lontra canadensis*)
River otter (*Lontra canadensis*)
Sugar glider (*Petaurus breviceps*)

Birds

African Gray parrot (*Psittacus erithacus*)
Atlantic puffin (*Fratercula arctica*)
Bald eagle (*Haliaeetus leucocephalus*)
Barn owl (*Tyto alba*)
Barred owl (*Strix varia*)
Black-neck stilt (*Himantopus mexicanus*)
Black-throated laughing thrush (*Garrulax chinensis*)
Blue and gold macaw (*Ara ararauna*)
Blue-fronted amazon parrot (*Amazona aestiva*)
Blue-headed pionus parrot (*Pionus menstruus*)
Blue-throated macaw (*Ara glaucogularis*)
Buderigar (*Melopsittacus undulatus*)
Burrowing owl (*Athene cunicularia*)
Cape parrot (*Poicephalus robustus*)
Caribbean flamingo (*Phoenicopterus ruber*)
Chinese crested goose (*Anser cygnoid*)
Chukar (*Alectoris chukar*)
Cockatiel (*Nymphicus hollandicus*)
Domestic chicken (*Gallus gallus domesticus*)
Domestic duck (*Anas platyrhynchos domestica*)
Domestic turkey (*Meleagris gallopova*)
Eclectus parrot (*Eclectus roratus*)
Emu (*Dromaius novaehollandiae*)
Ferruginous hawk (*Buteo regalis*)
Gannet (*Morus* sp.)
Gentoo penguin (*Pygoscelis papua*)
Goffin cockatoo (*Cacatua goffiniana*)
Golden eagle (*Aquila chrysaetos*)
Great horned owl (*Bubo virginianus*)
Greater Indian hill mynah (*Gracula religiosa intermedia*)
Green-cheeked conure (*Pyrrhura molinae*)
Green-wing macaw (*Ara chloropterus*)
Grey-cheeked parakeet (*Brotogeris pyrrhoptera*)
Gyrfalcon (*Falco rusticolus*)
Hyacinth macaw (*Anodorhynchus hyacinthinus*)
Java Rice bird (*Lonchura oryzivora*)
Kestrel (*Falco sparverius*)
Lesser sulfur crested cockatoo (*Cacatua sulphurea*)
Magpie (*Pica pica*)
Mallard duck (*Anas platyrhynchos*)
Military macaw (*Ara militaris*)
Moluccan (or salmon-crested) cockatoo (*Cacatua moluccensis*)
Northern flicker (*Colaptes auratus*)
Northern goshawk (*Accipiter gentilis*)
Orange-winged Amazon parrot (*Amazona amazonica*)
Peach-faced lovebird (*Agapornis roseicollis*)
Peregrine falcon (*Falco peregrinus*)
Pine siskin (*Carduelis pinus*)
Quail (*Colinus* sp.)
Red-tailed hawk (*Buteo jamaicensis*)
Rock dove, pigeon (*Columba livia*)
Rose-ringed parakeet (*Psittacula krameri*)
Skua (*Stercorarius* sp.)
Spectacled Amazon parrot (*Amazona albifrons*)
Sun conure (*Aratinga solstitialis*)
Swainson's hawk (*Buteo swainsoni*)

Thick-billed parrot (*Rhynchopsitta pachyrhyncha*)
Timneh African gray parrot (*Psittacus erithacus timneh*)
Turkey vulture (*Cathartes aura*)
Umbrella cockatoo (*Cacatua alba*)
Western screech owl (*Megascops kennicottii*)
White-winged wood duck (*Cairina scutulata*)
Wild turkey (*Meleagris gallopavo*)
Wrinkled hornbill (*Aceros corrugatus*)
Yellow-headed Amazon parrot (*Amazona oratrix*)
Yellow-naped Amazon parrot (*Amazona auropalliata*)

Reptiles
Bearded dragon (*Pogona vitticeps*)
Alligator snapping turtle (*Macrochelys temminckii*)
American alligator (*Alligator mississippiensis*)
Ball python (*Python regius*)
Burmese mountain tortoise (*Manouria emys*)
Burmese python snake (*Python bivittatus*)
California kingsnake (*Lampropeltis getula californiae*)
Common boa constrictor (*Boa constrictor*)
Common snapping turtle (*Chelydra serpentina*)
Corn snake (*Elaphe [Pantherophis] guttata*)
Cuvier's dwarf caiman (*Paleosuchus palpebrosus*)
Desert tortoise (*Gopherus agassizii*)
Emerald tree boa (*Corallus caninus*)
Gila monster (*Heloderma suspectum*)
Green iguana (*Iguana iguana*)
Green sea turtle (*Chelonia mydas*)
Green tree python (*Morelia viridis*)
Hognose snake (*Heterodon platirhinos*)
Jackson's chameleon lizard (*Trioceros jacksonii*)
Jungle carpet python (*Morelia spilota cheynei*)
Leopard gecko (*Eublepharis macularius*)
Leopard tortoise (*Stigmochelys pardalis*)
Loggerhead sea turtle (*Caretta caretta*)
Malayan box turtle (*Cuora amboinensis*)
New Guinea snapping turtle (*Elseya novaeguineae*)
Painted terrapin (*Batagur borneoensis*)
Ramsay's (or Woma) python (*Aspidites ramsayi*)
Red-eared slider (*Trachemys scripta elegans*)
Red-footed tortoise (*Chelonoidis carbonaria*)
Reeve's (or Chinese pond) turtle (*Chinemys reevesii*)
Spectacled caiman (*Caiman crocodilus*)
Spiny soft-shelled turtle (*Apalone spinifera*)
Spiny-tailed lizard (*Uromastyx* sp.)
Sulcata tortoise (*Centrochelys sulcata*)
Tegu (*Salvator merianae*)
Three-toed box turtle (*Terrapene carolina triunguis*)
Timber rattlesnake (*Crotalus horridus*)
Veiled chameleon (*Chamaeleo calyptratus*)
Water dragon (*Intellagama lesueurii*)
Western diamond back rattlesnake (*Crotalus atrox*)
Wood turtle (*Glyptemys insculpta*)
Yellow-footed tortoise (*Chelonoidis denticulata*)
Yellow pond turtle (*Mauremys mutica*)

Amphibians
African clawed frog (*Xenopus laevis*)
Argentine horned frog (*Ceratophrys ornate*)
Boreal toad (*Bufo boreas boreas*)
Colorado river toad (*Incilius alvarius*)
Cuban treefrog (*Osteopilus septentrionalis*)
Fire belly newt (*Cynops pyrrhogaster*)
Hellbender (*Cryptobranchus alleganiensis*)
Poison dart frog (family Dendrobatidae)
Rough skinned newt (*Taricha granulosa*)
Tiger salamander (*Ambystoma tigrinum*)
White's tree frog (*Litoria caerulea*)
Woodhouse toad (*Bufo woodhousii*)

Fish
Atlantic spadefish (*Chaetodipterus faber*)
Atlantic stingray (*Hypanus sabinus*)
Banded rainbow fish (*Melanotaenia trifasciata*)
Black surf perch (*Embiotica jacksoni*)
Black tip reef shark (*Carcharhinus melanopterus*)
Boeseman's rainbowfish (*Melanotaenia boesemani*)
Brook trout (*Salvelinus fontinalis*)
Carp, Koi (*Cyprinus carpio*)
Channel catfish (*Ictalurus punctatus*)
Clown knifefish (*Chitala chitala*)
Cownose ray (*Rhinoptera bonasus*)
Cutthroat trout (*Oncorhynchus clarkii*)
Damselfish (*Pomacentridae*)
Dwarf Gourami (*Trichogaster lalius*)
Electric yellow cichlid (*Labidochromis caeruleus*)
Flasher wrasse (*Paracheilinus carpenteri*)
French grunt (*Haemulon flavolineatum*)
Freshwater angelfish (*Pterophyllum scalare*)
Goldfish (*Carassius auratus*)
Green moray eels (*Gymnothorax funebris*)
Green sunfish (*Lepomis cyanellus*)
Guppy (*Poecilia reticulate*)
Iridescent shark catfish (*Pangasianodon hypophthalmus*)
Leopoldi stingray (*Potamotrygon leopoldi*)
Lionfish (*Pterois volitans/miles*)
Lumpfish (*Cyclopterus lumpus*)
Neon Tetra (*Paracheirodon innesi*)
Northern pike (*Esox lucius*)
Nurse shark (*Ginglymostoma cirratum*)
Oyster toadfish (*Opsanus tau*)
Orbicular batfish (*Platax orbicularis*)
Peacock flounder (*Bothus lunatus*)
Pepper cory catfish (*Corydoras paleatus*)
Plecostomus (*Hypostomus plecostomus*)
Rainbow trout (*Oncorhynchus mykiss*)
Red Oscar (*Astronotus ocellatus*)
Red-eye tetra (*Moenkhausia sanctaefilomenae*)
Red-tailed catfish (*Phractocephalus hemioliopterus*)
Regal tang (*Paracanthurus hepatus*)
Reticulate whipray (*Himantura uarnak*)
Round-tailed chub (*Gila robusta*)

Sandbar shark (*Carcharhinus plumbeus*)
Sand tiger shark (*Carcharias taurus*)
Seahorse (*Hippocampus* sp.)
Sharpnose puffer (*Canthigaster* sp)
Siamese fighting fish (*Betta splendens*)
Southern stingray (*Hypanus americanus* formerly *Dasyatis americana*)
Swordtail fish (*Xiphophorous hellerii*)
Tiger barb (*Puntigrus tetrazona*)
Tinfoil barb (*Barbonymus schwanenefeldii*)
Walleye (*Sander vitreus*)
White spotted bamboo shark (*Chiloscyllium plagiosum*)
White sturgeon (*Acipenser transmontanus*)
White tip reef shark (*Triaenodon obesus*)
Wolf eel (*Anarrhichthys ocellatus*)
Yellow tang (*Zebrasoma flavescens*)
Zebra shark (*Stegostoma fasciatum*)

SECTION I

Mammal

1 Blood and Bone Marrow Sample Collection and Preparation in Small Mammals

Blood Sample Collection

Blood sample collection is often challenging in small exotic mammals because they can be difficult to restrain, they lack superficial vessels, and the deeper vessels may be covered with fat. As many of these animals are prey species, the process of blood collection will be stressful to the patient. Successful blood collection from small rodents depends in part on successful restraint. Appropriate restraint is accomplished by either manual or chemical means. To reduce the amount of stress on the patient and if restraint is contraindicated, sedation or anesthesia is recommended. In some cases, chemical restraint may be required in order to safely handle the animal (e.g., primates) for blood collection. Injectable, inhaled, and topical approaches, independently or in combination depending on the conditions of the patient, should be considered. The use of chemicals for sedation or anesthesia can alter hematologic parameters, such as packed cell volume, and are discussed in more detail by animal type in Chapter 3. Formal training of the phlebotomist is desirable when obtaining blood samples from some animals in order to prevent the use of frequent or multiple anesthesia and blood sampling. A number of collection sites may be used to obtain blood from small exotic mammals.

Blood Volume Collection

Prior to blood collection, a physical examination should be performed, needed supplies should be gathered in advance, and sample processing and desired diagnostic tests should be determined. Determining and prioritizing diagnostic tests is important to provide a clear understanding of sample processing, given that only a small amount of blood may be obtained. The health status of the animal and its body weight will aid in the determination of the maximum amount of blood that can be safely collected. Often a total blood volume can be estimated given the body weight in kilograms of the animal (Table 1.1). For example, the blood volume of a healthy rabbit is between 5.5% and 7% of the body weight, and up to 10% of the total blood volume may be safely removed at any one time. In general, the maximum amount of blood that can be safely drawn from a patient during a single blood draw is about 10% of the total blood volume or approximately 1% of the total body weight. For example, a blood sample volume of 1.2 mL could be safely withdrawn from a healthy, adult sugar glider weighing 120 g (Johnson-Delaney, 2021). For compromised patients, it is recommended to collect a smaller sample size, such as 0.5% of the total body weight (Smith et al., 2015). The amount of the blood that may pool in a hematoma should also be considered as part of the amount of blood lost from the patient's total blood volume (Mitchell, 2011). The patient's total blood volume will be restored within 24 h of blood collection in most healthy mammals; however, it may take 2 weeks for all of the blood constituents to return to normal. If it is necessary to collect blood from a patient more frequently than every 2 weeks, a smaller sample size (such as 0.5% of the body weight) should be drawn. A maximum of 25% may be removed over a 2-week period (Cooke, 2000). The blood collected from small mammals is typically placed in lithium heparin because the blood sample volume is so small. The heparinized blood sample can then be used for both hematologic studies and clinical chemistries.

Exotic Animal Hematology and Cytology, Fifth Edition. Terry W. Campbell and Krystan R. Grant.

Companion website: www.wiley.com/go/campbell/exotic

Table 1.1. Blood collection sites and sample volumes for select small mammals.

Species and body weight (BW) range of adults	Collection sites	Blood volume (BV)	Maximum sample volume*
Mice *Mus musculus* (20–63 g)	Lateral saphenous vein Femoral vein Jugular vein Lateral tail vein Ventral tail artery	63–80 mL/kg	7.5–10% BV
Rats *Rattus norvegicus* (225–500 g)	Lateral saphenous vein Femoral vein Jugular vein Lateral tail vein Ventral tail artery Cephalic vein Dorsal tail vein Cranial vena cava	58–70 mL/kg	7.5–10% BV
Gerbils *Meriones unguiculatus* (70–130 g)	Cranial vena cava Lateral saphenous vein Cephalic vein Jugular vein	60–85 mL/kg	7.5–10% BV
Syrian hamsters *Mesocricetus auratus* (87–130 g)	Cranial vena cava Lateral saphenous vein Cephalic vein Jugular vein Gingival vein	65–80 mL/kg	7.5–10% BV
Rabbits *Oryctolagus cuniculus* (varies)	Lateral saphenous vein Cephalic vein Jugular vein Marginal ear vein Central ear artery	5.5–7% BW	7.7 mL/kg
Guinea pigs *Cavia porcellus* (700–1200 g)	Jugular vein Lateral saphenous vein Cephalic vein Gingival vein	70 mL/kg	7–10% BV
Chinchillas *Chinchilla lanigera* (450–900 g)	Jugular vein Lateral saphenous vein Cephalic vein Femoral vein	—	1% BW
Sugar gliders *Petaurus breviceps* (80–160 g)	Jugular vein Cranial vena cava Medial tibial artery Cephalic vein Lateral saphenous vein Femoral vein Ventral coccygeal vein	—	1% BW
Hedgehogs *Atelerix albiventris* (300–600 g)	Jugular vein Femoral vein Lateral saphenous vein Cephalic vein Cranial vena cava	—	1% BW
Ferrets *Mustela putorius furo* (500–2000 g)	Jugular vein Cranial vena cava Lateral saphenous vein Cephalic vein Tail artery (rarely used)	5–6% BW	7.5–10% BV

* From a healthy patient
Sources: Campbell (2015); Quesenberry et al. (2021); NIH (2019).

Restraint and Collection Sites

Myomorphs or True Rodents: Mice (*Mus musculus*), Rats (*Rattus norvegicus*), Gerbils (*Meriones unguiculatus*), Hamsters (*Mesocricetus auratus*)

Blood can be collected from most of the small rodents via the cephalic vein, lateral saphenous vein, lateral tail veins, ventral tail artery (rats), jugular veins, cranial vena cava, femoral vein, and gingival veins. When performing blood collection in small rodents, the patient should be sedated or immobilized, either manually or in some type of a restraint device (a plastic syringe case works well: the patient is placed headfirst into the case) (Machholz et al., 2012; Lindstrom et al., 2015; Frohlich, 2021; Miwa and Mayer, 2021). One hind limb can then be extended by firmly grasping the skin of the leg around the stifle. Simply grasping the skin in this manner often provides sufficient pressure to hold the saphenous vein for venipuncture. If possible, a tourniquet (using a rubber band and hemostat) may be applied to the leg of larger rodents, such as rats. Hair may be shaved from the lateral aspect of the tibia to expose the vein, or the hair may be wetted down with alcohol to facilitate visualization. The vessel is then either punctured with a small-gauge needle and blood is allowed to drip into microcapillary tubes or a microcontainer, or cannulated with a small-gauge needle. Following cannulation, blood is then allowed to drip from the needle hub into a microcollection device. The lateral saphenous vein is typically small and will easily collapse, making the collection of large sample volumes difficult. Similarly, the cephalic vein may be used for blood collection or catheter placement following the same approach used for other domestic mammals, like the dog or cat (Figures 1.1a and 1.1b).

The lateral tail veins can be used to collect blood from gerbils, mice, and rats. The animals need to be sedated or restrained as described above. Consideration must be taken when handling or restraining gerbils to avoid degloving their tails. The veins are located dorsolaterally on either side of the tail and can be dilated by placing the tail under a heat lamp or applying a warm compress prior to blood collection. Occlude the veins by placing a tourniquet at the base of the tail, and use a small-gauge needle attached to a small-sized syringe (e.g., an insulin syringe) to collect the blood sample (Figure 1.2). If the vessels are small, it may be necessary to simply cannulate the vessel with a small-gauge needle, and collect the blood sample in a microcollection device via the drip technique.

The ventral tail artery of rats may be used for blood collection. The rat must be adequately restrained or anesthetized and placed in dorsal recumbency in order to collect blood from this site. The artery is located slightly off the ventral midline of the tail and should be cannulated with a small-gauge needle attached to a 1- or 3-mL syringe with the plunger removed. Insert the needle at a 30° angle at a point approximately one-third the length of the tail from the base of the tail. Once the artery is entered, blood should enter the syringe barrel due to

(a) (b)

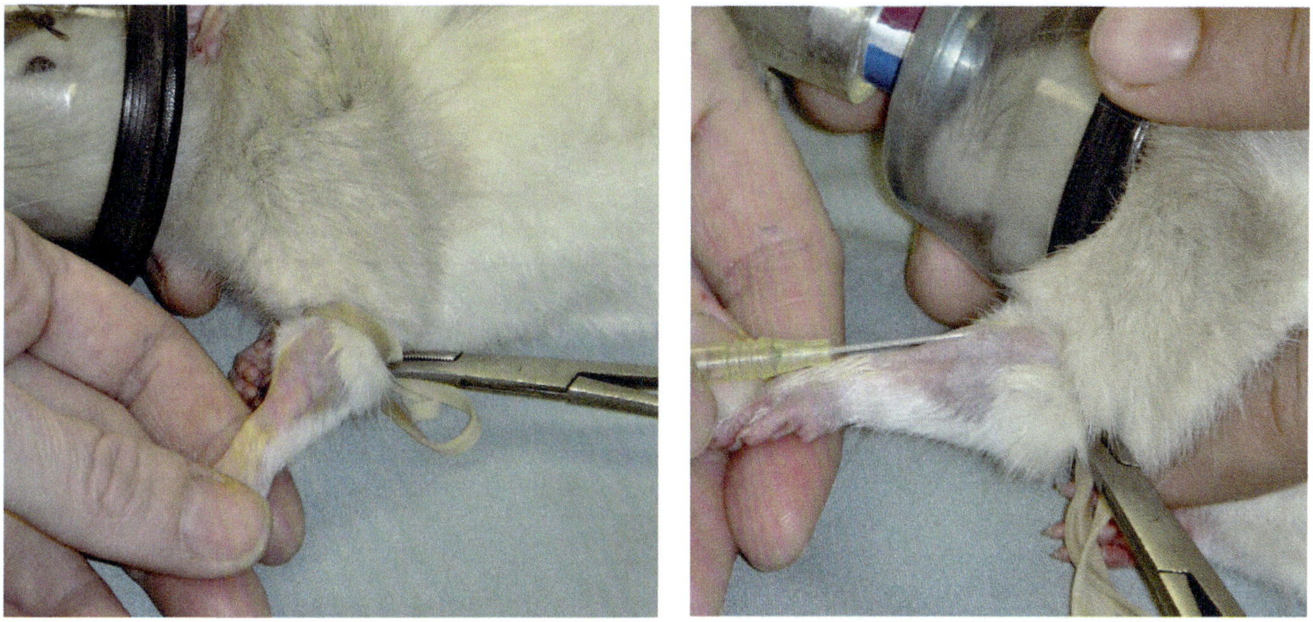

Fig. 1.1. This image shows the approach of using the cephalic vein for blood collection or catheter placement in a rat (*Rattus norvegicus*). (a) The rat is anesthetized, and the region of the forelimb over the cephalic vein is aseptically prepared for catheter placement. A rubber band and hemostat are used as a tourniquet. (b) A 24-gauge catheter is being placed in the cephalic vein of the rat in preparation for surgery.

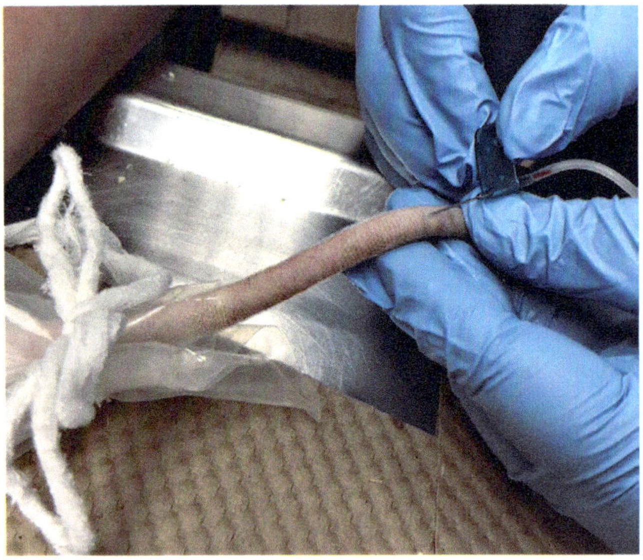

Fig. 1.2. Placement of a butterfly needle into the lateral tail vein for blood collection from a rat (*Rattus norvegicus*).

arterial pressure. After blood collection, apply direct digital pressure to the collection site for hemostasis.

The jugular veins can be used for blood collection and are realistically often the best site for blood collection in small exotic mammals because they are one of the largest accessible veins in a patient. In a laboratory environment, jugular venipuncture is often performed on unanesthetized animals, but in a clinical setting, sedation may be preferable in order to decrease stress on an animal that is often ill and a client's pet. After sedating or anesthetizing the patient, place it in dorsal recumbency and extend the head. The jugular vein is often not visible, but in all rodents lies along a line running from the manubrium toward the ear. The vessel may be occluded digitally at the manubrium, and a small-gauge needle attached to a small-sized syringe (insulin or tuberculin syringe) may be inserted to the hub at a 30° angle.

The cranial vena cava can be used for blood collection in hamsters, gerbils, and rats. This is often a desirable location due to the relatively large vessel size. The animal should be sedated or anesthetized when using this approach. In dorsal recumbency, the animal's forelimbs are held or secured along the sides of their body. The manubrium and first rib are palpated, and a small-gauge needle attached to a small-sized syringe is inserted just cranial to the first rib and within a half of a centimeter lateral to the manubrium (Picazo et al., 2009). The syringe is angled at about 30° from the patient (or table), toward the opposite hind limb, and gently advanced while applying negative pressure with the plunger of the syringe.

The gingival vein has been described for use in blood collection from small rodents in a laboratory setting and, due to the relatively mild traumatic outcome to the tissue and well-being of the animal, is also promising for the clinical setting (Teixeira de Oliveira et al., 2009; Rodrigues et al., 2017). For rodents with short tails or absent tails, such as hamsters and guinea pigs, it provides an additional anatomical location as an option for blood collection. The approach is described in an anesthetized animal in dorsal recumbency. With the lower lip retracted caudally, a 26-gauge needle attached to a 1-mL syringe is inserted just below the gingival-incisor margin along the midline between the two mandibular incisors at a 30–60° angle caudally. The needle is inserted 2–4 mm deep within the mucous membrane of the hamster (Figures 1.3a–1.3e).

Descriptions of blood collection from the retro-orbital venous plexus/sinus have been described in the literature. This method of blood collection is no longer recommended as a means of sample collection, even in laboratory settings, because trauma to the eye and surrounding structures is very common, and the sample volume that may be collected is very small. Because this procedure is no longer considered a viable means of blood collection, it will not be discussed further in this text.

Rabbit (*Oryctolagus cuniculus*)

The central auricular artery, marginal ear vein, jugular vein, cephalic vein, and lateral saphenous vein are the most used sites for venipuncture in rabbits. Rabbits can be timid patients and in general have a well-developed fight-or-flight response, making the need for adequate restraint an important part of blood collection. Because the rabbit skeleton makes up only approximately 8% of its total body mass, any rabbit that is inadequately restrained is at risk of fracturing its back or long bones. For this reason, the rabbit's hind limbs should never be unsupported or allowed to dangle during restraint. Nervous or intractable rabbits can be restrained using the "bunny burrito." A towel is placed on the exam tabletop, and the rabbit is placed on the towel in approximately the center, with its hindquarters angled into one of the corners of the towel. This corner is folded up over the hindquarters and back of the rabbit. One of the side corners is then folded snugly over the rabbit, followed by the other corner. The remaining corner of the towel can be folded over the rabbit's face. The rabbit can then be scooped up and held in the "football hold" for examination, treatment, or transport.

The lateral saphenous vein is readily accessible, and often a sizable volume of blood can be drawn quickly and easily (Figures 1.4a and 1.4b). Rabbits may be restrained in two ways for access to this vein:

1. The rabbit may be restrained on its side. The handler should scruff the rabbit and restrain it in lateral recumbency, bracing the rabbit's back against the forearm of the hand that is holding onto the scruff. The palm of the other hand should be placed around and over the ventral and caudal aspect of the rabbit's pelvis to stabilize

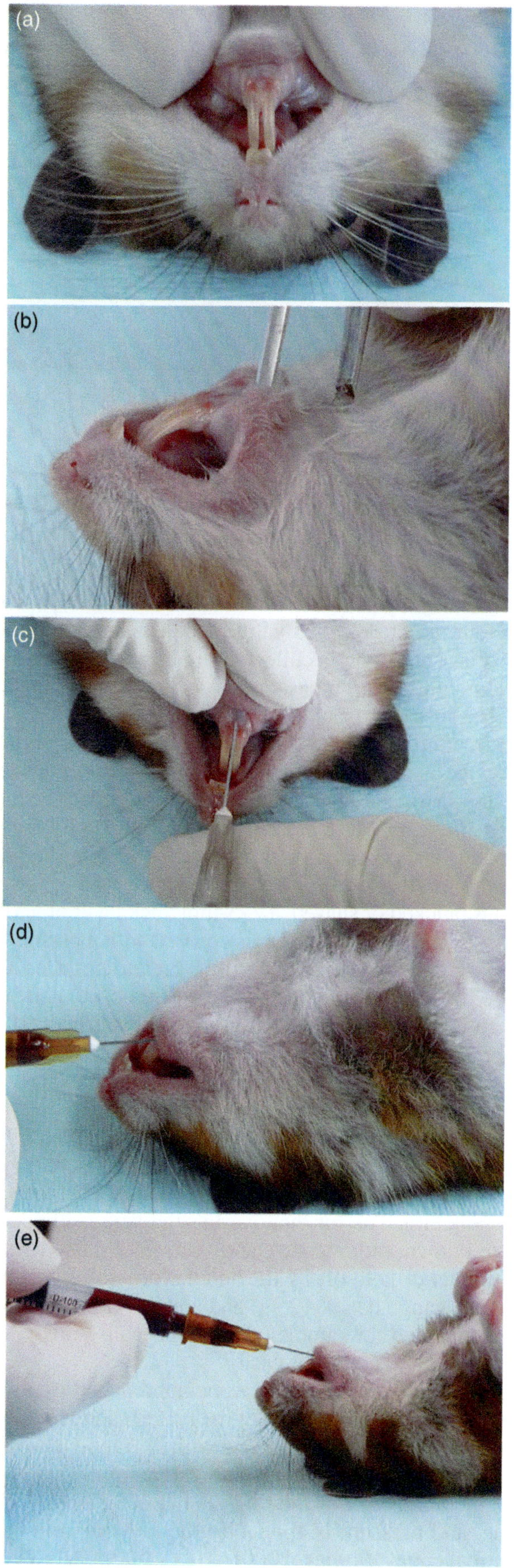

the hindquarters. The fingers of this hand then wrap around the upper hind limb to hold off the vein. The phlebotomist collecting the blood then extends the rabbit's leg for blood collection.

2. The rabbit is allowed to sit in sternal recumbency on the top of the examination table. The handler restraining the rabbit holds the rabbit's body against her/his own and tucks the rabbit's head into the crook of one arm. The other arm is placed around the rabbit for support. The handler performing the restraint then slides the rabbit toward the edge of the table until the hind leg closest to the edge of the table can drop off. The phlebotomist collecting the sample must kneel on the floor and gently restrain the hind leg in extension to draw the sample. Most rabbits, even intractable ones, will tolerate this method of sampling very well.

The fur over the lateral saphenous vein can be plucked and/or wetted to visualize the vessel. A small-gauge needle and 1- or 3-mL syringe are used to collect the sample. The vessel is superficial under a thin layer of skin, so a steady approach stabilizing the syringe or chemical restraint will help prevent hematoma formation.

The central auricular artery is another commonly used site for blood collection, and most rabbits will readily tolerate blood sampling from this site. The rabbit may be restrained on a tabletop in a "bunny burrito," as described previously, while the skin is prepared by wiping it with an alcohol wipe prior to the venipuncture. Often, application of alcohol will cause vasoconstriction of the auricular artery; however, a topical vasodilation agent such as oil of wintergreen may be applied over the artery, a warm compress applied over the vessel, or subcutaneous acepromazine (0.5–1.0 mg/kg) may also induce vasodilation (Moore et al., 2015). A 25-gauge needle is then introduced into the artery, and the blood is collected into Microtainer® tubes as it drips from the needle hub (Figure 1.5). Collection of blood using this technique is commonly preferred over other methods because the incidence of hematoma formation is relatively low. Some authors, however, do not recommend this method because blood collection from the central auricular artery of rabbits has the potential to cause

Fig. 1.3. Placement of a needle into the gingival vein for blood collection in an anesthetized Syrian hamster (*Mesocricetus auratus*). (a) and (b) Pull the lower lip away from the incisors to expose the vessel located along the midline below the mandibular incisors. (c) A 26-gauge needle on a 1-mL syringe is inserted in the gingival vein. (d) and (e) The lip is released and negative pressure is applied to collect the blood sample. Source: Images courtesy of Marcelo L. Santoro. Rodrigues et al. (2017). Used via license: https://creativecommons.org/licenses/by/4.0/

(a) (b)

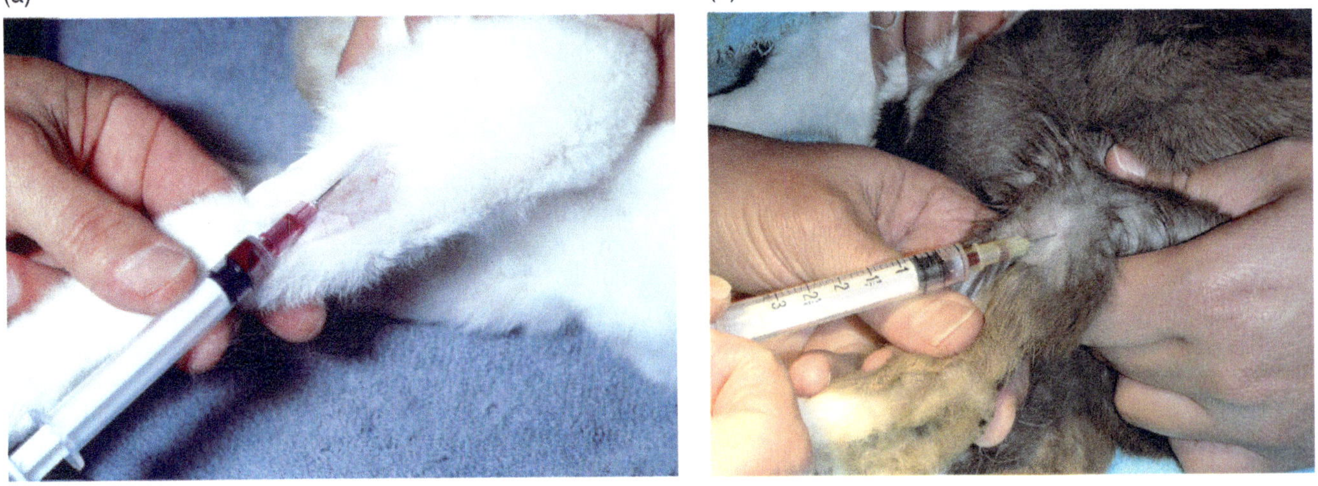

Fig. 1.4. Blood collection from a rabbit (*Oryctolagus cuniculus*) in lateral recumbency using the lateral saphenous vein. (a) The phlebotomist is supporting the syringe with their thumb and middle finger. (b) The phlebotomist is using their thumb as resting support for the syringe.

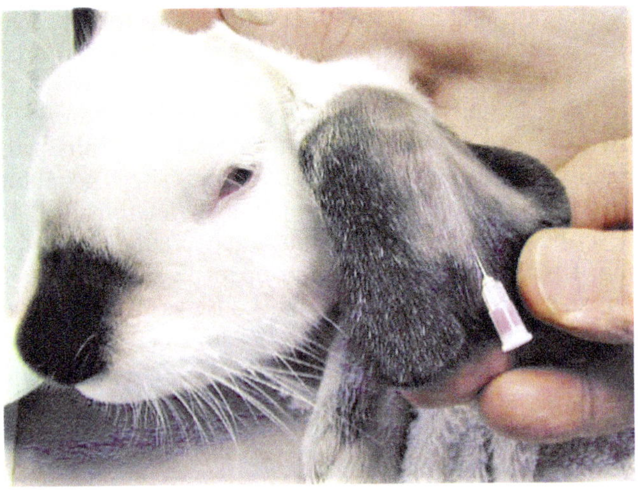

Fig. 1.5. Placement of a needle into the central auricular artery in preparation for blood collection from a rabbit (*Oryctolagus cuniculus*).

ischemic necrosis of most of the pinna (Malley, 2000). Alternative methods of blood collection from this site include use of a vacuum ear bleeder, or an evacuated glass tube with appropriate needle and needle holder; however, use of aspiration often results in collapse of the vessel in small rabbits. The vacuum ear bleeder method is performed by lacerating an ear vessel and placing the ear inside a flask with a side arm that is attached to a vacuum line and held firmly against the rabbit's head. This method is generally used for research rabbits, where large sample volumes are needed.

Another blood collection site from the ear of a rabbit is the marginal ear vein. Increased blood flow in the marginal ear vein to improve blood collection is made by the application of alcohol, oil of wintergreen, or petroleum jelly over the vein along with finger pressure as a tourniquet. A 23–25-gauge needle is introduced into the vein, and blood is collected directly from the needle hub into collection tubes.

Because some rabbits make a sudden movement as the vein or artery of the ear is punctured, collecting blood into a syringe is facilitated using a butterfly catheter, general anesthesia, or anesthesia of the skin. The skin can be anesthetized using EMLA cream (Astra Zeneca), a mixture of lidocaine and prilocaine that produces a full skin-thickness anesthesia (Flecknell, 2000). The fur overlying the ear vein is plucked or shaved, a 2–3-mm thick layer of EMLA cream is applied, and the ear is covered with a plastic film dressing and a bandage to hold the cream in place. After approximately 45 min, the bandage is removed, and venipuncture is performed. Since the skin is anesthetized, the rabbit does not react to the needle puncture.

Cephalic venipuncture may be performed on the rabbit in much the same manner described for dogs and cats (Figures 1.6a and 1.6b). The handler will restrain the rabbit in sternal recumbency using a "bunny burrito" and present the foreleg while the phlebotomist performs the venipuncture. The fur that overlies the vein is clipped or wetted down with alcohol, and the vein is raised with a tourniquet or held off by the handler providing restraint. A small-gauge needle (25 g) and small syringe (1 cc) are recommended for sample collection because this vein is very small and collapses easily.

Femoral venipuncture can be approached in a manner similar to venipuncture of the lateral saphenous vein. The femoral vein is approached with the rabbit restrained in lateral recumbency and the target leg slightly extended. The medial aspect of the thigh is clipped distally to the stifle, and pressure is applied to the femoral vein in the inguinal canal (Malley, 2000).

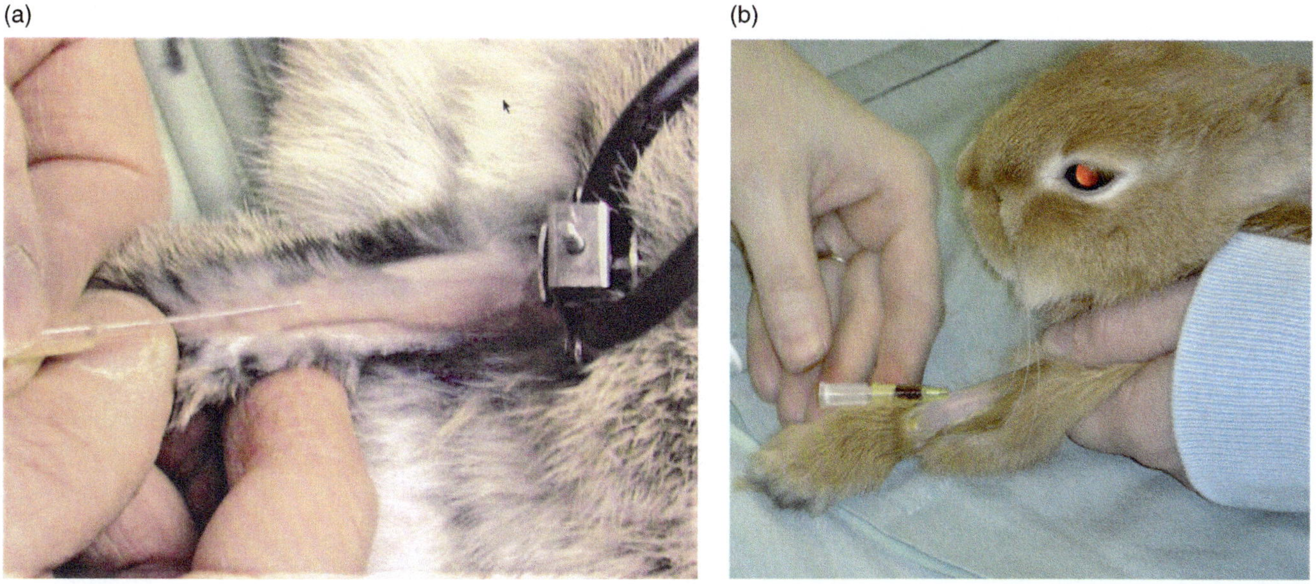

Fig. 1.6. (a) This image shows the cephalic vein of a rabbit (*Oryctolagus cuniculus*), which can be used to obtain blood for hematology studies or (b) the placement of an intravenous catheter.

Rabbits have large paired jugular veins; however, to collect blood from this site, some type of sedation is often necessary because many rabbits do not tolerate restraint and extension of the head. Light to moderate sedation using diazepam or midazolam at 0.5–1.0 mg/kg given intramuscularly 20 min prior to the procedure is recommended (Flecknell, 2000, 2016). Once sedated, the rabbit may be restrained in dorsal recumbency. The front feet are then retracted back alongside the thorax. The phlebotomist performing the venipuncture extends the rabbit's head and tips it back to expose the ventral neck region. Tractable rabbits may be restrained at the edge of a table with the front legs held down and the head extended up (Figure 1.7). If the rabbit struggles, it is best to abort the procedure to avoid back injury. An alternative is to perform jugular venipuncture on a rabbit under a general anesthetic.

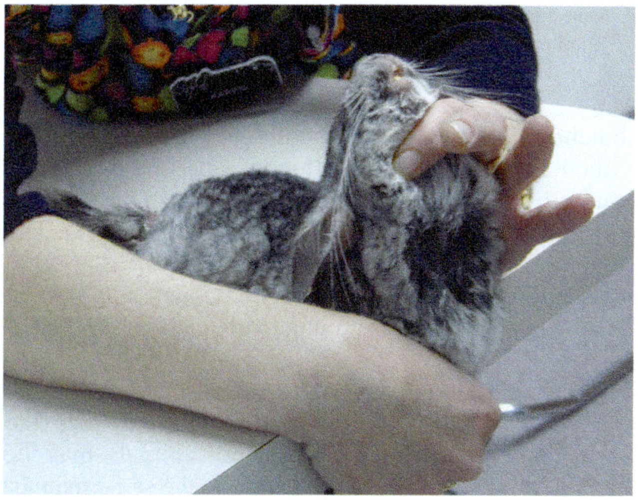

Fig. 1.7. Positioning of a chinchilla (*Chinchilla lanigera*) for jugular venipuncture. The animal is held in sternal recumbency at the edge of the table with the forelegs extended down as the head is held in extension.

Guinea Pig (*Cavia porcellus*) and Chinchilla (*Chinchilla lanigera*)

Venipuncture in guinea pigs and chinchillas can be difficult because many of the peripheral vessels are small and difficult to collect blood from. The jugular, lateral saphenous, and cephalic veins are the most used sites for blood collection in these animals. The femoral vein and ventral tail vein may be used for blood collection in the chinchilla as well. The gingival vein may be used in the guinea pig, but is not a reliable site for the chinchilla (Rodrigues et al., 2017; Mans and Donnelly, 2021; Pignon and Mayer, 2021). Warming the patient or applying a warm compress over the vessel may help induce vasodilation to assist with blood collection in guinea pigs (Zimmerman et al., 2015).

Guinea pigs and chinchillas may be restrained for jugular venipuncture in the same manner described for dogs and cats (Figure 1.7). The patient is held in sternal recumbency at the edge of the table with the forelegs extended down as the head is held in extension, and a small-gauge needle (25-gauge) attached to a 1–3-cc syringe is used to collect the sample. The jugular veins of the guinea pig are relatively deep due to the thick neck, and guinea pigs often become stressed during this procedure. It is often best to sedate these animals prior to attempting blood collection from this site. The jugular veins of chinchillas are relatively superficial, and most

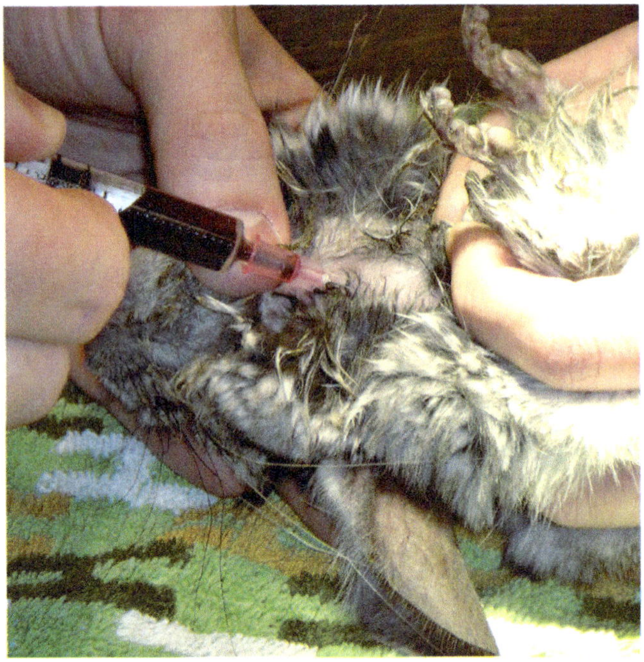

Fig. 1.8. The chinchilla (*Chinchilla lanigera*) is sedated or anesthetized and placed in dorsal recumbency for blood collection from the jugular vein.

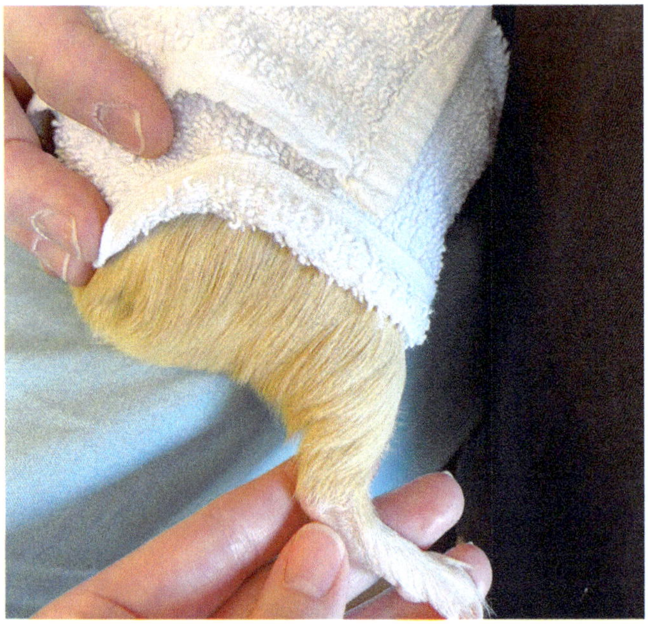

Fig. 1.9. A guinea pig (*Cavia porcellus*) restrained by wrapping in a towel (burrito) to aid preparation of blood collection from the lateral saphenous vein.

chinchillas will tolerate restraint for blood collection without sedation, but sedation or anesthesia may be required. In the chinchilla, the vein may also be accessed with the animal in dorsal recumbency (Figure 1.8). The vessels tend to be most accessible if the needle is inserted at a shallow angle just above the sternal notch of the first rib along a line of sight running from the sternal notch to the ear.

The lateral saphenous and cephalic veins are the most accessible veins, but are very small in both the guinea pig and the chinchilla. Both animals may be restrained for cephalic venipuncture in the same manner described for dogs and cats. Use of a guinea pig or chinchilla "burrito" often facilitates restraint during this procedure (Figure 1.9). When performing venipuncture of the lateral saphenous vein, these animals should be restrained in lateral recumbency. Small needles and insulin or tuberculin syringes must be used to prevent collapse of the vein.

The femoral vein may be used for blood collection in the chinchilla. Some form of sedation is recommended when performing venipuncture from this site. The sedated chinchilla may be placed in dorsal or lateral recumbency. Venipuncture is performed in the same manner described for cats using a small-gauge needle and syringe.

The ventral tail vein lies on the ventral midline of the tail and may be used for blood collection in the chinchilla. Anesthesia is recommended when collecting blood from this site. The anesthetized chinchilla is placed in dorsal recumbency and a small-gauge needle attached to a 1–3-cc syringe is inserted at a 30° angle at a point approximately one-third the length of the tail from the base of the tail. After the blood collection, apply direct digital pressure to the collection site for hemostasis.

As described for true rodents, the gingival vein may be used for blood collection in guinea pigs. The sedated or anesthetized guinea pig is placed in dorsal recumbency, and the inferior lip is retracted caudally to approach the vessel. A small-gauge needle attached to a 1-mL syringe is inserted just below the margin of the mucous membrane and mandibular incisors along the midline at a 30–60° angle. Negative pressure is applied as the needle is advanced 3–5 mm into the tissue (Figures 1.10a–1.10e) (Rodrigues et al., 2017).

Sugar Glider (*Petaurus breviceps*)

Blood collection in the sugar glider can be challenging and requires anesthesia. Venipuncture is limited primarily to the jugular veins or cranial vena cava due to the small size of the patient. To perform jugular venipuncture, the anesthetized sugar glider is placed in dorsal recumbency with the forelegs retracted back alongside the thorax. Insert a small-gauge needle (25-gauge or smaller) attached to a small syringe (insulin or tuberculin) along an imaginary line extending from the point of the shoulder toward the mandible. The needle should be inserted at a relatively steep angle along this line and is redirected as needed.

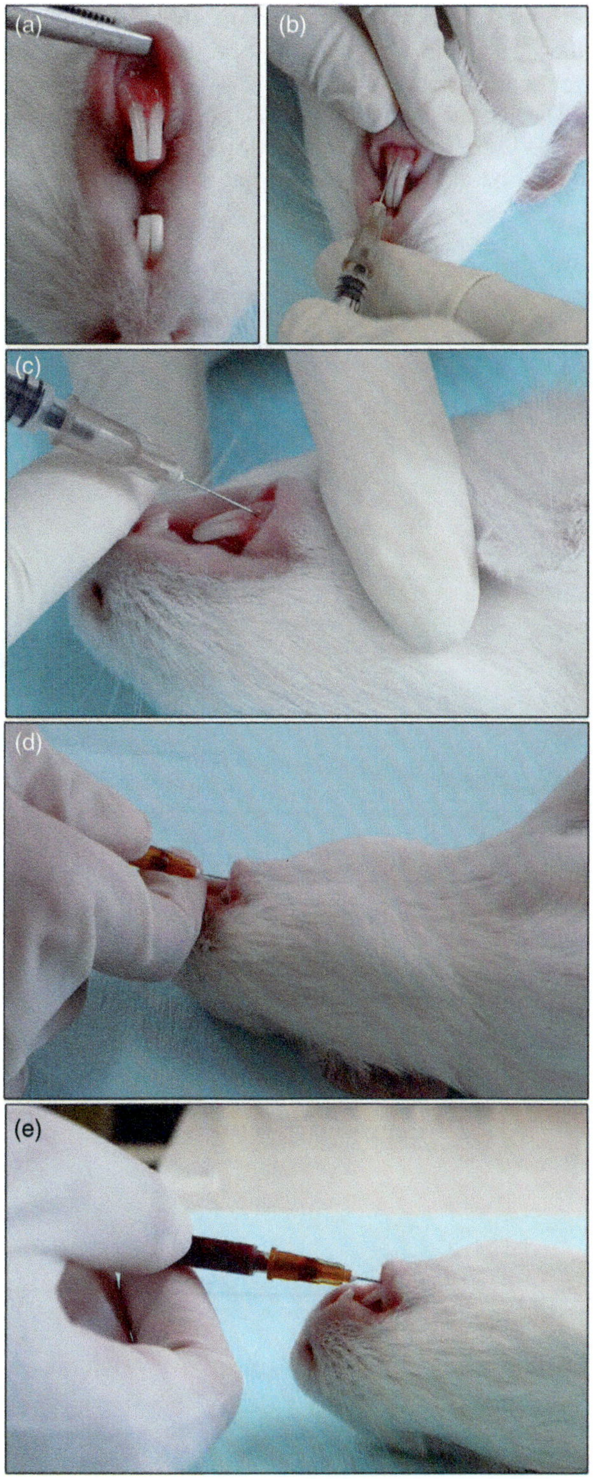

Fig. 1.10. Placement of a needle into the gingival vein for blood collection in an anesthetized guinea pig (*Cavia porcellus*). (a) and (b) Pull the lower lip away from the incisors to expose the vessel located along the midline below the mandibular incisors. (b) and (c) A 26-gauge needle on a 1-mL syringe is inserted in the gingival vein. (d) and (e) The lip is released, and negative pressure is applied to collect the blood sample. Source: Images courtesy of Marcelo L. Santoro. Rodrigues et al. (2017). Used via license: https://creativecommons.org/licenses/by/4.0/

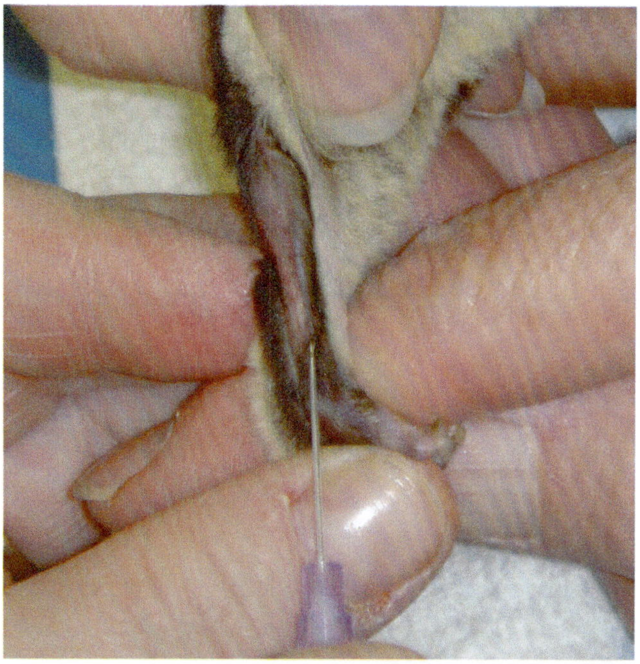

Fig. 1.11. This image shows the cephalic vein of a sugar glider (*Petaurus breviceps*), which can be used to obtain a very small blood sample for hematology or for placement of a 26-gauge intravenous catheter.

The cranial vena cava can be used for blood collection, and the approach is the same as with other small mammals. At the thoracic inlet, using the manubrium and first rib as the landmarks, insert a small needle attached to a small syringe at a 30° angle from the table aiming toward the opposite hind limb.

The peripheral vessels (cephalic vein, lateral saphenous vein, medial tibial artery, femoral vein, or coccygeal vein) may be used to collect very small samples, but may easily collapse (Figure 1.11). A 26-gauge or smaller needle should be used with a tuberculin syringe.

Hedgehog (*Atelerix albiventris*)

Anesthesia is almost always a requirement when performing venipuncture in the hedgehog, because even the tamest hedgehog will usually roll up at the veterinary clinic. Sites available for blood collection include the jugular veins, cranial vena cava, lateral saphenous and cephalic veins, and femoral veins.

Blood is typically collected from the jugular veins because these veins are the largest and most accessible veins present. To perform jugular venipuncture, place the anesthetized hedgehog in dorsal recumbency with the head extended. The jugular vein is rarely visible, but lies along a line of sight extending from the manubrium to the ear (Figure 1.12a). Insert a small-gauge needle (25-gauge or smaller) attached to a small syringe (insulin or tuberculin) along an imaginary line extending from the point of the shoulder toward the mandible (Figure 1.12b).

The cranial vena cava may be used for blood collection in hedgehogs. The approach is the same as described previously for other small mammals (Figures 1.13a and 1.13b). Caution should be taken with this approach due to the relatively short neck and the cranial position of the heart. Short needles may be used to avoid inadvertent cardiac puncture.

The lateral saphenous, cephalic, and femoral veins may be used for blood collection, but are very small, limiting the amount of blood that may be successfully

(a) (b)

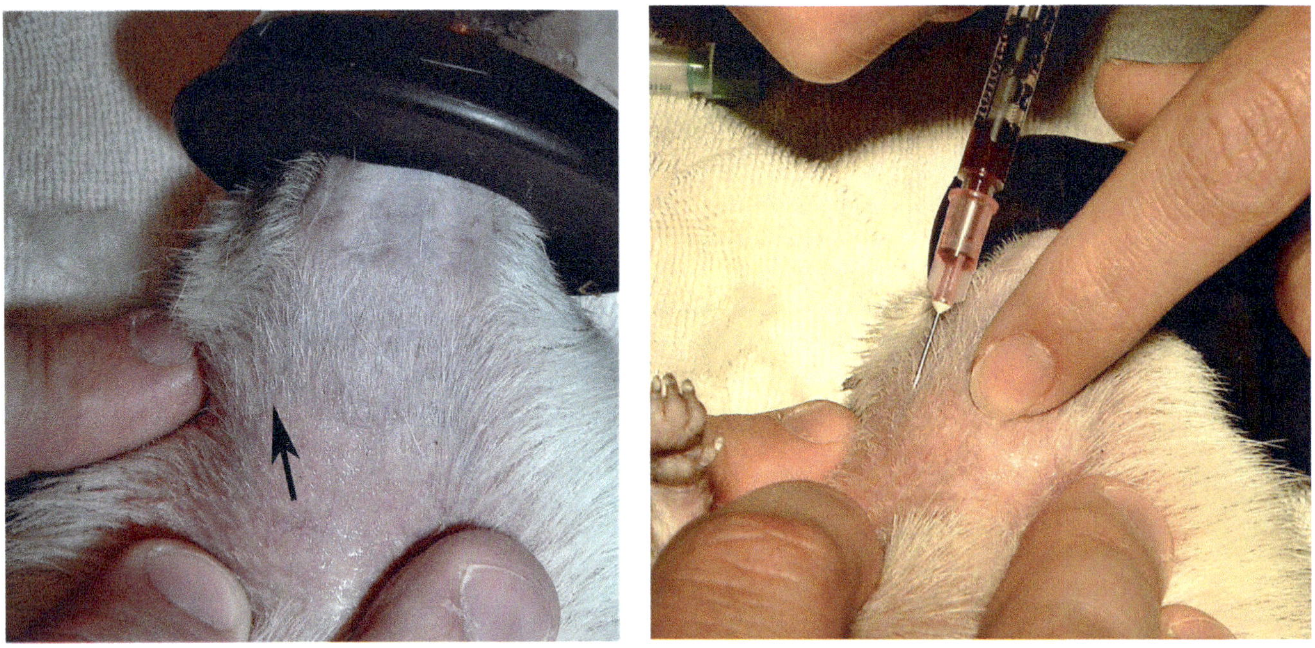

Fig. 1.12. The hedgehog (*Atelerix albiventris*) is anesthetized and placed in dorsal recumbency for blood collection from the jugular vein. (a) The jugular vein (arrow) is visualized in preparation for blood collection. (b) A 25-gauge needle on a 1-mL syringe is used to collect a blood sample.

(a) (b)

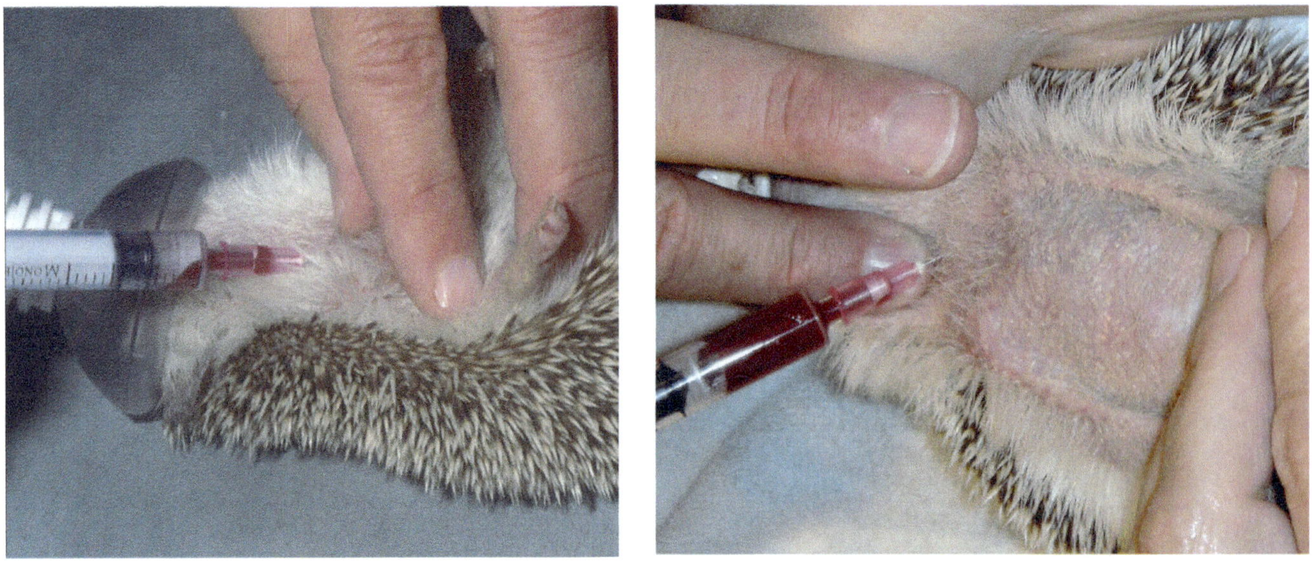

Fig. 1.13. Collection of blood from the cranial vena cava of a hedgehog (*Atelerix albiventris*) by inserting the needle in the "notch" where the first rib meets the manubrium. The jugular vein is also in this area in a shallower position, and a jugular venipuncture is often performed instead when using this method depending upon the depth of the needle insertion. (a) Lateral view, (b) ventral view.

collected from these sites. Blood may be collected using an insulin syringe, or via the drip technique after cannulation of the vessel with a small-gauge needle.

Ferret (*Mustela putorius furo*)

Venipuncture sites commonly used for blood collection in the ferret include the jugular vein, cephalic vein, lateral saphenous vein, tail artery, and cranial vena cava. Clipping a toenail to collect a blood sample should not be performed. It does not yield a viable laboratory sample, and it is painful to the patient.

Most ferrets can be manually restrained for blood collection. Aggressive or intractable ferrets may need to be anesthetized for sample collection; however, it is important to note that anesthesia can alter the hemogram (Marini et al., 1984; Quesenberry and de Matos, 2021). If anesthesia is used for blood collection, this information should be included on the laboratory requisition form.

Blood may be collected from the jugular vein via several techniques. Ferrets may be restrained using the same technique used for cats by holding the forelegs extended over the edge of a table with the neck extending up, or the ferret can be placed in dorsal recumbency and restrained using the same techniques described for the cranial vena cava. A third method of restraint involves wrapping the ferret in a towel with the front legs drawn back along the thorax, leaving only the head and neck extending from the towel. The ferret is then held by the scruff and placed in dorsal recumbency. The jugular veins lie more laterally in the neck compared to dogs and cats and are not always visible, so shaving the neck and applying pressure at the thoracic inlet may enhance the visibility for the phlebotomist (Figure 1.14). Blood samples may be collected with a 22- or 25-gauge needle on a 1–3-cc syringe. Ferrets that struggle or are excessively resistant to manual restraint should be anesthetized.

The cranial vena cava may be used for blood collection from ferrets; however, a jugular venipuncture is often performed when attempting to obtain blood from the anterior vena cava. The jugular vein is frequently encountered just under the skin in the same location as the approach to the cranial vena cava. Those unfamiliar with ferrets or having minimal experience in phlebotomy should perform this procedure on anesthetized ferrets until they become proficient with this technique, to avoid laceration of the vena cava and harm to the ferret. Restraint is very important and often requires two to three people when performing this method of blood collection on unanesthetized ferrets. One handler will restrain the forelimbs and head of the ferret while a second handler restrains the hind limbs and body. A phlebotomist draws the blood sample by palpating the "notch" where the first rib meets the manubrium and visualizing a line of sight running caudally from the "notch" across the midline of the ferret's body to the opposite hind leg. A 25-gauge needle attached to a 1–3-cc syringe is inserted at a 45° angle into the thoracic cavity (for a cranial vena cava blood collection) or just under the skin (for a jugular venipuncture) at the notch and aimed along the sight line toward the opposite hind limb (Figure 1.15). Negative pressure is applied to the syringe, and the needle is slowly withdrawn until blood begins to fill the syringe; at which point the needle is positioned in the vessel and should remain steady as the syringe fills with blood to the desired safe amount. If the ferret struggles, the syringe should be withdrawn

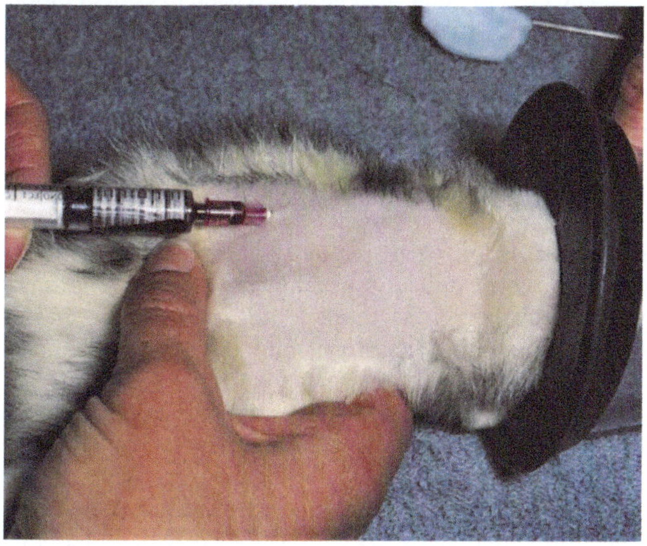

Fig. 1.14. Blood collection from a ferret (*Mustela putorius furo*) using the jugular venipuncture method.

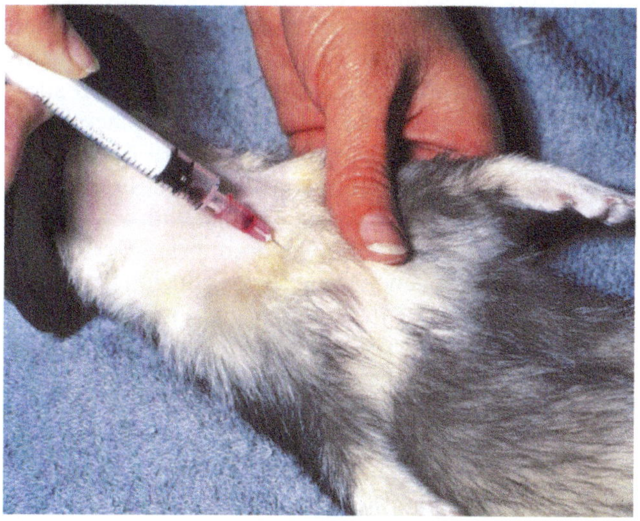

Fig. 1.15. Collection of blood from a ferret (*Mustela putorius furo*) using the cranial vena cava approach by inserting the needle in the "notch" where the first rib meets the manubrium. The jugular vein is also in this area in a shallower position, and a jugular venipuncture is often performed instead when using this method depending upon the depth of the needle insertion.

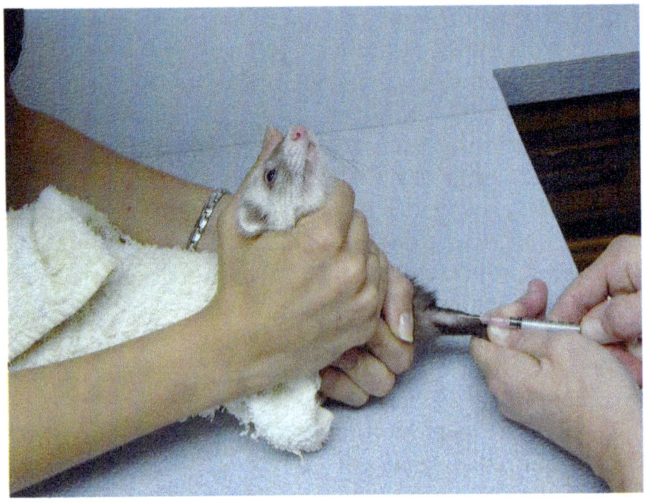

Fig. 1.16. Collection of a blood sample from the cephalic vein of a ferret (*Mustela putorius furo*).

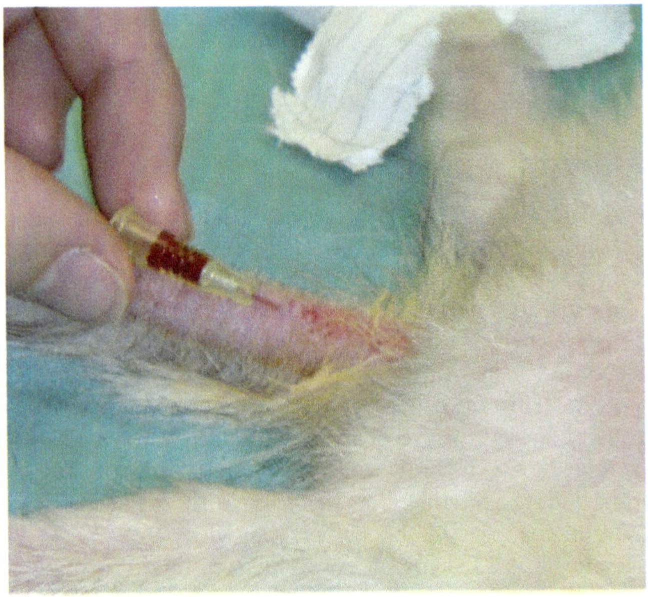

Fig. 1.17. A 24-gauge catheter placement in the ventral tail artery of a ferret (*Mustela putorius furo*).

quickly. A second attempt should not be made until the ferret is quiet. Any ferret that struggles excessively during this procedure should be sedated before attempting blood collection from this site.

The cephalic vein is located over the antebrachium, courses laterally, and may be used for the collection of small volumes of blood (up to 1 mL) using a 25-gauge needle attached to a 1-mL syringe. Ferrets may be restrained for cephalic venipuncture by wrapping them in a towel with the head and one foreleg free. The head should be restrained by extending it upward, while the foreleg is presented in extension (Figure 1.16). The vein may be occluded by simply placing the thumb or a finger over the dorsal surface of the elbow by the handler who is restraining the ferret. The cephalic vessel is small and easily collapses, so it is not necessary to roll this vessel as is commonly done with dogs and cats. If additional stability is required, the handler can place his or her forearms on the tabletop on each side of the ferret to support the body. Most ferrets will struggle briefly, and then will become quiet. A 1-cc syringe with a 25-gauge needle is used to collect the blood sample.

The lateral saphenous vein courses diagonally across the lateral surface of the hind leg just proximal to the hock and may be used for collecting small volumes of blood. A ferret may be restrained for blood collection from this site by scruffing it with one hand and laying it on its side. The handler then places the palm of the other hand over the sacrum and pelvis for support and holds off the vein by wrapping his or her fingers around the leg above the stifle. Occasionally, a second handler is needed to help restrain the ferret's body. A 25-gauge needle mounted on a 1-cc syringe is used for sample collection.

The tail artery may be used for venipuncture when necessary, but is not a common or preferred site for blood collection in the clinical setting. This site may be more painful for the ferret than other blood collection sites. The ferret may be restrained by either scruffing and restraining on its back, or by anesthetizing it and placing it in dorsal recumbency. A 25-gauge needle attached to a 1-mL syringe is then inserted at a 45° angle toward the body on the ventral midline of the proximal third of the tail and advanced until blood begins to fill the syringe (Figure 1.17). Direct digital pressure must be applied for at least 3 min after blood collection to provide adequate hemostasis.

Other Collection Sites and Considerations

The cranial vena cava has been used to collect blood from ferrets, small rodents, hedgehogs, sugar gliders, and other small exotic mammals, and many clinicians use this approach as a first choice of blood collection (Figures 1.13 and 1.15). This method of blood collection is very "safe"; however, there is high potential for complications such as intrathoracic bleeding, bleeding into the pericardial sac or mediastinum, or inadvertent cardiac puncture in small patients. The phlebotomist performing blood collection using the cranial vena cava must be aware of the thoracic anatomy of the animal they are intending to perform venipuncture on and must consider the size and length of the needle being used.

The femoral vein and artery are other considerations for blood collection in several mammals, such as rodents, sugar gliders, and other small mammalian species due to the potential of a relatively moderate volume collection. The animal may need to be sedated or placed under general anesthesia. In dorsal recumbency, the vessels are located on the medial aspect and proximal third of the

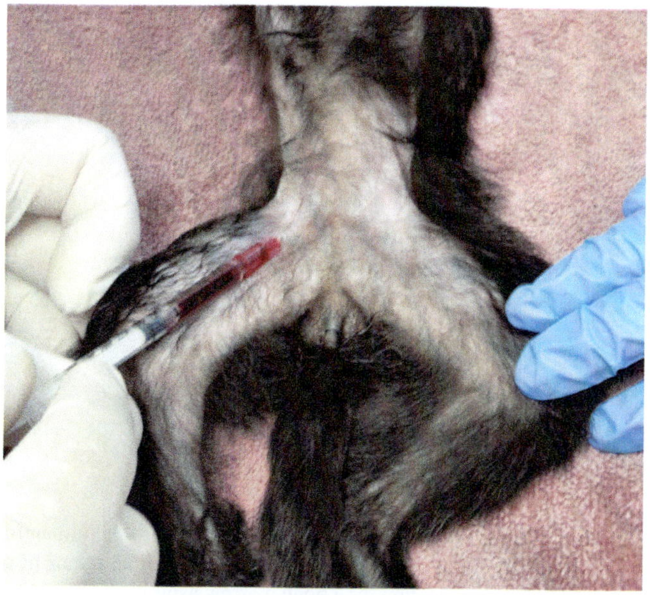

Fig. 1.18. Collection of a blood sample from the femoral vessel of a Goeldi's monkey (*Callimico goeldii*).

thigh. A small-gauge needle attached to a 1- or 3-mL syringe is inserted parallel to the femur just distal from the junction of the limb and body (Figure 1.18).

Cardiocentesis can be used to collect blood from small mammals, but is typically only performed for terminal procedures because of the risk of causing death during the procedure. Cardiocentesis must be performed under general anesthesia to ensure that there is no movement of the patient, and because the heart may move away from the needle during the procedure. To perform cardiocentesis, place the anesthetized animal in dorsal recumbency and locate the heart by palpation. Insert a needle attached to a syringe slightly to the left of the manubrium and advance it toward the heart.

Blood Sample Handling and Preparation

Blood for hematology is typically collected into tubes containing an anticoagulant, such as ethylenediaminetetraacetic acid (EDTA) or heparin. Blood collected for clinical biochemistry analysis is collected into tubes containing heparin or no anticoagulant. The blood sample from a small mammal is prepared for hematology studies in the same manner as described for domestic mammals (Weiser, 2012, 2022). Likewise, the hematologic methods used to evaluate the hemic cells in blood samples from these animals are the same as described for domestic mammals.

Bone Marrow Collection

Cytologic evaluation of a bone marrow aspiration biopsy is often performed as a diagnostic aid when an unexplained hematologic abnormality such as nonregenerative

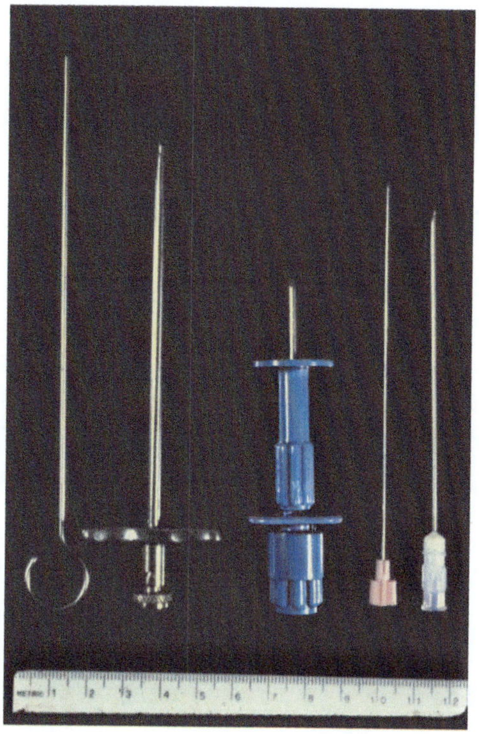

Fig. 1.19. Representative types of aspiration or core biopsy needles used to obtain bone marrow samples, including (left to right) pediatric Jamshidi bone marrow biopsy/aspiration needle (Kormed Corp., Minneapolis, MN), disposable Jamshidi Illinois sternal/iliac aspiration needle (Kormed Corp.), and disposable spinal needle.

anemia, neutropenia (heteropenia), thrombocytopenia, myeloproliferative or lymphoproliferative disorder (leukemia), gammopathy, or suspicion for neoplasia is present. Bone marrow biopsy needles or spinal needles are required for this procedure because they have a stylet to facilitate passage of the aspiration needle through the cortical bone into the marrow space. The type of biopsy needle used for aspiration depends upon the size of the animal, location of the biopsy site, and preference of the cytologist. Bone marrow biopsy needles commonly used for marrow collection in domestic mammals and humans can also be used for marrow collection in birds and reptiles (Jamshidi bone marrow biopsy/aspiration needles and disposable Jamshidi Illinois sternal/iliac aspiration needles, Kormed Corp., Minneapolis, MN) (Figure 1.19). The pediatric sizes are preferred because of the relatively small bone size of most small mammals, birds, and reptiles compared to the larger domestic mammals. Spinal needles containing a stylet can be used for marrow collection in very small animals as well.

The most common site for bone marrow aspiration biopsy or core biopsy in small exotic mammals is the proximal femur (Figures 1.20–1.25). Additional sites could include the proximal tibia, proximal humerus, and the ileum; however, the small body size of many small

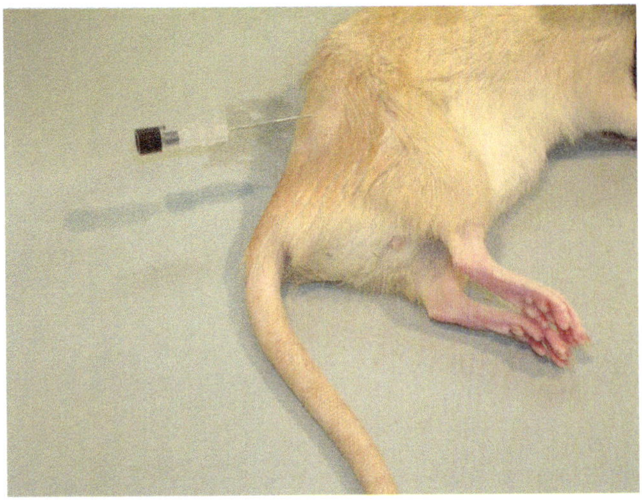

Fig. 1.20. Placement of a spinal needle into the proximal femur of a rat (*Rattus norvegicus*) for a bone marrow aspiration biopsy.

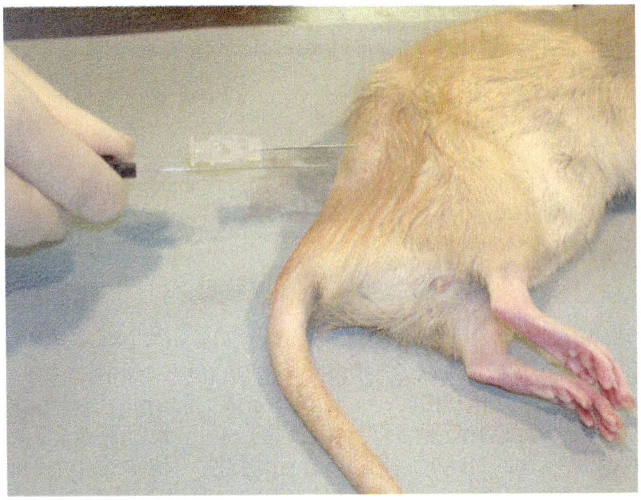

Fig. 1.21. Removal of the stylet from the spinal needle that was placed into the proximal femur of a rat (*Rattus norvegicus*) for a bone marrow aspiration biopsy.

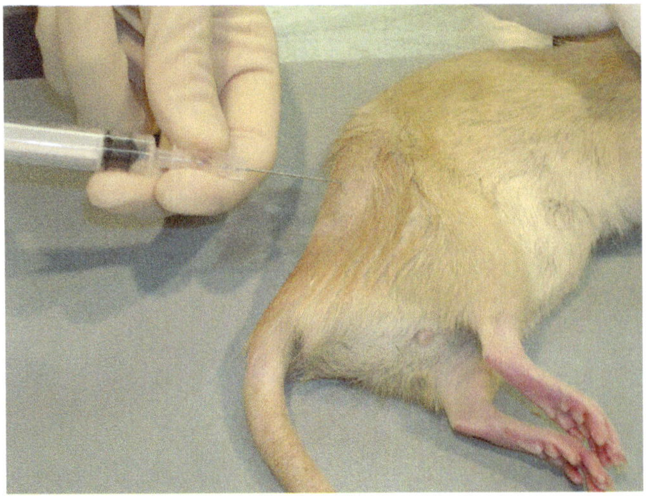

Fig. 1.22. Aspiration of the marrow sample into the lumen of the spinal needle that was placed into the proximal femur of a rat (*Rattus norvegicus*) for a bone marrow aspiration biopsy.

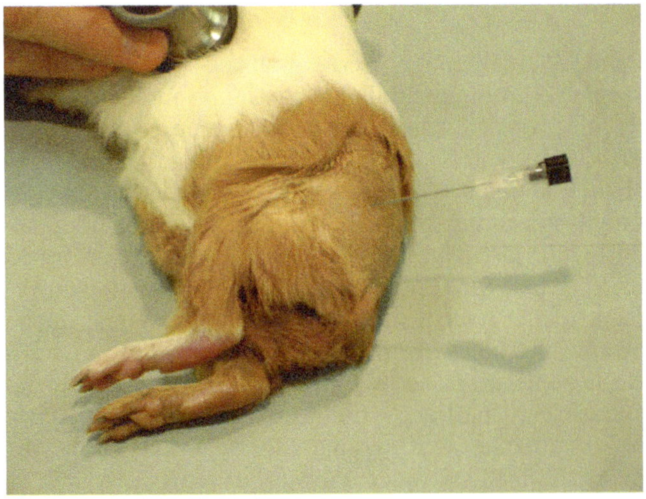

Fig. 1.23. Placement of a spinal needle into the proximal femur of a guinea pig (*Cavia porcellus*) for a bone marrow aspiration biopsy.

exotic mammals precludes the use of these sites for bone marrow collection.

When performing a bone marrow aspiration biopsy, a general anesthetic is recommended to facilitate restraint of the patient and to minimize the risk of stress and trauma to the patient. Infiltration of the subcutis and periosteum with a local anesthetic is also used to provide local analgesia. The anesthetized patient is placed in lateral recumbency, and the hair overlaying the greater trochanter is shaved. The skin is then surgically prepared, and a small incision is made to facilitate passage of the biopsy needle through the skin. The needle is advanced until it reaches the intertrochanteric fossa and is then seated and advanced through the cortical bone and into the marrow space by rotating it in a clockwise-counterclockwise manner.

Once seated within the marrow space, the stylet is removed, and a syringe is attached to the needle hub. Negative pressure is applied until marrow appears just beyond the hub of the needle. Excessive negative pressure and excessive sampling should be avoided to prevent peripheral blood contamination, because marrow samples that are diluted with peripheral blood are difficult to interpret. After collection, the marrow sample is immediately placed in EDTA and/or slides are made before clotting of the sample occurs. To prevent clotting of the sample, it may be advantageous to place two to three drops of 10% EDTA solution in the syringe prior to aspiration.

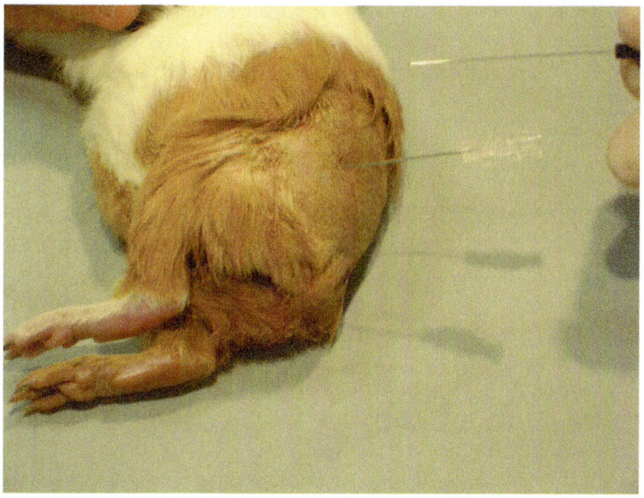

Fig. 1.24. This image shows the stylet removed from the spinal needle that was placed into the proximal femur of a guinea pig (*Cavia porcellus*) for a bone marrow aspiration biopsy.

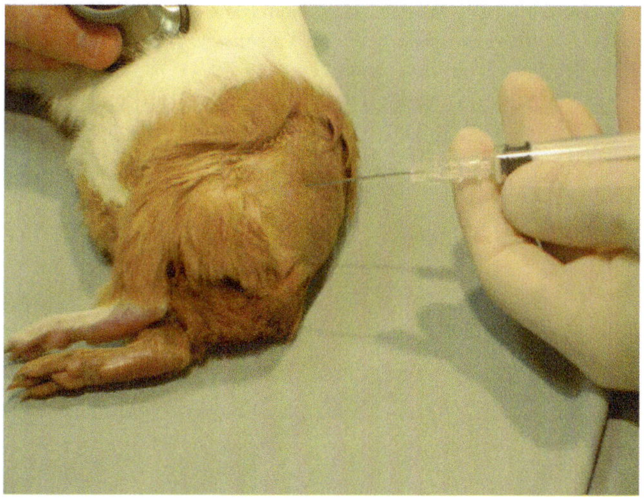

Fig. 1.25. Aspiration of the marrow sample into the lumen of the spinal needle that was placed into the proximal femur of a guinea pig (*Cavia porcellus*) for a bone marrow aspiration biopsy.

Bone marrow films are prepared by placing a drop of marrow on a glass slide, gently placing a spreader slide directly on top with a little or no manual pressure, and then pulling the two glass slides apart after the drop has been allowed to spread. Air-dried slides are stained with a Romanowsky stain.

Core biopsy samples may be obtained using a pediatric bone marrow biopsy needle. The same techniques described for bone marrow aspiration are used for core biopsy collection regarding patient preparation and introduction of the bone marrow needle into the marrow space. Once the marrow space has been entered, a core sample is obtained by advancing the biopsy needle through the marrow space to the opposite cortex after the stylet has been removed. A slight change in the direction of the needle tip movement is made once the end of the needle has reached the opposite cortex to "clip off" the marrow sample inside the needle. No aspiration is performed with this procedure; instead, the needle is withdrawn without replacing the stylet. After removing the needle from the marrow space, the stylet may be used to push the marrow sample out of the lumen of the needle. The core sample may then be rolled across the surface of a glass slide for cytological evaluation before placing it into formalin fixation for histopathology. Romanowsky-stained bone marrow films are evaluated for cellularity and the maturation of the myeloid and erythroid cells. Examination of other cells, such as macrophages, plasma cells, lymphocytes, megakaryocytes, osteoblasts, and osteoclasts, is also part of bone marrow evaluations in Chapter 4.

References

Campbell TW. 2015. Hematology. *Veterinary Clinics of North America: Exotic Animal Practice*. Philadelphia, PA: Elsevier.

Cooke SW. 2000. Clinical chemistry and haematology. In: Flecknell P (ed), *Manual of Rabbit Medicine and Surgery*. Gloucester: British Small Animal Veterinary Association.

Delk KW, Carpenter JW, Biller DS. 2013. Diagnostic challenge. *J Exot Pet Med* 22:409–412.

Flecknell PA. 2000. Anaesthesia. In: Flecknell P (ed), *Manual of Rabbit Medicine and Surgery*. Gloucester: British Small Animal Veterinary Association.

Flecknell PA. 2016. Anaesthesia of common laboratory species: special considerations. In: Flecknell PA (ed), *Laboratory Animal Anaesthesia*, 4th edn. Kidlington, Oxford: Academic Press, pp. 193–256.

Frohlich J. 2021. Rats and mice. In: Quesenberry KE, Orcutt CJ, Mans C, Carpenter JW (eds), *Ferrets, Rabbits, and Rodents Clinical Medicine and Surgery*, 4th edn. St. Louis, MO: Elsevier, pp. 345–367.

Garma-Aviña A. 2004. Cytology of the normal and abnormal choroid plexi in selected domestic mammals, wildlife species, and man. *J Vet Diagn Invest* 16:283–292. Doi-https://doi.org/10.1177/104063870401600405

Johnson-Delaney C. 2021. Sugar gliders. In: Quesenberry KE, Orcutt CJ, Mans C, Carpenter JW (eds), *Ferrets, Rabbits, and Rodents Clinical Medicine and Surgery*, 4th edn. St. Louis, MO: Elsevier, pp. 385–400.

Keller KA, Nevarez JG, Rodriguez D, Gieger T, Gumber S. 2014. Diagnosis and treatment of anaplastic mammary adenocarcinoma in a sugar glider (*Petaurus breviceps*). *J Exot Pet Med* 23:277–282.

Lindstrom NM, Moore DM, Zimmerman K, et al. 2015. Hematologic assessment in pet rats, mice, hamsters, and gerbils blood sample collection and blood cell identification. *Vet Clin Exot Anim* 18:21–32.

Machholz E, Mulder G, Ruiz C, et al. 2012. Manual restraint and common compound administration routes in mice and rats. *J Vis Exp* 67(e2771):1–8.

Malley D. 2000. Handling, restraint, and clinical techniques. In: Flecknell P (ed), *Manual of Rabbit Medicine and Surgery*. Gloucester: British Small Animal Veterinary Association.

Mans C, Donnelly TM. 2021. Chinchillas. In: Quesenberry KE, Orcutt CJ, Mans C, Carpenter JW (eds), *Ferrets, Rabbits, and Rodents Clinical Medicine and Surgery*, 4th edn. St. Louis, MO: Elsevier, pp. 298–322.

Marini RP, Jackson LR, Esteves MI, et al. 1984. Effect of isoflurane on hematologic variables in ferrets. *Am J Vet Res* 55:1479–1483.

Mitchell S. 2011. Venipuncture techniques in pet rodent species. *J Exot Pet Med* 20(4):284–293.

Miwa Y, Mayer J. 2021. Hamsters and gerbils. In: Quesenberry KE, Orcutt CJ, Mans C, Carpenter JW (eds), *Ferrets, Rabbits, and Rodents Clinical Medicine and Surgery*, 4th edn. St. Louis, MO: Elsevier, pp. 368–384.

Moore DM, Zimmerman K, Smith SA. 2015. Hematological assessment in pet rabbits blood sample collection and blood cell identification. *Vet Clin Exot Anim* 18:9–20.

NIH 2019. Guidelines for blood collection in mice and rats. *NIH Animal Research Advisory Committee* Guidelines. https://oacu.oir.nih.gov/sites/default/files/uploads/arac-guidelines/b2_blood_collection_in_mice_and_rats.pdf Accessed: September 5, 2020.

Picazo MG, Benito PJ, Garcia-Olmo DC. 2009. Efficiency and safety of a technique for drawing blood from the hamster cranial vena cava. *Lab Anim* 38:211–216.

Pignon C, Mayer J. 2021. Guinea pigs. In: Quesenberry KE, Orcutt CJ, Mans C, Carpenter JW (eds), *Ferrets, Rabbits, and Rodents Clinical Medicine and Surgery*, 4th edn. St. Louis, MO: Elsevier, pp. 270–297.

Quesenberry KE, de Matos R. 2021. Ferrets. In: Quesenberry KE, Orcutt CJ, Mans C, Carpenter JW (eds), *Ferrets, Rabbits, and Rodents Clinical Medicine and Surgery*, 4th edn. St. Louis, MO: Elsevier, pp. 13–26.

Quesenberry KE, Orcutt CJ, Mans C, Carpenter JW. 2021. Ferrets, Rabbits, and Rodents Clinical Medicine and Surgery. St. Louis, MO: Elsevier.

Rodrigues MV, Oliveira de Castro S, Zaccanini de Albuquerue C,et al. 2017. The gingival vein as a minimally traumatic site for multiple blood sampling in guinea pigs and hamsters. *PLOS One* 1–16.

Smith SA, Zimmerman K, Moore DM. 2015. Hematology of the domestic ferret (*Mustela putorius furo*). In: Campbell TW (ed), *Veterinary Clinics of North America: Exotic Animal Practice*. Philadelphia, PA: Elsevier, pp. 1–8.

Teixeira de Oliveira D, Souza-Silva E, Tonussi CR. 2009. Gingival vein punction: a new simple technique for drug administration or blood sampling in rats and mice. *Scand J Lab Anim Sci* 36(2):109–113.

Weiser G. 2012. Laboratory technology for veterinary medicine. In: Thrall M, Weiser G, Allison RW, Campbell TW (eds), *Veterinary Hematology and Clinical Chemistry*, 2nd edn. Ames, IA: Wiley-Blackwell, pp 3–33.

Weiser G. 2022. Laboratory technology for veterinary medicine. In: Thrall M, Weiser G, Allison RW, Campbell TW (eds), *Veterinary Hematology and Clinical Chemistry*, 3rd edn. Ames, IA: Wiley-Blackwell, in press.

Zimmerman K, Moore DM, Smith SA. 2015. Hematological assessment in pet guinea pigs (*Cavia porcellus*) blood sample collection and blood cell identification. *Vet Clin Exot Anim* 18:33–40.

2 Hematologic Techniques for Quantitative Assessment in Mammals

The in-house veterinary laboratory evaluation of the blood sample of mammals begins after the sample is prepared with preferred stains and solutions using a centrifuge, microhematocrit tube, refractometer, hemacytometer, and slides. The systematic approach to evaluating the mammalian hemogram involves an assessment of cell and plasma parameters, morphologic features of the cells, and intra- and extracellular parasites. This chapter is a synopsis on obtaining the sample parameter counts or concentrations with some interpretation of the mammalian hemogram. Details on procedures and instrument functionality are described elsewhere (Weiser, 2012, 2022). Chapter 3 will continue with procedures on the mammalian hemogram with a focus on evaluating the blood film by identifying the morphologic features of the cells and parasites as well as the interpretation of findings.

Erythrocyte and Plasma Parameters

The typical mammalian hematologic procedures include determination of packed cell volume (PCV) by centrifugation (or hematocrit by calculation), a plasma total protein estimation by refractometry, cell and platelet concentration by instrumentation, hemoglobin concentration by spectrophotometry, mean platelet volume by instrumentation, and a stained blood film evaluation. The secondary erythrocyte parameters include reticulocyte concentration, mean cell hemoglobin content (MCH), mean cell hemoglobin concentration (MCHC), and mean cell volume (MCV). Appendix B, Table B.1 provides guidelines for evaluating mammalian erythrocytes.

PCV

The PCV provides the percentage of whole blood that is composed of erythrocytes. Determination of the PCV via the microhematocrit method is the most used method for evaluating the red cell mass. The total erythrocyte count (TRBC) or erythrocyte concentration value, described later in the chapter, is commonly reported as well, but is not as useful for clinical interpretation and generally parallels the PCV and hemoglobin concentration (Weiser, 2012). The TRBC may be useful in calculating red cell indices or for calculating the hematocrit (HCT) when instrument determinations are used.

The HCT and PCV are often used interchangeably, but the HCT is calculated as a tenth of the product from the TRBC and MCV. The PCV is a direct method and therefore generally more accurate unless there are issues with the sample handling process or the centrifuge is not well maintained, not calibrated, or improper settings are used.

The PCV is determined using the standard manual technique that employs microhematocrit tubes, tube sealant, a microhematocrit centrifuge (12 000 *g* for 5 min), and a tube-reading card or device (Weiser, 2012, 2022). There are three distinct layers observed in the spun microhematocrit tube. The plasma column is located at the top of the tube, and the packed erythrocytes are located at the bottom. The buffy coat appears as a small, white band located just above the erythrocyte column and consists of leukocytes and platelets. The buffy coat typically increases in size when the leukocyte concentration increases.

The PCV is affected by the number and size of the erythrocytes, as well as changes in the plasma volume

Exotic Animal Hematology and Cytology, Fifth Edition. Terry W. Campbell and Krystan R. Grant.

Companion website: www.wiley.com/go/campbell/exotic

that do not affect the total cell mass. These changes include increased plasma volume (hemodilution), decreased plasma volume (hemoconcentration), improper blood sampling (hemodilution), and epinephrine administration and hypothermia, which may result in hemoconcentration (see Appendix B for PCV ranges of selected species). A PCV below the low end of the reference interval is suggestive of anemia and a PCV greater than the high end of the reference interval suggests dehydration or erythrocytosis (polycythemia). Anemia and erythrocytosis are described in more detail in Chapter 3.

Plasma Appearance and Protein

The color and clarity of the plasma column above the packed erythrocytes should be noted. Normal plasma is typically colorless and clear. Generally, in mammals, icteric plasma is yellow, lipemic plasma is white and opaque, and hemolytic plasma is red (Washington and Van Hoosier, 2012; Weiser, 2012, 2022). Lipemic samples may reflect disorders involving lipid metabolism. Hemolysis may occur and usually results from lysis of erythrocytes during blood collection or sample handling. Intravascular hemolysis may also cause hemolysis of the sample in some instances. If the PCV is normal, then the presence of the hemolysis is probably associated with artifactual lysis of erythrocytes.

Plasma protein concentration is typically determined using handheld refractometers, which have been the standard instruments for determining protein concentration in plasma and body cavity fluid samples since the 1960s (George and O'Neill, 2001). The microhematocrit tube is snapped above the buffer coat layer, and the isolated plasma can be loaded to the refractometer.

Hemoglobin

Hemoglobin is a protein with four iron-containing heme subunits that transports oxygen and carbon dioxide within circulation. Hemoglobin is usually determined by an automated analyzer with spectrophotometry. As with other mammals, hemoglobin is approximately one-third of the hematocrit. Hemolysis and lipemia may interfere with the hemoglobin concentration, resulting in a mismatch of hemoglobin to HCT.

Total Erythrocyte Concentration

The total erythrocyte concentration is usually determined using an automatic analyzer. Electronic impedance cell counters provide a rapid, reliable method for obtaining total red blood cell concentrations. Manual red blood cell counting is also an option and may be a more practical option given the small blood volume that is often obtained from some of the exotic or laboratory mammals. Previously, the method used to obtain total red blood cell counts was the erythrocyte Unopette (Unopette, Becton-Dickinson, Rutherford, NJ) method used in mammalian hematology. In 2009, the erythrocyte Unopette system was discontinued, but a similar kit is available for manual red cell counts in mammals (Erythro-pette™, Exotic Animal Solutions, Inc. Hueytown, AL).

Erythrocyte Indices

The erythrocyte indices help to classify anemia and include the MCV or mean erythrocyte volume (MEV), MCH or mean erythrocyte hemoglobin (MEH), and MCHC or mean erythrocyte hemoglobin concentration (MEHC). They can be provided with results from automatic analyzers or can be calculated using the PCV, erythrocyte concentration, and hemoglobin concentration. Depending on the sample volume, dilution of anticoagulants with small volumes may be a factor in altering results of the MCV and MCHC (Moorhead et al., 2016).

The MCV is an index of red cell volume and is calculated as follows:

$$\mathrm{MCV}\left(\mathrm{fL}\right)=\left(\mathrm{PCV}\left(\%\right)\times 10\right)/\ \mathrm{TRBC}$$

The MCH is an index of the hemoglobin content in an average red blood cell and is not commonly used (Weiser, 2012), but is calculated as follows:

$$\mathrm{MCH}\left(\mathrm{pg}\right)=\left(\mathrm{Hb}\left(\mathrm{g/dL}\right)\times 10\right)/\ \mathrm{TRBC}$$

The MCHC is an index denoting the proportion of hemoglobin present in an average erythrocyte and is calculated (Washington and Van Hoosier, 2012) as follows:

$$\mathrm{MCHC}\left(\mathrm{g/dL}\right)=\left(\mathrm{Hgb}\left(\mathrm{g/dL}\right)\times 100\right)/\ \mathrm{PCV}\left(\%\right)$$

Erythrocyte parameters for selected mammal species can be found in Appendix B, Table B.1.

Published MCV (femtoliters, μm^3) reference intervals for mammals vary and therefore should be reviewed based on species. The MCHC values are typically around 30 g/dL (Washington and Van Hoosier, 2012).

Reticulocytes

During the final stages of erythrocyte maturation in mammals (at the metarubricyte stage of development), the nucleus undergoes degeneration and is extruded from the cell. The reticulocyte represents the erythrocyte during the period between the loss of the nucleus and the loss of the ribosomes and mitochondria, at which time the cell becomes mature. Reticulocytes are identified by the presence of dark-staining organelles within supravitally stained erythrocytes.

Reticulocyte quantification is important for the evaluation of erythrocyte regeneration and the anemic patient. Microscopic counts of stained reticulocytes have been the standard quantification method since the 1940s; however, modern automated hematology analyzers have been developed and can quantify reticulocytes more accurately, faster, and at a reduced cost. (Riley et al., 2001). Initially developed to analyze human blood samples, these automated hematology analyzers have been adapted for veterinary use (Moritz et al., 2004). In general, the automated methods for obtaining absolute reticulocyte counts offer good correlation with manual counting for dogs, cats, rabbits, rats, and mice (Mathers et al., 2008; Kaufhold et al., 2018). However, microscopic confirmation of quantifications is recommended when high numbers of reticulocytes are observed when using automated methods, with ethylenediaminetetraacetic acid (EDTA) being the anticoagulant of choice (Kaufhold et al., 2018).

The manual reticulocyte counting method involves the counting of the number of reticulocytes in a supravitally stained (using brilliant cresyl blue or new methylene blue) blood film made from EDTA or lithium heparin blood. 50 µL of EDTA (or lithium heparin) blood and 50 µL of brilliant cresyl blue are mixed into an Eppendorf cup and incubated at room temperature for 30 min, before making the blood film. The number of reticulocytes in 1000 erythrocytes is counted twice using 1000× magnification (oil immersion).

Leukocyte Parameters

Total Leukocyte Concentration

Leukocyte counts may be obtained using manual and automated methods. In mammals, nucleated red blood cells appear in peripheral blood only during embryonic life. Afterward, these cells are absent from the blood of the healthy adult. Because the anucleated mammalian erythrocyte is unique among most animals, the presence of nucleated red blood cells in peripheral blood can result in an artificially elevated total leukocyte concentration of a blood sample. Therefore, recognizing the presence of nucleated red blood cells is important in various clinical settings (especially in mammals undergoing chemotherapy, where leukopenic patients may appear to have an elevated white blood cell count). Automated methods for obtaining total leukocyte counts may fail to recognize nucleated red blood cells; therefore, evaluation of the peripheral blood film becomes important (Simões et al., 2020).

Leukocyte Differential

The differential leukocyte count and leukocyte morphology are obtained by microscopic evaluation of stained blood films. A variety of hematologic stains are available (see Appendix A). Rapid stains (i.e., Diff–Quik, Dade Diagnostics, Aguada, Puerto Rico) or Hemacolor® (Miles Laboratories, Inc., Elkhart, IN) have a shorter staining time, but do not always provide adequate differentiation between the various leukocytes. Stains such as Wright's, Wright–Giemsa, and May–Grünwald–Giemsa stains are more time consuming, but provide better differentiation of the leukocytes and immature erythrocytes.

The leukocyte differential is performed during the microscopic evaluation of Romanowsky-stained blood films, typically from blood samples collected in EDTA as an anticoagulant. Blood samples collected into heparin make it necessary to prepare the blood films immediately following sample collection to decrease the incidence of cell clumping. Whenever possible, preparation of blood films using blood containing no anticoagulant is preferred. The differential leukocyte count is performed by counting a minimum of 100 leukocytes in a monocellular area in the blood film. The cells counted are those consecutively encountered as one moves from one counting field to the next. The cells are classified as neutrophils (Chapter 3: Figures 3.24, 3.43, and 3.50) or heterophils (Chapter 3: Figures 3.28, 3.35, and 3.37), eosinophils (Chapter 3: Figures 3.25, 3.30, and 3.44), basophils (Chapter 3: Figures 3.29, 3.39, and 3.52), lymphocytes (Chapter 3: Figures 3.23, 3.33, and 3.46), and monocytes (Chapter 3: Figures 3.26, 3.41, and 3.47). The number of each cell type becomes a fraction of the total or a percentage of the leukocyte population. Absolute numbers of each cell type are obtained by multiplying the total leukocyte concentration by the percentage of that type of leukocyte from the differential count.

Platelet Parameters

Platelet numbers in the blood can be counted using automated methods or manual techniques using a hemacytometer. Blood films may be used to assess thrombocyte numbers. A minimum of 5 platelets or 5–10 platelets per high-power field (1000× magnification or oil-immersion field) would be interpreted as an adequate number (Baker, 2004).

References

Baker DC. 2004. Diagnosis of disorders of hemostasis. In: Thrall MA, Baker DC, Campbell TW, et al. (eds), *Veterinary Hematology and Clinical Chemistry*. Philadelphia, PA: Lippincott Williams & Wilkins, pp. 179–196.

George JW, O'Neill SL. 2001. Comparison of refractometer and biuret methods for total protein measurement in body cavity fluids. *Vet Clin Pathol* 30:16–18.

Kaufhold AE, Hirschberger J, Reese S, et al. 2018. A comparison of manual counting of rabbit reticulocytes with ADVIA 2120i analyzer counting. *J Vet Diagn Invest* 30(3):337–341.

Mathers R, Evans GO, Bleby J, et al. 2008. Evaluation of the Sysmex XT-2000iV haematology analyser for rat, dog and mouse whole blood samples. *Comp Clin Pathol* 17:137–144.

Moorhead KA, Discipulo ML, Hu J, et al. 2016. Alterations due to dilution and anticoagulant effects in hematologic analysis of rodent blood samples on the Sysmex XT-2000iV. *Vet Clin Pathol* 45(2):215–224.

Moritz A, Meyer K, Failing K, et al. 2004. Canine and feline hematology reference values for the ADVIA 120 hematology system. *Vet Clin Pathol* 33:32–38.

Riley RS, Ben-Ezra JM, Goel R, et al. 2001. Reticulocytes and reticulocyte enumeration. *J Clin Lab Anim* 15:267–294.

Simões PB, Costa A, Santos A, et al. 2020. Blood from a "half-fish" dog: How modern analyzers deal with nucleated red blood cells. *Vet Clin Pathol* 49:8–10.

Washington IM, Van Hoosier G. 2012. Clinical biochemistry and hematology. In: Suckow MA, Stevens KA, Wilson RP (eds), *The Laboratory Rabbit, Guinea Pig, Hamster, and Other Rodents*. Oxford: Academic Press.

Weiser G. 2012. Laboratory technology for veterinary medicine. In: Thrall M, Weiser G, Allison RW, et al. (eds), *Veterinary Hematology and Clinical Chemistry*, 2nd edn, Ames, IA: Wiley-Blackwell, pp 3–33.

Weiser G. 2022. Laboratory technology for veterinary medicine. In: Thrall M, Weiser G, Allison RW, et al. (eds), *Veterinary Hematology and Clinical Chemistry*, 3rd edn, Ames, IA: Wiley-Blackwell, in press.

3 Evaluation and Interpretation of the Peripheral Blood of Mammals

The hematology of laboratory and exotic mammals is similar in many respects to that of domestic mammals. However, obtaining meaningful reference values can be difficult due to variations associated with blood collection, laboratory procedures, and intrinsic and extrinsic factors.

The hemograms of small mammals can vary dependent on age, sex, environmental conditions, and diet. Many of these animals are prey species with well-developed fight-or-flight responses. Any event that may be perceived as stressful by such an animal may result in excess catecholamine release, which will subsequently affect the hemograms. Often, the mere transportation of the patient to the veterinary hospital constitutes some type of stress, and the physical or chemical restraint that is sometimes required for blood collection adds to this response.

Interpretation of the hemograms of exotic animals can be challenging. In addition to the intrinsic and extrinsic factors directly associated with the exotic animal patient, other factors may affect interpretation of the hemograms as well. Laboratory procedures and sample handling are not standardized for most exotic animal species, which leads to variability between data sets from laboratory to laboratory.

Representative hemic cells found in mammalian blood films can be found in Appendix C.

Mammalian Erythrocytes

Erythrocyte evaluation is an integral part of the complete blood cell and morphology or hemic cytology of the blood film. Exotic and laboratory small mammal erythrocytes are similar in size (4–8 μm in diameter) and morphology compared to domestic mammals. Most mammalian erythrocytes are anucleate, round, and biconcave (Figure 3.1a). The biconcavity of the cell presents a central area of pallor, although species with smaller erythrocytes may have a more uniform appearance (Thrall, 2012d). The biconcavity allows for cell plasticity, thereby improving movement through vessels and decreasing the distance between hemoglobin and cell surface to promote efficient gas exchange. In general, the total erythrocyte count and mean cell volume vary among mammals, while the hemoglobin content and packed cell volume remain relatively constant. As a result, an inverse relationship between cell size and number exists. Mammals with smaller erythrocytes have a higher total erythrocyte count, and vice versa. The calculated relationship between these two parameters yields the hematocrit, which should be nearly equivalent to the packed cell volume.

Morphology and Color

The hemoglobin contained within erythrocytes provides oxygen to the tissues. Mammalian erythrocytes are efficient in making this exchange primarily based upon their shape. Erythrocytes in mammalian blood films are anucleated, round, and biconcave – except those from camelids, which are oval and flat. Romanowsky-stained blood films from mammals often reveal erythrocytes with a distinct area of central pallor resulting from their biconcavity. This shape provides for the efficient exchange of oxygen by allowing the red blood cell to deform its shape to enable travel through blood vessels

Exotic Animal Hematology and Cytology, Fifth Edition. Terry W. Campbell and Krystan R. Grant.

Companion website: www.wiley.com/go/campbell/exotic

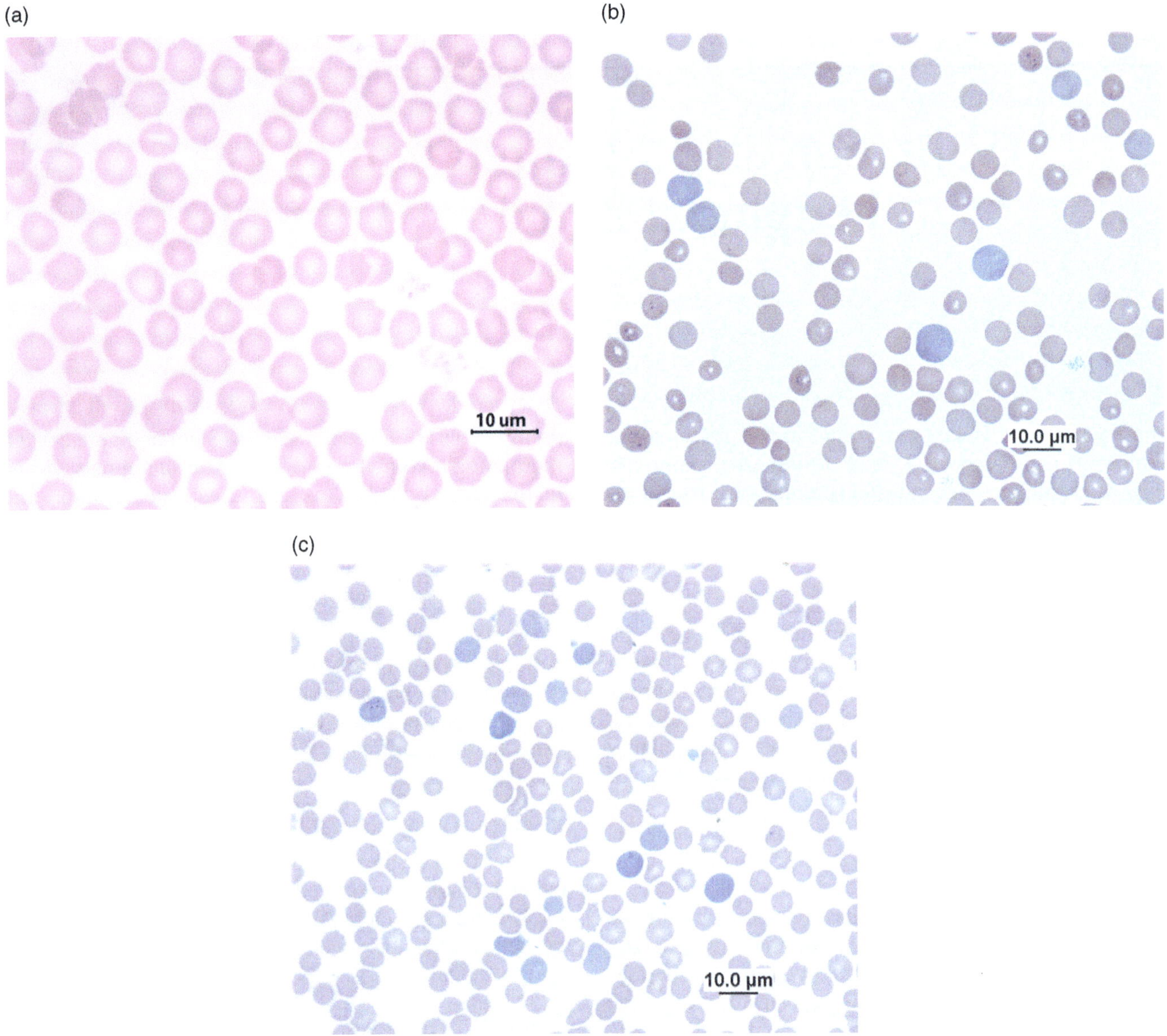

Fig. 3.1. (a) Normal erythrocytes in the blood film of a rabbit (*Oryctolagus cuniculus*), Wright–Giemsa stain. (b) Polychromasia in the blood film of an African hedgehog (*Atelerix albiventris*), Wright–Giemsa stain. (c) Polychromasia in the blood film of a ferret (*Mustela putorius furo*), Wright–Giemsa stain.

with a diameter smaller than its own. The morphology of the erythrocytes in the stained blood film is useful in providing clues as to the nature of red blood cell disorders, such an anemia.

Diagnostically, the important morphologic characteristics of mammalian erythrocytes include polychromatic, hypochromatic, microcytic, and macrocytic erythrocytes; poikilocytosis; and red blood cell inclusions. Appendix B, Tables B.1 and B.2 provide guidelines for the evaluation of mammalian erythrocytes. Important erythrocyte structures include Heinz bodies, basophilic stippling, nucleated erythrocytes, and Howell–Jolly bodies. Other abnormalities such as Rouleaux formation and red blood cell agglutination should also be reported.

Polychromasia and Hypochromasia

Polychromasia and hypochromasia are staining characteristics of erythrocytes that should be noted when evaluating erythrocyte morphology. Polychromatic erythrocytes (reticulocytes) are young erythrocytes that have been released into circulation early and are larger and more basophilic in color compared to mature erythrocytes (Figures 3.1b and 3.1c). The degree of polychromasia (total number of polychromatic erythrocytes) may aid the determination of the cause of an anemia. Polychromasia tends to occur in association with blood loss and blood destruction anemias. Polychromasia is not present in anemias caused by erythroid hypoplasia or in an aplastic anemia.

Polychromatic erythrocytes as seen in Romanowsky-stained blood films are considered the same as the reticulocytes seen on supravitally stained blood films, such as new methylene blue (see the section titled "Reticulocytes" in Chapter 2) (Figure 3.2). Both are used as a measure of the regenerative response of the erythrocytes; however, the reticulocytes are easier to differentiate from mature erythrocytes. An absolute reticulocyte count, therefore, is easier to obtain than an absolute polychromatic cell count.

Hypochromasia is indicated by pale-staining erythrocytes with an increased area of central pallor (Figure 3.3). Hypochromatic erythrocytes indicate a state of iron deficiency. Iron deficiency in adult mammals is generally the result of chronic blood loss caused by blood-sucking parasites, gastrointestinal ulcers, inflammatory bowel disease, or neoplasms. Iron-deficiency anemia in very young mammals is due to inadequate dietary iron.

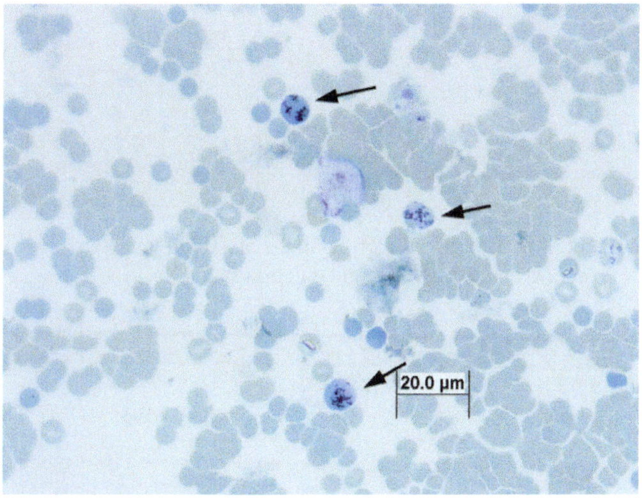

Fig. 3.2. Reticulocytes (arrows) in the blood film of a mammal, new methylene blue stain.

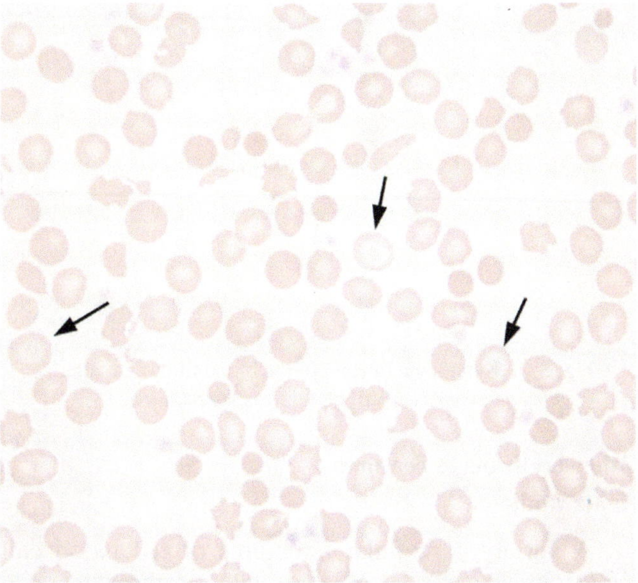

Fig. 3.3. Hypochromasia (arrows show hypochromic erythrocytes) in the blood film of an otter (*Lontra canadensis*), Wright–Giemsa stain (50×).

Size

Evaluation of erythrocyte size provides important hematologic clues to the process of some diseases. The mean cell volume (MCV) is a measure of the average size of the erythrocytes present in a blood sample. A low MCV is associated with microcytic erythrocytes, which are red blood cells that are smaller than normal cells (Figure 3.4). Microcytic erythrocytes are usually associated with iron-deficiency anemia. A high MCV is associated with macrocytic erythrocytes (red blood cells that are larger than normal cells). Macrocytic erythrocytes are made up of polychromatic erythrocytes associated with erythroid regeneration (Figures 3.1b and 3.1c).

Shape

Poikilocytosis is a general term used when erythrocytes with abnormal shapes are present in the blood film. Poikilocytosis can indicate a pathologic, physiological, or artifactual process. Erythrocyte shape is an important

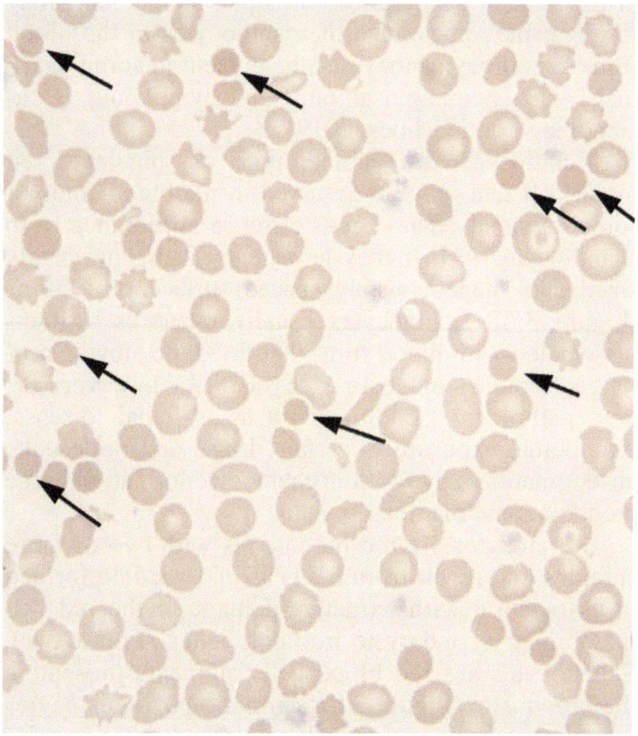

Fig. 3.4. Microcytic erythrocytes (arrows) in the blood film of an otter (*Lontra canadensis*), Wright–Giemsa stain (50×).

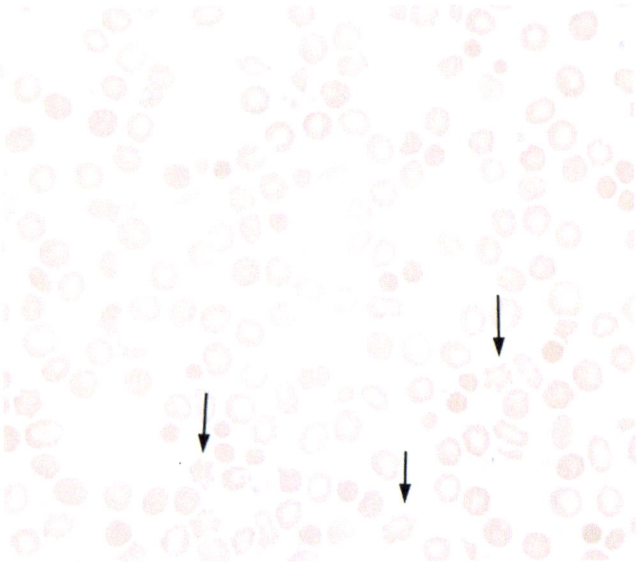

Fig. 3.5. Acanthocytes (arrows) in the blood film of an otter (*Lontra canadensis*), Wright–Giemsa stain (50×).

feature of the hemogram, and important shape abnormalities include acanthocytes, echinocytes, keratocytes, and schistocytes.

Acanthocytes are spiculated erythrocytes with irregularly spaced, spike-like surface projections that vary in length and thickness (Figure 3.5). The abnormal shape of the acanthocyte is associated with abnormal lipid content in the red cell membrane. Any disease-causing alterations in lipid metabolism may result in the appearance of acanthocytes in the blood film. Acanthocytes may also be present in some mammals with hemangiosarcoma and lymphoma (Bau-Gaudreault and Grimes, 2019).

Echinocytes are another type of spiculated red blood cell that may be observed in the blood films of some mammals. These cells differ in appearance from acanthocytes in that they have many short, uniformly sized and shaped, evenly spaced surface projections (Figure 3.6). Echinocytes usually occur as artifacts (associated with blood films that dried too slowly, prolonged sample storage, or excess EDTA); however, certain pathologic conditions such as renal disease, lymphoma, exposure to certain drugs, and rattlesnake envenomation may result in echinocyte formation in the blood of some mammal species.

Keratocytes are red blood cells with two or more spicules that result from the lysis of a vacuole formed in association with oxidative damage to the red cell membrane secondary to iron deficiency (Figure 3.7). Schistocytes are red blood cell fragments present in the blood film (Figure 3.8). Formation of schistocytes may be associated with disseminated intravascular coagulopathy (DIC), hemangiosarcomas, and iron deficiency.

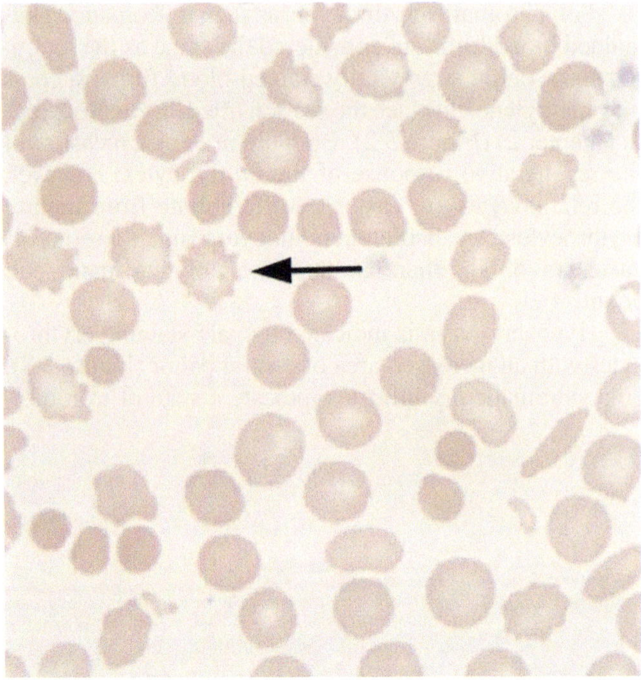

Fig. 3.6. Echinocyte (arrow) in the blood film of an otter (*Lontra canadensis*), Wright–Giemsa stain (50×).

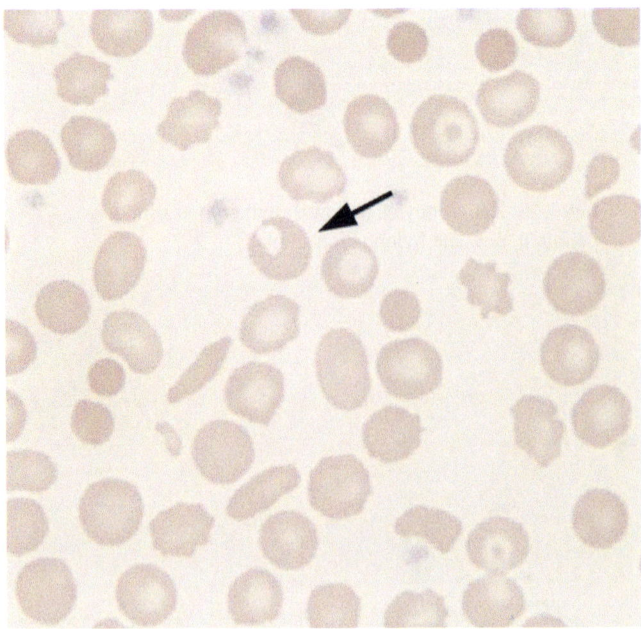

Fig. 3.7. Keratocyte (arrow) in the blood film of an otter (*Lontra canadensis*), Wright–Giemsa stain (50×).

Other Erythrocyte Features

Heinz Bodies

A variety of cellular structures or red blood cell inclusions can be associated with erythrocytes and should be noted. Heinz bodies are small, eccentric, single to multiple pale structures that often protrude slightly from the red cell margins (Figures 3.9a and 3.9b). They

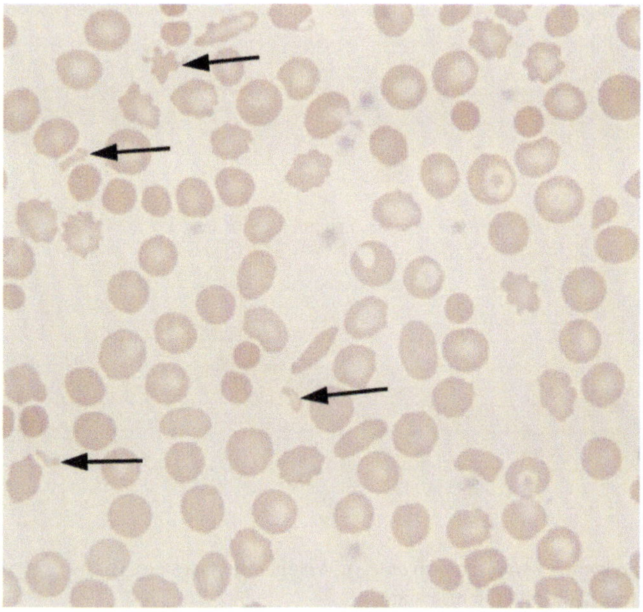

Fig. 3.8. Schistocytes (arrows) in the blood film of an otter (*Lontra canadensis*), Wright–Giemsa stain (50×).

are formed by oxidative denaturation of hemoglobin and can be associated with certain plant chemicals (onions and garlic), drugs (acetaminophen and propofol), and diseases such as lymphoma and hyperthyroidism.

Basophilic Stippling

Basophilic stippling appears in the erythrocyte as small basophilic granules present within the cytoplasm of the cell. Basophilic stippling is commonly associated with erythrocyte regeneration and is commonly found in blood films from healthy animals, such as gerbils. Basophilic stippling may also be associated with non-anemic animals with lead poisoning, but this is generally a rare finding.

Nucleated Red Blood Cells

Nucleated erythrocytes are immature red blood cells that are released in an early stage of maturation from the bone marrow usually as part of a regenerative response to anemia or hypoxia (Figures 3.10a and 3.10b). An inappropriate release of nucleated erythrocytes may be seen with lead poisoning or a myelodysplastic condition as well.

Howell–Jolly Bodies

Howell–Jolly bodies are small, variably sized, round, dark blue inclusions present in the cytoplasm of the erythrocyte (Figure 3.11). They represent nuclear remnants that occur as part of a regenerative response, or they may indicate suppressed splenic function.

Rouleaux

Rouleaux formation and red blood cell agglutination occur when red blood cells group together, and may be noted in the blood films of some animals. Rouleaux formation appears as linear stacking of erythrocytes and is often associated with increased plasma proteins, such as immunoglobulins, in domestic mammals. Erythrocyte agglutination may be identified by irregular to circular clumping of erythrocytes and is associated with immune-mediated hemolytic anemia. Rouleaux formation may

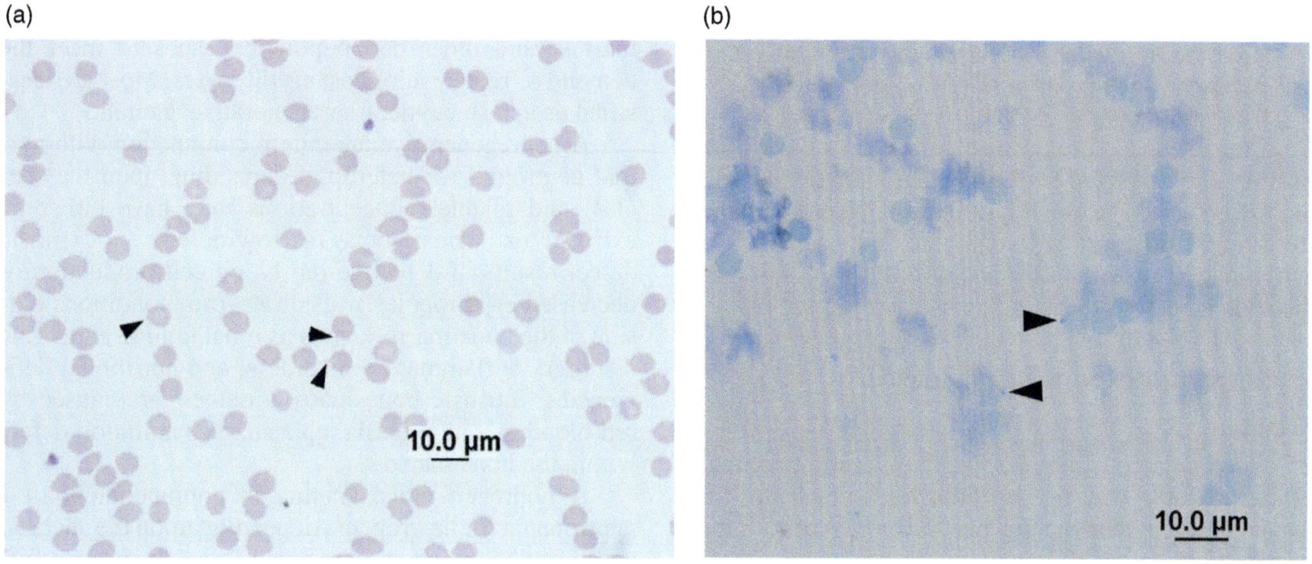

Fig. 3.9. (a) Heinz bodies (arrowheads) in the red blood cells of a ferret (*Mustela putorius furo*), Wright–Giemsa stain. (b) Heinz bodies (arrowheads) in the red blood cells of a ferret (*Mustela putorius furo*), new methylene blue stain.

(a) (b)

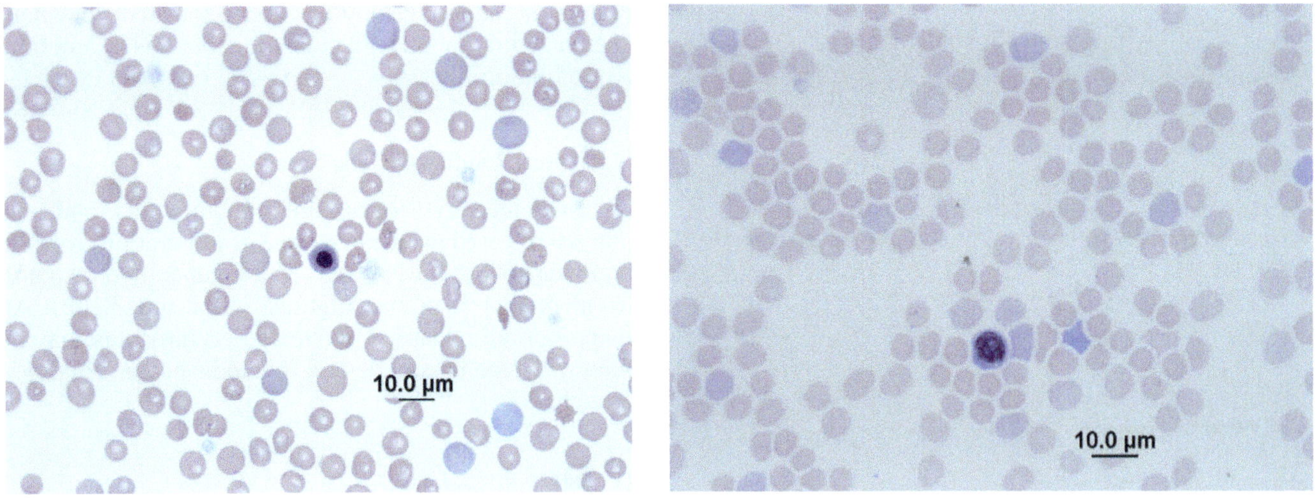

Fig. 3.10. (a) Nucleated erythrocyte in the blood film of an African hedgehog (*Atelerix albiventris*), Wright–Giemsa stain. (b) Nucleated erythrocyte in the blood film of a ferret (*Mustela putorius furo*), Wright–Giemsa stain.

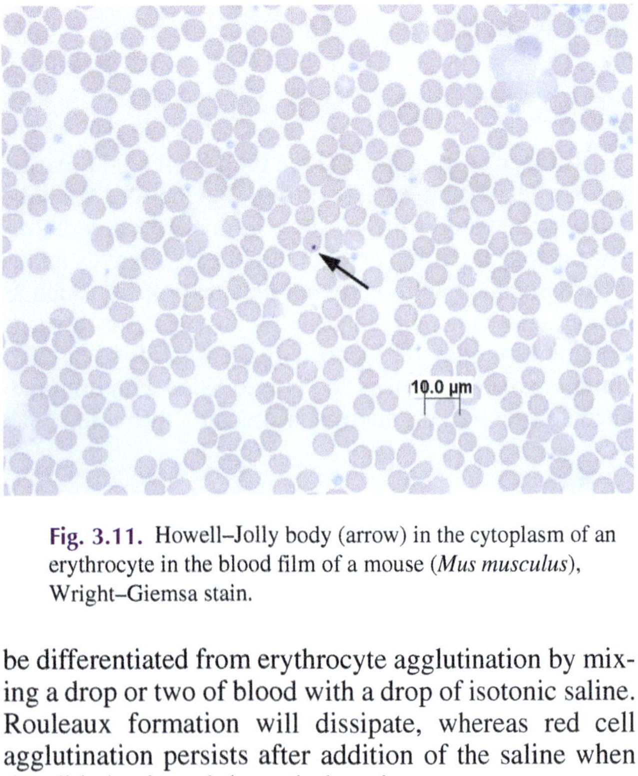

Fig. 3.11. Howell–Jolly body (arrow) in the cytoplasm of an erythrocyte in the blood film of a mouse (*Mus musculus*), Wright–Giemsa stain.

be differentiated from erythrocyte agglutination by mixing a drop or two of blood with a drop of isotonic saline. Rouleaux formation will dissipate, whereas red cell agglutination persists after addition of the saline when the slide is viewed through the microscope.

Erythrocyte Response to Disease

Anemias

Anemia is considered a reduction in the total mass of hemoglobin-bearing erythrocytes, which in turn results in a deficiency in oxygen transport. Anemias may be caused by many etiologies, but in general are caused by abnormal red blood cell loss that cannot be compensated by normal erythropoiesis, or decreased blood cell production, which cannot provide sufficient replacement of red cells that are lost normally.

Anemias are often classified according to their pathophysiology as hemolytic, hemorrhagic, or hypoplastic. Hemolytic anemia results from increased erythrocyte destruction. Hemorrhagic anemia results from erythrocyte loss via hemorrhage. Hypoplastic anemia results from decreased production of erythrocytes.

Nonregenerative Anemia

Anemia associated with the lack of a regenerative response in the form of circulating immature erythrocytes (polychromatophilic erythrocytes or reticulocytes) is indicative of a nonregenerative anemia. This is a result of the inability of the erythropoietic tissue in the bone marrow and other hematopoietic tissues to meet the demand of replenishing lost erythrocytes. Most are classified as a normocytic, nonregenerative anemia.

A nonregenerative anemia in conjunction with normal neutrophil (or heterophil depending upon the species) and platelet concentrations may have either an extrinsic or intrinsic bone marrow defect. An extrinsic defect results in defective red blood cell production or decreased erythropoiesis resulting from conditions outside of the bone marrow, such as renal failure, endocrine disorders, inflammatory disorders, and nutritional deficiencies. Intrinsic bone marrow defects are caused by red blood cell hypoplasia, aplasia, or maturation defect within the bone marrow.

A nonregenerative anemia in conjunction with a neutropenia (or heteropenia depending upon the species) and thrombocytopenia is referred to as a pancytopenia. Pancytopenia can indicate stem cell injury or myelophthisic disorder. Myelophthisic disorders occur when nonhematopoietic neoplastic cells (such as lymphomas) crowd out the hematopoietic tissue. Stem cell injury can be reversible or irreversible depending upon the etiology. Irreversible stem cell injuries result from an intrinsic defect in the proliferative behavior and/or regulation of stem cell ability to differentiate into the various cell types during hematopoiesis. Causes of irreversible stem cell injury include exposure to certain drugs, chemicals, viruses, and radiation, as well as immune-mediated stem cell injury. Injury to the stem cells can result in a general lack of cell production, resulting in aplastic anemia or an uncontrolled proliferation of neoplastic cells. Reversible stem cell injury, a transient condition, can also be caused by drugs, chemicals, viruses, radiation, and immune-mediated destruction of stem cells. Although reversible stem cell injury does not progress to neoplasia, it can lead to myelofibrosis.

Estrogen toxicosis is perhaps the most common cause of aplastic anemia (aplastic pancytopenia) in exotic mammals, especially intact female ferrets. Ferrets are induced ovulators, and when mating does not occur, the female will stay in estrus for an extended period, commonly resulting in marrow suppression from endogenous estrogen. This is a potentially fatal disorder. The exact mechanism of estrogen toxicosis is not known. One possible explanation is the secretion (possibly by thymic stromal cells) of an estrogen-induced substance that inhibits stem cells that causes an initial thrombocytosis and neutrophilia before the marrow suppression and aplastic anemia occur (Bernard et al., 1983). Myelosuppression may result from the administration of excessive amounts of estrogen or from an idiosyncratic sensitivity to estrogen. Bone marrow suppression resulting from excessive concentrations of endogenous estrogen can also occur in male animals with Sertoli cell tumors or in females with cystic ovaries or granulosa cell tumors (Thrall, 2012a).

A chemical agent, such as a drug used to create immunosuppression or to treat neoplasia, that commonly cause reversible stem cell damage in domestic mammals has a strong potential for creating the same disorders in nondomestic mammals. A list of these drugs can be found in clinical pathology references for domestic mammals (Thrall, 2012a). Likewise, stem cell destruction caused by drug-induced immune-mediated injury seen in domestic mammals may also occur in nondomestic mammals, resulting in aplastic anemia.

A nonregenerative anemia associated with normal neutrophil (or heterophil) and platelet concentrations in the peripheral blood and a marked decrease in the population of bone marrow erythroid precursors without a decrease in granulocyte precursors and megakaryocytes is a pure erythrocyte aplasia. In domestic mammals, especially the dog, this condition is nearly always the result of immune-mediated destruction of erythroid precursors (Thrall, 2012a). Affected animals often reveal an arrest at some stage of erythroid precursor maturation, but a complete absence of erythroid precursors may also be seen. The presence of phagocytized rubricytes or metarubricytes aids in the diagnosis.

Anemia of chronic disease (disorders) resulting in red cell hypoplasia is a common cause of nonregenerative anemia in exotic animals. This results from conditions that are extrinsic to the marrow, such as inflammatory disease, chronic renal failure, endocrine disease, and nutritional deficiencies (Campbell and Grant, 2010). Inflammatory diseases normally result in a mild-to-moderate, nonregenerative, normocytic anemia. Anemia can result from inflammation caused by infectious agents, trauma, or neoplasia. Chronic inflammation leads to a chain of events that limits the availability of iron for erythropoiesis and decreases erythrocyte production and red blood cell life span, resulting in anemia (Thrall, 2012a). The presence of an inflammatory leukogram, decreased serum iron concentration with a normal or increased serum ferritin concentration, or a normal or decreased total iron-binding capacity will aid the diagnosis. Chronic renal failure leads to a moderate-to-severe (depending upon the severity of the renal failure), nonregenerative, normocytic anemia. The failing kidneys quit producing erythropoietin, which in turn stops erythropoiesis. Domestic mammals, especially dogs, will demonstrate a mild, nonregenerative, normocytic anemia with various endocrine disorders, such as hypothyroidism and hypoadrenocorticism. These conditions have the potential for causing similar anemias in nondomestic mammals.

Common causes of nonregenerative anemia in nondomestic mammals include malignant neoplasia such as lymphoma, systemic infections, and hyperestrogenism (especially in the intact female ferret).

Regenerative Anemia and Reticulocytes

Regenerative anemia is indicated by the bone marrow's attempt to compensate for the loss of red blood cells by increased erythrocyte production and early release of immature red cells. This is indicated by an increase in the number of polychromatic red blood cells on the Wright's-stained blood film and increased reticulocyte concentration. The MCV may also be increased.

Reticulocytes are the stage of red blood cell maturation between metarubricytes and mature erythrocytes. They are evaluated by staining blood with a supravital dye, such as new methylene blue (1% in saline plus 1.6% potassium oxalate) or brilliant cresyl blue (1% in saline) to demonstrate ribosomal material in reticulocytes. Reticulocyte numbers in blood from exotic animals are generally counted manually on stained blood films and reported as a percentage of reticulocytes per 1000 red blood cells. Multiplying this percentage by the absolute erythrocyte count obtained by either the manual hemacytometer method or an automated method provides the absolute reticulocyte count.

Hemorrhagic Anemia

Blood loss anemia can occur from the acute or chronic loss of blood either externally or internally. Causes of acute hemorrhagic anemia include traumatic injury, blood loss during a surgical procedure, hemorrhagic ulcers (i.e., gastrointestinal ulcers or neoplasms), and bleeding disorders associated with coagulation defects. Such hemostatic disorders include thrombocytopenia, inherited coagulopathies, and acquired coagulopathies, such as warfarin toxicosis or disseminated vascular coagulopathy. Common causes of chronic blood loss include bleeding lesions, especially those within the gastrointestinal tract, and gastrointestinal or external parasites. Chronic blood loss from gastrointestinal ulcers is common in domestic ferrets and is generally associated with *Helicobacter mustelae*.

During external blood loss, blood components such as iron and plasma protein are lost. As a result, the laboratory findings generally include either a low-normal plasma protein concentration or hypoproteinemia coupled with a regenerative anemia. Hypoproteinemia, when present, implies a recent or severe blood loss because protein is replaced much faster than the red blood cells. However, hypoproteinemia caused by disorders other than blood loss should also be considered. These include decreased protein intake, such as malabsorption, maldigestion, and starvation; decreased production of protein, as seen in liver failure; or other types of protein loss, such as glomerulonephropathy and protein-losing enteropathy. Chronic external blood loss leads to iron-deficiency anemia.

Internal blood loss mimics hemolytic anemia because the red blood cells are broken down within the body, and the protein and iron are not lost. Blood loss within the body is more difficult to detect than the loss of blood outside the body.

Acute Blood Loss

Initially, during acute blood loss, the packed cell volume (PCV) remains normal because both cells and plasma proteins are lost. Within a few hours, the PCV and plasma protein decrease because of dilution, as interstitial fluid is added to blood to restore normal vascular volume. This is followed by a pre-regenerative period, because it generally takes 1–2 days following the acute blood loss for a regenerative response in the form of increased numbers of polychromatophilic erythrocytes (reticulocytes) to appear in the blood. Dehydration can delay the decrease in the hematocrit, and hemodilution by excessive fluid therapy can reduce the hematocrit, clouding the assessment of the true severity of the anemia. The presence of macrocytic, hypochromic erythrocytes indicates prior red blood cell regeneration.

In some animals, such as the dog, the presence of acanthocytes and schistocytes is associated with acute blood loss associated with a hemangiosarcoma. Laboratory findings associated with hemangiosarcomas include increased polychromasia (reticulocytosis), a transient hypoproteinemia, and a mild-to-moderate thrombocytopenia.

Chronic Blood Loss and Iron-Deficiency Anemia

Iron-deficiency anemia in adult animals is usually associated with chronic blood loss when iron stores are quickly depleted. Gastrointestinal bleeding, such as occurs with ulcers, neoplasms, or internal parasites, or heavy infestations of blood-sucking ectoparasites, leads to iron-deficiency anemia. Because iron is required for hemoglobin synthesis, iron deficiency results in a deficiency in hemoglobin production, and iron-deficient erythrocytes undergo one or two additional cell divisions resulting in the formation of microcytes (Weiss, 2010). Therefore, laboratory findings associated with iron-deficiency anemia include a decreased MCV or the presence of microcytosis. The mean corpuscular hemoglobin concentration (MCHC) tends to decrease following the decrease in the MCV; however, it is commonly within the reference interval. Examination of the blood film reveals hypochromatic (pale) erythrocytes with increased central pallor (often only a narrow rim of lightly stained hemoglobin is present) and poikilocytosis. Keratocytes and schistocytes are common because of increased membrane susceptibility to oxidative damage. Initially, the erythrocyte develops a blister or vacuole where inner membrane surfaces are cross-linked across the cell, which eventually expands and breaks open to form the "apple-stem cells" and keratocytes (spiculated erythrocytes with two or more pointed projections) (Campbell and Grant, 2010; Thrall, 2012a). Projections from the keratocytes fragment from the cell to form schistocytes (cytoplasmic fragments). Iron-deficiency anemia usually demonstrates a regenerative response.

A thrombocytosis is present in some patients with iron-deficiency anemia. The mechanism for this is not known (it may be associated with increased erythropoietin or other cytokines) (Thrall, 2012a).

Iron deficiency is associated with a decreased serum iron concentration and low iron storage. Transferrin (a plasma glycoprotein that transports iron) saturation as measured by the total iron-binding capacity is usually increased in most species with iron deficiency, but may decrease in others. Assessment of iron storage can be determined by measuring serum ferritin (an acute phase protein); however, measuring serum ferritin can be difficult as it is a species-specific test and may be increased with iron deficiency in some species. Examination of a bone marrow aspirate for its iron content can also be used to assess iron storage. Bone marrow aspirates can be stained with Prussian blue to detect hemosiderin stored in macrophages. The absence of hemosiderin in macrophages when examining a bone marrow aspirate indicates low iron storage; however, there is species variability with this method as some noniron-deficient animals may lack stainable iron in their bone marrow. Thus, the determination of low serum iron and a decreased MCV in an anemic patient is usually adequate to diagnose iron-deficiency anemia.

Hemolytic Anemia

Blood destruction (hemolysis) may be either intravascular or extravascular. This may occur because of an intrinsic (primary) defect, such as hereditary membrane defects or enzyme deficiencies, or of extrinsic (secondary) causes, such as erythrocyte parasites or immune-mediated destruction. Intravascular hemolysis occurs when there is actual lysis of erythrocytes within the vascular system. Extravascular hemolysis occurs when abnormal erythrocytes are phagocytized by macrophages, usually within the spleen or liver. Common causes of hemolytic anemia include immune-mediated mechanisms, erythrocyte parasites, and Heinz body formation because of oxidative damage caused by exposure to certain drugs and chemicals. Hemolytic anemia is a typically regenerative type of anemia characterized by increased anisocytosis, macrocytosis, polychromasia, nucleated erythrocytes, and Howell–Jolly bodies in the blood film (Figure 3.12).

Heinz Body Anemia

Heinz bodies form in red blood cell following oxidative damage that denatures and precipitates hemoglobin. Heinz bodies are detected in the blood stained with the same supravital dyes, such as new methylene blue and brilliant cresyl blue, used to demonstrate ribosomal material in reticulocytes (Campbell and Grant, 2010). Romanowsky-stained blood films may reveal Heinz bodies as bulges from the surface of red blood cells, lighter and refractile bodies compared to the rest of the hemoglobin of the red blood cell, or round bodies the color of hemoglobin in ghost cells (pale erythrocytes). Heinz bodies stained with supravital stains are lighter blue compared to the ribosomal material of reticulocytes and appear as large, round bodies (e.g., 1–2 μm in diameter in guinea pigs and rabbits) or multiple, small granular bodies depending upon the species.

Immune-Mediated Anemia

Immune-mediated hemolytic anemia (IMHA) is caused by red cell destruction due to antibodies directed against erythrocytes or immune complexes attached to erythrocytes. This typically results in a regenerative anemia unless antibodies are formed against red blood cell precursors causing destruction of polychromatophilic erythrocytes or earlier erythrocytes. In domestic animals, this type of anemia can be related to disorders such as infections, vaccinations, neoplasia, and administration of certain drugs (Thrall, 2012b).

The presence of spherocytes in the blood film because of partial erythrophagocytosis by macrophages is indicative of IMHA. Spherocytes are small erythrocytes that appear dense because they lack an area of lack central pallor (Figure 3.13). Spherocytes are difficult to detect in species in which the red cells normally lack central pallor. Red blood cell agglutination, another indication of IMHA, occurs when the cells are coated with autoantibody.

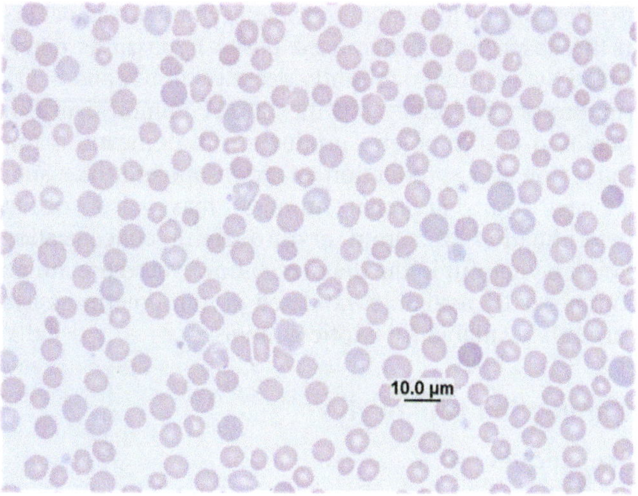

Fig. 3.12. Anisocytosis, macrocytosis, polychromasia in the blood film of an African hedgehog (*Atelerix albiventris*), Wright–Giemsa stain.

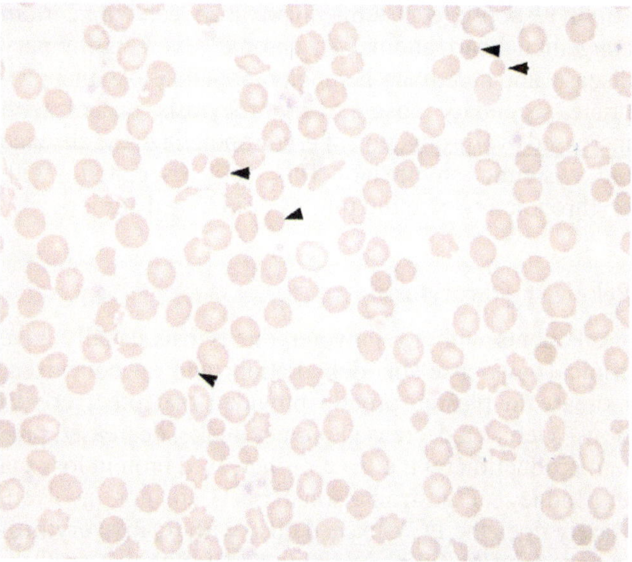

Fig. 3.13. Spherocytes (arrowheads) in the blood film of an otter (*Lontra canadensis*), Wright–Giemsa stain (50×).

Hemoparasites

Microorganisms, such as blood parasites, that infect erythrocytes may cause intravascular hemolysis or extravascular hemolysis, resulting in a hemolytic anemia. Most of these microorganisms that cause anemia do so by immune-mediated extravascular hemolysis. This occurs when antibodies against the organism, immune complexes, or complement bind to infected erythrocytes, which are removed from the blood by macrophages (erythrophagocytosis).

Erythrocytosis (Polycythemia)

The terms polycythemia and erythrocytosis are often used interchangeably by clinicians; however, erythrocytosis refers to an increase in the PCV (or hematocrit), red blood cell count, and hemoglobin concentration, whereas polycythemia implies that all blood cells, including leukocytes, are increased in concentration. A relative erythrocytosis refers to an increase in the PCV due to a decrease in plasma volume and hemoconcentration, as seen with dehydration. In some domestic species, this can also occur with erythrocyte redistribution and body fluid shifts, as seen with splenic contraction commonly associated with excitable animals. Absolute erythrocytosis refers to a true increase in the red cell mass. Primary absolute erythrocytosis (i.e., polycythemia vera) is a rare well-differentiated chronic myeloproliferative disorder (of humans, dogs, and cats) resulting in an autonomous proliferation of erythroid precursors independent of the erythropoietin concentration. Diagnosis of primary erythrocytosis is typically made by excluding causes of secondary erythrocytosis. Secondary absolute erythrocytosis results from excessive production of erythropoietin. This can be an appropriate overproduction of erythropoietin in response to systemic hypoxia as seen with certain congenital heart anomalies, chronic severe pulmonary disease, and hereditary hemoglobinopathies. An inappropriate secondary absolute erythrocytosis occurs with increased overproduction of erythropoietin in the absence of systemic hypoxia. This is associated with erythropoietin-secreting tumors or kidney disorders.

Relative Erythrocytosis

Patients with a relative erythrocytosis usually have clinical evidence of dehydration and a concurrent increase in plasma protein provided that other conditions, such as a decreased protein intake, decreased protein production by the liver, or increased protein loss via the kidney or gastrointestinal tract, are not involved. Rarely does the PCV exceed 60% with relative erythrocytosis (Hasler, 2000; Watson, 2000). Relative erythrocytosis resolves with treatment using replacement of fluids and electrolytes.

Effects of splenic contraction are typically seen only in those species of domestic mammals with normal high PCVs in association with exertion or excitement (epinephrine release). Splenic contraction results in a mild increase in the PCV with no increase in the plasma protein concentration. Presence of an excitement leukogram (a mature neutrophilia and lymphocytosis) is supportive of this type of relative erythrocytosis.

Primary Absolute Erythrocytosis

Unlike most other types of hematopoietic neoplasia, this myeloproliferative disorder exhibits normal-appearing erythroid cells with a normal maturation sequence. The human form of polycythemia vera is also associated with an abnormal proliferation of neutrophils (causing a leukocytosis) and platelets (thrombocytosis), and therefore is referred to as a primary absolute polycythemia. Abnormal proliferation of cells other than red blood cells is a rare occurrence in domestic animals with this disorder. Primary erythrocytosis has been reported in dogs, cats, horses, cattle, and llamas (Thrall, 2012c). It is likely that this disease occurs in exotic species as well, but may be under reported.

Secondary Absolute Erythrocytosis

Physiologically appropriate erythrocytosis occurs with generalized hypoxia. When available, arterial blood gas analysis showing reduced arterial partial pressure of oxygen (PaO_2) or determination of hemoglobin oxygen saturation (SaO_2) is helpful in the detection of hypoxemia. Inadequate tissue oxygenation as detected by StO_2 less than 60 mmHg or SaO_2 less than 95% at sea level triggers an increase in erythropoietin production, which in turn stimulates erythrocyte production and release so that more oxygen can be carried to the tissues (Thrall, 2012c).

Physiologically inappropriate erythrocytosis occurs in the absence of generalized tissue hypoxia as determined by a normal or slightly decreased StO_2 and SaO_2. Tumors of the kidney are the most common cause of increased erythropoietin production in domestic mammals; however, production of erythropoietin-like substances from nonrenal tumors may also occur. Determination of serum erythropoietin concentration would be helpful in the diagnosis; however, there are no commercially available validated erythropoietin assays currently available for exotic animals.

Mammalian Leukocytes

Granulocytes

The granulocytes of nondomestic mammals vary in appearance, but can be classified as neutrophils or heterophils, eosinophils, and basophils (Hawkey, 1975; Hawkey et al., 1989; Campbell and Ellis, 2007).

Neutrophils/Heterophils

There are two types of neutrophils commonly found in normal blood samples of most exotic mammal species. These cells include segmented neutrophils and small numbers of band neutrophils. Band neutrophils are immature neutrophils and contain a smooth nucleus that has parallel sides and no constrictions in the nuclear membrane. Segmented neutrophils develop from band neutrophils. The nuclei of these cells have varying degrees of indentations and constrictions in the nuclear membrane, which causes the nucleus to fold into lobes of various shapes that are connected by filaments. Neutrophils contain numerous small granules that vary from colorless to pale-staining to dark-staining among different species of mammals. The neutrophil of some mammals is generally referred to as a heterophil when it contains cytoplasmic granules that do not stain neutral with Romanowsky stains, but are distinctly eosinophilic. Cytochemical and ultrastructural features of cells often differ among species. For example, lysozyme activity is lacking in the neutrophils of hamsters, and alkaline phosphatase activity is less in the neutrophils of mice (Parmley, 1988). Neutrophils of mammals are phagocytic, and one of their primary functions is to destroy microorganisms. Circulating neutrophil concentration increases with inflammation, especially when associated with invading microorganisms, such as bacteria.

Eosinophils

The granules of eosinophils become intensely eosinophilic with maturation because of the changes in the basic protein content. The ultrastructure of the granules in mammalian eosinophils reveals a distinct crystalline shape (an electron-dense axial crystalloid that does not seem to be a constant feature of the eosinophils of other vertebrates) that varies with species; for instance, a trapezoidal pattern is found in the eosinophils of guinea pigs and true rodents, and a needle-shaped pattern is found in rabbit eosinophils (Kelenyi and Nemeth, 1969; Parmley, 1988). Eosinophils contain large cytoplasmic granules that become increasingly eosinophilic in color as the cell matures because of the changes in the basic protein content of the granule. Mammalian eosinophils have phagocytic activity similar to that of neutrophils, but are less effective. Eosinophils are particularly numerous in the peripheral blood when antigens are continually being released, as occurs in parasitic disease (especially those involving larvae of helminths) and allergic reactions (especially those associated with mast cell and basophil degranulation). In general, the presence of an eosinophilia is suggestive of one of these processes; however, extreme eosinophilias may indicate eosinophilic leukemia (Nakamura et al., 2020).

Basophils

Mammalian basophils have characteristic cytoplasmic granules that are strongly basophilic in Romanowsky-stained blood films. Some species variation in the color of the granules does occur. For example, the granules present in guinea pig basophils often stain reddish-purple to black. Unlike basophils of lower vertebrates, those of mammals tend to have lobed nuclei. The ultrastructural appearance of the granules varies with species; for instance, a coiled threaded pattern is observed in basophil granules from primates and rabbits, and a homogeneous pattern is observed in rodents (Parmley, 1988). Basophils participate in allergic and delayed hypersensitivity reactions.

Although rare, mast cells may occur in the peripheral blood and must be differentiated from basophils. Mast cells may be most frequently encountered when evaluating blood films of rodents if cardiocentesis is performed.

Mononuclear Cells

Monocytes

Mammalian monocytes generally are the largest leukocytes in peripheral blood films and do not vary grossly in appearance with species. The monocyte nucleus varies in shape (round or oval to lobed), and the moderately abundant cytoplasm is typically light blue-gray in color and may be vacuolated. The granules, when present, are very fine and appear azurophilic in Romanowsky-stained preparations. Monocytes engulf and degrade microorganisms, abnormal cells, and cell debris. Monocytes also regulate immune responses and myelopoiesis.

Lymphocytes

The appearance of mammalian lymphocytes varies depending upon the species, lymphocyte type, and degree of activation. Mammalian lymphocytes vary in size, color of cytoplasm (light to dark blue), and degree of nuclear chromatin condensation. Variability depends on the degree of antigenic stimulation and type of lymphocyte. The size of lymphocytes ranges from the size of an erythrocyte to the size of a neutrophil. The small lymphocytes are the inactive forms. Reactive lymphocytes have a slightly more abundant cytoplasm that stains basophilic and nuclei that have clefts or are irregular in shape. These cells are the B cells involved in immunoglobulin production (Weiser, 2012a). Large lymphocytes that have an increased amount of light-blue cytoplasm, and azurophilic granules that vary in size are the T cells or natural killer cells (Weiser and Thrall, 2004).

Leukocyte Response to Disease

Inflammatory Leukogram in Mammals

Mediators of Inflammation

Mammalian neutrophils and heterophils are the first line of defense against any inciting inflammatory signal, such as occurs with the invasion of microorganisms or tissue trauma (Appleberg, 2006). Cytochemical and ultrastructural features of these cells differ among species (Parmley, 1988). These cells contain a variety of granules that contain antimicrobial proteins, proteases, components of the respiratory burst (the release of chemically active oxygen molecules designed to kill invading organisms), and mediators of inflammation (Faurschou and Borregaard, 2003). The granule types have been best described in humans; however, although poorly studied, a large degree of species variability exists among other mammals (Nabity and Ramaian, 2010). In general, the neutrophils or heterophils of most mammalian species studied contain both primary and secondary granules that contain the same most frequently encountered enzymes within those granules. Many species of mammals, such as the rabbit, rat, and guinea pig, also have neutrophils/heterophils that contain a tertiary granule, but it may not necessarily correlate with that granule in human neutrophils. Studies involving the enzyme content of the entire neutrophil/heterophil have also shown marked variation among mammalian species (Rausch and Moore, 1975). In these studies, myeloperoxidase and beta-glucuronidase were present in varying degrees of activity (generally lower when compared to humans) in all species of mammals. Small amounts of lysozyme activity were detected in these cells in rats and guinea pigs, but not in hamsters. Rabbit heterophils contain large amounts of elastase activity when compared to other mammalian species. Alpha-defensins have been detected in the neutrophils/heterophils of rabbits, guinea pigs, and hamsters, but not in the neutrophils of mice. Cathelicidins are found in the neutrophils/heterophils of rabbits, guinea pigs, rats, and mice (Linde et al., 2008).

Neutrophil/Heterophil Inflammatory Response

Inflammation is the most common blood leukocyte response in mammals. The inflammatory process involves the consumption, production, and release of neutrophils or heterophils. During this process, these cells are released from the bone marrow and delivered via the blood to the inflammatory lesion until it resolves. Peripheral blood concentrations of neutrophils or heterophils vary from severely decreased to markedly increased depending upon the balance between consumption at the site of the lesion and production and release by the bone marrow. In small mammals, most inflammatory processes result in some degree of neutrophilia or heterophilia, indicating that marrow releases more cells into the blood than are consumed at the site of inflammation. The inflammatory leukogram may be classified as mild to severe depending upon the number of neutrophils or heterophils and their morphology, such as the presence of a left shift and toxic changes. Severe (usually acute) inflammation is indicated by a neutropenia or heteropenia with a left shift because more of these cells are consumed than can be delivered to the blood. The balance between neutrophil/heterophil consumption and delivery by bone marrow is affected by species differences as to the amount of these cells in reserve and the proliferative capacity of the marrow (Weiser, 2012b). These differences translate into magnitudes of neutrophilia/heterophilia that can occur with inflammatory disease in each species. Species with large reserves would be expected to deliver large numbers of neutrophils/heterophils into peripheral circulation and therefore would be expected to exhibit neutrophilia/heterophilia during acute inflammation. Species with small reserves may exhibit an initial neutropenia/heteropenia until bone marrow production has had time to catch up. For example, healthy rabbits are primarily lymphocytic, meaning that small and large lymphocytes are the predominant leukocytes in the normal blood film. As a result, infections rarely cause a significant leukocytosis (>15 000 cells/μL) and acute infections may cause a leukopenia (<5000 cells/μL) with a normal differential or heterophilia, thrombocytopenia, and increase in nucleated erythrocytes in the peripheral blood (Vennen and Mitchell, 2009).

In general, changes in the leukocyte morphology of nondomestic mammals are a reliable indication of disease. Given the amount of information known about the different small exotic mammal species, strains, and breeds, the most reliable criteria for infectious disease appear to be the presence of immature leukocytes, toxic neutrophils, and Döhle bodies, and not necessarily the total leukocyte and differential counts.

Mammalian neutrophils/heterophils found in the peripheral blood are present in either the circulating pool or the marginating pool. The circulating pool occurs in large blood vessels and consists of neutrophils/heterophils that do not interact with the endothelial wall of the vessel. Blood collected by venipuncture consists of samples taken from the circulating pool. The marginating pool consists of neutrophils/heterophils that are interacting with the endothelium of small blood vessels and capillaries.

Left Shift

The term *left shift* refers to an increased concentration of immature neutrophils or heterophils in blood. The immature cells usually consist of bands, but also could include increased numbers of metamyelocytes and myelocytes (Figure 3.14). A left shift with neutrophilia/heterophilia indicates the presence of marked inflammation. A left shift

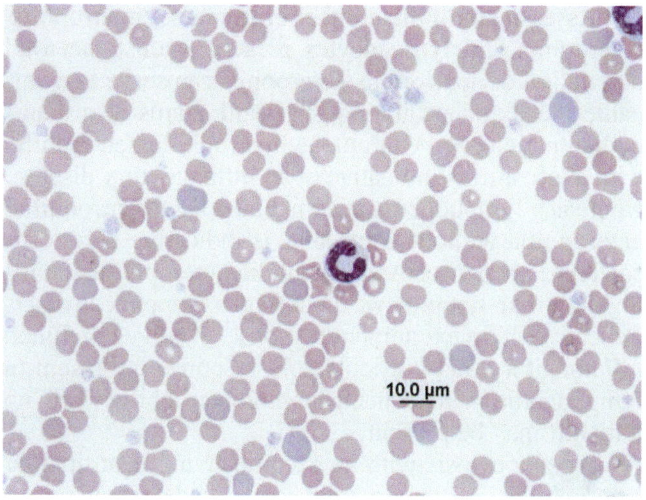

Fig. 3.14. Band cell in the blood film of an African hedgehog (*Atelerix albiventris*), Wright–Giemsa stain.

with neutropenia/heteropenia indicates severe consumption of neutrophils. This is seen with overwhelming infections where peripheral utilization of these cells is greater than their replacement.

Toxic Change

Toxic change in neutrophils/heterophils refers to morphologic changes associated with inflammatory diseases that alter bone marrow production of these types of cells. In response to the inflammatory disease, an acceleration of neutrophil/heterophil production occurs, resulting in the production and release of early-stage neutrophils/heterophils with retained organelles such as ribosomes. Retention of these organelles results in cytoplasmic basophilia and the presence of cytoplasmic vacuolation (Figures 3.15a–3.15c). Döhle bodies may also be present. They are composed of aggregates of endoplasmic reticulum and appear as gray-blue cytoplasmic inclusions.

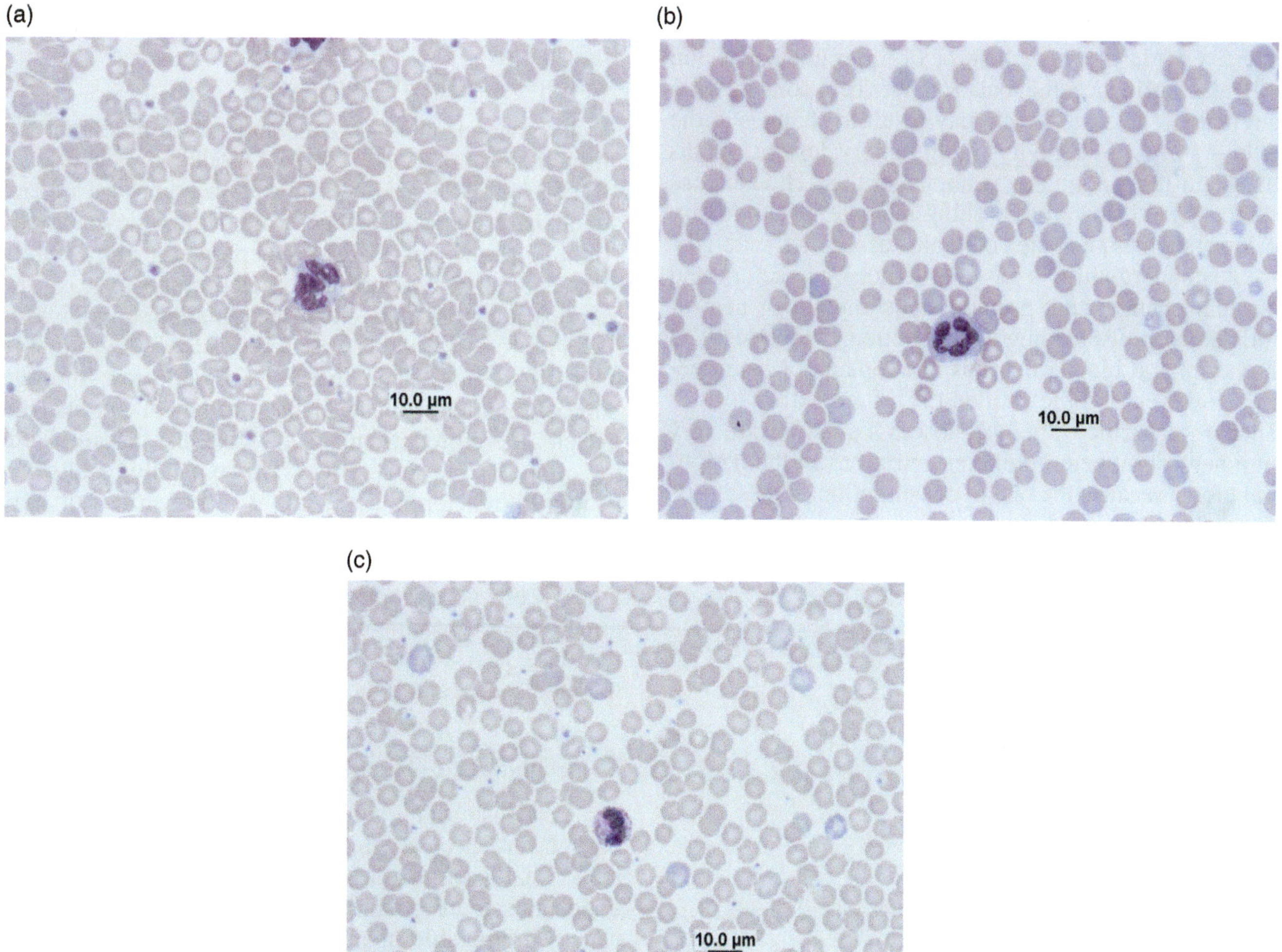

Fig. 3.15. (a) Toxic neutrophil in the blood film of a ferret (*Mustela putorius furo*), Wright–Giemsa stain. (b) Toxic neutrophil in the blood film of an African hedgehog (*Atelerix albiventris*), Wright–Giemsa stain. (c) Toxic heterophil in the blood film of a rabbit (*Oryctolagus cuniculus*), Wright–Giemsa stain.

Neutrophil/Heterophil Degeneration

The term *neutrophil/heterophil degeneration* is used to describe the cellular changes in cytologic samples that have been exposed to an unhealthy microenvironment, such as those produced by bacterial toxins or exposed epithelial surfaces. Degenerate neutrophils/heterophils found in peripheral blood films, therefore, are created by artifacts of sample preparation, such as prolonged storage of blood prior to preparing a blood film. Degenerate neutrophils/heterophils exhibit cytoplasmic vacuolation and nuclear swelling, which may be described cytologically as a pale-staining nucleus that has lost chromatin definition. Cell lysis can also occur with extreme degeneration. Pyknosis or karyorrhexis of leukocytes can occur with natural disease and toxicosis (e.g., xenobiotic administration) (Rovira and Kreklau, 2012) (Figure 3.16).

Types of Inflammation

Besides species differences in the amount of neutrophils/heterophils held in reserve and the proliferative capacity of the marrow, the type of inflammatory lesion will also influence the balance between consumption and marrow release, which may result in changes to the leukogram. Closed-cavity inflammatory lesions versus diffuse inflammation are examples of this. The increase in local blood flow and swelling in acute inflammatory lesions (such as an acute coelomitis associated with gastrointestinal rupture) leads to chemotactic factors and vascular changes that promote consumption of neutrophils/heterophils, leading to a reduction of these cells in the peripheral blood, and thus neutropenia or heteropenia. However, chronic, walled-off inflammatory lesions (such as a chronic walled-off abscess) often lead to very high neutrophil/heterophil concentrations in the peripheral blood because the rate of consumption of these cells is less than their production.

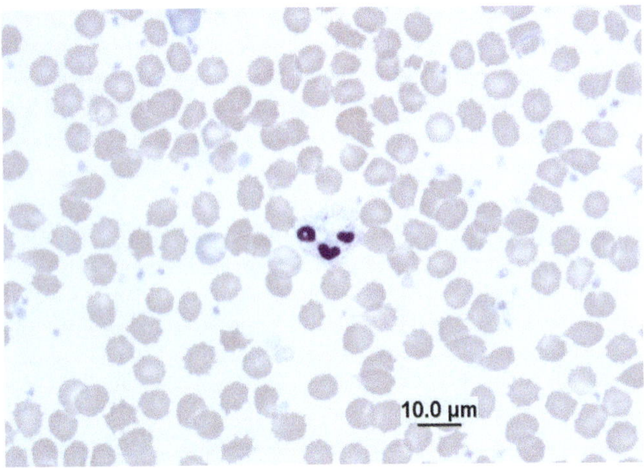

Fig. 3.16. Pyknosis of a heterophil in the blood film of a guinea pig (*Cavia porcellus*), Wright–Giemsa stain.

Assessment of the number of immature neutrophils/heterophils and lymphocytes present against the total population of neutrophils/heterophils can serve as a valuable means of evaluating the health status of a mammalian patient. For example, a neutrophilia/heterophilia with a left shift is indicative of an inflammatory disease, whereas a lymphopenia accompanied by a neutrophilia/heterophilia without a left shift is indicative of a corticosteroid response. A neutrophilia/heterophilia with a high normal lymphocyte count or a lymphocytosis is indicative of an excitement response. When a combined inflammatory and corticosteroid response is present, a lymphopenia with a neutrophilia/heterophilia with no left shift may be present.

A leukocytosis with an accompanying neutrophilia/heterophilia indicates a mild to marked response to a managed inflammatory condition. Severe inflammatory responses are indicated by the presence of a left shift and toxic neutrophils/heterophils. Some animals may not exhibit a leukocytosis, but will still demonstrate changes in the neutrophil/heterophil population and morphology.

Neutrophilia of Excitement

In general, leukocytosis and neutrophilia/heterophilia indicate that bone marrow production and release of neutrophils/heterophils are exceeding peripheral demands. However, during excitement (known as the "fight-or-flight" response), epinephrine is immediately released, causing neutrophils (heterophils) to leave the marginating pool and enter the circulating pool as a response to increased heart rate and blood flow through microcirculation. This increased blood flow through microcirculation is especially prominent in skeletal muscle; therefore, strenuous exercise just before bleeding often has the same effect. This typically results in a neutrophilia/heterophilia without a left shift, but may also result in a lymphocytosis. Depending upon the species, the numbers of these leukocytes nearly double as mature cells in microcirculation are swept from the marginating pool into the circulating pool. This excitement response is a common finding in many small exotic mammals, especially those not accustomed to handling.

Neutrophilia of Corticosteroid Excess

Corticosteroid excess resulting from endogenous corticosteroid release in association with the physiologic stress that accompanies systemic disease or from an exogenous source, such as a therapeutic administration, causes predictable changes in the leukogram of most mammals. In response to major systemic illnesses (such as renal failure, dehydration, and inflammatory disease), metabolic disturbances (such as diabetic ketoacidosis), and pain (such as pain associated with trauma), cortisol is released from the adrenal gland following the release of adrenocorticotropic hormone from the pituitary gland. Other endogenous sources for an increase in plasma corticosteroids in small mammals include physical restraint, transport, a change in the cage population density, extremes in temperature, and loud sounds (Drozdowicz et al., 1990).

Corticosteroids, generated by endogenous corticosteroid excess or introduced by therapeutic administration of exogenous corticosteroids, typically result in predictable changes in the leukogram of small exotic mammals. Lymphopenia is the most consistent change observed because corticosteroids induce lymphocyte apoptosis (cell self-destruction) and may affect the recirculation of lymphocytes (Campbell and Grant, 2010). A mature neutrophilia/heterophilia (often doubling of these cells) is also commonly observed in the leukogram because corticosteroids cause a decrease in the stickiness of these leukocytes, decreasing the marginating pool. These leukocytes also stay in circulation longer than they normally would, which results in hypersegmentation.

Nuclear hypersegmentation (five or more segments or lobes) is a normal state in the progression of nuclear maturation in the neutrophil/heterophil and commonly occurs after the neutrophil/heterophil has left circulation (Figure 3.17). The presence of cells exhibiting hypersegmentation in the peripheral blood is an indication that the neutrophils/heterophils are staying in circulation longer than normal. This morphologic condition is typically associated with prolonged corticosteroid effects on the neutrophils or heterophils.

A left shift is not associated with a corticosteroid affect unless there is coexisting inflammation. Less commonly seen changes to the leukogram may also include eosinopenia and monocytosis, but some species variability does occur among the small exotic mammals. For example, in the rabbit, a mature heterophilia and lymphopenia characterize glucocorticoid-mediated changes in the leukogram, which normally has more circulating lymphocytes than heterophils.

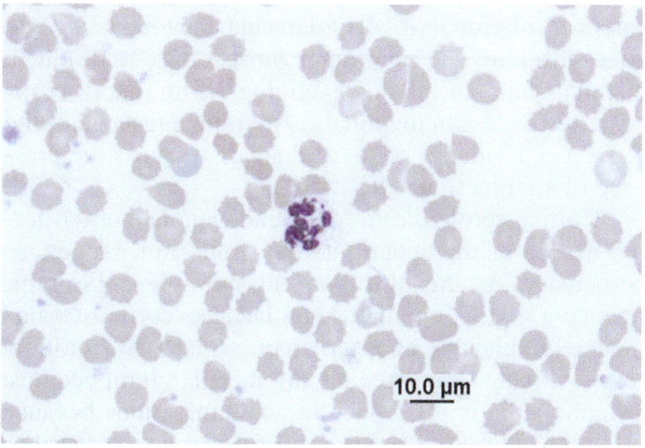

Fig. 3.17. Nuclear hypersegmentation in a heterophil in the blood film of a guinea pig (*Cavia porcellus*), Wright–Giemsa stain.

An inflammatory disorder is often accompanied by a steroid response. Assessment of the number of immature neutrophils/heterophils and lymphocytes present against the total population of neutrophils/heterophils can serve as a valuable means of evaluating the health status of a mammalian patient. For example, a neutrophilia/heterophilia with a left shift is indicative of an inflammatory disease, whereas a lymphopenia accompanied by a neutrophilia/heterophilia without a left shift is indicative of a corticosteroid response. A neutrophilia/heterophilia with a high normal lymphocyte count or a lymphocytosis is indicative of an excitement response. When a combined inflammatory and corticosteroid response is present, a lymphopenia with a neutrophilia/heterophilia with or without a left shift may be present.

Neutropenia/Heteropenia

Neutropenia/heteropenia occurs when neutrophils/heterophils are overwhelmingly consumed at a faster rate than they are being produced and released into the peripheral circulation, and is often associated with an acute inflammatory disease or a disease of marked severity. This is especially notable with infections by pyogenic bacteria that often cause a degenerative left shift (where the number of immature neutrophils/heterophils is greater than that of mature cells). A neutropenia/heteropenia with a left shift and toxic changes that occurs in the absence of anemia and a normal platelet count is indicative of an acute inflammatory response associated with excessive peripheral utilization of neutrophils/heterophils. Toxic changes may occur within a few days of the onset of the process (Weiser, 2012b).

A neutropenia/heteropenia with no left shift, no anemia, and an adequate platelet count is indicative of an acute viral infection or injury to rapidly dividing stem cells in the bone marrow. For example, ferrets with canine distemper typically exhibit leukopenia and neutropenia (Wolf, 2009). Because neutrophils/heterophils have a higher turnover in circulating blood when compared to other hemic cells, neutropenia/heteropenia develops before thrombocytopenia and nonregenerative anemia. A neutropenia/heteropenia associated with a nonregenerative anemia and possibly thrombocytopenia is indicative of a chronic bone marrow injury.

Reversible stem cell injury associated with an acute neutropenia/heteropenia that occurs without a left shift will frequently be brief (e.g., lasting only for 24–48 h) as the marrow repopulates. This is followed by a left shift with progressively increasing mature neutrophil/heterophil concentrations leading to an inflammatory pattern that consists of a neutrophilia/heterophilia and left shift. Depending upon the cause, a neutropenia/heteropenia associated with a reversible stem cell injury with a longer duration (e.g., several days or longer) will also result in thrombocytopenia and a nonregenerative anemia. Certain chemotherapeutic agents, total body ionizing radiation therapy, or estrogen toxicity can damage hematopoietic stem and progenitor cells or inhibit cell replication, resulting in this type of hemogram.

Therefore, a neutropenia/heteropenia associated with a left shift and toxic change is likely associated with inflammatory disease (Campbell and Grant, 2010). However, if the neutropenia/heteropenia is not associated with a left shift but there is a combination of thrombocytopenia and nonregenerative anemia, then stem cell injury in the bone marrow should be considered.

Other miscellaneous causes of neutropenia/heteropenia may occur in small exotic mammals. Immune-mediated neutropenia/heteropenia is a rare condition that results in a profound neutropenia/heteropenia in the peripheral blood and depletion of the maturation pool in the bone marrow.

Eosinophil Response

Eosinophilia

Eosinophilia is a nonspecific response that could be associated with parasite infestation, hypersensitivity reactions, or other agents chemotactic for eosinophils (Campbell and Grant, 2010; Weiser, 2012b). A peripheral eosinophilia does not always occur in the presence of tissue eosinophilic inflammation. Although the exact mechanism of eosinophilic inflammation in not well understood, it appears to be associated with eosinophil chemoattractants, such as interleukin-5 released from T cells sensitized by parasite antigens (both endoparasites and ectoparasites) or allergens and mast cell degranulation. (Herndon and Kayes, 1992). Eosinophilia is more likely to occur when parasites are present in tissues rather than in the lumen of the gastrointestinal tract (Young and Meadows, 2010).

Chronic eosinophilia mediated by mast cell degranulation is often associated with inflammation involving tissues that normally contain a high concentration of mast cells. Such tissues are species specific, but generally include the skin, lung, gastrointestinal tract, and female reproductive tract. For example, eosinophilic inflammatory bowel disease, a poorly characterized gastroenteritis that may have an allergic component, of ferrets will occasionally produce a peripheral eosinophilia.

Eosinopenia

Eosinopenia has limited significance as healthy animals often have no eosinophils identified in their 100-cell leukocyte differential counts. However, it is known that corticosteroids cause eosinopenia. This is likely due to inhibition of mast cell degranulation, neutralization of circulating histamine, sequestration of eosinophils, and delayed release of eosinophils from the bone marrow (Young and Meadows, 2010). Catecholamines may also induce an eosinopenia by a β-adrenergic effect. Thus, during acute inflammation, eosinopenia may occur due to increased corticosteroids and catecholamine release.

Basophilia in Mammals

The number of circulating basophils in any given species is, as a rule, inversely proportional to the tissue mast cell concentration (Fortman et al., 2002). Basophilia has limited significance as healthy animals often have no basophils identified in their 100-cell leukocyte differential counts. Mammalian basophils participate in allergic and delayed hypersensitivity reactions; therefore, basophilia is usually associated with eosinophilia. The exact interpretation of basophilia is usually unknown (Weiser, 2012b). Rabbits typically have more basophils than other exotic animal species. Often, 5% of the leukocytes in the total leukocyte count are basophils, but they can be as high as 30% in rabbits with no apparent abnormalities (Campbell and Ellis, 2007).

Lymphocyte Response

Lymphopenia in Mammals

Lymphopenia is generally indicative of corticosteroid excess, but may occur as a relative change in the neutrophil/heterophil to lymphocyte ratio in association with some inflammatory disease in some animals. For example, rabbits do not develop an overall leukocytosis with bacterial infections but will develop an increase in the absolute heterophil concentration and decrease in the absolute lymphocyte concentration. Therefore, in the rabbit, the H:L ratio and absolute heterophil and lymphocyte concentrations appear to be more reliable indicators of inflammatory disorders than the total leukocyte concentration. The neutrophil morphology may aid in distinguishing an infectious etiology from that of corticosteroid excess in mammals exhibiting a reversal of the N:L ratio. Evidence of toxic changes supports the presence of an infectious etiology.

Corticosteroids, caused by endogenous corticosteroid excess or therapeutic administration of exogenous corticosteroids, create a transient and predictable lymphopenia. Lymphopenia occurs because corticosteroids induce lymphocyte apoptosis (cell self-destruction) and may affect the recirculation of lymphocytes. Lymphopenia is often seen in acute infections because of stress-induced corticosteroid release and redistribution of lymphocytes where lymphocytes become trapped in lymphoid tissue or circulating lymphocytes migrate to antigenically stimulated lymph nodes (reactive lymph nodes) (Jain, 1993; Latimer, 1995). Lymphopenia may also be caused by viral diseases (Müller et al., 2009).

Reactive lymphocytes, also called immunocytes and transformed lymphocytes, are antigenically stimulated lymphocytes in the peripheral blood. They vary in size, nuclear chromatin pattern, number of visible nucleoli, and amount of cytoplasmic vacuolation; however, they are identified by their deeply basophilic cytoplasm (Figures 3.18a–3.18c). Some resemble lymphoblasts, and those with a prominent perinuclear halo or Golgi resemble plasma cells.

Lymphadenitis may also cause lymphopenia as the efferent lymph flow from the inflamed lymph node prevents lymphocyte recirculation (Hopkins and McConnell, 1984). Loss of lymphocyte-rich fluid within the lumen of the intestine associated with a protein-losing enteropathy or ulcerative enteritis may also explain lymphopenia (Kull et al., 2001). Likewise, loss of lymphocyte-rich fluid into a body cavity, such as chylothorax or chyloperitoneum, can result in sequestration of lymphocytes causing lymphopenia (Schultze, 2010).

Lymphocytosis in Mammals

Lymphocytosis in the mammalian patient is usually associated with an excitement response or lymphocytic leukemia. An excitement response results in a moderate increase in the number of circulating normal-appearing small, mature lymphocytes. A marked increase in the lymphocyte count should be viewed with suspicion for a lymphoproliferative disorder such as lymphocytic leukemia. In general, a lymphoproliferative disorder is a lymphoid cell neoplastic disorder in the blood or bone marrow.

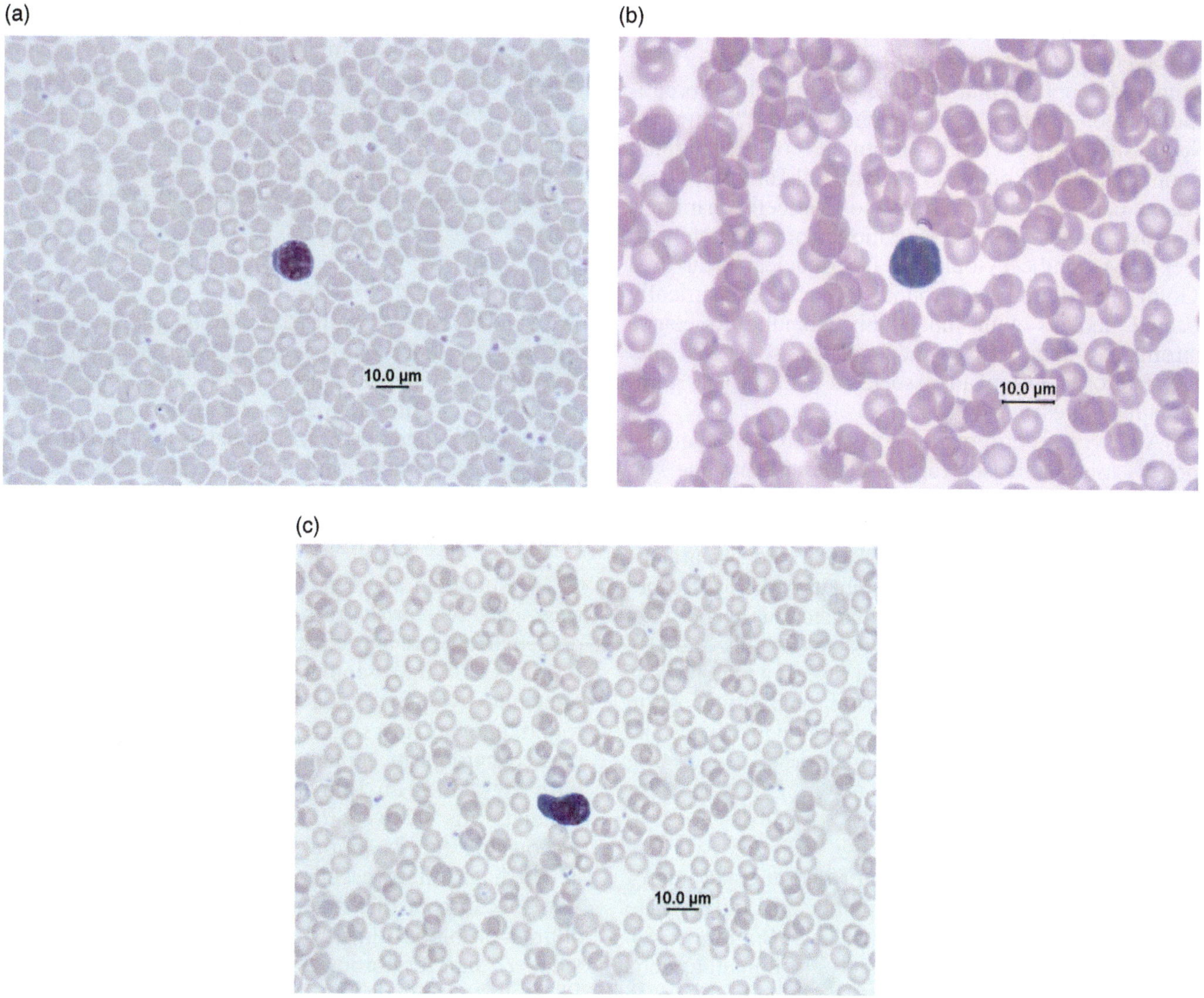

Fig. 3.18. (a) Reactive lymphocyte in the blood film of a ferret (*Mustela putorius furo*), Wright–Giemsa stain. (b) Reactive lymphocyte in the blood film of a guinea pig (*Cavia porcellus*), Wright–Giemsa stain. (c) Reactive lymphocyte in the blood film of a cottontail rabbit (*Sylvilagus floridanus*), Wright–Giemsa stain.

Lymphoma is a term used to describe lymphoid neoplasia involving solid tissue. *Lymphocytic leukemia* is the term used to describe lymphoid neoplasia involving blood or bone marrow. Lymphocytic leukemia is indicated by a marked increase in lymphocytes and is often accompanied by the presence of abnormal lymphocyte morphology. Lymphocytic leukemia is not commonly reported in small exotic mammals, but has been reported in the rabbit and ferret (Finnie et al., 1980; Toth et al., 1990; Boone et al., 1995).

Important lymphocyte morphology changes associated with lymphoid neoplasia include the presence of large lymphocytes (larger in size than neutrophils/heterophils) with a pale-staining nucleus containing fine nuclear chromatin. The presence of a prominent nucleolus and increased cytoplasmic volume are additional supportive features of malignant lymphocytes. Occasionally, lymphocytes exhibit cytoplasmic vacuolation. Lymphocyte vacuolation can also be associated with toxins or storage disorders (Weiser, 2012b).

Myeloma is a term referring to a specific form of lymphoid neoplasia that involves plasma cell differentiation (see Chapter 7, sections titled "Malignant Neoplasia," "Structural Features of Malignant Neoplasia," and "Round or Discrete Cell Tumor"). These plasma cells are discrete round to oval cells characterized by a moderate to large amount of moderately to deeply basophilic cytoplasm, a perinuclear clear area (Golgi), medium-sized round to oval eccentrically located nucleus with moderately granular to coarse chromatin, and mild-to-moderate anisocytosis and anisokaryosis. Often an associated monoclonal gammopathy is present as well.

A rare cause of lymphocytosis is chronic inflammatory disease. The reason for this is that the immune system responds to the inflammation with lymphoid hyperplasia in lymphoid tissues, but it rarely manifests as lymphocytosis in blood (Weiser, 2012b). Persistent antigenic stimulation in chronic inflammatory diseases, especially those associated with certain infectious agents, may be more likely to cause a lymphocytosis (Schultze, 2010). In such cases, the blood film often reveals a high proportion of large granular lymphocytes (chronic ehrlichiosis in the dog is an example of this). Such findings may also be seen occasionally in small exotic mammals.

Monocytosis

Mammalian monocytes engulf and degrade microorganisms, abnormal cells, and cell debris, and regulate immune responses and myelopoiesis (Figure 3.19). Monocytes in the peripheral blood are immature cells that migrate to inflammatory lesions in body tissues to become macrophages. Therefore, a monocytosis may be interpreted as a response to increased tissue demand for macrophages during acute and chronic inflammatory conditions and is typically associated with neutrophilia/heterophilia. A monocytosis can be associated with necrosis, suppuration, malignant neoplasia, pyogranulomatous lesions, internal hemorrhage, hemolysis, immune-mediated disease, and trauma (Latimer, 1995). A corticosteroid response may also cause a monocytosis in some species. A monocytosis can also be associated with certain viral infections (Müller et al., 2009).

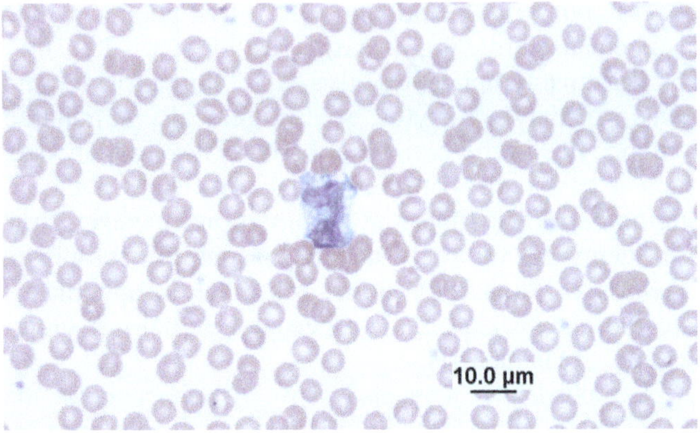

Fig. 3.19. A monocyte with numerous cytoplasmic vacuoles (reactive monocyte) in the blood film of a ferret (*Mustela putorius furo*), Wright–Giemsa stain.

Myeloproliferative Diseases

Myeloproliferative diseases are neoplastic diseases affecting the bone marrow with unregulated proliferation of clonal hematopoietic stem cells. This uncontrolled cell proliferation leads to reduction of normal hematopoiesis and invasion of other tissues. Granulocytic leukemia is a variant of myeloproliferative disease.

Platelets of Mammals

Mammalian platelets are composed of cytoplasmic fragments that arise from megakaryocytes within the bone marrow and participate in hemostasis. Platelets are flat disks of the cytoplasm that contain cytoplasmic organelles (Figures 3.20a and 3.20b). They tend to be round, but can vary slightly in shape and size. The anucleated cytoplasm contains variable amounts of small purple granules on Romanowsky-stained blood films. Platelets are involved in the clotting process and are responsible for the initial hemostatic plug to prevent hemorrhage after vascular injury to the microcirculation. Because of this function, they are often found in clumps on blood films. Mammalian platelets are much smaller than erythrocytes in the same blood film. Platelets that are larger in size than erythrocytes are occasionally noted in the blood film. These cells are called macroplatelets or shift platelets (Figure 3.21). These large platelets may indicate an accelerated

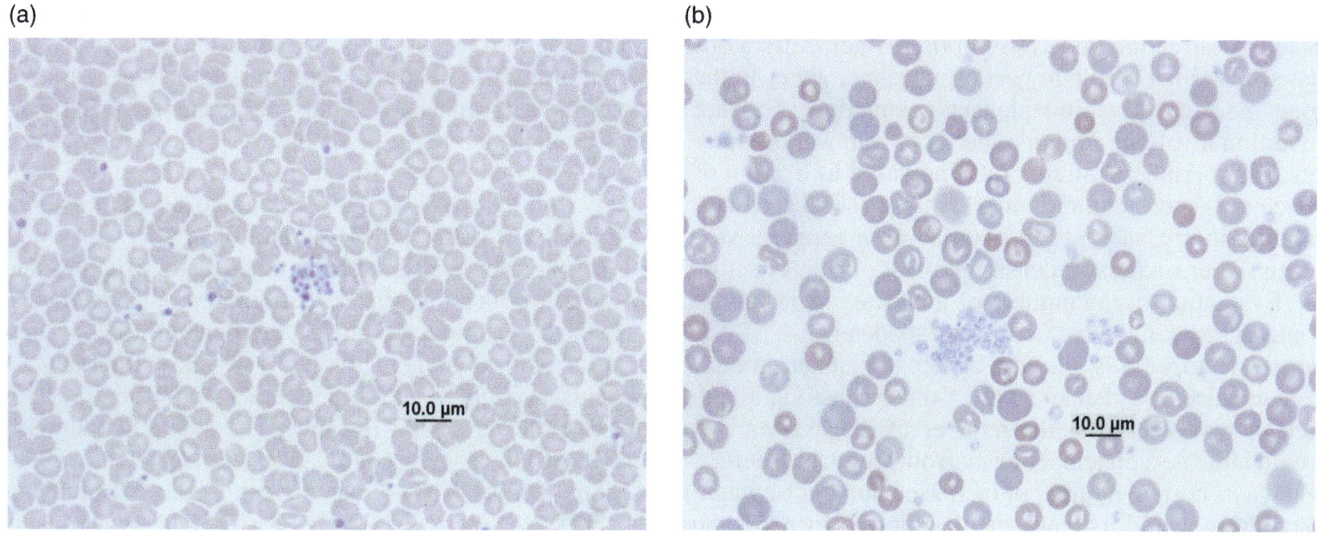

Fig. 3.20. (a) Platelets in the blood film of a ferret (*Mustela putorius furo*), Wright–Giemsa stain. (b) Platelets in the blood film of an African hedgehog (*Atelerix albiventris*), Wright–Giemsa stain.

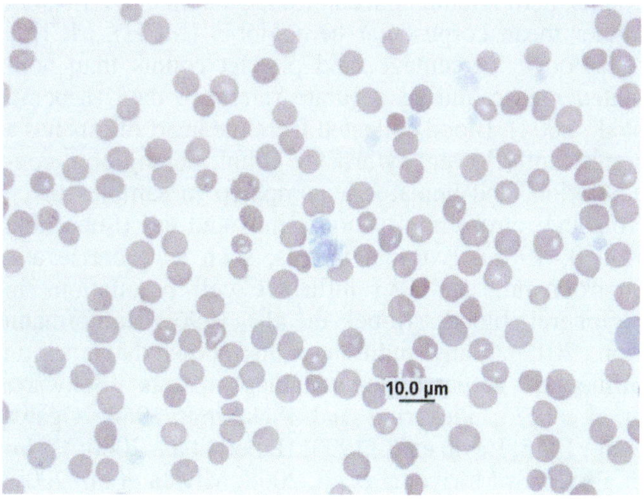

Fig. 3.21. Large platelets in the blood film of an African hedgehog (*Atelerix albiventris*), Wright–Giemsa stain.

thrombocytopoiesis with early release of immature forms into the circulating blood; therefore, they are an indication of platelet regeneration in some species.

Platelet numbers in the blood can be counted using automated methods or manual techniques using a hemacytometer. The number of platelets present in a blood film can be determined manually by counting the number of platelets per high-power field. A minimum of 5 platelets or a range of 5–10 platelets per high-power field (1000× magnification or oil-immersion field) would be interpreted as an adequate number (Baker, 2004). Normal platelet concentrations for most mammals are greater than 100 000/mL of blood. If excessive platelet clumping is present, the platelet count may appear to be lower than normal. The presence of clumping and its artifactual effect on the platelet count can be confirmed by identifying clumps of platelets at the feathered edge of the smear.

Platelet concentrations in rodents tend to be high compared with those of larger domestic mammals, and platelet concentrations greater than 1×10^6 per µL are common. The total platelet count of hamsters and gerbils is similar to that of other rodents with an expected range of $400–600 \times 10^3$/µL. A normal physiologic decrease in the total platelet count may occur as seen in hibernating hamsters (Reznik, 1975; Deveci et al., 2001).

Thrombocytopenia and Thrombocytosis in Mammals

Thrombocytopenia occurs because of decreased platelet production, increased platelet destruction, or increased platelet utilization (consumption). Thrombocyte concentrations below 25 000/mL of blood may result in bleeding.

Decreases in platelet production are indicated by a decrease in the number of megakaryocytes in the bone marrow. Toxicities, whole-body irradiation, infectious agents, neoplastic conditions, and immune-mediated disorders can cause decreased-platelet-production thrombocytopenias in domestic mammals and are likely factors involved with such conditions in the small exotic mammals, as well (Baker, 2010). Chemicals that attack dividing cells will have a detrimental effect on all the dividing cells in the bone marrow, including megakaryocytes. For example, ferret bone marrow is highly susceptible to estrogen-induced suppression. This is commonly seen in the panhypoplasia created by estrogen toxicity of intact female ferrets suffering from prolonged estrus. The mechanism for this is complex and poorly understood, but may involve serum inhibitors of hematopoiesis derived from T cells (Farris and Benjamin, 1993).

A thrombocytopenia associated with increased platelet destruction and consumption is generally associated with increased numbers of megakaryocytes in the bone marrow. Increased platelet destruction is a rare condition involving immune-mediated removal of platelets from peripheral circulation. Increased utilization of platelets is more common and is often associated with vascular injury, such as DIC, hemangiosarcoma, or vasculitis, where excessive consumption of platelets occurs.

Evaluation of the number of megakaryocytes in the bone marrow may be necessary to determine if the thrombocytopenia is due to a defect in platelet production or caused by platelet destruction or consumption. A lack of or decrease in the number of megakaryocytes would indicate a platelet bone marrow production defect, whereas a normal number or increased number of megakaryocytes would indicate that thrombocytopenia is the result of platelet destruction or consumption.

Blood loss alone does not result in significant thrombocytopenia since the platelet concentration rarely is less than 100 000/μL following hemorrhage (Baker, 2010).

A pseudothrombocytopenia is an in vitro condition resulting from platelet clumping as identified by platelet clumps found on the feathered edge of the blood film. Excessive platelet clumping typically results from poor to difficult venipuncture (a common occurrence when dealing with small exotic mammals) that subsequently initiates platelet activation (Russell, 2010).

A general guideline to estimate the platelet count from a blood film is to count the number of platelets in ten 100× (oil-immersion) fields and multiply that number by 15 000 to obtain an estimated platelet count/μL (Russell, 2010). Another method to assess whether there are an adequate number of platelets on a blood film is to obtain the average number of platelets per oil-immersion field (magnification, 1000×). With this approach, the number of platelets is adequate if there are at least five platelets per oil-immersion field (Baker, 2010).

Thrombocytosis is a rare condition where an excessive number of platelets is present in the peripheral blood. The cause of increased platelet concentrations in the peripheral blood is a nonspecific condition that is generally not associated with clinical signs of disease. Examples of conditions associated with thrombocytosis in domestic mammals include iron-deficiency anemia, inflammatory diseases, and epinephrine effects.

Hemogram Evaluation of Specific Species

Myomorphs or True Rodents (Mice, Rats, Gerbils, Hamsters)

The hematology of rodents commonly seen in veterinary practices is like that of domestic mammals. Extensive reference values based on age, sex, diet, housing, supplier, and collection site are available for rodents used as laboratory animals (Leonard and Ruben, 1986; Moore, 2000a, b; Bolliger et al., 2010). These reference values should be used as a tool when evaluating the hematology of pet rodents and not as the sole guide to determine if values are abnormal, because the parameters upon which these published reference intervals are based and laboratory instrument and methodology used likely will vary from those obtained for the patient (Appendix B, Tables B.1, B.2, and B.3).

It has been well established that factors such as site of sample collection, age, sex, strain, reproductive status, anesthesia, method of restraint, temperature, season, and stress may alter hematologic reference intervals in rodents (Wright et al., 1983; Suber and Kodell, 1985; Jackson et al., 1988; Turton et al., 1989; Drozdowicz et al., 1990; Robel et al., 1996; Alemán et al., 1998; Moore, 2000a; Nahas and Provost, 2002; Kampfmann et al., 2012; Xu and Hu, 2020). For example, male rodents tend to have higher erythrocyte concentrations than female rodents, but these differences are not clinically significant. Pregnant rats tend to have lower erythrocyte counts, hemoglobin concentrations, and hematocrits, but higher mean corpuscular hemoglobin (MCH), MCHC, reticulocyte percentage, and platelet counts than nonmated rats, requiring separate reference data (Liberati et al., 2004). Blood collected from the heart of rats has a significantly lower erythrocyte count, hemoglobin concentration, and hematocrit compared to samples taken from the retro-orbital venous sinus and tail (Suber and Kodell, 1985). External factors, such as exercise and environment, can also influence cell populations in peripheral blood (Robel et al., 1996; Kampfmann et al., 2012). Many studies have also shown that nutrition influences hematologic variables in rats (Schwartz et al., 1973; Pickering and Pickering, 1984; Ogawa et al., 1985; Levin et al., 1993; Hubert et al., 2000; Yoshii et al., 2003; Moriyama et al., 2008; Miyata et al., 2009; Asanuma et al., 2011). A distinct circadian rhythm affects peripheral leukocyte concentration with an increase in circulating leukocyte concentration occurring during the light phase and a decrease during the dark phase. In mice, a distinct decrease in the total leukocyte concentration, which is directly associated with a decrease in total lymphocyte numbers, occurs following stress.

Erythrocytes of Myomorphs

The Romanowsky-stained erythrocytes of true rodents (rats, *Rattus norvegicus*; mice, *Mus musculus*; gerbils, *Meriones unguiculatus*; and hamsters, *Mesocricetus auratus*) are round, anucleated, pink, biconcave disks with a central pale area and a mean diameter between 5 and 7 μm. The erythrocytes of these animals have a relatively short half-life (45–68 days) compared to the larger domestic mammals, such as dogs and cats, and as a result, their blood generally has a higher concentration of reticulocytes compared to other

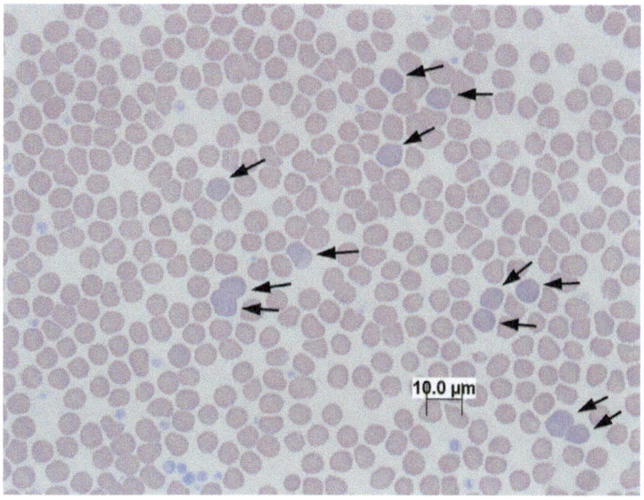

Fig. 3.22. Polychromatic erythrocytes (arrows) in the blood film of a mouse (*Mus musculus*), Wright–Giemsa stain.

mammals; therefore, the presence of a greater degree of polychromasia and anisocytosis on the blood film is expected (Ringer and Dabich, 1979; Moore, 2000a, b; Everds, 2006) (Figure 3.22). Polychromatic cells represent 1–18% of the erythrocyte population in healthy rats and mice (Ringer and Dabich, 1979). In general, 1–5% reticulocytes are expected in adult non-anemic rodents. However, when evaluating the erythropoietic response in rodents, an actual reticulocyte count offers a better assessment compared to the relative percentages of these cells. For comparison, an absolute reticulocyte count between 150 000/µL and 300 000/µL is expected for non-anemic adult mice and rats. The presence of a low number (usually less than 2% of erythrocytes) of Howell–Jolly bodies, basophilic stippling, and nucleated red blood cells is also common in rodent blood films. Nucleated red blood cells may account for up to 2% of erythrocytes in blood films of normal hamsters (Criswell et al., 2000; Car et al., 2006). Basophilic stippling and polychromasia are features of normal gerbil blood films. Rouleaux formation of erythrocytes is rarely seen in rodents, even with inflammatory disease.

Adult rats and mice normally have a high degree of reticulocytosis with means that average between 2% and 7%, and the young have even higher numbers that range between 10% and 20%. In general, a normal hematocrit range for rodents ranges between 35% and 55% based on the normal hematocrit ranges of 38–51% for rats, 35–52% for mice (Bolliger et al., 2010), 35–50% for gerbils (Wagner and Farrar, 1987), and 36–55% for hamsters (Harkness and Wagner, 1989; Johnson-Delaney, 1995). The hemoglobin concentration of rodents generally ranges between 10 and 17 g/dL based on the normal hemoglobin ranges of 12–16 g/dL for rats, 10–17 g/dL for mice (Bolliger et al., 2010), 10–17 g/dL for gerbils (Wagner and Farrar, 1987), and 10–16 g/dL for hamsters (Harkness and Wagner, 1989; Johnson-Delaney, 1995). The MCV of rodents generally ranges between 45 and 62 fL based on the normal MCV of 55–62 fL for rats (Moore, 2000a), 45–55 fL for mice, and 46–60 fL for gerbils (Mitruka and Rawnsley, 1981). The normal MCV of 65–78 fL for hamsters is higher than that of the other true rodents (Mitruka and Rawnsley, 1981). The red blood cell distribution width (RDW) obtained by calculation from automated hematology analyzers is a reliable indicator of variation in the size of red blood cells; however, the normal values are instrument dependent. The MCHC of rodents generally ranges between 30 and 37 g/dL based on the normal MCHC of 30–34 g/dL for rats (Moore, 2000a), 30–38 g/dL for mice, 30–33 g/dL for gerbils (Mitruka and Rawnsley, 1981), and 28–37 g/dL for hamsters (Mitruka and Rawnsley, 1981). For best results in measuring hematologic analytes in rodents, the blood samples should be processed in a timely manner, preferably within 1 h after collection (Ameri et al., 2011).

Leukocytes of Mice (*Mus musculus*) and Rats (*Rattus norvegicus*)

Lymphocytes are the predominant leukocytes in the blood of healthy mice and rats, and they represent 70–80% and 60–75% of the leukocyte population, respectively (Bolliger et al., 2010; Campbell, 2012). The size of lymphocytes ranges from the size of erythrocytes to the size of neutrophils (Figures 3.23a and 3.23b). The cytoplasm of lymphocytes stains light blue, and azurophilic cytoplasmic granules are occasionally found in large lymphocytes.

Granulocytes of mice and rats often have nuclei without distinct lobes and typically exhibit a horseshoe, sausage, or ring (doughnut) shape (Campbell and Ellis, 2007; Bolliger et al., 2010) (Figures 3.24a and 3.24b). The ring shape results from a gradually increasing hole that develops in the nucleus during maturation of the granulocyte. Nuclear segmentation occurs as the ring breaks during maturation and begins to form constrictions; therefore, an increase in nuclear ring forms is suggestive of accelerated granulopoiesis.

Neutrophils represent 12–38% of the leukocyte differential in rats and 20–30% in mice. Neutrophils generally have a colorless cytoplasm, but the cytoplasm of mice and rat neutrophils may contain dust-like red granules, creating a diffusely pink appearance with Romanowsky stains. The nucleus of the typical rat neutrophil has few segments, but it has numerous indentations that make them appear hypersegmented. The nucleus of the mouse neutrophil is often segmented with fine connecting threads of chromatin. Rat neutrophils measure 11 µm in diameter.

(a) (b)

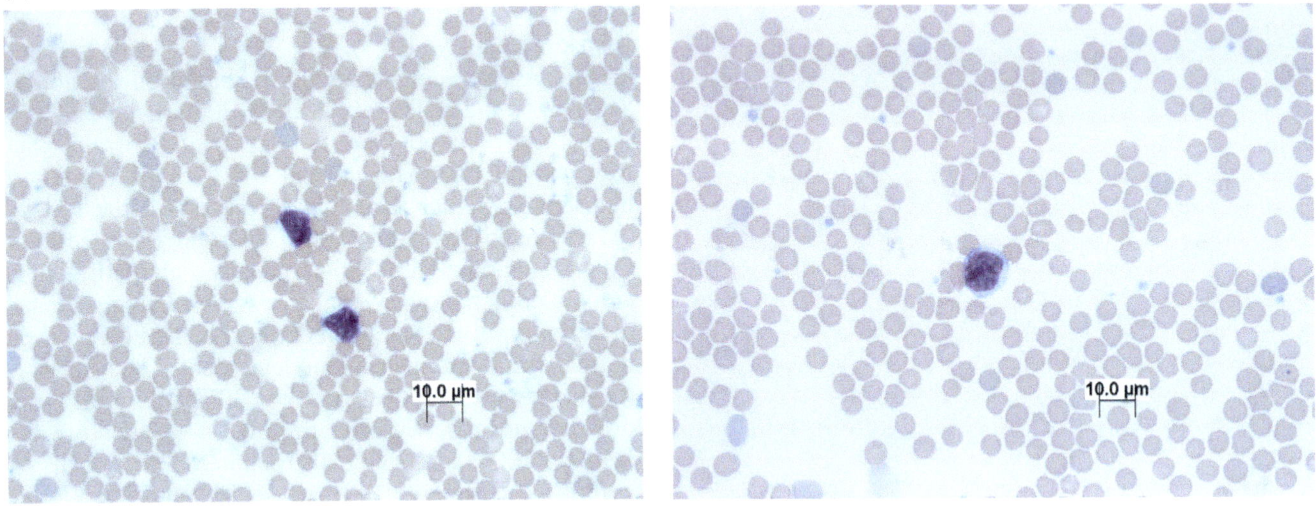

Fig. 3.23. (a) Small lymphocytes in the blood film of a mouse (*Mus musculus*), Wright–Giemsa stain. (b) Large lymphocyte in the blood film of a mouse (*Mus musculus*), Wright–Giemsa stain.

(a) (b)

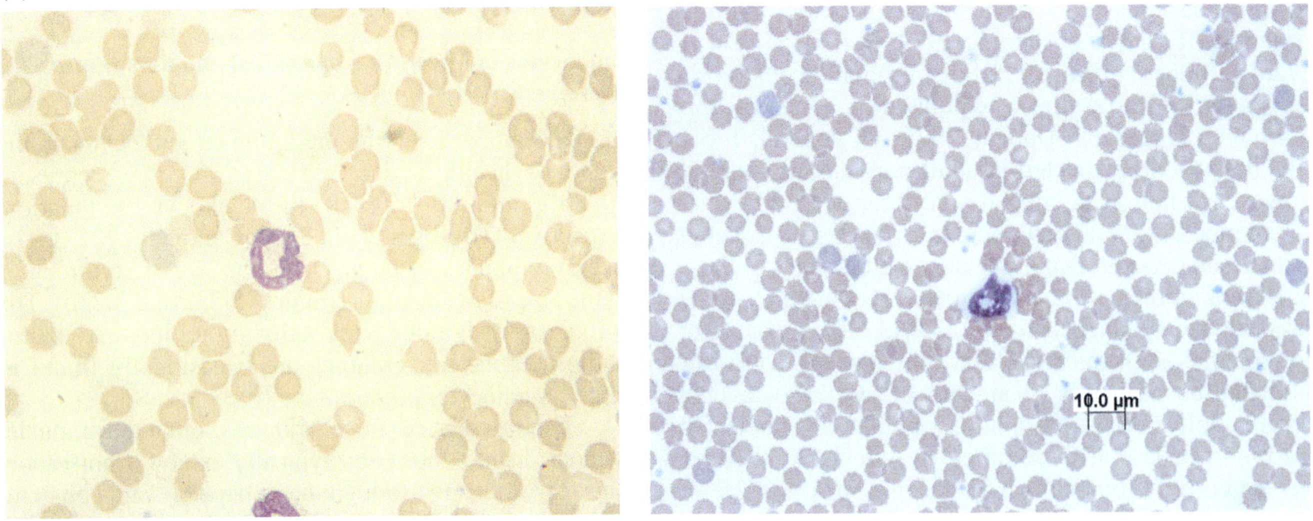

Fig. 3.24. (a) Neutrophil in the blood film of a domestic rat (*Rattus norvegicus*), Wright–Giemsa stain (100×, oil). (b) Neutrophil in the blood film of a mouse (*Mus musculus*), Wright–Giemsa stain.

Eosinophils generally comprise 0–7% of the leukocyte differential in the mouse and 1–4% in the rat. They have a ring- or U-shaped nucleus, a basophilic cytoplasm, and numerous round, eosinophilic cytoplasmic granules that may be arranged in small clumps (Figures 3.25a and 3.25b). The granules found in the eosinophils of mice are large and uniform with indistinct margins, whereas those of rats are small and numerous.

Basophils are present in small numbers (0–1% of the leukocyte differential) in the blood of mice and rats. They often contain numerous large, round, purple cytoplasmic granules. Basophils with their lobed nuclei should be differentiated from mast cells with their nuclei without lobulation that may appear in peripheral blood, especially when cardiocentesis is performed. Basophil numbers appear higher in blood collected from the tail of mice and rats when excessive trauma is involved, such as the laceration technique and tail compression to facilitate blood flow (Moore, 2000a).

Monocytes, measuring 17 µm in diameter, are the largest leukocytes found in the peripheral blood of rats and mice. They account for 1–6% of the leukocyte population in rats and 0–2% in mice. Monocytes have a variably shaped (round, indented, or lobulated) nucleus with the kidney-bean shape being the most common form (Figure 3.26). The abundant blue-gray cytoplasm often contains fine azurophilic granules and occasional vacuoles (Fredrickson and Harris, 2000).

(a) (b)

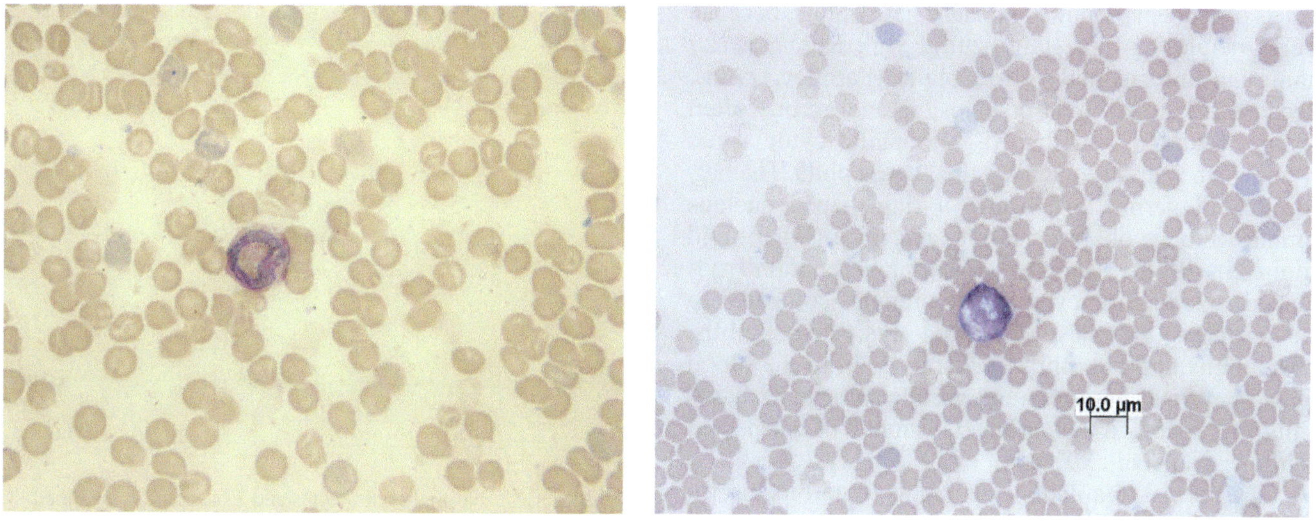

Fig. 3.25. (a) Eosinophil in the blood film of a domestic rat (*Rattus norvegicus*), Wright–Giemsa stain (100×, oil). (b) Eosinophil in the blood film of a mouse (*Mus musculus*), Wright–Giemsa stain.

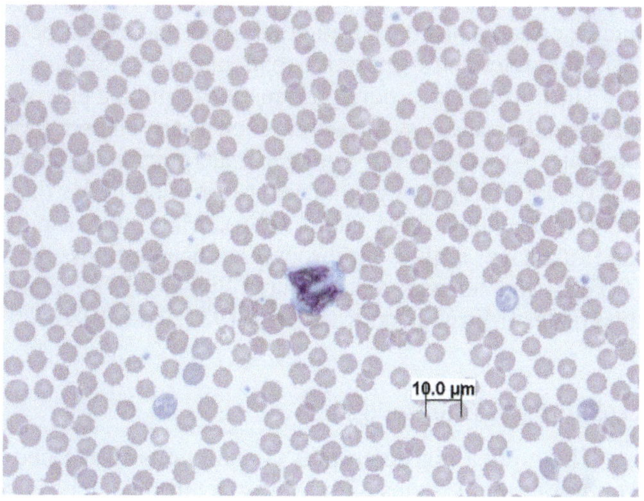

Fig. 3.26. Monocyte in the blood film of a mouse (*Mus musculus*), Wright–Giemsa stain.

Leukocyte concentrations of mice and rats not only demonstrate a distinct diurnal variation, but also vary markedly between strains and reproductive status (Wright et al., 1983). A distinct circadian rhythm affects peripheral leukocyte concentrations with an increase in circulating leukocyte concentration occurring during the light phase and a decrease during the dark phase. Pregnant rats tend to have higher leukocyte, segmented neutrophil, lymphocyte, and monocyte counts than nonmated rats, requiring separate reference data (Liberati et al., 2004). There is also an age-dependent variation in the neutrophil to lymphocyte ratio, with the lymphocyte concentration decreasing and neutrophil concentration increasing as a rodent ages. A distinct decrease in the total leukocyte count associated with a decrease in lymphocytes occurs in mice following the stress, such as occurs during transportation (Bean-Knudsen and Wagner, 1987; Drozdowicz et al., 1990). Thus, it is difficult to establish reference hematologic values for mice and rats because of the large number of strains and variations in blood collection methods, handling techniques, and environmental conditions.

Leukocytes of Mongolian Gerbils (*Meriones unguiculatus*) and Hamsters (*Mesocricetus auratus*)

The hematologic features of hamsters and gerbils resemble those of mice and rats (Moore, 2000c, d). As with rats and mice, polychromasia/reticulocytosis and anisocytosis are normal findings in blood film from these rodents. Howell–Jolly bodies and nucleated red blood cells are commonly found, especially in the hamster; nucleated erythrocytes can represent up to 2% of the red blood cells in healthy adults (Harkness and Wagner, 1989). Stippled basophilia (remnant of cytoplasmic ribonucleoprotein) is a prominent feature of gerbil red blood cells (George et al., 1983). The red blood cell indices, such as MCV, hemoglobin concentration (Hgb), hematocrit (Hct), and MCHC, have been reported to be higher in adult male gerbils compared with adult females; however, the differences may not be clinically significant (Zimmerman et al., 2010c). The total erythrocyte count of male hamsters decreases by 25–30% following castration and will return to normal following testosterone supplementation (Smith et al., 2010). The red blood cell count and hemoglobin concentration increase with no change in the MCV in hibernating hamsters, which is likely associated with a near doubling of the red blood cell lifespan during this period (Reznik, 1975).

The neutrophils of some rodents were previously called pseudoeosinophils and later, heterophils, because their granules do not stain neutral with Romanowsky stains but are distinctly eosinophilic (Parmley, 1988). Because the neutrophils of hamsters and gerbils often contain round to rod-shaped, acidophilic cytoplasmic granules, they are frequently called heterophils. The heterophils of gerbils often have a ring-shaped nucleus similar to those observed in rats and mice (Weeks and Glomski, 1978). Hamster eosinophils contain rod-shaped, eosinophilic cytoplasmic granules compared to the rounder granules of mice, rats, and gerbils. Eosinophils and basophils are rarely seen in the blood films of normal hamsters and gerbils. Whenever basophils are found, a nematodiasis should be suspected (Zimmerman et al., 2010c).

The normal total leukocyte counts of gerbils resemble those of mice rather than those of hamsters. The nocturnal habit of the hamster affects the white blood cells, causing an increase in circulating heterophils (neutrophils) and thus the total leukocyte count when the animal is more active (Smith et al., 2010). The total leukocyte count of hibernating hamsters decreases with a shift to an even heterophil:lymphocyte ratio from that of non-hibernating hamsters, where lymphocytes represent 60–80% of the leukocyte differential (Reznik, 1975). Gerbils normally exhibit a high degree of polychromasia, circulating reticulocytes, and stippled basophilia owing to the short red cell life span of 9–10 days. The normal hemogram of the gerbil is influenced by sex and age. Gerbils less than 8 weeks of age exhibit a macrocytosis, a panleukopenia, and an erythrocyte count that is half that of a normal adult, and male gerbils generally have higher MCV, Hb, PCV, and MCHC as well as higher leukocyte counts with higher absolute lymphocytes compared to females (Heatley and Harris, 2009). Thus, the lymphocyte:neutrophil ratio of gerbils is generally considered to be 6.1:1 for males and 3.2:1 for females (Mays, 1969).

Guinea Pigs (*Cavia porcellus*)

Erythrocytes of Guinea Pigs

The Romanowsky-stained erythrocytes of guinea pigs (*Cavia porcellus*) are round, anucleated, pink, biconcave disks with a central pale area and a mean diameter between 6.6 and 7.9 μm, larger than those of most other rodents (Moore, 2000e) (Figure 3.27). Polychromasia is commonly observed on guinea pig blood films, which like those of true rodents, is directly related to the short half-life of the erythrocytes. The normal degree of polychromasia is 1.5% in adult guinea pigs, but is much higher in young guinea pigs (4.5% in juveniles) (Zimmerman et al., 2010b). The red blood cell indices, such as the total erythrocyte count, PCV, and hemoglobin concentration, of guinea pigs are generally lower than those of true rodents (Marshall, 2008). Increased polychromasia/reticulocytosis and a macrocytosis characterize regenerative responses to anemia.

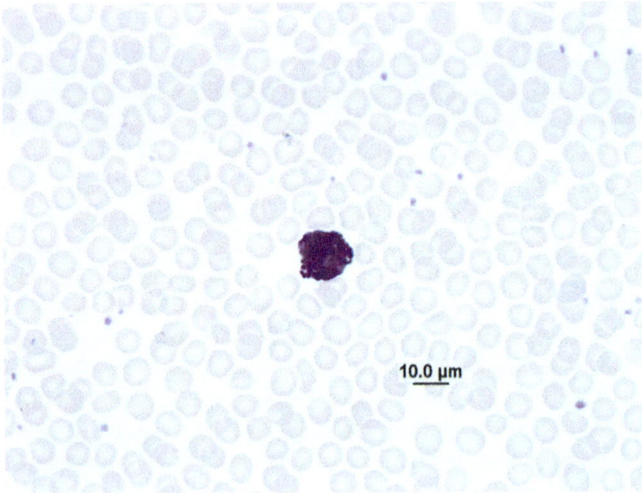

Fig. 3.27. Normal erythrocytes and a basophil in the blood film of a guinea pig (*Cavia porcellus*), Wright–Giemsa stain.

The normal erythrocyte parameters of guinea pigs are influenced by a variety of factors, such as age and sex. For example, 1-month-old or younger male guinea pigs tend to have lower erythrocyte concentrations and PCVs than older male guinea pigs (Jain, 1986). Male guinea pigs tend to have higher erythrocyte concentrations than females, and females tend to have higher MCV values than males (Mitruka and Rawnsley, 1981; Jain, 1986).

Leukocytes of Guinea Pigs

The guinea pig heterophil is analogous to the neutrophil of other species. Guinea pig heterophils measure 10–12 μm in diameter, have a pyknotic segmented nucleus, and contain cytoplasmic granules that stain eosinophilic, because of which they were often referred to as pseudoeosinophils in older references (Figures 3.28 and 3.29).

Guinea pig eosinophils (10–15 μm in diameter) tend to be slightly larger than the heterophils in the same blood film (Figure 3.30). They contain large, round to rod-shaped, bright-red cytoplasmic granules. The granules of eosinophils are larger than the granules of heterophils, making eosinophils easy to differentiate from heterophils.

Guinea pig basophils are nearly the same size of heterophils. Their cytoplasm is densely packed with reddish-purple to black granules of variable sizes (Figures 3.27 and 3.29).

Lymphocytes are the predominant leukocytes in the differential of healthy guinea pigs (Figures 3.28, 3.29, and 3.31). Small lymphocytes (approximately the size of

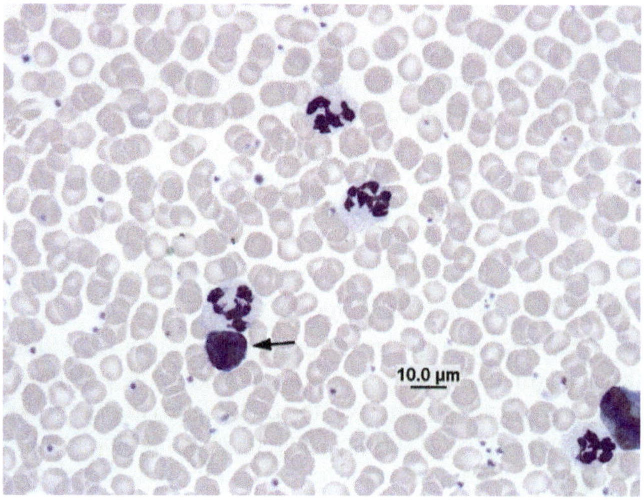

Fig. 3.28. Heterophils and lymphocyte (arrow) in the blood film of a guinea pig (*Cavia porcellus*), Wright–Giemsa stain.

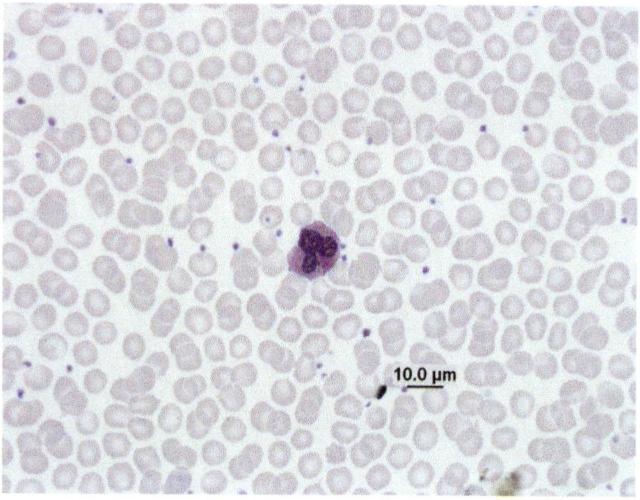

Fig. 3.30. Eosinophil in the blood film of a guinea pig (*Cavia porcellus*), Wright–Giemsa stain.

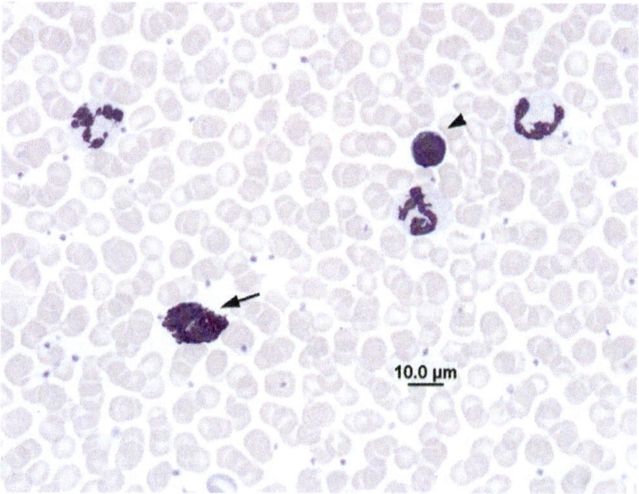

Fig. 3.29. Basophil (arrow), heterophils, and lymphocyte (arrowhead) in the blood film of a guinea pig (*Cavia porcellus*), Wright–Giemsa stain.

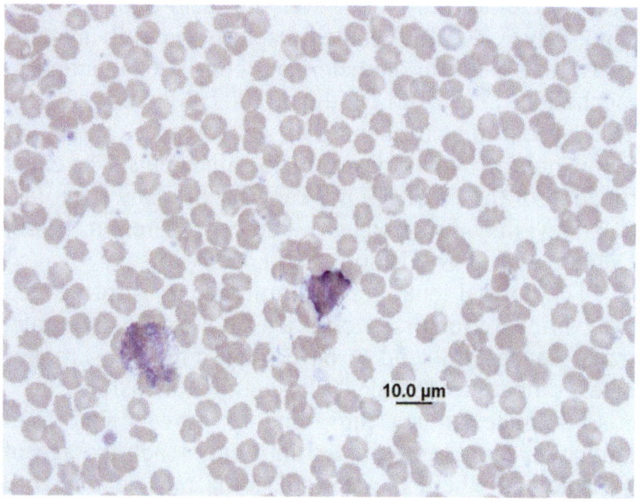

Fig. 3.31. Large lymphocyte with azurophilic granules in the blood film of a guinea pig (*Cavia porcellus*), Wright–Giemsa stain.

erythrocytes) are the most common form. They have a round nucleus with condensed nuclear chromatin that is surrounded by a narrow band of light-blue cytoplasm with the Romanowsky stains. Large lymphocytes that are almost twice the size of small lymphocytes occur in fewer numbers. Large lymphocytes have a slightly smaller nucleus:cytoplasmic ratio, less condensed nucleus, and more abundant blue cytoplasm that often contains azurophilic granules (Figure 3.31).

Because guinea pigs are normally lymphocytic, the response in early inflammation reveals an increase in heterophils and decrease in lymphocytes with either a normal leukocyte count or a leukopenia. Often, the total platelet count is an important marker of inflammation in guinea pigs as well as other small mammals, where a large increase in the platelet count (>1000 000/μL) can be seen without a change in total white blood cell count (Riggs, 2009; Riggs and Mitchell, 2009).

Monocytes in guinea pig blood films are large mononuclear leukocytes with an abundant blue-gray cytoplasm that tends to be darker than that of large lymphocytes (Figure 3.32). The nuclear chromatin of monocytes is usually more dispersed compared to that of large lymphocytes.

Approximately 3–4% of the leukocytes in the peripheral blood of adult guinea pigs are large mononuclear cells that contain a single large cytoplasmic inclusion referred to as a Kurloff body (Jain, 1986) (Figures 3.33a and 3.33b). These Foà-Kurloff cells are unique to cavies, such as guinea pigs and capybaras. The finely granular and occasionally vacuolated Kurloff bodies stain homogeneously red with Romanowsky stains and stain positive

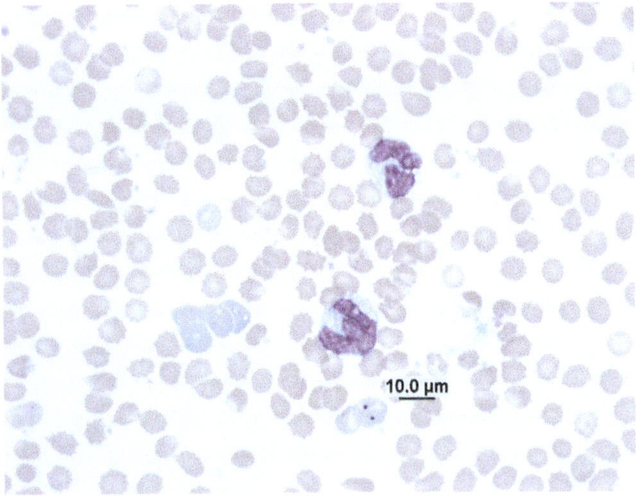

Fig. 3.32. Monocytes in the blood film of a guinea pig (*Cavia porcellus*), Wright–Giemsa stain.

with toluidine blue and Periodic acid-Schiff (PAS) (Jain, 1993). Kurloff bodies displace the cell nucleus, measure 1–8 µm in diameter, and consist of mucopolysaccharide (Percy and Barthold, 2007; Marshall, 2008). They appear to be influenced by sex hormones and occur in low numbers in immature male guinea pigs. The exact function of these cells is not known, but many speculate that they may function as killer cells (Eremin, 1980; Debout et al., 1999; Moore, 2000e).

The normal leukogram of guinea pigs is influenced by a variety of factors, such as age and sex. For example, male guinea pigs tend to have more circulating monocytes compared to females (Mitruka and Rawnsley, 1981). Also, female guinea pigs tend to have higher total leukocyte counts than males until they reach the age of 4–6 months where the sexes become more equal until they reach 12 months of age, when males tend to have the higher counts (Jain, 1986).

The bone marrow evaluation of guinea pigs is the same as that of other rodents and domestic mammals. The normal myeloid:erythroid (M: E) ratio for these animals generally ranges between 1.2:1 and 1.6:1 (Marshall, 2008; Zimmerman, 2010b).

Chinchillas (*Chinchilla lanigera*)

The hematologic features of chinchillas resemble those of mice and rats. As with rats and mice, polychromasia is a normal finding on the blood film (Figure 3.34). The neutrophils of chinchillas have faint acidophilic cytoplasmic granules and therefore are often referred to as heterophils, but should not be confused with eosinophils (Campbell and Grant, 2010). The nuclei of the neutrophils are polymorphic and typically hyposegmented, often resembling neutrophils of dogs with the Pelger–Huët anomaly (Figure 3.35). Like the guinea pig, the chinchilla is normally lymphocytic; therefore, the hemic response in early inflammation often reveals an increase in neutrophils and a decrease in lymphocytes with either a normal leukocyte count or leukopenia.

Rabbits (*Oryctolagus cuniculus*)

Erythrocytes of Rabbits

The Romanowsky-stained erythrocytes of rabbits are round, anucleated, pink, biconcave disks with an average diameter of 6.8 µm; however, the presence of erythrocytes with a range of 5.0–7.8 µm makes reporting of a significant anisocytosis, a common finding in the hemogram of normal rabbits (Figure 3.36). The PCV of

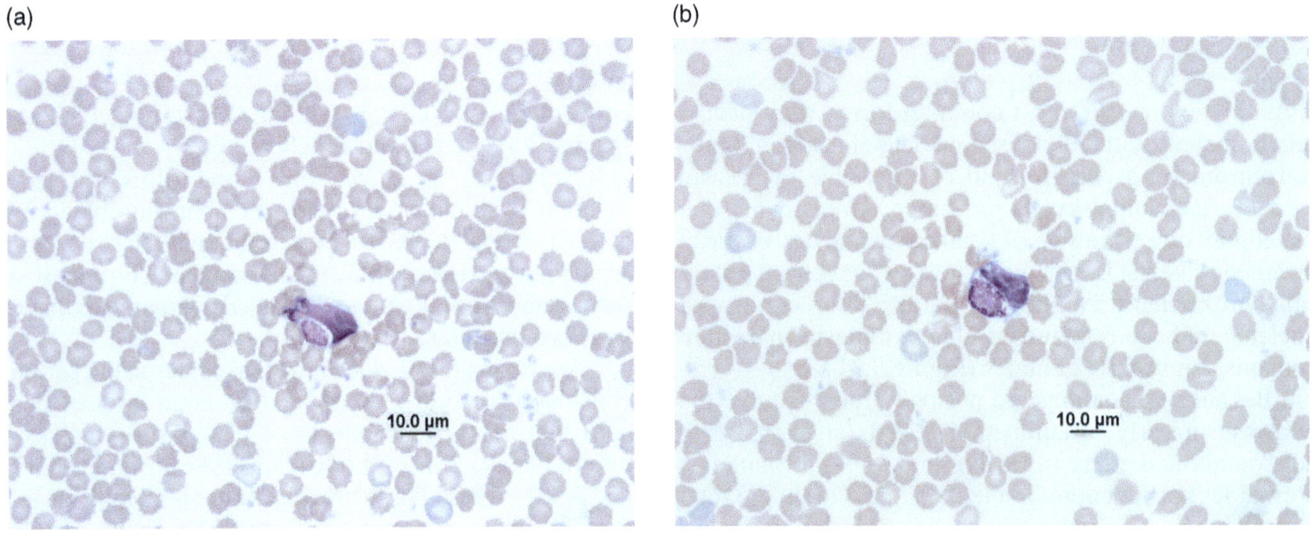

Fig. 3.33. (a) Lymphocyte with Kurloff body in the blood film of a guinea pig (*Cavia porcellus*), Wright–Giemsa stain. (b) Lymphocyte with Kurloff body in the blood film of a guinea pig (*Cavia porcellus*), Wright–Giemsa stain.

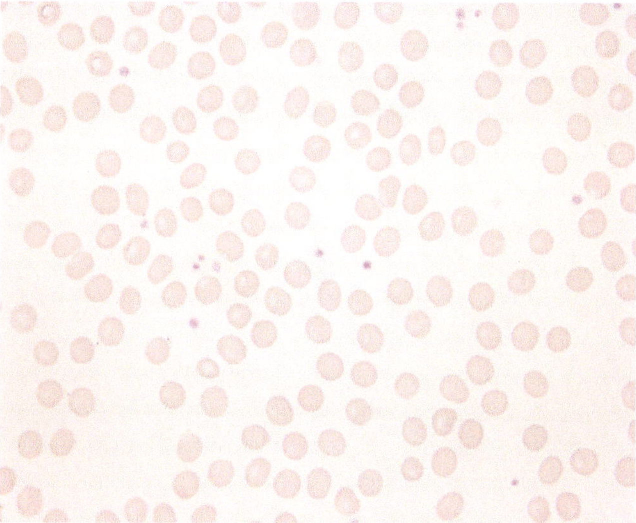

Fig. 3.34. Normal erythrocytes in the blood film of a chinchilla (*Chinchilla lanigera*), Wright–Giemsa stain (100×, oil).

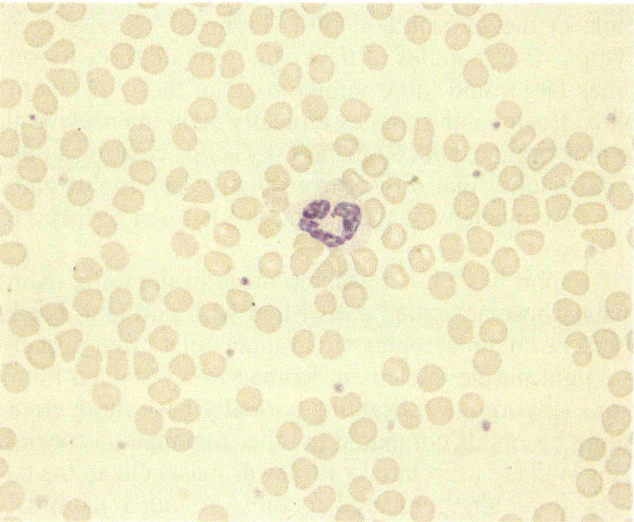

Fig. 3.35. Neutrophil (heterophil) in the blood film of a chinchilla (*Chinchilla lanigera*), Wright–Giemsa stain (100×, oil).

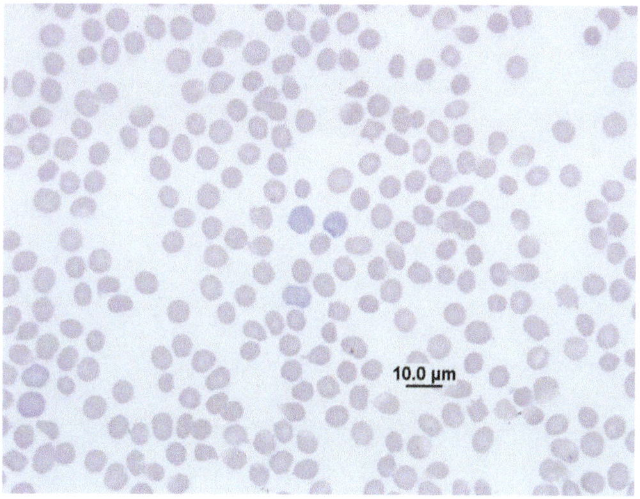

Fig. 3.36. Normal erythrocytes in the blood film of a rabbit (*Oryctolagus cuniculus*), Wright–Giemsa stain.

healthy rabbits generally ranges between 30% and 50%. Polychromatic erythrocytes and reticulocytes are common features of normal rabbit blood films. The estimated half-life of rabbit erythrocytes is between 45 and 70 days (Vacha, 1983; Zimmerman et al., 2010a). Polychromasia is typically observed in 2–4% of the erythrocyte population of healthy adult rabbits. The percentage of reticulocytes can be high (2.7–12.1%) in rabbits less than 2 months of age, but drops to 50% by 3 months of age, eventually leveling to 1.7–4.3% in adults (Jacobson, 1978). Nucleated erythrocytes and Howell–Jolly bodies are occasionally observed in blood films from healthy rabbits (Moore, 2000f).

A general anesthetic is often used in clinical practice to restrain rabbits for obtaining blood samples, but this practice does not appear to influence the hematologic test results (Melillo, 2007). However, the normal erythrocyte parameters of rabbits can be influenced by a variety of other factors, such as age, sex, and reproductive status. For example, rabbits less than 6 months of age have lower red blood cell counts and higher MCV and MCH values when compared to adults (Bartolotti et al., 1989; Marco et al., 2003). Male rabbits tend to have slightly higher erythrocyte counts and hemoglobin concentrations than females (Zimmerman et al., 2010a). The total erythrocyte count, hemoglobin concentration, and hematocrit values can be significantly lower in the pregnant rabbits in the third trimester compared to nonpregnant rabbits; however, the MCV value increases (Kim et al., 2002). For best results in measuring hematologic analytes in rabbits, the blood samples should be processed in a timely manner, preferably within 1 h after collection (Ameri et al., 2011).

Anemia is commonly associated with a variety of diseases in rabbits. A regenerative response to an anemia in the rabbit patient is characterized by increased anisocytosis, polychromasia, nucleated erythrocytes, and presence of Howell–Jolly bodies. Infectious diseases often result in increased number of nucleated erythrocytes. Acanthocytes are more frequently observed in rabbits suffering from inflammatory or neoplastic diseases (Christopher et al., 2014). Erythrocyte fragility studies used as a diagnostic aid in the detection of IMHA in rabbits is based upon the sodium chloride concentrations, whereby the first detectable hemolysis in normal rabbits occurs at 0.5–0.3% NaCl (McLaughlin and Fish, 1994).

Leukocytes of Rabbits

The rabbit neutrophil is generally referred to as a heterophil because the cytoplasm typically stains diffusely pink with Romanowsky stains due to the fusion of

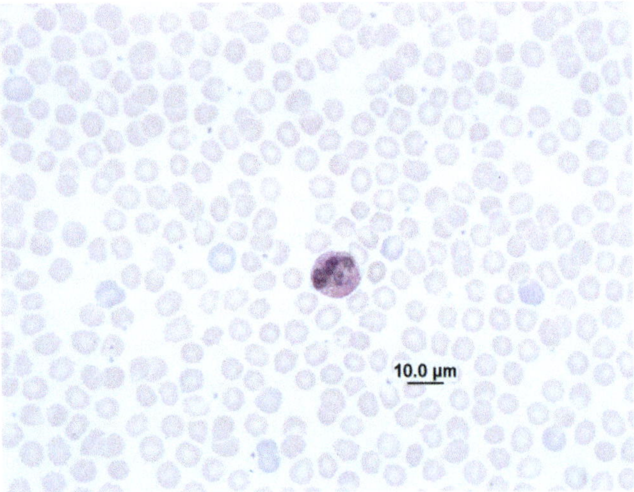

Fig. 3.37. Heterophil in the blood film of a rabbit (*Oryctolagus cuniculus*), Wright–Giemsa stain.

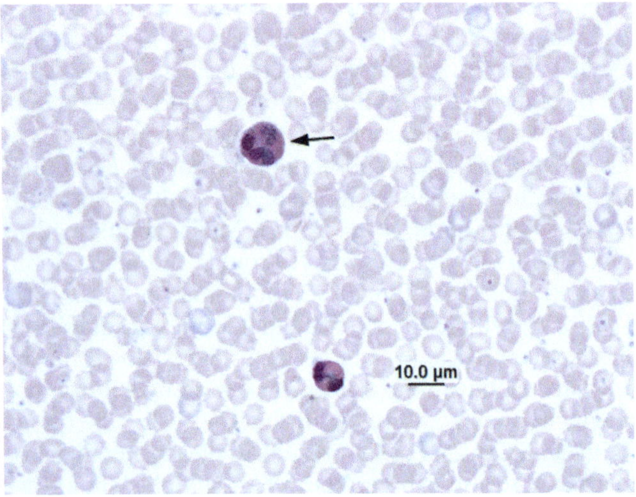

Fig. 3.38. Eosinophil (arrow) and heterophil in the blood film of a rabbit (*Oryctolagus cuniculus*), Wright–Giemsa stain.

many small acidophilic granules (primary granules) (Figure 3.37 and Figure 3.38). A variable number of larger eosinophilic granules are also present. The heterophils of rabbits and some rodents were previously called pseudoeosinophils because their granules (the larger secondary granules) do not stain neutral with Romanowsky stains, but are distinctly eosinophilic. The rabbit heterophil normally measures between 10 and 15 µm in diameter. The polymorphic nucleus stains light blue to purple with Romanowsky stains. Rabbit heterophils are ultrastructurally, functionally, and biochemically equivalent to neutrophils from other domestic mammals and humans (Parmley, 1988). An occasional heterophil with characteristics of the Pelger–Huët anomaly may be observed in blood films from normal rabbits. Rabbit heterophils are easily distinguished from the eosinophils, which have large eosinophilic granules.

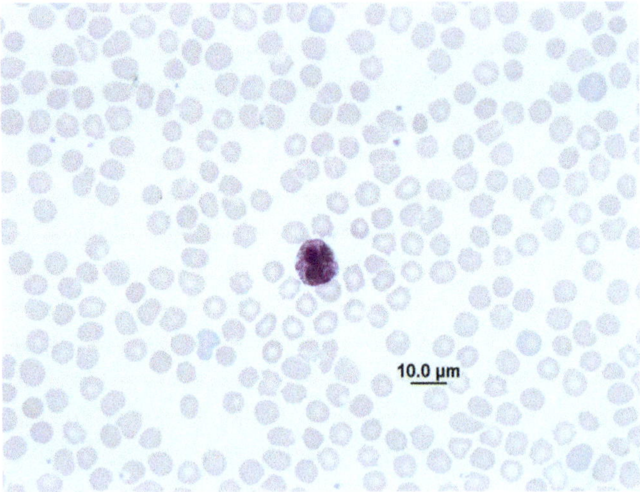

Fig. 3.39. Basophil in the blood film of a rabbit (*Oryctolagus cuniculus*), Wright–Giemsa stain.

Rabbit eosinophils measure between 12 and 16 µm in diameter; therefore, they are larger than the heterophils in the same blood film (Figure 3.38). Also, the cytoplasmic granules of the eosinophil are three to four times larger and more numerous than those of heterophils. Eosinophil granules typically stain intensely pink to pink orange, with Romanowsky stains creating a tinctorial quality that differs from that of heterophil granules. The nucleus of the eosinophil is often bi-lobed to U-shaped.

Rabbit basophils resemble those of domestic mammals. These are round cells filled with purple to black, metachromatic cytoplasmic granules that often obscure the light purple nucleus in Romanowsky-stained blood films (Figure 3.39). Rabbits typically have more circulating basophils compared to other mammalian species. This is likely associated with fewer mast cells in the tissues of rabbits compared to those of other mammals (Jain and Zinkl, 1981). Basophils commonly represent 5% of the leukocytes in the differential white blood cell count of healthy rabbits, but they can also be as high as 30% in rabbits with no apparent abnormalities (Campbell and Ellis, 2007).

Rabbit lymphocytes are morphologically similar to those of other domestic mammals and humans (Figure 3.40). They have a round nucleus with condensed nuclear chromatin that is surrounded by a narrow band of blue cytoplasm. Most lymphocytes in healthy rabbit blood films are small (between 7 and 10 µm in diameter); however, large lymphocytes (between 10 and 15 µm in diameter) may also be present (Reagan et al., 2008). The large lymphocytes commonly demonstrate azurophilic granules in the cytoplasm.

Likewise, rabbit monocytes are morphologically like those found in other domestic mammals (Figure 3.41). These are large cells (15–18 µm in diameter) with a nuclear pattern that varies from lobulated to

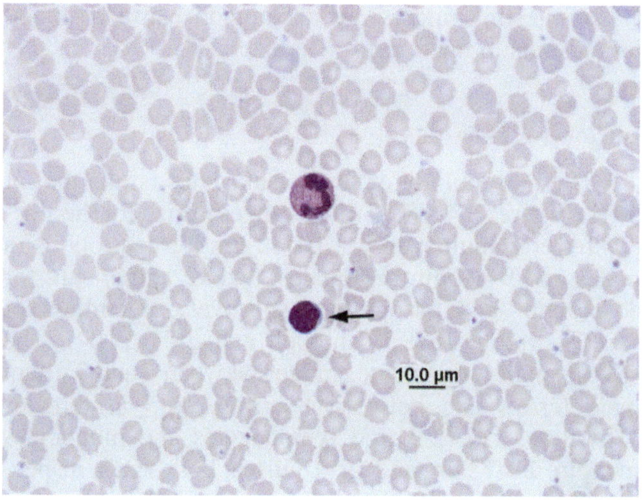

Fig. 3.40. Lymphocyte (arrow) and heterophil in the blood film of a rabbit (*Oryctolagus cuniculus*), Wright–Giemsa stain.

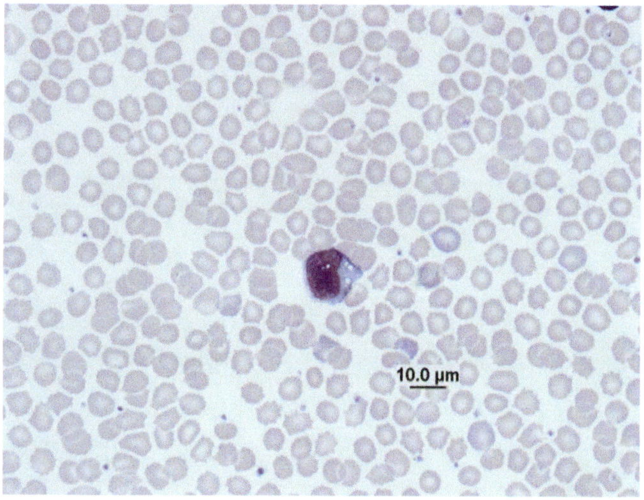

Fig. 3.41. Monocyte in the blood film of a rabbit (*Oryctolagus cuniculus*), Wright–Giemsa stain.

bean-shaped with a diffuse chromatin that stains light compared to that of lymphocytes. The monocyte cytoplasm typically stains blue and may contain a few vacuoles.

The normal leukocyte concentration of rabbits is typically reported to range between 7000/μL and 9000/μL. Variations occur with age, restraint methods, pregnancy, and methods of blood collection that may alter the heterophil:lymphocyte (H:L) ratio. A bimodal increase in the leukocyte concentration is seen with increasing age, with the highest lymphocyte concentration occurring at 3 months of age and then slowly declining, and the highest heterophil concentrations occurring in older animals (Moore, 2000f). The normal H:L ratio of 33:60 at 2 months of age changes to 45:45 by 12 months of age. Therefore, rabbits younger than 12 months are expected to have lower H:L ratios than do older rabbits, which typically have equal numbers of heterophils and lymphocytes. A stress response associated with restraint during blood collection procedures can result in a decrease in the total leukocyte count of as much as 15–30% (Drozdowicz et al., 1990).

A mature heterophilia and lymphopenia characterize glucocorticoid-mediated changes in the leukogram. Pregnant rabbits demonstrate a slight increase in total leukocyte counts during the first half of gestation due to an increase in lymphocyte numbers; however, a significant decrease can occur in the second half due to a decrease in lymphocytes and/or heterophil numbers (Kim et al., 2002). Rabbits generally do not develop a strong leukocytosis with bacterial infections, but will demonstrate a reversal of the H:L ratio; therefore, the H:L ratio appears to be a more reliable indicator of inflammatory disorders than total leukocyte concentrations. However, a reversal of the H:L ratio can also be associated with increases in serum cortisol concentrations (Toth and January, 1990).

Inflammation in Rabbits

As mentioned earlier, in the normal healthy rabbit, lymphocyte concentrations are higher than heterophil concentrations, and rabbits do not typically develop a leukocytosis when bacterial infections are present, but will exhibit an increase in the absolute heterophil concentration and possibly a decrease in the absolute lymphocyte concentration (Stieve-Caldwell et al., 2009; Campbell and Grant, 2010). This reversal of the H:L ratio is also associated with increases in serum cortisol concentrations where there is a decrease in the lymphocyte concentration. The presence of toxic changes in the heterophils is an important clue to an inflammatory response in the rabbit. Therefore, the H:L ratio, the absolute heterophil and lymphocyte concentrations, and heterophil morphology appear to be more reliable indicators of inflammatory disorders in the rabbit than total leukocyte concentrations.

Platelets of Rabbits

Rabbit platelets resemble those of other mammals. They appear as small pale blue cytoplasmic fragments that contain small clusters of azurophilic granules. The normal total platelet count of rabbits varies, but generally is between 200 000 and 1000 000/μL (Harkness and Wagner, 1995).

Ferrets (*Mustela putorius furo*)

Erythrocytes of Ferrets

Romanowsky-stained erythrocytes of ferrets are round, anucleated, pink, biconcave disks with an

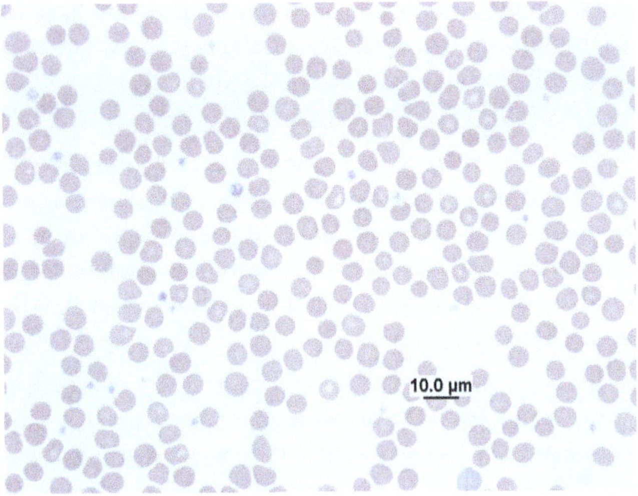

Fig. 3.42. Erythrocytes in the blood film of a ferret (*Mustela putorius furo*), Wright–Giemsa stain.

average diameter of 5.94 μm for males and 6.32 μm for females; however, the normal range for both sexes is 4.6–7.7 μm (Hillyer and Quesenberry, 1997; Marini et al., 2002; Siperstein, 2008) (Figure 3.42). In general, the hematology of ferrets resembles that of domestic carnivores except that the hematocrit values and total red blood cell counts tend to be higher (Fox and Marini, 1998; Moore, 2000g; Yuschenkoff et al., 2021).

Ferrets are commonly anesthetized to restrain them for blood collection; however, the use of inhalant anesthetics such as isoflurane, enflurane, and halothane can result in significant and rapid decreases in the red blood cell count, hematocrit, and hemoglobin concentration. As much as a 33% decrease in the hemoglobin concentration has been reported with the use of these inhalant anesthetics (Marini et al., 1994). Splenic sequestration and anesthetic-induced hypotension are possible causes for this response in ferrets. The erythron returns to normal within 45 min of recovery from the anesthetic. Either the use of manual restraint or injectable anesthesia such as ketamine or rapid blood collection following anesthetic induction (less than 3 min) is required to avoid this effect in the erythron.

The hemogram of domestic ferrets is influenced by sex and age. Young male ferrets have lower red blood cell counts, hematocrits, and hemoglobin concentrations than do adult males, and young females and females show a decrease in the hematocrit with increasing age (Fox, 1988).

Ferrets with lymphoma are more likely to exhibit schistocytes and acanthocytes in their peripheral blood films (Bau-Gaudreault and Grimes, 2019). Common causes of nonregenerative anemia in domestic ferrets include malignant neoplasia (such as lymphoma), systemic infections, and hyperestrogenism in intact females. Gastrointestinal ulcers are a common cause of blood loss anemia in the ferret.

Leukocytes of Ferrets

The morphology of ferret leukocytes is like that of dogs (Figures 3.43–3.47). The ranges in size for the various ferret granulocytes are 10–13 μm for neutrophils in males and 9–10 μm in females; and 12 and 14 μm for eosinophils and basophils, respectively, regardless of sex (Thornton, 1979; Campbell and Ellis, 2007). The size of small lymphocytes ranges between 6 and 9 μm in male ferrets and between 8 and 10 μm in females (Thornton, 1979). Large lymphocytes and monocytes measure 11–12 μm and 12–18 μm in both sexes, respectively (Thornton, 1979).

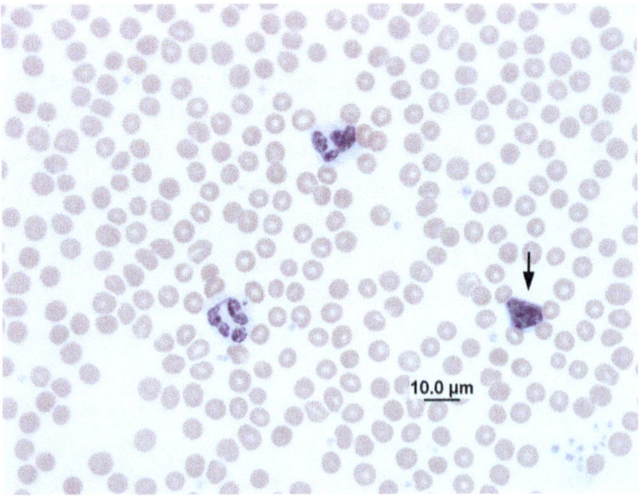

Fig. 3.43. Neutrophils and a lymphocyte (arrow) in the blood film of a ferret (*Mustela putorius furo*), Wright–Giemsa stain.

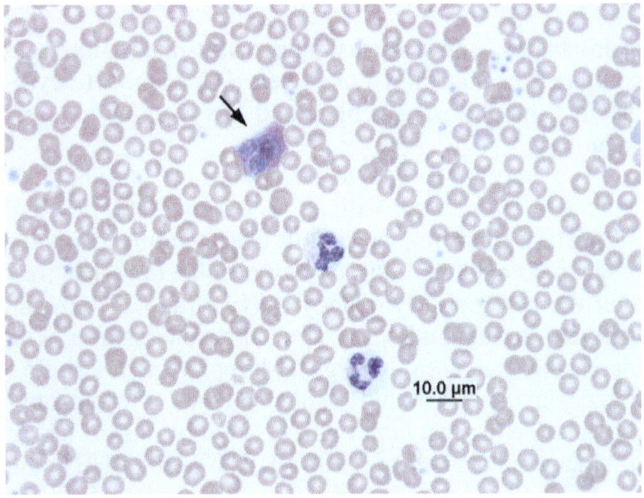

Fig. 3.44. Eosinophil (arrow) and neutrophils in the blood film of a ferret (*Mustela putorius furo*), Wright–Giemsa stain.

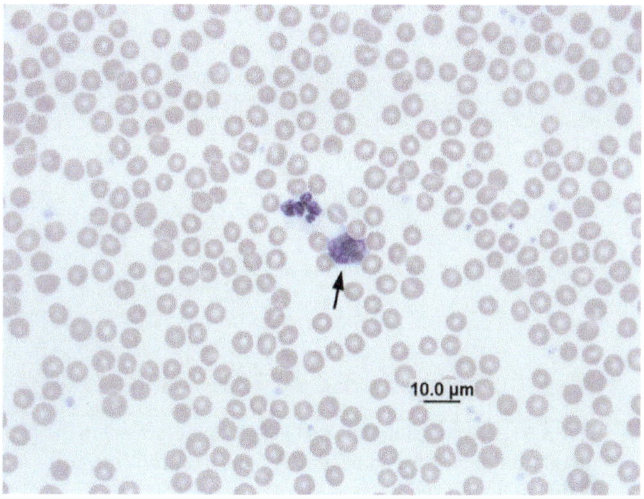

Fig. 3.45. Neutrophil and a large lymphocyte (arrow) in the blood film of a ferret (*Mustela putorius furo*), Wright–Giemsa stain.

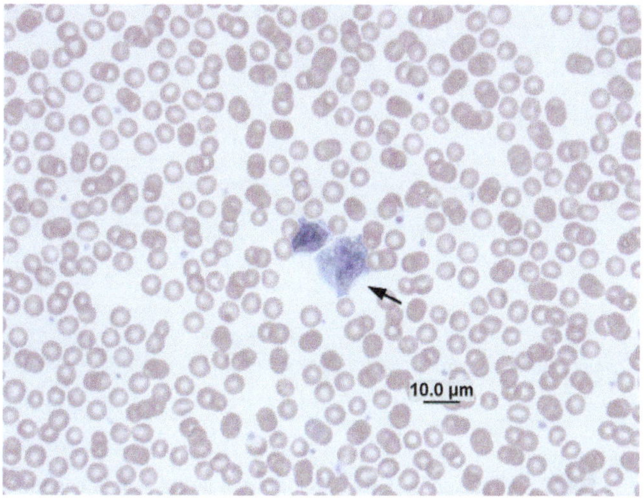

Fig. 3.46. Lymphocyte and monocyte (arrow) in the blood film of a ferret (*Mustela putorius furo*), Wright–Giemsa stain.

Inflammation in Ferrets

In the normal healthy ferret, neutrophil concentrations are higher than lymphocyte concentrations, and they demonstrate an increase in neutrophil concentration and a decrease in the lymphocyte concentration with increasing age (Kawasaki, 1994; Moore, 2000g). The total leukocyte count of healthy ferrets can be as low as 3000/µL (Lee et al., 1982; Kawasaki, 1994). Ferrets are unable to develop a marked leukocytosis with inflammatory disease; therefore, a concentration greater than 20 000/µL is unusual and a left shift is rare (Kawasaki, 1994).

Lymphoma in Ferrets

The total leukocyte count and the lymphocyte count are often used as a means of monitoring ferrets for lymphoma. The total leukocyte count of ferrets with

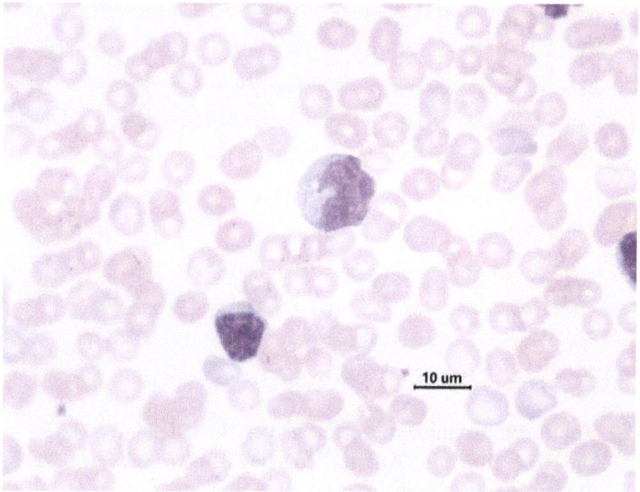

Fig. 3.47. Lymphocyte (smaller of the two leukocytes) and monocyte in the blood film of a ferret (*Mustela putorius furo*), Wright–Giemsa stain.

lymphoma may be normal or may demonstrate an absolute or relative lymphocytosis. Marked leukocytosis (leukocyte count greater than 20 000/µL) is often associated with lymphocytic leukemia or lymphoma (Erdman et al., 1992; Brown, 1997). Anemia, leukopenia, and thrombocytopenia may also be noted in some cases. Abnormal lymphocytes occasionally appear in the differential. As a general rule, a persistent absolute lymphocyte count greater than 3500/µL or a relative lymphocytosis (>60%) is considered suspicious, even if the total leukocyte count is normal.

Platelets of Ferrets

Ferret platelets resemble those of other mammals. They appear as small, pale blue cytoplasmic fragments that contain small clusters of azurophilic granules. The normal total platelet count of ferrets varies with the references, but generally lies between 245 000/µL and 910 000/µL (Thornton, 1979; Besch-Williford, 1987; Kawasaki, 1994).

African Hedgehogs (*Atelerix albiventris*)

The hematology of African hedgehogs resembles that of domestic carnivores, such as the dog and cat. The morphology of the hemic cells is like that of other small mammals (Figures 3.48–3.54). Likewise, interpretation of the hemic response is based upon that of other small mammals.

Eosinophilic leukemia is a rare form of myeloproliferative disease and a variant of granulocytic leukemia that has been described in African hedgehogs (Higbie et al., 2016; Martínez-Jiménez et al., 2017). Eosinophilic leukemia must be differentiated from other conditions

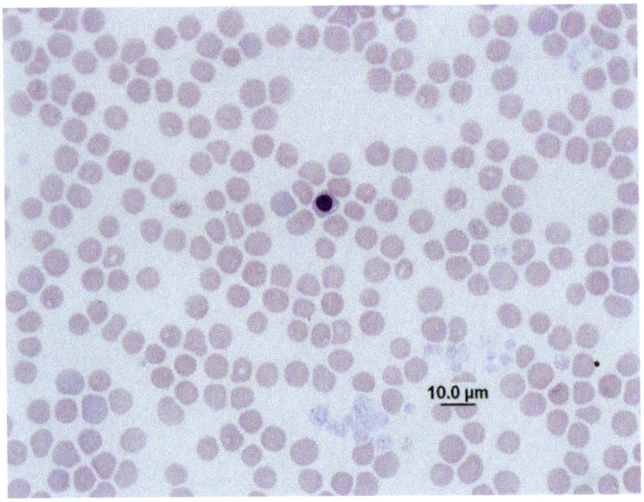

Fig. 3.48. Erythrocytes, nucleated erythrocyte, and platelets in the blood film of an African hedgehog (*Atelerix albiventris*), Wright–Giemsa stain.

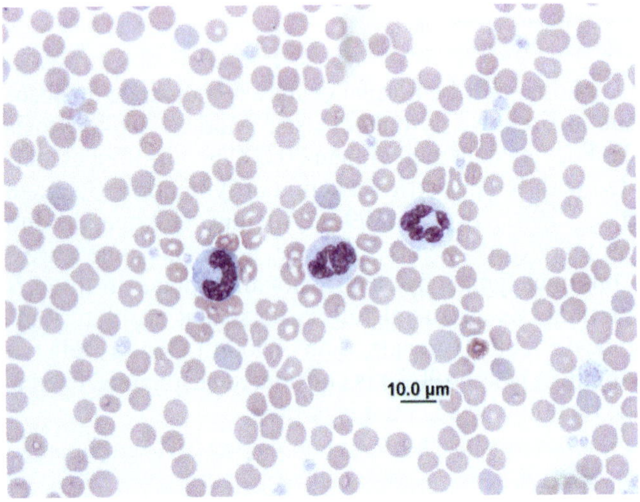

Fig. 3.49. Neutrophils in the blood film of an African hedgehog (*Atelerix albiventris*), Wright–Giemsa stain.

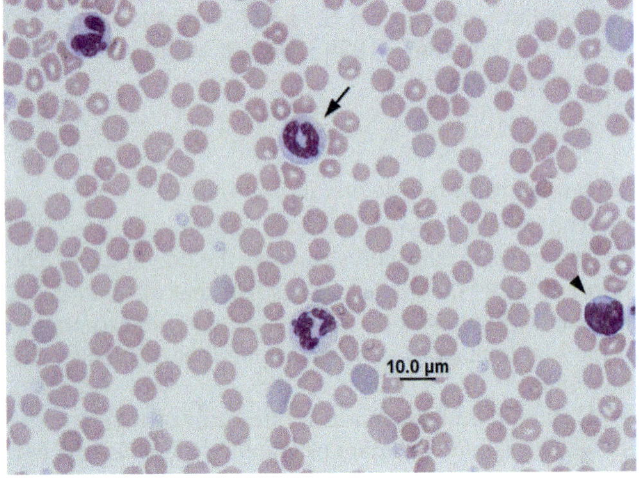

Fig. 3.50. Neutrophils, one band cell (arrow), and lymphocyte (arrowhead) in the blood film of an African hedgehog (*Atelerix albiventris*), Wright–Giemsa stain.

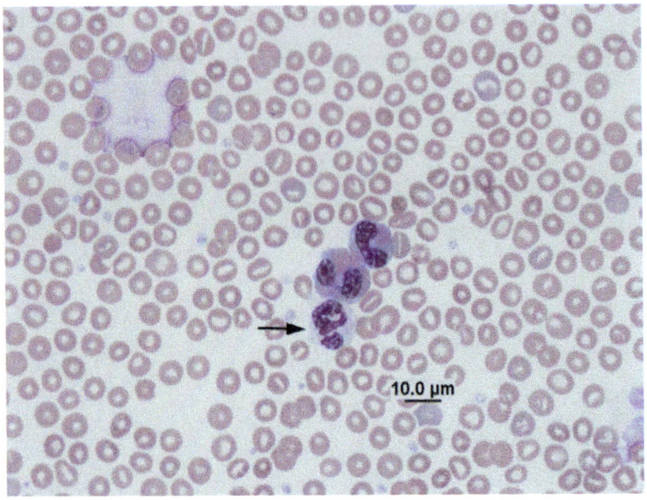

Fig. 3.51. Two eosinophils and a neutrophil (arrow) in the blood film of an African hedgehog (*Atelerix albiventris*), Wright–Giemsa stain.

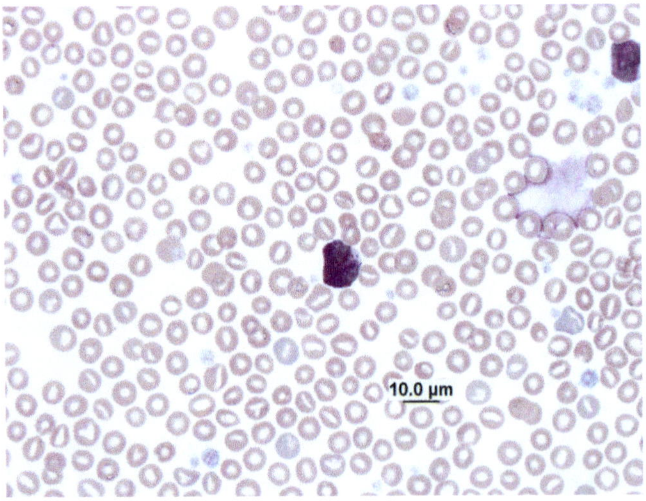

Fig. 3.52. Basophil in the blood film of an African hedgehog (*Atelerix albiventris*), Wright–Giemsa stain.

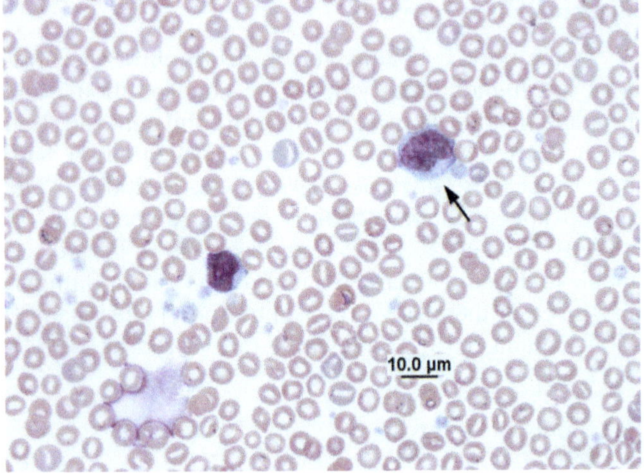

Fig. 3.53. Lymphocyte and monocyte (arrow) in the blood film of an African hedgehog (*Atelerix albiventris*), Wright–Giemsa stain.

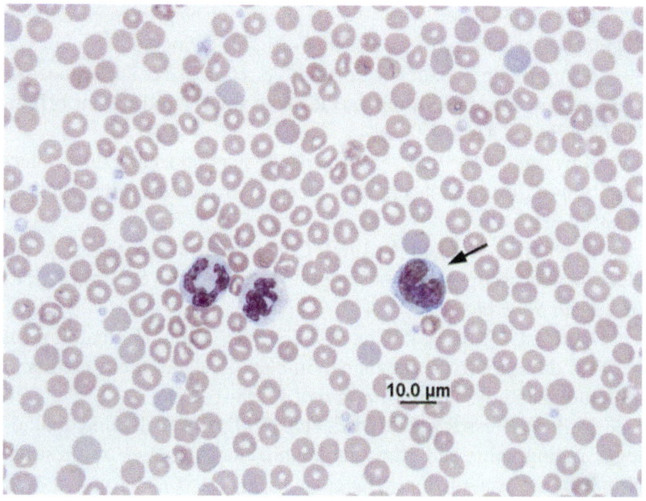

Fig. 3.54. Neutrophils and monocyte (arrow) in the blood film of an African hedgehog, Wright–Giemsa stain.

such as hypereosinophilic syndrome, a chronic idiopathic condition in which high numbers of mature eosinophils are seen in the peripheral blood and infiltrating various organs. In hypereosinophilic syndrome, most of the eosinophils are mature, and no atypical cells are seen, whereas in eosinophilic leukemia, immature cells can be present in increased numbers in circulation and in tissues, and they predominate in the bone marrow. Although eosinophils are easily recognized in cytologic and hematologic specimens, staining blood films with Luna stain (originally developed to detect the cytoplasmic granules within eosinophils in histologic sections) can also be used to detect eosinophils in hedgehogs (Martínez-Jiménez et al., 2017).

References

Alemán CL, Más RM, Rodeiro I, et al. 1998. Reference database of the main physiological parameters in Sprague-Dawley rats from 6 to 32 month. *Lab Anim* 32:457–466.

Ameri M, Schnaars HA, Sibley JR, et al. 2011. Stability of hematologic analytes in monkey, rabbit, rat, and mouse blood stored at 41C in EDTA using the ADVIA 120 hematology analyzer. *Vet Clin Pathol* 40(2):188–194.

Appleberg R. 2006. Neutrophils and intracellular pathogens: beyond phagocytosis and killing. *Trends Microbiol* 15:87–92.

Asanuma F, Miyata H, Iwaki Y, et al. 2011. Feature on erythropoiesis in dietary restricted rats. *J Vet Med Sci* 73:89–96.

Baker DC. 2004. Diagnosis of disorders of hemostasis. In: Thrall MA, Baker DC, Campbell TW, et al. (eds), *Veterinary Hematology and Clinical Chemistry*. Philadelphia, PA: Lippincott Williams & Wilkins, pp. 179–196.

Baker DC. 2010. Diagnosis of disorders of hemostasis. In: Thrall MA, Weiser G, Allison RW, et al. (eds), *Veterinary Hematology and Clinical Chemistry*, 2nd edn. Ames, IA: Wiley-Blackwell, pp. 185–204.

Bartolotti A, Castelli D, Bonati M. 1989. Hematology and serum chemistry values of adult, pregnant and newborn New Zealand rabbits (*Oryctolagus cuniculus*). *Lab Anim Sci* 39:437–439.

Bau-Gaudreault L, Grimes C. 2019. Evaluation of erythrocyte morphology and prevalence of poikilocytes in peripheral blood of sick domestic ferrets (*Mustela putorius furo*). *J Exotic Pet Med* 31: 86–90.

Bean-Knudsen DE, Wagner JE. 1987. Effect of shipping stress on clinicopathologic indicators in F344/N rats. *Am J Vet Res* 48(2):306–308.

Bernard SL, Leather CW, Brobst DF, et al. 1983. Estrogen-induced bone marrow depression in ferrets. *Am J Vet Res* 44:657–661.

Besch-Williford CL. 1987. Biology and medicine of the ferret. *Vet Clin N Am Small Anim Pract* 17:1155–1183.

Bolliger AP, Everds NE, Zimmerman KL, et al. 2010. Hematology of laboratory animals. In: Weiss DJ, Wardrop KJ (eds), *Schalm's Veterinary Hematology*, 6th edn. Ames, IA: Wiley-Blackwell, pp. 852–887.

Boone LI, Barthel R, Helman RG, et al. 1995. Large granular lymphocytic leukemia in a ferret. *Vet Clin Pathol* 24(1):6–10.

Brown SA. 1997. Neoplasia. In: Hillyer E, Quesenberry K (eds), *Ferrets, Rabbits, and Rodents: Clinical Medicine and Surgery*. Philadelphia, PA: WB Saunders.

Campbell TW. 2012. Mammalian hematology: laboratory animals and miscellaneous species. In: Thrall MA, Weiser G, Allison RW, et al. (eds), *Veterinary Hematology and Clinical Chemistry*, 2nd edn. Ames, IA: Wiley-Blackwell, pp. 225–237.

Campbell TW, Ellis CK. 2007. *Avian and Exotic Animal Hematology and Cytology*, 3rd edn. Ames, IA: Blackwell Publishing Ltd.

Campbell TW, Grant KR. 2010. *Clinical Cases in Avian and Exotic Animal Hematology and Cytology*. Ames, IA: Wiley-Blackwell.

Car BD, Eng VM, Everds NE, et al. 2006. Clinical pathology of the rat. In: Suckow MA, Weisbroth SH, Franklin CL (eds), *The Laboratory Rat*, 2nd edn. Amsterdam: Elsevier, pp. 127–146.

Christopher MM, Hawkins MG, Burton AG. 2014. Poikilocytosis in rabbits: prevalence, type, and association with disease. *PLoS One* 9:e112455.

Criswell KA, Sulkanene AP, Hochbaum AF, et al. 2000. Effects of phenylhydrazine or phlebotomy on peripheral blood, bone marrow, and erythropoietin in Wistar rats. *J Appl Toxicol* 20:25–34.

Debout C, Quillec M, Izard J. 1999. New data on the cytolytic effects of natural killer cells (Kurloff cells) on a leukemic cell line (guinea pig 1.2C). *Leuk Res* 23:137–147.

Deveci D, Stone PC, Egginton S. 2001. Differential effect of cold acclimation on blood composition in rats and hamsters. *J Comp Physiol B* 171:135–143.

Drozdowicz CK, Bowman TA, Webb ML, et al. 1990. Effect of in-house transport on murine plasma corticosterone concentration and blood lymphocyte populations. *Am J Vet Res* 51(11): 1841–1846.

Erdman SE, Moore FM, Rose R, et al. 1992. Malignant lymphoma in ferrets: clinical and pathological findings in 19 cases. *J Comp Pathol* 106:37–47.

Eremin O. 1980. Antibody-dependent cellular cytotoxicity in the guinea pig: the role of the Kurloff cell. *Cell Immunol* 55:312–327.

Everds NE. 2006. Hematology of the laboratory mouse. In: Foster HL, Small JD, Fox JC (eds), *The Mouse in Biomedical Research*, 2nd edn., Vol. 3. Amsterdam: Elsevier, pp. 133–170.

Farris GM, Benjamin SA. 1993. Inhibition of myelopoiesis by conditioned medium from cultured canine thymic cells exposed to estrogen. *Am J Vet Res* 54:1366–1373.

Faurschou M, Borregaard N. 2003. Neutrophil granules and secretory vesicles in inflammation. *Microbes Infect* 5:1317–1327.

Finnie RW, Bostock DE, Walden NB. 1980. Lymphoblastic leukaemia in a rabbit: a case report. *Lab Anim* 14:49–51.

Fortman JD, Hewett TA, Bennet BT. 2002. *The Laboratory Nonhuman Primate*. Boca Raton, FL: CRC Press, pp. 16–22.

Fox JG. 1988. Normal clinical and biologic parameters. In: Fox JG (ed), *Biology and Diseases of the Ferret*. Philadelphia, PA: Lea & Febiger, pp. 159–173.

Fox JG, Marini R. 1998. Diseases of the endocrine system. In: Fox JG (ed), *Biology and Diseases of the Ferret*. Baltimore, MD: Williams & Wilkins, pp. 291–305.

Fredrickson TN, Harris AW. 2000. *Atlas of Mouse Hematopathology*. Amsterdam: Harwood Academic.

George JW, Duncan JR, Mahaffey EA. 1983. Comparison of pyrimidine 5′ nucleotidase activity in erythrocytes of sheep, dogs, cats, horses, calves and Mongolian gerbils. *Am J Vet Res* 44:1968–1970.

Harkness JE, Wagner JE. 1989. *The Biology and Medicine of Rabbits and Rodents*, 3rd edn. Philadelphia, PA: Lea & Febiger, p. 230.

Harkness JE, Wagner JE. 1995. *The Biology and Medicine of Rabbits and Rodents*, 4th edn. Baltimore, MD: Williams & Wilkins, p. 372.

Hasler AH. 2000. Polycythemia. In: Ettinger SJ, Felman EC (eds), *Textbook of Veterinary Internal Medicine*, 6th edn. St Louis, MO: Elsevier Saunders, pp. 216–218.

Hawkey CM. 1975. *Comparative Mammalian Haematology*. London: William Heinemann Medical Books Ltd.

Hawkey CM, Dennett TB, Peirce MA. 1989. *Color Atlas of Comparative Veterinary Hematology*. London: Wolfe Medical Publications Ltd.

Heatley JJ, Harris MC. 2009. Hamsters and gerbils. In: Mitchell MA, Tully TN (eds), *Manual of Exotic Pet Practice*. St. Louis, MO: Saunders Elsevier, pp. 406–432.

Herndon FJ, Kayes SG. 1992. Depletion of eosinophils by anti-IL-5 monoclonal antibody treatment of mice infected with *Trichinella spiralis* does not alter parasite burden or immunologic resistance to reinfection. *J Immunol* 149:3642–3647.

Higbie CT, Eshar D, Choudhary S, et al. 2016. Eosinophilic leukemia in a pet African hedgehog (*Atelerix albiventris*). *J Exotic Pet Med* 25: 65–71.

Hillyer EV, Quesenberry KE. 1997. *Ferrets, Rabbits, and Rodents: Clinical Medicine and Surgery*. Philadelphia, PA: WB Saunders, p. 432.

Hopkins J, McConnell I. 1984. Immunological aspects of lymphocyte recirulation. *Vet Immunol Immunopathol* 6:3–33.

Hubert MF, Laroque P, Gillet LP, et al. 2000. The effects of diet, ad libitum feeding, and moderate and severe dietary restriction on body weight, survival, clinical pathology parameters, and cause of death in control Sprague-Dawley rats. *Toxicol Sci* 58:195–207.

Jackson CW, Hutson NK, Stewart SA, et al. 1988. The Wistar Furth rat: an animal model of hereditary macrothrombocytopenia. *Blood* 71:1676–1686.

Jacobson HA. 1978. Hematologic comparisons of shot and live trapped cottontail rabbits. *J Wildlife Dis* 14:82–88.

Jain NC. 1986. *Schalm's Veterinary Hematology*, 4th edn. Philadelphia, PA: Lea & Febiger.

Jain NC. 1993. *Essentials of Veterinary Hematology*. Philadelphia, PA: Lea & Febiger.

Jain NC, Zinkl JG. 1981. Symposium on clinical hematology. *Vet Clin N Am Small Anim Pract* 187–438.

Johnson-Delaney CA. 1995. *Exotic Companion Medicine Handbook for Veterinarians*. Lake Worth, FL: Wingers.

Kampfmann I, Bauer N, Johannes S, et al. 2012. Differences in hematologic variables in rats of the same strain but different origin. *Vet Clin Pathol* 41(2):228–234.

Kawasaki TA. 1994. Normal parameters and laboratory interpretation of disease states in the domestic ferret. *Semin Avian Exotic Pet Med* 3:40–47.

Kelenyi G, Nemeth A. 1969. Comparative histochemistry and electron microscopy of the eosinophil leucocytes of vertebrates. *Acta Biol Acad Sci Hung* 20:405–417.

Kim J-C, Yun H-I, Cha S-W, et al. 2002. Haematological changes during normal pregnancy in New Zealand white rabbits: a longitudinal study. *Comp Clin Pathol* 11:98–106.

Kull PA, Hess RS, Craig LE, et al. 2001. Clinical, clinicopathologic, radiographic and ultrasonographic characteristics of intestinal lymphangiectasia in dogs: 17 cases (1996–1998). *J Am Vet Med Assoc* 219:197–202.

Latimer KS. 1995. Leukocytes in health and disease. In: Ettinger SJ, Feldman EC (eds), *Textbook of Veterinary Internal Medicine. Diseases of the Dog and Cat*, 4th edn. Philadelphia, PA: WB Saunders, pp. 1892–1946.

Lee EJ, Moore WE, Fryer HC, et al. 1982. Haematological and serum chemistry profiles of ferrets (*Mustela putorius furo*). *Lab Anim* 16:133–137.

Leonard R, Ruben Z. 1986. Hematology reference values for peripheral blood of laboratory rats. *Lab Anim Sci* 36:277.

Levin S, Semler D, Ruben Z. 1993. Effects of two weeks of feed restriction on some common toxicologic parameters in Sprague-Dawley rats. *J Toxicol Pathol* 21:1–14.

Liberati TA, Sansone SR, Feuston MH. 2004. Hematology and clinical chemistry values in pregnant Wistar Hannover rats compared with nonmated controls. *Vet Clin Pathol* 33(2):68–73.

Linde A, Ross CR, Davis EG, et al. 2008. Innate immunity and host defense peptides in veterinary medicine. *J Vet Intern Med* 22:247–265.

Marco I, Cuenca R, Pastor J, et al. 2003. Hematology and serum chemistry values of the European Brown hare. *Vet Clin Pathol* 32(4):195–198.

Marini RP, Jackson LR, Esteves MI, et al. 1994. Effect of isoflurane on hematologic variables in ferrets. *Am J Vet Res* 55:1479–1483.

Marini RP, Otto G, Erdman S. 2002. Biology and diseases of the ferret. In: Fox JG, Anderson L, Lowe F (eds), *Laboratory Animal Medicine*. London: Academic Press, pp. 483–517.

Marshall KL. 2008. Clinical hematology of rodent species. *Vet Clin N Am Exotic Anim Pract* 11:523–533.

Martínez-Jiménez D, Garner B, Coutermarsh-Ott S, et al. 2017. Eosinophilic leukemia in three African pygmy hedgehogs (*Atelerix albiventris*) and validation of Luna stain. *J Vet Diagn Invest.* 29(2): 217–223.

Mays A Jr. 1969. Baseline hematological and blood biochemical parameters of the Mongolian gerbil (*Meriones unguiculatus*). *Lab Anim Care* 19:838–842.

McLaughlin RM, Fish RE. 1994. Clinical biochemistry and hematology. In: Manning PJ, Ringler DH, Newcomer CE (eds), *The Biology of the Laboratory Rabbit*. San Diego, CA: Academic Press, p. 483.

Melillo A. 2007. Rabbit clinical pathology. *J Exotic Pet Med* 16:135–145.

Mitruka BM, Rawnsley HM. 1981. *Clinical Biochemical and Hematological Reference Values in Normal Experimental Animals and Normal Humans*, 2nd edn. New York: Masson, p. 413.

Miyata H, Asanuma F, Iwaki Y, et al. 2009. Evaluation of myelotoxicity in dietary restricted rats. *J Toxicol Pathol* 22:53–63.

Moore DM. 2000a. Hematology of the rat (*Rattus norvegicus*). In: Feldman BF, Zinkl JG, Jain NC (eds), *Schalm's Veterinary Hematology*, 5th edn. Philadelphia, PA: Lippincott Williams & Wilkins, pp. 1210–1218.

Moore DM. 2000b. Hematology of the mouse (*Mus musculus*). In: Feldman BF, Zinkl JG, Jain NC (eds), *Schalm's Veterinary Hematology*, 5th edn. Philadelphia, PA: Lippincott Williams & Wilkins, pp. 1219–1224.

Moore DM. 2000c. Hematology of the Mongolian gerbil (*Meriones unguiculatus*). In: Feldman BF, Zinkl JG, Jain NC (eds), *Schalm's Veterinary Hematology*, 5th edn. Philadelphia, PA: Lippincott Williams & Wilkins, pp. 1111–1114.

Moore DM. 2000d. Hematology of the Syrian (Golden) hamster (*Mesocricetus auratus*). In: Feldman BF, Zinkl JG, Jain NC (eds), *Schalm's Veterinary Hematology*, 5th edn. Philadelphia, PA: Lippincott Williams & Wilkins, pp. 1115–1119.

Moore DM. 2000e. Hematology of the guinea pig (*Cavia porcellus*). In: Feldman BF, Zinkl JG, Jain NC (eds), *Schalm's Veterinary Hematology*, 5th edn. Philadelphia, PA: Lippincott Williams & Wilkins, pp. 1107–1110.

Moore DM. 2000f. Hematology of rabbits. In: Feldman BF, Zinkl JG, Jain NC (eds), *Schalm's Veterinary Hematology*, 5th edn. Philadelphia, PA: Lippincott Williams & Wilkins, pp. 1100–1106.

Moore DM. 2000g. Hematology of the ferret (*Mustela putorius-furo*). In: Feldman BF, Zinkl JG, Jain NC (eds), *Schalm's Veterinary Hematology*, 5th edn. Philadelphia, PA: Lippincott Williams & Wilkins, pp. 1096–1099.

Moriyama T, Tsujioka S, Ohira T, et al. 2008. Effects of reduced food intake on toxicity study parameters in rats. *J Toxicol Sci* 33: 537–547.

Müller K, Fuchs W, Heblinski N, et al. 2009. Encephalitis in a rabbit caused by human herpesvirus-1. *Am Vet Med Assoc* 235:66–69.

Nabity MB, Ramaian SK. 2010. Neutrophil structure and biochemistry. In: Weiss DJ, Wardrop KJ (eds), *Schalm's Veterinary Hematology*, 6th edn. Ames, IA: Wiley-Blackwell, pp. 263–267.

Nahas K, Provost J-P. 2002. Blood sampling in the rat: current practices and limitations. *Comp Clin Pathol* 11:14–37.

Nakamura S, Yasuda M, Ozaki K, et al. 2020. Eosinophilic leukaemia and systemic *Mycobacterium marinum* infection in an African pygmy hedgehog (*Atelerix albiventris*). *J Comp Pathol* 181: 33–37.

Ogawa Y, Matsumoto K, Kamata E, et al. 1985. Effect of food restriction on peripheral blood and bone marrow cell count of Wistar rats. *Exp Anim* 34:407–416.

Parmley RT. 1988. Mammals. In: Rowley AF, Ratcliffe NA (eds), *Vertebrate Blood Cells*. Cambridge: Cambridge University Press, pp. 337–424.

Percy DH, Barthold SW. 2007. *Pathology of Laboratory Rodents and Rabbits*. Ames, IA: Blackwell, p. 325.

Pickering RG, Pickering CE. 1984. The effects of reduced dietary intake upon the body and organ weights, and some clinical chemistry and hematological variants of the young Wistar rat. *Toxicol Lett* 21:271–277.

Rausch PG, Moore TG. 1975. Granule enzymes of polymorphonuclear neutrophils: a phylogenic comparison. *Blood* 46:913–919.

Reagan WJ, Irizarry Rovira AR, DeNicola D. 2008. Normal white cell morphology. In: *Veterinary Hematology: Atlas of Common Domestic and Non-Domestic Species*. Ames, IA: Blackwell, pp. 29–35.

Reznik G. 1975. Comparative studies of blood from hibernating and nonhibernating European hamsters (*Cricetus cricetus* L). *Lab Anim Sci* 25:210–215.

Riggs SM. 2009. Guinea pigs. In: Mitchell MA, Tully TN (eds), *Manual of Exotic Pet Practice*. St. Louis, MO: Saunders Elsevier, pp. 456–473.

Riggs SM, Mitchell MA. 2009. Chinchillas. In: Mitchell MA, Tully TN (eds), *Manual of Exotic Pet Practice*. St. Louis, MO: Saunders Elsevier, pp. 474–492.

Ringer DH, Dabich L. 1979. Hematology and clinical biochemistry. In: Baker HJ, Lindsey JR, Weisbroth SH (eds), *The Laboratory Rat, Volume 1, Biology and Disease*. New York: Academic Press, pp. 105–121.

Robel GL, Lochmiller RL, McMurry ST, et al. 1996. Environmental, age, and sex effects on coton rat (*Sigmodon hispidus*) hematology. *J Wildlife Dis* 32:390–394.

Rovira ARI, Kreklau E. 2012. What is your diagnosis? CBC and cytogram data from a Sprague-Dawley rat. *Vet Clin Pathol* 41(1):164–165.

Russell KE. 2010. Platelet kinetics and laboratory evaluation of thrombocytopenia. In: Weiss DJ, Wardrop KJ (eds), *Schalm's Veterinary Hematology*, 6th edn. Ames, IA: Wiley-Blackwell, pp. 576–585.

Schultze AE. 2010. Interpretation of canine leukocyte responses. In: Weiss DJ, Wardrop KJ (eds), *Schalm's Veterinary Hematology*, 6th edn. Ames, IA: Wiley-Blackwell, pp. 321–334.

Schwartz E, Tornaben JA, Boxill GC. 1973. The effect of food restriction on hematology, clinical chemistry and pathology in the albino rat. *Toxicol Appl Pharmacol* 25:515–524.

Siperstein LJ. 2008. Ferret hematology and related disorders. *Vet Clin N Am Exotic Anim Pract* 11:535–550.

Smith SA, Zimmerman KL, Moore DM. 2010. Hematology of the Syrian (Golden) hamster. In: Weiss DJ, Wardrop KJ (eds), *Schalm's Veterinary Hematology*, 6th edn. Ames, IA: Wiley-Blackwell, pp. 904–909.

Stieve-Caldwell EL, Morandi F, Souza M, et al. 2009. Vet med today: what is your diagnosis? *J Am Vet Med Assoc* 235(6):665–666.

Suber RL, Kodell RL. 1985. The effect of three phlebotomy techniques on hematological and clinical chemical evaluation in Sprague-Dawley rats. *Vet Clin Pathol* 14:23–30.

Thornton PC. 1979. The ferret *Mustela putorius furo*, as a new species in toxicology. *Lab Anim* 13:119–124.

Thrall MA. 2012a. Classification of and diagnostic approach to anemia. In: Thrall MA, Weiser G, Allison RW, et al. (eds), *Veterinary Hematology and Clinical Chemistry*, 2nd edn. Ames, IA: Wiley-Blackwell, pp. 75–86.

Thrall MA. 2012b. Regenerative anemia. In: Thrall MA, Weiser G, Allison RW, et al. (eds), *Veterinary Hematology and Clinical Chemistry*, 2nd edn. Ames, IA: Wiley-Blackwell, pp. 87–113.

Thrall MA. 2012c. Classification of and diagnostic approach to polycythemia. In: Thrall MA, Weiser G, Allison RW, et al. (eds), *Veterinary Hematology and Clinical Chemistry*, 2nd edn. Ames, IA: Wiley-Blackwell, pp. 114–122.

Thrall MA. 2012d. Erythrocyte morphology. In: Thrall MA, Weiser G, Allison RW, et al. (eds), *Veterinary Hematology and Clinical Chemistry*, 2nd edn. Ames, IA: Wiley-Blackwell, pp. 61–74.

Toth LA, January B. 1990. Physiological stabilization of rabbits after shipping. *Lab Animal Sci* 40: 384–387.

Toth LA, Olson GA, Wilson E, et al. 1990. Lymphocytic leukemia and lymphosarcoma in a rabbit. *J Am Vet Med Assoc* 197(5):627–629.

Turton JA, Hawkey CM, Hart MG, et al. 1989. Age-related changes in the hematology of female F344 rats. *Lab Anim* 23:295–301.

Vacha J. 1983. Red cell life-span. In: Agar NS, Board PG (eds), *Red Blood Cells of Domestic Mammals*. Amsterdam: Elsevier, p. 420.

Vennen KM, Mitchell MA. 2009. Rabbits. In: Mitchell MA, Tully TN (eds), *Manual of Exotic Pet Practice*. St. Louis, MO: Saunders Elsevier, pp. 375–405.

Wagner JE, Farrar PL. 1987. Husbandry and medicine of small rodents. *Vet Clin N Am Small Anim Pract* 17:1061–1087.

Watson ADJ. 2000. Erythrocytosis and polycythemia. In: Feldman BF, Zinkl JG, Jain NC (eds), *Schalm's Veterinary Hematology*, 5th edn. Philadelphia, PA: Lippincott Williams & Wilkins, pp. 216–221.

Weeks AM, Glomski CA. 1978. Cytology of the bone marrow in the Mongolian gerbil. *Lab Anim* 12:195–202.

Weiser G. 2012a. Introduction to leukocytes and the leukogram. In: Thrall MA, Weiser G, Allison RW, et al. (eds), *Veterinary Hematology and Clinical Chemistry*, 2nd edn. Ames, IA: Wiley-Blackwell, pp. 118–122.

Weiser G. 2012b. Interpretation of leukocyte responses in disease. In: Thrall MA, Weiser G, Allison RW, et al. (eds), *Veterinary Hematology and Clinical Chemistry*, 2nd edn. Ames, IA: Wiley-Blackwell, pp. 127–139.

Weiser G, Thrall MA. 2004. Introduction to leukocytes and the leukogram. In: Thrall MA, Baker DC, Campbell TW, et al. (eds), *Veterinary Hematology and Clinical Chemistry*. Philadelphia, PA: Lippincott Williams & Wilkins, pp. 125–130.

Weiss DJ. 2010. Iron and copper deficiencies and disorders of iron metabolism. In: Weiss DJ, Wardrop KJ (eds), *Schalm's Veterinary Hematology*, 6th edn. Ames, IA: Wiley-Blackwell, pp. 167–171.

Wolf TM. 2009. Ferrets. In: Mitchell MA, Tully TN (eds), *Manual of Exotic Pet Practice*. St. Louis, MO: Sanders Elsevier, pp. 345–374.

Wright JR, Yates AJ, Shah NT, et al. 1983. Hematological characteristics of the BB Wistar rat. *Vet Clin Pathol* 12:9–13.

Xu DL, Hu XK. 2020. Season and sex have different effects on hematology and cytokines in striped hamsters (*Cricetulus barabensis*). *J Comp Physiol B* 190:87–100.

Yoshii A, Shiraishi Y, Ogawa S, et al. 2003. Effects of food restriction of hematology examination and urinalysis in CD(SD)IGS rats – a four-week restricted feeding examination with two-week recovery period in six weeks old rats. In: Maeda Y, Shibuya K (eds), *Biological Reference Data on CD(SD)IGS Rats*. Tokyo, Japan: CD(SD) IGS Study Group 2002/2003, pp. 73–84.

Young KM, Meadows RL. 2010. Eosinophils and their disorders. In: Weiss DJ, Wardrop KJ (eds), *Schalm's Veterinary Hematology*, 6th edn. Ames, IA: Wiley-Blackwell, pp. 281–289.

Yuschenkoff D, Graham J, Sharkey L, et al. 2021. Reference interval determination of venous blood gas, hematologic, and biochemical parameters in healthy sedated, neutered ferrets (*Mustela putorius furo*). *J Exotic Pet Med* 36: 25–27.

Zimmerman KL, Moore DM, Smith SA. 2010a. Hematology of laboratory rabbits (*Oryctolagus cuniculus*). In: Weiss DJ, Wardrop KJ (eds), *Schalm's Veterinary Hematology*, 6th edn. Ames, IA: Wiley-Blackwell, pp. 862–869.

Zimmerman KL, Moore DM, Smith SA. 2010b. Hematology of the guinea pig. In: Weiss DJ, Wardrop KJ (eds), *Schalm's Veterinary Hematology*, 6th edn. Ames, IA: Wiley-Blackwell, pp. 893–898.

Zimmerman KL, Moore DM, Smith SA. 2010c. Hematology of the Mongolian gerbil. In: Weiss DJ, Wardrop KJ (eds), *Schalm's Veterinary Hematology*, 6th edn. Ames, IA: Wiley-Blackwell, pp. 899–903.

4 Evaluation of Mammalian Bone Marrow

Mammalian Hematopoiesis

The production of cells found in peripheral blood, or hematopoiesis, occurs primarily in the bone marrow, which is referred to as medullary hematopoiesis. Blood cell production occurring outside the bone marrow, most notably in the spleen, liver, and lymph nodes, is called extramedullary hematopoiesis. Extramedullary hematopoiesis commonly occurs in several healthy mammals, such as rodents and ferrets.

Hematopoiesis begins with the pluripotent stem cell that produces the committed progenitor cells that differentiate into the different cell lines: erythrocytes, granulocytes, megakaryocytes, monocytes, and lymphocytes. Because the pluripotent stem cells resemble lymphocytes on films stained with routine Romanowsky stains, the bone marrow examination evaluates only differentiated cells, such as erythrocytic cell lines, granulocytic cell lines, and megakaryocytes.

Mammalian Erythropoiesis

Erythropoiesis, the production of erythrocytes, in small exotic mammals appears to be the same process as that in domestic mammals. Erythroid precursors tend to be round cells (the largest typically being 20–30 μm in diameter) that have round nuclei with coarsely granular chromatin, and blue cytoplasm (darker blue when compared to granulocytic precursors). As these cells mature, their nuclei decrease in size, nuclear chromatin condenses, and the cytoplasm becomes less blue and redder (due to hemoglobin production). Erythropoiesis ends with the production of mature erythrocytes, the biconcave discoid red blood cells that lack a nucleus with a red-orange cytoplasm found in peripheral blood and cytology specimens.

Erythroid precursors that are capable of dividing are the cells in the early stages of erythropoiesis. These include the rubriblasts, prorubricytes, and rubricytes. The rubriblast is a relatively large, round cell with a high N:C ratio (Figures 4.1a and 4.1b). The cytoplasm is scant and deeply basophilic (blue). The round nucleus is large and contains coarsely granular chromatin and prominent nucleoli.

The prorubricyte resembles the rubriblast and is of equal or slightly larger size. Major defining factors that distinguish prorubricytes from rubriblasts include the lack of nucleoli and the presence of perinuclear clear areas in the blue cytoplasm (Figures 4.2a and 4.2b).

The rubricyte is smaller than the rubriblast and prorubricyte. The round nucleus contains coarsely granular chromatin that is more condensed compared to its precursors (Figures 4.3a and 4.3b). The small amount of cytoplasm stains blue to reddish blue (the blue-pink of a polychromatic cytoplasm).

Maturing erythrocyte precursors that are incapable of dividing include the metarubricytes and polychromatic erythrocytes. Metarubricytes are smaller than rubricytes (Figures 4.3b, 4.4a, and 4.4b). They have a very small, dark, dense (highly condensed and pyknotic), round to slightly oval nucleus and a cytoplasm that is moderately blue to reddish blue (polychromatophilic).

Polychromatophilic erythrocytes are anucleated cells that contain a blue-pink cytoplasm (Figures 3.1b and 3.1c). These cells may be slightly larger than mature erythrocytes and may contain nuclear remnants (Howell–Jolly bodies). When stained with supravital stains (new methylene blue or brilliant cresyl blue), polychromatic erythrocytes are called reticulocytes and demonstrate blue-staining reticulum, which is caused by clumping of their organelles and mRNA (Figure 3.2).

Exotic Animal Hematology and Cytology, Fifth Edition. Terry W. Campbell and Krystan R. Grant.

Companion website: www.wiley.com/go/campbell/exotic

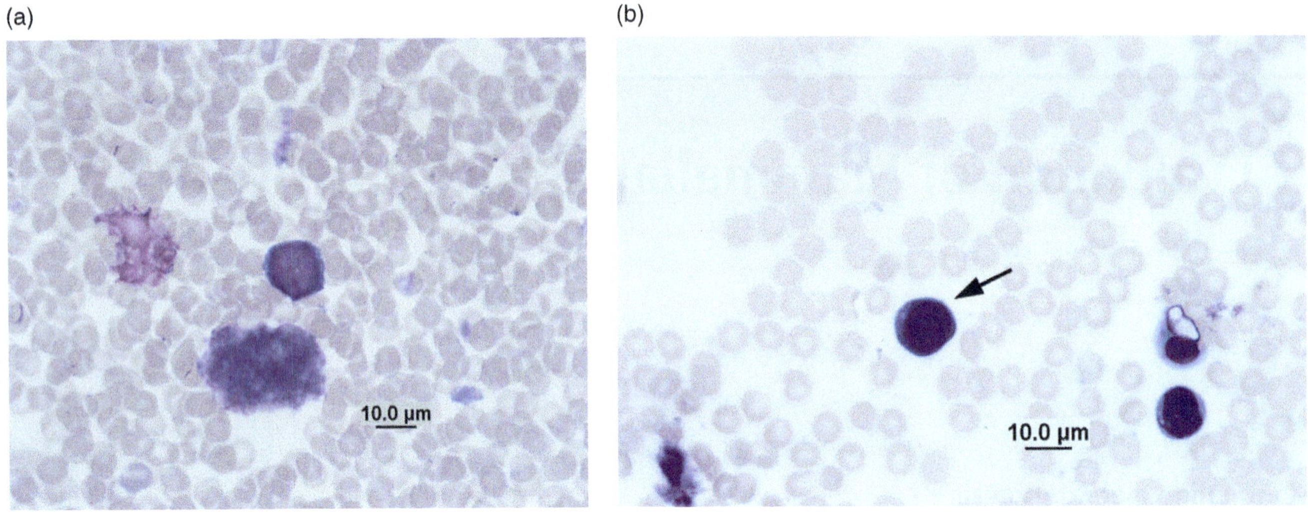

Fig. 4.1. (a) Rubriblast in the bone marrow of a guinea pig (*Cavia porcellus*), Wright–Giemsa stain. (b) Rubriblast (arrow) in the bone marrow of a domestic rat (*Rattus norvegicus*), Wright–Giemsa stain.

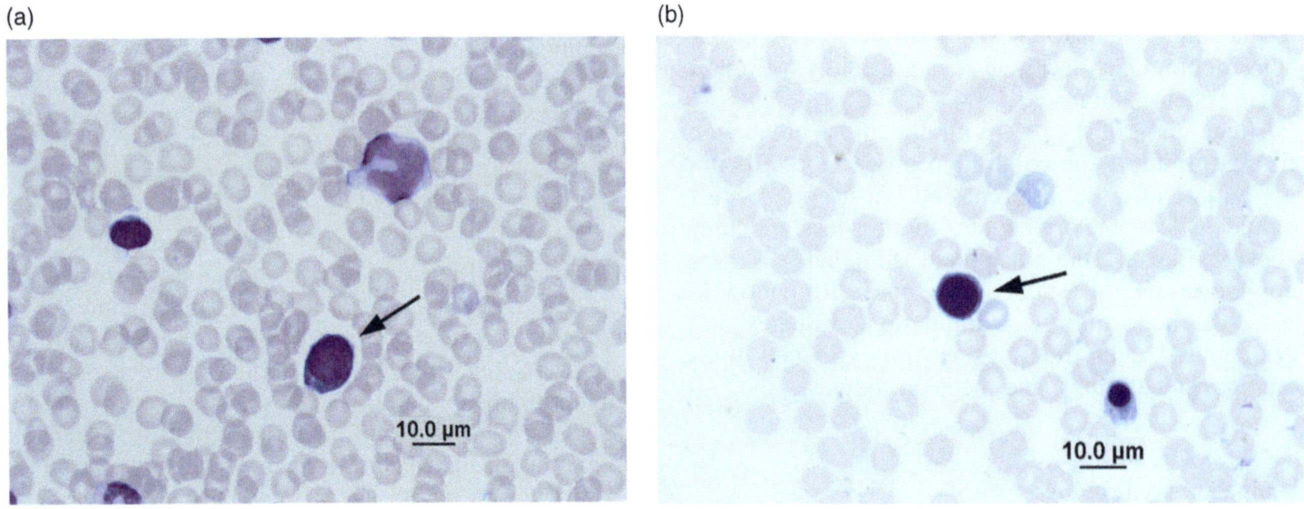

Fig. 4.2. (a) Prorubricyte (arrow) in the bone marrow of a guinea pig (*Cavia porcellus*), Wright–Giemsa stain. (b) Prorubricyte (arrow) in the bone marrow of a domestic rat (*Rattus norvegicus*), Wright–Giemsa stain.

Mammalian Granulopoiesis

Subpopulations of the granulocytic stem cells will then differentiate into the neutrophils (heterophils), eosinophils, and basophils found in the peripheral blood. Granulocytic cells are identified as round cells with abundant lavender-colored cytoplasm (less blue than erythrocytic precursors) and irregularly shaped and sometimes eccentric nuclei that contain fine to stippled chromatin. Granulocytes follow a characteristic maturation sequence that begins with the myeloblast, and continues through the promyelocyte, myelocyte, metamyelocyte, and band cell. Myeloblasts, promyelocytes, and myelocytes are capable of cell division and have a high ribosome content that gives the cytoplasm of these cells a blue tint with Romanowsky stains. Metamyelocyte and band cells are not capable of division and make up the final maturation stages. They are smaller than their precursors and their cytoplasm is less blue.

Myeloblasts are large cells with high N:C ratios that resemble the blast cells of other cell lines (Figures 4.5a and 4.5b). These cells have round to oval nuclei with finely stippled or smooth nuclear chromatin, an irregular nuclear margin, one or more nucleoli, and a scant amount of moderately blue cytoplasm with a ground-glass appearance. The cytoplasm of myeloblasts may contain rare small vacuoles. Myeloblasts may be broken down into two cell groups. Type I myeloblasts contain a centrally positioned nucleus and have no cytoplasmic

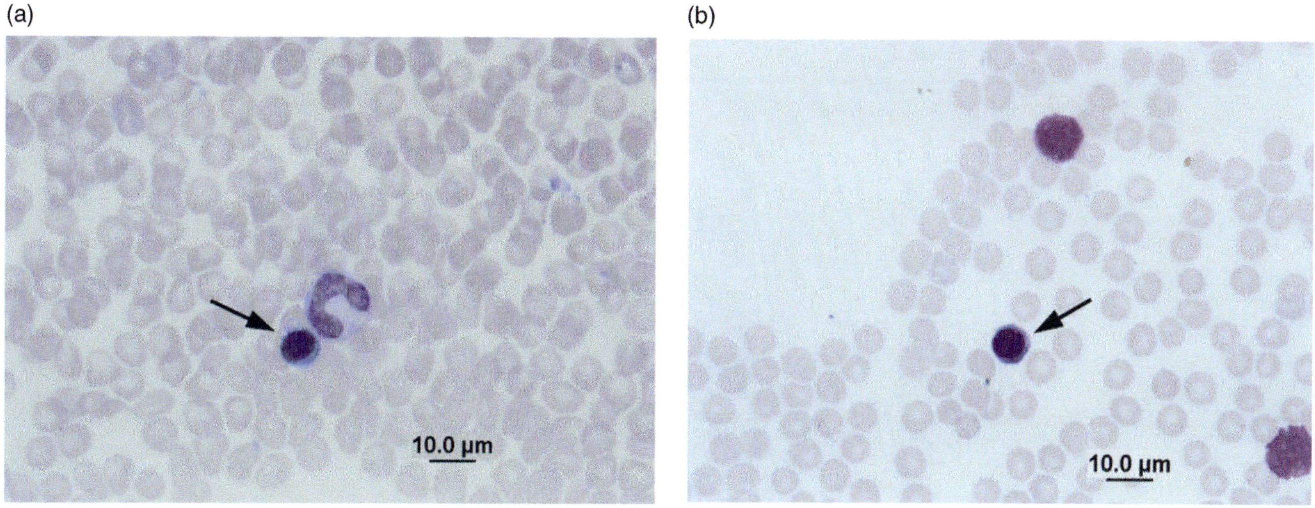

Fig. 4.3. (a) Rubricyte (arrow) and band cell in the bone marrow of a guinea pig (*Cavia porcellus*), Wright–Giemsa stain. (b) Rubricyte (arrow) in the bone marrow of a domestic rat (*Rattus norvegicus*), Wright–Giemsa stain.

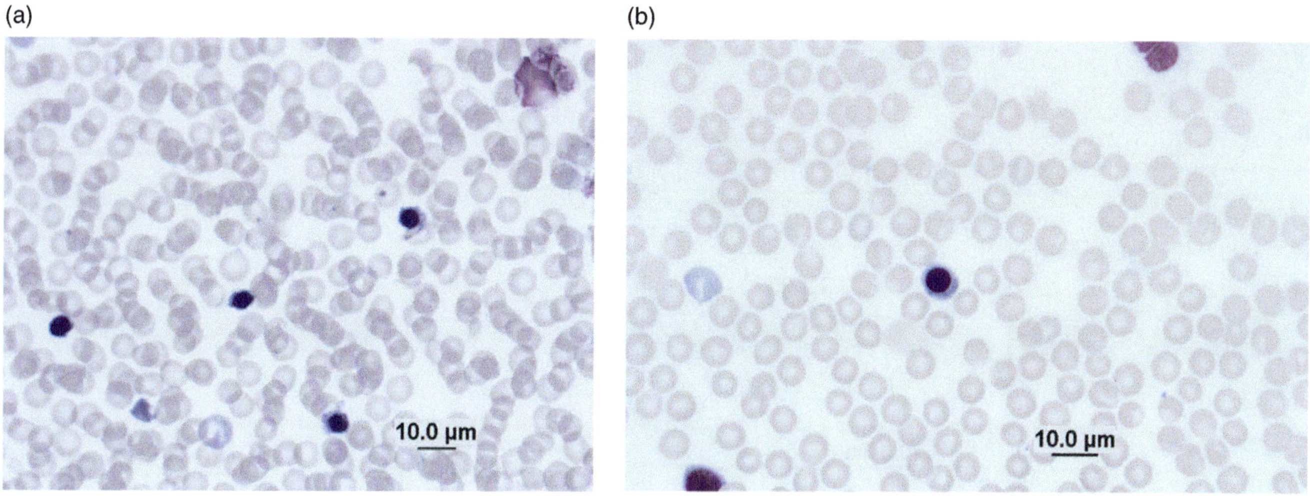

Fig. 4.4. (a) Metarubricytes in the bone marrow of a guinea pig (*Cavia porcellus*), Wright–Giemsa stain. (b) Metarubricyte in the bone marrow of a domestic rat (*Rattus norvegicus*), Wright–Giemsa stain.

azurophilic granules. Type II myeloblasts may have an eccentric nucleus and cytoplasm that contains small azurophilic granules (primary granules).

Promyelocytes (progranulocytes) develop from myeloblasts and appear as large cells with a central or eccentric nucleus containing smooth to slightly stippled chromatin that lacks nucleoli. Promyelocytes are recognized by the presence of many distinct, small pink to purple cytoplasmic granules (primary granules or azurophilic granules) (Figures 4.6a and 4.6b). A clear Golgi zone may also be present.

The myelocyte makes up the third stage of development. This cell is smaller than the promyelocyte and contains a round to oval (occasionally slightly indented) nucleus with fine to moderately granular chromatin (Figure 4.7). The cytoplasm stains light blue and contains no primary granules because the primary granules have been replaced by the larger secondary granules characteristic of the type of granulocyte that the cell represents. For example, eosinophil myelocytes have prominent pink granules, and basophil myelocytes have azurophilic to dark purple granules (Figures 4.8a and 4.8b). The cytoplasmic granules of neutrophil myelocytes are difficult to see (Figure 4.7).

The next stage of development is the metamyelocyte stage. It is at this stage that the nucleus begins to significantly change shape by becoming indented and taking on the classic kidney bean appearance and contains nuclear chromatin that has become more condensed and clumped. Metamyelocytes also contain cytoplasm that is no longer basophilic in color and contains secondary granules (Figures 4.9a and 4.9b).

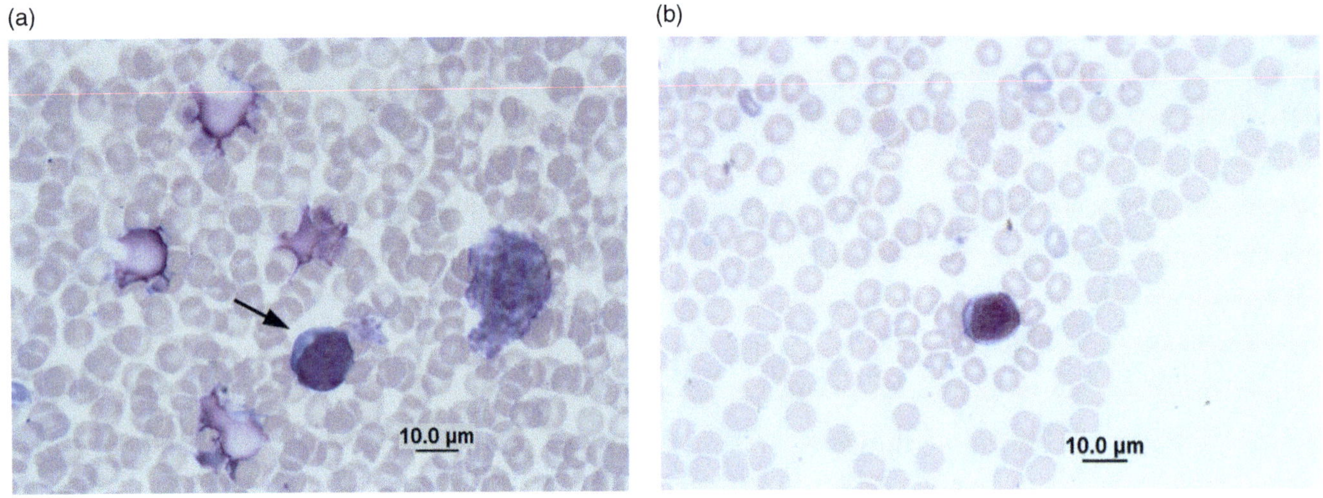

Fig. 4.5. (a) Myeloblast (arrow) in the bone marrow of a guinea pig (*Cavia porcellus*), Wright–Giemsa stain. (b) Myeloblast in the bone marrow of a domestic rat (*Rattus norvegicus*), Wright–Giemsa stain.

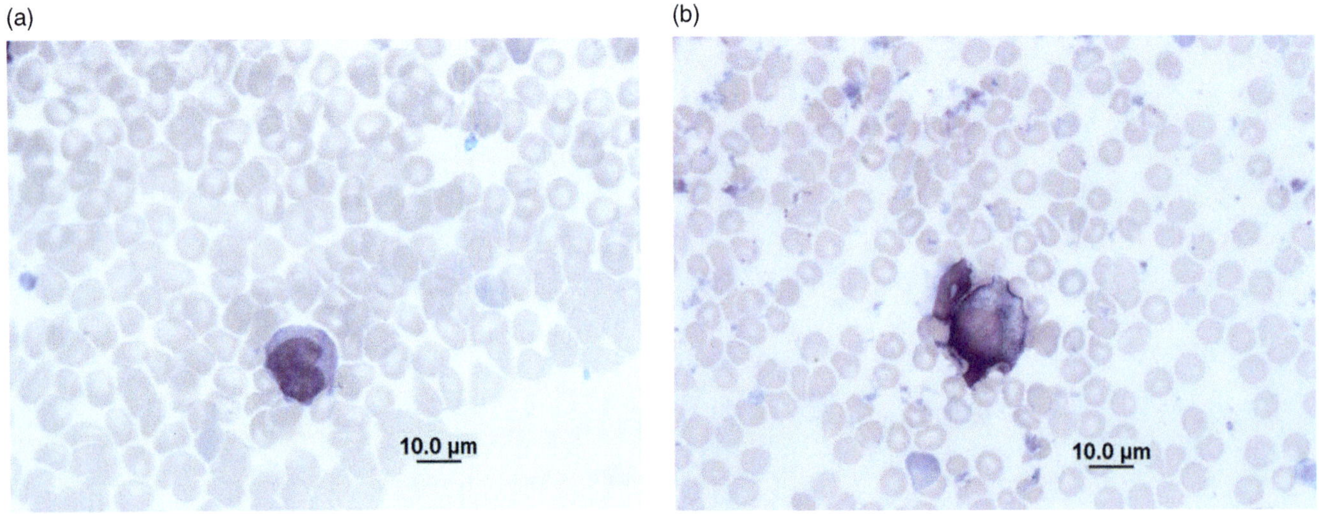

Fig. 4.6. (a) Promyelocyte in the bone marrow of a guinea pig (*Cavia porcellus*), Wright–Giemsa stain. (b) Promyelocyte in the bone marrow of a domestic rat (*Rattus norvegicus*), Wright–Giemsa stain.

The band cell is the penultimate stage of granulocyte development. The classic band cell nucleus has coarsely granular and clumped chromatin and a horseshoe shape; the nucleus is curved and elongated with parallel sides and no constrictions in the nuclear membrane (Figures 4.3a, 4.9a, and 4.10). The cytoplasm of band cells is characteristic of the cytoplasm of the definitive granulocyte.

The final stage of granulocyte maturation is the mature or segmented granulocyte. These are the cells found in the peripheral blood. The mature or segmented granulocyte has a lobulated or markedly constricted nucleus containing large, coarse chromatin clumps.

Granulocyte production in the normal bone marrow is predominated by the neutrophil lineage. Normal granulopoiesis reveals a progressive increase in the relative cell numbers with each stage of maturation. As a result, normal bone marrow reveals small numbers of proliferating cells, such as myeloblasts and progranulocytes; larger numbers of metamyelocytes; and numerous band cells and mature granulocytes. The bone marrow can be viewed as consisting of various compartments or pools depending upon the stage of development. These include the stem cell pool, the proliferative pool, and the maturation and storage pool. The proliferative pool consists of those cells capable of division, which would include the myeloblasts, progranulocytes, and myelocytes. The maturation and storage pool consists of cells that are incapable of division and would include the metamyelocytes, band cells, and mature granulocytes. The sizes of the maturation and storage pools vary with species in domestic mammals, and the same is likely true of small exotic mammals as well (Weiser, 2012).

When the maturation process of the neutrophil occurs at a faster rate than normal (i.e., because of inflammation), the cytoplasm is more basophilic and sometimes vacuolated. Such cells are identified as toxic neutrophils in the evaluation of Romanowsky-stained peripheral blood films (Figures 3.15a, 3.15b, and 3.15c).

Mammalian Platelet Production

The platelets found in the peripheral blood are derived from the cytoplasm of megakaryocytes, which reside within the bone marrow. The developmental stages of megakaryocytes that are present in mammalian bone marrow include the megakaryoblast, promegakaryocyte, and megakaryocyte. In general, megakaryoblasts and promegakaryocytes are much larger than the myeloblasts and rubriblasts.

The megakaryoblast is a very large cell that appears denser than other types of blast cells and contains a single large nucleus with a prominent nucleolus and deeply basophilic cytoplasm. These cells develop into the larger promegakaryocytes (typically 100–200 µm), cells with deep blue agranular cytoplasm and two to four nuclei connected by thin strands of nuclear material. Mature megakaryocytes arise from promegakaryocytes (Figures 4.11a–4.11c). They are very large cells containing abundant granular light blue cytoplasm that often stains light pink when compared to megakaryoblasts and promegakaryocytes. These cells contain numerous nuclei that form a multilobulated structure in the center of the cell. Cytoplasmic fragments from megakaryocytes become the platelets seen in peripheral blood. Platelets are small anucleated discoid cells with light pink cytoplasm often with purple granules (Figures 3.20a, 3.20b, and 3.21).

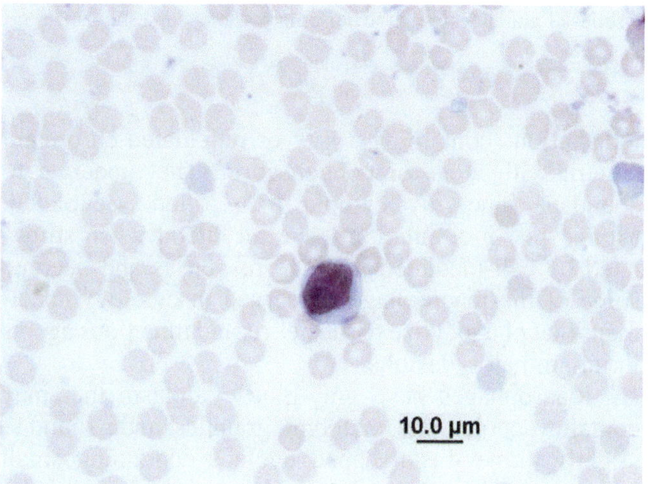

Fig. 4.7. Myelocyte in the neutrophil series of granulocytes in the bone marrow of a domestic rat (*Rattus norvegicus*), Wright–Giemsa stain.

Other Cells in the Mammalian Bone Marrow

Cells of the monocyte series comprise the monoblast, promonocyte, and mature monocyte. These cells are few in number and are often difficult to distinguish from other cells of the myeloid series. In general, these cells have irregular nuclear outlines, which aid in their differentiation from other myeloid cells.

Monoblasts are large cells that resemble myeloblasts, and contain round, irregular, or folded nuclei with fine reticular nuclear chromatin, and one or more prominent nucleoli. Monoblasts have a moderate amount of

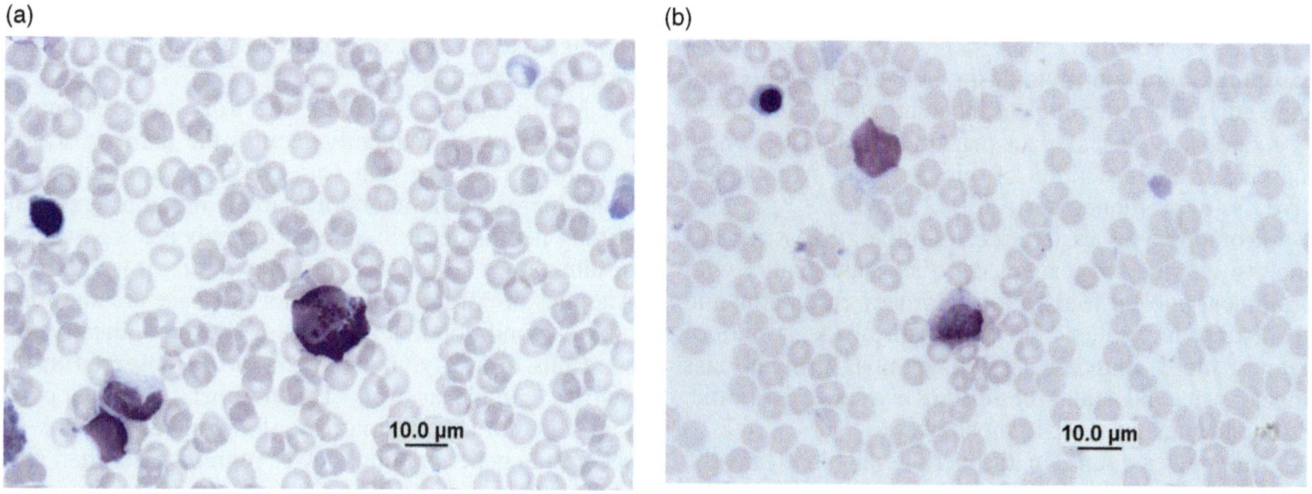

Fig. 4.8. (a) Myelocyte in the basophil series of granulocytes in the bone marrow of a guinea pig (*Cavia porcellus*), Wright–Giemsa stain. (b) Myelocyte in the eosinophil series of granulocytes in the bone marrow of a domestic rat (*Rattus norvegicus*), Wright–Giemsa stain.

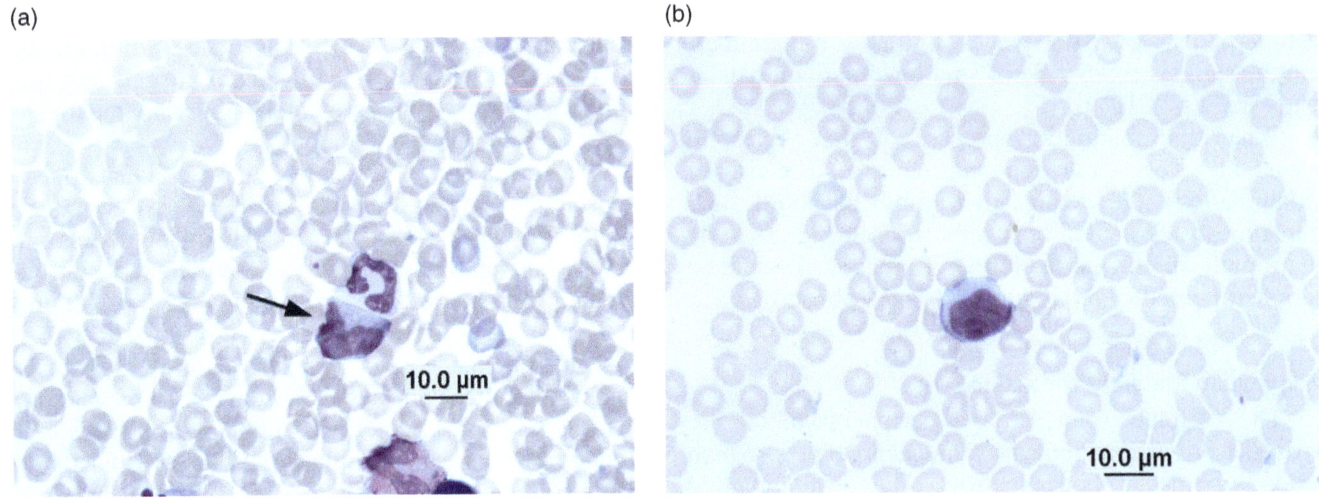

Fig. 4.9. (a) Metamyelocyte (arrow) in the neutrophil series of granulocytes and a band cell in the bone marrow of a guinea pig (*Cavia porcellus*), Wright–Giemsa stain. (b) Metamyelocyte in the neutrophil series of granulocytes in the bone marrow of a domestic rat (*Rattus norvegicus*), Wright–Giemsa stain.

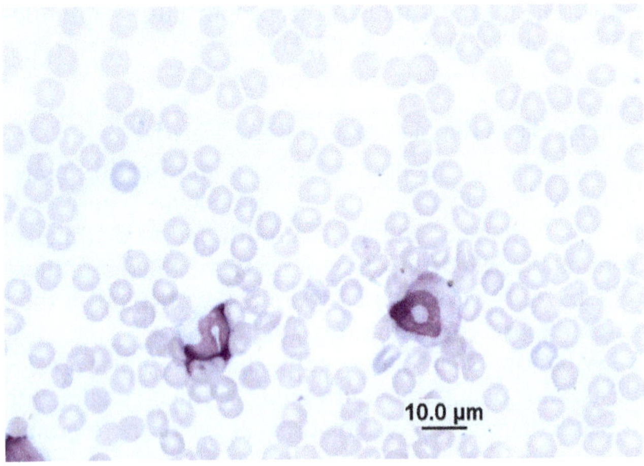

Fig. 4.10. A band eosinophil forming a ring-shaped nucleus in the bone marrow of a domestic rat (*Rattus norvegicus*), Wright–Giemsa stain.

basophilic agranular cytoplasm and may have a Golgi zone adjacent to the nuclear indentation. The N:C ratio of monoblasts is less than that of myeloblasts, which may aid in identification of this cell type. Monoblasts give rise to promonocytes.

Promonocytes are large cells similar in gross appearance to myelocytes, except that they have nuclei with prominent nuclear folds, stippled or lacy chromatin, and no distinct nucleolus. The cytoplasm of the promonocyte is more abundant, has a granular ground-glass appearance, and stains comparatively less basophilic. Promonocytes give rise to monocytes.

Monocytes found in the peripheral blood are the definitive cell of this cell line. Monocytes are generally the largest leukocytes found in peripheral blood. They have a variable-shaped nucleus that typically has multiple indentations containing a lacy or reticulated chromatin pattern with areas of condensation. The moderate to abundant blue-gray cytoplasm is often vacuolated. Monocytes in circulation leave the blood when stimulated by cell-mediated immune responses and become some of the macrophages observed in cytology specimens that phagocytize tissue debris and infectious agents in inflammatory lesions.

Macrophages have gray-blue cytoplasm that may contain vacuoles and small pink granules, and a round to slightly kidney-bean-shaped nucleus containing small inconspicuous nucleoli. Macrophages may occasionally contain phagocytized material as well. Macrophages generally represent less than 1% of the nucleated cell population of a normal bone marrow. Macrophages may increase in number (1% of the nucleated cells) with immune-mediated disorders or necrosis of the marrow. Increased numbers of macrophages exhibiting erythrophagocytosis indicate immune-mediated destruction of red blood cells.

Macrophages containing the iron storage pigment hemosiderin are frequently seen in the marrow of normal mammals, although some species variability does exist. Increased numbers of marrow macrophages containing hemosiderin in anemic animals is suggestive of inflammatory disease with increased iron storage. Anemias of chronic inflammatory disease are an example of a condition that this finding may be indicative of.

Cells of the lymphocyte series are observed in the marrow sample as well. The number of lymphocytes found in the normal marrow of mammals varies with species. In general, lymphocytes represent less than 20% of the nucleated cells; however, they appear in greater numbers in the bone marrow of rodents (Reagan et al., 2008).

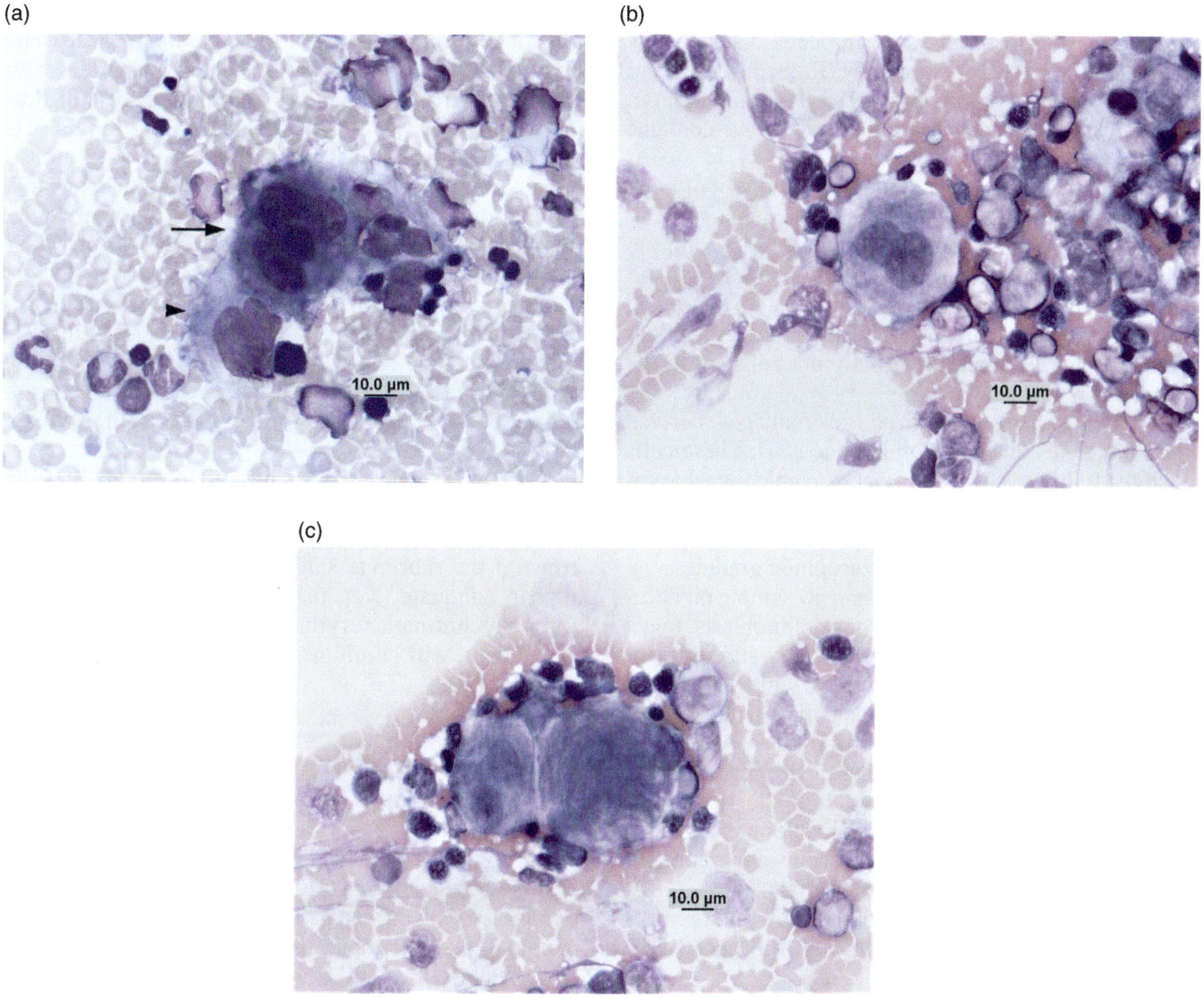

Fig. 4.11. (a) A promegakaryocyte (arrowhead) and a megakaryocyte (arrow) in the bone marrow of a guinea pig (*Cavia porcellus*), Wright–Giemsa stain. (b) A promegakaryocyte in a fine-needle aspiration biopsy of the spleen in a domestic ferret (*Mustela putorius furo*), Wright–Giemsa stain. (c) Megakaryocytes in a fine-needle aspiration biopsy of the spleen in a domestic ferret (*Mustela putorius furo*), Wright–Giemsa stain.

Lymphoblasts appear as small to large cells with a high N:C ratio. These cells contain a small to moderate amount of pale blue cytoplasm that contains no azurophilic granules. The nucleus is round to oval and contains fine stippled to slightly coarse nuclear chromatin and one or more nucleoli. The nuclear margins may be slightly indented or irregular. Lymphoblasts are often confused with myeloblasts and rubriblasts. These cells may be differentiated from rubriblasts by a comparison of the nucleus. The nucleus of the rubriblast is more rounded than that of the lymphoblast. Lymphoblasts may be distinguished from myeloblasts based on the appearance of the chromatin (which is slightly coarser), the smaller cytoplasmic volume, and the absence of azurophilic granules.

Small, mature lymphocytes may be noted in the marrow sample and appear as round cells that are smaller than neutrophils. The cytoplasm is scant and light blue in color, and the nucleus is typically round or slightly indented and contains diffuse chromatin and no nucleolus.

Plasma cells generally represent less than 2% of the nucleated cells in the bone marrow of normal mammals, are similar in size to neutrophils, and resemble rubricytes. Plasma cells may be differentiated from rubricytes based on the appearance of the cytoplasm and the nucleus. The cytoplasm of the plasma cell is light blue in color, is more abundant, and contains a clear Golgi zone adjacent to the eccentric nucleus. Variations of the plasma cell may be occasionally seen. Plasma cells distended by eosinophilic staining amorphous material are often referred to as "flame cells." Plasma cells distended by round, clear to light blue structures (Russell bodies) are often referred to as Mott cells (Figures 15.33 and 15.34). The nucleus of the plasma cell is round and contains dense, coarse chromatin and no nucleoli.

Osteoblasts are rarely found in the cytology of bone marrow aspirates. Osteoblasts resemble plasma cells, but are larger in size and contain an eccentric, round to oval nucleus that is pushed to the margins of the cell. Osteoblasts have an abundant basophilic cytoplasm and small, pink or azurophilic cytoplasmic granules. A clear Golgi area that is small and usually not adjacent to the nucleus is present as well.

Osteoclasts are specialized macrophages derived from monocytes that function in bone lysis. These cells are large, multinucleated cells that resemble megakaryocytes, except that their nuclei are individual and are not connected. Osteoclasts contain a basophilic cytoplasm that may contain a few pink to azurophilic granules.

Other cells seen in the bone marrow sample on occasion include mast cells and fibrocytes or fibroblasts. Intact mast cells are recognized on Romanowsky-stained cytologic specimens as discrete, round cells with pale, eccentric nuclei and inconspicuous nucleoli. The cytoplasm contains numerous small, distinct, purple or metachromatic cytoplasmic granules ranging in size from 0.2 to 5 μm in diameter. In some specimens, the nuclei of the cells may be obscured by the number of granules present in the cytoplasm. For example, the bone marrow of rats contains many mast cells and free mast cell granules from disrupted cells in the background (Bolliger, 2004). Fibrocytes are spindle-shaped cells with round to oval nuclei. The cytoplasm is lightly basophilic.

Mammalian Bone Marrow Responses in Disease

Hypoplasia and Hyperplasia

Complete examination of bone marrow should include determination of the myeloid:erythroid (M:E) ratio, with or without a 200- or 500-cell differential count. This is used to compare to the normal range of the M:E ratio of the species. For example, the normal M:E ratio in rat bone marrow varies from 1.07 to 1.93 (Bolliger, 2004).

The maturation index (proliferation index or the ratio of proliferating:non-proliferating cells) is also important. This has been calculated for rats and appears to be stable, and is useful for characterizing abnormalities of maturation and to verify subjective interpretations of ineffective hematopoiesis. The accuracy of these calculations can be ensured only when the same individual performs the bone marrow examinations on high-quality smears (Bolliger, 2004).

Hypoplasia of the bone marrow can result from infectious disease, estrogen toxicity, chemical toxicity, myelofibrosis, or immune-mediated disorders. For example, estrogen toxicity is a common cause of bone marrow hypoplasia in intact female (jill) ferrets. The lack of cells from all the cell lines is an indication of bone marrow aplasia. Most cases of bone marrow aplasia in domestic mammals are associated with either immune-mediated disease or immunosuppressive therapy (Thrall and Weiser, 2012, 2022).

Hyperplasia of the marrow sample can occur as a regenerative response to the peripheral loss of cells. The response may be either myeloid or erythroid depending on the type of cells lost. Hyperplasia can also result from neoplastic disorders, such as lymphoproliferative or myeloproliferative diseases.

Maturation arrest is identified by a cell line that stops development at a certain stage. For example, immune-mediated anemia may reveal a maturation arrest at the rubricyte stage, where rubricyte numbers appear adequate, yet there are few metarubricytes and polychromatic erythrocytes. A similar situation may occur with immune-mediated disease affecting granulocytes.

Mammalian Myeloid Neoplasms

Classification of myeloid neoplasms in veterinary medicine has undergone several changes since its early modeling in the 1990s. Guidelines developed by World Health Organization (WHO) standards direct veterinary terminology involving myeloid neoplasia for domestic mammals. For example, the WHO revisions have lowered the blast threshold from 30% to 20% for diagnosing acute myeloid leukemia (AML) and expanded and redefined AML categories. Currently, the AML alphanumeric designations, such as M1, M2, and so on, have been discontinued in favor of subdivision into four broad groups: (1) AML with recurrent genetic abnormalities, (2) AML with multilineage dysplasia, (3) AML with previous chemotherapy and/or radiation, and (4) AML, not otherwise specified (McManus, 2005; Arber et al., 2016). The new classification eliminates the category of myelodysplastic syndrome (MDS) – refractory anemia with excess blasts in transformation and replaces it with a new MDS category – refractory cytopenia with multilineage dysplasia (RCMD), where at least 10% of cells from each of two lineages must display atypia for a diagnosis of RCMD. That threshold is 50% for diagnosing AML with multilineage dysplasia. Chronic myelomonocytic leukemia has been removed from the MDS category and included in a new category of diseases that have features of both MDS and chronic leukemia (McManus, 2005). Classification of myeloid neoplasms in nondomestic mammals should follow the current guidelines whenever possible.

Bone Marrow Evaluation

Bone Marrow Evaluation of Rodents

The bone marrow evaluation of rodents is the same as that of domestic mammals, such as the dog and cat. The M:E ratio for these animals generally ranges between 0.6:1 and 3.6:1 based on the ranges reported for mice, rats, gerbils, and hamsters (Bolliger et al., 2010; Smith et al., 2010; Zimmerman et al., 2010). The erythropoiesis maturation process begins with the rubriblast followed by the prorubricyte, rubricyte (early, basophilic, and polychromatic), metarubricyte and the reticulocyte before reaching maturity. Erythrocyte basophilic stippling is commonly seen in bone marrow samples from gerbils, where 18.5–33.7% of the erythrocytes exhibit stippling (Zimmerman et al., 2010).

Myeloid precursors include the myeloblast, promyelocyte, myelocyte, metamyelocytes, and band granulocyte. The nucleus of these cells progresses from round to segmented with maturation. In mice, rats, and to a lesser extent, gerbils, the nucleus of the promyelocyte appears as a ring of nuclear chromatin. The center of this ring becomes progressively larger and the nucleus thinner with maturation. The ring form of the nucleus is often maintained in neutrophils and eosinophils, but not in basophils in peripheral blood. In general, erythrocyte precursors represent 20–40% and myeloid precursors represent 34–52% of the nucleated cells in rodent bone marrow smears (Bolliger, 2004). The number of lymphocytes observed in the bone marrow can vary. References indicate that lymphocytes represent 1.4–20.1% of the nucleated cells in gerbils and 7.3–21.1% of the nucleated cells in rat bone marrows (Bolliger, 2004; Zimmerman et al., 2010). Lymphocyte percentages likely will vary with age, with young animals having higher percentages (Saad et al., 2000). The variability in lymphocyte numbers may also be due to the inability to differentiate metarubricytes from lymphocytes.

Megakaryocytes are more numerous in the bone marrow smears of rodents when compared to domestic mammals (e.g., dogs and cats). Mast cells are also commonly found, especially in the rat (Bolliger et al., 2010).

Bone Marrow Evaluation of Rabbits

The bone marrow evaluation of rabbits is the same as that of other mammals, such as the dog and cat (McLaughlin and Fish, 1994). The erythropoiesis maturation process begins with the rubriblast followed by the prorubricyte, rubricyte (early, basophilic, and polychromatic), metarubricyte, and the reticulocyte before reaching maturity. Granulocyte development begins with the myeloblast followed by the promyelocyte, myelocyte, metamyelocytes, and band cell before becoming the mature granulocyte. The nucleus of these cells progresses from round to segmented with maturation. The normal M:E ratio for rabbits is 1:1 (Sanderson and Phillips, 1981).

Bone Marrow Evaluation of Ferrets

The bone marrow evaluation of ferrets is the same as that of other mammals. The erythropoiesis maturation process begins with the rubriblast followed by the prorubricyte, rubricyte (early, basophilic, and polychromatic), metarubricyte, and the reticulocyte before reaching maturity. Granulocyte development begins with the myeloblast followed by the promyelocyte, myelocyte, metamyelocytes, and band cell before becoming the mature granulocyte. The nucleus of these cells progresses from round to segmented with maturation. The normal M:E ratio for ferrets is 2.3–4.5:1 (Sherrill and Gorham, 1985). Hyperestrogenism in female ferrets undergoing prolonged periods of estrus results in depletion of erythroid and granulocytic precursors and megakaryocytes (Sherrill and Gorham, 1985).

References

Arber DA, Orazi A, Hasserjian R, et al. 2016. The 2016 revision of the World Health Organization classification of myeloid neoplasms and acute leukemia. *Blood* 127(20):2391–2405. https://doi.org/10.1182/blood-2016-03-643544

Bolliger AP. 2004. Cytologic evaluation of bone marrow in rats: indications, methods, and normal morphology. *Vet Clin Pathol* 33:58–67.

Bolliger AP, Everds NE, Zimmerman KL, et al. 2010. Hematology of laboratory animals. In: Weiss DJ, Wardrop KJ (eds), *Schalm's Veterinary Hematology*, 6th edn. Ames, IA: Wiley-Blackwell, pp. 852–887.

McLaughlin RM, Fish RE. 1994. Clinical biochemistry and hematology. In: Manning PJ, Ringler DH, Newcomer CE (eds), *The Biology of the Laboratory Rabbit*. New York: Academic Press, pp. 111–127.

McManus PM. 2005. Classification of myeloid neoplasms: a comparative review. *Vet Clin Pathol* 34:189–212.

Reagan WJ, Irizarry Rovira AR, DeNicola DB. 2008. *Veterinary Hematology: Atlas of Common Domestic and Non-Domestic Species*, 2nd edn. Ames, IA: Wiley-Blackwell.

Saad A, Palm M, Widell S, et al. 2000. Differential analysis of rat bone marrow by flow cytometry. *Comp Haematol Intl* 10:97–101.

Sanderson JH, Phillips CE. 1981. *An Atlas of Laboratory Animal Haematology*. Oxford: Oxford University Press, p. 473.

Sherrill A, Gorham J. 1985. Bone marrow hypoplasia associated with estrus in ferrets. *Lab Anim Sci* 35:280–286.

Smith SA, Zimmerman KL, Moore DM. 2010. Hematology of the Syrian (Golden) hamster. In: Weiss DJ, Wardrop KJ (eds), *Schalm's Veterinary Hematology*, 6th edn. Ames, IA: Wiley-Blackwell, pp. 904–909.

Thrall MA, Weiser G. 2012. Laboratory evaluation of bone marrow. In: Thrall MA, Weiser G, Allison RW, et al. (eds). *Veterinary Hematology and Clinical Chemistry*, 2nd edn. Philadelphia, PA: Lippincott Williams & Wilkins, pp. 150–165.

Thrall MA, Weiser G. 2022. Laboratory evaluation of bone marrow. In: Thrall MA, Weiser G, Allison RW, et al. (eds). *Veterinary Hematology and Clinical Chemistry*, 3rd edn. Philadelphia, PA: Lippincott Williams & Wilkins, in press.

Weiser G. 2012. Neutrophil production, trafficking, and kinetics. In: Thrall MA, Weiser G, Allison RW, et al. (eds). *Veterinary Hematology and Clinical Chemistry*, 2nd edn. Philadelphia, PA: Lippincott Williams & Wilkins, pp. 123–126.

Zimmerman KL, Moore DM, Smith SA. 2010. Hematology of the Mongolian gerbil. In: Weiss DJ, Wardrop KJ (eds), *Schalm's Veterinary Hematology*, 6th edn. Ames, IA: Wiley-Blackwell, pp. 899–903.

5 Mammalian Hematology and Clinical Chemistry: Clinical Case Presentations

Case 1: Chinchilla with Dental Disease

Signalment

7-year-old female chinchilla (*Chinchilla lanigera*)

History

The chinchilla had a history of moderate dental disease, which was managed with several teeth trims over the last one and a half years. Six months prior to presentation, the chinchilla presented with pain, anorexia, and drooling. At that time, mandibular molar roots were palpated; therefore, radiographs of the skull were taken. The radiographs at that time revealed right mandibular apical irregularity to the teeth, presumably representative of a tooth root abscess, and a triangular osseous body in the mandible, possibly representing a tooth fracture. A CT was recommended but declined. The chinchilla was managed with a dental trim, antibiotics, pain medications, and critical care feeding supplementation. The chinchilla returned for a dental trim.

Physical Examination

Upon physical examination, the chinchilla was slightly underconditioned and had lost approximately 20% of its body weight since the examination six months prior. The chinchilla was otherwise quiet, alert, and responsive therefore was prepared for the dental trim. She was anesthetized with gas induction but intubation was unsuccessful, and therefore the procedure was cancelled. The chinchilla was housed in the hospital overnight. The following day she was more lethargic than expected, had labored breathing, and harsh lower airway sounds were noted on auscultation (upper airway sounds were noted as normal). The labored breathing improved with oxygen supplementation. To differentiate between aspiration pneumonia, noncardiogenic pulmonary edema, or some other underlying lung pathology, whole body radiographs were taken. The radiographs revealed bronchial changes, specifically a pattern of peribronchial cuffs, distributed in all lung lobes consistent with bronchitis. Blood was collected for a CBC (Table 5.1) and evaluation of the blood film (Figures 5.1a–5.1d).

Table 5.1. Chinchilla hematology results (Case 1).

		Reference[a]
WBC $\times 10^3/\mu L$	6.2	2.1–17.6
Neutrophils $\times 10^3/\mu L$	5.0	—
%	81	4–58
Lymphocytes $\times 10^3/\mu L$	0.4	—
%	7	31–95
Monocytes $\times 10^3/\mu L$	0.7	—
%	11	0–14
Eosinophils $\times 10^3/\mu L$	0.1	—
%	1	0–3
Basophils $\times 10^3/\mu L$	0	—
%	0	0–1
Plasma protein g/dL	6.0	4.1–6.7 (biuret)
RBC $\times 10^6/\mu L$	7.1	5.8–9.2
Hb g/dL	12.2	10.5–15.2
PCV %	42.0	33–48
MCV fL	59.0	49–59
MCHC g/dL	29.0	29.3–36.0
RDW	13.0	—
Platelets $10^3/\mu L$	577	208–867
MPV fL	8.2	—

[a] Mans (2021).

Exotic Animal Hematology and Cytology, Fifth Edition. Terry W. Campbell and Krystan R. Grant.

Companion website: www.wiley.com/go/campbell/exotic

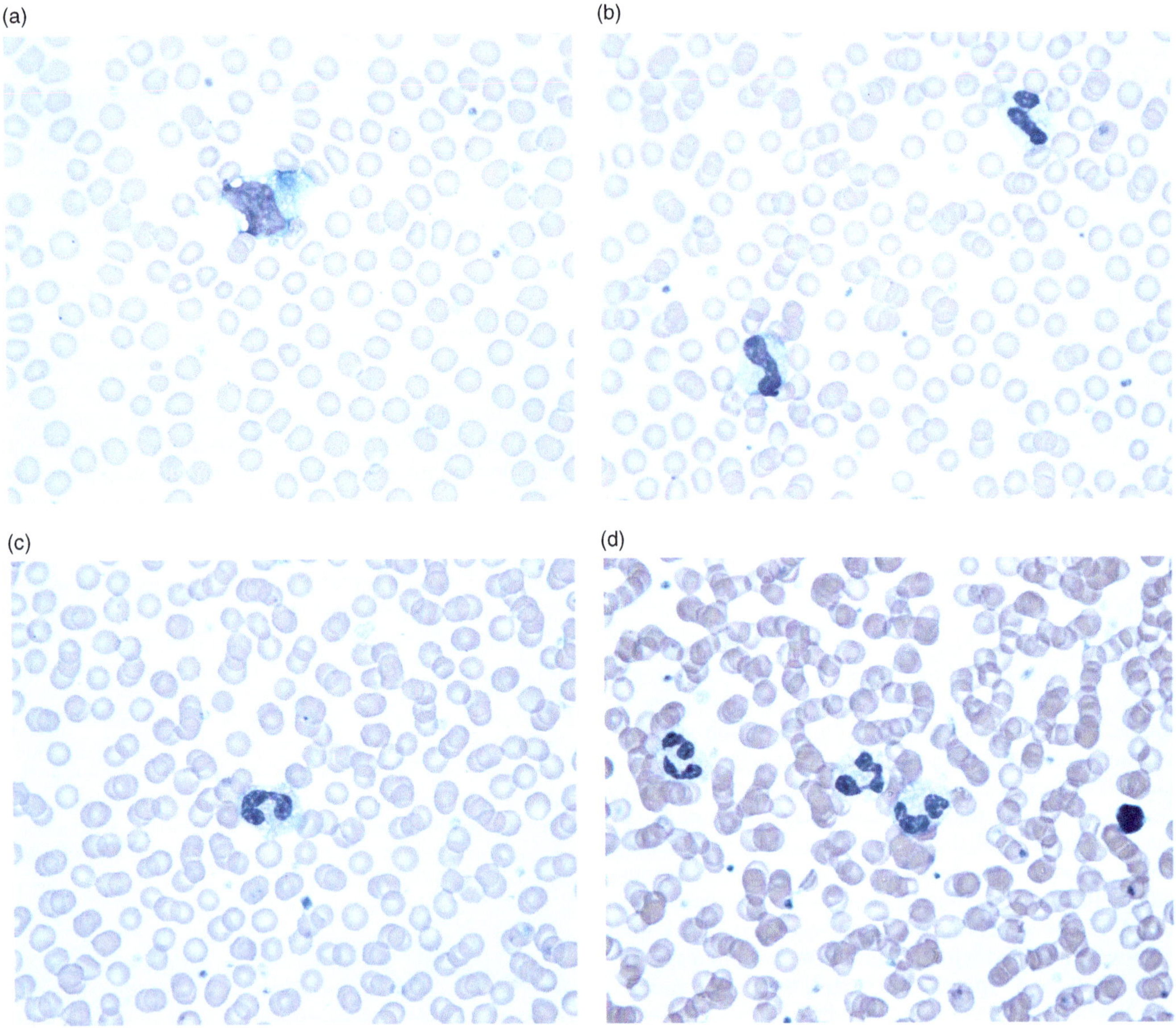

Fig. 5.1. (a), (b), (c), (d) Blood films (Wrights–Giemsa stain, 100× oil).

Interpretive Discussion

Although the CBC revealed a total leukocyte count within the normal reference interval, there were other indications of inflammation and disease. Chinchillas tend to be more lymphocytic, and this case demonstrated neutrophilia, lymphopenia, and monocytosis. The distribution of these cells, along with other features of morphology, such as band neutrophils and toxic neutrophils, indicated an inflammatory leukogram. Figure 5.1a revealed a reactive monocyte. Figure 5.1b revealed a toxic neutrophil and band neutrophil. Figure 5.1c revealed a toxic band neutrophil. Figure 5.1d revealed three toxic neutrophils and a lymphocyte. Marked toxic neutrophils were reported on the hematology form from the laboratory.

Summary

This case was a referral for review of the blood film, and therefore only portions of the record were available. In addition to the radiographs and CBC, a plasma biochemistry panel, ultrasound, and fine needle aspirates of the liver were performed. The plasma biochemistry panel revealed elevated liver enzymes. The ultrasound showed a diffusely homogenous and hyperechoic liver and multiple fluid-distended loops of bowel. These findings were most likely consistent with hepatic lipidosis, although other infiltrative disease could not be ruled out, and ileus. Cytology of the liver aspirates showed numerous hepatocytes (mostly ruptured) admixed with blood and lipid droplets, consistent with the suspicion of hepatic lipidosis reported from the ultrasound examination. The case was lost to follow-up, but it appeared as though the dental disease was worsening; the chinchilla was having difficulty eating and therefore losing weight and in a negative metabolic state. The severity of the disease precluded continued management with dental trims due to the progression and prolonged recovery from the anesthetic event. The degree and severity of the toxic changes and the increased number of band cells on the blood film are indicative of a poor prognosis. The additional steps of reviewing the blood film, evaluating the relative count of band cells, and quantifying the grade of toxicity of neutrophils have been helpful in assessing horses with inflammatory disease (Lambert et al., 2016).

Case 2: Guinea Pig with Gastric Stasis

Signalment

2.5-year-old intact female guinea pig (*Cavia porcellus*)

History

The guinea pig presented to the urgent care/emergency service for acute onset lethargy, inappetence, and bloat. Earlier the evening of presentation, the owner reported that the guinea pig was not interested in eating. She appeared lethargic and hid in the corner of the habitat in her plastic castle. When the owner picked up the guinea pig, her abdomen was wet and bloated. The guinea pig was last reported eating the morning of presentation and the owner also stated that the guinea pig appeared normal at that time. The guinea pig is housed in a five-and-a-half by two-foot enclosure with another female guinea pig indoors. The bedding used in the enclosure was triple filtered aspen shavings. The diet consisted of continuous timothy hay, ¼ cup Sunburst Fiesta guinea pig pellets twice daily, and ½–1 cup green bell peppers and other vegetables daily. The owner also added vitamin C drops to the water. There was another pet in the house, a cat, but there were no known interactions that day.

Physical Examination

Upon physical examination during the urgent care visit, the 1.2-kg guinea pig was described as depressed and lethargic. Other findings on exam included palpation of a firm, distended abdomen and a small, firm, freely moveable mass on the right submandibular region; borborygmic was present on abdominal auscultation; AFAST (brief ultrasound assessment) showed multiple gas-filled bowel loops that made evaluation of other organ systems difficult. Radiographs were recommended to rule out obstruction and volvulus, and the owner agreed. The guinea was placed under general anesthesia to perform diagnostics and supportive treatment. Radiographs were taken first to help guide the treatment plan (Figures 5.2a–5.2c). Blood was collected after the radiographs were taken and during the initiation of supportive treatment. Only enough blood was obtained for a CBC (Table 5.2; Figures 5.3a–5.3d).

Interpretive Discussion

Overall, the radiographs revealed a markedly gas-distended stomach and multiple gas-filled loops of intestine which were also subjectively dilated. The cecum was filled with a moderate amount of heterogeneous soft tissue opacity and gas. There were two small, oval, smoothly marginated mineral opacities superimposed over the soft tissues caudal and ventral to the pelvis. There was ill-defined mineral opacity in the caudoventral abdomen in the region of the urinary bladder. There were triangular mineral opacities cranial to the greater trochanters bilaterally. The intestines were superimposed over the kidneys on the lateral projections, but the left kidney was within normal limits on the ventrodorsal projection. The forelimbs were superimposed over the caudal thorax on the lateral projections, but the thorax was within normal limits on the ventrodorsal projection. There were triangular mineral opacities within the stifle joints. The remaining osseous and soft tissue structures were within normal limits. The conclusions of the findings were gastric dilatation with small intestinal segmental functional ileus, dystrophic mineralization within vulvar recess or less likely urethroliths, mineralized meniscus or synovial osteochondroma bilateral on the stifles, dystrophic mineralization of the soft tissues cranial to the coxofemoral joints bilaterally, and possible sand-like cystic calculi.

The hemogram results revealed a leukocytosis with a left-shift heterophilia and lymphopenia. The hematology results along with the morphology revealing moderate numbers of toxic heterophils indicated a severe inflammatory disease. Figures 5.3a–5.3c revealed examples of toxic band heterophils and toxic heterophils. A small amount of polychromasia is commonly observed in guinea pigs due to the short half-life of the erythrocytes. Figure 5.3d revealed two monocytes. Moderate toxic neutrophils were reported on the hematology form from the laboratory.

Summary

The guinea pig was hospitalized in the critical care unit and supportive care, and treatment included buprenorphine (0.3 mg/kg) gastric decompression, fluid therapy with LRS (60 mL SC), enrofloxacin (10 mg/kg SC),

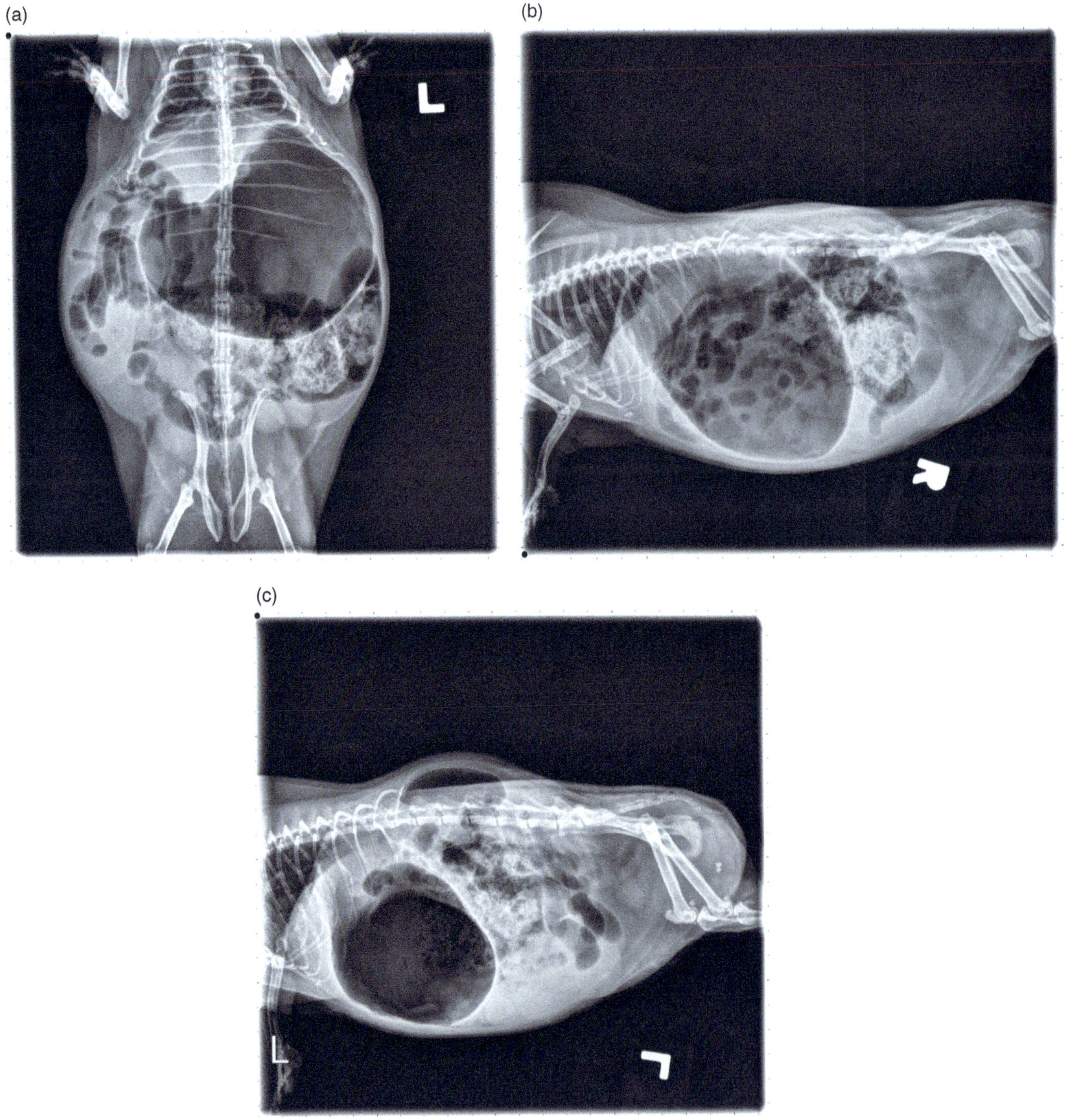

Fig. 5.2. (a) Whole body radiograph (ventrodorsal view). (b) Whole body (radiograph right lateral view). (c) Whole body (radiograph left lateral view).

sucralfate, critical care syringe feeding, and oxygen as needed. During the gastric decompression, precautions were taken to prevent aspiration by positioning the guinea pig's head over the edge of the table; however, increased lung sounds were auscultated immediately following decompression. Generally, gastric decompression is risky and only done when gastric tympany is noted in emergency situations (Pignon and Mayer, 2021). Based on the radiographs, it appeared that the stomach and small intestines were in the position consistent with gastrointestinal stasis. In cases of guinea pigs with gastric dilatation and volvulus (GDV), the stomach is often positioned to the right and may be displaced caudally, allowing the intestines to reposition between it and the liver (Pignon and Mayer, 2021). The findings on the radiographs in this case did not appear to be consistent with a GDV.

Table 5.2. Guinea pig hematology results (Case 2).

		Reference[a]
WBC $\times 10^3/\mu L$	21.4	2.9–14.4
Bands $\times 10^3/\mu L$	0.9	—
%	4	—
Heterophils $\times 10^3/\mu L$	18.6	—
%	87	12–63
Lymphocytes $\times 10^3/\mu L$	1.3	—
%	6	28–84
Monocytes $\times 10^3/\mu L$	0.6	—
%	3	0–9
Eosinophils $\times 10^3/\mu L$	0	—
%	0	0–14
Basophils $\times 10^3/\mu L$	0	—
%	0	0–2
Plasma protein g/dL	NR	4.4–6.6 (biuret)
RBC $\times 10^6/\mu L$	5.81	4.5–6.4
Hb g/dL	16.1	—
HCT %	46.0	39–55
MCV fL	79.0	80–89
MCHC g/dL	34.0	29–32
RDW	14.9	—
Platelets $10^3/\mu L$	558	273–745
MPV fL	8.4	—

[a] Pignon (2021).

The condition of the guinea pig declined overnight, and the next morning it was transferred to the exotics service. An intraosseous catheter was immediately placed to deliver IO fluids and buprenorphine, and oxygen were continued. Unfortunately, a few hours later, the guinea pig died.

Gastrointestinal stasis (or hypomotility, ileus) is a common condition in small herbivores and may occur for a variety of reasons. Underlying disease, dental problems, pain, stress, inappropriate oral antibiotics, or nutritional deficiency (fiber insufficiency) may all be predisposing factors to gastrointestinal stasis. The general approach to this condition is to rule out any underlying disease and identify potential root cause(s). Supportive care is aimed at rehydration (fluid therapy, 100 mL/kg), pain management, and nutrition (critical care syringe feeding).

Case 3: Hedgehog with Anorexia

Signalment

3-year-old intact male African pygmy hedgehog (*Atelerix albiventris*)

History

The hedgehog presented with anorexia and ongoing skin issues. The owner reported that the hedgehog had not eaten for about two days, was lethargic, and not exercising on his wheel. The owner also stated that he had been losing spines for several months, within the week prior to presentation two lumps were noticed on his hind end, and he seemed to have an odor coming from him, prompting concern of an underlying skin condition. Approximately one month prior to the visit, the hedgehog was on antibiotics (orbifloxacin) for a primary gastrointestinal problem. The owner reported that he responded well to the antibiotics; however, since stopping the medications, the spine and skin issues progressively worsened.

Physical Examination

Upon physical examination, the hedgehog was slightly underconditioned with a body condition score of 2/5, although he had gained 5 g since the visit one month earlier. Because he was agitated during the examination, he was placed under gas anesthesia. His heart and respiratory rates were monitored during anesthesia and remained within normal limits. His heart and lungs sounds were normal; there were no abnormal findings with his eyes, ears, nose, teeth, or gingiva. He had peri-anal fecal staining, presumably from diarrhea, and there was a small raised, white, cauliflower-like lesion near his anus. Abdominal palpation revealed a large, firm mass.

Cytology of the skin mass revealed no inflammatory or neoplastic cells, and the mass was likely a benign epithelial cyst. A skin scraping was also done, but there were no significant findings. Further diagnostics included a CBC (Table 5.3 and Figures 5.4, 5.5a–5.5d, 5.6), plasma biochemical profile (Table 5.4), and radiographs (Figures 5.7a and 5.7b).

Interpretive Discussion

The only parameter outside the reference interval on the plasma biochemistry profile results was total protein, which was slightly below the low end. The hypoproteinemia (hypoalbuminemia) may be due to the hedgehog's recent anorexia or previous primary gastrointestinal issue (unresolved or chronic malnutrition or protein-losing enteropathy). The fecal staining around the anus may be an indication of diarrhea, which may fit with protein-losing enteropathy, malabsorption, or maldigestion.

The hemogram revealed a moderate leukocytosis with a left-shift neutrophilia, lymphopenia, and monocytosis. Figure 5.4 shows the blood film at lower power to appreciate the leukocytosis. There were also a moderate number of toxic neutrophils observed on the blood film. Figure 5.5a revealed a band neutrophil, two neutrophils, and a lymphocyte. Figure 5.5b revealed a neutrophil, lymphocyte, and eosinophil. Figure 5.5c

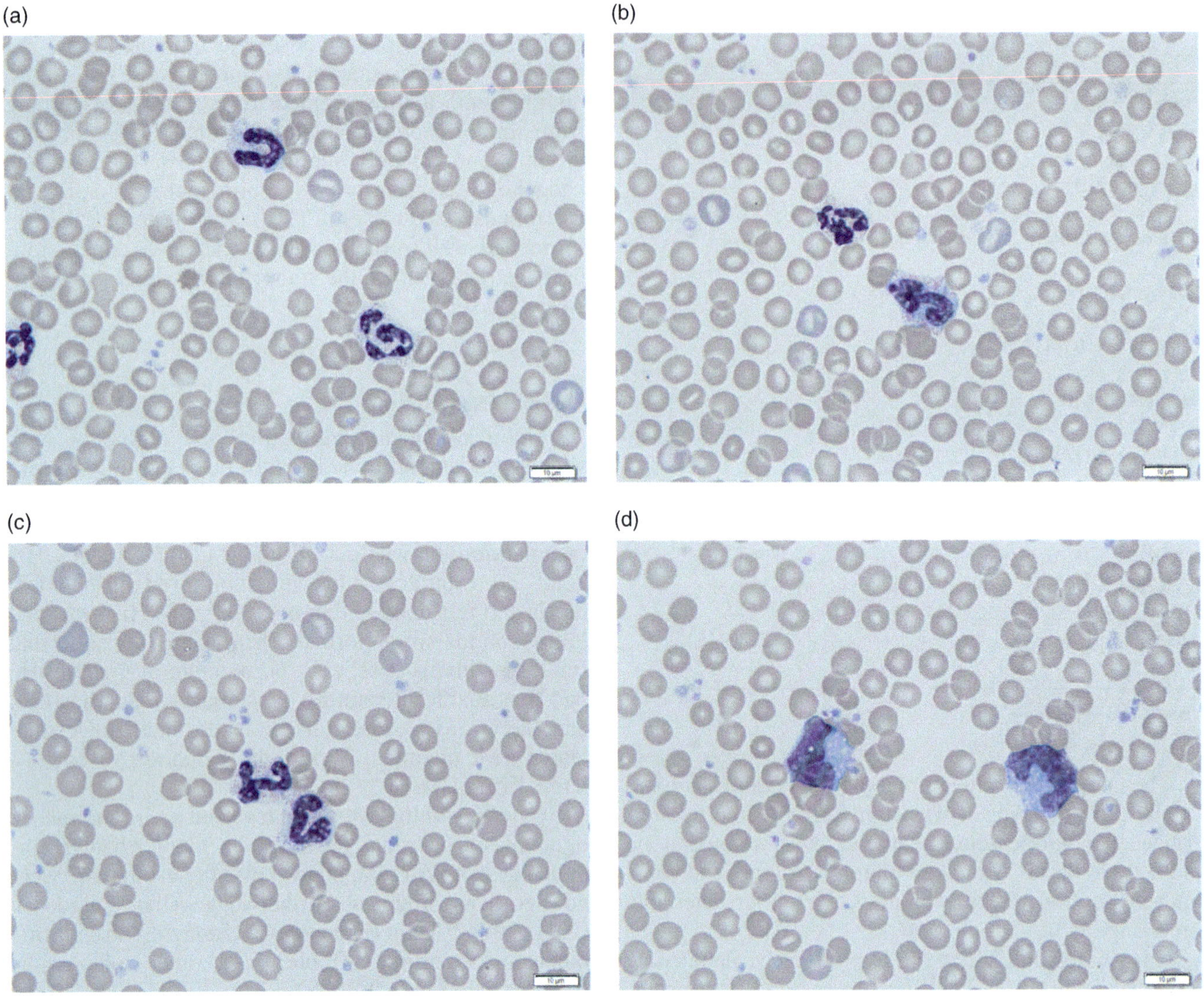

Fig. 5.3. (a), (b), (c), (d) Blood film (Wrights–Giemsa stain, 100× oil).

revealed a large lymphocyte (left) and monocyte (right). Figure 5.5d revealed a basophil. Figure 5.6 revealed a nucleated red blood cell and a neutrophil. The hemogram also reported reticulocytes with a PCV within the normal reference interval. European hedgehogs (*Erinaceus europaeus*) commonly have some nucleated erythrocytes and reticulocytes in circulation after overwintering in rehabilitation centers, so perhaps this may not be an unusual finding (Rossi et al., 2014). These findings indicated an inflammatory leukogram with possibly an infectious etiology. Moderate toxic neutrophils were reported on the hematology form from the laboratory.

Whole body radiographs showed several changes. The radiology report revealed that there was a bronchointerstitial pattern throughout the pulmonary parenchyma, which becomes more interstitial within the left lung lobes. There was heterogeneity of the humeri and femurs with areas of increased lucency, intermixed with mineral opacity. The remaining distal bones of the limbs were normal. There was spondylosis deformans of the lumbar spine. Within the right stifle, there were multiple variably sized, irregularly marginated, osseous bodies with the largest measuring 1.1 × 1 mm. There were osteophytes on the base and apex of the right patella. There was subluxation of the distal interphalangeal joint of the right second front toe. Nails were missing on the first, fourth, and fifth left front digits. The conclusions of these findings were a bronchointerstitial pattern (more so on the left lung) that could represent an interstitial pneumonia and chronic, allergic, or infectious bronchitis; osteochondromas and moderate degenerate changes of the right stifle; and subluxation and the distal interphalangeal join of the right second front toe.

Table 5.3. Hedgehog hematology results (Case 3).

		Reference[a]	Reference[a]
WBC ×10³/μL	27.7	11±6(3–43)	15±0.7(11.5–21.7)
Bands ×10³/μL	1.7	—	—
%	6	—	—
Neutrophils ×10³/μL	23.0	5.1±5.2(0.6–37.4)	9.5±0.5(6.1–14.6)
%	83	—	—
Lymphocytes ×10³/μL	1.1	4±2.2(0.9–13.1)	5.2±0.4(3.3–8.9)
%	4	—	—
Monocytes ×10³/μL	0.8	0.3±0.3(0–1.6)	0.2±0.1(0–0.8)
%	3	—	—
Eosinophils ×10³/μL	0.8	1.2±0.9(0–5.1)	0.2(0–0.3)
%	3	—	—
Basophils ×10³/μL	0.3	0.4±0.3(0–1.5)	0.1(0–0.2)
%	1	—	—
Plasma protein g/dL	4.5	—	—
RBC × 10⁶/ μL	6.1	6±2(3–16)	5.0±0.1(4.3–6.0)
Hb g/dL	13.6	12±2.8(7–21.1)	13.1±0.3(10.7–14.9)
PCV %	42.0	36±7(22–64)	42.0±0.9(33.5–47.0)
MCV fL	69.0	67±9(41–94)	87.8±1.8(76.3–99.8)
MCHC g/dL	33.0	34±5(17–48)	30.9±0.5(27.7–35.2)
Reticulocytes/μL	515,100	—	—
%	8.5%	—	—
Cell Hgb Retic pg	24.8	—	—
MCV Retic fL	85.0	—	—
RDW	18.2	—	—
Platelets 10³/μL	421.0	226±108(60–347)	—
MPV fL	16.1	—	—

[a] Doss (2021).

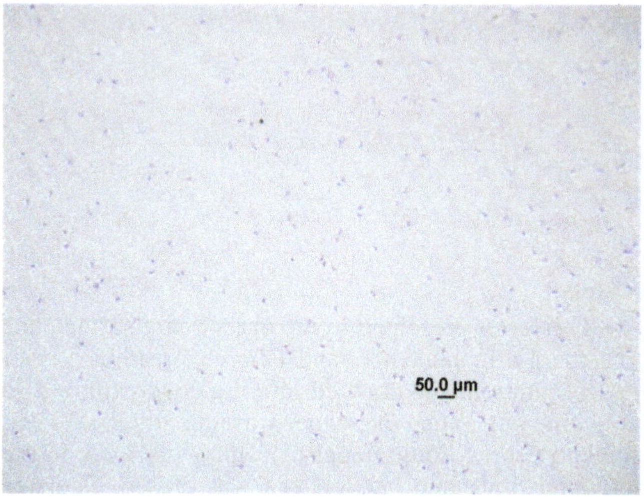

Fig. 5.4. Blood film (Wrights–Giemsa stain, 10×).

Summary

The primary diagnosis of concern was the pneumonia; therefore, it was decided to treat the pneumonia first and further evaluate the skin masses and recheck the alopecia/spine loss during the follow-up visit. Because the hedgehog responded to orbifloxacin after the last visit, it was prescribed again (10 mg/kg PO q24h × 14d). The hedgehog was also given an injection of ivermectin (0.3 mg/kg SC repeat in 10 days) for presumptive mites. The owner was instructed to monitor the hedgehog as some improvement was expected within the next two days. If improvement was not observed, additional therapy could be added, such as nebulization, which could be done at the hospital or at home with a portable nebulizer. Another recommendation made was to ensure the environment was clean, at the appropriate temperature, and free of any source of dust or other irritants. The owner was also provided some suggestions on different foods to offer to encourage eating, such as canned cat food, and syringe feeding meat-flavored baby food was also an option. Hill's a/d canned food was sent home with the hedgehog. The plan for the follow-up appointment was to recheck radiographs and repeat the ivermectin injection.

Case 4: Ferret with Lethargy, Inappetence, and Labored Breathing

Signalment

1-year-old intact female ferret (*Mustela putorius furo*)

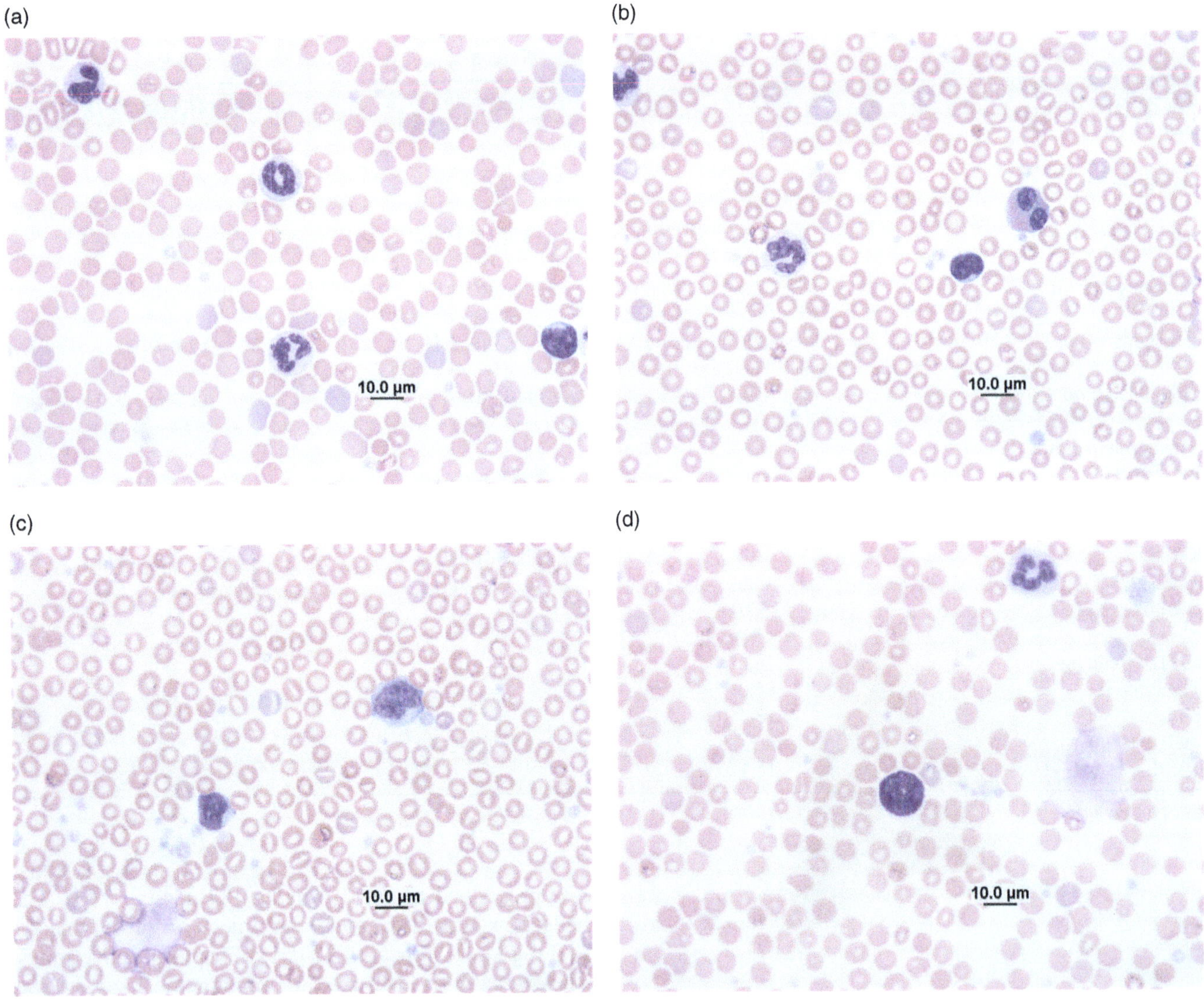

Fig. 5.5. (a), (b), (c), (d) Blood film (Wrights–Giemsa stain, 100× oil).

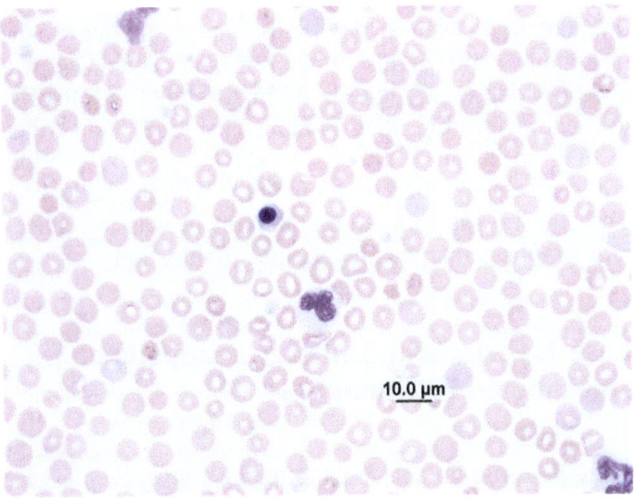

Fig. 5.6. Blood film (Wrights–Giemsa stain, 100× oil).

History

The ferret presented to the urgent care service due to lethargy, inappetence, and labored breathing. Prior to presentation, she crawled into the couch and would not come out. When the owner was able to retrieve her, she had yellow liquid under her chin, was weak in her left hind limb, and her left eye was closed. She was taken to an emergency veterinarian, where a blood glucose was taken, whole body radiographs were obtained, and a FAST scan was performed with no remarkable findings. At the emergency hospital, she was hypothermic at 93 °F and received subcutaneous fluids. She deteriorated overnight, but urinated normally at home and drank some water. She had not eaten since the morning prior to presentation. The ferret had been previously healthy, although she had always had mildly abnormal stools that reportedly had been normal

Table 5.4. Hedgehog plasma biochemical results (Case 3).

	Results	Reference[a]	Reference[a]
Glucose mg/dL	94	89±30	86.1±4.7(60–125)
BUN mg/dL	39	27±9(13–54)	47.1±2.3(34.3–57.3)
Creatinine mg/dL	0.2	0.4±0.2(0–0.8)	0.7±0.1(0.5–1.0)
Phosphorus mg/dL	3.9	5.3±1.9(2.4–12)	—
Calcium mg/dL	9.2	8.8±1.4(5.2–11.3)	9.7±0.3(8.6–11.4)
Total protein g/dL	4.2	5.8±0.7(4–7.7)	6.0±0.2(4.6–6.9)
Albumin g/dL	1.9	2.9±0.4(1.8–4.2)	3.4±0.2(2.7–3.9)
Globulin g/dL	2.3	2.7±0.5(1.6–3.9)	2.6±0.2(1.9–3.6)
A/G ratio	0.8	—	—
Cholesterol mg/dL	80	131±25(86–189)	132.5±5.3(100–150)
T. Bilirubin mg/dL	0.0	0.3±0.3(1–1.3)	—
CK IU/L	914	863±413(333–1964)	—
ALP IU/L	42	51±21(8–92)	22.4±1.0(18.2–25.5)
ALT IU/L	29	53±24(16–134)	22.8±1.4(15.2–28.8)
AST IU/L	33	34±22(8–137)	33.5±3.5(19.0–65.6)
GGT IU/L	0	4±1(0–12)	—
Sodium mEq/dL	140	141±9(120–165)	—
Potassium mEq/dL	4.9	4.9±1(3.2–7.2)	—
Chloride mEq/dL	111	109±10(92–128)	—
Bicarbonate mEq/dL	27.3	—	—
Anion gap	7	—	—
Calc. osmolality	289	—	—
Lipemia mg/dL	9	—	—
Hemolysis mg/dL	7	—	—
Icterus mg/dL	0	—	—

[a] Doss (2021).

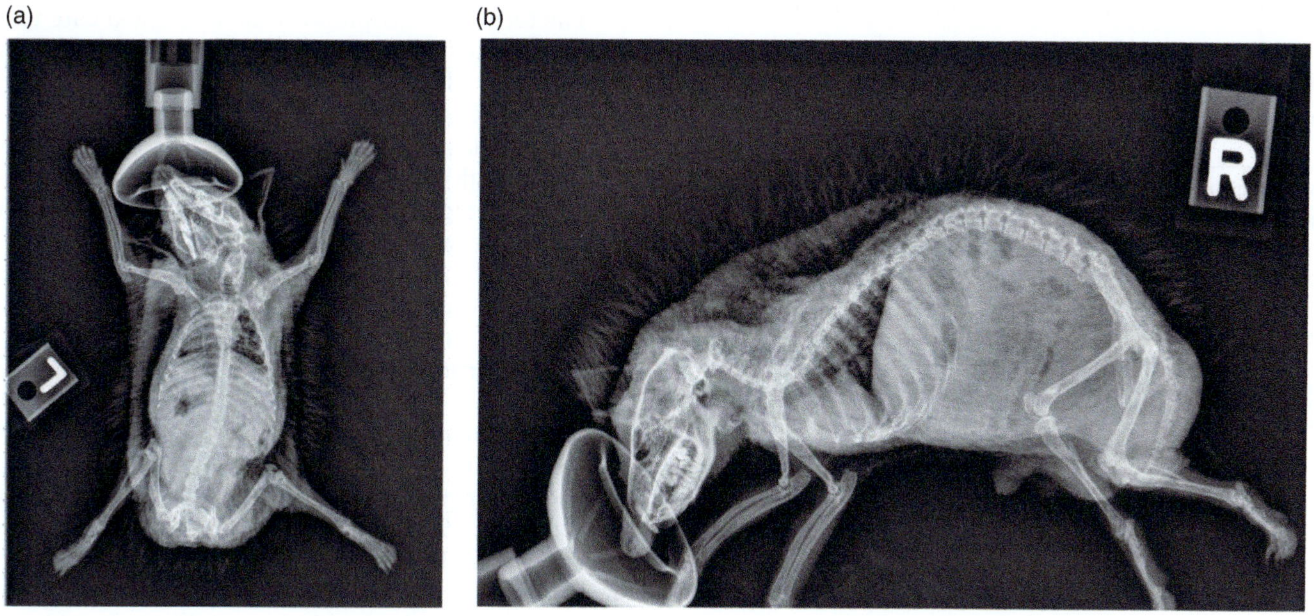

Fig. 5.7. (a) Whole body radiograph (ventrodorsal view). (b) Whole body radiograph (right lateral view).

on cytology. She lived with another ferret at home that was apparently healthy. Both ferrets were offered a diet of Totally Ferret, and they lived in a cage but had free access around the house when the owners were home and able to supervise them.

Physical Examination

Upon physical examination, the 800 g ferret appeared to be mildly hyperventilating. Her temperature and pulse were within normal limits, but her respiratory rate was 152 bpm. She exhibited blepharospasm

OS, had moderate hind limb paresis bilaterally, tachypnea, a large firm urinary bladder on palpation, and a 1–2 cm mass palpated in her mid-abdomen that was moderately painful. She urinated and defecated during the examination on her own. Her urine was markedly green in color (suspected biliverdin), and her feces were soft and green.

She managed to settle down after the examination, and her breathing stabilized to 30–35 bpm. A FAST scan ultrasound was performed with notable findings that included a large urinary bladder, and the palpable mass did not image with soft tissue echogenicity. An ultrasound-guided cystocentesis was performed, and green urine was obtained. Blood was collected for a CBC (Table 5.5; Figures 5.8a–5.8d) and plasma biochemistry profile (Table 5.6). Because multiple attempts to place an IV catheter failed, subcutaneous fluids were given, and the ferret was treated for pain (buprenorphine) and with an antibiotic (Clavamox) for possible urinary tract infection.

Interpretive Discussion

The hemogram revealed a mild leukocytosis with neutrophilia, lymphopenia, and monocytosis. Her PCV was also slightly outside and below the reference interval for female ferrets. There were no significant findings on the blood film, other than reactive monocytes. Figure 5.8a revealed two neutrophils and an eosinophil.

Table 5.5. Ferret hematology results (Case 4).

		Reference[a]
WBC $\times 10^3/\mu L$	11.4	2.5–8.6
Bands $\times 10^3/\mu L$	0.1	0–0.248
%	1	—
Neutrophils $\times 10^3/\mu L$	8.7	0.725–2.409
%	76	18–47
Lymphocytes $\times 10^3/\mu L$	1.6	1.475–5.590
%	14	41–73
Monocytes $\times 10^3/\mu L$	0.9	0.1–0.372
%	8	0–4
Eosinophils $\times 10^3/\mu L$	0.1	0.050–0.516
%	1	0–4
Basophils $\times 10^3/\mu L$	0	0–0.172
%	0	0–2
Plasma protein g/dL	5.5	—
RBC x $10^6/\mu L$	8.5	7.01–9.65
Hb g/dL	14.2	15.2–17.4
PCV %	43.0	47–51 (HCT)
MCV fL	51.0	50–54
MCHC g/dL	33.0	32–35
RDW	13.2	—
Platelets $10^3/\mu L$	370.0	200–459
MPV fL	8.1	—

[a] Quesenberry (2021).

Figure 5.8b revealed a lymphocyte and a monocyte. Figure 5.8c revealed a neutrophil and a large lymphocyte. Figure 5.8d revealed a reactive monocyte (vacuolated).

The most significant finding on the plasma biochemistry profile was the markedly elevated liver enzymes, AST and ALT. There was also a hypoalbuminemia and hypophosphatemia. These findings along with the diarrhea, age of ferret, hemogram results, and physical exam findings (greed urine and feces) led to a primary suspicion of enteric coronavirus or epizootic catarrhal enteritis (ECE). Other gastrointestinal diseases that were also possible or concurrent included foreign body and *Helicobacter mustelae* gastritis.

Summary

Because a small mass was palpated that was not consistent with soft tissue echogenicity on ultrasound, an exploratory laparotomy was performed. During surgery, all organs appeared grossly normal. There was no evidence of a foreign body; however, the spleen appeared slightly enlarged and with 180-degree torsion, but did not appear congested. There was one large mesenteric lymph node (perhaps the palpable mass), but all other lymph nodes appeared to be normal. A liver biopsy was obtained and submitted for histologic evaluation.

The ferret was hospitalized in the critical care unit overnight and maintained on fluid therapy and pain medications. The ferret recovered uneventfully. Histopathology revealed a multifocal mild to moderate lymphoplasmacytic portal hepatitis, which was consistent with the suspicion of ECE. All of the ferret's clinical signs were consistent with ECE except the issues she was having with her left eye. An ophthalmologic examination revealed a mild uveitis. The uveitis may be associated with the systemic inflammation from the presumed ECE. Ophthalmic drops containing a corticosteroid were given to reduce the inflammation. The ferret was discharged with Tramadol (3 mg/kg PO up to TID for pain), Clavamox (13 mg/kg PO BID × 14d), Meloxicam (0.1 mg/kg PO q24h × 5d for pain and inflammation), and prednisolone acetate 1% for the left eye. Other discharge instructions included monitoring her feed intake and encouraging her to eat as much as possible due to the concern of weight loss with this condition. It was also recommended to keep her relatively inactive while she recovered from surgery.

Ferrets presenting with diarrhea may be affected by one or more of several gastrointestinal diseases or conditions (Figure 5.9). General considerations are shown in Figure 5.9, but are not absolute. This was demonstrated in this case, where a foreign body was highly suspected;

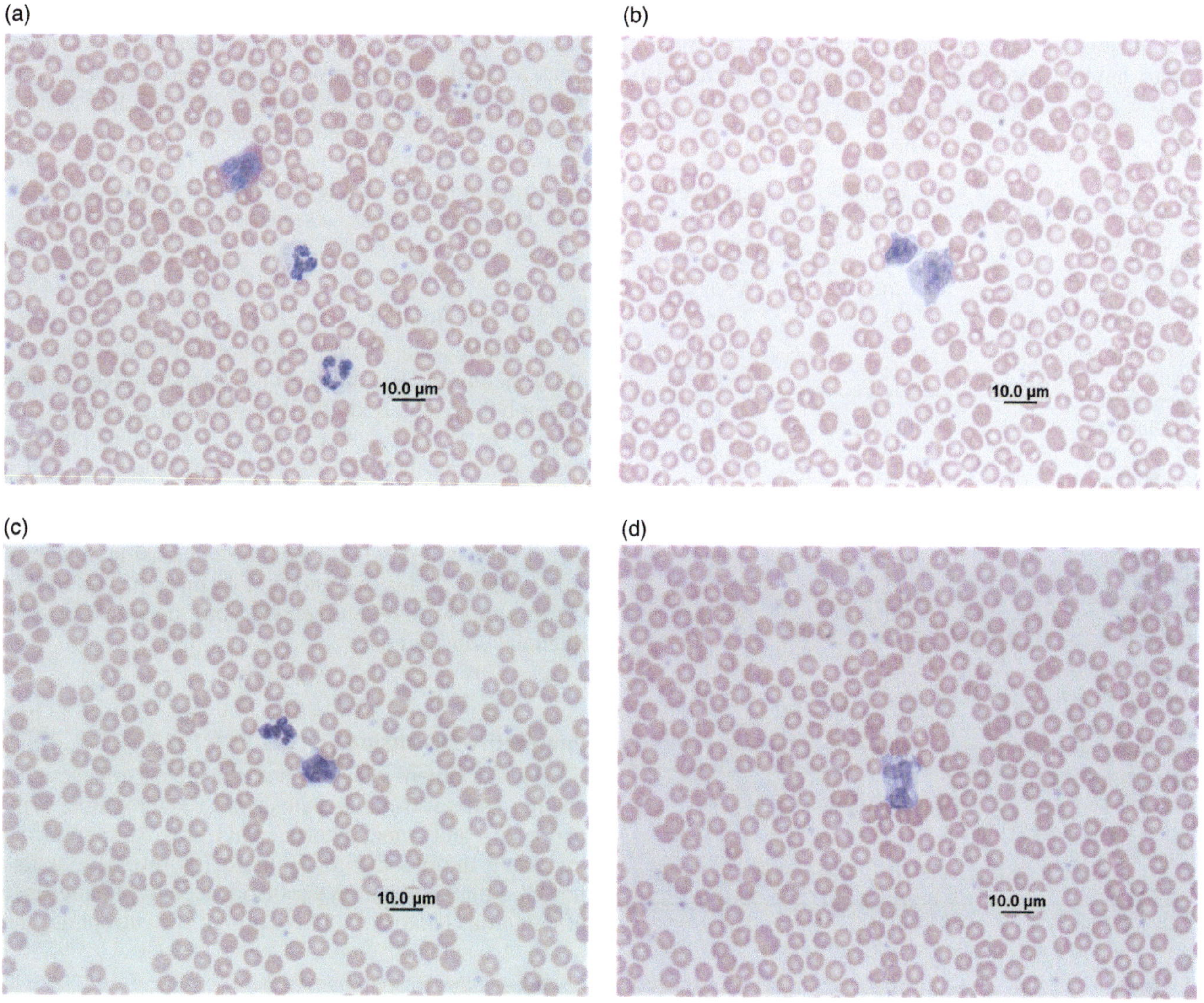

Fig. 5.8. (a), (b), (c), (d) Blood film (Wrights–Giemsa stain, 100× oil).

however, ECE was more likely. ECE is recognized as a ferret enteric coronavirus. It is highly contagious and causes diarrhea, often green with mucus, and in chronic conditions a bird-seed-like appearance. It is common in young ferrets, but also in any aged ferret that may have interacted with a new or young ferret. Clinical signs and physical exam findings often include lethargy, anorexia, enlarged mesenteric lymph nodes, dehydration, and diarrhea (green with mucus and/or bird-seed consistency). Other findings may include green urine, jaundice, bruxism, or rectal prolapse, but are less common (Kiupel and Perpiñan, 2014). Coronavirus can be identified by polymerase chain reaction (PCR) testing from tissue or feces at the Diagnostic Center for Population and Animal Health (Michigan State University) or at Charles River Laboratory (Greenacre, 2020; Hoefer, 2020). Treatment is supportive with fluid therapy, antibiotics, and nutritional support.

Case 5: Ferret with Lethargy and Weakness

Signalment

5-year-old castrated male ferret (*Mustela putorius furo*)

History

Eight months prior to presentation, the ferret was presumptively diagnosed with adrenal gland disease and insulinoma. As part of the treatment plan, the ferret had been receiving monthly Lupron injections for the adrenal disease and prednisone to help regulate his blood glucose for the insulinoma. Four months later, flutamide was added to the treatment plan as an aid to combat potential prostatitis, a side effect of the adrenal gland disease. Five days prior to presentation, a melatonin implant was administered subcutaneously to replace the monthly Lupron injections, for the adrenal gland disease. During that visit, his blood glucose was 103 mg/dL despite having fasted for eight hours. The ferret also exhibited severe hind end weakness. During presentation, the owner reported that the ferret continued to be weak and lethargic at home. He had a good appetite, but was also being syringe-fed every 4–6 h. It was also reported that he exhibited polyuria and polydipsia, and the owner expresses large amounts of normal urine prior to syringe feeding. The ferret was reported to occasionally sneeze and develop a serous nasal discharge.

Table 5.6. Ferret plasma biochemical results (Case 4).

	Results	Reference[a]
Glucose mg/dL	156	80–117
BUN mg/dL	20	18–32
Creatinine mg/dL	0.2	0.2–0.5
Phosphorus mg/dL	3.1	5.1–6.5
Calcium mg/dL	8.4	8.1–9.5
Total protein g/dL	4.8	4.5–6.2
Albumin g/dL	1.9	2.5–4.0
Globulin g/dL	2.9	—
A/G ratio	0.7	—
Cholesterol mg/dL	137	119–163
T. Bilirubin mg/dL	0.4	0.2–0.5
CK IU/L	5177	55–93
ALP IU/L	24	25–60
ALT IU/L	536	65–128
AST IU/L	515	70–100
GGT IU/L	5	8–34
Sodium mEq/dL	147	142–148
Potassium mEq/dL	3.8	4.5–6.1
Chloride mEq/dL	112	—
Bicarbonate mEq/dL	27.7	—
Anion gap	11	—
Calc. osmolality	296	—
Lipemia mg/dL	20	—
Hemolysis mg/dL	19	—
Icterus mg/dL	0	—

[a]Quesenberry (2021).

Physical Examination

Upon physical examination, the ferret was quiet and mildly lethargic, but did respond when handled. He did not ambulate. His body weight was 960 g (down from his weight of 1045 g five days earlier). Other physical exam findings included decreased muscle tone and a thin, patchy hair coat. No discharge was observed from the nose, and there was no urine staining. Blood was collected for a complete blood count and plasma biochemistry panel (Tables 5.7 and 5.8; Figures 5.10a–5.10c). Ultrasound was recommended, but declined due to financial constraints.

Interpretive Discussion

The complete blood count revealed a regenerative anemia and severe leukocytosis with heterophilia, lymphopenia, and monocytosis. This was supported by reviewing the blood film. Figure 5.10a revealed, at low power, a marked leukocytosis evidenced by the presence of numerous leukocytes, likely primarily neutrophils, and

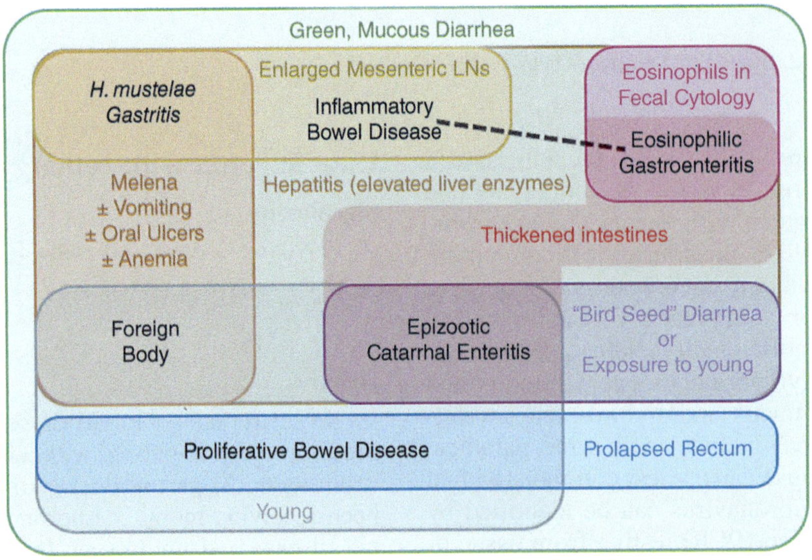

Fig. 5.9. Diagram illustrating the differentiation and commonalities of the ferret gastrointestinal diseases and conditions presenting with green and/or mucoid diarrhea (large green box). The color-coded blocks with same color text represent clinical signs, physical exam findings, or diagnostic findings. The bold black text at the intersection or overlapping of the blocks represents a likely gastrointestinal disease or condition. The dotted line indicates that eosinophilic gastroenteritis is a type of inflammatory bowel disease. The clinical signs or findings are not all-encompassing as they may be present with other diseases or conditions. LNs = Lymph Nodes.

Table 5.7. Ferret hematology results (Case 5).

		Reference[a]
WBC $\times 10^3/\mu L$	48.5	2.5–8.6
Neutrophils $\times 10^3/\mu L$	47.0	0.725–2.409
%	97	18–47
Lymphocytes $\times 10^3/\mu L$	0.5	1.475–5.590
%	1	41–73
Monocytes $\times 10^3/\mu L$	1.0	0.1–0.372
%	2	0–4
Eosinophils $\times 10^3/\mu L$	0	0.050–0.516
%	0	0–4
Basophils $\times 10^3/\mu L$	0	0–0.172
%	0	0–2
Plasma protein g/dL	8.8	—
RBC x $10^6/\mu L$	6.4	7.01–9.65
Hb g/dL	11.2	15.2–17.4
PCV %	34.0	47–51 (HCT)
MCV fL	53.0	50–54
MCHC g/dL	33.0	32–35
Reticulocytes	25 520	—
Cell Hgb Retic pg	18.5	—
MCV Retic fL	65.0	—
RDW	12.1	—
Platelets $\times 10^3/\mu L$	517.0	200–459
MPV fL	8.1	—
Comments	Moderately lipemic, rouleaux, clumped platelets exist	

[a] Quesenberry (2021).

Table 5.8. Ferret plasma biochemical results (Case 5).

	Results	Reference[a]
Glucose mg/dL	155	80–117
BUN mg/dL	65	18–32
Creatinine mg/dL	0.6	0.2–0.5
Phosphorus mg/dL	7.4	5.1–6.5
Calcium mg/dL	8.0	8.1–9.5
Total protein g/dL	7.8	4.5–6.2
Albumin g/dL	1.2	2.5–4.0
Globulin g/dL	5.6	—
A/G ratio	—	—
Cholesterol mg/dL	—	119–163
T. Bilirubin mg/dL	0.4	0.2–0.5
CK IU/L	—	55–93
ALP IU/L	38	25–60
ALT IU/L	—	65–128
AST IU/L	—	70–100
GGT IU/L	—	8–34
Sodium mEq/dL	136	142–148
Potassium mEq/dL	1.6	4.5–6.1
Chloride mEq/dL	—	—
Bicarbonate mEq/dL	—	—
Anion gap	—	—
Calc. osmolality	—	—
Lipemia mg/dL	—	—
Hemolysis mg/dL	—	—
Icterus mg/dL	—	—

[a] Quesenberry (2021).

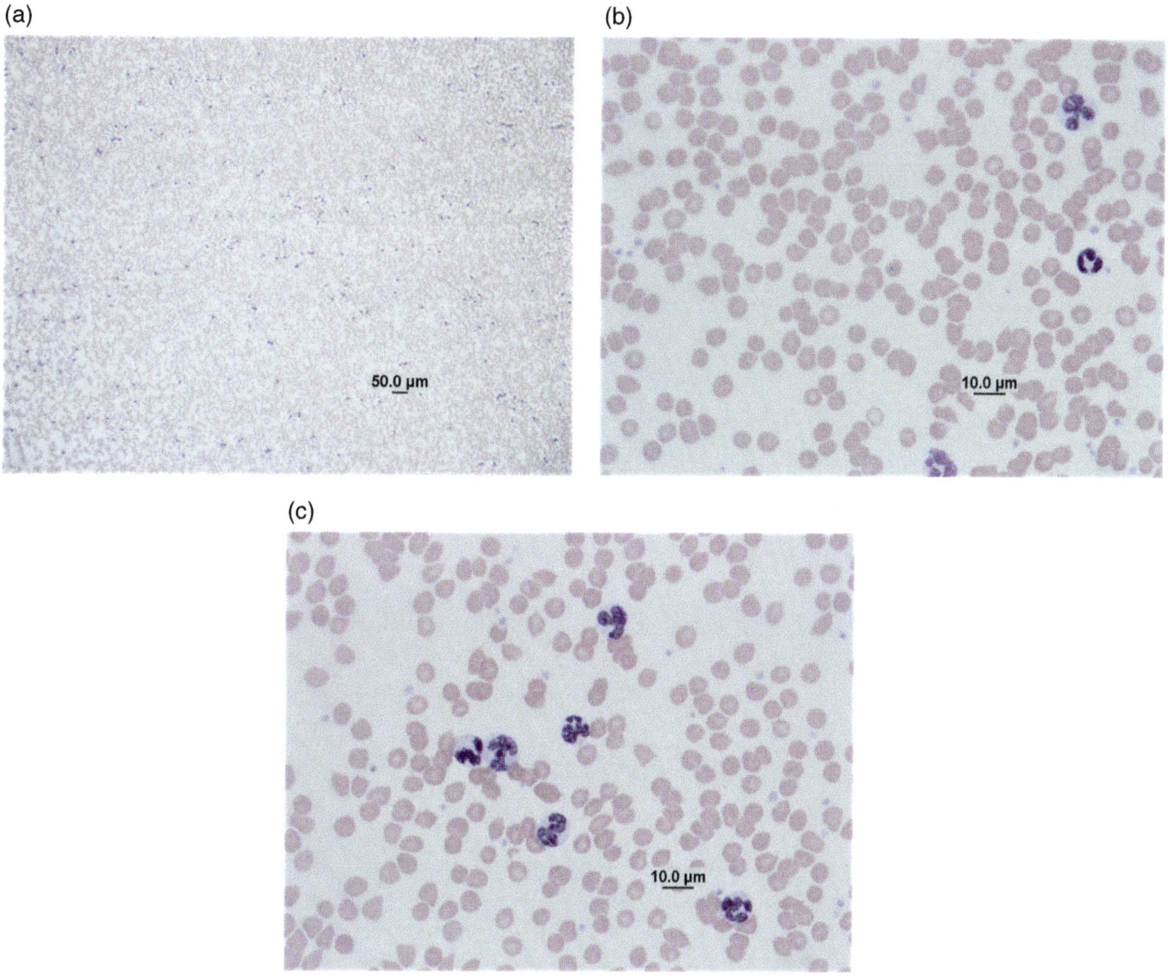

Fig. 5.10. (a) Blood film (Wrights–Giemsa stain, 10×). (b), (c) Blood film (Wrights–Giemsa stain, 100× oil).

some monocytes. Figure 5.10b shows a single erythrocyte with a Howell–Jolly body in the center of the image, along with two neutrophils on the right. Figure 5.10c shows six neutrophils in one field supporting the hemogram result of neutrophilia. These results suggest possibly an inflammatory and likely infectious process.

The plasma biochemical profile revealed hyperglycemia, azotemia, hyperproteinemia (hypoalbuminemia), hyperphosphatemia, and hypokalemia. The hyperglycemia may have been due to the chronic use of glucocorticoid or due to another undiagnosed condition. The other parameters noted outside of the reference interval support the diagnosis of chronic renal disease, but an infection in the kidney was also suspected, like pyelonephritis.

Summary

The ferret was prescribed an antibiotic, orbifloxacin (30 mg/kg PO q24h), for suspected pyelonephritis. Unfortunately, the ferret's condition continued to decline over the following 24 h, and he died on the way back to the hospital the following day. His body was submitted to the diagnostic lab for necropsy and histopathology. The results from the histopathology review included hypersplenism, bilateral adrenal endocrine neoplasia (right cortical carcinoma and left cortical nodular hyperplasia), and chronic kidney disease (moderate to severe chronic glomerulopathy) with acute and severe pyelonephritis (severe, acute, bilateral suppurative and necrotizing pyelo- and tubulointerstitial nephritis with intralesional coccoid bacteria). The kidney pathology was most likely the cause of death and of the leukemoid response present histologically throughout the tissues.

References

Doss GA, Carpenter JW. 2021. Africa pygmy hedgehogs. In: Quesenberry KE, Orcutt CJ, Mans C, et al. (eds), *Ferrets, Rabbits, and Rodents Clinical Medicine and Surgery*, 4th edn. St. Louis: Elsevier Saunders, p. 406.

Greenacre CB. 2020. Ferrets. In: Heatley JJ, Russell KE (eds), *Exotic Animal Laboratory Diagnosis*. Hoboken, NJ: Wiley & Sons, Inc., pp. 17–44.

Hoefer HL. 2021. Gastrointestinal diseases of Ferrets. In: Quesenberry KE, Orcutt CJ, Mans C, et al. (eds), *Ferrets, Rabbits, and Rodents Clinical Medicine and Surgery*, 4th edn. St. Louis, MO: Elsevier, pp. 27–38.

Kiupel M, Perpiñan D. 2014. Viral diseases of Ferrets. In: Fox JG, Marini RP (eds), *Biology and Diseases of Ferrets*, 3rd edn. Ames, IA: Wiley Blackwell, pp. 439–517.

Lambert JL, Fernandez NJ, Roy M-F. 2016. Association of presence of band cells and toxic neutrophils with systemic inflammatory response syndrome and outcome in horses with acute disease. *J Vet Intern Med* 30(4):1284–92.

Mans C, Donnelly TM, Mayer J. 2021. Chinchillas. In: Quesenberry KE, Orcutt CJ, Mans C, et al. (eds), *Ferrets, Rabbits, and Rodents Clinical Medicine and Surgery*, 4th edn. St. Louis: Elsevier Saunders, p. 307.

Pignon C, Mayer J. 2021. Guinea pigs. In: Quesenberry KE, Orcutt CJ, Mans C, et al. (eds), *Ferrets, Rabbits, and Rodents Clinical Medicine and Surgery*, 4th edn. St. Louis, MO: Elsevier, pp. 270–297.

Rossi G, Mangiagalli G, Paracchini G,et al. 2014. Hematologic and biochemical variables of hedgehogs (*Erinaceus europaeus*) after overwintering in rehabilitation centers. *Vet Clin Pathol* 43(1):6–14.

Quesenberry KE, De Matos R. 2021. Basic approach to veterinary care of ferrets. In: Quesenberry KE, Orcutt CJ, Mans C, et al. (eds), *Ferrets, Rabbits, and Rodents Clinical Medicine and Surgery*, 4th edn. St. Louis: Elsevier Saunders, p.19–20.

6 Sample Collection for Mammalian Cytodiagnosis

Diagnostic cytology plays a major role in the diagnosis and management of diseases affecting domestic mammals. It is also an important diagnostic tool in the management of diseases involving nondomestic small exotic mammalian (i.e., rabbits, rodents, ferrets, hedgehogs) and lower vertebrate patients, especially birds and reptiles. There has been limited use of cytology in other vertebrates, such as amphibians and fish. Even so, diagnostic microscopy using wet-mount techniques are routinely used in the management of amphibian and fish patients.

Cytology Sampling and Evaluation Techniques

Cytology is a rapid, simple, diagnostic procedure requiring little in terms of equipment and cost to the veterinarian. The basic equipment needed to perform cytology includes a microscope with good resolution (especially at 20×, 40×, 50×, and 100× or oil-immersion), clean microscope slides with frosted ends, coverslips, and cytologic stains (i.e., Wright's and Stat stains). If pre-cleaned microscope slides are not used, the slides should be routinely dry-wiped to remove glass particles that often remain on the glass surface and interfere with sample preparation. Cytodiagnosis is typically made using 40× (high-dry) or 50× or 100× oil-immersion objectives. Placement of a glass coverslip on top of an air-dried stained smear provides optimal microscopic resolution when using a 40× (high-dry objective) because that objective is manufactured to require a coverslip for a focused view. If a coverslip is not applied to the glass slide, then the field of view will be hazy and appear as if immersion oil is on the objective of the 40× lens (Meuten and Meichner, 2022).

Sample Locations

The Integument

Examination of the skin during the routine physical examination of mammalian patients may reveal macules, papules, nodules, vesicles, bullae, pustules, or ulcers. Cytological examination of smears made from swabbing or a scraping of the lesion will often prove the presumptive or definitive diagnosis (Figure 6.1). Masses found in the skin can be aspirated or excised to obtain a cytological sample. A touch imprint of a biopsy sample can also provide a cytologic sample.

Alimentary Tract

Examination of the oral cavity during the routine physical examination of mammalian patients may reveal plaques, nodules, or ulcers. Cytological examination of smears made from swabbing or a scraping of the lesion will often prove the presumptive or definitive diagnosis. Masses found in the oral cavity can be aspirated or excised to obtain a cytological sample.

Cytological samples of the esophagus are indicated whenever lesions are detected by palpation or by endoscopy. A cytologic sample can be obtained by a touch imprint of a biopsy sample or a brush cytologic preparation. A sample can also be obtained by passing a sterile cotton swab through the oral cavity into the esophageal lumen. An oral speculum or general anesthesia should be used in animals capable of biting and breaking the swab.

Cytologic evaluation of the stomach and intestines is complicated by the presence of many bacteria

Exotic Animal Hematology and Cytology, Fifth Edition. Terry W. Campbell and Krystan R. Grant.

Companion website: www.wiley.com/go/campbell/exotic

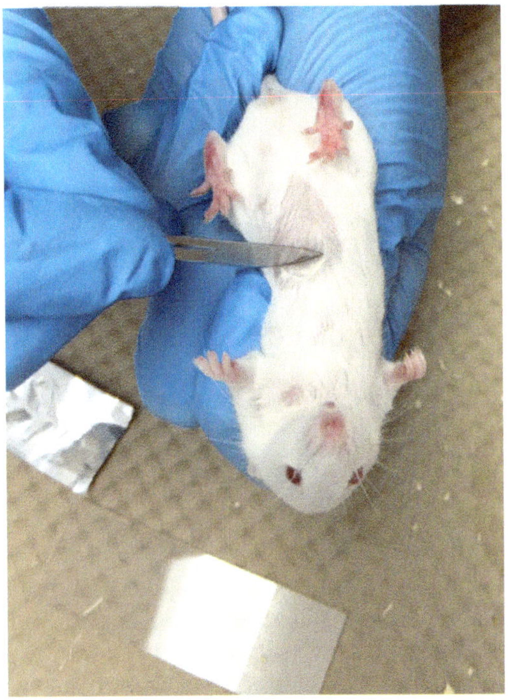

Fig. 6.1. Collection of a cytologic sample using a sterile scalpel blade to gently rub along the cutaneous lesion. The collected sample is applied to a microscope slide.

and much cell debris. Samples are obtained by gastric washes, endoscopy, or exploratory surgery.

Dry-mount fecal cytology is commonly used in the diagnostic evaluation of gastrointestinal disease. The fecal sampling technique influences the quality of the sample. For example, in the dog, sampling methods differ in their sensitivity to detect abnormalities in fecal cytology, where digital examination and rectal scraping have a higher sensitivity compared to rectal lavage (Frezoulis et al., 2017).

Respiratory Tract

Cytological evaluation of samples obtained from the nasal cavity, sinuses, larynx, trachea, and lungs support other clinical diagnostics to produce a diagnosis in mammals with respiratory disease. The upper respiratory tract of mammals consists of the nasal cavity, which begins at the nares. The mammalian nasal cavity is composed of bony and cartilaginous sinuses divided by a nasal septum and ends at the ethmoid plate.

Keratinized squamous epithelium lines the external part of the nares, but transitions into a nonkeratinized squamous epithelial lining inside the nares. Ciliated pseudostratified columnar epithelium makes up the mucous membrane that lines most of the nasal cavity. Paranasal sinuses, serous glands, mucous glands, and lymphoid tissue are associated with the nasal cavity of mammals. The larynx of mammals is the part of the upper respiratory tract that is associated with the vocal cords, arytenoids cartilage, and glottis. The larynx is lined by stratified squamous epithelium and is associated with lymphoid tissue. The trachea extends from the larynx to the bronchi. Both structures are lined by ciliated pseudostratified columnar epithelium with goblet cells. Beyond the bronchi, the smaller airways, the bronchioles, are lined by ciliated and nonciliated cuboidal epithelium. The airways continue to become smaller until they reach the alveolar ducts, alveolar sacs, and alveoli. The mammalian alveoli are lined by flattened epithelium, type I pneumocytes, and rounded epithelium, type II pneumocytes (Burkhard et al., 2001).

Cytological samples of the nasal cavity can be obtained in larger mammals during rhinoscopy when a biopsy or brush sample can be obtained for impression cytology. However, nasal swabs and flush methods are used on small mammals or when endoscopy is unavailable. Nasal swabs are easily obtained and are relatively nontraumatic. Nasal flush sampling may also provide a diagnostic cytological sample (Smallwood and Zenoble, 1993). A nasal flush is obtained by inserting an appropriately sized soft polypropylene or red rubber feeding tube or urinary catheter into the nasal cavity. Sterile physiologic saline (non-bacteriostatic) is used to flush the nasal cavity. A traumatic nasal flush can be used to increase the cellularity of the sample by scraping the mucous membrane with the tip of the tube, which has been beveled to create a rough point. Penetration of the cribriform plate should be avoided by prior measurement of, or cutting the tube at, the length between the nares and the medial canthus of the eye (Burkhard et al., 2001). Small amounts of saline are flushed into the nasal cavity using alternating positive and negative pressure on the syringe attached to the tube. The tubing is moved back and forth during the process to encourage exfoliation of cells and tissue fragments. The cytologic specimen is either aspirated into the syringe or collected on a gauze pad held at the end of the nares. The sample is prepared as for other fluid samples. Any tissue particles retrieved during the process are prepared as squash preparations.

In larger mammals, laryngoscopy can be used to directly visualize the larynx and provide a means for sampling either by biopsy or brush preparation. Ultrasound-guided fine-needle aspiration can also be used to sample laryngeal masses (Rudorf and Brown, 1998).

A tracheal wash is a sampling technique used to obtain cytological specimens from mammals suspected of lower respiratory tract disease. General anesthesia is required for this procedure in mammals because placement of an endotracheal tube is recommended whenever possible. Contamination of the tip of the endotracheal tube with the oropharynx should be avoided as much as possible because this material will be picked up by the collection tube as it passes through the endotracheal tube. After intubation and inflation of the endotracheal tube cuff, the small mammal is placed in lateral recumbency. A small sterile tube (i.e., urinary or intravenous catheter) is inserted into the endotracheal tube and extended to the distal end of the trachea (Smallwood and Zenoble, 1993). This is quickly followed by the infusion of warm, sterile, non-bacteriostatic saline (1.0–2.0 mL/kg bodyweight), leaving enough air in the attached syringe to completely clear the tube. The fluid sample is immediately re-aspirated back into the tube and syringe. The caudal end of the animal can be elevated to facilitate aspiration of the wash fluid. An alternative method is to use half the volume of saline to rapidly inject into the trachea and replace the syringe with an empty syringe for aspiration (Burkhard et al., 2001). The procedure is repeated a second time with the remainder of the saline. The wash sample is processed in the manner of fluid samples.

Cytologic evaluation of the lungs of animals can be performed on samples obtained using a fine-needle aspiration technique. Indications for doing this include diffuse lung disease or a discrete mass or masses revealed by radiographic or ultrasound evaluations (Wood et al., 1998). There are some risks to the patient with this technique depending upon the location of the mass, especially in critically ill patients and those with coagulopathies. However, fine-needle aspiration has the least risk when compared to other sources of samples, such as tissue biopsy (Teske et al., 1991). When possible, coagulation screening should be performed prior to fine-needle aspiration of the lung. This includes platelet or thrombocyte counts, prothrombin time, and activated partial thromboplastin time (Burkhard et al., 2001).

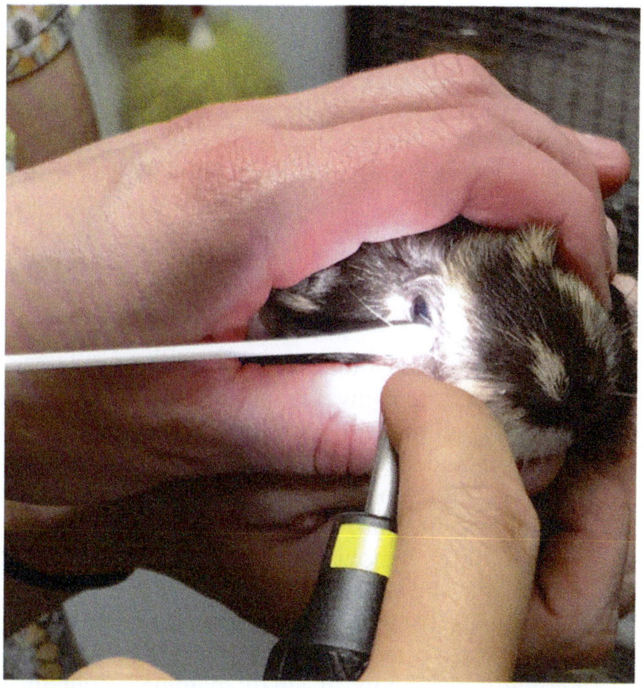

Fig. 6.2. Collection of a conjunctival sample using a sterile, moist cotton swab to gently rub along the inner eyelid.

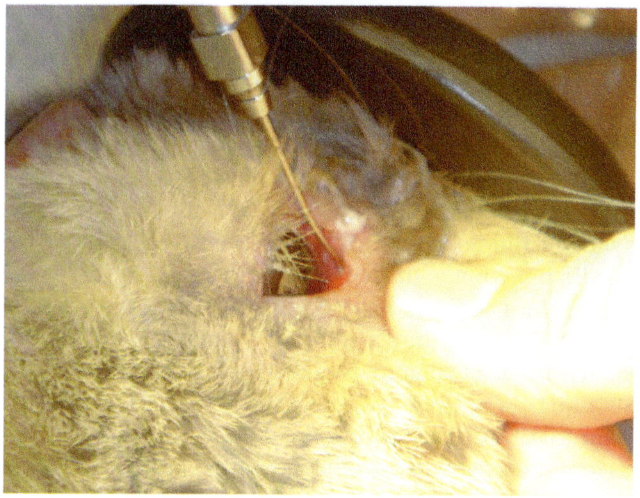

Fig. 6.3. A nasolacrimal duct flush.

Conjunctiva and Cornea

Exotic animals often present with clinical signs of conjunctivitis or keratoconjunctivitis. Evaluation of the cellular content of samples obtained from ocular lesions may be useful in the evaluation of the disease process involved. Samples can be obtained by using sterile, moist cotton swab, soft brush, or a metal ophthalmic spatula to gently scrape the margins of the cornea or conjunctiva (Figure 6.2) (Martin, 1973; Willis et al., 1997).

Collection of a cytologic sample of the nasolacrimal duct is performed using manual restraint and applying a drop of topical ophthalmic anesthetic (proparacaine hydrochloride 0.5% ophthalmic solution) into the eye. A nasolacrimal duct flush is performed using a 22-gauge, 2.5 cm, over-the-needle type intravenous catheter introduced without a stylet into the nasolacrimal duct punctum (Figure 6.3). In the rabbit, use of a rigid metal cannula is discouraged because it can potentially perforate through the wall of the duct; instead, soft Teflon catheters (27G) are preferred and should be introduced into the nasolacrimal puncta carefully to avoid causing trauma (Bedard, 2019). A syringe containing 3 mL of 0.9% sterile saline is used to flush the nasolacrimal duct, and the fluid dripping from the nose is collected into a sterile specimen container.

Cytocentrifuged preparations of nasolacrimal duct flushes are used to evaluate the cytology (Lopez et al., 2020). With an appropriate number of cells, a 100-leukocyte and 500-epithelial cell differential is performed. A total nucleated cell count can be estimated from the direct preparations of the sample using the equation 5000 × (average number of cells in ten 10× fields) = (number of cells/μL) when using a 10× objective with a field number of 26.5 mm (Lopez et. al., 2020). When more than 25 leukocytes are available on the prepared slides, a 100-leukocyte differential is performed at 50× magnification. Epithelial cells are characterized as columnar epithelial cells, intermediate cells, nucleated keratinized squamous epithelial cells, anucleated keratinized squamous epithelial cells, and goblet cells.

Synovial Fluid

Cytologic examination of the synovial fluid is part of the diagnostic steps involved in the determination of joint disease in animals. A complete synovial fluid analysis should include assessment of appearance, such as color and turbidity, protein content, viscosity, mucin clot test, nucleated cell count, differential, and cell morphology (Fisher, 2001). Synovial fluid is evaluated much like fluid evaluation; however, because of the small size of most exotic pets, the sample volume (usually limited to one or two drops) often limits the available tests.

Normally, the joints of small mammals contain a fluid volume that is too small for sampling or proper evaluation. Fluid distension of a joint may occur with certain arthropathies, allowing for collection of enough synovial fluid for evaluation. Collection of synovial fluid often requires sedation or anesthesia, and the amount required depends upon the needed restraint and comfort of the animal. The skin over the joint at the sampling site is prepared using aseptic techniques as one would use for surgery. A 22-gauge (or smaller) needle and syringe (usually a 3-cc syringe) is used to obtain the synovial fluid sample. Identification of the best site for needle insertion is made by palpation and flexion of the joint. The needle is inserted through the joint capsule and fluid is withdrawn into the syringe once the joint cavity has been entered. Negative pressure in the syringe should be removed by releasing the plunger prior to removal of the needle from the joint. The sample is then used to prepare direct films using glass microscope slides for microscopic evaluation.

Lacking a significant concentration of fibrinogen, normal synovial fluid does not clot; however, it may gel to a semisolid state when left standing at room temperature, a process termed *thixotropy* (Walberg and Loar, 2004; Meinkoth, 2022). Thixotropy will be reversed when the sample is warmed and remixed. Clotting occurs with peripheral blood contamination or marked inflammation.

The color and character of the synovial fluid should be noted during the aspiration procedure. A reddish tinge or grossly bloody color indicates either hemorrhage into the joint (hemarthrosis) or peripheral blood contamination of the sample during collection.

If blood suddenly appears in the sample, then peripheral blood contamination has likely occurred. Peripheral blood contamination of the sample will cause the sample to clot, making evaluation difficult. Placement of samples contaminated with blood into an EDTA tube to prevent clotting is advised, keeping in mind that EDTA interferes with mucin clot tests and cultures. Although EDTA is considered the best anticoagulant to prevent clot formation and preserve cell morphology, heparin can also be used if a mucin clot test is desired, also keeping in mind that it is not a permanent anticoagulant and that after 24 h cell counts may significantly decrease (Meinkoth, 2022).

Normal synovial fluid is clear or straw-colored and is viscous. A simple viscosity test can be performed on the synovial fluid sample by placing a drop of fresh fluid onto a clean glass slide. Once the fluid sample is touched with a finger or wooden applicator stick, the length of the strand formed as the fluid is lifted from the surface of the slide is measured (Figure 6.4). The viscosity of the fluid is considered reduced if the strand breaks before reaching 2 cm in length from the slide surface. Synovial fluid with poor viscosity indicates a decreased hyaluronic acid content or dilution of the fluid with an effusion, as seen in inflammatory disease.

A mucin clot test is a semiquantitative assessment of the mucin quality or the amount of polymerized hyaluronic acid in the synovial sample. One or two drops of the joint fluid are added to four to eight drops of 2% glacial acetic acid (Fisher, 2001). The mixture is allowed to stand for 1 min. If there is a normal hyaluronic acid concentration, then a firm, thick, homogenous clot (tight, ropey clot) will form (Figure 6.5). If the test is performed on a microscope slide, the clot should remain attached to the slide when the slide is inverted. Synovial fluid with reduced hyaluronic acid concentration will not form a firm, homogenous, adherent clot. The test is typically scored as good, fair, or poor with normal synovial fluid receiving a good score. Accumulation of effusion dilutes the hyaluronic acid content of the joint, resulting in a fair mucin clot score. A poor mucin clot test results with

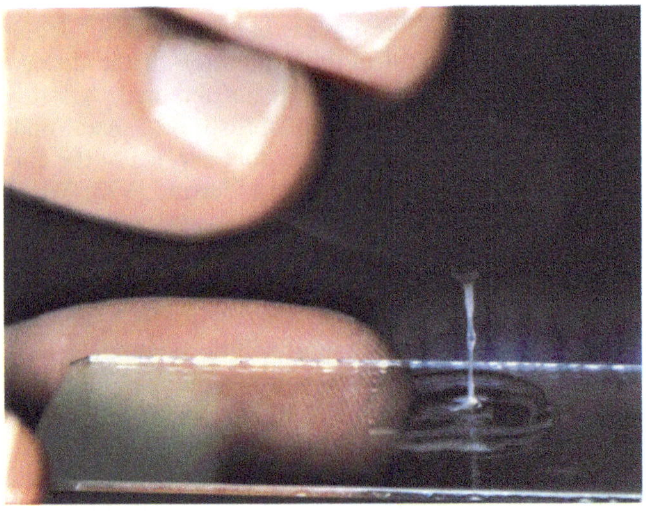

Fig. 6.4. A simple viscosity test.

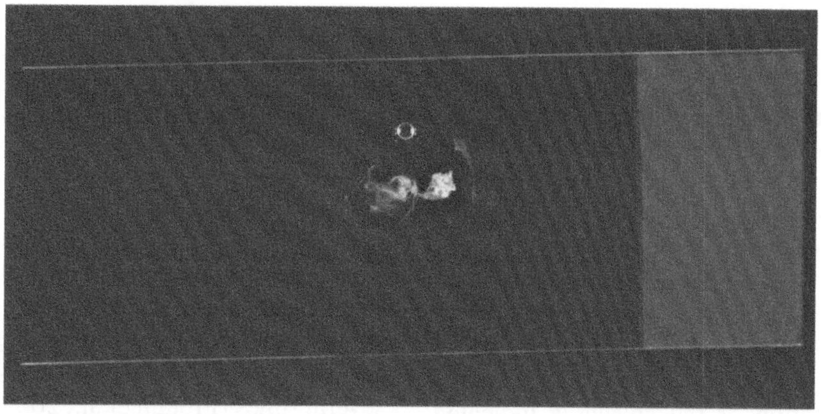

Fig. 6.5. A normal mucin clot test.

neutrophilic (heterophilic) inflammation, as the proteolytic enzymes in the inflammatory cells degrade hyaluronic acid. It should be noted that a mucin clot test is no longer run by most commercial laboratories, which prefer to assess the presence of inflammation within the joint using actual cell counts or simple direct examination of direct smears of synovial fluid (Meinkoth, 2022).

The protein content of synovial fluid is measured by refractometry. Normal synovial fluid has a low protein concentration (<2.5 g/dL). Protein content increases with inflammatory joint disease. Refractometry can significantly overestimate the protein concentration when an insufficient amount of sample is placed in an EDTA tube, resulting in high refractive index caused by the excessive amount of EDTA (Meinkoth, 2022).

Synovial fluid turbidity typically results from increased cellularity. If enough sample volume can be collected, then a cell count can be performed using the same methods as performed with peripheral blood. The cellularity of normal synovial fluid in all species is extremely low (e.g., less than 1000/μL). The total nucleated cell count of synovial fluid can be determined by (a) use of an automated hematology analyzer, (b) manual counts via the hemocytometer method, or (c) subjective assessment of cellularity based on an examination of direct smears (Dusick et al., 2014; Meinkoth, 2022). Cell counts obtained by either automated analyzers or hemocytometers can be falsely decreased due to cell clumping in the diluent due to the viscosity of the synovial fluid (Froom et al., 2013). Often, hyaluronidase is added to the synovial fluid to reduce the cell viscosity and prevent clotting to provide a more accurate cell count (Fisher, 2001).

If only a small sample volume is obtained, then an estimated cell count (subjective assessment of cellularity) can be performed on a synovial fluid film. Fluid from normal joints contains less than three cells per high-power field depending upon the thickness of the smear, which can be used as a guideline. A direct smear also allows for the evaluation of cell morphology and presence of infectious organisms.

Direct smears of synovial fluid are made by placing a small drop of well-mixed sample at one end of a glass slide and using a second spreader slide to spread out the sample in the same way that a blood film is prepared (Dusick et al., 2014). Viscous samples that spread poorly using the blood film preparation method require placing a slide on top of the slide with the sample and pulling the slides apart.

A portion of the sample should be used to inoculate culture media immediately following sampling whenever infectious joint disease is likely. If sufficient sample remains after making direct smears and inoculating culture systems, the remaining sample can be placed into either a serum tube or an EDTA tube to obtain a total nucleated cell count (Meinkoth, 2022).

Lymph Nodes

The lymphoid organs, especially the lymph nodes of mammals, are commonly sampled for cytologic examination. Biopsy of lymph nodes is indicated when the nodes are enlarged or for the evaluation of metastatic disease. Lymph nodes selected for sampling may include the submandibular (ventral to the angle of the mandible), prescapular (in front of the supraspinatus muscle on the scapula), axillary (caudal and medial to the shoulder joint), and popliteal (behind the stifle) in most mammals.

Lymph node aspirates are performed using a 22-gauge needle either alone or attached to a 3- or 6-mL syringe. The unattached needle is inserted into the lymph node and moved in several different planes to obtain a small sample inside the needle's lumen. The needle is removed from the node, and an air-filled syringe is attached to expel the sample onto the center of a glass microscope slide. If an attached syringe is used, multiple withdrawal motions of the plunger are made to create negative pressure during the sampling process. The negative pressure is released prior to withdrawal of the needle from the node to prevent the sample from entering the syringe. The syringe is removed and filled with air before reattaching it to the needle to expel the sample onto the glass slide. The sample is carefully squashed between two microscope slides before sliding them apart horizontally to prepare the cytologic specimen to minimize rupture of the lymphocytes.

Imprints of excisional biopsy samples provide a higher cellular yield and better cell preservation than do aspirates. Excessive fluid should be blotted from the freshly cut surface before making the imprint onto a glass microscope slide.

Spleen

Cytologic examination of the spleen is indicated with the presence of splenomegaly as detected by palpation, radiography, or ultrasound examination and abnormal splenic imaging. Ultrasound-guided splenic biopsy or biopsies performed during laparoscopy are two common methods for obtaining splenic samples for cytologic examination. Aspirations should be performed using a needle and syringe coated with 4% disodium EDTA to reduce the potential of sample clotting.

Liver

Cytological evaluation of hepatic tissue can provide supportive information concerning the nature of liver disease in animals. Liver biopsy provides hepatic specimens for cytological and histological evaluation to obtain a diagnosis for the clinical findings of hepatomegaly or abnormal hepatic imaging. Samples for cytologic examination are obtained using ultrasound-guided liver biopsy methods or biopsies performed during laparoscopy or celiotomy procedures. Cytologic specimens are obtained by imprints of core samples using biopsy forceps or by aspirates using fine-needle biopsy. Fine-needle aspiration biopsy techniques are performed using either a non-aspiration or an aspiration procedure.

Kidney

Cytologic examination of the kidney is performed to evaluate the cause of renomegaly or abnormal renal imaging. Samples for cytologic examination are obtained using ultrasound-guided kidney biopsy methods or biopsies performed during laparoscopy or celiotomy procedures. Cytologic specimens are obtained by imprints of samples using biopsy forceps or by aspirates using fine-needle biopsy.

Kidney aspirates are usually poorly cellular and contain peripheral blood contamination. Renal tubular epithelial cells exfoliate in clusters or as individual cells. They are round to columnar cells with abundant basophilic cytoplasm that may contain vacuoles. The nucleus is round and slightly eccentric. The nuclei of normal renal tubular epithelial cells are uniform in appearance.

Reproductive Tract

Vaginal cytology samples are typically obtained from a swab of the vagina. The sample is rolled across the surface of a glass microscope slide and allowed to air-dry prior to staining.

A preputial lavage sample is obtained for cytologic examination by gently cleansing the preputial opening prior to sample collection. In the ferret, for example, a preputial lavage is accomplished with 20 μL of sterile physiologic saline (0.9% NaCl) solution, which was introduced into the external preputial opening with a flame-smoothed pipette tip and subsequently aspirated several times (Protain et al., 2009). The preputial lavage fluid is dispensed onto a glass microscope slide, allowed to dry, and then stained with a Romanowsky stain.

Preparation for Cytologic Examination

Köhler Illumination

Critical evaluation of the hemic and cytologic specimen under the microscope requires proper illumination of the sample. Without proper alignment of the light passing through the microscope, the sample will be unevenly illuminated, creating artifacts, such as visualization of the bulb filament, glare, and shadowing, that make clear examination of the cells difficult. When the image of the light source (i.e., light bulb) is in the same plane as the image of the specimen, the uneven illumination that is created will result in areas of the viewing field being more brightly illuminated than others.

A method of illumination that uses a defocused image of the light source to illuminate the sample, commonly referred to as Köhler illumination, has been in use for decades (Köhler, 1894). The primary advantage of Köhler illumination is the reduction of image artifacts while providing high sample contrast.

Köhler alignment is the adjustment of the optical components to optimize the light and specimen image plane as viewed through the microscope. When using a binocular microscope, Köhler alignment begins by turning on the light source to a comfortable level of illumination intensity. After adjusting the inter-pupillary distance so that images from the right and left eyepieces merge into one, proceed as follows:

1. Place a microscope slide containing the stained specimen onto the microscope stage, and focus the cells using the 10× objective with the coarse focus knob of the microscope; then use the fine focus to reveal the smallest visible detail. Next, using the fine focus adjustment, focus on the cells with the 40× objective.
2. Using the substage or field diaphragm control ring, close the field diaphragm to its smallest size. (The collector (and/or field lenses) collects light from the light source and focuses it at the plane of the condenser diaphragm; thus, the light is not focused through the sample.) Bring the image of

the field diaphragm into focus with the condenser focus knob. The edges of the diaphragm should be in the same conjugate image planes as the specimen and therefore should appear in focus. The image should be a tight circle of light with the cells in focus in the center of the field. If the circle of light (position of the field diaphragm) is not centered, then use the condenser centering mechanism on the microscope (i.e., adjustment screws) to bring the light into proper position into the center of the field of view. Finally, the field diaphragm is reopened to just beyond the field of view.

3. Centering the illumination is not required for microscopes with pre-centered illumination systems. Otherwise, remove the diffuser filter from the microscope; close the aperture diaphragm on the condenser; and using a neutral density filter as a mirror to observe the filament image on the underside of the condenser, focus the filament image by moving the lamp housing in or out until it comes into sharp focus. After the filament is in focus and centered, the diffuser is replaced.

4. To adjust the condenser diaphragm, remove one of the eyepieces to allow visualization through the eyepiece tube and down toward the back of the objective. Next, adjust the aperture diaphragm so that it is just inside the exit pupil of the objective.

Köhler alignment allows the amount of light entering the sample to be adjusted without altering the wavelengths of light, which occurs when the power to the light source is reduced.

When using a microscope for cytology, the Köhler illumination should be routinely checked for correct alignment. To test the alignment of components on the light source image plane, the eyepiece is removed to observe the position of the eyepiece diaphragm. The light bulb filament and the edges of the condenser diaphragm should appear in focus.

Sample Collection

The basic equipment needed for the collection of cytologic samples includes syringes (3–12 cc), fine-gauge needles (23–20 gauge, 5/8–1.5 inch), scalpel blades (No. 10 or 11), sterile cotton swabs, sterile rubber or soft plastic tubes (i.e., feeding tubes), sterile physiologic saline, and EDTA and serum tubes without separator gel.

The techniques used for sample collection in domestic mammals also apply to exotic animals. The common cytologic techniques used in avian and reptilian medicine typically include aspirates, imprints of biopsy material, tracheal washes, crop (ingluvies) aspirates or washes in birds, gastric washes in reptiles, sinus aspirates, lung washes in reptiles, aspiration of coelomic fluid, and fecal smears.

Poor sample preparations that exhibit poor cellularity (noted as QNS, or quantity not sufficient, on cytology reports), lysed cells, excessive amounts of blood, artifacts, under-stained slides, and thick smears are not diagnostic (Meuten and Meichner, 2022). Likewise, a diagnosis is difficult to achieve when using a poorly maintained and adjusted microscope.

Sample Collection Techniques

Fine-Needle Aspiration Biopsy

Fine-needle aspiration biopsy is a cost-effective procedure that can be performed on cutaneous, subcutaneous, or internal masses and internal organs such as the liver, spleen, and kidney. The procedure can provide a cytologic sample for a rapid presumptive or definitive diagnosis and often can be repeated if necessary, with minimal trauma to the patient. Two basic techniques are typically used for this procedure: aspiration and non-aspiration. Both techniques require the following materials: a hypodermic needle (22-gauge, 1 inch is commonly used although a range of 25–20 gauge is acceptable), a syringe (3 mL or larger), and glass microscope slides.

Prior to the aspiration biopsy of vascular tissues, coating the lumen of the needle and syringe with sterile 4% disodium EDTA will reduce the risk of clot formation, which would compromise the quality of the cytologic sample (Meyer, 2001). Heparin is not recommended for use because it will alter the cell morphology of the sample (Baker and Lumsden, 2000).

When aspirating any mass, the gross morphology, location, estimated thickness, consistency, and adherence to the skin or surrounding tissues should be noted. The skin over the aspiration site should be cleansed using an alcohol swab (excessive application of alcohol should be avoided), and the alcohol is allowed to dry.

When using the aspiration technique for fine-needle aspiration biopsy, the mass is stabilized by firmly grasping it with the fingers of the free hand, and the needle with the attached syringe is quickly inserted into the mass. The syringe plunger is then retracted slightly to provide 0.5–1 cc of vacuum. While maintaining slight negative pressure (a pumping action should be avoided), the needle is advanced and retracted at different angles within the mass to ensure an adequate harvest of cells. The needle direction is changed by partially withdrawing the needle to avoid laceration of the tissue that occurs when moving the needle's direction while it is advanced (Baker and Lumsden, 2000). It is important to keep the needle tip within the lesion or tissue during sample collection.

The aspiration is completed when the sample appears in the needle hub, or when several passes within the tissue have been made and the sample is in the lumen of the needle. Avoid aspirating the sample into the lumen of the syringe because when this happens, it is often not possible to retrieve the cells for examination. When the sample has been successfully collected, release the vacuum and withdraw the needle from the tissue. If vacuum pressure is applied to the syringe during withdrawal of the needle, the sample will be aspirated into the syringe barrel, making it difficult to retrieve.

The aspirated sample is then deposited onto a glass microscope slide by detaching the needle from the syringe, filling the syringe with air, reattaching the needle, and forcing the air through the needle with the syringe. The needle point should lie against the microscope slide surface to place a small drop of the sample onto the slide. A second slide is placed onto the first, and the sample is spread between the two flat glass surfaces by pulling the slides apart in a manner similar to making bone marrow aspirate smears. Two smears containing monolayer fields of cells can be obtained using this technique.

If fluid is present during the fine-needle aspiration biopsy, the site should be completely drained, and the needle should be withdrawn. The fluid specimen should be placed in an EDTA tube for cytologic examination and other diagnostic procedures, such as bacterial culture and sensitivity testing. After the fluid has been removed from the mass, repeat the fine-needle aspiration procedure using a new needle and syringe to collect a cytologic sample from the firm tissue.

The second method of obtaining a fine-needle biopsy is sometimes referred to as the "fine-needle capillary sampling" technique or the non-aspiration fine-needle biopsy method (Orell et al., 1992; Cowell et al., 1999; Meyer, 2001). The site to be sampled is alcohol cleansed and stabilized as previously described, and a cytologic sample is obtained by inserting a needle into the lesion without an attached syringe. The needle is advanced and retracted at different angles within the tissue several times; the tip of the needle is never removed from the lesion while changing the direction (Figure 6.6). The cells are exfoliated into the lumen of the needle with this technique by capillary action.

When sampling is completed, the needle is completely withdrawn, and a syringe is attached to expel the sample from the needle lumen onto a glass slide as previously described. The advantage of this method over the aspiration method is the reduction of blood contamination when sampling highly vascular tissues. This method is especially useful for obtaining cytologic specimens from the liver, spleen, and kidney using ultrasound-guided techniques.

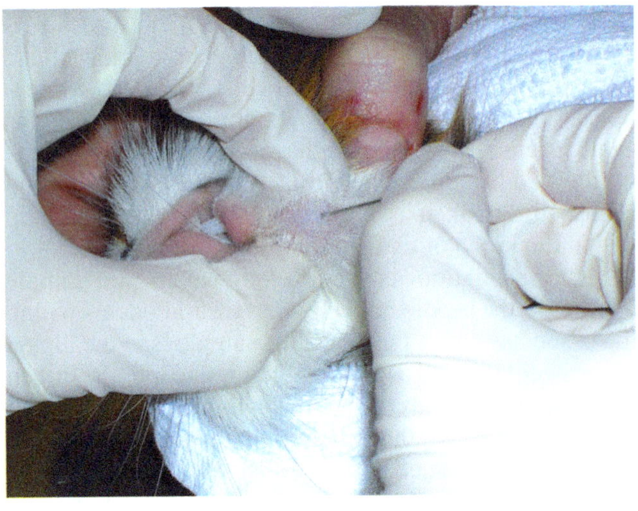

Fig. 6.6. Fine-needle biopsy, non-aspiration method.

Ultrasound-Guided Fine-Needle Aspiration

Ultrasound-guided fine-needle aspiration has been used successfully in exotic animal medicine for obtaining cytology samples in small exotic mammals, birds, and reptiles (Ramiro et al., 1993; Nordberg et al., 2000; Hauptman et al., 2001; Rademacher et al., 2012). For cytological sampling, the needle (1.5-inch, 22-gauge) can be attached to a 3-mL syringe with the plunger pulled back to 1 mL to prevent positive pressure. To visualize the needle path in the ultrasound image, the plane of the needle insertion should be brought to a 45° angle with the midline plane of the transducer. Ensure that the bevel of the needle faces the transducer as gas trapped in the bevel aids visibility. Needle visibility can be further maximized by moving the needle slightly in and out under the skin or by gently rocking the transducer to and fro to find the needle. The needle should only enter a single body cavity or organ and never cross one organ to sample another. The needle is guided to the region of interest, the sample is taken by stabbing the needle in and out of the intended lesion two to three times, and the needle removed. The needle is detached from the syringe, after which the plunger pulled back and then reattached to the needle, and the contents sprayed onto the slide and smeared. Alternatively, suction (three to four gentle suctions when the needle tip is in the area of interest) can be performed instead of the stab technique if the latter does not result in an adequate sample on the glass slide; however, this method often results in a greater degree of blood contamination in the sample. It is important not to maintain suction when removing the needle as this will result in aspirations of tissues along the needle tract.

Brush Cytology

Brush cytology is a useful, reliable, and routinely applicable method for diagnosis of the upper gastrointestinal and respiratory tract (Nishino et al., 2018). Cytology samples are obtained by gentle brushing the mucosal surfaces while avoiding bleeding under endoscopy. Whereas mucosal biopsy is invasive and increases the risk of unexpected bleeding, the use of endoscopic brush samples is noninvasive and makes it possible to avoid massive contamination of the sample (Muniraj et al., 2016).

Contact Smears (Touch Imprints or Impression Smears) and Squash Preparations (Compression Preparations)

The cells will frequently exfoliate onto a glass microscope slide from the freshly cut surface of an excised mass or tissue when contact between the slide and tissue is made. This is the basic principle used to prepare contact smears for cytologic evaluation. In general, contact smears are made by imprinting the cut surfaces of the removed masses or tissues or the cellular material obtained from the scraping of an exposed lesion in situ onto a glass microscope slide (Perman et al., 1979; Cowell et al., 1999). This technique is also useful for obtaining cytologic specimens from semisolid and mucoid samples or sample pellets obtained by centrifugation.

Imprints of solid masses should be made from a freshly cut surface that is relatively dry and free of blood. This can be achieved by using a scalpel blade to prepare a freshly cut surface, then lightly blotting the cut surface on a clean paper towel to remove excess blood and exudates. Imprint slides are then made by lightly touching the glass microscope slide to the surface of the mass to obtain monolayers of cells (Figure 6.7).

The glass slide should be lightly rolled over the tissue surface to produce a good cytologic specimen. Several imprints should be made on each slide. Avoid sliding the tissue across the slide surface or creating suction between the sample and the slide when lifting the slide from the sample in a perpendicular manner (Baker and Lumsden, 2000). The slide should be "touched" to the surface of the mass, not vice versa; the smears will often be too thick if the tissue is pressed onto the glass slide to make the imprint.

If the imprint is acellular, the cellularity of the sample may be improved by scraping the cut surface of the mass with a scalpel blade to increase the cellular exfoliation. The imprint procedure can then be repeated, or imprints can be made from the material remaining on the scalpel blade.

Cells can also be collected from tissues or exposed lesions by rubbing a dry or saline-dampened cotton swab on the surface of the lesion. The cotton swab containing the sample is then gently rolled across the surface of a glass microscope slide in one direction using light pressure to obtain the smear (Figure 6.8). This can be repeated several times across the same slide, creating several separate lines of specimen. One should avoid rolling the swab back and forth across the slide to avoid creating thick preparation or disrupting the cells.

Cytologic preparation for semisolid, mucoid, or pelleted samples involves the use of the "squash" preparation method. It should also be noted here that use of a needle greater than 21 gauge in size for fine-needle aspiration biopsy frequently results in small core biopsy that requires use of the "squash" method (Baker and Lumsden, 2000).

To perform a "squash prep," a small amount of the sample is placed on a glass microscope slide, and a second glass slide is placed over the specimen at a right angle. The specimen is gently but firmly compressed between the flat sides of the two glass slide surfaces, and then with a continuous gliding motion, the top slide is moved along the surface of the first slide carrying the material with it. This creates a smear where the sample is distributed across the first slide to create areas of cellular monolayer for cytologic evaluation.

A modification of this technique involves the placement of the upper spreader slide at a right angle to the specimen, compressing the sample as previously described, and then rotating the spreader slide 90° so that the long dimensions of the glass slides are now parallel to each other (Figures 6.9 and 6.10). Spreading of the sample is completed with a continuous motion by moving the spreader slide along the length of the bottom slide, keeping it in the same plane as where it started. This method often creates two slides for examination; however, there is a greater risk of creating cell lysis and an uneven spread of the specimen (Meyer, 2001).

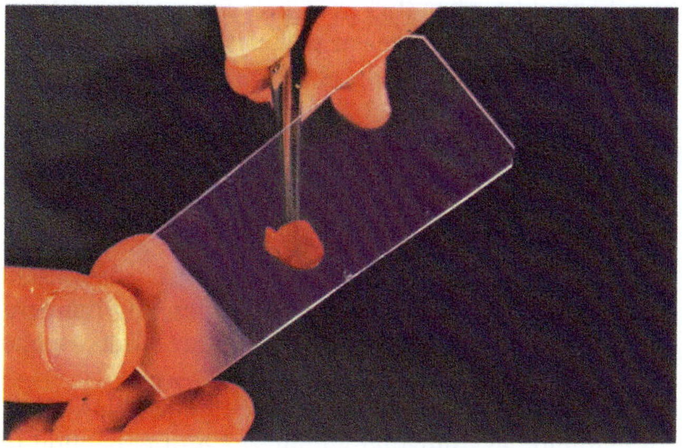

Fig. 6.7. To make a contact smear, the freshly cut surface of a tissue is imprinted onto a slide.

Fig. 6.8. A swab sample is rolled in one direction across the slide and repeated several times to create lines of the cytologic specimen.

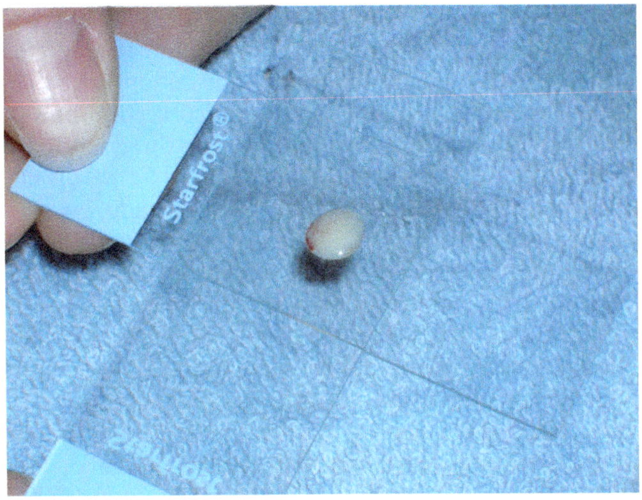

Fig. 6.9. To perform the "squash prep method," a second slide is placed at a right angle on top of the slide containing the specimen.

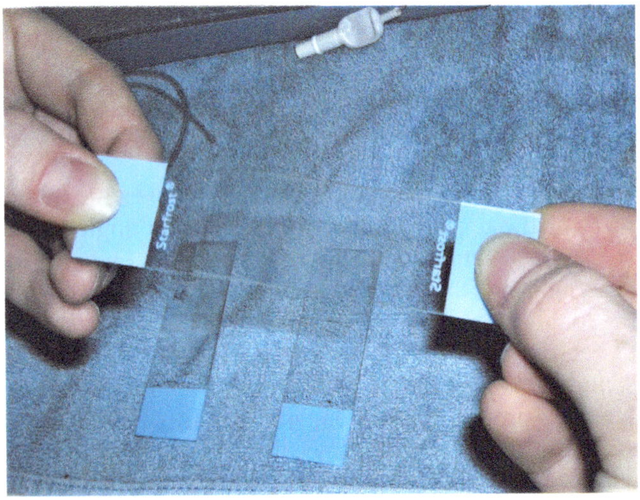

Fig. 6.10. A modification of the method shown in Figure 6.9 is to pull the two slides apart after rotating the top slide 90°.

Fluid Samples

Prior to the preparation of fluid samples for cytologic examination, macroscopic observations of fluid samples should be made and recorded. These include the source, color, appearance (e.g., bloody, mucoid, serosanguinous, watery, milky, or cloudy), and refractometer-determined total solute (protein) concentration of the fluid, as well as the presence of any odor, clots, or tissue fragments. This information will facilitate classification of effusions, such as transudates, modified transudates, or exudates.

Fluid samples are usually obtained by aspiration methods (Figure 6.11). Fluid samples should be collected using aseptic technique and an aliquot placed into two tubes: a tube containing EDTA after collection to prevent clotting of the sample and a sterile red top blood

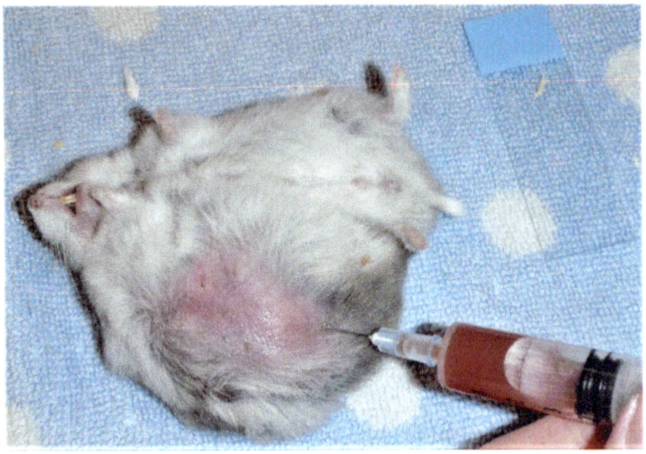

Fig. 6.11. Fine-needle aspiration biopsy from a soft tissue, fluid-filled mass from a hamster after euthanasia.

collection tube (Allison, 2022). Fluid from the EDTA tube is best for cytologic evaluation, nucleated cell counts, and total protein estimation. Fluid from the sterile red top tube may be used for bacterial or fungal culture and ancillary biochemical testing, if needed. Fluids that have a plasma-like consistency should be handled in the same manner as preparing a blood film. Direct smears should be made quickly after fluid collection from aspirated fluids with good cellularity (i.e., 10 000 cell/mL or greater) and can be prepared using the conventional wedge method or the cover-glass method commonly used for making blood films.

Mucoid samples or fluids containing clots or solid tissue fragments should be prepared using the "squash prep" method, which is described above. When preparing mucoid samples, it may be necessary to pull the slides apart using a wavy motion while separating them in order to break apart the tenacious fluid. Raised tissue fragments and clots should be removed from the surface of the slide to avoid problems with overstaining and placement of a cover slip.

Fluid samples that are composed predominantly of blood should be handled as if preparing a blood film. Preparing a buffy coat smear will also improve the diagnostic yield of such samples. To prepare a buffy coat smear, first transfer part of the sample from the EDTA tube to a microhematocrit tube. The microhematocrit tube is centrifuged in the same way that a microhematocrit is prepared in order to concentrate the buffy coat. After centrifugation, the tube is broken at the cell–plasma interface to obtain the concentrated cells located in the buffy coat area. The sample containing the concentrated cells is applied to two or three microscope slides and spread as direct smears.

Fluids with low specific gravity should be prepared for cytologic examination within 2–3 h of collection to reduce the risk of cell lysis (Meyer, 2001). If the protein content of the fluid is low, the cells may be easily washed off the slides during the staining process. Use of serum-coated slides for the preparation of such samples will facilitate the fixing of the cells to the slide (Meyer, 2001). Serum-coated slides can be made in advance by applying several drops of serum across the surface of glass microscope slides to create a film and allowing the slides to dry. After drying, the slides may be stored in the freezer to prevent bacterial growth. Slides are thawed and allowed to reach room temperature before using them to prepare cytologic specimens to prevent condensation, which will cause cell lysis.

Fluids, especially of low cellularity, should be processed immediately after collection to avoid degenerative cellular artifacts. Fluids with low cellularity may be clear or hazy, in which case both a direct smear and a concentrated preparation should be evaluated (Allison, 2022). Poorly cellular fluids and wash samples require concentration methods in order to increase the sample cellularity, which will in turn increase the number of cells available for microscopic examination. Several methods of cell concentration may be used to improve the cellularity of the sample and include margination of the cells, preparation of a sediment smear, cytocentrifugation, and sedimentation.

The first method of cell concentration would be to marginate the cells while making the smear, using the conventional two-slide wedge technique. Samples are prepared using the same two-slide wedge technique previously described for preparing blood films except that the spreader slide is advanced more slowly and is abruptly lifted from the surface of the slide near the end of the smear. It is important that the entire fluid sample applied to the slide should remain on the slide; the fluid should not be allowed to go off the end of the slide during sample preparation. If sample is lost from the end of the slide, there is a potential for the loss of diagnostic cellular material, such as clumps of neoplastic cells and large infectious agents. Marginated cells will be concentrated at the feathered end of the smear. The thinner area of the stained smear can be used to estimate cell numbers, while the thicker part near the end of the slide is used to evaluate the cell types.

The second method of concentrating cells is provided by preparation of a sediment smear following centrifugation. Following the preparation of a direct smear, an aliquot of the fluid sample is transferred to a plastic conical tube or test tube and centrifuged at a relative centrifugal force of 600 × G (gravity) for 10 min. The concentrated preparation is used to evaluate cell populations, and the direct smear is used to estimate the total nucleated cellularity. If possible, use disposable centrifuge tubes with plastic screw tops to prevent aerosolization of the sample during centrifugation. Glass tubes should not be used for the sample preparation because cells often adhere to glass surfaces and will be lost for sampling.

During centrifugation, the cellular content of the fluid is concentrated at the bottom of the tube and forms a button or pellet. After centrifugation, the clear supernatant is discarded, and the sediment is either aspirated from the tube using a disposable pipette or syringe; collected on a wire loop or cotton-tipped swab that has been premoistened by the supernatant fluid; or re-suspending the cell pellet and making a smear from the sediment in the same way that a urine sample is processed. When a pipette or syringe is used to obtain the concentrated sample, a few drops are placed on the surface of the slide and another slide is used to make the smear. If a cotton swab is used, the swab is gently rolled in one direction across the slide.

A third technique for cell concentration of fluid samples involves the use of cytocentrifugation: either a commercially available dedicated automated centrifuge, a manual converted salad spinner, or a hand-powered centrifuge used in molecular biology is employed to concentrate cells on a microscope slide (Brown et al., 2011; Moran and Galindo, 2011; Marcos et al., 2016) (Figure 6.12). This method involves the use of centrifugation to directly deposit the concentrated cells onto the glass slide while absorbing the noncellular fluid onto filter paper. The concentrated cells are located in a small circular area in the center of the slide.

A fourth cell-concentrating method is based on sedimentation (Garma-Avinã, 2004). For example, filter paper (e.g., Whatman no. 2 filter paper, Whatman International Ltd., Middlesex, UK) is cut in the shape of the slide, and a standard 2 mm paper punch is used to create a hole in the center of the filter paper. The filter paper is then placed on the slide with the hole centered on the slide. A sedimentation device is made using a base to support the microscope slide, and a clamping mechanism to firmly support a fluid column is made

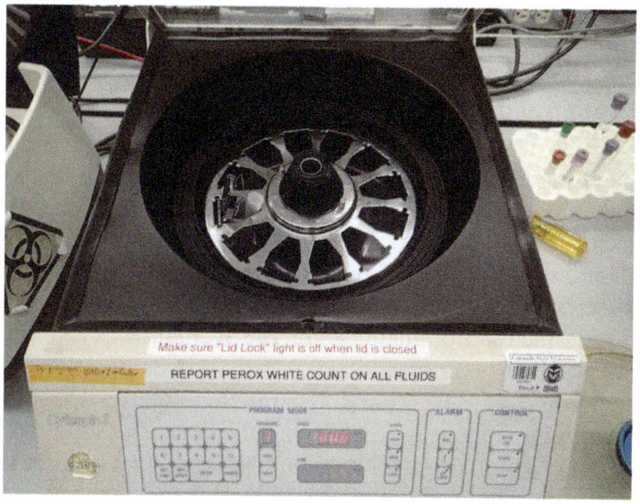

Fig. 6.12. A cytocentrifuge (Cytospin, Shandon Southern Instruments, Inc., Sewickley, PA) is designed to concentrate cells in fluid samples onto a microscope slide.

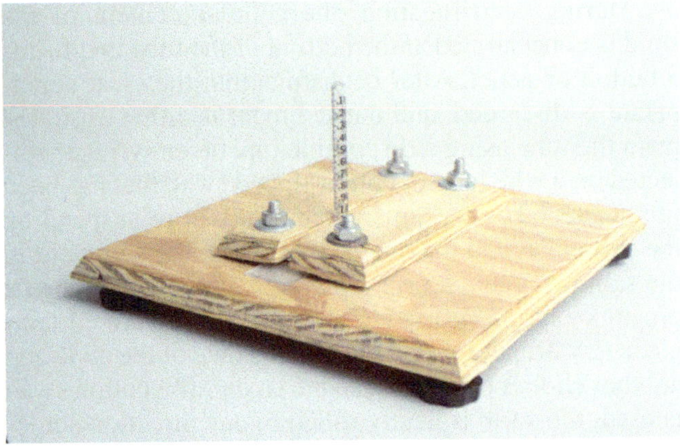

Fig. 6.13. A sedimentation apparatus made by the author using a 1-cc syringe barrel as a column to hold the liquid sample and to concentrate the cells onto a glass microscope slide. The supportive structure is made of wood, and the clamping component is made of wood, small bolts, and nuts.

from the barrel of an 1-mL syringe (which has a 2 mm diameter equal to that of the hole in the filter paper) with the tip removed (Figure 6.13). The base of the syringe barrel is positioned with the opening superimposed over the hole in the filter paper and secured to the slide with a tight seal. A small amount of fluid (e.g., 0.5 mL or less) is placed in the syringe column, and the apparatus is allowed to stand undisturbed. As the fluid falls in the column by gravity, it is absorbed by the filter paper. The cells adhere to the surface of the exposed glass slide.

After the fluid has drained, the apparatus is disassembled, and the cellular sample remaining in the 2 mm circle created by the hole in the filter paper is allowed to air-dry before staining. This method is somewhat complicated and time consuming, but has the advantage that cell morphology is better preserved compared to that of the cells concentrated using centrifugation.

Sample Preparation and Evaluation

Fixation and Staining

Once the sample has been collected and a smear has been made, the specimen must be properly fixed to the slide. The method of fixation will depend on the staining procedure used (Clark, 1981). Whenever possible, more than one smear should be made per sample to allow for specific staining procedures. For example, fresh air-dried smears are adequate for the Romanowsky stains (i.e., Wright–Giemsa stains), but proper fixation is required for other stains, as directed by the specific staining procedures. Slides should be air-dried completely, kept at room temperature, protected from formalin fumes, and stained within three days to prevent cell deterioration and staining artifacts (Allison, 2022).

A variety of stains and staining methods have been used by veterinary cytologists. Stains commonly used in veterinary medicine include Romanowsky stains, new methylene blue, and tri-chrome stains (such as Papanicolaou's and Sano's stains) (Andrews, 1971; Perman et al., 1979; Cowell et al., 1999; Baker and Lumsden, 2000).

Romanowsky-type stains (Wright's, Giemsa, Wright–Giemsa, Leishman's, and May–Grünwald–Giemsa stains) are polychromatic stains made up of a mixture of basic and acidic dyes dissolved in methyl alcohol that are especially useful in practice settings. Wright's stain (Wright's Stain Solution, Fisher Scientific) is the standard stain used to evaluate blood films in human and veterinary medical laboratories. Other Romanowsky-type stains used either alone or in combination include the so-called quick or stat stains. Advantages of the quick or stat stains include a simple staining procedure, rapid staining time (usually 20 s, which allows for rapid examination of the specimen), and good staining quality. The slides produced may be retained as permanent slides to be used as references for comparison with other cytologic samples.

Whereas the Romanowsky-type stains are commonly used in veterinary cytopathology, the tri-chrome Papanicolaou and bi-chrome hematoxylin and eosin (H&E) stains are more commonly used in human cytopathology. Romanowsky-type stains are composed of reduced eosin and methylene blue in various buffer formulations, and highlight the cytoplasm and extracellular matrix well, but provide little nuclear detail. By contrast, Papanicolaou stains are composed of hematoxylin, Orange G, eosin, and Light Green SF in proportions that vary depending on the manufacturer and require cell fixation for adequate stain penetration and provide excellent nuclear and nucleolar detail, but do not stain the cytoplasm well (Jorundsson et al., 1999; Bienzle et al., 2012).

New methylene blue stain is an inexpensive stain used as a wet-mount preparation. This stain is often used for the evaluation of urine sediment and cytologic specimens and is an excellent stain for evaluating cell nuclei, bacteria, fungal hyphae, yeast, and lipids. It is also useful for the detection of reticulocytes. New methylene blue will not stain erythrocyte cytoplasm or eosinophil granules, making it difficult to evaluate those cells. New methylene blue does not provide for a permanent slide to preserve cytologic specimens.

Special staining procedures may be required to demonstrate specific etiologic agents or cellular structures. Commonly used special stains include Gram's stain for bacteria, acid-fast stain for mycobacteria and cryptosporidium, Giménez stain for chlamydia, and rickettsiae, Macchiavello's stain for chlamydia, and Sudan stains for fat. Staining procedures for the stains used in this text are listed in Appendix A.

When using stains, especially the quick stains, the solutions should be changed frequently. The frequency of refreshing the staining solutions will depend upon the number of slides being stained and the amount of contamination appearing in the staining solution as a result of cells and debris coming off the slides. For this reason, two sets of staining stations are recommended: one for relatively "clean" samples, such as blood films, wash samples, effusions, and organ biopsies, and a second set for "dirty" specimens, such as abscesses, fecal samples, and skin scrapings.

Evaluation of the Cytologic Sample

Once the smears have been stained, they are ready for microscopic examination. Scanning (40× or 100×) and low (200×) magnifications are used initially to obtain a general impression of the smear quality. At these magnifications, the examiner can estimate the smear cellularity, examine cellular aggregates, identify large infectious agents (e.g., yeast and fungal elements), and determine the best locations for examination at higher magnifications (monolayers of cells). High-dry (400× or 500×) and oil-immersion (500× and 1000×) magnifications are used to examine cell structure, bacteria, and other small structures (e.g., cellular inclusions).

Cellular distribution should also be noted when scanning the entire smear. The conventional blood film technique for making cytology slides often causes margination of bacteria, macrophages, and large neoplastic cells at the periphery of the smear. For this reason, the peripheral margins of smears made from fluid samples should be examined closely.

Cellular interpretation is best made in monolayer areas of cells because the thickness of the smear will affect the appearance of the cells and the quality of the cellular sample. Areas containing a heavy accumulation of cells and background material will not allow the cells to expand on the slide, and the cells appear smaller and denser compared to the same cell type in thinner areas of the smear.

Optimum evaluation of cytologic specimens requires knowledge of the origin of the sample, the method of sample collection, and normal cellular morphology. Knowledge of the origin of the sample is required since cytologic specimens lack the tissue architecture used to identify the specimen during histologic evaluation. Knowledge of the method of sample collection is beneficial since contact smears tend to provide samples with higher cellularity and better cellular association than do smears made from aspirates. Knowledge of normal cellular morphology is important because the detection of abnormal cellular responses requires knowledge of normal cellular components. Establishing a reference file of contact and aspirate smears from various normal tissues and of normal and abnormal cellular responses is a good way to familiarize oneself with cellular morphology and cytodiagnosis.

Cytodiagnosis involves the examination of individual cells in the smear, with an emphasis on the general cellular and nuclear features. Important cellular features include the sample cellularity (the number of cells seen in the sample), cellular distribution, size, and shape of the various cells, and the cytoplasmic appearance of the cells.

The number of cells in a sample depends on the origin of the sample (e.g., epithelial tissue tends to provide samples higher in cellularity than samples from mesenchymal tissue), sampling technique (e.g., contact smears are more cellular than aspirates), use of concentration procedures, and the nature of the lesion.

Cellular distribution is important to note when performing cytodiagnosis. Certain cells tend to occur singly (e.g., mesenchymal cells), and others occur in aggregates (e.g., epithelial cells). Cells may occur in different types of aggregates. Cells regularly arranged in relationship to each other occur in sheet-like aggregates, suggesting normal cellular polarity in the parent epithelium. Cells with indistinct cell boundaries that are irregularly arranged in relationship to each other have a syncytial arrangement. This arrangement is suggestive of altered polarity in the parent epithelium and is considered an abnormal finding.

The size and shape of the cells are important, but can be affected by the quality of the smear. In general, monolayer areas of cells provide the best locations for evaluating cell size and shape. Cells may be larger or smaller than normal in diseased states, and a variation in the size of cells in aggregates is characteristic of some neoplastic conditions. It is not uncommon to refer to cell size in association with cells of known sizes (e.g., erythrocytes or granulocytes).

The shape of the cell is related to function, cell membrane "rigidity," cytoplasmic viscosity, surface tension, microtubules in the cell, and pressures exerted by adjacent cells. Some cells have a relatively constant shape (e.g., epithelial cells), whereas others have a variable shape (e.g., macrophages). The shape of cells can appear polygonal, spherical, cuboidal, columnar, prismatic, spindle-shaped, or elongated. For example, epithelial cells are usually polygonal, spherical, cuboidal, or columnar, whereas connective tissue cells tend to be long and thin (spindle-shaped and elongated) (Figure 6.14). The epithelial cells obtained from traumatic exfoliation may differ in shape from the same cells that have spontaneously shed from the surface (these tend to be spherical). Abnormal cells may or may not resemble their normal precursor cells.

The cytoplasmic features of a cell indicate the origin, function, and differentiation of that cell. Important features of the cytoplasm that should be evaluated include the cytoplasmic margin, color, and inclusions. A distinct cell margin is a feature of epithelial cells, whereas an indistinct margin is the characteristic of connective tissue cells. Poorly differentiated epithelial cells tend to have poorly defined cellular margins. The color

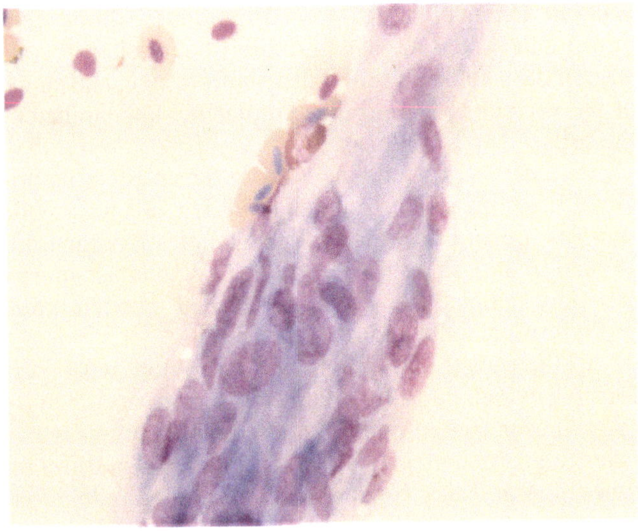

Fig. 6.14. Mesenchymal cells from a sarcoma as an example of connective tissues cells, which tend to be long and thin (spindle-shaped and elongated), Wright–Giemsa stain (100× oil).

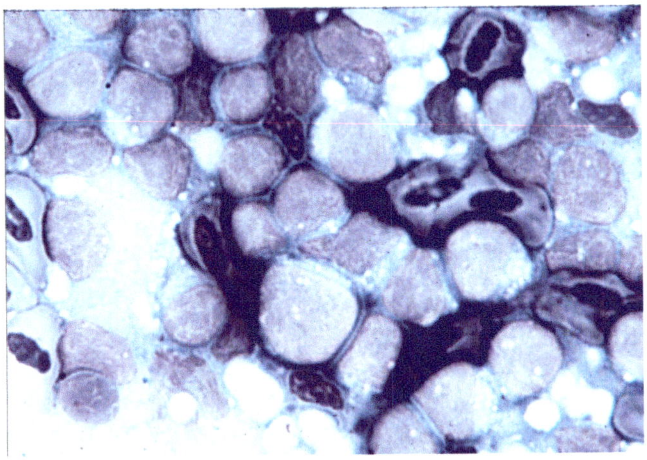

Fig. 6.15. The large lymphocyte in the lower center part of the image reveals a uniformly finely granular nuclear chromatin pattern, Wright–Giemsa stain (100× oil).

and appearance of the cytoplasm may be affected by the metabolic status of the cell, age, method of fixation, and staining method. Cytoplasmic granulation and vacuolation are seen in secretory cells and are suggestive of the cell origin.

All cells from lower vertebrates, such as birds and reptiles, contain a nucleus except for the squamous cells originating from the surface of stratified squamous epithelium. The appearance of the nucleus reflects the reproductive potential of the cell; therefore, important nuclear features to note include the size, shape, and position of the nucleus within the cell, the number of nuclei present, the chromatin pattern present within the nucleus, the appearance of the nucleoli, and the presence of mitotic figures.

The nuclear size is often evaluated in relation to the amount of cytoplasm and is indicated as the nuclear to cytoplasmic ratio (N:C ratio). Mature, well-differentiated epithelial cells tend to have small nuclei (a low N:C ratio), whereas malignant, poorly differentiated epithelial cells frequently have large nuclei (a high N:C ratio).

The shape of the nucleus is often related to the shape of the cell (e.g., an elongated cell tends to have an elongated or compressed nucleus). The nuclear shape of some cells, however, is unrelated to the cell shape (e.g., neutrophils and heterophils with lobed nuclei). The nucleus is frequently centrally located in epithelial cells, but may be eccentric if displaced by secretory granules or vacuoles. Most normal cells have a single nucleus; however, some normal cells may contain multiple nuclei (e.g., hepatocytes are often binucleated and osteoclasts are multinucleated).

The nuclear chromatin patterns should be described when performing cytodiagnosis. The nuclear chromatin pattern that is present may indicate cellular immaturity or an abnormality (e.g., neoplasia). The patterns commonly noted include uniformly fine granular chromatin, finely granular chromatin with irregular distribution, uniformly coarse granular chromatin, and coarsely granular chromatin with irregular distribution (Figure 6.15). The finer chromatin patterns generally indicate nuclear immaturity. Some nuclei (e.g., the nuclei of mature lymphocytes) often contain one or larger, prominent chromatin clumps called chromocenters or false nucleoli.

Mitotic figures indicate cells undergoing active division. The appearance of mitotic figures can be a normal cellular feature of some tissues (e.g., bone marrow and liver) if found in low numbers. The characteristic arrangement of the chromatin indicates the stage of mitosis (i.e., prophase, metaphase, or anaphase).

The appearance of the nucleoli should be noted during cellular interpretation. Nucleoli appear as clear, circular spaces inside the nucleus of the cells stained with Wright's stain. Many normal cells often contain one or more small nucleoli. Large or irregular nucleoli are considered abnormal. Nuclei with numerous nucleoli (i.e., greater than five) are also considered to be abnormal.

The staining quality of the background of the slide should be noted, because the characteristics of the noncellular background of a smear may provide clues to the nature of the material being examined. Smears containing many secretory cells may have heavy background material due to the accumulation of the secretory product. A finely granular background in the smears of the inflammatory exudates stained with new methylene blue suggests an increase in protein content. A coarsely granular background is present in the smears containing high amounts of mucopolysaccharides (e.g., mucin) when stained with Wright's stain. The presence of bacteria, crystals, lipid droplets, nuclear materials from ruptured cells, and foreign material (e.g., plant cells, pollen, talcum, or starch crystals) should be noted as well.

Cytologic samples often contain variable amounts of peripheral blood. Excessive peripheral blood contamination of the sample will dilute and mask the diagnostic cells, making the cytologic interpretation difficult.

Basic Cytologic Responses

Many veterinarians are familiar with mammalian cytodiagnosis, especially with the common domestic species, and much has been written on the subject. The cytologic responses of lower vertebrates, especially birds and reptiles, are similar to those of mammals. When examining a cytologic specimen, the cytologist attempts to classify the predominant cellular response as a representative of inflammation, malignant neoplasia, tissue hyperplasia or benign neoplasia, or normal cellular elements. Two or more basic types of cellular responses may occur simultaneously. An example is the appearance of a secondary inflammatory response superimposed on a primary neoplastic lesion, which is seen in a cytologic sample from an ulcerated neoplasm. Once the basic cytologic response has been determined, an attempt to classify the response in a subcategory should be made. For example, inflammatory lesions of birds and reptiles have subcategories of heterophilic, mixed-cell, or macrophagic inflammation. Neoplastic lesions can be further classified as mesenchymal tissue-derived, epithelial-glandular tissue-derived, a discrete cell, or poorly differentiated neoplasm.

References

Allison RW. 2022. Inflammation and infectious agents. In: Thrall MA (ed), *Veterinary Hematology, Clinical Chemistry, and Cytology*, 3rd edn. Ames, IA: Wiley-Blackwell, in press.

Andrews GS. 1971. Exfoliative cytology. In: Andrews GS (ed), *Exfoliative Cytology*. Springfield, IL: Charles C. Thomas.

Baker R, Lumsden JH. 2000. Cytopathology techniques and interpretation. In: Baker R, Lumsden JH (eds), *Color Atlas of the Dog and Cat*. St. Louis, MO: Mosby.

Bedard KM. 2019. Ocular surface disease of rabbits. *Vet Clin Exot Anim* 22:1–14.

Bienzle D, Wood D, Jacobs RM. 2012. What's in a stain? *Vet Clin Pathol* 41(1):6–7.

Brown J, Theis L, Kerr L, et al. 2011. A hand-powered, portable, low-cost centrifuge for diagnosing anemia in low-resource settings. *Am J Trop Med Hyg* 85:327–332.

Burkhard, MJ, Valenciano A, Barger A. 2001. *Respiratory tract*. In: Raskin RE, Meyer D (eds), *Atlas of Canine and Feline Cytology*. Philadelphia, PA: WB Saunders.

Clark G. 1981. Staining. In: Clark G (ed), *Staining Procedures*, 4th edn. Baltimore, MD: Williams & Wilkins.

Cowell RL, Tyler RD, Meinkoth JH. 1999. Diagnostic cytology and hematology of the dog and cat. In: Cowell RL, Tyler RD, Meinkoth JH (eds), *Diagnostic Cytology and Hematology of the Dog and Cat*, 2nd edn. St. Louis, MO: Mosby.

Dusick A, Young KM, Muir P. 2014. Relationship between automated total nucleated cell count and estimation of cells on direct smears of canine synovial fluid. *Vet J* 202:550–554.

Frezoulis PS, Angelidou E, Diakou A, et al. 2017. Optimization of fecal cytology in the dog: comparison of three sampling methods. *J Vet Diagn Invest* 29(5):767–771.

Fisher, DJ. 2001. *Musculoskeletal system*. In: Raskin RE, Meyer D (eds), *Atlas of Canine and Feline Cytology*. Philadelphia, PA: WB Saunders.

Froom P, Diab A, Barak M. 2013. Automated evaluation of synovial fluid and ascitic fluid with the ADVIA 2120 hematology analyzer. *Am J Clin Pathol* 140:828–830.

Garma-Avinã A. 2004. An inexpensive sedimentation chamber for the preparation of cytologic specimens of cerebrospinal fluid. *J Vet Diagn Invest* 16:585–587.

Hauptman K, Tichy F, Knotek Z. 2001. Clinical diagnostics of hepatopathies in small mammals: evaluation of importance of individual methods. *Acta Vet Brno* 70:297–311.

Jorundsson E, Lumsden JH, Jacobs RM. 1999. Rapid staining techniques in cytopathology: a review and comparison of modified protocols for hematoxylin and eosin, Papanicolaou and Romanowsky stains. *Vet Clin Pathol* 28:100–108.

Köhler A. 1894. New method of illumination for photomicrographical purposes. *J Roy Microsc Soc* 14:261–262.

Lopez GT, Moore AR, Rao S, et al. 2020. Characterization of cells collected from nasolacrimal duct flush samples in healthy rabbits (*Oryctolagus cuniculus*). *J Exotic Pet Med* 35:58–62.

Marcos R, Santos M, Marrinhas C, et al. 2016. Technical report: Cytocentrifuge preparation in veterinary cytology: a quick, simple, and affordable manual method to concentrate low cellularity fluids. *Vet Clin Pathol* 45(4):725–731.

Martin, CL. 1973. Conjunctivitis differential diagnosis and treatment. *Vet Clin North Am (Small Anim Pract)* 3:367.

Meinkoth J. 2022. Cytology of synovial fluid. In: Thrall MA (ed), *Veterinary Hematology, Clinical Chemistry, and Cytology*, 3rd edn. Ames, IA: Wiley-Blackwell, in press.

Meuten DJ, Meichner K. 2022. Inflammation and infectious agents. In: Thrall MA (ed), *Veterinary Hematology, Clinical Chemistry, and Cytology*, 3rd edn. Ames, IA: Wiley-Blackwell, in press.

Meyer DJ. 2001. The acquisition and management of cytology specimens. In: Raskin R, Meyer D (eds), *Atlas of Canine and Feline Cytology*. Philadelphia, PA: WB Saunders.

Moran P, Galindo J. 2011. A practical home-made microcentrifuge for teaching purposes. *Biochem Mol Biol Educ* 39:298–299.

Muniraj F, Siddaraju N, Sistla SC. 2016. Role of brush cytology in the diagnosis of neoplastic and nonneoplastic upper gastrointestinal lesions. *Cytopathology* 27(6):407–417.

Nishino K, Nishida A, Inoue R, et al. 2018. Analysis of endoscopic brush samples identified mucosa-associated dysbiosis in inflammatory bowel disease. *J Gastroenterol* 53:95–106.

Nordberg C, O'Brian RT, Paul-Murphy J, et al. 2000. Ultrasound examination and guided fine-needle aspiration of the liver in Amazon parrots (*Amazona* species). *J Avian Med Surg* 14:180–184.

Orell SR, Sterrett GF, Walters M, et al. 1992. Manual and atlas of fine needle aspiration cytology. In: Orell SR, Sterrett GF, Walters M, et al. (eds), *Manual and Atlas of Fine Needle Aspiration Cytology*. New York: Churchill Livingstone.

Perman V, Alsaker RD, Riis RC. 1979. Cytology of the dog and cat. In: Perman V, Alsaker RD, Riis RC (eds), *Cytology of the Dog and Cat*. South Bend, IN: American Animal Hospital Association.

Protain HJ, Kutzler MA, Valentine BA. 2009. Assessment of cytologic evaluation of preputial epithelial cells as a diagnostic test for detection of adrenocortical disease in castrated ferrets. *Am J Vet Res* 70(5):619–623.

Rademacher N, Gaschen L, Tully TN. 2012. Clinical technique: Ultrasound-guided fine-needle aspirate in ferrets *J Exotic Pet Med* 21:235–237.

Ramiro I, Ackerman N, Schumacher J. 1993. Ultrasound-guided percutaneous liver biopsy in snakes. *Vet Radiol Ultrasound* 34:452–454.

Rudorf H, Brown P. 1998. Ultrasonography of laryngeal masses in six cats and one dog. *Vet Radiol Ultrasound* 39:430–434.

Smallwood CJ, Zenoble RD. 1993. Biopsy and cytologic sampling of the respiratory tract. *Semin Vet Med Surg* 8:250–257.

Teske E, Stokhof AA, Van Den Ingh TSGAM. 1991. Transthoracic needle aspiration biopsy of the lung in dogs with pulmonic diseases. *J Am Animal Hosp Assoc* 27:289–285.

Walberg J, Loar AS. 2004. Cytology and hematology of small mammals. In: Carpenter J, Quesenberry K (eds), *Ferrets, Rabbits, and Rodents Clinical Medicine and Surgery*. St. Louis: Saunders Elsevier.

Willis M, Bounous DI, Hirsh S, et.al. 1997. Conjunctival brush cytology: evaluation of a new cytological collection technique in dogs and cats with a comparison to conjunctival scraping. *Vet Comp Ophthalmol* 7:74–81.

Wood EF, O'Brien RT, Young KM. 1998. Ultrasound-guided fine-needle aspiration of focal parenchymal lesions of the lung in dogs and cats. *J Vet Intern Med* 12:338–342.

7 Mammalian Cytodiagnosis

Normal Mammalian Cytology

Proper evaluation of cytologic preparations is dependent upon the quality of the sample. Important features of high-quality preparations include adequate thickness providing plenty of monocellular areas for evaluation, good cell morphology, and proper staining (Sapierzyński et al., 2017).

Cells observed in cytological specimens can generally be classified by origin into one of four tissue groups: hemic, epithelial-glandular, connective, or nervous. Cells derived from hemic (blood and blood-forming) tissue are found in peripheral blood, bone marrow, and ectopic hematopoietic sites in various organs (e.g., the spleen and liver). The evaluation of cells from hemic tissue has been previously discussed in the hematology and bone marrow sections of this text (Chapters 3 and 4). It is important that the cytologist become familiar with cells from hemic tissue since many of these cells are important features of various cytological responses.

Cells from epithelial and glandular tissues tend to exfoliate easily and provide a cytological specimen of good cellularity. These cohesive cells often appear in tight sheets or clumps, are relatively uniform in appearance, and have distinct cell boundaries (Figures 7.1 and 7.2). Epithelial cells can vary in shape, but in general they tend to have abundant cytoplasm, distinct cytoplasmic borders, and small nuclei. The nucleus tends to be round or oval with a uniformly finely granular chromatin, and prominent small nucleoli may be present. Mature squamous epithelial cells from the outer layer of stratified squamous epithelium are polygonal, whereas other epithelial cells may be round, oval, cuboidal, or columnar. Epithelial cells that have shed spontaneously from epithelial surfaces often appear round or oval instead of polygonal. Epithelial cells from secretory epithelium tend to be cuboidal or columnar in shape and contain cytoplasmic granules or vacuoles. Cuboidal epithelial cells have comparable height and width, whereas columnar epithelial cells are taller than they are wide.

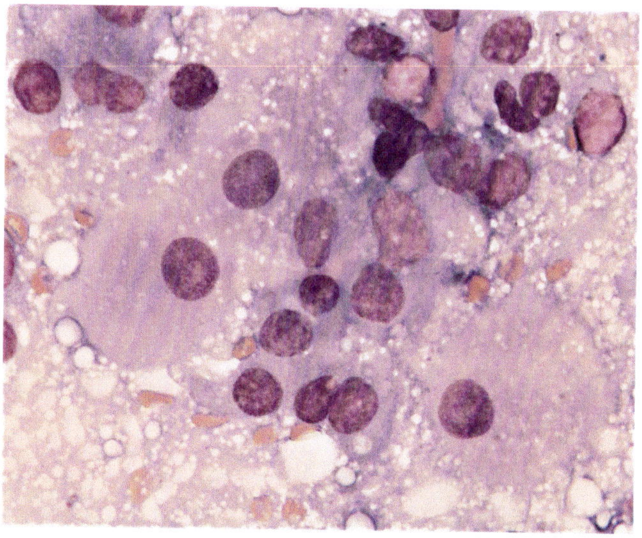

Fig. 7.1. Epithelial cells in an imprint of an adrenal mass in a ferret (*Mustela putorius furo*), Wright–Giemsa stain (100× oil).

Mesenchymal cells tend to exfoliate poorly and provide poorly cellular cytological specimens. In normal tissue and benign lesions, it is not uncommon to see only one or two cells on a slide. Mesenchymal cells typically exfoliate singly rather than in cellular aggregates. Traumatic exfoliation is often required to obtain a significant number of cells for proper evaluation. Connective tissue cells have variable shapes, indistinct cytoplasmic margins, and variable cytoplasmic volumes and nuclear shapes, depending on their origin (Figures 7.3a and 7.3b).

Exotic Animal Hematology and Cytology, Fifth Edition. Terry W. Campbell and Krystan R. Grant.

Companion website: www.wiley.com/go/campbell/exotic

They are commonly spindle shaped with wispy cytoplasmic borders and an oval nucleus. Cells derived from the nervous system are rarely seen on cytological specimens. Deeply basophilic stellate cells with cytoplasmic projections may be of nervous tissue origin.

Round cells, such as lymphocytes, readily exfoliate resulting in highly cellular samples. These cells are round with a scant to moderate rim of basophilic cytoplasm. Although unlike epithelial cells, round cells are not cohesive; however, at times, they can occur in sheets that resemble those of epithelial cells.

Digestive Tract

The oral cavity is lined with cornified squamous epithelium, and the esophagus with noncornified stratified squamous epithelium. Normal cytology of the mouth and oropharynx is predominated by superficial and intermediate squamous epithelial cells. These cells have keratinized cytoplasm and may be anucleate or contain a small, round nucleus (Figure 7.4). These cells often exfoliate singly, are angular, polygonal in shape, contain a condensed pyknotic nucleus, and demonstrate varying degrees of cornification. Cells that are highly cornified typically possess angular or folded cytoplasmic margins and are typically anucleated (Figure 7.5). Intermediate squamous epithelial

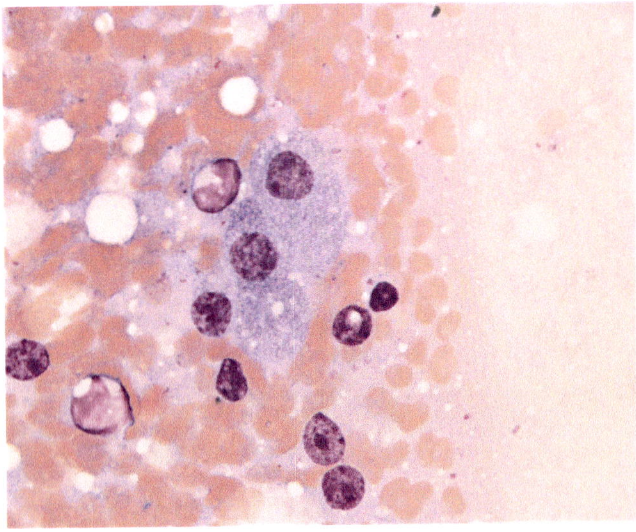

Fig. 7.2. Hepatocytes in a fine-needle aspiration biopsy of the liver in a ferret (*Mustela putorius furo*), Wright–Giemsa stain (100× oil).

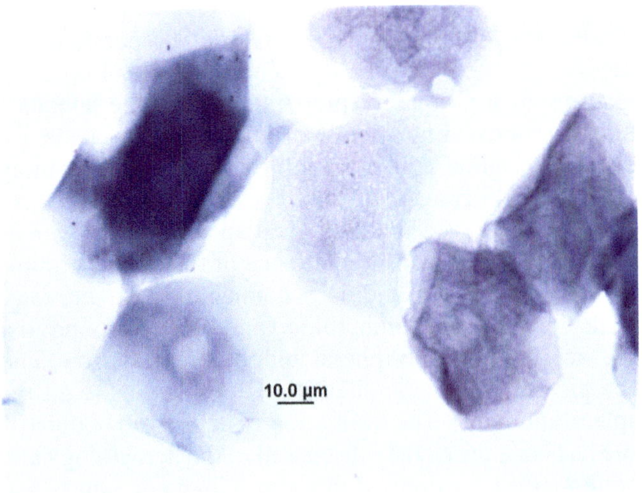

Fig. 7.4. Mature squamous epithelial cells, Wright–Giemsa stain (100× oil).

(a) (b)

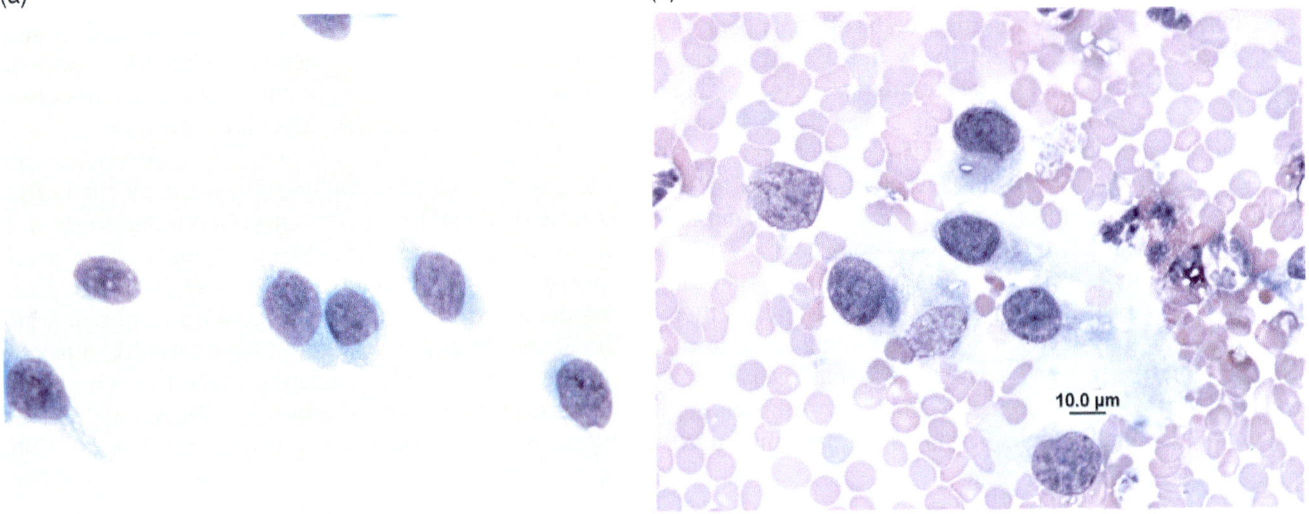

Fig. 7.3. (a) Mesenchymal cells in a fine-needle aspiration biopsy of a mass on the lip of a rabbit (*Oryctolagus cuniculus*), Wright–Giemsa stain (100× oil). (b) Mesenchymal cells in a fine-needle aspiration biopsy of a uterine mass in an African hedgehog (*Atelerix albiventris*), Wright–Giemsa stain (100× oil).

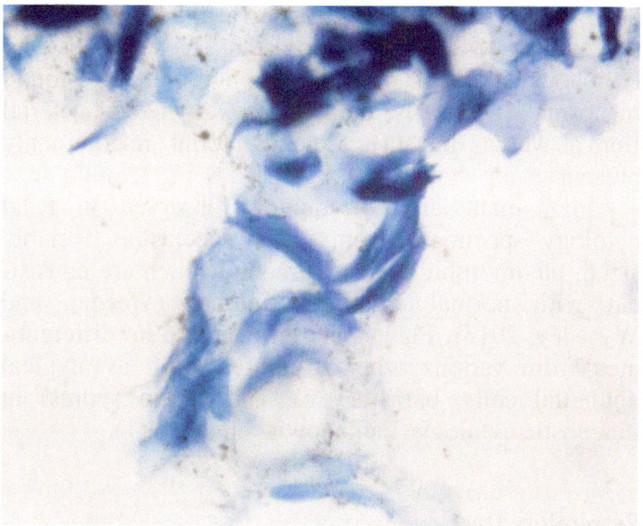

Fig. 7.5. Highly cornified squamous epithelial cells that have exfoliated as elongated clusters of cells called keratin bars, Wright–Giemsa stain (100× oil).

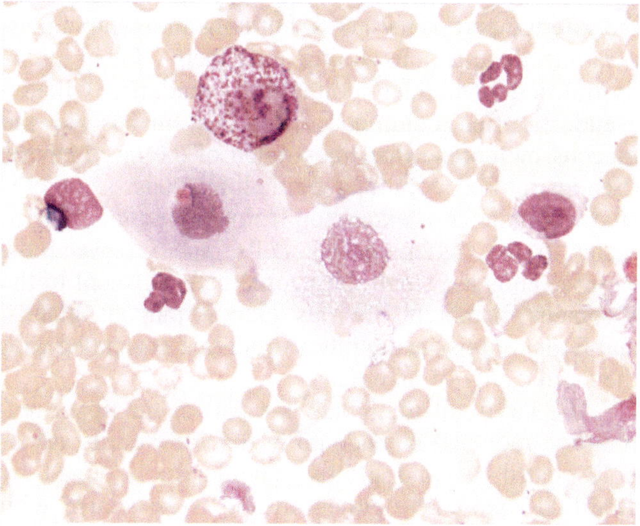

Fig. 7.6. Intermediate squamous epithelial cells as contaminates likely from the oral cavity in a tracheal wash from a guinea pig (*Cavia porcellus*), Wright–Giemsa stain (100× oil).

cells are common in normal esophageal specimens. Intermediate squamous epithelial cells often occur in sheets and are oval to polygonal in shape, have a low nuclear to cytoplasmic (N:C) ratio, and possess an oval, centrally located vesicular nucleus with a finely granular chromatin (Figure 7.6). These cells typically do not have folded cytoplasmic margins. Basal cells may be seen in normal cytology samples if traumatic exfoliation occurs during sample collection. Basal cells are cells that are normally found adjacent to the basement membrane and are smaller in size than intermediate cells. These cells are typically round and contain a deeply basophilic cytoplasm, eccentric nuclei, and a high N:C ratio.

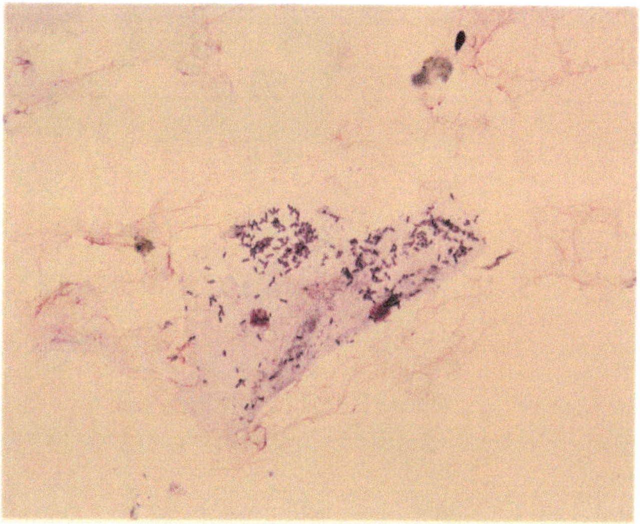

Fig. 7.7. Extracellular bacteria associated with squamous epithelial cells, Wright–Giemsa stain (100× oil).

The oropharynx has normal flora as part of its normal cytology; therefore, it is common to identify bacteria in the cytologic sample. Generally, a mixed population of bacteria is observed, and several extracellular bacteria made up of a variety of morphological types are often associated with squamous epithelial cells in normal cytological samples from the upper alimentary tract (Figure 7.7). Additionally, a moderate amount of background debris and foreign material (e.g., plant fibers and other material entering the mouth) is often present in samples obtained from the alimentary tract of animals.

A healthy stomach consists of an epithelial lining with a cytology that reveals mucosal epithelial cells. The mucosa of the stomach is lined with columnar epithelial cells containing moderate amounts lightly basophilic or eosinophilic cytoplasm, and oval to round nuclei with dispersed chromatin. Columnar epithelial cells tend to exfoliate in clusters of uniform-appearing cells. These cells produce mucin; therefore, a variable amount of mucus is usually found in the background, which appears as variably staining amorphous material. The fundic region of the stomach consists of round epithelial cells (the parietal and chief cells). Thus, in mammalian gastric samples, the larger, rounded parietal cells, which contain abundant pale eosinophilic cytoplasm, and the smaller chief cells, which contain lightly basophilic granular or microvesicular cytoplasm, may be seen (Andreasen et al., 2001). These cells may also be identified in gastric samples of other animals. Mucus mixed with normal flora is a common finding. Spiral bacteria, which may potentially be *Helicobacter*-like (e.g., H. *mustelae* of ferrets) bacteria, are rarely associated with the cells or mucus in the sample.

Cytological specimens of the intestinal mucosa are obtained by biopsy via endoscopy or exploratory

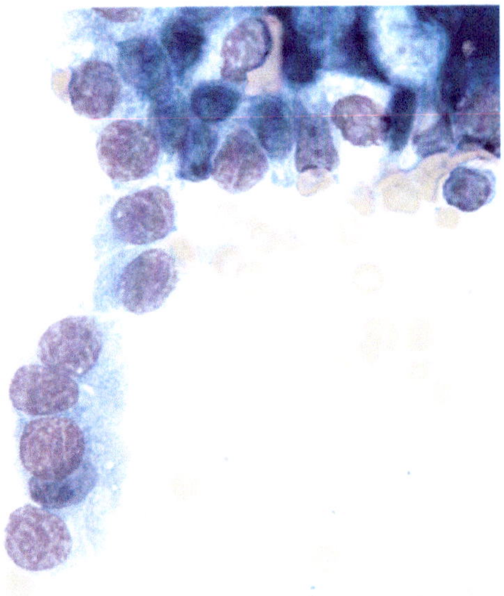

Fig. 7.8. Columnar epithelial cells in an intestinal biopsy from a lion (*Panthera leo*), Wright–Giemsa stain (100× oil). Source: Image from Campbell and Grant (2010, p. 153).

surgery. Ultrasound-guided fine-needle aspiration biopsy of intestinal lesions is another possible sampling method (Bertram et al., 2019). The small intestine is composed of columnar epithelial cells (frequently containing small, discrete vacuoles), goblet cells, and occasionally lymphoid cells from Peyer's patches. Therefore, the normal cytologic specimens contain columnar epithelial cells and goblet cells. The mucosal columnar epithelial cells often exfoliate in uniform clusters with the nuclei lined in rows (Figure 7.8). Individual cells contain a moderate amount of lightly basophilic cytoplasm, round to oval basophilic nuclei, and smooth to finely granular nuclear chromatin; they may have indistinct cell margins. Large, clear cytoplasmic vacuoles representing apical mucus vacuoles may be associated with cell clusters. The goblet cell is another type of columnar epithelial cell. Goblet cells produce mucus, which appears as distinct basophilic granules or diffuse basophilia. Small mature lymphocytes are frequently noted on normal intestinal cytology samples because lymphoid aggregates make up part of the normal intestinal mucosa. Low numbers of bacteria represented by a wide variety of morphological types can be observed and are part of a normal flora. Plant material is frequently observed in fecal cytology specimens from many species as variably sized, pleomorphic plant fragments, which is consistent with normal cytologic findings (Weeden and Wamsley, 2015).

Normal colonic, rectal, and fecal cytology consists of uniform-appearing columnar epithelial cells that often occur in clusters or sheets. These cells may be found occasionally in fecal samples as they exfoliate, especially in association with diarrhea; however, it may be difficult to identify their origin. Goblet cells and lymphocytes (small, medium, and large) are also found in normal specimens, but are rare. A mixed bacterial flora as well as digesta and plant material are commonly present.

Plant material is frequently observed in fecal cytology specimens from many species as variably sized, pleomorphic plant fragments, which are consistent with normal cytologic findings (Weeden and Wamsley, 2015). Plant material needs to be differentiated from various other structures, such as atypical epithelial cells, parasite ova, and pollen spores) in diagnostic cytology (Pantanowitz et al., 2011).

Respiratory Tract

The upper respiratory tract of mammals consists of the nasal cavity, which begins at the nares. The mammalian nasal cavity is composed of bony and cartilaginous sinuses divided by a nasal septum and ends at the ethmoid plate. Keratinized squamous epithelium lines the external part of the nares, but transitions into a nonkeratinized squamous lining and then ciliated pseudostratified columnar epithelium caudally. Ciliated pseudostratified columnar epithelium makes up the mucous membrane that lines much of the nasal cavity. Pseudostratified columnar epithelium consists of ciliated columnar cells extending from the basement membrane to the lumen, goblet cells, and reserve cells. Reserve cells are small, polygonal cells adjacent to the basement membrane. Serous glands, mucous glands, and lymphoid tissue are other structures associated with the nasal cavity of mammals.

The larynx of mammals is a part of the upper respiratory tract, and is made up of the vocal cords, arytenoids cartilage, and glottis. The larynx is lined by stratified squamous epithelium and is associated with lymphoid tissue. The trachea extends from the larynx to the bronchi. The larynx and bronchi are lined by ciliated pseudostratified columnar epithelium with goblet cells. Beyond the bronchi lie the bronchioles, which are lined by ciliated and nonciliated cuboidal epithelium. The airways continue to become smaller until they reach the alveolar ducts, alveolar sacs, and alveoli. Mammalian alveoli are lined by flattened epithelium (type I pneumocytes) and rounded epithelium (type-II pneumocytes) (Burkhard et al., 2001).

Samples collected from the respiratory system of normal healthy animals tend to be poorly cellular; however, when present, normal respiratory cells typically include ciliated epithelial cells, round to cuboidal epithelial cells, and macrophages (Burkhard et al., 2001). Other cells that may occur less frequently in normal respiratory tract samples include neutrophils (or heterophils), lymphocytes, eosinophils (depending upon the

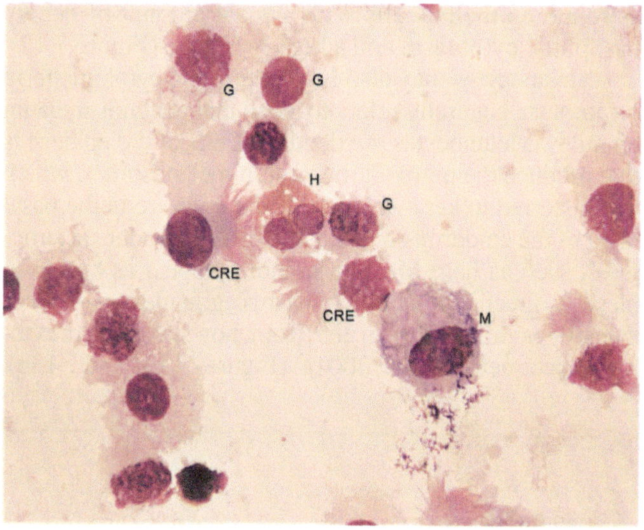

Fig. 7.9. Cytospin preparation of a tracheal wash from a healthy guinea pig (*Cavia porcellus*) reveals normal cellular structures that include ciliated respiratory epithelial cells (CRE), goblet cells (G), a heterophil (H), and a macrophage (M), Wright–Giemsa stain (100× oil).

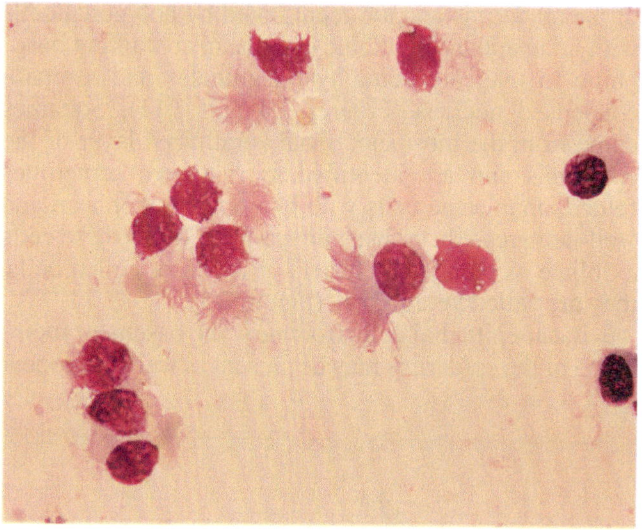

Fig. 7.10. Ciliated respiratory cells in a tracheal wash from a guinea pig (*Cavia porcellus*), Wright–Giemsa stain (100× oil).

species), goblet cells, and mast cells (Rebar et al., 1980a; Padrid et al., 1991; Vail et al., 1995; Baker and Lumsden, 2000) (Figure 7.9).

Squamous epithelial cells may also be observed routinely as contaminants in tracheal wash fluids because these cells readily exfoliate from the oral mucosa onto the catheter or bronchoscope. These cells are large cells with abundant blue-gray cytoplasm and a central pyknotic nucleus, and often have adherent bacteria (Figure 7.7). Some epithelial cells may be keratinized and have abundant hyalinized, basophilic cytoplasm with angular borders. Small, occasionally pyknotic or karyorrhectic nuclei are usually seen. The macrophages present in samples collected from the respiratory tract are typically large, highly vacuolated cells that may contain phagocytized material.

Ciliated respiratory epithelial cells are derived from the trachea and bronchi, and tend to exfoliate singly or in clusters. These cells may vary in size and shape, but generally appear as elongated columnar cells with a round to oval nucleus at one pole of the cell, and an abundant basophilic, often granular cytoplasm (Figures 7.9 and 7.10). Prominent eosinophilic cilia are present at the large end of the cell. The nucleus contains finely granular chromatin with prominent nucleoli and lies on the small pole of the cell opposite the cilia. These cells tend to be fragile and may appear as cellular fragments in the cytologic specimen (Figure 23.7 in Chapter 23).

Goblet cells exfoliate singly or in clusters and appear as columnar cells that resemble ciliated respiratory epithelial cells, but lack the cilia (Figure 7.9). The cytoplasm is abundant and contains vacuoles and round, uniform eosinophilic granules that frequently distend the cytoplasmic borders. The nucleus is large, round to oval, and basilar in location within the cell. Goblet cells secret mucin, which often appears in the background of air-dried smears stained with Romanowsky stains as amorphous ribbons of lightly basophilic or eosinophilic material. Mucus often entraps cells, making them difficult to identify. Spiral casts of basophilic mucus, called Curschmann's spirals, are seen in association with excessive mucus production (Baker and Lumsden, 2000).

Skin

The skin is composed of the epidermis and dermis. The epidermis is composed of a basal layer, intermediate layer, and a transitional layer (stratum corneum), which is composed of the cornified cells that contain keratin (Raskin, 2001a). The underlying dermis contains adnexal structures, connective tissue, smooth muscle, blood vessels, lymphatic vessels, and nerves. Adipose tissue may be located below the dermis in some animals. The adnexal structures of mammalian skin include hair follicles, sweat glands, and sebaceous glands.

The cytology of normal skin is predominated by mature, anucleated, keratinized squamous epithelial cells from the epidermis with fewer cells from the dermis, such as glandular and basal epithelial cells and a few stromal connective tissue cells. A variable amount of debris and extracellular bacteria is often present as well. The debris often includes fragments of adnexal structures, such as hair. The bacteria are represented by a variety of morphological types.

Keratinocytes, which are composed primarily of keratin, include keratin bars, squames, and superficial squamous epithelial cells (Raskin, 2001a). Superficial squamous epithelial cells arise from the granular layer of the epidermis and are represented by polygonal cells with an abundant light blue cytoplasm containing basophilic to magenta keratohyalin granules and a small, condensed nucleus (Figures 7.4 and 7.11). Squames come from the most superficial keratinized layer of the epidermis and are identified as flattened, sometimes folded, anucleated cells with blue-green cytoplasm and well-demarcated cytoplasmic margins. When these cells exfoliate as elongated clusters of rolled or coiled cells, they are called keratin bars (Figure 7.5).

Basal epithelial cells from near the basement membrane of the epidermis may be present as well and appear as round epithelial cells with a scant amount of deeply basophilic cytoplasm and a high N:C ratio (Figure 7.12).

Melanocytes may also be present. The cytologic term *melanocyte* generally refers to a cell that contains melanin granules. Melanocytes are dendritic cells of the epidermis that produce the pigment melanin in melanosomes, which is transferred to keratinocytes. These cells are in the basal layer of the epidermis or are associated with adnexal structures, such as hair. Melanin granules appear as brownish black to greenish black cytoplasmic granules in melanocytes or keratinocytes in the Romanowsky-stained cytologic specimen (Raskin, 2001a) (Figures 7.13a and 7.13b).

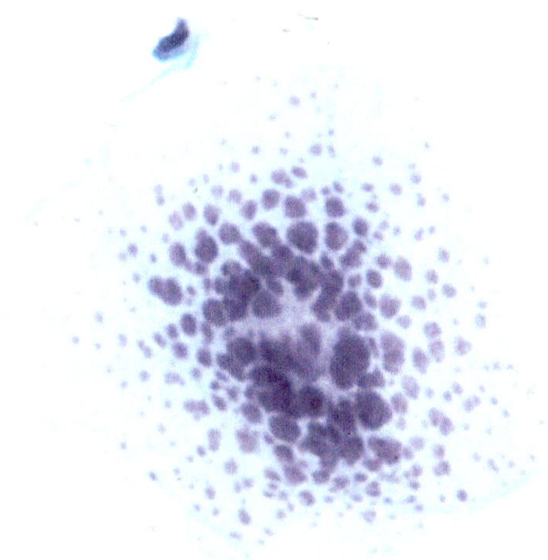

Fig. 7.11. Superficial squamous epithelial cell with magenta keratohyalin granules, Wright–Giemsa stain (100× oil).

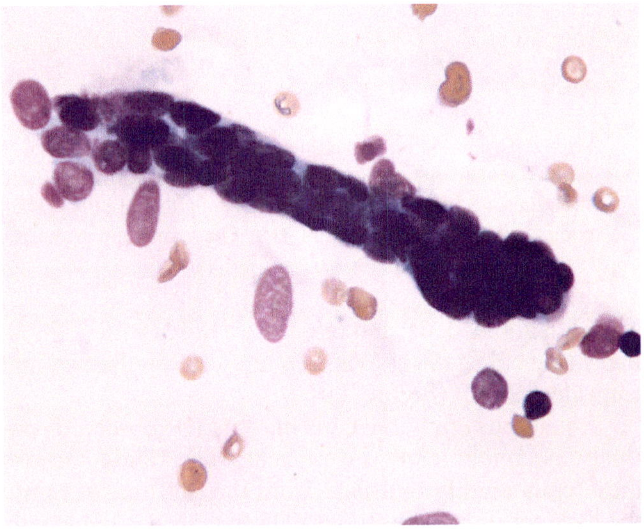

Fig. 7.12. Basal epithelial cells that have exfoliated into a tight linear cluster in a fine-needle aspiration biopsy of a basal cell tumor in a rabbit (*Oryctolagus cuniculus*), Wright–Giemsa stain (100× oil).

(a)

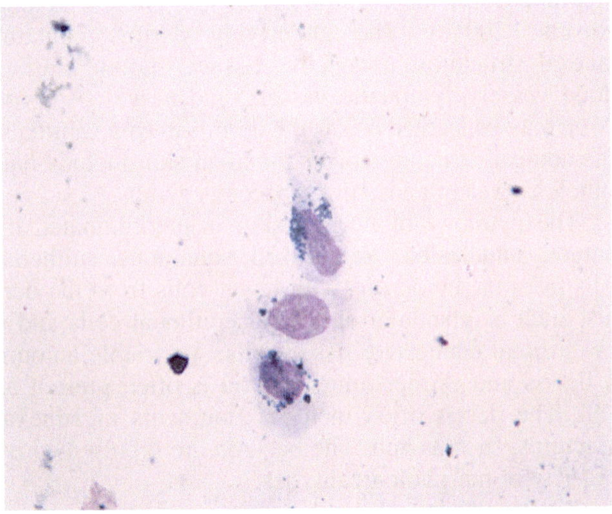

(b)

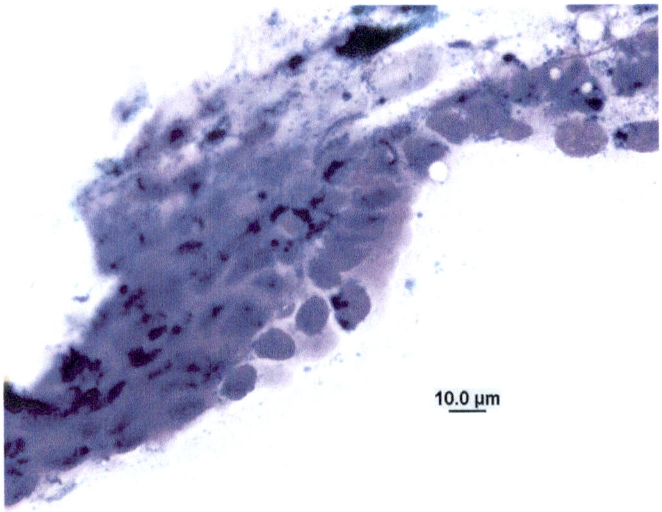

Fig. 7.13. (a) Melanocytes likely from the cutaneous edge of the eyelid in a conjunctival scraping from a guinea pig (*Cavia porcellus*), Wright–Giemsa stain (100× oil). (b) Melanocytes likely from the cutaneous edge of the eyelid in a conjunctival scraping from a guinea pig (*Cavia porcellus*), Wright–Giemsa stain (100× oil).

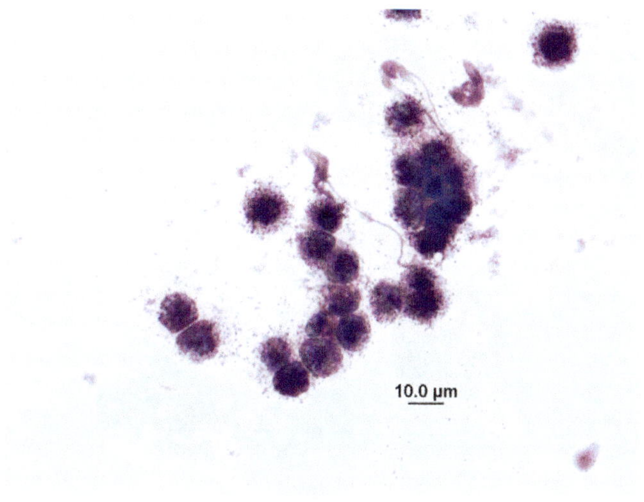

Fig. 7.14. Mast cells in a fine-needle aspiration biopsy of a skin lesion in a ferret (*Mustela putorius furo*), Wright–Giemsa stain (100× oil).

Mast cells may be present in mammalian skin specimens. These are mesenchymal cells that contain basophilic, metachromatic (variable staining with the same stain) cytoplasmic granules with Romanowsky stains (Figure 7.14). The mast cell granules contain histamine, heparin, and in some rodents, serotonin.

Central Nervous System

Cerebrospinal fluid (CSF) analysis is a critical tool in the evaluation of central nervous system disease in mammals with signs of neurologic disease. The analysis includes obtaining a total nucleated cell count, total protein concentration, and red blood cell count as well as a fluid concentration method, such as use of a cytospin preparation, for a microscopic cell differential used to determine inflammatory or noninflammatory responses.

In the dog, occasional neutrophils, eosinophils, mitotic figures, phagocytic cells, and ependymal cells are seen in many low-cellularity CSF samples, while mild increases in neutrophils, eosinophils, and mononuclear cells (lymphocytes and monocytes) or the presence of unusual cells (e.g., plasma cells, neoplastic cells) will result in the classification of a sample as abnormal even if the total cell count is normal (Krimer et al., 2016).

Because 90% of the CSF is produced by the choroid plexi cells, it is important to recognize these cells in CSF cytologic preparations. Impression smears of the choroid plexi of various mammals reveal four different morphologic types of epithelial cells that are consistently found in all the species. These include deeply basophilic alpha cells, beta cells with a neutral to weakly acidophilic cytoplasm, gamma cells that contains inclusions (vesicles) filled with many tiny pale tan to pink granules, and Kolmer cells (Garma-Aviña, 2004) (Figures 7.15–7.22).

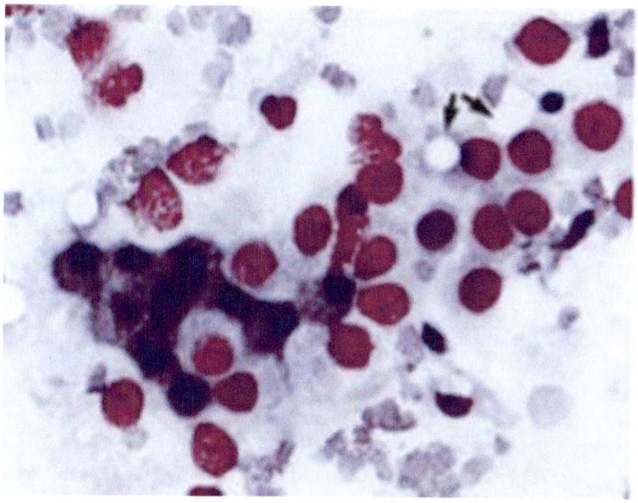

Fig. 7.15. Imprint of the choroid plexi from a horse revealing a raft of choroid plexi cells. Alpha cells have dark blue cytoplasm and densely stained nuclei, and beta cells have paler nuclei with a cribriform chromatin distribution. Two gamma cells with intracellular vesicles are seen (arrows). Wright–Giemsa stain (540×). Source: Garma-Aviña (2004).

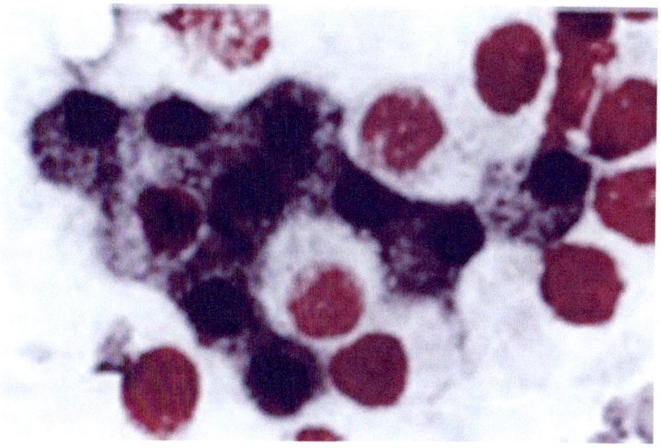

Fig. 7.16. Higher magnification of the cells in Figure 7.15 reveals the deeply basophilic cytoplasm of alpha cells and the paler beta cells with larger nuclei. Wright–Giemsa stain (1,080×). Source: Garma-Aviña (2004).

Eye

The conjunctival mucosa is composed of pseudostratified columnar epithelium with numerous goblet cells (Banks, 1974; Raskin, 2001b). The portion of the conjunctiva that lines the fornix (the junction of the upper and lower conjunctiva) is lined with stratified cuboidal epithelium. The portion of the conjunctiva (bulbar conjunctiva) that is continuous with the corneal epithelium consists of stratified nonkeratinized epithelium.

The nictitating membrane of mammals is covered by nonkeratinized stratified squamous epithelium on the palpebral and bulbar surfaces. Variable quantities of lymphoid aggregates are found on the bulbar surface.

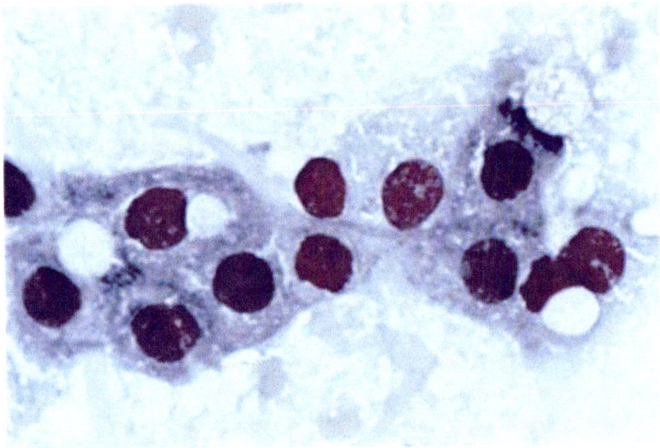

Fig. 7.17. Imprint of the choroid plexus from a dog reveals three gamma cells with intracytoplasmic vesicles with a larger fourth extracellular vesicle. Delicate linear granular material is present. Wright–Giemsa stain (1,080×). Source: Garma-Aviña (2004).

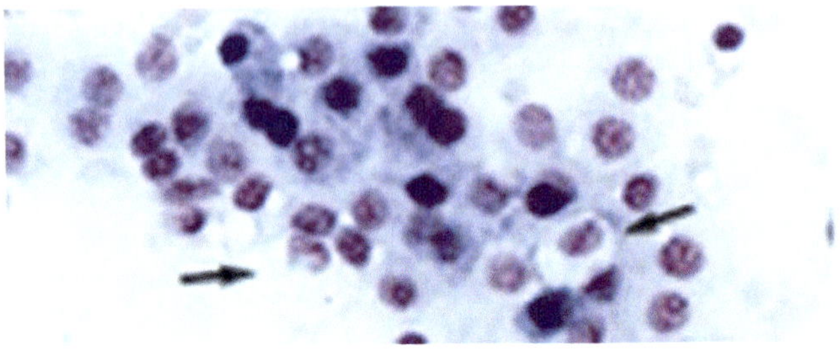

Fig. 7.18. Raft of choroid plexus cells from a horse revealing two pale Kolmer or epiplexus cells (arrows). Wright–Giemsa stain (540×). Source: Garma-Aviña (2004).

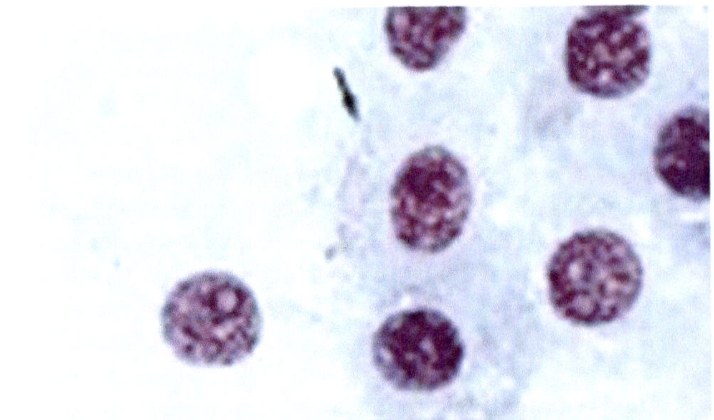

Fig. 7.19. Imprint of the choroid plexus from a dog revealing a cell with reddish granules (arrow) and a nucleus resembling that of other choroid plexus cells. Wright–Giemsa stain (1080×). Source: Garma-Aviña (2004).

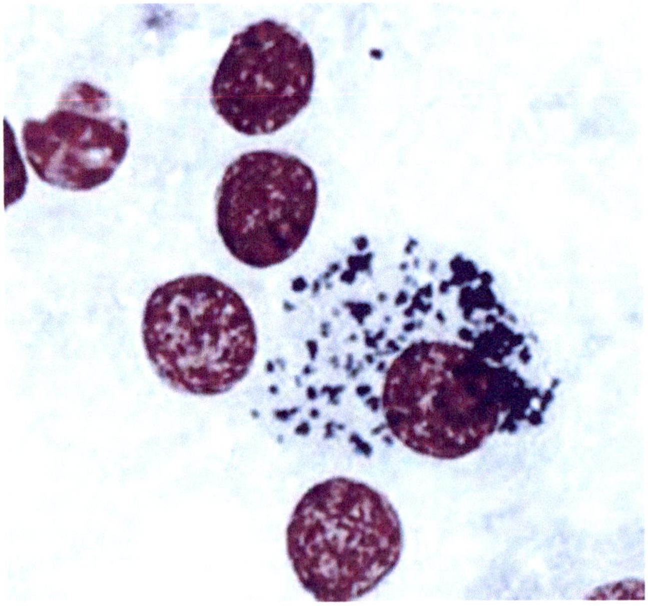

Fig. 7.20. Choroid plexi imprint from a dog revealing a cell with dark blue-green intracytoplasmic bile crystals and nuclear features resembling those of epithelial choroid plexus cells. Wright–Giemsa stain (1080×). Source: Garma-Aviña (2004).

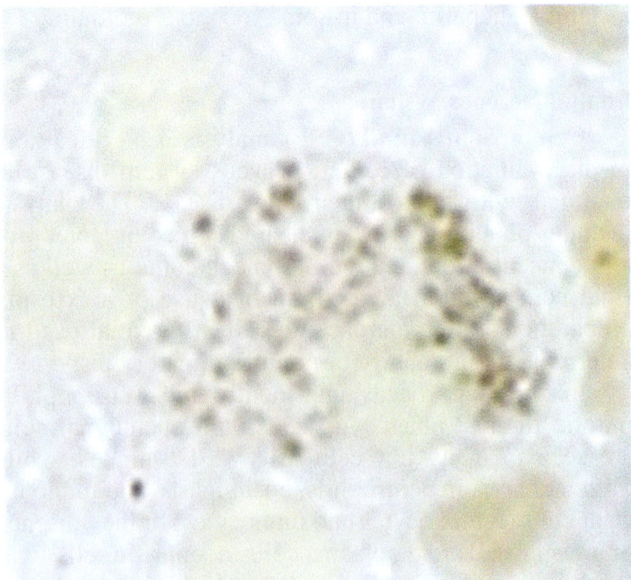

Fig. 7.21. The same cell as shown in Figure 7.22 stained with a stain for bile indicating the crystals that stained pale green were bile. Hall stain (1080×). Source: Garma-Aviña (2004).

The normal cytology of a conjunctival scraping or brush specimen consists of epithelial cells and goblet cells. The background may contain variable amounts of mucus, which appears as strands of lightly basophilic amorphous material. The epithelial cells present in the sample appear uniformly polygonal, and contain basophilic cytoplasm and large, round nuclei (Figure 7.23).

The goblet cells typically exfoliate singly or in aggregates and contain abundant foamy cytoplasm and large secretory vacuoles. Some goblet cells contain purple cytoplasmic granules. The nuclei are located next to the cell margin.

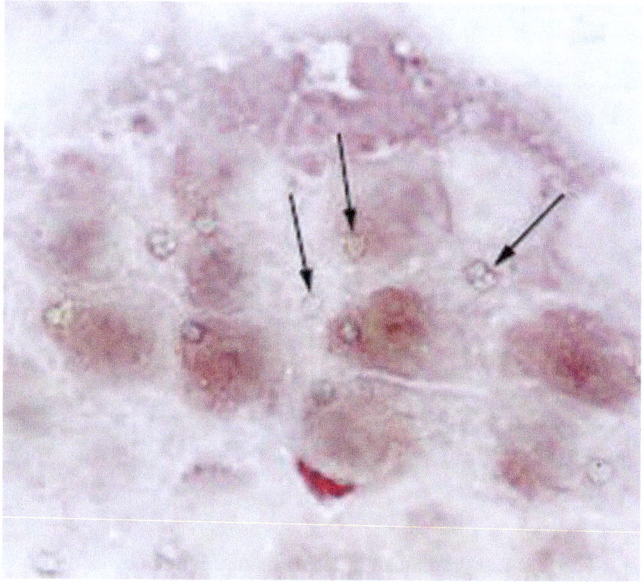

Fig. 7.22. The same cells as shown in Figure 7.21 at higher magnification and after being stained for bile reveal the crystals to be bile crystals (arrows). Hall stain (1080×). Source: Garma-Aviña (2004).

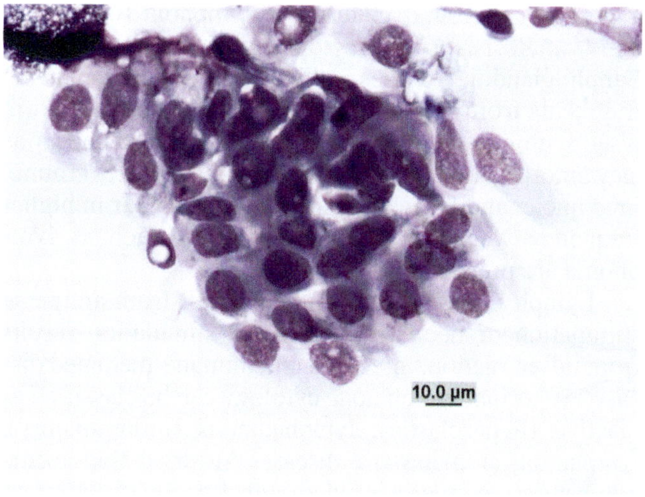

Fig. 7.23. Conjunctival epithelial cells from a conjunctival scraping guinea pig (*Cavia porcellus*), Wright–Giemsa stain.

The cornea is composed of nonkeratinized, stratified squamous epithelium (Banks, 1974). Cytologic specimens are obtained by gently scraping corneal lesions using an ophthalmic spatula or cotton-tipped applicator. The normal cytology of the cornea reveals a poorly cellular sample consisting of nonkeratinized squamous epithelial cells with central vesicular nuclei.

Ocular sampling may also be obtained by flushing the nasolacrimal duct. A normal nasolacrimal flush cytology from a rabbit is represented by 56.4 ± 31.5% heterophils, 29.5 ± 26.3% lymphocytes, 30.9 ± 23.6% columnar cells, 8% large mononuclear cells, 16.7% anucleate keratinized epithelial cells, 18.4% nucleated epithelial cells, 2.4% intermediate epithelial cells, and 1.7% goblet cells (López et al., 2020). Epithelial cells were characterized as anucleate keratinized squamous cells, nucleated keratinizing squamous cells, intermediate cells, columnar cells, and goblet cells.

Joint Fluid

Cytologic examination of the synovial fluid is the most valuable part of the diagnostic process involved in the determination of joint disease in animals. The amount of synovial fluid obtained in a healthy joint is dependent not only on the joint size but also on the animal species (Brombini et al., 2017). The interpretation of synovial fluid cell analysis should be done within hours of collection; otherwise, the sample should be refrigerated.

A complete synovial fluid analysis should include assessment of appearance (volume, color, clarity, turbidity, and presence of clots), protein content, viscosity, a mucin clot test, and a nucleated cell count, differential, and cell morphology (see Chapter 6). Under normal conditions, the joints of most small mammals contain a fluid volume that is too small for sampling or complete evaluation. Fluid distension of a joint may occur when certain arthropathies are present, which will allow for collection of enough synovial fluid for evaluation. Even when significant joint distention is present, however, often only a few drops of synovial fluid can be collected for cytologic evaluation.

A cell count may be performed on synovial if enough sample volume can be collected (see Chapter 6). Because synovial fluid often turns into a gel at room temperature (called thixotropism), obtaining an accurate cell count can be difficult (Walberg and Loar, 2004). Hyaluronidase can be added to the synovial fluid to reduce the fluid viscosity and prevent clotting to provide a more accurate cell count (Fisher, 2001). If only a small sample volume is obtained, then an estimated cell count can be performed on a synovial fluid film. Fluid from normal joints is poorly cellular and contains less than five cells per 200× magnification (20× objective field) depending upon the thickness of the smear.

An estimated white cell count can be obtained by taking the average number of cells seen per 20× objective field and multiplying it by 500, the goal being not to obtain a precise number of cells/µL but to differentiate normal cellularity, mildly increased cellularity, and markedly increased cellularity (Dusick et al., 2014; Meinkoth, 2022). It is important to be in a thin area that would be equivalent to the monolayer of a blood film when estimating cellularity as well as when evaluating the density of the noncellular background, which is often (but not always) stippled eosinophilic with a normal amount of hyaluronic acid in the joint fluid.

Synovial joints are composed of articular cartilage and an articular capsule, which is composed of a fibrous layer and a synovial membrane. The synovial membrane is composed of flat cells that produce the synovial fluid that lubricates the joint. Normal synovial fluid is poorly cellular and contains primarily small and large mononuclear cells (macrophages and synovial lining cells), and granulocytes (neutrophils or heterophils) on a granular background with Wright's stain. Synovial lining cells (synoviocytes) are large mononuclear cells with eccentric nuclei and abundant vacuolated cytoplasm that often contains pink-staining granules.

The percentages of the different mononuclear cells (small lymphocytes, macrophages, and synovial lining cells) present vary and are not diagnostically significant. The granulocytes account for less than 10% of the cell differential in normal synovial fluid. The amount of granular background material indicates the amount of mucin present in the fluid. Cells in highly viscous synovial fluid tend to line up in parallel rows, called "wind rowing of cell," when the cytological slide is prepared (Walberg and Loar, 2004).

Macrophages in normal synovial fluid do not have distended, vacuolated cytoplasm or show evidence of phagocytosis of other material (Meinkoth, 2022). Although vacuolated macrophages are often associated with inflammatory or degenerative arthropathies, they may occur whenever there is a delay between sample collection and slide preparation; therefore, it is recommended to prepare smears for cytology immediately following collection to avoid any artifacts associated with cellular aging.

Lymphoid Tissue/Lymph Nodes

Lymphoid cells found in lymph node aspirates include small lymphocytes, intermediate-sized lymphocytes, and large lymphocytes. Small lymphocytes are round cells (7–10 μm in diameter) with scant blue cytoplasm and large nuclei with densely clumped chromatin and no visible nucleoli. Intermediate-sized lymphocytes (10–14 μm in diameter) are nearly twice the size of the small lymphocytes with a round nucleus without a nucleolus and basophilic cytoplasm. Large lymphocytes (14–21 μm in diameter) have an eccentrically located round to oval nucleus with coarse chromatin and often one to multiple visible nucleoli and deeply basophilic cytoplasm that is slightly greater in amount than is seen with small and intermediate-sized lymphocytes. Other cells that may be present in low numbers include plasma cells, macrophages, neutrophils, and mast cells (Figure 7.24). Plasma cells have an eccentrically positioned nucleus with densely clumped chromatin, abundant deeply basophilic cytoplasm, and a distinct perinuclear halo (Golgi area). A normal lymph node has 75–95% small lymphocytes, less than 5% of large lymphocytes, and less than 5% plasma cells (Barrios-Arpi and Morales-Cauti, 2020).

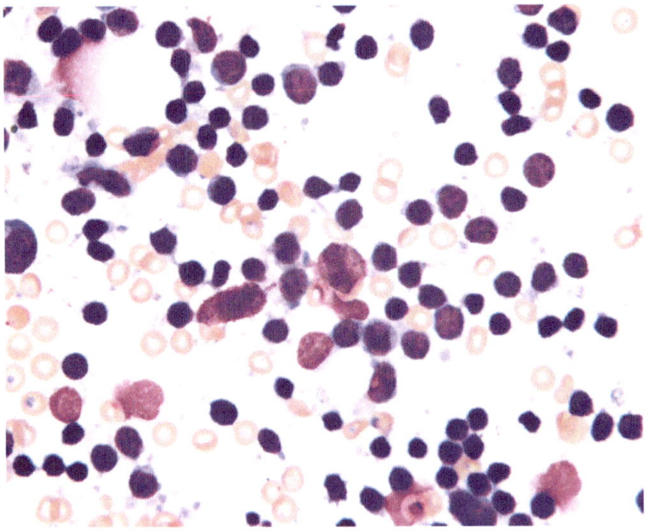

Fig. 7.24. Predominantly small mature lymphocytes and two mast cells (center) in a fine-needle aspiration biopsy of a lymph node in a ferret (*Mustela putorius furo*), Wright–Giemsa stain (100× oil).

The background material of lymphoid tissue contains small basophilic cytoplasmic fragments called lymphoglandular bodies, which represent cytoplasmic fragments from ruptured lymphocytes. Free nuclei from lysed lymphocytes may be present as well and appear as lacy amorphous eosinophilic material in the background. Free nuclei and lymphoglandular bodies occur in higher frequency when lymph node disorders such as lymphoma are present.

Lymph node enlargement can result from antigenic stimulation or neoplasia. Antigenic stimulation results from inflammation, infection, and immune-mediated disease. Abnormal lymph node cytology can be classified as reactive (hyperplastic), lymphadenitis (inflammatory), lymphoma, or metastatic disease. Air-dried fine-needle non-aspiration smears stained with Romanowsky stains offer a fast and simple method for the evaluation of enlarged lymph nodes. For example, in a clinical study involving guinea pigs with cervical lymphadenopathy, such samples revealed that 64.5% of the cases were compatible with pseudo-eosinophilic (heterophilic) lymphadenitis, 22.6% with reactive lymphatic node, 6.45% with lymphoma, and 6.45% with Hodgkin's-like lymphoma (Barrios-Arpi and Morales-Cauti, 2020).

Spleen

The spleen is a blood-forming and blood-destroying organ; therefore, imprints of normal spleen biopsies or aspirates contain a marked amount of peripheral blood contamination typified by large numbers of intact mature erythrocytes and platelet or thrombocyte clumps. The spleen is also a major lymphoid organ; therefore, many lymphocytes are present as well. The distribution of the lymphocytes in normal splenic samples should be the same as those described for normal lymph nodes in mammals. Low numbers of macrophages showing varying degrees of erythrophagocytosis are expected. Splenic samples contain many free nuclei.

The evaluation of the lymphoid elements of the spleen provides an indication of the overall status of the animal's immune system and lymphoid tissues. A reactive or hyperplastic spleen reveals a predominance of small mature lymphocytes with an increase in the number of medium and large lymphocytes. Macrophages and plasma cells may be easily identified in reactive spleens.

Extramedullary hematopoiesis may at first glance resemble splenitis; however, closer inspection will reveal precursors of erythroid, myeloid, and thrombocyte or platelet (megakaryocytes in the case of mammals) cell lines. Erythrophagocytosis and excessive iron storage within macrophages may be associated with hemolytic anemias. Systemic infections may sometimes be detected by the presence of the etiologic agent in splenic samples.

Liver

The normal liver provides highly cellular samples that contain hepatocytes and variable amounts of hemic cells from peripheral blood contamination of the sample. Hepatocytes are large (25–30 μm), slightly oval to polygonal cells with distinct cell margins that occur singly or in sheets and clusters (Figure 7.2). The cytoplasm is abundant and lightly basophilic, and fine eosinophilic granulation may be seen occasionally with Wright's stain. The nuclei are round to oval, uniform in appearance, and are slightly eccentric in location within the cells. The nuclei contain coarse chromatin and one or two prominent nucleoli. Binucleation is occasionally seen. Hepatocytes are easily damaged, resulting in numerous free nuclei scattered throughout the smear and a background that resembles the cytoplasm of intact hepatocytes. Degenerative hepatocytes may be seen with hepatic disease or postmortem autolysis.

Biliary epithelial cells, mesothelial cells, lymphocytes, plasma cells, macrophages, and spindle-shaped cells are occasionally seen in normal smears. Blue-green bile pigment may occasionally be identified among the cells as well (Figure 7.25). Biliary epithelial cells are present as clusters of uniform-appearing, small, round cells with round nuclei, dense granular to homogenous chromatin, and a scant amount of poorly staining cytoplasm. Mesothelial cells are angular cells that typically are present in sheets, possibly because they were traumatically exfoliated during the sampling procedure. Discrete mesothelial cells have an oval appearance with

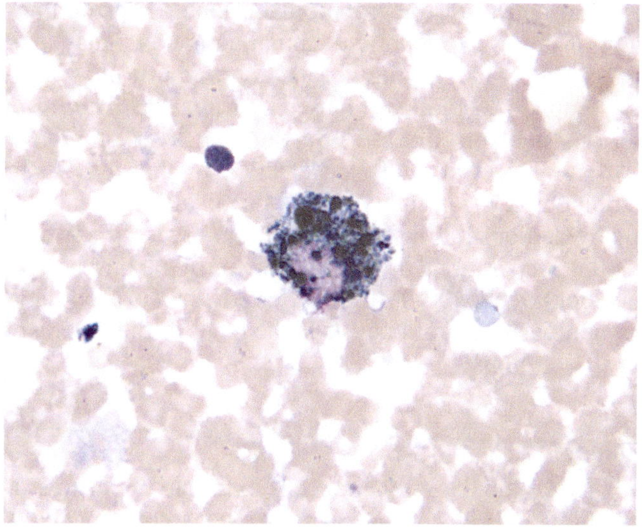

Fig. 7.25. Intracytoplasmic bile pigment in a fine-needle aspiration biopsy of the liver in a ferret (*Mustela putorius furo*), Wright–Giemsa stain (100× oil).

scalloped or villus-like eosinophilic cytoplasmic margins (pink to red fringe). The macrophages present within the cytology sample often contain iron pigment (hemosiderin), indicating hemoglobin catabolism. Excessive iron pigment within many macrophages may be associated with hemolytic anemias or iron storage secondary to chronic inflammatory disorders.

Hydropic degeneration of hepatocytes may occur when hypoxia, toxic insult, or corticosteroid-induced hepatopathy is present, and is indicated by cytoplasmic rarefaction of hepatocytes in the cytology sample. Cytoplasmic rarefaction is indicated by swollen (ballooning) cytoplasm that has less density than normal and does not form discrete vacuoles owing to an increase in glycogen and water content (Meyer, 2001b).

In the dog and cat, cytologic examination of the liver can be useful in the identification of hepatic diseases, such as acute and chronic cholestasis, chronic cholangitis, feline lymphoplasmacytic cholangitis, and cholangiocellular neoplasms. The accumulation of dark green to black granules within hepatocytes is a consequence of cholestasis. Cholangiocytes (cells from the biliary ducts of the liver) are rarely seen in normal hepatic cytology; therefore, their presence in large numbers is suggestive of biliary disease (Masserdotti, 2020). Cholangiocytes appear as clusters or sheets of cuboidal to columnar cells with high N:C ratios, scant pale blue cytoplasm, and a round, central nucleus with dense, smooth chromatin (Arndt and Shelly, 2014). Cells from the terminal bile ducts are cuboidal with scant light blue cytoplasm and round nuclei (slightly larger than those of hepatocytes) with densely granular to homogenous cytoplasm, whereas large bile ductular cells are columnar with ciliated brush borders (Masserdotti, 2020). Together with clinical and ultrasonographic data, cytologic examination of the liver of exotic mammalian patients may also be useful for identifying hepatic abnormalities.

Hepatic coccidiosis (caused by *Eimeria stiedae*) is a serious parasitic disease affecting the liver of rabbits (Al-Rukibat et al., 2001). Detection of this disease in rabbit colonies is usually made as a postmortem diagnosis by demonstration of the coccidian organism on wet-mount preparations of liver lesions or bile from the gall bladder (Deeb, 2000). Antemortem diagnosis is possible by demonstration of oocysts in the feces or the organism in a liver biopsy.

Kidney

Renal tubular epithelial cells exfoliate in clusters or as individual cells and appear as round to columnar cells with abundant basophilic cytoplasm that may contain vacuoles. The nuclei of normal renal tubular epithelial cells are uniform in appearance and appear round and slightly eccentric.

Reproductive Tract

Vaginal cytology of the black-footed ferret (*Mustela nigripes*), Siberian polecat (M. *eversmanni*), and domestic ferret (M. *putorius furo*) is similar, where proestrus is characterized by an increasing percentage of superficial epithelial cells and estrus is identified by fully keratinized epithelial cells in vaginal lavage preparations (Williams et al., 1992). Cytologic characteristics indicative of estrus (≥90% cornified epithelial cells) results as a response to a high serum 17β-estradiol concentration (Lipman et al., 1993). Neutrophils are more common during all stages of the estrous cycle in domestic ferrets than they are in the other species. Following copulation, the percentage of superficial cells in the vagina declined.

Preputial lavage samples obtained from male ferrets reveal preputial epithelial cells morphologically like vaginal epithelial cells in female ferrets (Williams et al., 1992). Parabasal cells, intermediate cells, superficial cells, and anuclear squamous cells are found in preputial lavage samples of male ferrets with the number of each cell type expected to vary among samples. Parabasal and intermediate cells are deeply basophilic, whereas superficial cells are lighter stained, contained evidence of degenerative nuclear changes (pyknosis or karyorrhexis) with angled cytoplasmic margins, and have a larger cytoplasm-to-nucleus ratio (Protain et al., 2009). Anuclear squamous cells are larger, have angled cytoplasmic margins, and lack nuclei.

Inflammation

The inflammatory response of mammals can be classified as either neutrophilic/heterophilic, eosinophilic, mixed cell, or macrophagic depending upon the predominant cell type. Inflammatory cells arrive at the lesion by active migration in response to various chemotactic factors, and the type of inflammatory response present may suggest a possible etiology and pathogenesis. Inflammation may be caused by living organisms (microorganisms), nonliving (traumatic, thermal, or chemical) agents, or neoplastic processes.

Neutrophilic/Heterophilic Inflammation of Mammals

Inflammation occurs whenever chemotactic factors for inflammatory cells, such as vasoactive amines (i.e., 5-hydroxy-tryptamine from mast cell granules) are released. The most common causes are microbes and their toxins, physical and chemical trauma, death of cells from circulatory insufficiency, and immune reactions. The rate of the inflammatory response in the endothermic mammals is consistent and predictable. The inflammatory process begins with the acute phase. Acute inflammation is initiated by the action of vasoactive amines and cell breakdown products released by the damaged tissue on the microcirculation of the affected tissue. These chemicals and products cause capillary dilatation, increased blood flow into the area, and increased lumen diameter of the capillaries, which allows the large serum proteins (such as fibrinogen and immunoglobulins normally confined within circulation) to exude into the tissues. Leukocytes actively migrate into the affected tissue. The degree of the leukocyte migration depends on the stimulus, which is particularly marked in certain bacterial infections. The cells that leave the blood include neutrophils or heterophils (depending upon the species), monocytes, and lymphocytes.

Neutrophils/heterophils are typically the first cells to arrive at the scene, where they destroy ingested organisms. Lysosomes are released when the neutrophil/heterophil dies, causing lysis of surrounding tissues and recruitment of other neutrophils/heterophils to form an abscess (a focal accumulation of neutrophils/heterophils, tissue fluids, fibrin, and necrotic tissue). Monocytes in circulation in conjunction with local tissue macrophages (which have multiplied at the site of inflammation) begin to phagocytize tissue debris and infectious agents as the inflammation becomes established. Monocytes and macrophages are stimulated by the cell-mediated immune response; they are the dominant inflammatory cell in most cellular inflammatory responses and can develop into epithelioid and multinucleated giant cells. As the inflammatory process continues and becomes chronic, granulomas may develop as the macrophages form layers that resemble epithelium, and this is the reason for the term *epithelioid cells*. As the lesion matures, fibroblasts proliferate and begin to lay down collagen. These proliferating fibroblasts appear large compared to the small, densely staining fibroblasts of normal fibrous tissue. Lymphocytes appear within the stroma and participate in the cell-mediated immune response. Fusion of macrophages into giant cells occurs in association with material that is not readily digested by macrophages. Therefore, the results of acute inflammation may be complete resolution, development of an exudative or necrotic lesion with continuation of the inflammatory response, or progression to chronic inflammation.

Neutrophilic/heterophilic inflammation of mammals is also referred to as purulent or suppurative inflammation and is represented by a predominance of neutrophils/heterophils (greater than 85% of the inflammatory cells) in the cytologic sample (Figures 7.26 and 7.27). Neutrophilic/heterophilic inflammation is classified by the presence or absence of degeneration of these granulocytes (Raskin, 2001c; Campbell and Grant, 2010). Degenerate heterophils have similar characteristics to degenerate mammalian neutrophils. Infectious agents produce toxins and induce cytokine activation, resulting in cell chemotaxis and degenerative changes in the neutrophils or heterophils. Some aerobic bacteria and fungi cause degenerative cell changes, whereas many anaerobic bacteria and mycoplasma initiate chemotaxis, but do not affect the morphology of the neutrophils or heterophils (Baker and Lumsden, 2000).

The nuclear features of degenerate neutrophils/heterophils include swelling, karyorrhexis, and karyolysis (Figures 7.28 and 7.29). A nucleus that appears larger than normal is swollen. Karyorrhexis, or rupture of the nuclear membrane and fragmentation of the nuclear chromatin, indicates the end stage of cell death and is represented by multiple pyknotic nuclear segments

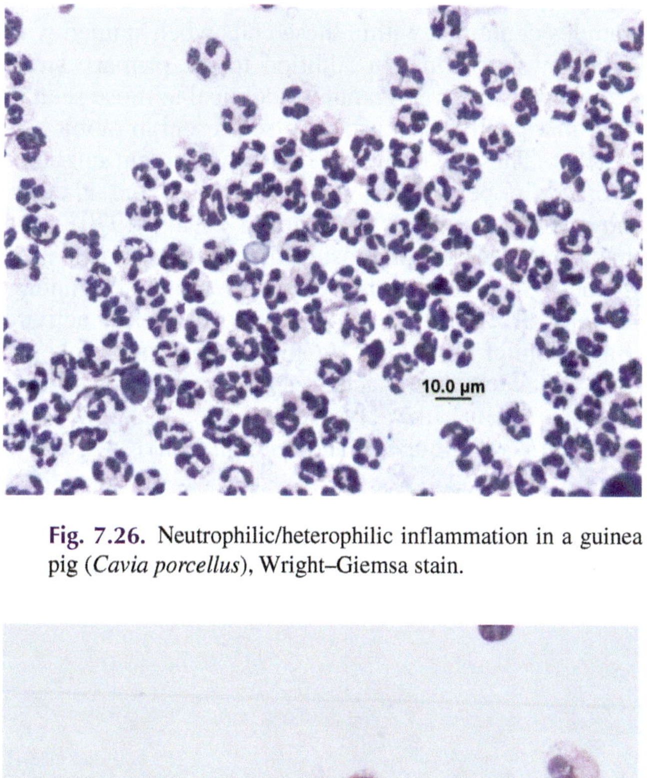

Fig. 7.26. Neutrophilic/heterophilic inflammation in a guinea pig (*Cavia porcellus*), Wright–Giemsa stain.

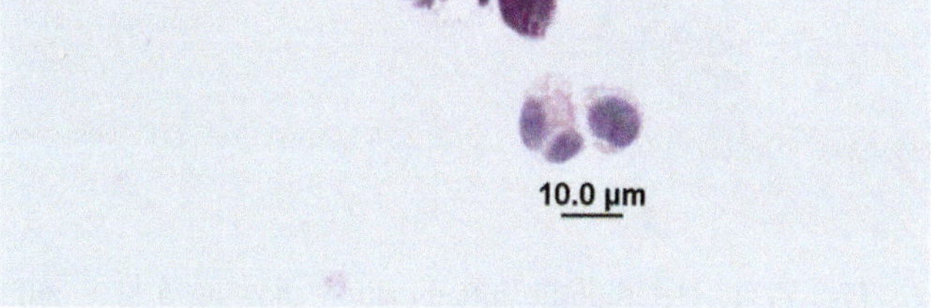

Fig. 7.27. Heterophilic inflammation in a rabbit (*Oryctolagus cuniculus*) with rhinitis, Wright–Giemsa stain.

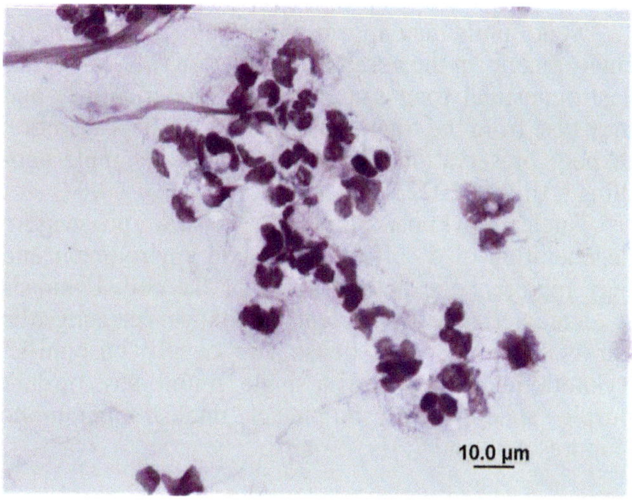

Fig. 7.28. Neutrophilic inflammation showing degenerate neutrophils in a rat (*Rattus norvegicus*) with an ulcerative skin lesion, Wright–Giemsa stain.

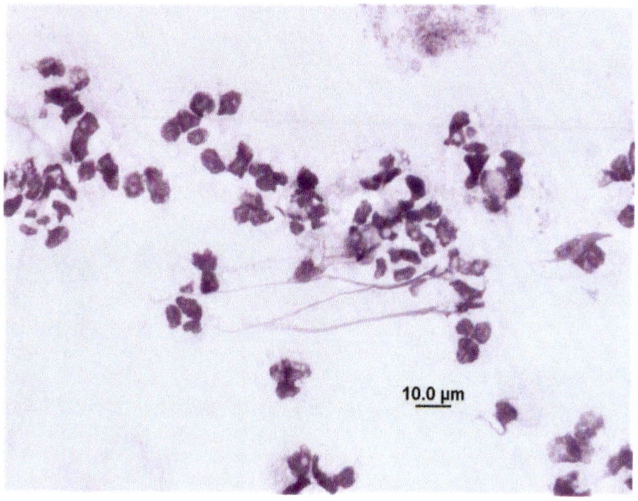

Fig. 7.29. Neutrophilic inflammation showing degenerate neutrophils in a sugar glider (*Petaurus breviceps*) abscess, Wright–Giemsa stain.

(representing nuclear fragmentation) in the center of the cell. Therefore, karyorrhexis is seen as multiple dark, dense, round structures that were once the cell nucleus. Karyolysis occurs as the nucleic acids are hydrolyzed, and the nucleus loses its basophilia and appears swollen with poorly defined homogenous pink chromatin with Romanowsky stains.

The cytoplasmic features of degenerate neutrophils/heterophils include increased basophilia, vacuolization, and the presence of Döhle bodies. Degenerate neutrophils/heterophils represent rapid cell death and suggest the presence of toxins, such as bacterial toxins, in the microenvironment (Perman et al., 1979). These changes occur during formation of the neutrophil in the marrow and suggest altered development; therefore, toxic changes to neutrophils in the peripheral blood films would be expected (Bellows, 2011).

Neutrophils may appear degenerate in some microenvironments in the absence of infection (i.e., airway or gastrointestinal tract samples, exposure to urine) and may lyse from the trauma of improper slide preparation or poor preservation caused by improper sample handling (Allison, 2022).

Nuclear pyknosis indicates a slow progressive degeneration of a cell in a nontoxic environment and may represent the natural aging of the cell. Pyknosis is characterized by nuclear shrinkage, causing the chromatin to become dense and deeply basophilic. Pyknotic nuclei appear as a single, round mass or dark purple spheres with an intact nuclear membrane (Figures 7.30 and 7.31).

Neutrophilic/heterophilic inflammation in mammals is associated with a suppurative inflammatory process that is often associated with infectious agents, especially bacteria. These leukocytes are often degenerate with bacterial infections. Close examination of the neutrophils/heterophils for infectious agents should be made when this type of inflammation is present. A bacterial infection often reveals neutrophils with karyolysis where the nucleus appears pale and swollen. These cells are called degenerative neutrophils. These cells should be closely examined for intracytoplasmic microorganisms. Neutrophilic/heterophilic inflammation can also be associated with noninfectious agents, such as tissue inflammation secondary to neoplasia, necrosis, trauma, and immune-mediated disease (Allison, 2022).

The primary granulocyte in rabbits is the heterophil, which is homologous to the neutrophil of other mammals, such as dogs and cats. They are named heterophils due to the staining property of the small acidophilic granules contained within these cells when stained with Romanowsky stains. In addition to the primary small granules, fewer large granules, identical to those seen in other mammalian species, are also present in rabbit heterophils. These cytoplasmic granules contain enzymes involved in peroxidase, acid hydrolase, and alkaline phosphatase activities (Baggiolini et al., 1970). The small granules contain most of the alkaline phosphatase and acid hydrolase of the cell, while the large granules account for most of the cell's myeloperoxidase activity (Baggiolini et al., 1969). Rabbit heterophils are phagocytic and show chemotactic response to sites of inflammation where the lysosomal granules degrade phagocytized pathogens and foreign material through

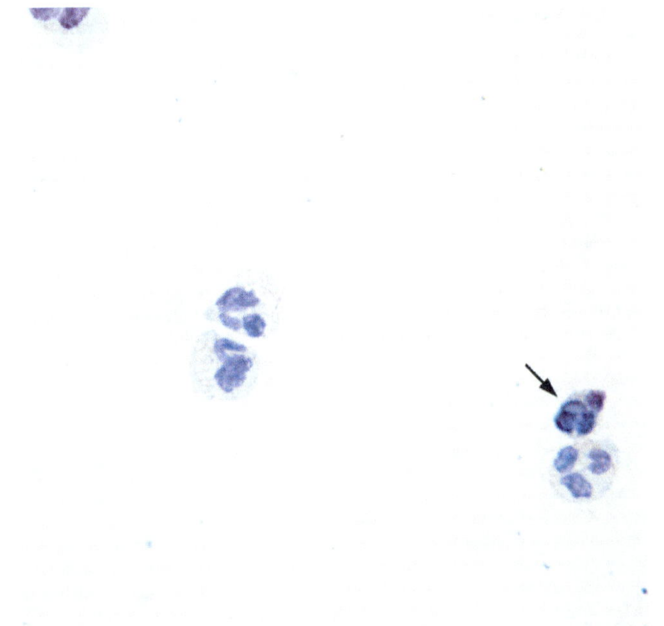

Fig. 7.30. Neutrophilic inflammation showing a neutrophil with a pyknotic nucleus (arrow) in a conjunctival scraping from a chinchilla (*Chinchilla lanigera*), Wright–Giemsa stain (100× oil).

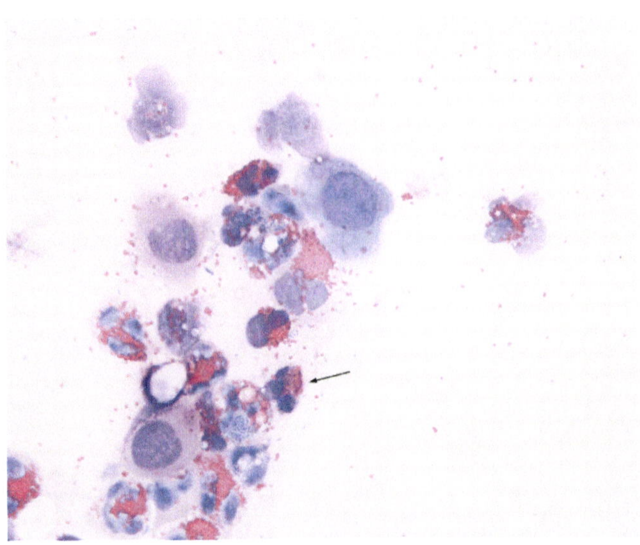

Fig. 7.31. Heterophilic inflammation showing a heterophil with a pyknotic nucleus (arrow) in a conjunctival scraping from a rabbit (*Oryctolagus cuniculus*), Wright–Giemsa stain (100× oil).

enzymatic digestion (Marshall, 2008). Because there are fewer large granules in rabbit heterophils, the degradative activity associated with myeloperoxidase activity is limited; therefore, a thick caseous suppurative purulent material develops whenever there is an infection or tissue damage. The abscess, typical for rabbits, develops as the suppurative reaction progresses and becomes walled off from the surrounding tissue as fibroblasts, inflammatory cells, and blood vessels respond to the insult (Harcourt-Brown, 2002b).

Septic Inflammation

Septic inflammation is indicated by the presence of intracellular bacteria (Figures 7.32 and 7.33). Bacteria that have been phagocytized by leukocytes often appear within vacuoles called phagosomes, which are membrane-bound vesicles formed by invagination of the cell membrane. Most bacteria stain blue with Romanowsky stains.

Mixed Cell Inflammation

A mixed inflammatory cell population composed predominantly of neutrophils and macrophages may be termed either *mixed* (preferred for cytology) or *pyogranulomatous*. Such mixed inflammatory processes may also contain small numbers of lymphocytes and plasma cells.

When there is an influx of macrophages and lymphocytes into the inflammatory lesion, a *mixed cell inflammation* (pyogranulomatous) is created (Figures 7.34a, 7.34b, and 7.35). Mixed cell inflammation (the preferred term

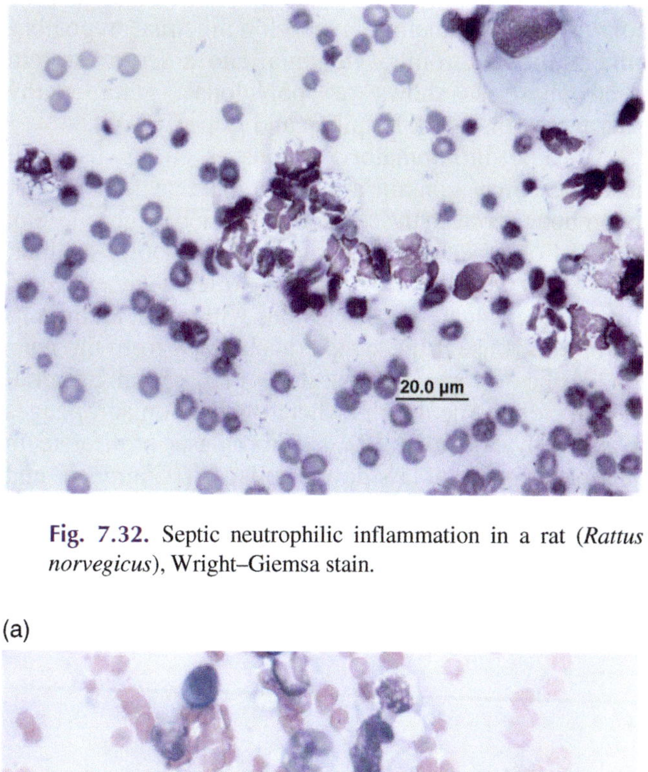

Fig. 7.32. Septic neutrophilic inflammation in a rat (*Rattus norvegicus*), Wright–Giemsa stain.

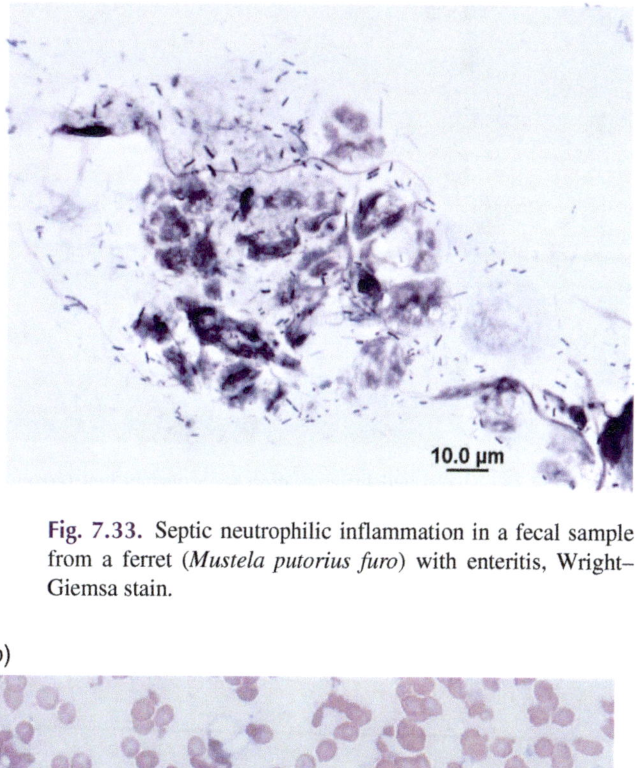

Fig. 7.33. Septic neutrophilic inflammation in a fecal sample from a ferret (*Mustela putorius furo*) with enteritis, Wright–Giemsa stain.

(a) (b)

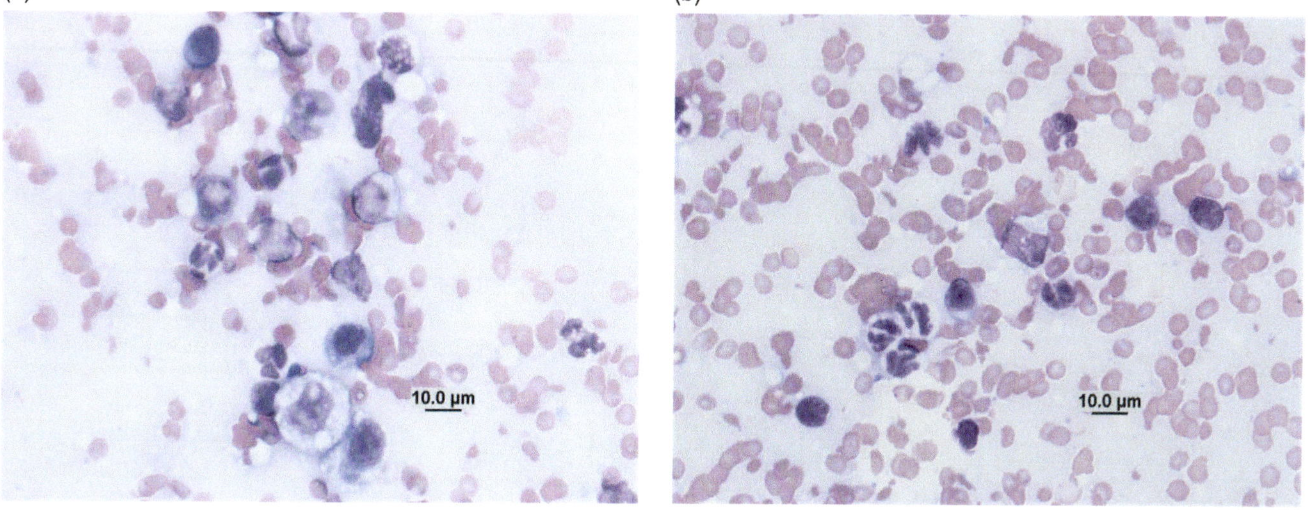

Fig. 7.34. (a), (b) Mixed cell inflammation (pyogranulomatous) in a ferret (*Mustela putorius furo*) with steatitis, Wright–Giemsa stain.

for cytology) is composed predominantly of neutrophils and macrophages (Allison, 2022). A pyogranulomatous response consists of a mixture of neutrophils, epithelioid macrophages, and multinucleated giant cells. A mixed cell inflammation indicates an established, active inflammatory lesion (originally known as chronic active inflammation). Mixed cell inflammation is typically represented by a predominance of neutrophils/heterophils (greater than 50% of the inflammatory cells) with an increased number of mononuclear leukocytes. Neutrophils/heterophils in mixed cell inflammatory lesions are usually normal and nondegenerate in appearance. Lymphocytes and plasma cells are often associated with acute neutrophilic/heterophilic granulomas, whereas the presence of epithelioid cells (macrophages that contain no vacuoles or phagocytized material) and connective tissue cells (i.e., fibroblasts) suggests chronic granulomas. Frequently, the epithelial and mesenchymal cells adjacent to inflammatory lesions proliferate, resulting in the presence of features of tissue hyperplasia in these cell types. This type of inflammatory response is commonly observed with a variety of infectious (i.e., bacterial and fungal) and noninfectious (i.e., traumatic and foreign body) etiologies.

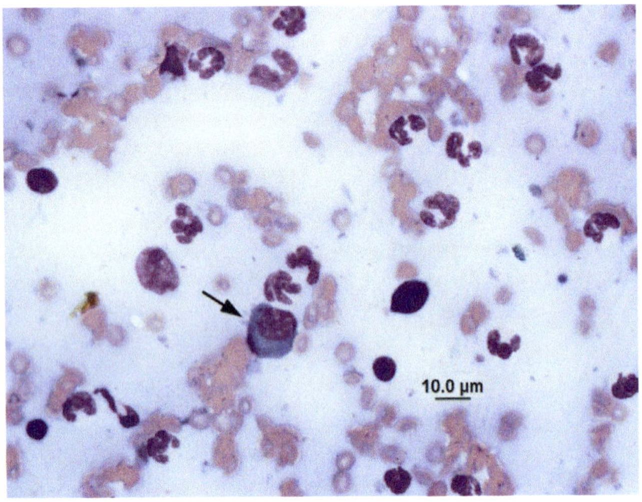

Fig. 7.35. Mixed cell inflammation with plasma cell (arrow) and neutrophils in a hedgehog (*Atelerix albiventris*) with stomatitis, Wright–Giemsa stain.

Ferret systemic coronavirus is responsible for the pyogranulomatous disease that closely resembles feline infectious peritonitis. Clinical signs include chronic weight loss, diarrhea, and a palpable abdominal mass. Abdominal ultrasonography examination reveals a hypoechoic abdominal mass, and a fine-needle aspiration cytology reveals a pyogranulomatous inflammation consisting of macrophages, neutrophils, and lymphocytes (Shigemoto et al., 2014). This disease has mostly been reported in young ferrets (18 months of age or younger). Typical associated hematologic signs include nonregenerative anemia, hyperglobulinemia, hypoalbuminemia, and thrombocytopenia, and a serum protein electrophoresis shows a polyclonal gammopathy (Garner, et al., 2006; Perpiñán and López, 2008).

Chronic inflammatory lesions, such as bacterial abscesses, may contain a large amount of noncellular, amorphous debris in the center of the lesion (Figure 7.36a). Material obtained from this area will be poorly cellular, and the few cells that are present are often degenerate and difficult to evaluate. Active lesions will reveal an inflammatory response if the sample is obtained from the margin of the lesion. Septic lesions may reveal bacterial phagocytosis in neutrophils (heterophils) or macrophages (Campbell and Grant, 2010). Fibroblasts proliferate in mature lesions to lay down collagen (Campbell and Ellis, 2007) (Figure 7.36b).

(a) (b)

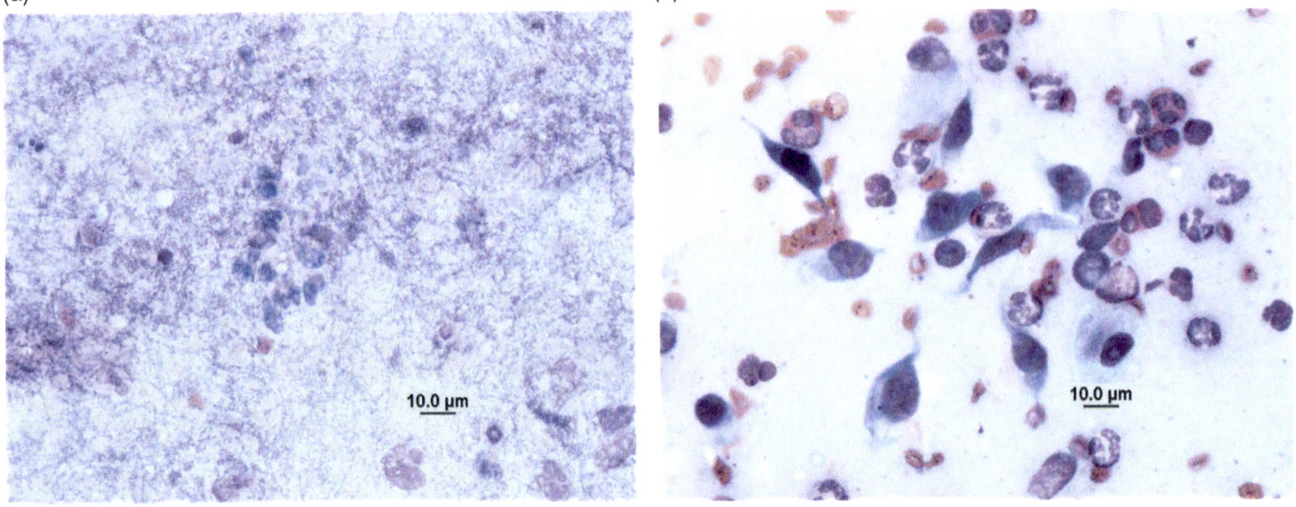

Fig. 7.36. (a, b) Cellular debris, erythrocytes, fibroblasts, and numerous bacteria in an aspirate from the center of an abscess from a hamster (*Mesocricetus auratus*), Wright–Giemsa stain (100× oil).

Lymphocytic and plasmacytic infiltration, also referred to as lymphocytic inflammation, is indicated by increased numbers of small and intermediate-sized lymphocytes and plasma cells in the cellular response, along with neutrophils and macrophages (Raskin, 2001c; Allison, 2022) (Figure 7.35). Conditions that are often associated with this type of cellular response include early viral infections, immune-mediated disorders, and chronic inflammation. The lymphocyte population is composed of small and intermediate-sized mature lymphocytes and plasma cells. Plasma cells are large, round to oval lymphocytes with an abundant, deeply basophilic cytoplasm. The nucleus is eccentrically located and appears mature. A prominent Golgi apparatus is found adjacent to the nucleus. Plasma cells distended by round, clear to light blue structures (Russell bodies) are often referred to as Mott cells (Cazzini et al., 2013) (Figure 7.37). The nucleus of the plasma cell is round and contains dense, coarse chromatin and no nucleoli.

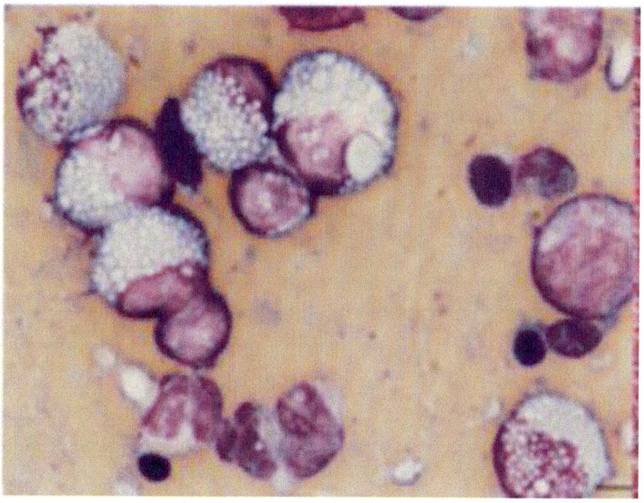

Fig. 7.37. A population of neoplastic Mott cells with numerous intracytoplasmic Russell bodies. Wright–Giemsa. Bar = 20 mm. Source: Gupta et al. (2010).

Macrophagic Inflammation

Macrophages are important in antigen presentation, production, and secretion of cytokines, phagocytosis, and bacterial killing by the production of reactive oxygen radicals and nitrogen intermediates (Quereshi, 1998). Inflammation characterized by a predominance of macrophages is termed *histiocytic*, *granulomatous*, or *macrophagic* inflammation (Allison, 2022). Macrophagic inflammation consists primarily of macrophages with multinucleated giant cells and lesser numbers of other inflammatory cells, such as lymphocytes and plasma cells. This type of inflammatory response does not always exfoliate well and may be of low cellularity.

Macrophage morphology can vary considerably in cytologic samples, where they may resemble monocytes in peripheral blood: large, round cells with oval to indented nuclei and abundant lightly basophilic cytoplasm. Activated macrophages are vacuolated and often contain phagocytized cells or cell debris, erythrocytes, or hemosiderin (evidence of previous hemorrhage), or microorganisms (Allison, 2022). Epithelioid macrophages (epithelioid cells) are non-vacuolated and tend to cluster. Macrophages may fuse to become multinucleated inflammatory giant cells. Because macrophages are capable of proliferating in tissues, mitotic figures may be observed.

Macrophagic inflammation in mammals is suggestive of chronic inflammation and is often seen with foreign body reactions and mycobacterial infections (Raskin, 2001c; Campbell and Grant, 2010) (Figures 7.38a and 7.38b). Large activated macrophages resembling

(a) (b)

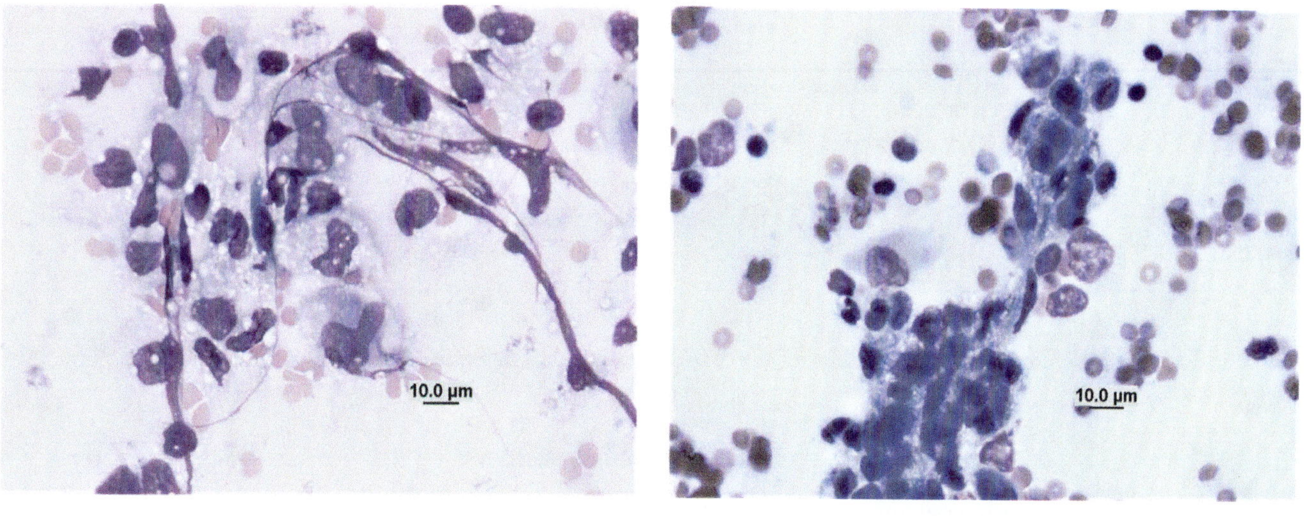

Fig. 7.38. (a), (b) Macrophagic inflammation in a ferret (*Mustela putorius furo*) with peritonitis, Wright–Giemsa stain.

epithelial cells (epithelioid macrophages) that later develop into multinucleated giant cells, apparently responding to necrotic tissue, are a feature of this type of inflammation (Campbell and Grant, 2010). Epithelioid cells often appear as clusters of macrophages with non-vacuolated blue-gray to pink cytoplasm, and distinct cytoplasmic margins (Burkhard et al., 2001).

Macrophages can normally have features consistent with criteria of malignancy, such as anisocytosis, multinucleation, prominent nucleoli, and mitotic figures; therefore, caution is warranted when considering a diagnosis of malignant neoplasia in the face of inflammation (Allison, 2022).

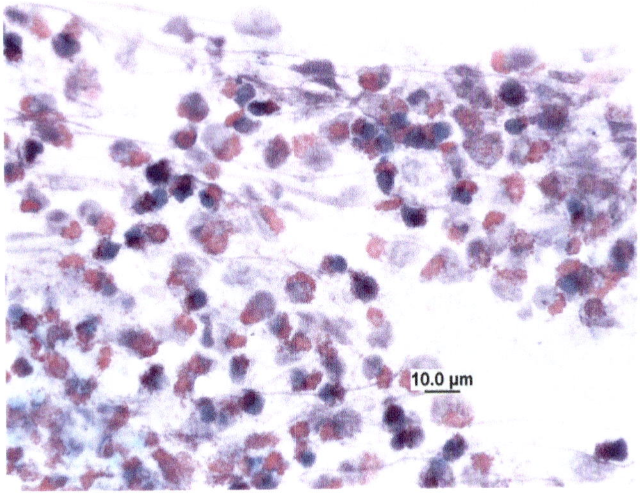

Fig. 7.39. Eosinophilic inflammation in the skin of a hedgehog (*Atelerix albiventris*), Wright–Giemsa stain.

Eosinophilic Inflammation

In mammals, an increased number of eosinophils (10% of the inflammatory cells or greater) in the inflammatory response is indicative of an eosinophilic inflammation (Figures 7.39, 7.40a, and 7.40b). The eosinophils resemble those found in peripheral blood and contain an abundant amount of eosinophilic cytoplasmic granules.

Low numbers of mast cells often accompany eosinophils in inflammatory conditions. Mast cells are round cells with round nuclei and moderately abundant cytoplasm that contains abundant dark purple (metachromatic) granules. Mast cell granules may stain poorly, if at all, with aqueous Romanowsky stains.

Eosinophils phagocytize antibody/antigen complexes and therefore may have a role in maintaining homeostasis during infection. They are particularly numerous when antigens are continually being released, as in parasitic disease. Thus, eosinophilic inflammation is often associated with hypersensitivity or allergic reactions, parasitic infestation, mast cell tumors, and eosinophilic granulomas or paraneoplastic responses. Eosinophilic inflammation associated with an allergic response (type I hypersensitivity reaction) may also demonstrate increased numbers of mast cells, lymphocytes, and plasma cells.

Inflammatory Lesions of the Alimentary Tract

Inflammatory lesions involving the upper alimentary tract (i.e., stomatitis and esophagitis) can be caused by traumatic injury, foreign bodies, chemical irritation (e.g., silver nitrate used for hemostasis) and infectious agents (Campbell, 1983; Campbell, 1995). The cytology reveals an increased number of inflammatory cells and a variable

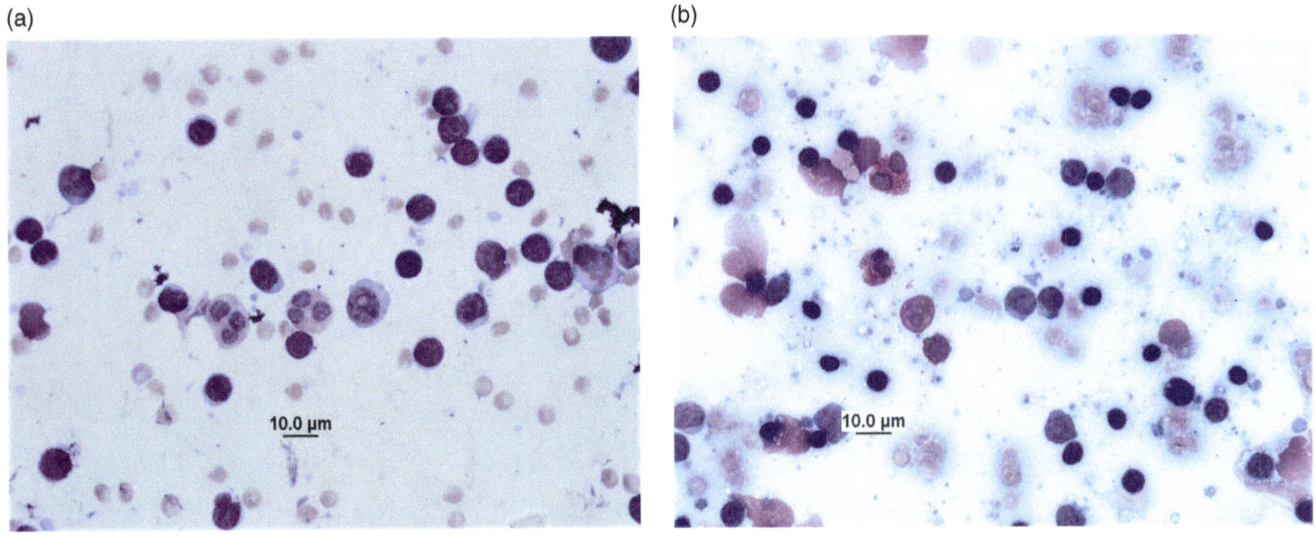

Fig. 7.40. (a) Eosinophils associated with a reactive lymphadenitis in a lymph node from a ferret (*Mustela putorius furo*), Wright–Giemsa stain. (b) Eosinophils associated with a reactive lymphadenitis in a lymph node from a lion (*Panthera leo*), Wright–Giemsa stain.

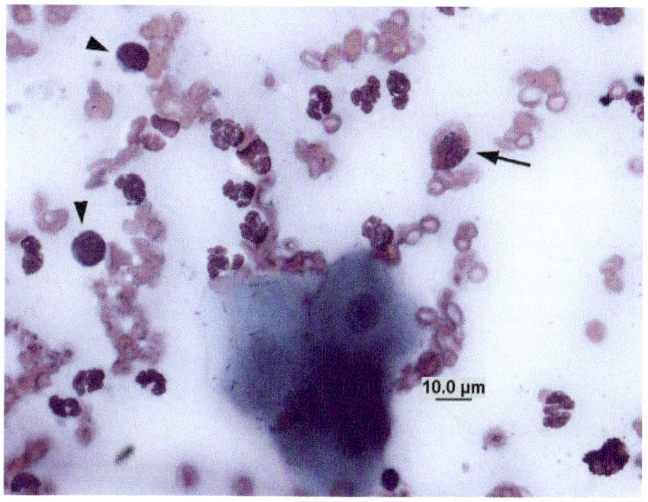

Fig. 7.41. Neutrophils, an eosinophil (arrow), lymphocytes (arrowheads), and squamous epithelial cells from the oral cavity of a hedgehog (*Atelerix albiventris*) with stomatitis, Wright–Giemsa stain.

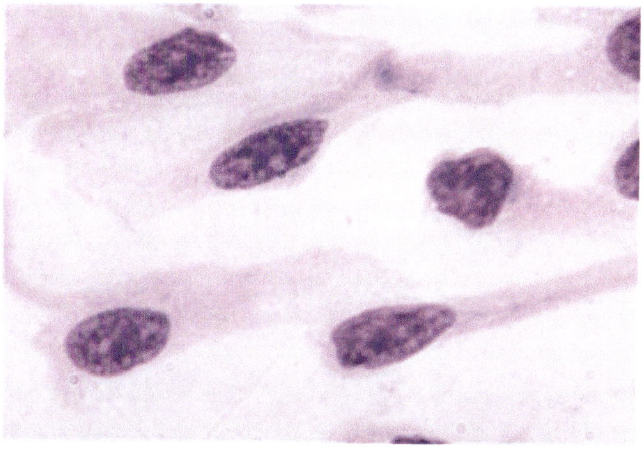

Fig. 7.42. Fibroblasts appear as discrete, spindle-shaped cells characterized by a moderate amount of basophilic cytoplasm and indistinct cytoplasmic margins. The nuclei reveal slight anisokaryosis and granular chromatin, Wright–Giemsa stain (100× oil).

number of squamous epithelial cells (Figures 7.35 and 7.41). An increased amount of background debris and lightly basophilic proteinaceous material may be present as well. Basal cells are present in inflammatory lesions when ulceration of the epithelium is present (Green, 1992). Septic lesions reveal inflammatory cells (heterophilic or mixed cell inflammation) containing intracytoplasmic bacteria (either primary or secondary pathogens) and may contain degenerate leukocytes (primarily neutrophils/heterophils).

Chronic inflammatory lesions may reveal many epithelial cells with a high N:C ratio, multiple prominent nucleoli, and abnormal chromatin patterns. These cells represent a reactive epithelial response to the inflammation and should not be confused with a neoplastic condition. In such cases, it is important to correlate the clinical and the cytological findings to arrive at a reasonable interpretation of the cellular response. When deeply ulcerated lesions or chronic inflammatory lesions are present, fibroblasts may be present in the cytology specimen. Fibroblasts appear as spindle-shaped cells with single, oval to elongated nuclei (occasional multinucleation occurs during rapid proliferation) (Figure 7.42).

Eosinophilic granulomatous stomatitis is a condition that commonly reported in domestic cats (*Felis catus*). It can also occur in captive exotic cats, such as tigers. The cytology typically reveals a mixed cell inflammation with a predominance of eosinophils and occasional mast cell (Figures 7.43a and 7.43b).

Gastritis and enteritis are indicated by the presence of inflammatory cells along with bacteria and cell debris. Acute inflammatory lesions exhibit primarily neutrophils/heterophils. A mixed cell inflammation indicates an established lesion. Chronic gastritis and enteritis are indicated by the presence of lymphocytic or lymphoplasmacytic inflammation. *Helicobacter mustelae* is a common cause of gastroenteritis in ferrets (Hoefer and Bell, 2004). *Helicobacter*, curved to spiral shaped, gram-negative bacteria, are often seen in gastric samples of dogs and cats; however, the organism is difficult to detect in gastric samples of affected ferrets (Walberg and Loar, 2004).

Eosinophilic gastroenteritis is an inflammatory bowel disease that may be associated with a peripheral eosinophilia in ferrets (Hoefer and Bell, 2004). This disorder has an unknown etiology; however, food allergies have been suggested. The diagnosis is made by demonstration of an eosinophilic inflammation in biopsy specimens. Eosinophils are rarely found in fecal cytology samples, but when present are supportive of this disease (Campbell and Grant, 2010) (Figure 7.44).

Fecal cytology has very low numbers of inflammatory cells. Even rectal scrapes in mammalian patients will reveal a rare neutrophil, so any number of inflammatory cells on a fecal smear is significant. Neutrophils and eosinophils are the most common inflammatory cells seen and therefore are considered abnormal and reflect an inflammatory lesion involving the recto-colon or anal area. Ulcerative lesions may reveal basal epithelial cells and numerous erythrocytes along with the inflammatory cells (Figure 7.8). Septic inflammation is indicated by leukocytic phagocytosis of bacteria (Figure 7.33).

In domestic mammals, a pyogranulomatous inflammatory response can be seen with histoplasmosis; however, the quality of the rectal scrape is determined by the presence of epithelial cells. If no epithelial cells are identified, then histoplasmosis likely cannot be diagnosed from the rectal scrape.

(a) (b)

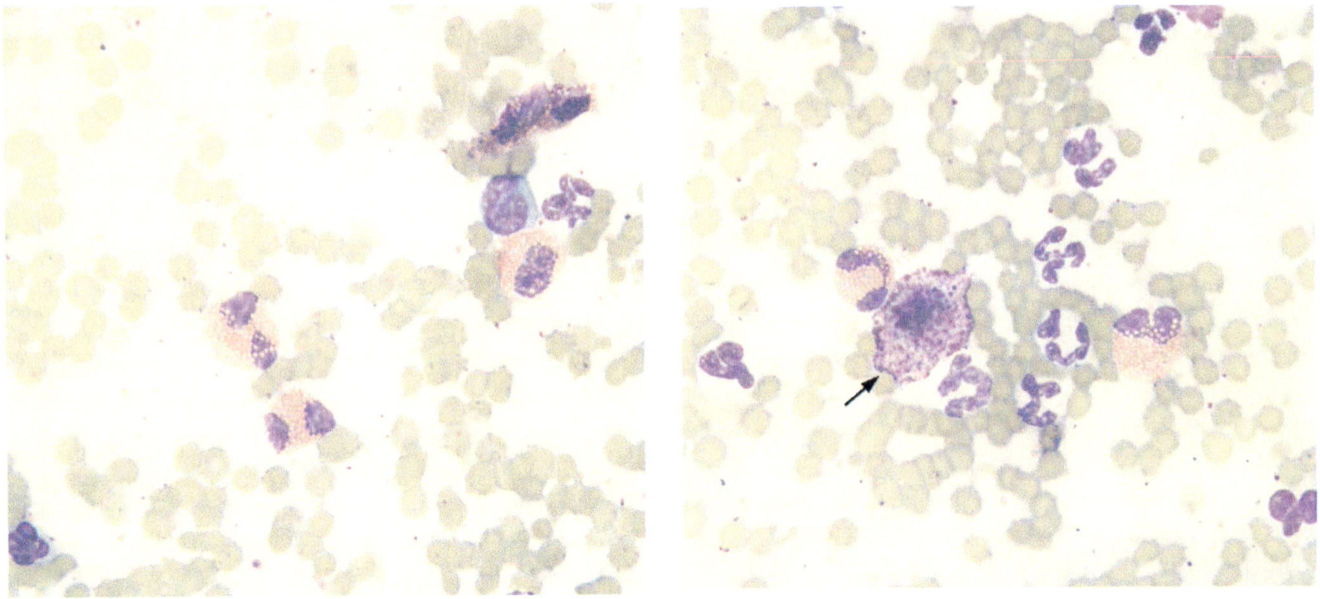

Fig. 7.43. (a) An aspirate of a lesion on the soft palate revealing numerous eosinophils from a tiger (*Panthera tigris tigris*), Wright–Giemsa stain (100× oil). Source: Image from Campbell and Grant (2010, p. 148). (b) An aspirate of a lesion on the soft palate revealing numerous neutrophils, eosinophils, and a mast cell (arrow) from a tiger (*Panthera tigris tigris*), Wright–Giemsa stain (100× oil). Source: Image from Campbell and Grant (2010, p. 148).

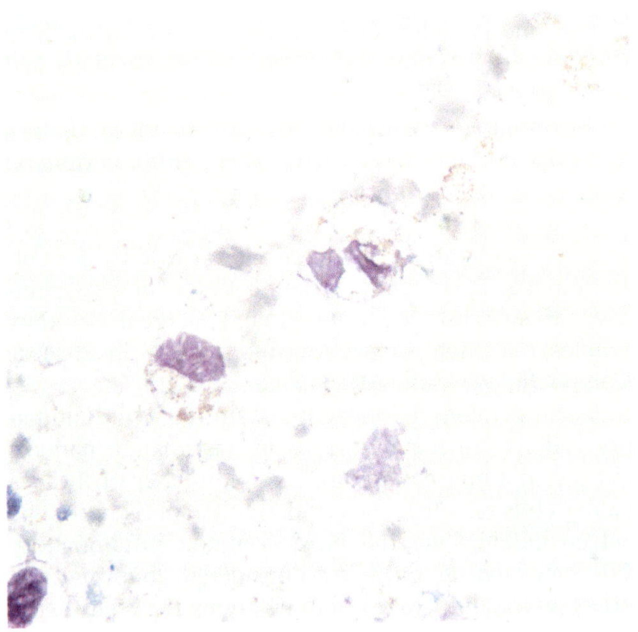

Fig. 7.44. Eosinophils in a fecal smear from a ferret (*Mustela putorius furo*), Wright–Giemsa stain (100× oil). Source: Image from Campbell and Grant (2010, p. 188).

Part of the evaluation of feces is the evaluation of the flora. A mixed population of bacteria is expected. Therefore, a predominance of one type of bacteria (uniform population) is suggestive of bacterial overgrowth and indicates a need for bacterial culture, as this may represent an acute bacterial infection before the inflammatory response or the inflammatory response has been overwhelmed. Low numbers of *Clostridium*-like organisms are acceptable for most domestic mammals; however, the presence of more than three to five suggests a *Clostridium* sp. overgrowth. The presence of *Campylobacter* sp. organisms is also a significant finding, especially if the patient has diarrhea. The appearance of *Candida* sp. and *Saccharomyces* sp. yeast organisms are common findings in the feces of domestic mammals and are not generally considered to be nonpathogenic. See the section titled "Infectious Agents" later in this chapter.

Inflammation of the Respiratory Tract

The presence of inflammatory cells in the cytology sample supports the diagnosis of respiratory tract inflammation, and the type of inflammation present may reveal the etiology. For example, a sample containing mixed cell (pyogranulomatous) inflammation with evidence of foreign material would support the diagnosis of a respiratory foreign body. Primary and secondary bacterial infections are indicated by neutrophilic/heterophilic (suppurative) or mixed cell inflammation with evidence of bacterial phagocytosis (Figure 7.27). Allergic rhinitis is indicated by a sample containing a predominance of eosinophils, and possibly increased numbers of goblet cells as well. Mast cells and plasma cells may also be present in low numbers (Burkhard et al., 2001).

Along with the inflammatory response, severe infections of the respiratory tract may reveal degenerate ciliated respiratory epithelial cells. These cells exhibit losses of cilia, cytoplasmic vacuolation, cell lysis, and karyolysis. Septic lesions are confirmed by the presence of leukocyte phagocytosis of bacteria. Ulcerative lesions may show an increase in erythrocytes and cellular debris. Immune-mediated tracheobronchitis and/or allergic responses should be suspected when many eosinophils, goblet cells, and increased mucin in the background are present in the cytology sample.

The cytology of sinusitis is represented by an increase in inflammatory cells in the sinus aspirate smear. The number and type of inflammatory cells depend on the nature of the infectious agent, severity of the inflammation, and duration of the disease. A moderate to marked amount of background debris, and the causative agent, either primary or secondary, may be present as well. Septic sinusitis is indicated by the presence of a relatively monomorphic population of bacteria, and intracytoplasmic bacteria within leukocytes (typically neutrophils or heterophils). Bacterial sinusitis may not reveal the microorganisms on the cytology specimen; however, a positive culture would support the diagnosis.

Chronic irritation or inflammation affecting the respiratory tract leads to cellular hyperplasia, which results in numerous clusters and sheets of epithelial cells in the cytologic sample. These epithelial cells contain features of tissue hyperplasia, which include increased N:C ratios, increased cytoplasmic basophilia, and mild nuclear anisocytosis. Increased numbers of normal mitotic figures may also be seen.

Tracheal wash samples of mammals that exhibit many neutrophils or heterophils and macrophages, increased numbers of goblet cells, and increased mucin in the background indicate a tracheobronchitis or pneumonia. Neutrophils or heterophils are more predominant in acute lesions. When chronic inflammation is present, increased numbers of macrophages, lymphocytes, and plasma cells are present. Macrophages associated with chronic inflammation of the lower respiratory tract are often large and multinucleated. Degenerate ciliated respiratory epithelial cells (i.e., loss of cilia, cytoplasmic vacuolation, cell lysis, and karyolysis) may be seen with severe infections. Fragmented ciliated respiratory epithelial cells associated with a mononuclear leukocytic inflammatory response are suggestive of a viral etiology. Septic lesions are confirmed by the presence of leukocyte phagocytosis of bacteria.

A foreign body reaction or aspiration tracheobronchitis associated with the lower respiratory tract may reveal large reactive macrophages that form giant cells containing phagocytized foreign material.

Macrophagic inflammation associated with the tracheobronchial tract and lungs is often associated with fungal, foreign body, or mycobacterial lesions. The macrophages present may appear as reactive multinucleated giant cells, or as epithelioid cells. Epithelioid cells often appear as clusters of macrophages with blue-gray to pink cytoplasm, and distinct cytoplasmic margins (Burkhard et al., 2001).

Verminous pneumonia is a common clinical problem in the European hedgehog, most commonly by both nematodes, *Eucoleus aerophilus* (syn. *Capillaria aerophila*) and *Crenosoma striatum*. Cytologic preparations of lungs with mixed infection reveal mixed cell inflammation with a background of proteinaceous debris and rod-shaped bacteria along with morulated nematode eggs and larvae and barrel-shaped bipolar plugs, typical of trichuroid/capillarid morphology (Manzocchi et al., 2016).

Inflammation of the Skin

Fine-needle aspiration cytology is a rapid, efficient, cost-effective, relatively painless procedure and produces a speedy result with high diagnostic accuracy. In human studies, it has high rates of sensitivity and specificity in diagnosing papulonodular lesions of skin. In one study compared to histopathologic results, fine-needle aspiration cytology demonstrated a 100% correlation in cases of epidermal cyst, leprosy, tuberculosis, actinomycosis, and acute and chronic inflammatory lesions, and therefore is a valuable tool in the diagnosis and management of patients with papulonodular skin lesions (Patel et al., 2016).

Lesions involving the skin and subcutis can be classified using the basic categories of cytodiagnosis: inflammatory, hyperplasic, and neoplastic. Inflammatory lesions can have an infectious or a noninfectious etiology. Suppurative inflammation of the skin and subcutaneous tissue is common because bacterial infections of the skin and subcutaneous usually result in this type of inflammation where intracellular bacteria are often easy to find and the neutrophils/heterophils often appear degenerate (Figures 7.26–7.29). Thus, bacterial infections are characterized cytologically by numerous degenerate neutrophils/heterophils, cellular debris, and bacteria (Figures 7.28 and 7.45). Septic inflammation is indicated by the presence of intracellular bacteria. The appearance of the bacteria may suggest the etiology; however, bacterial culture is necessary for a definitive diagnosis. For example, slender, filamentous and branching bacterial rods that stain slightly basophilic and contain red spotted areas are suggestive of *Nocardia* spp. or *Actinomyces* spp. (Raskin, 2001a).

Granulomas in the skin are represented cytologically by the presence of a macrophagic inflammation with epithelioid cells (epithelial macrophages) and giant cells (Baker and Lumsden, 2000). Granulomas are often caused by noninfectious agents, such as foreign bodies, or infectious agents, such as fungi or mycobacterium. Pyogranulomatous inflammation is often caused by

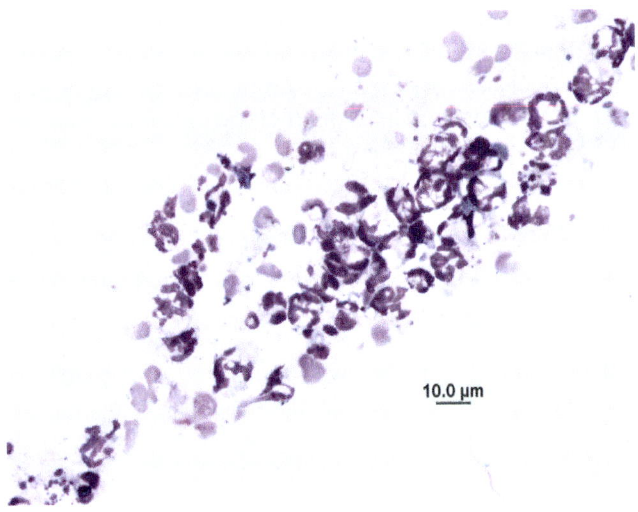

Fig. 7.45. Degenerate neutrophils in a swab of an ulcerative skin lesion in a rat (*Rattus norvegicus*), Wright–Giemsa stain.

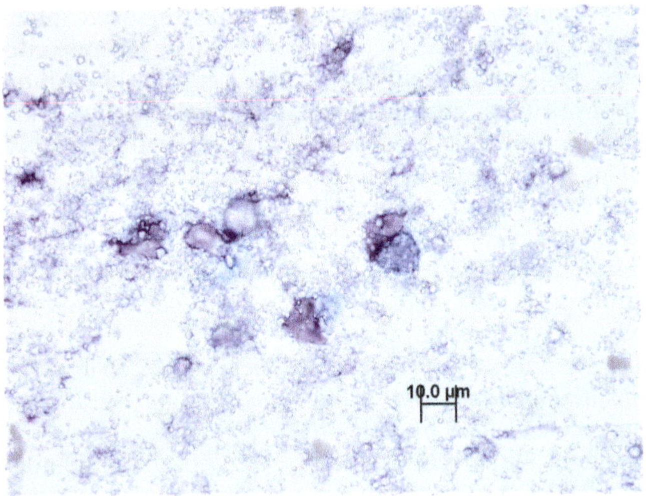

Fig. 7.46. Numerous refractile crystals of various shapes and sizes along with an inflammatory response that consists predominantly of macrophages in a fine-needle aspiration biopsy from a cutaneous calcinosis circumscripta lesion in a sugar glider (*Petaurus breviceps*), Wright–Giemsa stain (100× oil).

fungal organisms, though sterile pyogranulomatous inflammation can also occur.

Mycotic infections are indicated by the presence of mixed cell or macrophagic inflammation and fungal elements. Macrophages, neutrophils or heterophils, lymphocytes, plasma cells, and fibroblasts are typically part of the cellular response to dermal fungal infections. Fungal hyphae may stain poorly in some specimens and appear as large, negative-staining structures among the inflammatory cells (Figures 15.134, 15.138 in Chapter 15; Figure 23.33 in Chapter 23).

Noninfectious inflammatory lesions of the skin and subcutaneous tissues include foreign body reaction, xanthomatosis, epidermal cysts (follicular cysts or feather follicle cysts), calcinosis circumscripta, and hematoma. Foreign bodies in the skin or subcutis cause mixed cell inflammation or macrophagic inflammation with multinucleated giant cells. The macrophages present in the cytology sample may contain phagocytized material. A secondary septic inflammation may also be present.

In mammals, xanthomas may form secondary to primary or secondary hyperlipidemia, with high plasma concentrations of cholesterol or triglyceride-containing lipoproteins. Cutaneous xanthomatosis is a rare granulomatous inflammation of the skin of domestic cats (Grieshaber et al., 1991; Raskin, 2001c). Cutaneous xanthomatosis results from the accumulation of excess lipid material (cholesterol and triglycerides) and an associated macrophagic inflammation in the skin. Lesions occur as discrete yellow nodules or plaques, or may appear as a diffuse thickening of the skin. The lesions can be locally invasive.

Cytological features of xanthomatosis include numerous highly vacuolated (foamy) macrophages, multinucleated giant cells, and cholesterol crystals (Figures 15.47–15.52 in Chapter 15). The background of the cytologic sample is often heavy with round, clear areas that resemble fat droplets. Cholesterol crystals appear as angular, variable-shaped, negative-staining (clear), notched plates that often appear stacked in the noncellular background. These crystals will often dissolve in the alcohol fixatives of some stains and subsequently appear as a negative image in the cytology sample. The foamy macrophages (highly vacuolated) will stain positive with lipid stains.

The cytologic findings of xanthomatosis reflect what is observed on histology. Histological characteristic of cutaneous xanthogranulomas have features of both xanthomas and granulomas with numerous highly vacuolated, lipid-laden macrophages (called foam or xanthoma cells), cholesterol clefts, fibroblasts, and multinucleated giant cells.

Calcinosis circumscripta is a benign lesion presumed to be associated with mineralization of necrotic tissue secondary to trauma or inflammation. This condition has been primarily reported in mammals. Cytological features of the lesions reveal numerous refractile crystals of various shapes and sizes along with an inflammatory response that consists predominantly of macrophages and fibroblasts (Figure 7.46).

Inflammation of Synovial Joints

Inflammatory joint disease (suppurative arthropathies) can be caused by infectious agents such as bacteria, fungi, parasites, mycoplasma, and viruses, or by noninfectious etiologies such as gout and immune-mediated disease. Cytology of inflammatory joint disease reveals an increase in the total nucleated cell count (e.g., 20 000 to greater than 100 000 μL), increased percentage of neutrophils/heterophils (e.g., greater than 50%), abnormal color and clarity, and reduced viscosity and mucin quality. A concurrent increase in the large vacuolated macrophages may also be present. The background of smears made from synovial fluid with poor mucin quality lacks the granular appearance (stippled eosinophilic background) of normal joint fluid. An increase in the refractometric total protein concentration (e.g., 4.5–7.5 g/dL) is expected (Meinkoth, 2022). The presence of multinucleated osteoclasts or spindle-shaped fibroblasts indicates erosion of the articular cartilage, exposing underlying bone, or erosion into the fibrous layer of the articular capsule.

Septic arthritis is indicated by a high total nucleated cell count (e.g., greater than 50 000/μL) and the presence of high numbers of neutrophils/heterophils. The neutrophils/heterophils in bacterial arthritis are often uncharacteristically nondegenerate because the viscosity of the synovial fluid is protective to cell morphology (Meinkoth, 2022). Extracellular bacteria are suggestive of bacterial involvement, and bacterial phagocytosis is considered diagnostic for septic joint disease. Bacteria often are not inherently obvious on the slide; however, the presence of degenerative neutrophils/heterophils is suggestive of a septic lesion.

A marked increase in both the absolute number and percentage of neutrophils/heterophils is expected with septic or immune-mediated arthropathies; however, only a modest increase in these cells is typically associated inflammation resulting from joint trauma, periarticular inflammation, chronic hemarthrosis, or intra-articular injections.

Traumatic injury to the joint (traumatic arthritis) may reveal an increase in the number of inflammatory leukocytes, primarily neutrophils/heterophils in cases of acute trauma. Depending upon the degree of joint injury, synoviocytes and mesenchymal cells representing exfoliation of cells from the underlying cartilage may be present. Cartilage fragments may also be found. These are represented by the presence of amorphous material with variable staining characteristics on the Romanowsky-stained smear. The mucin clot test and viscosity of synovial fluid associated with acute traumatic arthritis is typically normal if hemarthrosis is not involved.

Joints affected by immune-mediated disease exhibit increased numbers of nondegenerate neutrophils/heterophils. Increased numbers of lymphocytes and plasma cells may also be seen.

Degenerative joint disease (degenerative arthropathies or noninflammatory arthropathies) is a gradual breakdown of articular cartilage with periarticular bony proliferation most often related to joint laxity. Degenerative joint disease is represented by synovial fluid with mild increases in cell numbers (e.g., 5000–10 000/μl) compared to the marked increases observed with inflammatory joint disease. The cells in synovial fluid from a degenerative joint are represented primarily by mononuclear cells (greater than 90% of the cells), such as macrophages, lymphocytes, and synovial cells. An increased number of macrophages (activated) with vacuolated cytoplasm and phagocytized material may be found. Joint aspirates associated with degenerative joint disease often reveal synoviocytes, and mesenchymal cells representing exfoliation of cells from the underlying cartilage may be present. Severely damaged joints may reveal multinucleated osteoclasts in the joint fluid. Cartilage fragments may also be found. These are represented by the presence of amorphous material with variable staining characteristics on the Romanowsky-stained smear. The viscosity and mucin clot tests may be normal or reduced with degenerative joint disease.

Fine-needle aspiration cytology is a simple and effective technique for the diagnosis of periarticular nodules. Crystal deposition joint disease includes deposition of uric acid crystals (articular gout) or calcium pyrophosphate deposition (pseudogout). Among primates, gout appears to be a uniquely human malady; however, pseudogout has been reported in a variety of nonhuman primates (Lowenstine et al., 2016). Aspirates of gouty tophi (see avian and herptile cytodiagnosis) in most cases reveal a chalky white particulate that tends to wash off microscope slides. The cytology reveals negatively birefringent needle-shaped crystals consistent with monosodium urate crystals in amorphous granular debris on cytology. Crystals can also be demonstrated in wet-mount preparations from needle washings made by flushing the aspirating needle with absolute alcohol (Nasser et al., 1994). In some cases, microscopy will also show erythrocytes, foamy macrophages, multinucleated giant cells, neutrophils, and epithelioid cells. Crystal identification can sometimes be obscured by background blood and inflammatory exudate. Paucity of crystalline material with an intense inflammatory reaction may also mask the true nature of the lesion. Presence of amorphous or granular material should alert the cytopathologist to examine the smear under a polarizing microscope. Calcium pyrophosphate deposition crystals in pseudogout lesions are shorter, more often rhomboid than needle shaped and show positive birefringence (Agarwal, et al., 2007).

Inflammation of Lymphoid Tissue

Lymphadenitis is represented by an increase in the number of inflammatory cells in the cytology sample from the mammalian lymph node. Inflammation is indicated when the population of neutrophils/heterophils is greater than 5% of the population of cells. The type of inflammatory cell population present is used to classify the lymphadenitis. Neutrophilic/heterophilic (purulent or suppurative) lymphadenitis is indicated by a predominance of neutrophils/heterophils in the inflammatory cell population, and is typically associated with bacterial infection, neoplasia, and immune-mediated disease.

Pyogranulomatous lymphadenitis is indicated by increased numbers of macrophages and neutrophils/heterophils. Therefore, pyogranulomatous lymphadenitis is represented by more than 40% of macrophages, multinucleated giant cells, and epithelioid macrophages, and many neutrophils (Messick, 2014; Barrios-Arpi and Morales-Cauti, 2020).

Granulomatous inflammation (macrophagic (histiocytic) lymphadenitis) is represented an abundance of inflammatory giant cells and epithelioid macrophages with a small number of neutrophils (heterophils) (Messick, 2014; Barrios-Arpi and Morales-Cauti, 2020). Granulomatous lymphadenitis is associated with diseases such as fungal infections and mycobacteriosis.

A cytodiagnosis of eosinophilic lymphadenitis is made when the population of eosinophils is greater than 3% of the cells in the lymph node aspirate (Messick, 2014; Barrios-Arpi and Morales-Cauti, 2020) (Figures 7.39, 7.40a, 7.40b, 7.47a, and 7.47b). Eosinophilic lymphadenitis is associated with hypersensitivity and neoplastic disorders.

Splenitis is indicated by the presence of increased numbers of inflammatory cells in the splenic sample. When evaluating a splenic sample for splenitis, it is important to differentiate between true inflammatory changes in the spleen and contamination of the sample with peripheral blood that contains a peripheral leukocytosis. Cytologic specimens, splenic or otherwise, that are contaminated with peripheral blood having a marked leukocytosis appear to have an inflammatory response; however, the majority of neutrophils/heterophils present have originated from the blood and not from the tissue being examined.

Inflammation of the Liver

Hepatitis (inflammatory responses involving the liver) is indicated by the presence of numerous leukocytes in the cytology specimen. Suppurative inflammation – that is, neutrophilic/heterophilic inflammation – is suggested when high numbers of mature neutrophils/heterophils are observed relative to the red blood cell numbers. The presence of neutrophils/heterophils associated with aggregates of hepatocytes provides further cytologic support of suppurative inflammation. Septic inflammation is indicated by the presence of bacteria within leukocytes. Extracellular bacteria must be differentiated from "cadaver" bacteria or bacterial contamination of the sample when the sample is obtained during necropsy.

Mixed cell or macrophagic inflammation of the liver can be associated with mycotic, parasitic, or mycobacterial infections (Figure 7.48). Granulomatous lesions reveal macrophages that are often vacuolated and multinucleated giant cells.

Ophthalmic Inflammation

Conjunctivitis is a common cause for sampling the conjunctiva for cytologic examination and is recognized by the presence of many inflammatory cells (Figures 7.49 and 7.50). Neutrophilic/heterophilic inflammation of the

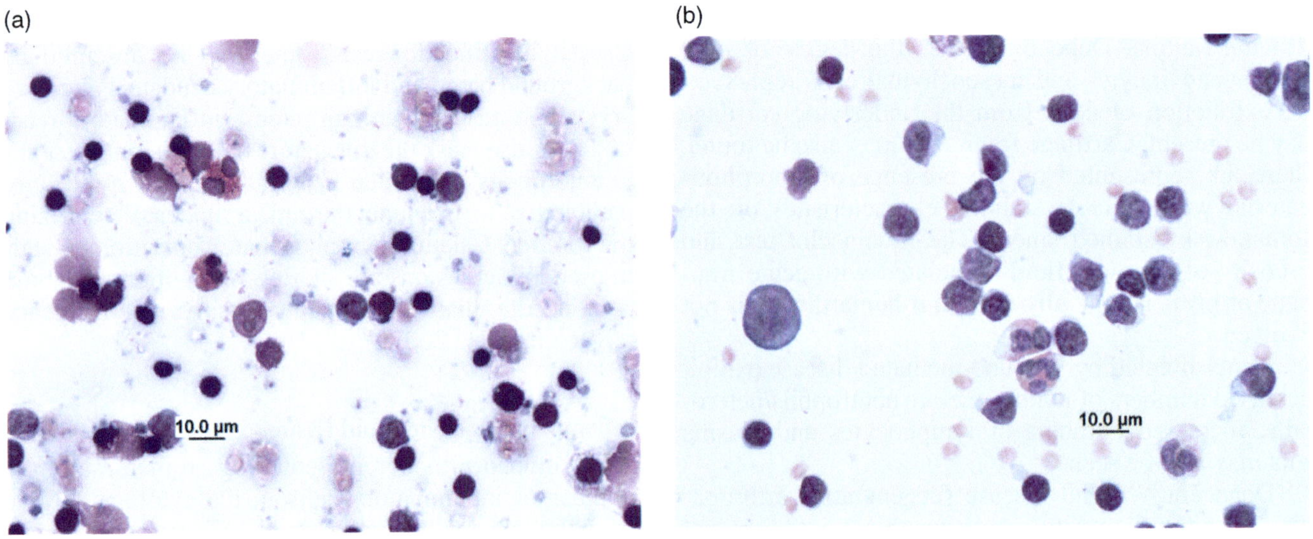

Fig. 7.47. (a) A mesenteric lymph node aspirate revealing predominantly small, mature lymphocytes with an increase in the eosinophil population (greater than 3% of the cells) from a lion (*Panthera leo*) with eosinophilic gastroenteritis, Wright–Giemsa stain. (b) A lymph node aspirate from a ferret (*Mustela putorius furo*) revealing predominantly small mature lymphocytes with an increase in the medium lymphocytes, lymphoblasts, and eosinophils, Wright–Giemsa stain.

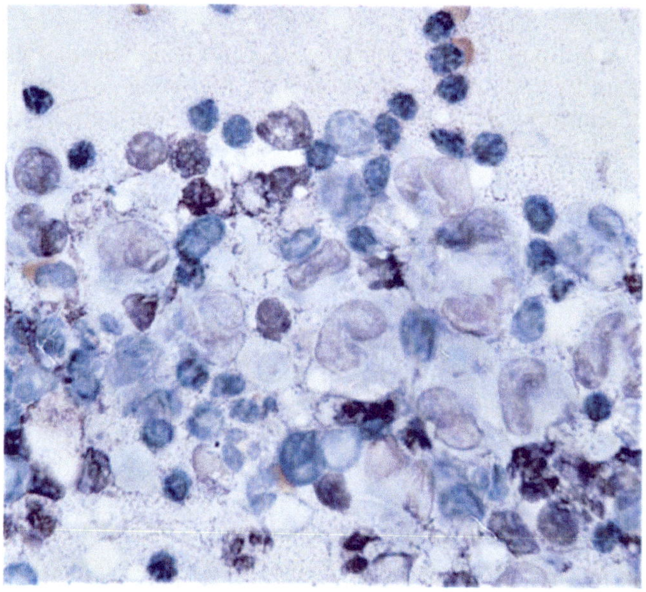

Fig. 7.48. A contact smear of a liver revealing a macrophagic inflammation with a predominance of macrophages and lymphocytes from a ferret (*Mustela putorius furo*) with a *Mycobacterium goodii* infection, Wright–Giemsa stain (100× oil). Source: Image from Campbell and Grant (2010, p. 184).

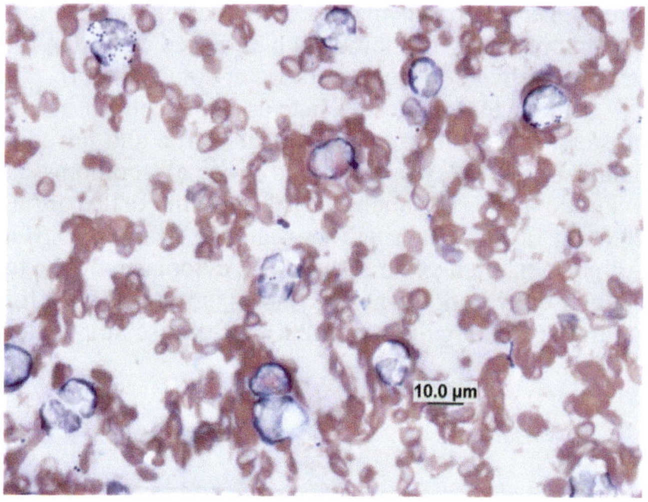

Fig. 7.49. Septic neutrophilic inflammation in a fine-needle aspiration biopsy of a conjunctival mass from an African hedgehog (*Atelerix albiventris*), Wright–Giemsa stain.

conjunctiva can be caused by bacteria, viruses, or noninfectious agents, such as trauma, foreign bodies, and environmental irritants.

Degenerate neutrophils or heterophils are often associated with bacterial infections.

Bacterial conjunctivitis is common in small mammals, such as rodents and rabbits. Common bacterial isolates in rabbits include *Pasteurella multocida*, *Staphylococcus aureus*, *Bordetella* spp., and *Bacillus subtilis* (van der Woerdt, 2004). Common bacterial isolates from

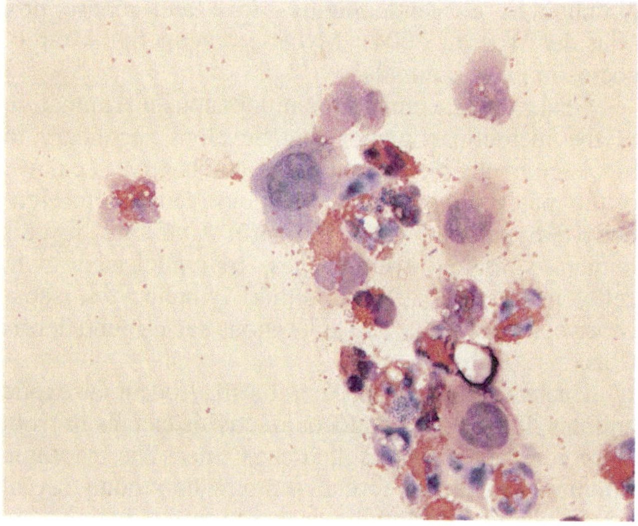

Fig. 7.50. Heterophilic inflammation with epithelial cells in a conjunctival swab from a rabbit (*Oryctolagus cuniculus*) with conjunctivitis, Wright– Giemsa stain (100× oil).

conjunctival lesions in rodents include *Pseudomonas aeruginosa*, *P. pneumotropica*, *Salmonella* spp., *Streptobacillus moniliformis*, and *Corynebacterium kutscheri* (van der Woerdt, 2004). *Chlamydophila psittaci* is a common cause of conjunctivitis in guinea pigs (Kern, 1989).

Skinny pigs, nearly hairless guinea pigs, were found to be at higher risk for *Pasteurellaceae*-associated conjunctivitis (Wu et al., 2019). Bacterial conjunctivitis in mammals is often associated with a mucopurulent discharge. Septic conjunctivitis is confirmed cytologically by the presence of phagocytosis of the bacterial pathogens. The epithelial cells in septic lesions may show degenerative changes such as cytoplasmic vacuolation, karyolysis, or karyorrhexis.

Chlamydia organisms may be seen on cytologic specimens from conjunctival scrapings. They appear as intracytoplasmic inclusion bodies in epithelial cells (see Chapter 15).

Mycoplasma infections are common causes of conjunctivitis in rats and possibly other rodents and occasionally in rabbits (Kern, 1989; van der Woerdt, 2004). Mycoplasma is frequently overlooked as a cause for conjunctivitis because it can be difficult to diagnose. Mycoplasmal inclusions appear as small basophilic granules on the surface of epithelial cells (Campbell et al., 1973).

Viral agents associated with conjunctivitis have been reported in small mammals. Myxoma virus infections can cause conjunctivitis in rabbits; however, as with viral etiologies of other animals, conjunctivitis is not the only clinical sign (van der Woerdt, 2004). Canine distemper virus causes a mucopurulent conjunctivitis in ferrets (Kern, 1989). Several viruses can cause conjunctivitis in rodents. These include Sendai virus, lymphocytic choriomeningitis virus, and mouse pox (van der Woerdt, 2004). Mycotic conjunctivitis rarely occurs in exotic animals.

Chalazion is a chronic granulomatous inflammation of the meibomian glands that develops secondary to blockage of the ductules into the conjunctiva. Leakage of the material in the meibomian cyst causes a foreign-body-like inflammatory response. Cytology reveals numerous foamy macrophages, multinucleated giant cells, neutrophils or heterophils, lymphocytes, sebaceous epithelial cells, and amorphous background debris (Raskin, 2001b).

Bacterial and fungal keratitis may occur in exotic animals. In rodents, keratoconjunctivitis can result from ammonia vapors from soiled cage litter. The cytologic samples obtained by corneal scraping commonly reveal a neutrophilic/heterophilic or mixed inflammation. The etiologic agent, such as bacteria or fungal elements, may be present as well.

Hyperplasia/Benign Neoplasia

Tissue hyperplasia is a proliferative process of tissues responding to cellular injury or chronic stimulation (i.e., glandular hyperplasia). Neoplasia is the proliferation of cells under conditions that lack the normal controls that would result in the cessation of the multiplication of normal cells. Therefore, benign neoplasia consists of cells that are not malignant.

Based upon cytomorphology alone, tissue hyperplasia and benign neoplasia are indistinguishable. Cells representative of tissue hyperplasia or benign neoplasia exhibit uniformity in overall appearance. Cells typically have an immature appearance and exhibit an increased cytoplasmic basophilia with pale vesicular nuclei (Rebar, 1978). They are similar in size with similar N:C ratios and nuclear features. Cells associated with cellular hyperplasia may exhibit an increase in normal mitotic figures, which is indicative of the proliferative nature of the tissue.

A survey of over 1500 histopathologic samples of cutaneous tumors in ferrets, rabbits, and guinea pigs revealed that most of them are benign (Kanfer and Reavill, 2013). That study found the most common skin tumors of guinea pigs in 133 samples were, in order of frequency, trichofolliculomas, lipomas, trichoepitheliomas, and mammary gland adenocarcinomas. According to the same study, the most common skin tumors in rabbits from 672 cases in order of frequency were basal cell tumors, spindle cell sarcomas, collagenous hamartomas, squamous papillomas, and mammary gland adenocarcinomas. The study revealed that out of 763 cases in ferrets, the most common skin tumors, in order of frequency, were mast cell tumors, sebaceous epitheliomas, cutaneous hemangiomas, preputial gland tumors, and lymphoma.

Adipose

A lipoma is an example of benign neoplasia frequently encountered in domestic mammals. It is an uncommon benign mesenchymal cell skin tumor of small exotic mammals. Lipomas have been occasionally reported in the guinea pig (Scott et al., 2001). Lipomas are benign, encapsulated tumors of adipose tissue that are composed of normal, mature adipocytes (fat cells). Grossly, lipomas typically appear as pale yellow, soft, often freely movable subcutaneous masses that occur singly or as multiple masses. Lipomas are slow growing and can become quite large. Because it is often difficult to differentiate a lipoma from normal adipose tissue cytologically, accidental aspiration of normal adipose tissue should be ruled out whenever lipocytes are identified in a cytology sample. The gross appearance of the tissue sample may aid in the diagnosis in some cases. Grossly, unstained aspirated material from a lipoma has a "greasy" appearance and does not dry completely on the slide due to the lipid content.

Lipid and adipose cells often disappear when stains containing alcohol or alcohol fixatives (Romanowsky stains) are used. Cytologic specimens prepared with an alcohol fixative reveal a slide with numerous background fat droplets that appear as small, clear, unstained circles. Lipid droplets may be easily detected in a cytology sample using fat stains, such as oil red O, Sudan IV, or new methylene blue stain (a water-soluble stain).

Adipocytes tend to exfoliate as single cells or in cell clusters. Mammalian adipocytes are large and have an abundant clear cytoplasm and a small compressed pyknotic-appearing nucleus pushed to the cell margin, creating a "signet ring" appearance (Figure 7.51). Adipocytes often exhibit a wrinkled cytoplasm owing to cellular dehydration when alcohol fixatives are used for staining (Walberg and Loar, 2004). Because adipocytes

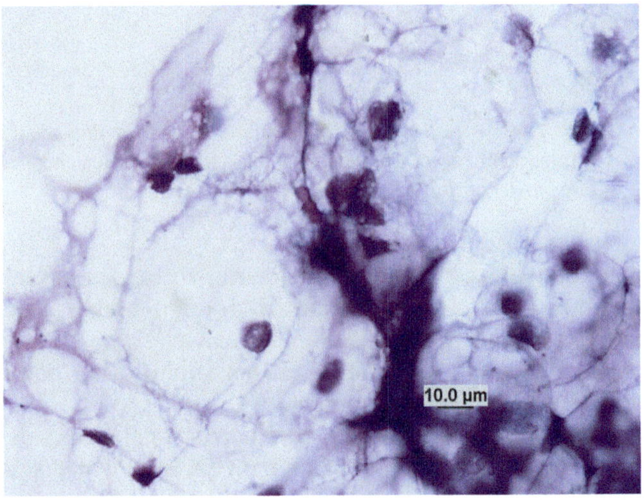

Fig. 7.51. Adipocytes in a fine-needle aspiration biopsy from a lipoma in rat (*Rattus norvegicus*), Wright–Giemsa stain.

are large cells with a thin cytoplasmic membrane, they tend to rupture easily during slide preparation, leaving free nuclei and fat droplets in the noncellular background. Fat stains can confirm lipid content, but are seldom required for routine interpretation.

Liposarcomas are differentiated from benign lipomas based on the cytologic appearance of the adipocytes. Cells from liposarcomas appear as dense aggregates of highly pleomorphic mesenchymal cells with variable amounts and sizes of the intracytoplasmic lipid vacuoles. The pleomorphic adipocytes vary in size, ranging from large cells with a low N:C ratio and abundant cytoplasm to small cells with high N:C ratios and a small amount of basophilic cytoplasm.

Fine-needle aspirate cytology of lipomas and liposarcomas usually cannot provide a definitive diagnosis, because the lipid droplets within the adipocytes (lipomas) or neoplastic cells (liposarcomas) will be dissolved by the alcohol associated with the staining procedure. However, cytology is helpful in distinguishing between lipomas, abscesses, or hematomas, and it is helpful in identifying adipocytes, if these cells are present (Liptak and Forrest, 2007).

Hepatic Lipidosis

Cytology is routinely used to diagnose hepatic lipidosis in companion animals (Arndt and Shelly, 2014; Barger and MacNeill, 2016; Meyer, 2016; Fry et al., 2018). Hepatic lipidosis (fatty liver syndrome or steatosis) is represented by the appearance of hepatocytes with many small or large, clear cytoplasmic vacuoles, which represent lipid that has dissolved during the staining process. Unstained smears made from livers with fatty change may appear "greasy" on gross inspection of the slide. Hepatic lipidosis may represent a lipid storage disorder (usually seen in young animals). Hepatic lipidosis is relatively common in small mammals, such as rodents, hedgehogs, and rabbits. Hepatic lipidosis develops rapidly in anorectic rabbits, especially if they are overweight (Deeb, 2000). In dairy cattle, hepatic lipidosis has been evaluated microscopically using a novel ordinal scale (0–4) based on the estimated percentage of hepatocytes with discrete cytoplasmic vacuolation and on the estimated mean percentage of cytoplasm occupied by vacuoles on Wright–Giemsa-stained imprints (Fry et al., 2018).

Epidermal Cyst

Epidermal inclusion cysts are common masses on older dogs. Cytologically they consist of mature squamous epithelial cells and thick aggregates of keratinaceous debris. Occasionally, cholesterol crystals are identified. When these cysts rupture, they elicit a marked inflammatory response that appears as a suppurative to pyogranulomatous inflammation where the inflammatory cells are observed surrounding aggregates of keratinaceous material. In mammals, an epidermal cyst associated with a hair follicle is called a follicular cyst, and those lacking adnexal differentiation and a connection to the skin surface histologically are called epidermal inclusion cysts (Raskin, 2001a). Cytologically, epidermal inclusion cysts and follicular cysts contain squames, keratin bars, and keratinized epithelial cells with pyknotic nuclei all distributed in a background of basophilic amorphous cellular debris (Raskin, 2001a) (Figures 7.4 and 7.5). As the cells degenerate, cholesterol crystals appear. Because the cholesterol crystals often dissolve in the alcohol in Romanowsky types of stains, only their negative images (cholesterol clefts) may be present on the slide. Rupture of the cyst wall sometimes occurs and leads to a mixed cell inflammatory response with a predominance of neutrophils and macrophages.

Sebaceous Cysts

Sebaceous cysts and sebaceous hyperplasia consist of clusters of sebaceous epithelial cells. The cytology reveals aggregates of cells with a moderate rim of cytoplasm filled with distinct cytoplasmic vacuoles. It is difficult to differentiate sebaceous hyperplasia from an adenoma based on cytology alone.

Trichoepitheliomas

Trichoepitheliomas originate in the hair follicle and are characterized as well-demarcated, encapsulated, round to ovoid dermal masses in rabbits, guinea pigs, and rodents, such as hamsters (Greenacre, 2004; Heatley and Smith, 2004; Garner, 2007). Benign trichoepitheliomas appear on the head, thorax, limb, perineum, and ischium of rabbits (Budgeon et al., 2014). Fine-needle aspiration samples stained with a Romanowsky-type stain reveal keratinized squamous cells and glandular epithelial cells of sebaceous gland origin (Martorell and Melero, 2013). Epithelioma/trichoepithelioma has been related to hamster polyomavirus (HaPV), specifically in Syrian hamsters (Donnelly, 2004; Orr, 2009).

Papillomas

Papillomas are difficult to diagnose by cytology alone because they reveal predominantly cornified squamous epithelial cells on the cellular sample. Oral papillomas occur in rabbits, where they are more common in young rabbits (Harcourt-Brown, 2002a). The main differential diagnoses for such growths in domestic rabbits include cottontail rabbit (Shope) papillomavirus, spontaneous nonviral squamous papillomas, and rabbit (Shope) fibroma virus infection (Kerr and Donnelly, 2013). Surgical mass excision or biopsy with histological examination is required to make the final diagnosis for most epithelial lesions.

Histiocytoma

A histiocytoma is a benign round cell (discrete cell) neoplasm of the integument that has been reported in ferrets (Scott et al., 2001). Grossly, the lesion may appear as a small, red, solitary, well-circumscribed, dome-shaped mass that may be ulcerated (Raskin, 2001a). A fine-needle aspirate yields a sample of low to moderate cellularity with a uniform to mildly pleomorphic population of mononuclear cells (Tyler et al., 1999). Cytologic specimens reveal round cells demonstrating moderate anisocytosis. The cytoplasm of the cells is abundant, and clear to lightly basophilic in color (Figures 7.52a and 7.52b). The cytoplasmic margins may be variably distinct, and the nuclei typically appear round, oval, or sometimes indented. The nuclear chromatin is finely granular in appearance, and nucleoli are rare.

Chordomas

Chordomas are benign tumors that originate from notochordal remnants in the nucleus pulposus of the intervertebral disk. (Goad and Fox, 1988; Cantile and Youssef, 2016; Cole et al., 2020). The notochord regresses after completing its function of axial positioning in the developing embryo. It is then replaced by the nucleus pulposus of the intervertebral disks. However, a small portion of notochordal cells can still be found as notochordal remnants in adults (Vujovic et al., 2006). The location of chordomas follows the anatomic distribution of notochordal remnants. In ferrets, chordomas are relatively commonly reported and frequently appear as hairless swelling at the tip of the tail; however, they can occur in other locations along the spine (Camus et al., 2009; Fox et al., 2014) (Figure 7.53). In rodents, the location of the tumor varies among the cranial, cervical, thoracic, lumbar, sacral, and coccygeal segments of the axial skeleton.

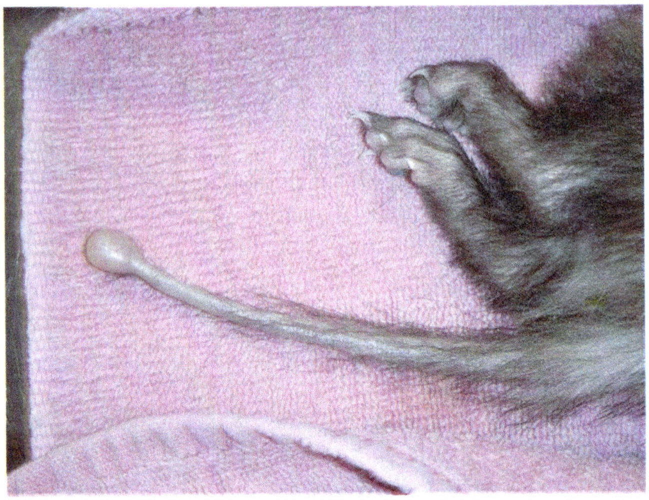

Fig. 7.53. A ferret (*Mustela putorius furo*) with a chordoma on the tail tip. The ferret also has alopecia, likely from a concurrent adrenal disease.

(a)

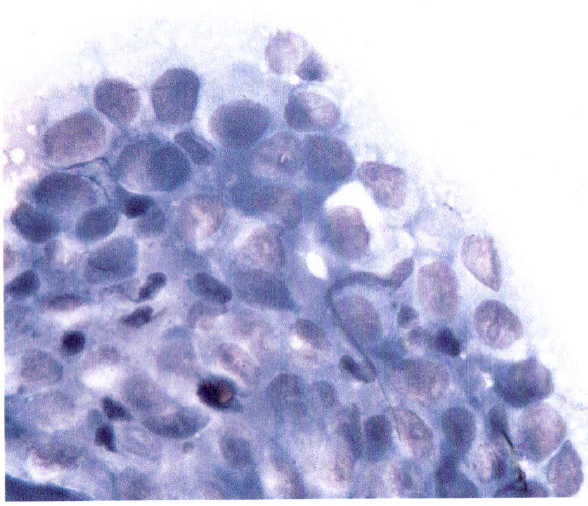

(b)

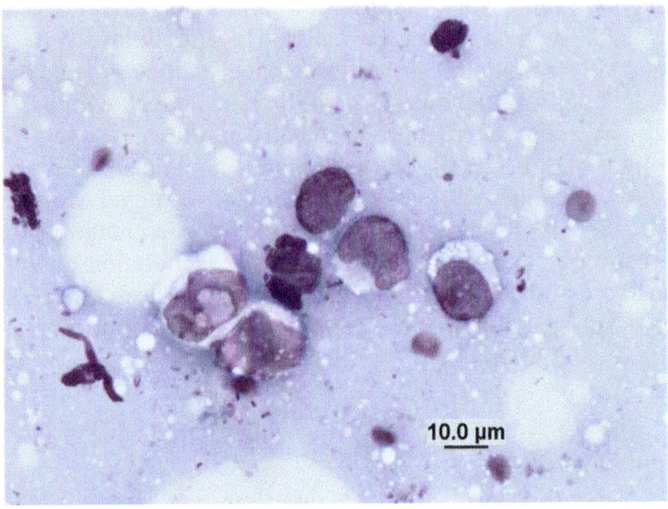

Fig. 7.52. (a) A cluster of round cells with variably distinct, abundant, light blue cytoplasm and round to oval nuclei with finely granular nuclear chromatin in a fine-needle aspiration biopsy of a histiocytoma in a ferret (*Mustela putorius furo*), Diff–Quik stain (100× oil). (b) A fine-needle aspiration biopsy of a histiocytoma in a ferret (*Mustela putorius furo*) revealed a sample with low cellularity consisting of mild pleomorphic mononuclear cells, Diff–Quik (100×, oil).

Chordomas have been reported in several species: humans, in which both sporadic and familial forms have been identified; dogs; cats; mink; ferrets; Perdido Key beach mice (*Peromyscus polionotus trissyllepsis*); rats (Sprague-Dawley and Fischer); a degu (*Octodon degus*); a tiger; and zebrafish (Kuramochi et al., 2015; Yui T et al., 2015; Taylor et al., 2016; Tauziede-Espariat et al., 2016; Kondo et al., 2018; Sautier et al., 2019, Cole et al., 2020). These tumors are locally expansile and invasive masses of large physaliferous (vacuolated) cells with small, round, hyperchromatic nuclei, like the "classic" form of chordomas described in humans. Histologically, these tumors feature intracellular, bubble-like vacuoles that are uniquely described as physaliferous. Cytology of chordomas reveals large, foamy cells (physaliphorous or physaliferous cells) that are pathognomonic for this neoplasm (Walberg and Loar, 2004) (Figures 7.54a, 7.54b, and 7.54c). The large pleomorphic physaliphorous cells are found individually and in small clusters. They typically have a large amount of moderately basophilic foamy cytoplasm; one to two medium- to large-sized round nuclei with coarse granular chromatin; one to two medium-sized, round to angular nucleoli; and moderate anisocytosis and anisokaryosis. The cytology may also exhibit a background of mucinous pinkish material representing an amphophilic (staining with both acidic and basic dyes) cartilaginous matrix among the cells on the specimen. Neoplastic cells contained abundant granules positive by the periodic acid–Schiff reaction.

Zymbal Gland Adenoma

Zymbal glands (auditory sebaceous glands) are small, bilateral sebaceous glands located ventral to the orifice of the external ear canal. Zymbal gland tumors arise from acini or ductal epithelium and may be

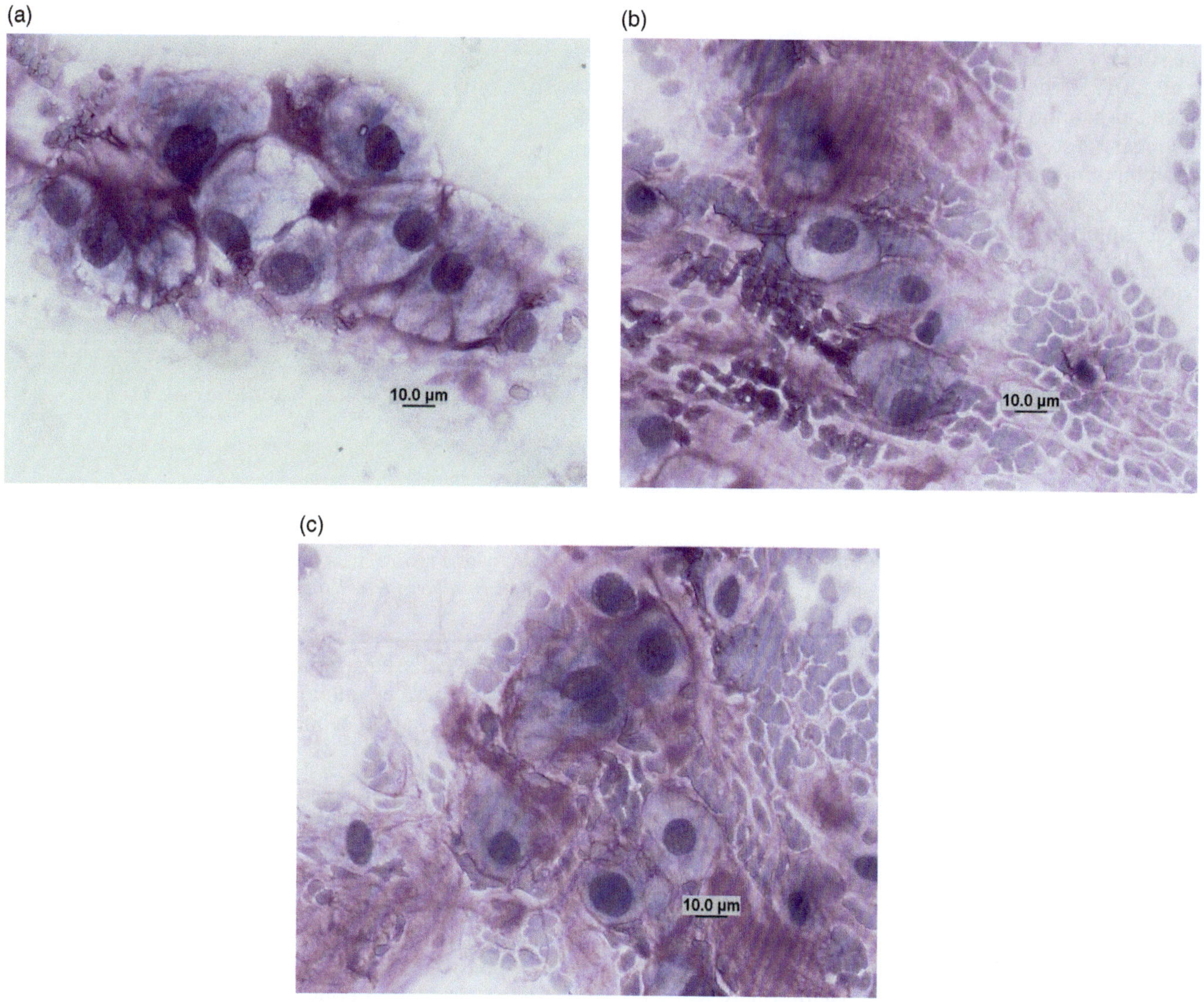

Fig. 7.54. (a)–(c) Large foamy physaliphorous cells with a background of mucinous pinkish material from a fine-needle aspiration biopsy of a chordoma on the tail of in a ferret (*Mustela putorius furo*). See Figure 7.58, Wright–Giemsa stain.

(a) (b)

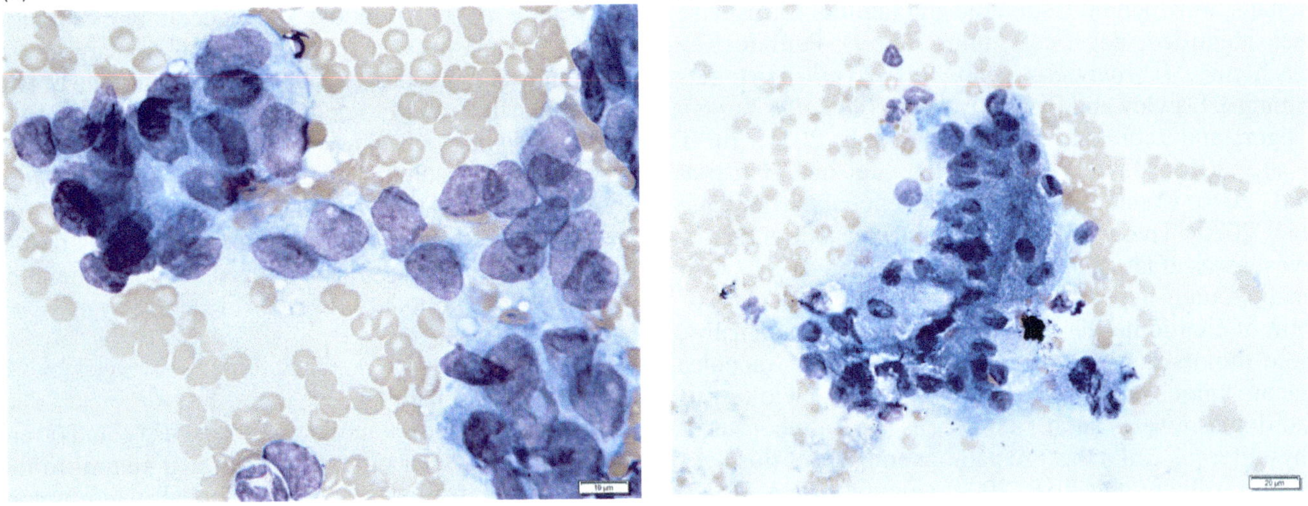

Fig. 7.55. (a), (b) Cells from a fine-needle aspiration biopsy of a Zymbal gland adenoma in the ear of a rat (*Rattus norvegicus*), Wright–Giemsa stain (100× oil).

classified as adenomas or adenocarcinomas (Grandi et al., 2012). The Zymbal gland is a frequent target for chemical carcinogens for evaluation in toxicology and chemical safety screening studies and the fourth most common tumor site in rats (Pucheu-Haston et al., 2016).

Cytologic preparations typically reveal abundant extracellular keratin and small, three-dimensional clusters of basaloid round to oval cells with orangeophilic cytoplasm and round to oval, monomorphic nuclei with a smooth chromatin in a pale basophilic background (Grandi et al., 2012) (Figures 7.55a and 7.55b). Differential diagnoses included epidermal inclusion cyst, basal cell tumor, Zymbal gland ductular hyperplasia, and Zymbal gland adenoma.

Leiomyoma

Leiomyomas are benign submucosal tumors that arise from smooth muscle cells and are generally small, localized, and well encapsulated. Leiomyomas most commonly develop in the gastrointestinal tract, but have also been identified in the spleen, liver, genitourinary tract, retroperitoneal space, and subcutaneous tissue (Gardhouse et al., 2016). The mucosa over the tumor usually remains intact, and gastric ulceration and hemorrhage are uncommon. The cytology alone does not provide enough information for a definitive diagnosis as it generally reveals numerous mesenchymal cells with few features of neoplasia (Figures 7.3b and 7.56). Cytologic evaluation of smears made from fine-needle aspirates often reveals a purple background that contained scattered free cell nuclei and erythrocytes. A few intact spindle cells with elongated nuclei (with finely stippled chromatin, and indistinct to occasionally prominent nucleoli) arranged in poorly defined aggregates may be present.

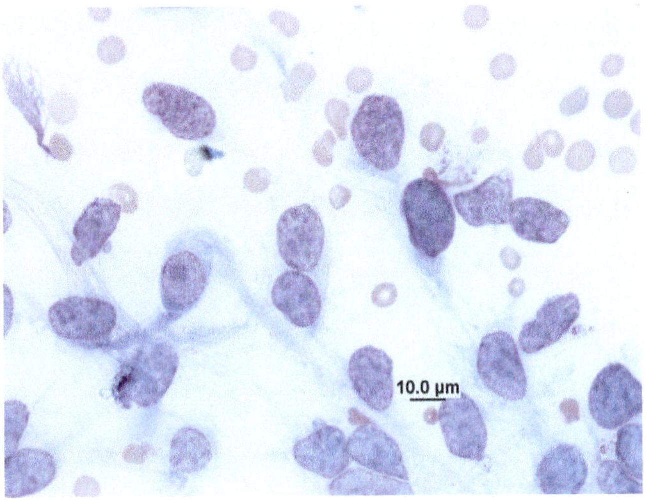

Fig. 7.56. Mesenchymal cells in a fine-needle aspiration biopsy of a uterine mass (leiomyoma) in an African hedgehog (*Atelerix albiventris*), Wright–Giemsa stain (100× oil).

The spindle cells have mild to moderate anisokaryosis, small to moderate amounts of moderately basophilic cytoplasm, and indistinct borders (Gardhouse et al., 2016).

Squamous Hyperplasia/Metaplasia

Hypovitaminosis A causes hyperkeratosis and hyperplasia of squamous epithelium and squamous metaplasia of nonsquamous epithelium in all species. Metaplasia is the transformation of nonsquamous epithelium into squamous epithelium.

High circulating concentrations of sex-related steroids (e.g., estradiol and androstenedione) may also result in squamous metaplasia of tissues, such as the prostate.

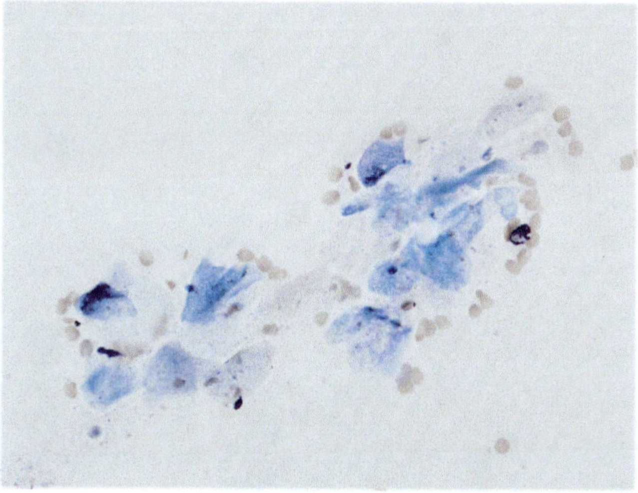

Fig. 7.57. Squamous metaplasia of a prostate gland in a ferret (*Mustela putorius furo*), Wright–Giemsa stain (100× oil).

This is sometimes seen in domestic ferrets and secondary to adrenocortical hyperplasia, adenoma, or adenocarcinoma (Bau-Gaudreault and Grimes, 2017).

Hyperplasia of the conjunctival epithelium can be associated with hypovitaminosis A, chronic inflammation, and mechanical or chemical irritants. Cytologic specimens reveal increased numbers of keratinized epithelial cells and goblet cells (Murphy, 1988). Hyperpigmentation is a frequent finding in inflammatory lesions of the conjunctiva and is indicated by increased numbers of epithelial cells containing intracytoplasmic melanin granules.

Cytologic preparations of early squamous hyperplasia and metaplasia lesions reveal a highly cellular content with individual and clustered large, round to polygonal cells with distinct cell margins (Figure 7.57). These cells have pale blue keratinized cytoplasm, and rarely, an ovoid central nucleus containing granular chromatin and no visible nucleolus. Moderate anisocytosis and mild anisokaryosis are often observed. There is little background debris and no evidence of inflammation, yeast, or protozoa.

Chronic lesions are often characterized by the presence of secondary infection and an associated neutrophilic, heterophilic, or mixed cell inflammatory response in addition to the squamous hyperplasia or metaplasia. The background may contain abundant granular, basophilic to gray, amorphous material compatible with necrosis (Bau-Gaudreault and Grimes, 2017).

Lymphoid Hyperplasia

Small, mature lymphocytes predominate in the cytology of reactive lymph nodes; however, there is an increase in the number of medium and large lymphocytes and plasma cells as well (Figures 7.58a–7.58d, 7.59a, and 7.59b). Therefore, lymphoid hyperplasia is indicated by more than 50% of small lymphocytes, 10–25% large lymphocytes, and more than 5% of plasma cells (Raskin and Meyer, 2016). Along with the increased numbers of plasma cells, the Mott cell variant of plasma cells may also be observed. Mott cells are typically seen after antigen-related stimulation or neoplastic proliferation of plasma cells.

Mott cells are plasma cells characterized by cytoplasmic globules consisting of retained immunoglobulins, termed *Russell bodies*. Russell bodies can vary greatly in shape, size, and staining properties, and may appear as multiple small spheres, single large inclusions displacing the nucleus, or needle-like inclusions, resulting in bulging of the cytoplasmic membrane (Cazzini et al., 2013). In cytologic specimens, Russell bodies have a waxy or glassy appearance and generally stain basophilic with Romanowsky stains.

Macrophages, neutrophils, eosinophils, and mast cells may also be seen more frequently in reactive lymph nodes; however, their numbers are lower than expected with lymphadenitis (Figure 7.58d).

Thyroid Hyperplasia

Hyperplasia or benign neoplasia (adenoma) of the thyroid gland often reveals a highly cellular sample containing primarily epithelial cells occurring in adherent groups (Campbell and Grant, 2010; Gibbons, et al., 2012). The round or cuboidal epithelial cells generally have round to oval nuclei, exhibit mild nuclear pleomorphism, and show prominent, multiple nucleoli (Figures 7.60a and 7.60b). Blue-black granules can be found within cells as well as in the noncellular background. The blue-black granules associated with the epithelial cells stained with Wright–Giemsa–Romanowsky stain are indicative of colloid associated with cells from the thyroid gland.

Ferret Adrenocortical Disease

Clinically normal ferrets have a significantly lower percentage of cornified preputial epithelial cells in preputial lavage samples compared to those with clinical signs of adrenocortical disease.

The increased cornification of preputial epithelial cells correlates with an increase in serum 17-hydroxyprogesterone concentration as well as clinical signs of adrenocortical disease in castrated ferrets (Protain et al., 2009).

Malignant Neoplasia

Neoplasia is the proliferation of cells under conditions that lack the normal controls that would result in the cessation of the multiplication of normal cells. Neoplasia is a common disorder of exotic animals and is

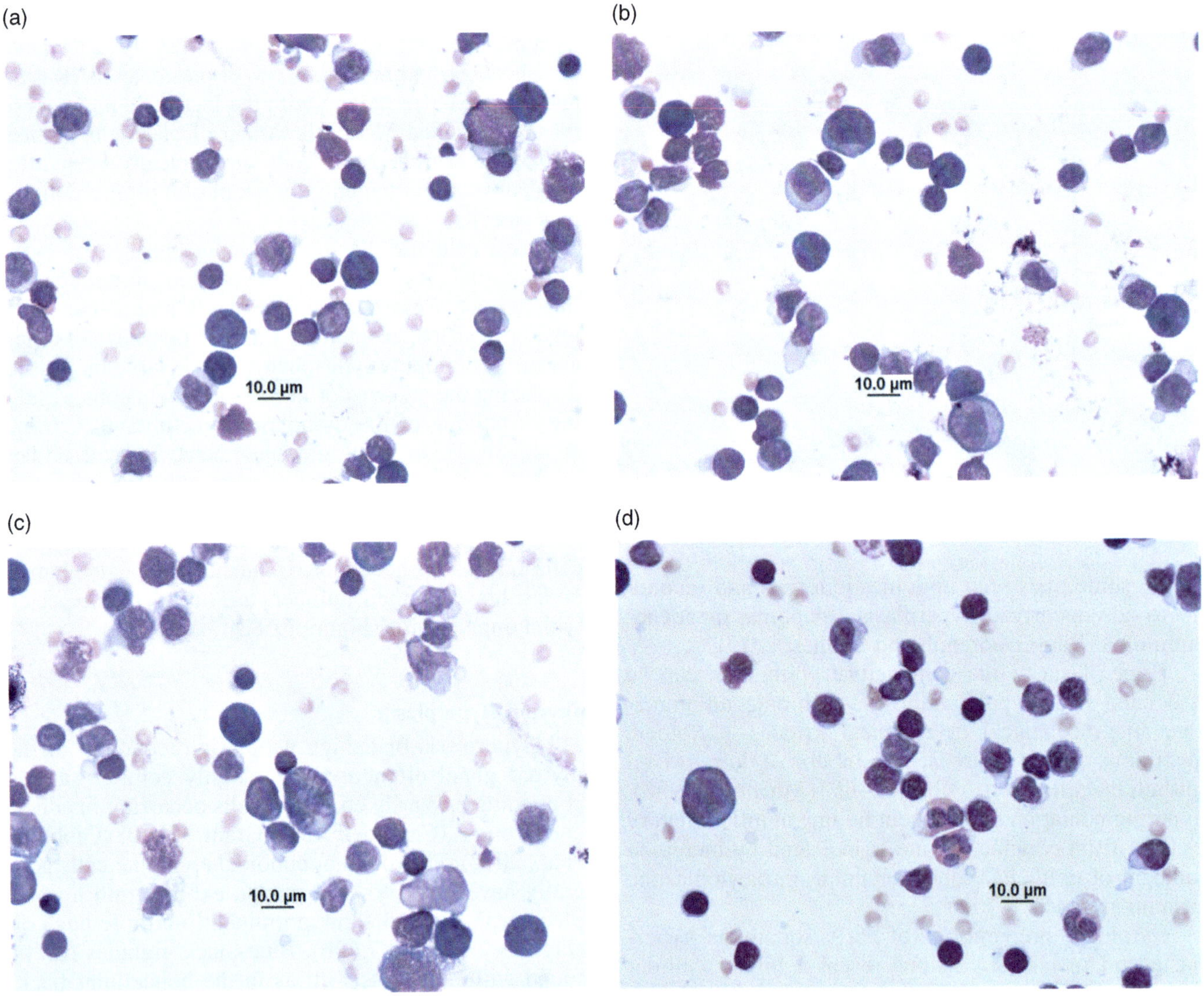

Fig. 7.58. (a) An increased number of large and medium lymphocytes are indicative of a reactive lymph node in a lymph node aspirate from a ferret (*Mustela putorius furo*), Wright–Giemsa stain (100× oil), (b) image also reveals an increased number of large and medium lymphocytes from the sample in Figure 7.58a, (c) A mitotic figure along with increased numbers of medium and large lymphocytes are indicative of a reactive lymph node in a lymph node aspirate from a ferret (*Mustela putorius furo*), Wright–Giemsa stain (100× oil), (d) Eosinophils, a lymphoblast and medium and large lymphocytes indicating a reactive lymph node in a lymph node aspirate from a ferret (*Mustela putorius furo*), Wright–Giemsa stain (100× oil).

frequently encountered in small mammalian patients, such as rodents, rabbits, African pygmy hedgehogs, ferrets, and sugar gliders (Weisbroth, 1994; Hoefer, 1994; Donnelly, 1997; Schaeffer and Donnelly, 1997; Raymond and White, 1999; Williams and Weiss, 2004; Williams and Wyre, 2021). Neoplastic lesions can be classified as mesenchymal tissue-derived, epithelial-glandular tissue-derived, a discrete cell, or poorly differentiated neoplasm. Frequently, a correlation between the clinical and cytological findings is needed to arrive at a diagnosis of malignant neoplasia. It should be noted here that a false-negative diagnosis of malignant neoplasia is often less harmful to the patient than a false-positive diagnosis.

The number of neoplastic cells and their appearance will vary with the type and location of the neoplasm and the sampling technique; therefore, a combination of cytological features (usually three or more criteria) from many cells in the sample is required for the diagnosis of malignant neoplasia. The criteria for the cytologic diagnosis of malignant neoplasia can be divided into four categories: general cellular, cytoplasmic, nuclear, and structural features.

Although the term *criteria of malignancy* in cytopathology implies that a tumor is malignant when these features are present, a tumor may have these features and not actually be malignant (Meuten and Meichner, 2022). For example, inflammatory cells,

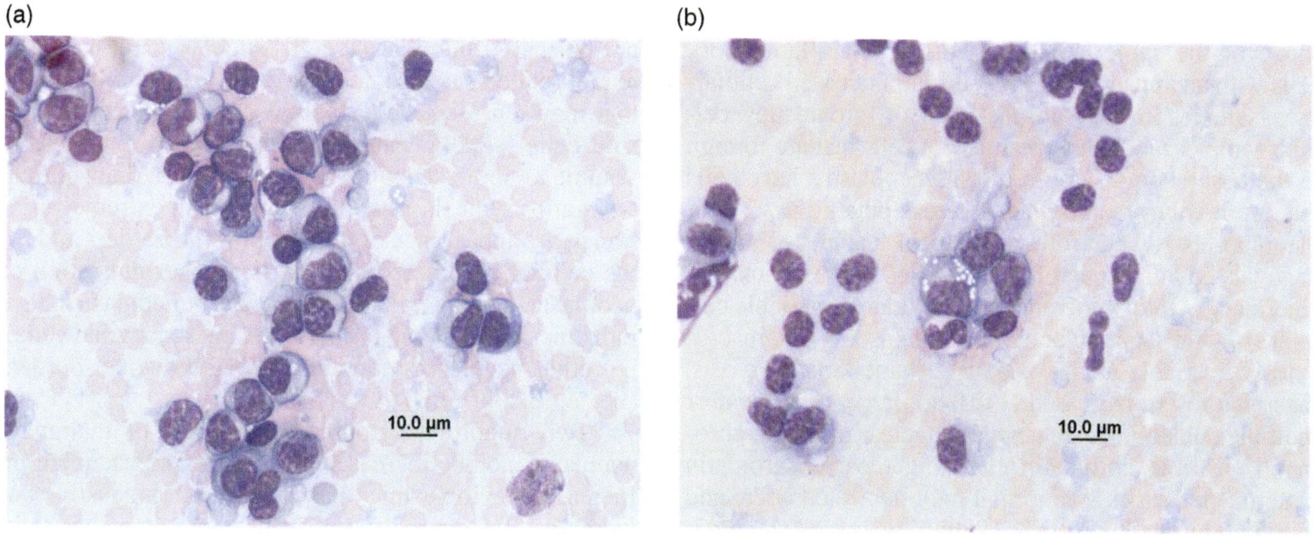

Fig. 7.59. (a) Increased number of plasma cells in a fine-needle aspiration biopsy of the spleen from a ferret (*Mustela putorius furo*) with multiple myeloma, Wright–Giemsa stain (100× oil). (b) Same sample as in Figure 7.59a revealing plasma cells: one is a Mott cell variant, in a fine-needle aspiration biopsy of the spleen from a ferret (*Mustela putorius furo*) with multiple myeloma, Wright–Giemsa stain (100× oil).

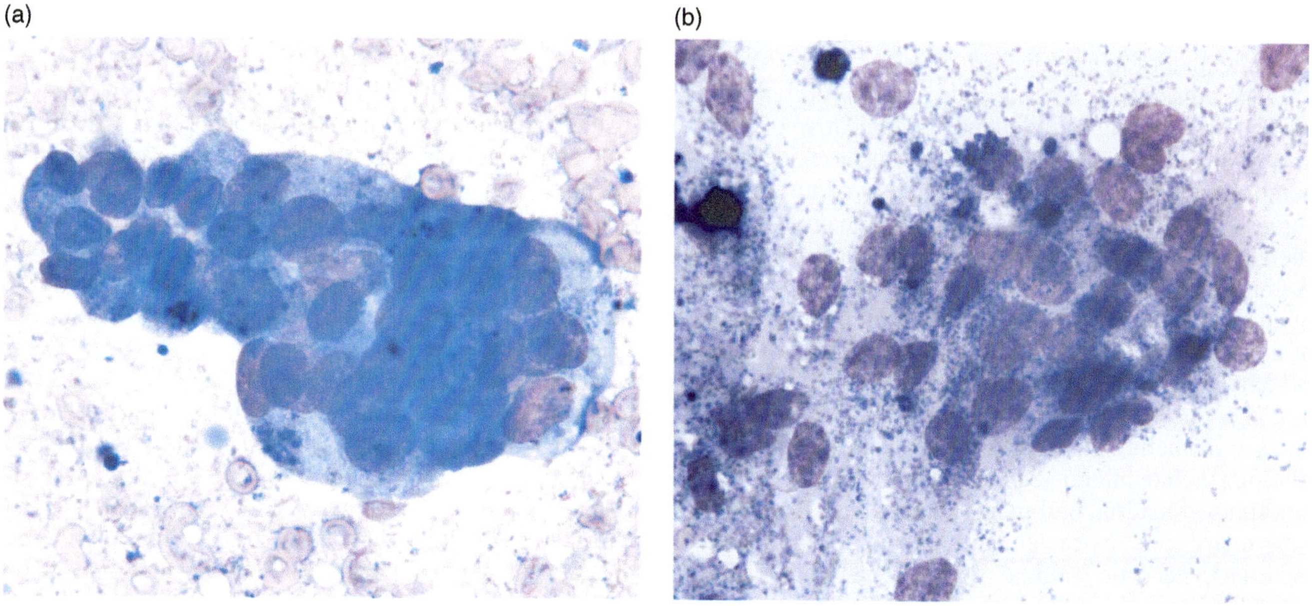

Fig. 7.60. (a) Tightly adherent epithelial cells with round to oval nuclei showing mild nuclear pleomorphism and prominent nucleoli with blue-black granules (colloid) in the cells and the background in a fine-needle aspiration biopsy of a thyroid adenoma in a guinea pig (*Cavia porcellus*), Wright–Giemsa stain (100× oil). Source: Image from Campbell and Grant (2010, p. 138). (b) Epithelial cells with round to oval nuclei showing mild nuclear pleomorphism and blue-black granules (colloid) in the cytoplasm and the background in a fine-needle aspiration biopsy of a thyroid adenoma in a guinea pig (*Cavia porcellus*), Wright–Giemsa stain (100× oil). Source: Image from Campbell and Grant (2010, p. 138).

reactive fibroblasts, and cells from young blood vessels can possess nuclear features of malignancy. Also, an aggressive, metastatic tumor that invades adjacent tissues may not possess any of these cytologic criteria of malignancy.

General Cellular Features of Malignant Neoplasia

General cellular features of malignant neoplasia refer to the appearance of the cell population present in the cytology sample. This would include the presence of a monomorphic cell population in the absence of inflammation, pleomorphism (variability in the size and shape of the same cell type) among noninflammatory cells with an apparent common origin, increased cellularity in samples from tissues that normally provide low cellular samples, and the appearance of cells that are foreign to the tissue being sampled. Some neoplasms have cells that are highly pleomorphic, whereas others show slight pleomorphism. Therefore, cytological features of malignancy listed in most cytological studies and textbooks for veterinary cytology include hypercellularity, variable cellular size and shape (pleomorphism; anisocytosis, macrocytosis), variable nuclear size and shape (anisokaryosis, macrokaryosis), increased N:C ratio; large, prominent or multiple nucleoli, anisonucleosis, nuclear molding; chromatin clearing, chromatin clumping (coarse chromatin pattern); presence of abnormal multinucleated cells, and mitotic figures (Allen et al., 1986; Meinkoth et al., 2007; Yildirim and Gurel, 2012).

In general, the best cytological feature to estimate behavior is uniformity versus variability (pleomorphism) in cells, nuclei, and nucleoli (Meuten and Meichner, 2022). The more uniform the cell size and shape, the more likely the tumor is benign. Therefore, uniformity is associated with benign behavior, and variable sizes, numbers, and shapes of nuclei and nucleoli are indicative of aggressive behavior.

The presence of ectopic cells or cells foreign to the normal tissue being sampled may be indicative of a metastatic malignant neoplasm. Cytological evidence of hemorrhage in an area without a history of trauma may suggest an erosive neoplasm. Erythrophagocytosis in such lesions would be indicative of chronic hemorrhage. A chronic hemoperitoneum with radiographic evidence of an abdominal mass leads to the presumptive diagnosis of a neoplasm, although there may be no direct cellular evidence of malignant cells in the fluid.

The background material may provide important clues to the nature of the malignant neoplasm. Important findings include muco-secretory material (i.e., light blue amorphous material and foamy macrophages), extracellular matrix (i.e., extracellular eosinophilic, osteoid-like material), necrotic cellular debris (i.e., fragments of fragile cells, cells without recognizable features, basophilic blue-gray amorphous debris), inflammatory cells, and red blood cells (Karim et al., 2008).

Cytoplasmic Features of Malignant Neoplasia

The appearance of the cytoplasm may also aid in the diagnosis of malignant neoplasia. Cytoplasmic features suggestive of malignant neoplasia include basophilia, vacuolation, variations in staining quality, inclusions, small cytoplasmic volume, and variable cytoplasmic margins. Variations in staining quality refer to areas of the cytoplasm that stain differently or variation in staining of the cytoplasm between cells of the same type. Cytoplasmic inclusions include a variety of structures not normally found in the cells, such as small pieces of nuclei (called satellite nuclei); dark, irregular structures that may represent degenerate organelles; or phagocytized cells (cellular cannibalism). A small cytoplasmic volume is indicated by cells with higher than normal N:C ratios typical of neoplastic cells. An extreme variation in the appearance of the cytoplasmic borders adds to the cellular pleomorphism and is another indication of neoplasia. Certain cells from malignant neoplasms have indistinct cytoplasmic borders (i.e., mesenchymal cells), but other neoplasms contain cells with distinct borders (i.e., epithelial cells).

Two important cytoplasmic features of malignant neoplasia include increased basophilia and vacuolation. Increased cytoplasmic basophilia is suggestive of increased RNA activity typical of young, metabolically active cells. However, the color of the cytoplasm alone cannot be used to predict biological behavior (Meuten and Meichner, 2022). Increased cytoplasmic vacuolation could suggest cellular degeneration, especially if the vacuoles are small. Neoplastic cells originating from secretory tissue (adenocarcinomas) often produce large secretory vacuoles.

Nuclear Features of Malignant Neoplasia

The morphology of the cell nucleus can be an important cytological feature in the diagnosis of malignant neoplasia. The most frequently observed nuclear criteria for malignant neoplasia include nuclear hypertrophy, anisokaryosis, variable N:C ratios, nuclear pleomorphism, abnormal mitoses, abnormal chromatin patterns, multinucleation, irregular nuclear membrane, and abnormal nucleoli.

Cells in cellular aggregates that exhibit varying and unusual nuclear chromatin patterns should also be viewed with suspicion for neoplasia. Irregular, coarse, hyperchromatic chromatin with clear parachromatin spaces is especially suggestive of neoplasia. Coarse chromatin pattern refers to a nuclear chromatin that appears coarser than normal and is abnormal. The abnormal chromatin may appear ropelike (ropy) or cordlike.

Cells with very large nuclei should be viewed with suspicion of neoplasia. Large nuclei that occur in cells exposed to hypotonic solutions (e.g., use of water instead of isotonic saline for wash samples) appear swollen and degenerate with pale pink homogenous chromatin, and should not be confused with nuclear features of malignancy.

Anisokaryosis (variation in nuclear sizes) is an important feature of neoplasia, especially in cellular aggregates. This is represented by cells that resemble each other but exhibit varying sizes of nuclei. This also translates into variable N:C ratios.

A variable or high N:C ratio in cells that normally have a low ratio is suggestive of malignancy, although some cells (such as lymphocytes) normally have a high N:C ratio and should not be considered neoplastic based on that alone. Generally, the greater the N:C ratio, the more aggressive the tumor, and cells with a paucity of cytoplasm and large nuclei that nearly fill the entire cell are often aggressive, for example, lymphoma (Meuten and Meichner, 2022). Aggregates of like cells that exhibit variable N:C ratios should be viewed with suspicion for neoplasia.

Nuclear molding refers to the deformation of nuclei by other nuclei within the same cell or adjacent cells.

Nuclear pleomorphism may indicate a rapid mitotic rate or abnormal mitosis. This is represented by aggregates of like cells having nuclei of varying shapes. The nuclei of these cells have irregular nuclear membranes creating the nuclear pleomorphism. Cells with abnormally lobed nuclei with deep clefts are especially suggestive of neoplasia.

Mitotic figures are associated with neoplasia and linked to more aggressive tumors; however, it should be considered that mitoses are part of normal cell replication, and certain tissues proliferate at faster rates with mitotic figures appearing in those samples, such as non-neoplastic bone marrow, lymph nodes, and intestines (Meuten and Meichner, 2022). Also, young granulation tissue with proliferating fibroblasts (reactive fibroblasts) and endothelial cells (angiogenesis) will contain mitotic figures in cytological preparations; therefore, finding a mitotic figure does not confirm a diagnosis of malignant neoplasia.

Mitotic figures are nuclear aggregates containing short rods or spikes of chromosomes unbound by a nuclear membrane after prophase, and their appearance varies depending on the phase of mitosis (Donovan et al., 2021). Prophase (the first stage of mitosis) is identified by condensed and duplicated chromosomes with no projections of individual chromosomes. Prometaphase is characterized by a dark, round cluster of chromosomes with short rods/spikes or projections: a ring or rosette may also be visible. Metaphase is the most easily recognized phase of mitosis and is represented by a plate, band, or ring of chromosomes with easily visible rods or spikes (the ring form or rosette/starburst occurs when the metaphase plate of chromosomes is parallel to the spindle). Anaphase is recognized by duplicated chromosomes formed during mitosis that are separated by variable distances (the aggregates have visible irregular rods, spikes, or projections). Telophase (uncommonly seen in cytologic specimens) exhibits two genomes at opposite ends of the cell with formation of a nuclear envelope and cleavage furrows (separating the two daughter cells).

Increased mitotic activity is a feature of malignant neoplasia as mitosis is rarely found in cytologic preparations of normal tissue. Cells usually divide evenly in two; any increase in the presence of mitotic figures or cells that are not dividing equally would be considered malignant criteria. Abnormal mitotic figures are cells that appear to have more than two poles of nuclear division (multipolar), resulting in bizarre mitotic figures. Aggregates of cells exhibiting a high mitotic index are also suggestive of a malignant neoplasm.

The number and type of mitoses observed in cytologic preparations are often used as criteria of malignancy. Cells exhibiting mitoses in clinical samples are often seen in metaphase (Tvedten, 2009). When the metaphase plate is viewed to be linear and perpendicular to the long axis of the spindle apparatus, the mitosis is normal. If the metaphase plate is in a parallel view (head-on) to the axis with chromosomes, thus forming a ring or round layer, the mitosis is often misinterpreted as atypical and called a *starburst* form.

Abnormal mitotic figures can be an indicator of malignant neoplasia: however, they can also be an artifact of sample preparation. For example, the process of cells drying and collapsing on a glass slide may distort chromosomes and the spindle apparatus, producing what look like abnormal mitotic figures (Tvedten, 2009).

Abnormal mitosis identified based upon chromosome segregation errors at mitosis are defined in terms of spindle symmetry, such as spindle multipolarity; size asymmetry of anaphase-telophase poles; and in abnormal sister chromatid segregation (i.e., chromosome bridges, chromatid bridges, chromosome lagging, and acentric fragment lagging). Multipolarity and lagging chromosomes are often detected on routine cytological specimens, but anaphase bridges are not.

Polar asymmetry is indicated with the occurrence of uneven division of chromosomes to either pole, resulting in hyperploidy or hypoploid poles. Multipolar mitoses have more than the normal two spindle poles at any stage of the mitotic cycle; therefore, tripolar or more mitosis is easily detected in routine cytologic specimens (even monopolar mitoses with one centriole can be identified) (Donovan et al., 2021).

The morphology of cells at interphase can indicate evidence of mitotic errors, such as micronuclei, nuclear strings, and nuclear blebs. A micronucleus is a rounded chromatin fragment located near a nucleus and with a diameter no more than 1/3 the nucleus (Tvedten, 2009). A nuclear string is a thread of chromatin connected to the membrane(s) of one or two nuclei. A nuclear bleb is a round or oval protrusion of the nuclear membrane connected to the main part of the nucleus by a thinner chromatin segment. These nuclear changes correlate strongly with anaphase bridges that can affect cytokinesis and lead to the formation of double nuclei.

Cells in cellular aggregates that exhibit varying and unusual nuclear chromatin patterns should also be viewed with suspicion for neoplasia. Irregular, coarse, hyperchromatic chromatin with clear parachromatin spaces is especially suggestive of neoplasia.

Multinucleated giant cells, especially cells with an uneven number of nuclei, may indicate asynchronous cell division. Multinucleated giant cells from malignant lesions often have nuclei that are irregularly arranged, enlarged, and pleomorphic. These should not be confused with multinucleated giant cells associated with inflammation that possess even numbers of uniforml-appearing nuclei. The appearance of multinucleated giant cells in a cytological specimen that lacks evidence of inflammation is also supportive of neoplasia.

Although multinucleated giant cells are a prominent and common histological feature of many mesenchymal neoplasms (i.e., anaplastic sarcoma, fibrosarcoma, myxosarcoma, giant cell tumor of soft parts, peripheral nerve sheath tumors, perivascular wall tumors, pleomorphic liposarcoma, rhabdomyosarcoma, osteosarcoma, giant cell glioblastoma, osteoclastoma, histiocytic sarcoma, mast cell tumors, extramedullary plasmacytoma, and deciduosarcoma), they are rarely reported in epithelial neoplasms (i.e., anaplastic mammary carcinomas and undifferentiated thyroid carcinomas (Bertram et al., 2020b). Multinucleation of neoplastic cells is caused by endomitosis, which represents an abortive mitosis without cell division into two daughter cells (cytokinesis), due to physiological or pathological stress (Bertram et al., 2020b). Mesenchymal neoplasms with multinucleated giant cells for which the cell lineage is unclear are generally referred to as giant cell sarcomas.

Abnormal nucleoli that vary in shape (especially angular nucleoli), size (anisonucleosis), number, and staining quality are additional features of neoplasia. Large (greater than one-third the diameter of the nucleus), pleomorphic, or multiple (greater than four) nucleoli should be viewed with suspicion of malignancy.

It should be noted that nuclear and nucleolar pleomorphism are more important to assess than cellular features when evaluating cells for evidence of malignancy (Meuten and Meichner, 2022). Multiple nucleoli of various sizes is a widely used cytological feature associated with aggressive tumors.

Structural Features of Malignant Neoplasia

Structural features of malignant neoplasia refer to those features that may aid in the identification of the neoplasm, such as epithelial neoplasia (carcinomas), mesenchymal neoplasia (sarcomas), discrete cell neoplasia (round cell neoplasms), or neuroendocrine. The most significant cytological features within each category are round cell tumors, which are made up of individualized cells with a round shape; epithelial tumors have large cells that are adhered in clusters or morulae; mesenchymal tumors have spindle-shaped cells; and neuroendocrine tumors produce cells with uniform nuclei that often appear without surrounding cytoplasm (Meuten and Meichner, 2022).

Round or Discrete Cell Tumor

The cytologic category of round or discrete cell tumor is a term that is applied to tumors that exfoliate as individual (discrete) cells, which are generally round. Round cell tumors (discrete cell neoplasia) result from abnormal development of cells that have no normal structural interaction. The cells tend to be round or oval, have distinct cytoplasmic margins and low to moderate cytoplasmic volume, are generally smaller than epithelial cells, and typically exfoliate well, producing many individual cells. The nuclei are generally round.

In domestic animals, such as dogs and cats, round cell tumors include mast cell tumors, histiocytic tumors (histiocytoma and histiocytic sarcoma), lymphoma, plasma cell tumors (plasmacytomas), and transmissible venereal tumors (Baker and Lumsden, 2000). All but the transmissible venereal tumors occur in small exotic mammals. Cytology is considered one of the best diagnostic tests for the identification and classification of round cell tumors (Cian, 2014).

Mast cell tumors are one of the most frequent cutaneous neoplasms of ferrets; however, they are rarely reported in other exotic mammals, including squirrels, llama, and hedgehogs (Scott et al., 2001; Williams and Weiss, 2004; Lin et al., 2010; Vilalta et al., 2016). Mast cell tumors of ferrets typically appear as solitary or multiple skin nodules or papules that may wax and wane. Grossly, the tumors can vary in color from pale to red, and may be firm, soft, or cystic in texture. Most mast cell tumors in ferrets are benign.

Mast cells are mesenchymal cells that contain basophilic, metachromatic (variable staining with the same stain) cytoplasmic granules with Romanowsky stains (Figures 7.61a and 7.61b, and 7.62). The mast cell granules contain histamine, heparin, and in some rodents, serotonin. Mast cells exfoliate easily, but are fragile and often rupture during preparation of cytology slides, where the released granules are found scattered throughout the background. Intact mast cells are recognized on Romanowsky-stained cytologic specimens as discrete, round cells (sometimes in non-cohesive aggregates) with well-defined margins; clear and finely vacuolated or granular cytoplasm; pale, eccentric, round nuclei with finely stippled to coarse chromatin; and inconspicuous nucleoli. The cytoplasm contains numerous distinct purple or metachromatic cytoplasmic granules ranging in size from 0.2 to 5.0 mm in diameter. In some specimens, the nuclei of the cells may be obscured by the number of granules present in the cytoplasm. Moderate anisocytosis and anisokaryosis; nuclear pleomorphism; binucleated cells; and mitotic figures may be seen occasionally. Eosinophils may be present in the cytology preparation as well.

The staining technique used will affect the intensity and color of mast cell granules. Because they are

(a) (b)

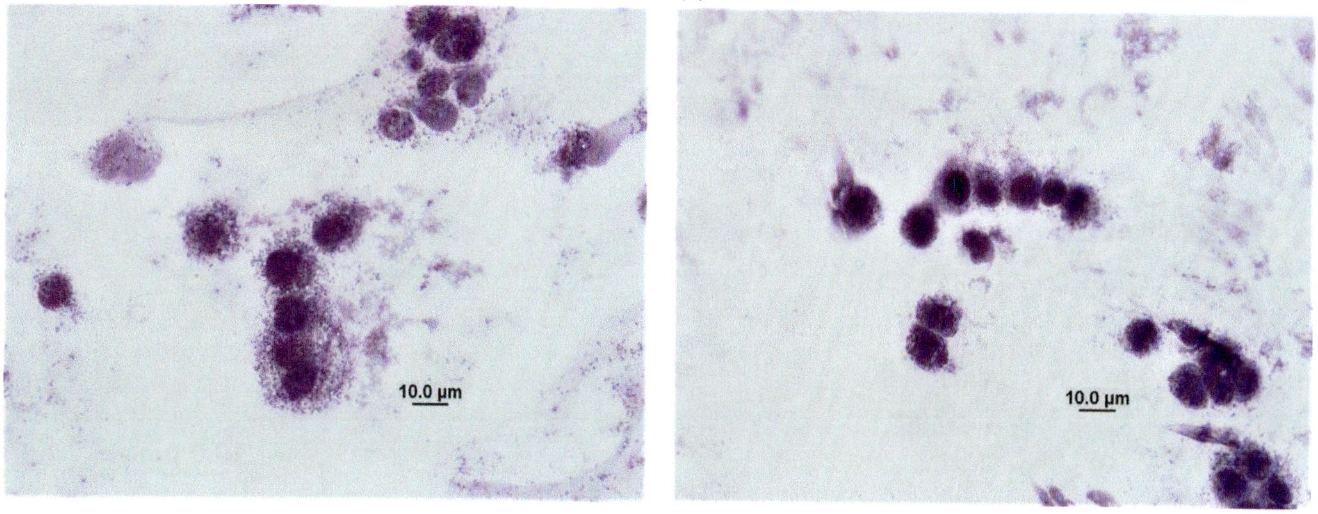

Fig. 7.61. (a), (b) Round cells with distinct cell borders, a medium-sized round to oval eccentrically placed nucleus with granular chromatin, occasional poorly defined nucleoli, and moderate anisocytosis and anisokaryosis in a fine-needle aspiration biopsy from a skin lesion in a ferret (*Mustela putorius furo*). The cells contain basophilic granules characteristic of fully granulated, well-differentiated mast cells. The background contains numerous mast cell granules that have escaped from ruptured cells. Wright–Giemsa stain.

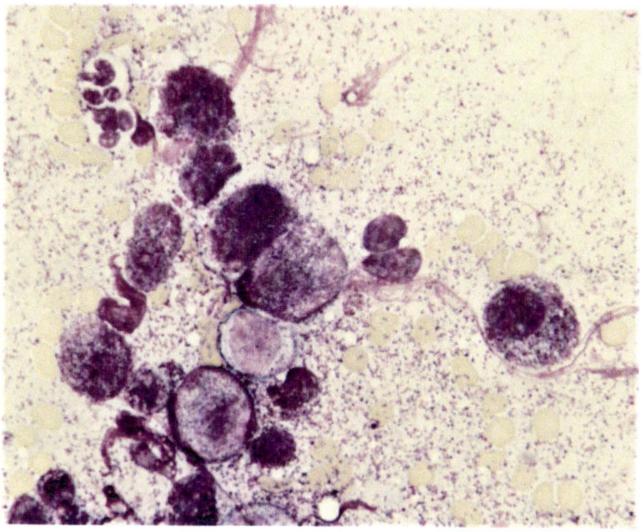

Fig. 7.62. Round cells with basophilic granules characteristic of fully granulated, well-differentiated mast cells along with a background containing numerous mast cell granules that have escaped from ruptured cells from a fine-needle aspiration biopsy of a cutaneous mass in a tiger cub (*Panthera tigris tigris*). Wright–Giemsa stain (100× oil).

inexpensive, readily available, and easy to prepare, maintain, and use, Romanowsky-type stains are commonly used in veterinary practice. Romanowsky stains may be either aqueous (e.g., Diff–Quik and Hema 3) or methanol based (e.g., Wright and Giemsa stains). However, even though aqueous-based stains are the most used in private practice, they may fail to stain the granules of mast cells, basophils, and large granular lymphocytes (Figures 7.63a and 7.63b). Toluidine blue is an acidophilic metachromatic dye that selectively stains acidic tissue components. It has been used to highlight mast cell granules, mucins, and cartilage. Mast cell granules stain purple with toluidine blue due to the presence of heparin and histamine (Vilalta et al., 2016).

A two-tiered histologic grading scheme for cutaneous mast cell tumors based on morphologic characteristics of neoplastic cells that include karyomegaly, multinucleation, nuclear pleomorphism, and mitotic figures was the basis for the development of a grading scheme of cytologic preparations of aspirated samples from dogs (Camus et al., 2016). Aspirates from cutaneous mast cell tumors provide the same information more quickly, inexpensively, and less invasively. A cutaneous mast cell tumor is classified as high grade if it is poorly granulated or had at least two of four findings: mitotic figures, binucleated or multinucleated cells, nuclear pleomorphism, or >50% anisokaryosis. This grading scheme may provide useful for exotic animal patients as well.

Histiocytic tumors, such as histiocytic sarcomas, are part of a spectrum of several histiocytic diseases in the dog. Cells of histiocytic lineage include both professional antigen-presenting cells in the innate immune system such as dendritic cells as well as macrophages specialized for phagocytosis (Affolter and Moore, 2002; Fulmer and Mauldin, 2007; Leissinger et al., 2013). Histopathological and immunohistochemical studies of histiocytic sarcomas of hedgehogs (*Atelerix albiventris*) suggest that the tumor cells have variable features of histiocyte origin, including dendritic cells, Langerhans cells, and macrophages (Son et al., 2020; Sirivisoot et al., 2021). The histiocytic diseases in dogs include

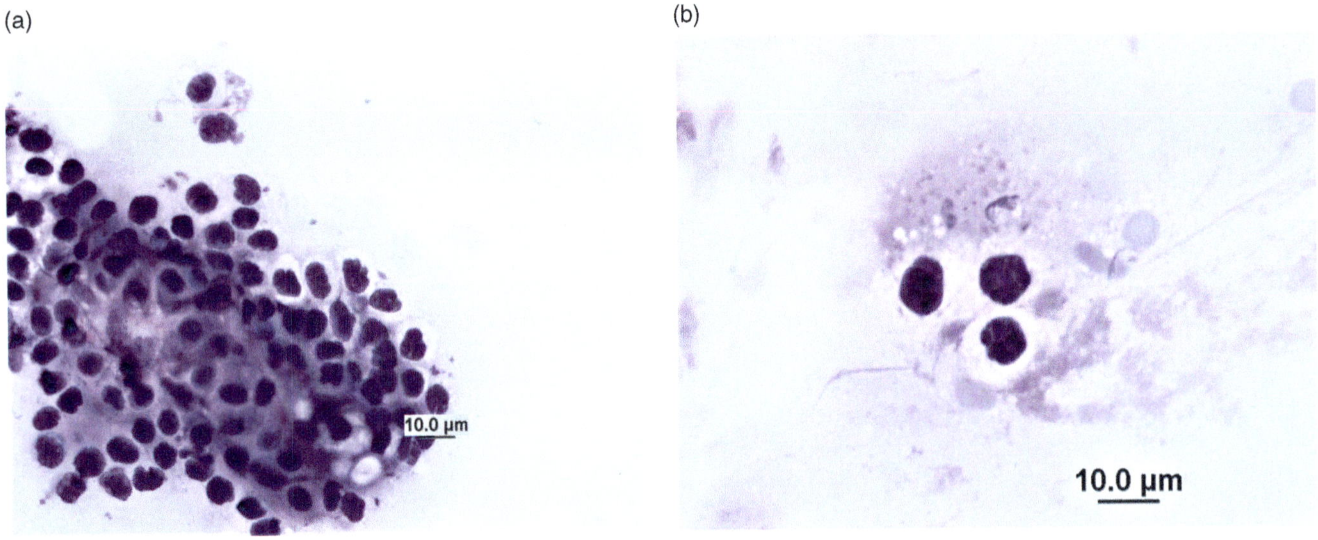

Fig. 7.63. (a), (b) A fine-needle aspiration biopsy from a skin lesion in a ferret (*Mustela putorius furo*) reveals round cells with distinct cell margins with slight anisocytosis and anisokaryosis. The medium-sized oval nucleus of the cells frequently has irregular margins, can be eccentrically positioned, contains granular chromatin, and has poorly defined nucleoli. The cytologic features are consistent with a discrete cell or round cell tumor, which include a histiocytoma, mast cell tumor, and lymphoma. If this were a canine patient, a transmissible venereal tumor would also be included in the list. These cells are from the same lesion as in Figures 7.66a and 7.66b, but stained with Diff–Quik stain.

nonmalignant non-neoplastic (cutaneous and systemic histiocytosis), nonmalignant neoplastic (histiocytoma), and malignant neoplastic (local and systemic histiocytic sarcoma) diseases. Histiocytic sarcoma has been reported in exotic mammals, including the mouse, rabbit, hedgehog, and the rat (Leissinger et al., 2013; Ogihara et al., 2016; Ogihara et al., 2017; Karim et al., 2017). In the rat, histiocytic sarcoma is the most common hematopoietic malignancy.

Histiocytic sarcoma is classified as a mesenchymal tumor, but the cells resemble that of a pleomorphic round cells tumor instead of spindle-shaped mesenchymal cells (Meuten and Meichner, 2022). Cytologic samples often reveal moderate numbers of round cells that occur individually or occasionally in loosely adherent clusters. On Wright–Giemsa-stained cytological preparations, the cells tend to have moderate to large amounts of lightly basophilic cytoplasm with indistinct cytoplasmic borders and low to moderate numbers of clear punctate vacuoles (Figures 7.52a, 7.52b, 7.64, 7.65a, and 7.65b). The nuclei typically measure 5–20 μm in diameter and have coarsely clumped to stippled chromatin and inconspicuous nucleoli. The cells usually displayed several criteria of malignancy, including a low N:C ratio, marked anisocytosis, marked anisokaryosis, variably sized and shaped nucleoli, abnormal mitotic figures, and macronucleoli. The abundant cytoplasm typically favors histiocytic tumors over other malignant round cell tumor types.

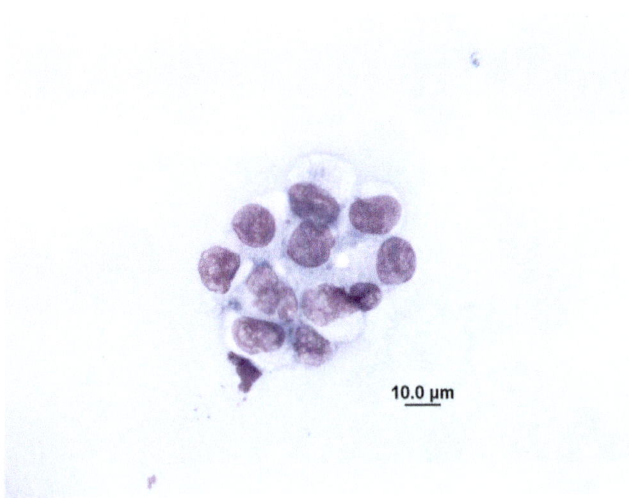

Fig. 7.64. Cells with round to irregular to indented eccentric nuclei and a moderate to abundant amount of light blue pink to purple cytoplasm that often contains low discrete vacuoles from a ferret (*Mustela putorius furo*) diagnosed with malignant histiocytosis, Wright–Giemsa stain.

A poorly differentiated malignant plasma cell tumor and a histiocytic sarcoma may appear microscopically similar with both having individualized cells with abundant cytoplasm, one to numerous nuclei, and highly variable nuclei and nucleoli regarding number, size and shape (Meuten and Meichner, 2022). The presence of numerous giant cells, multinucleation, and bizarre nuclei and nucleoli favors a diagnosis of histiocytic sarcoma. Likewise, granulomatous or pyogranulomatous inflammation may be confused with histiocytic sarcoma (and

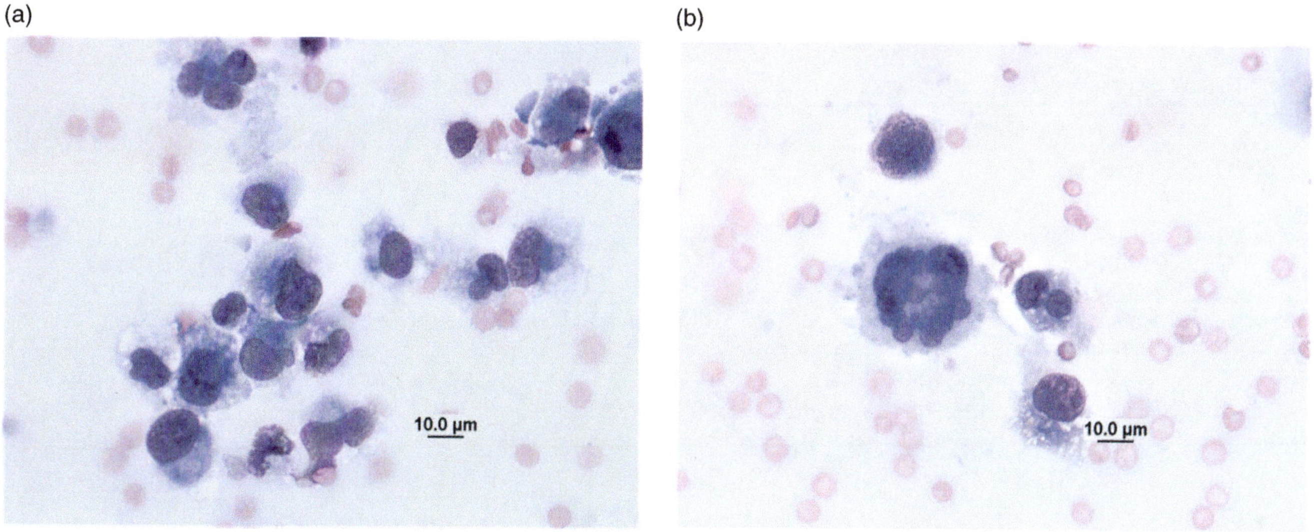

Fig. 7.65. (a) Cells with round to irregular to indented eccentric nuclei and a moderate to abundant amount of light blue, pink to purple cytoplasm that often contains low discrete vacuoles from a rat (*Rattus norvegicus*) diagnosed with histiocytic sarcoma, Wright–Giemsa stain. (b) Multinucleated giant cell in the same sample as in Figure 7.70a. Wright–Giemsa stain.

squamous cell carcinoma) because of the presence of macrophages (histiocytes) and multinucleated giant cells exhibiting cytological features characteristic of malignant neoplasia, such as large nuclei, prominent nucleoli, and multinucleation (Meuten and Meichner, 2022). The cytologic diagnosis can be confirmed using a cytochemical stain – α-naphthyl butyrate esterase (ANBE) – that detects the presence of intracellular esterase enzymes, enzymes present in cells of dendritic or monocytic origin. Neoplastic cells can also be categorized as histiocytic based on characteristic morphology and positive immunohistochemistry for vimentin (Leissinger et al., 2013). Although immunohistochemistry may be helpful in identifying histiocytes, lesion localization, cell morphology, and tissue architecture are also required to distinguish among the various histiocytic diseases and to differentiate them from histiocytic inflammation (Son et al., 2020).

Lymphoid neoplasia or *lymphomas* are characterized by the maturation arrest of a malignant clone of lymphoid cells. Lymphoma is a common neoplastic disease in exotic mammals and has been classified into multicentric, gastrointestinal, mediastinal, cutaneous, and extra-nodal forms according to the site of origin (Gupta et al., 2010; Chung et al., 2014; Nagata et al., 2019).

Lymphoma is the third most common neoplastic disease in ferrets, following adrenal tumors and insulinomas (Gupta et al., 2010; Mayer et al., 2014). The chronic lymphocytic lymphoma that involves visceral organs (especially the spleen, liver, kidneys, and lymph nodes) is the most common form and affects ferrets older than 2 years of age. The acute lymphoblastic variant, which typically involves mediastinum, thymus, spleen, liver, and bone marrow, occurs in younger ferrets (Long et al., 2016). An immunoblastic polymorphous type can occur at all ages and has varying degrees of peripheral lymphadenopathy and visceral organ involvement (Gupta et al., 2010). There is no definitive cause of lymphoma in ferrets, although a possible viral or infectious etiology has been hypothesized (Delk et al., 2013).

Lymphoma is the primary neoplasia of lymphocytes, and the cytology indicative of lymphoma reveals a predominance of medium or large lymphocytes representing 60–90% of the cell population (Figures 7.66a–7.66c, 7.67, and 7.68). The neoplastic lymphocytes are often immature and are represented by lymphoblasts and prolymphocytes. Numerous classification schemes have been applied to lymphoid tumors in dogs; however, no standardized classification scheme has been developed for exotic mammals (Baker and Lumsden, 2000; Delk et al., 2013). Hypercalcemia and hyperglobulinemia associated with paraneoplastic syndrome is commonly reported in domestic mammals with malignant lymphoma and may also occur with exotic mammals with the same condition.

Cytological findings associated with lymphoid neoplasia are typically characterized by a monotypic, homogenous, or heterogeneous population of lymphocytes devoid of inflammatory cells. Cells from malignant lymphoid tissue exhibit a marked increase in the number of large lymphocytes, such as lymphoblasts; nuclear and cytoplasmic pleomorphism; cytoplasmic basophilia; and mitotic figures. Abnormal or multiple nucleoli are also frequently seen. At times, lymphomas may resemble histiocytic sarcomas (Figures 7.69 and 7.70)

Cytoplasmic features of the abnormal lymphocytes are evaluated for cytoplasmic volume, quantity and color (basophilic intensity), the positioning of the cytoplasm

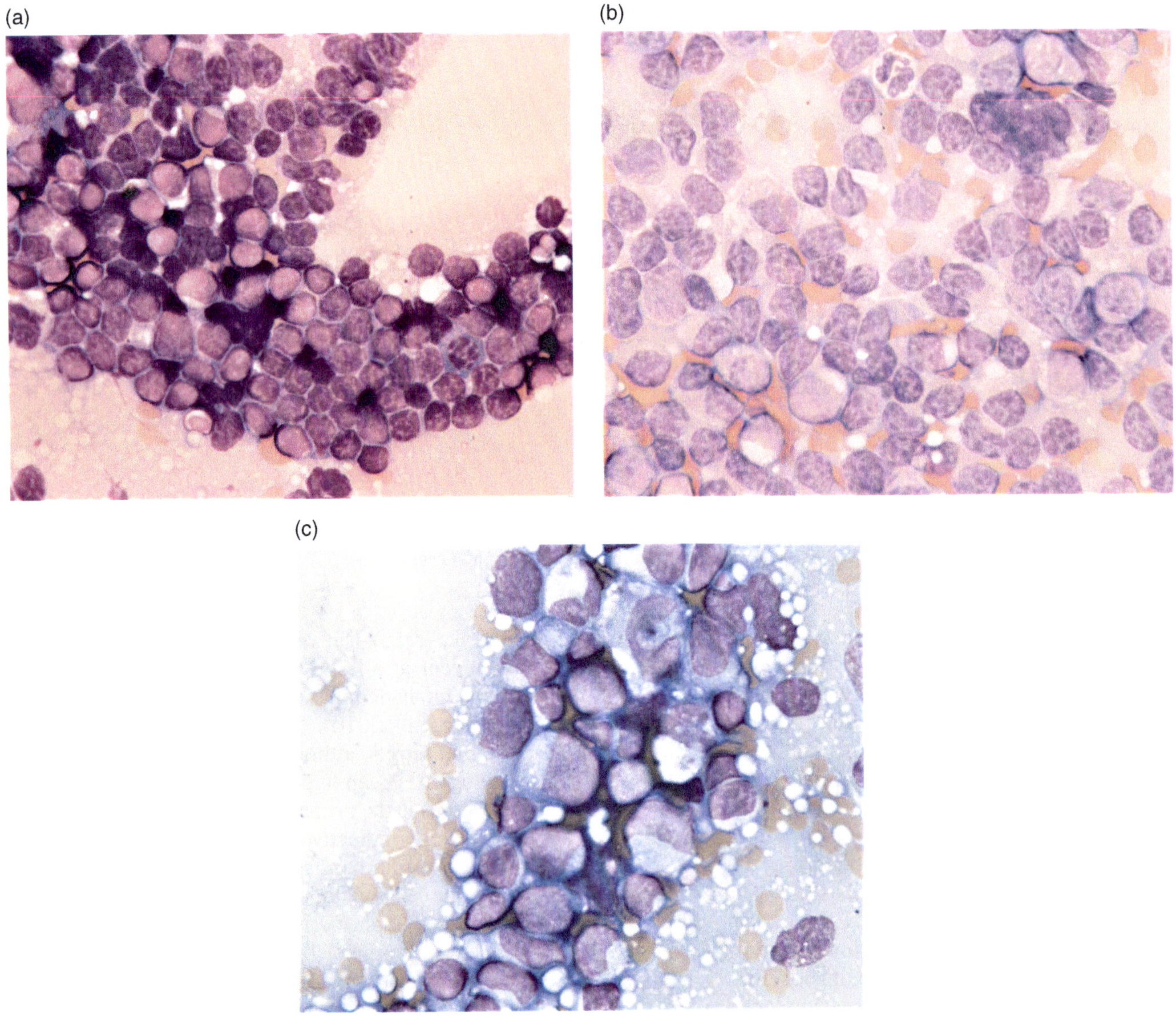

Fig. 7.66. (a) A predominance of large lymphocytes with moderate nuclear and cytoplasmic pleomorphism and cytoplasmic basophilia in a fine-needle aspiration biopsy of a lymph node from a ferret (*Mustela putorius furo*) diagnosed with lymphoma, Wright–Giemsa stain (50×). (b) A preponderance of large lymphocytes (>90% of the cells) that are 1.0–1.25 times the size of the neutrophil in a fine-needle aspiration biopsy of a lymph node from a ferret (*Mustela putorius furo*) diagnosed with lymphoma, Wright–Giemsa stain (100× oil). (c) A preponderance (>90% of the cells) of large lymphocytes (lymphoblasts and prolymphocytes) in an imprint of a lymph node obtained during exploratory surgery from a ferret (*Mustela putorius furo*) diagnosed with lymphoma, Wright–Giemsa stain (100× oil).

around the nucleus, and the presence/absence of vacuolation and granules. A scant cytoplasm is indicated by a narrow rim of cytoplasm around the nucleus as seen in normal, small, mature lymphocytes. Abundant cytoplasm is indicated by a cytoplasmic volume nearly twice the nuclear volume, whereas moderate cytoplasmic volumes are between scant and abundant. Normal, small, mature lymphocytes have a pale blue to nearly clear cytoplasm, whereas a dark blue cytoplasm is typical of immature lymphocytes, such as lymphoblasts.

Nuclear pleomorphism should be evaluated. The general shape of the nucleus of lymphoma cells is classified as round (circular with no indentations) as seen in normal lymphocytes, irregularly round (circular with indentations or convolutions), convoluted (nuclei with many deep indentations), and clefted (nucleus with a single deep indentation). The nuclei are also classified as central or eccentric in position within the cell. Anisokaryosis is a common feature of lymphoma cells.

Nuclear chromatin is described as fine, pinpoint, stippled, aggregated or clumped, and woven or reticulated. Normal, small lymphocytes (slightly smaller than heterophils) have a round to slightly indented nucleus, heavily clumped or reticulated chromatin pattern without visible nucleoli, and scant pale blue cytoplasm. The nuclear chromatin pattern of lymphoma cells varies

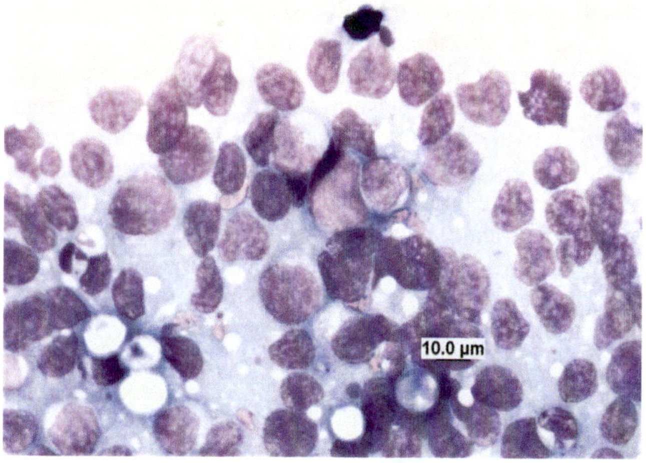

Fig. 7.67. Large immature lymphocytes and free nuclei in a fine-needle aspiration biopsy of a skin mass in a gerbil (*Meriones unguiculatus*) diagnosed with lymphoma, Wright–Giemsa stain (100× oil).

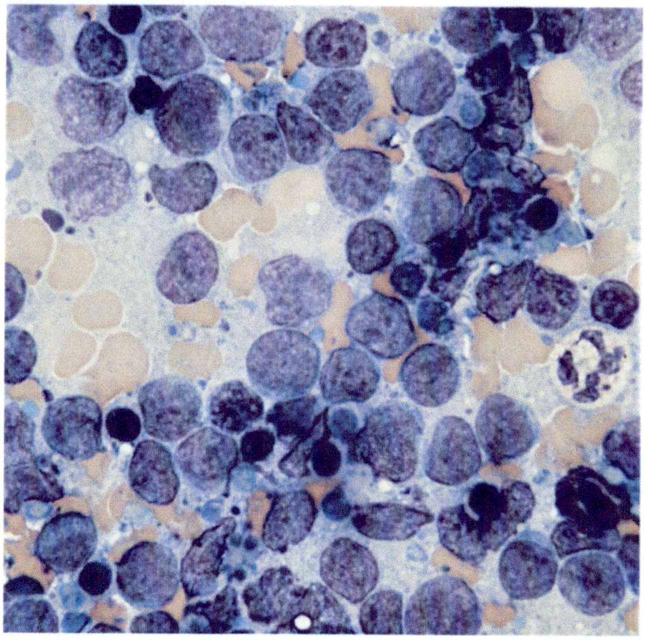

Fig. 7.68. A preponderance of large lymphocytes (>90% of the cells) that are 1.0–1.25 times the size of the heterophil in a fine-needle aspiration biopsy of a lymph node from a guinea pig (*Cavia porcellus*) diagnosed with lymphoma, Wright–Giemsa stain (100× oil).

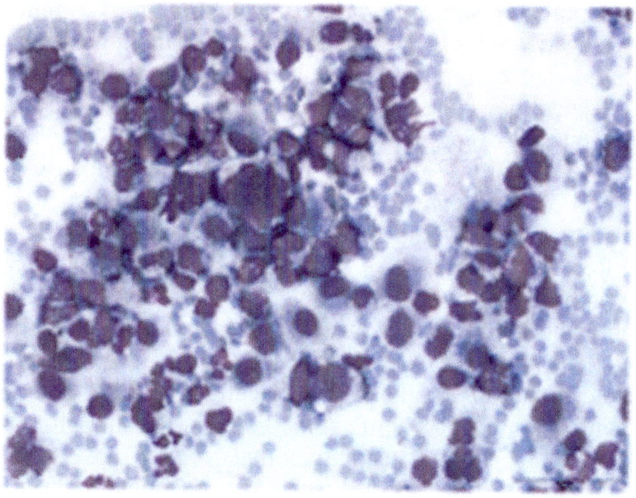

Fig. 7.69. Pleomorphism within the population of neoplastic cells in an imprint of an abdominal mass from a ferret (*Mustela putorius furo*) diagnosed with T-cell lymphoma. Note the variation in cell size, as well as nuclear size and shape between the neoplastic cells. These cells also exhibit significant variation of the nuclear to cytoplasmic (N:C) ratio. Other nucleated cells include frequent neutrophils and two eosinophils. There are scattered RBCs in the background. Modified Wright Stain (600×). Source: Delk et al. (2013).

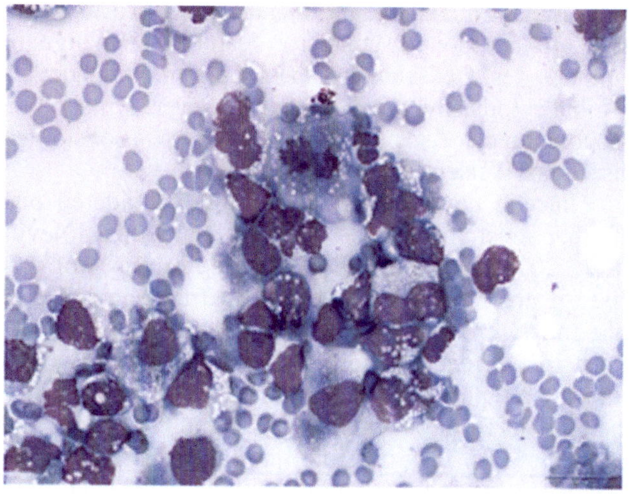

Fig. 7.70. Pleomorphic neoplastic cells, a mitotic figure, ruptured cells, and a neutrophil among red blood cells in an imprint of an abdominal mass from a ferret (*Mustela putorius furo*) diagnosed with T-cell lymphoma. Modified Wright Stain (1,000×). Source: Delk et al. (2013).

from stippled to irregularly or uniformly clumped chromatin. Clumping of the nuclear chromatin is generally regarded as a sign of lymphocyte maturity.

Features of the nucleoli such as the size, number, and location within the nucleus should be documented as well. In general, nucleoli are noted as being single or multiple, large or small, indistinct or prominent, and central or marginated. It should be noted that nucleoli are absent in normal, small, mature lymphocytes.

The mitotic index is a final feature that should be noted and serves as an estimate of the average number of mitotic figures observed per 100× or oil-immersion field.

Other cellular features associated with lymphoma include the presence of lymphoglandular bodies (small basophilic cytoplasmic fragments from ruptured lymphocytes) and tangible body macrophages. Lymphoglandular bodies are commonly associated with lymphoid tissue; however, they increase in number with degenerating lymphocytes as occurs with lymphomas.

Lymphomas of exotic mammals are typically of T-cell origin; however, the plasmacytoid appearance of the lymphocytes and presence of Mott cells provide a differential diagnosis of extramedullary plasmacytoma, lymphoplasmacytic lymphoma, and signet ring cell lymphoma (where a single, large, clear vacuole displaces the nucleus to the periphery of the cell) (Gupta et al., 2010). Determination of either a T- or B-cell origin can be made using immunocytochemical methods for immunophenotyping of lymphomas in mammals, which have been validated in some species, such as the guinea pig (Harr et al., 2018).

Lymphocytic leukemia is the term used to describe lymphoid neoplasia involving blood or bone marrow. A marked increase in lymphocytes in the peripheral blood should be viewed with suspicion for lymphocytic leukemia. Lymphocytic leukemia is indicated by a marked increase in lymphocytes, especially with the presence of abnormal lymphocyte morphology. Important morphology includes large lymphocytes (larger than heterophils) with fine nuclear chromatin and a pale-staining nucleus. A prominent nucleolus and increased cytoplasmic volume are additional supportive features of malignant lymphocytes. Occasionally, the neoplastic lymphocytes exhibit cytoplasmic vacuolation; however, lymphocyte vacuolation can also be associated with toxins or storage disorders (Weiser, 2012).

Chronic lymphocytic leukemia is considered one of the most frequent forms of leukemia (Nevitt et al., 2014). In domestic dogs, three subtypes of this disease are reported in decreasing frequency: T cell (the most common form, with CD8 granular lymphocytes most frequently affected), B cell, and atypical chronic lymphocytic leukemia; however, in humans, the B-cell form is the most common (Vernau and Moore, 1999). It is possible that nondomestic canids, like domestic dogs, are more commonly affected with the T-cell form (Nevitt et al., 2014).

In domestic dogs and possibly exotic mammals, mild lymphocytosis can be observed with hypoadrenocorticism; however, few diseases, other than lymphoproliferative disorders, result in persistent lymphocytosis with counts greater than 13 000 lymphocytes/μL (Avery and Avery, 2007). In exotic mammals, a presumptive diagnosis of chronic lymphocytic leukemia is made based on lymphocyte morphology, negative results of serologic tests for infectious diseases, lack of clinical signs of illness, response to treatment, and lack of postmortem findings suggestive of other chronic inflammatory diseases. Immunophenotype markers are generally species specific and may not be helpful; however, the presence of a monoclonal gammopathy is indicative of this disease (Nevitt et al., 2014).

Multiple myeloma is a term referring to a specific form of lymphoid neoplasia that involves plasma cell differentiation. These plasma cells are seen as discrete, round to oval cells characterized by a moderate to large amount of moderately to deeply basophilic cytoplasm; a perinuclear clear area (Golgi); a medium-sized, round to oval, eccentrically located nucleus with moderately granular to coarse chromatin; and mild to moderate anisocytosis and anisokaryosis (Figures 7.71 and 7.72). Often, there is an associated monoclonal gammopathy. Multiple myeloma has been reported in exotic mammal patients,

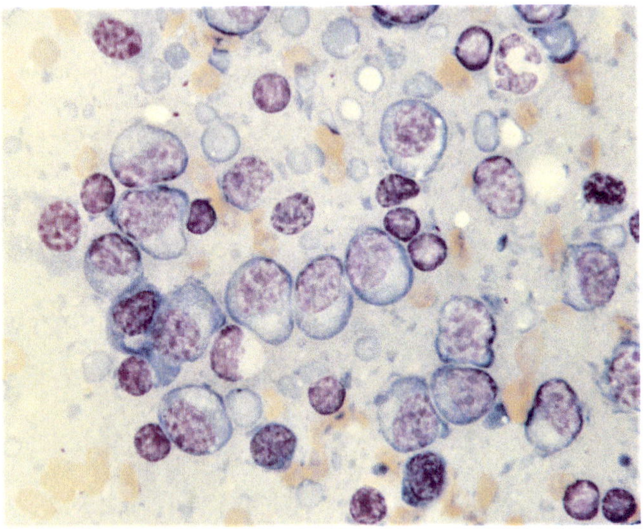

Fig. 7.71. Predominance of plasma cells in a bone marrow aspirate from a ferret (*Mustela putorius furo*) with multiple myeloma, Wright–Giemsa stain (100× oil).

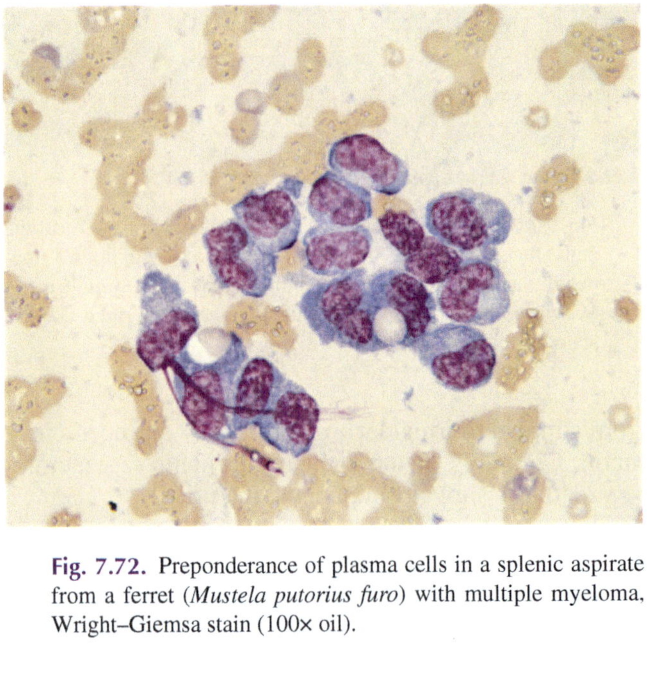

Fig. 7.72. Preponderance of plasma cells in a splenic aspirate from a ferret (*Mustela putorius furo*) with multiple myeloma, Wright–Giemsa stain (100× oil).

and there is no clear etiology; however, genetic, viral, and environmental carcinogens have all been suggested as possible contributing factors (Snow et al., 2018).

Myelogenous Leukemia

Chronic myelogenous leukemia (CML) is a rare disease in both domestic animals and wildlife species. Myelogenous leukemia is a neoplastic disorder of the multipotent stem cell characterized by the purposeless production or accumulation of differentiated hematopoietic precursors or both (Raskin, 1996).

Carcinoma

Carcinomas are epithelial cell tumors with nuclear criteria of malignancy, such as anisokaryosis, nuclear gigantism (macrokaryosis, macronuclei), multinucleation, coarse nuclear chromatin, large bizarre or angular nucleoli, multiple nucleoli, nuclear molding high N:C ratios, numerous mitotic figures, as well as anisocytosis, basophilic cytoplasm, and abnormal cytoplasmic vacuolation (Figures 7.73a, 7.73b, 7.74a, and 7.74b). Cluster formation is common with carcinomas. This type of neoplasm tends to provide highly cellular samples containing large round, cuboidal, columnar, or polygonal cells with distinct cytoplasmic margins depending on the cell type. Epithelial cells adhere to each other, typically exhibit common adjoining borders (tight junctions called desmosomes), and often produce cells that exfoliate in cellular aggregates (sheets or clusters) (Baker and Lumsden, 2000).

Adenocarcinomas (malignant neoplasia of glandular epithelium) reveal epithelial cells occurring singly and in clusters of variable size (Figures 7.75a and 7.75b). Cells are usually round, with round to oval, eccentrically placed nuclei, and variable quantities of basophilic cytoplasm that contains vacuoles that may be filled with secretory product. Cell borders are usually distinct. Cellular aggregates occurring in balls, rosettes, or loose cellular groupings are suggestive of adenocarcinomas, and the arrangement of these cells may suggest acinar, tubular, or papillary formation (Figures 7.75a, 7.75b, 7.76, and 7.77). Adenocarcinomas also have the cytological features of large cytoplasmic secretory vacuoles and giant cell formation (Figures 7.77–7.81). Binucleated or multinucleated cells may be seen (Figures 7.73a and 7.73b). Mesenchymal cells may be present in variable numbers.

Squamous cell carcinomas are frequently observed in mammals, especially domestic dogs and cats (Mauldin and Peters-Kennedy, 2016; Goldschmidt and Goldschmidt, 2017; Naylor et al., 2018). Development of squamous cell carcinomas has been associated with papillomavirus infection and prolonged exposure to ultraviolet light in multiple species (Mauldin and Peters-Kennedy, 2016; Goldschmidt and Goldschmidt, 2017). Squamous cell carcinoma is a malignant neoplasm of epithelial cells in which the cells show differentiation to keratinocytes of the epidermis. During normal maturation, the nucleus of a squamous epithelial cell undergoes pyknosis and karyorrhexis and eventually disappears, leaving an anuclear squame. As the nuclear chromatin condenses, the cells undergo keratinization, and as the

(a) (b)

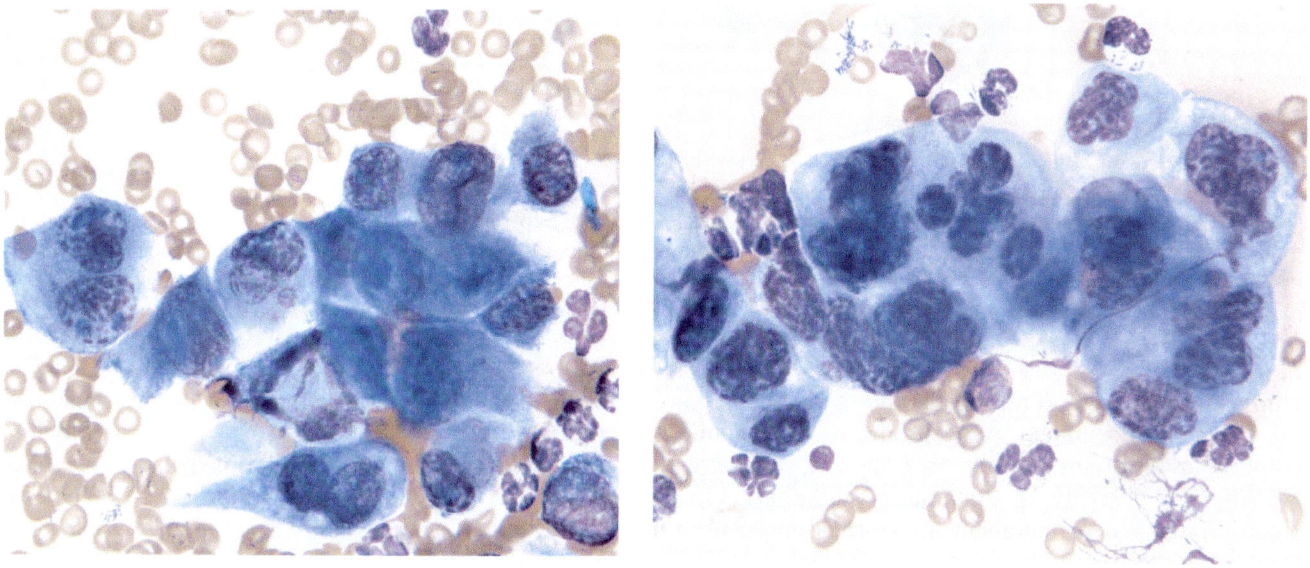

Fig. 7.73. (a), (b) Aggregates of large, often multinucleate epithelial cells showing moderate anisocytosis, significant pleomorphism, high nuclear to cytoplasm (N:C) ratios, and large nucleoli in a fine-needle aspiration biopsy of poorly differentiated carcinoma in a ferret (*Mustela putorius furo*), Wright–Giemsa stain (100× oil). Source: Image from Campbell and Grant (2010, p. 160).

(a) (b)

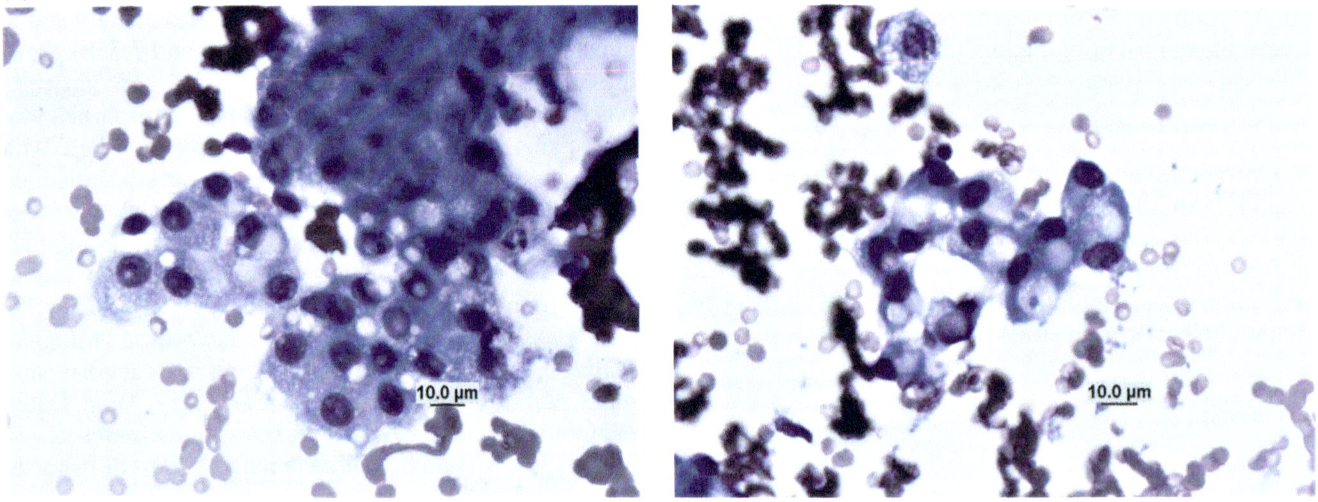

Fig. 7.74. (a), (b) Aggregates of large, often multinucleate, epithelial cells showing moderate anisocytosis, significant pleomorphism, high nuclear to cytoplasm (N:C) ratios, and large nucleoli in a fine-needle aspiration biopsy of poorly differentiated carcinoma in a ferret (*Mustela putorius furo*), Wright–Giemsa stain (100×, oil). Source: Image from Campbell and Grant (2010, p. 160).

(a) (b)

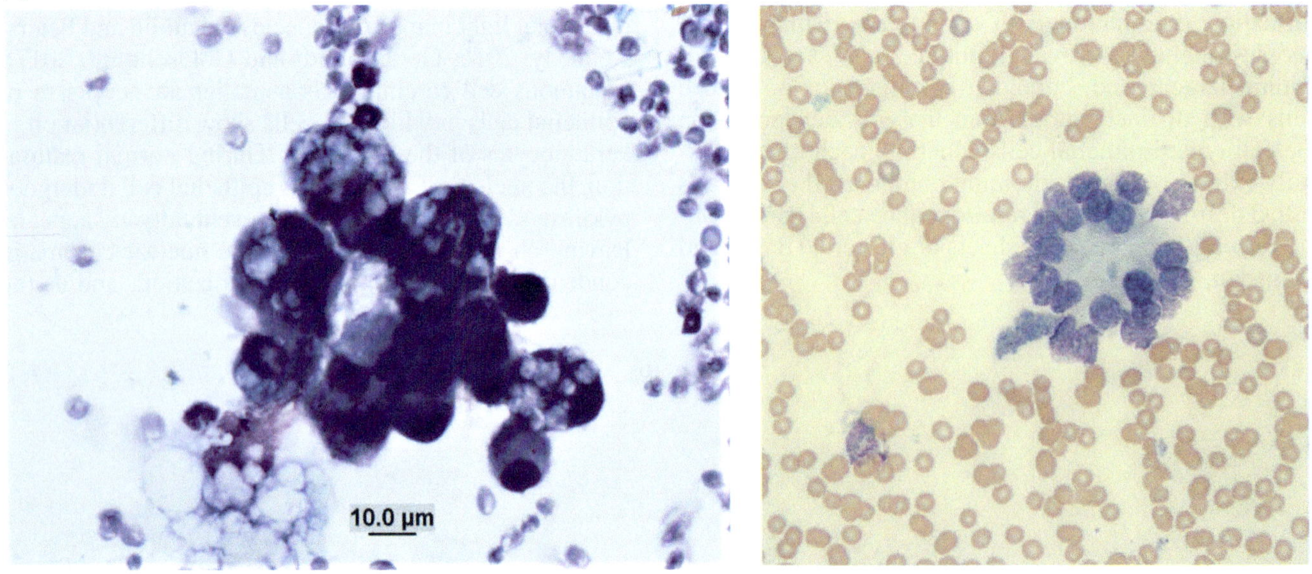

Fig. 7.75. (a) Aggregate of epithelial cells with moderate anisocytosis and deeply basophilic cytoplasm with vacuolated cytoplasm in a fine-needle aspiration biopsy of a mammary adenocarcinomas from a hamster (*Mesocricetus auratus*), Wright–Giemsa stain. (b) Cohesive cluster of epithelial cells in an acinar formation in a fine-needle aspiration biopsy of a mammary adenocarcinoma from a guinea pig (*Cavia porcellus*) Wright–Giemsa stain (100× oil). Source: Image from Campbell and Grant (2010, p. 196).

cytoplasm becomes keratinized, the cell becomes blue-green in appearance. Asynchrony in nuclear and cytoplasmic differentiation is an important indicator of malignancy involving squamous epithelial cells (Figure 7.82). When malignant transformation occurs, normal progressive differentiation disappears, and the resultant dysplastic squamous epithelial cells exhibit cellular and nuclear pleomorphism. Atypical cells exhibit a dysmaturation between the cell nucleus and cytoplasm (nuclear–cytoplasmic asynchrony), resulting in round to oval cells with high N:C ratios and hyalinized cytoplasm, or angular squamous cells with atypical nuclei. Cells may have open vesicular or vacuolated nuclei despite having a highly keratinized cytoplasm or may contain small pyknotic nuclei in parabasal or early intermediate squamous epithelial cells (Baker and Lumsden, 2000). The cytoplasm may be vacuolated with distinct perinuclear vacuolation, which represents

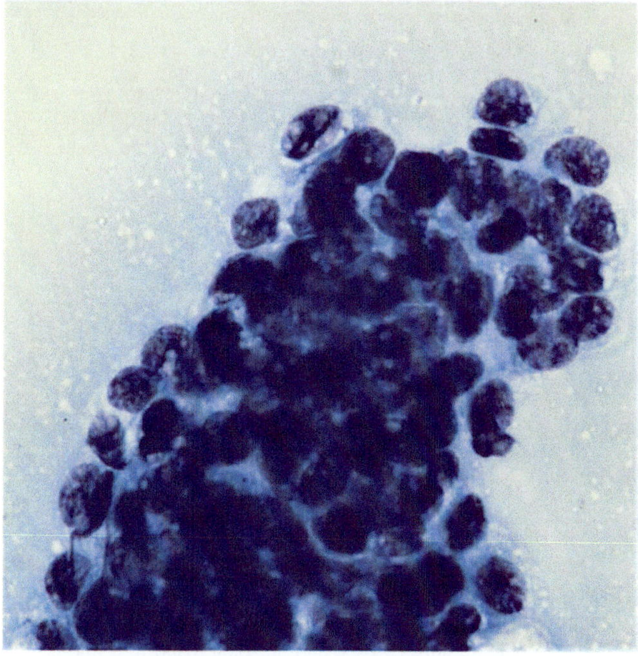

Fig. 7.76. Cohesive clusters of epithelial cells exhibiting features of malignancy (moderate anisocytosis, high nucleus to cytoplasmic (N:C) ratio, and scant deeply basophilic cytoplasm) in a fine-needle aspiration biopsy of a cutaneous adenocarcinomas from a gerbil (*Meriones unguiculatus*), Wright–Giemsa stain (100× oil). Source: Image from Campbell and Grant (2010, p. 194).

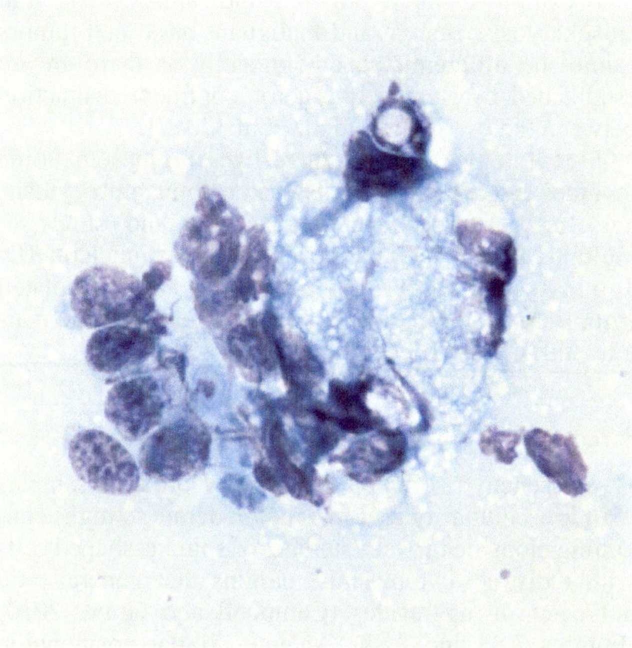

Fig. 7.77. Cohesive clusters of epithelial cells exhibiting features of malignancy (marked anisocytosis and high nucleus to cytoplasmic ratio except for the vacuolated giant cells) in a fine-needle aspiration biopsy of a cutaneous adenocarcinomas from a gerbil (*Meriones unguiculatus*), Wright–Giemsa stain (100× oil). Source: Image from Campbell and Grant (2010, p. 194).

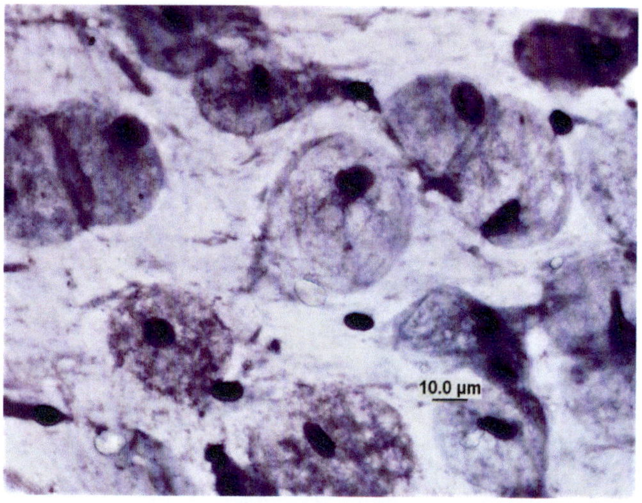

Fig. 7.78. Aggregate of large epithelial cells with features of malignant neoplasia (marked anisocytosis, multinucleation, and deep cytoplasmic basophilia) in an impression of the uterus from a guinea pig (*Mesocricetus auratus*) with an endometrial adenoma, Wright–Giemsa stain.

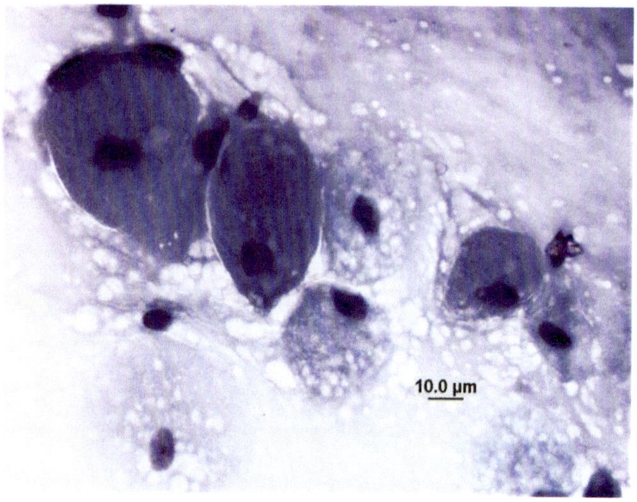

Fig. 7.79. Giant cells with features of malignant neoplasia (marked anisocytosis, mild pleomorphism, and deep cytoplasmic basophilia) in an impression of the uterus from a guinea pig (*Mesocricetus auratus*) with an endometrial adenoma, Wright–Giemsa stain.

colorless keratohyalin granules (Raskin, 2001c). Abnormal squamous epithelial cells may exfoliate as single cells or in cell clusters. Intracellular bridges representing desmosomes may be visible, especially in wet fixation and trichrome stains (Baker and Lumsden, 2000).

The presence of dysplastic squamous cells differentiates squamous cell carcinomas from benign lesions, such as papillomas; however, the degree of atypical squamous cells can vary. A heterophilic inflammation may be associated with squamous cell carcinomas, which can create a diagnostic challenge in the differentiation of the dysplastic squamous cells of malignant

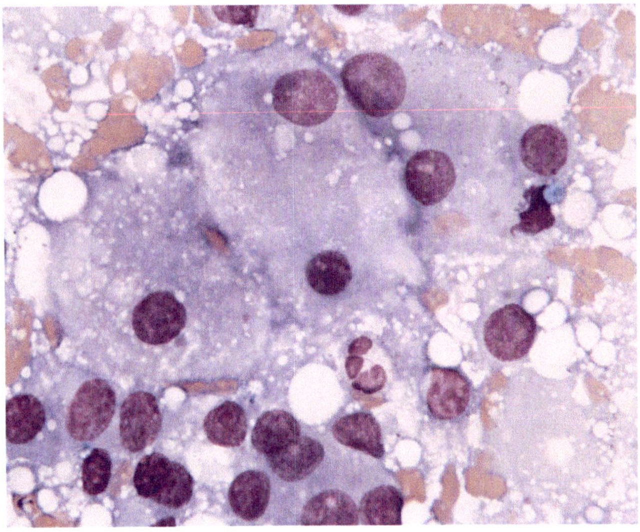

Fig. 7.80. Epithelial cells with features of malignant neoplasia (marked anisocytosis, mild pleomorphism, granular nuclear chromatin, large nucleoli, and giant cell formation) in an impression of an adrenal adenocarcinoma from a ferret (*Mustela putorius furo*), Wright–Giemsa stain (100× oil).

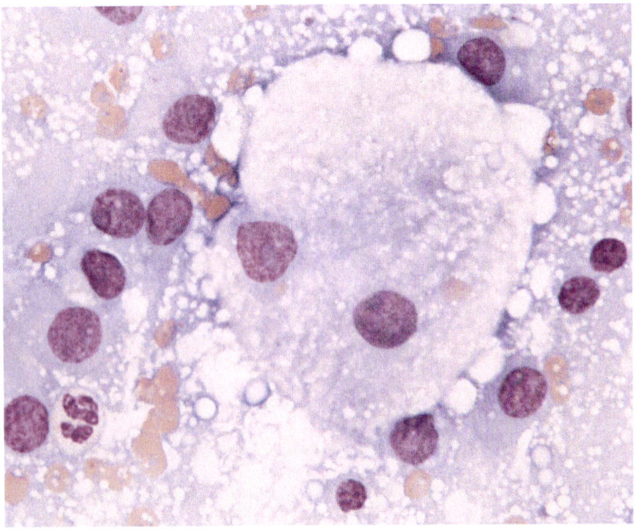

Fig. 7.81. Epithelial cells with features of malignant neoplasia (marked anisocytosis, mild pleomorphism, granular nuclear chromatin, large nucleoli, and giant cell formation) in an impression of an adrenal adenocarcinoma from a ferret (*Mustela putorius furo*), Wright–Giemsa stain (100× oil).

neoplasia from those associated with a chronic inflammatory response.

Basal cell tumors (cutaneous basilar epithelial neoplasm) are dermal tumors seen commonly in mammals. Basal cell tumors contain uniform small, round to polygonal-shaped cells with round to oval nuclei, sometimes with a prominent single nucleolus and a high N:C ratio (1:1 ratio) (Baker and Lumsden, 2000). Exfoliated basal epithelial cells occasionally occur in rows or

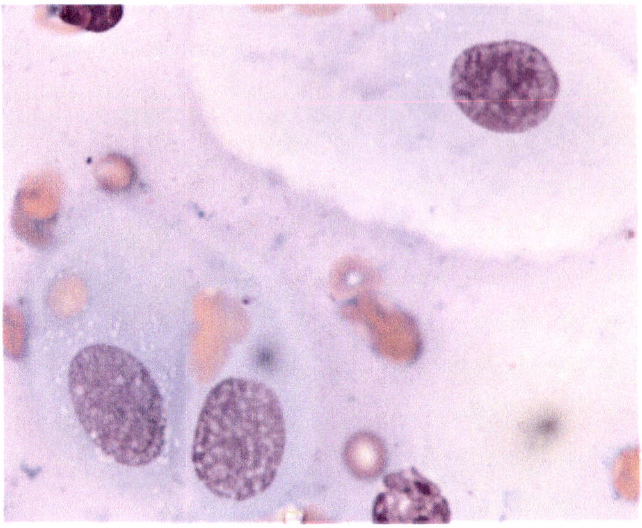

Fig. 7.82. Squamous epithelial cells with features of malignant neoplasia (high nucleus to cytoplasmic (N:C) ratio, large nuclei with coarse granular chromatin, prominent multiple nucleoli, macronucleoli, anisocytosis, and anisokaryosis) in a fine-needle aspiration biopsy of an oral squamous cell carcinoma from a hedgehog (*Atelerix albiventris*), Wright–Giemsa stain (100× oil).

ribbons of cells (Barton, 1987) (Figure 7.12). The basophilic cytoplasm may contain vacuoles, fine blue granules (keratohyalin), or melanin pigment. There may be atypical basal cells among the uniform cells in a cluster that exhibit a three- to fourfold anisocytosis and anisokaryosis. Benign and malignant basal cell tumors cannot be differentiated cytologically as there are no established cytologic criteria for confident distinction between the two (Munasinghe et al., 2017).

A cytological pattern suggestive of a mesothelioma includes aggregates of cells that exhibit anisocytosis, aniso-macrokaryosis, multinucleation, and single to multiple prominent and variably shaped nucleoli (Di Tommaso et al., 2015). Some cells may have vacuolated cytoplasm and villus-like eosinophilic cytoplasmic margins (thick brush border).

Sarcoma

Mesenchymal neoplasms usually produce samples with low cellularity (but may be moderate to high) containing elongated (oval), stellate, or spindle-shaped cells with indistinct cytoplasmic margins that generally do not occur in aggregates (Campbell and Grant, 2010) (Figures 7.83 and 7.84). An intercellular eosinophilic matrix may be observed. The cells often appear as individual cells in the cytology sample and are generally smaller than epithelial cells. The shape of the nuclei can vary from round to elliptical and fusiform. An example of a commonly occurring mesenchymal neoplasm is the fibrosarcoma.

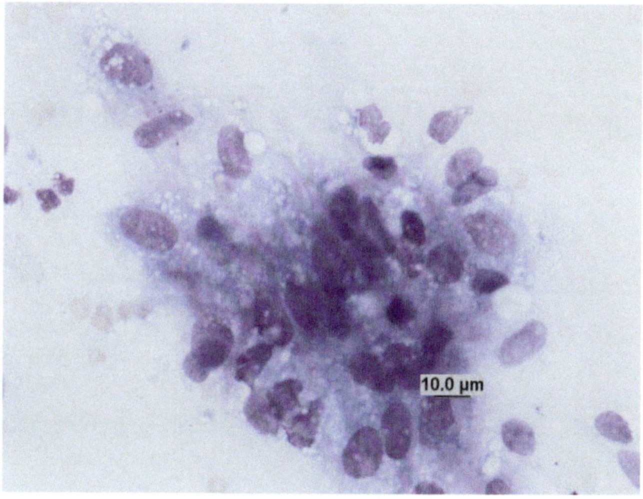

Fig. 7.83. Pleomorphic mesenchymal cells in an imprint from a poorly differentiated cutaneous sarcoma from a hamster (*Mesocricetus auratus*), Wright–Giemsa stain.

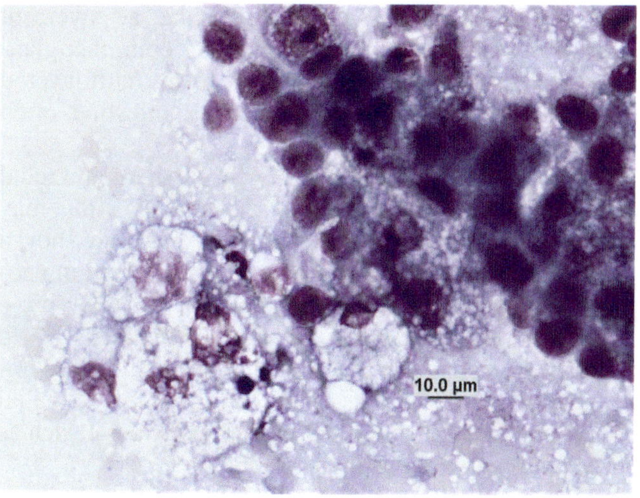

Fig. 7.84. Pleomorphic mesenchymal cells in an imprint from a poorly differentiated abdominal sarcoma from a gerbil (*Meriones unguiculatus*), Wright–Giemsa stain.

The cytology of a fibrosarcoma reveals large, plump, spindle-shaped mesenchymal cells that have exfoliated singly or in aggregates within a pink amorphous background substance (collagenous material) (Figure 7.84). In general, these cells appear less uniform than normal fibroblasts, have high N:C ratios, and contain lightly to deeply basophilic cytoplasm with indistinct margins. Nuclear pleomorphism is often present and aids in the differentiation of the malignant fibroblasts from the benign cells of a fibroma or fibrous hyperplasia. Multinucleated giant cells may also be part of the cytologic findings.

Osteosarcomas are rare in exotic mammalian pets, such as ferrets, rabbits, and chinchillas; however, they are commonly found in hedgehogs (Reyes-Matute et al., 2017). Microscopic examination of cytologic preparations reveals a mixture of individual and multinucleated cells. The individual cells (osteoblasts) may be round to oval with variably shaped nuclei, prominent and multiple nucleoli, and dark blue vacuolated cytoplasm containing fine, pink granules (Di Tommaso et al., 2015). Other samples may exhibit polygonal to fusiform cells (osteoblasts) with indistinct cytoplasmic margins that exhibit mild pleomorphism, a clear distinct Golgi apparatus, multiple cytoplasmic punctate vacuoles, variable N:C ratio, and moderate anisocytosis and anisokaryosis with clumped nuclear chromatin and multiple nucleoli (Conrado et al., 2013). The osteoblasts are associated with an amorphous eosinophilic background material (osteoid). Large multinucleated osteoclasts may also be present.

Chondromas and chondrosarcomas are neoplasia of cartilage (chondrocytes and cartilaginous cells). The cytology often reveals mesenchymal cells embedded in a bright, pink, smooth to slightly granular background material (chondroid). The cells look similar to those found in osteosarcomas (primary neoplasia of bone) and can vary from round to fusiform with large nuclei and deeply basophilic cytoplasm. Like cells from osteosarcomas, chondrosarcomas can contain small intracytoplasmic vacuoles and fine eosinophilic granules.

Peripheral nerve sheath tumors (neurofibromas, schwannomas, neurilemmomas, and perineuromas) reveal neoplastic spindle cells on cytologic preparations. The pink background (matrix) typically contains free cell nuclei. The cells are spindle- to stellate-shaped with light blue, wispy cytoplasm and high N:C ratios with nuclei having finely stippled chromatin with multiple inconspicuous nucleoli (Reimnitz et al., 2019). Moderate anisocytosis and anisokaryosis are expected (de Cecco et al., 2018).

Cytologic diagnosis of hemangiosarcoma can be challenging; therefore, histopathology and immunohistochemistry are useful for establishing a definitive diagnosis. Erythrophagia and low numbers of mesenchymal cells with features of malignancy, such as increased N:C ratio, macrokaryosis, anisokaryosis, anisonucleosis, and distinct multiple nucleoli, may be seen.

Neuroendocrine

Neoplasia involving endocrine or neuroendocrine tissue has characteristic cytologic features that include cells that easily exfoliate (exfoliate moderate to high number of cells), are fragile, and are easily disrupted (cells not intact with bare nuclei devoid of encompassing cytoplasm or embedded in a sea of cytoplasm) during the collection process. Therefore, cytological preparations are highly cellular with loosely cohesive sheets of small, cuboidal epithelial cells, typically surrounded by abundant bare nuclei (Figures 7.85a and 7.85b). The

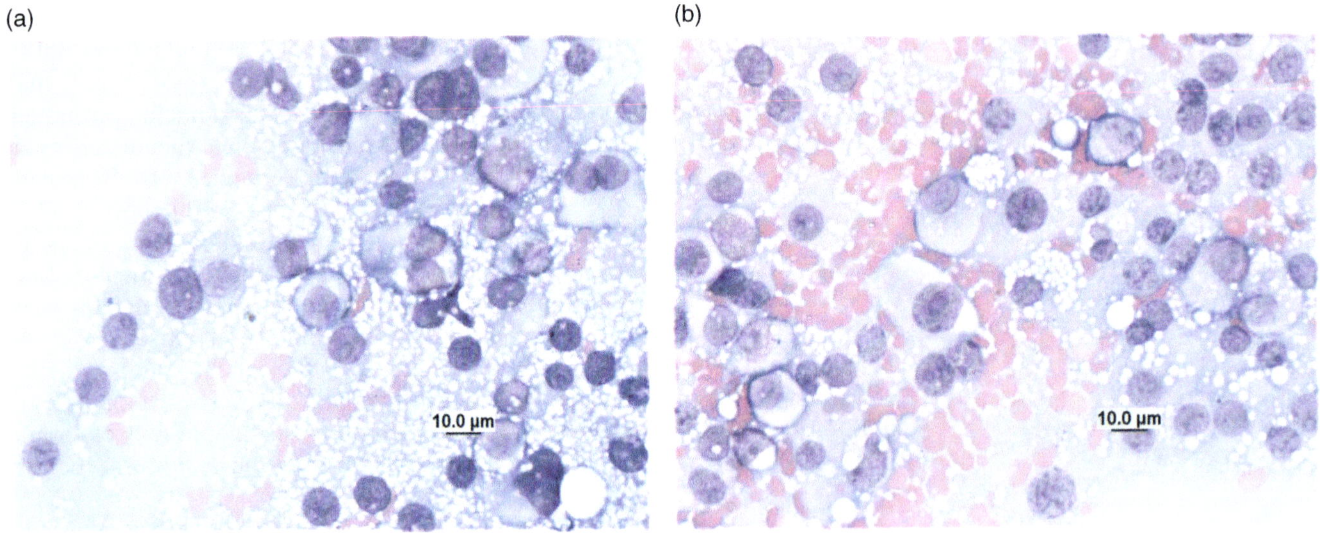

Fig. 7.85. (a), (b) Imprint of an adrenal mass from a ferret (*Mustela putorius furo*) with adrenal gland disease, Wright–Giemsa stain (100× oil).

bare, round, and uniform nuclei of ruptured cells generally have intact outlines, are distorted, and exhibit streaming chromatin. The intact cells are often uniform and well differentiated, with minimal cytologic atypia, even in biologically aggressive lesions, making it difficult to determine malignancy (Anderson et al., 2019).

Cellular Arrangements

Exfoliated cells on the cytology preparation may be found in different types of arrangements that may provide additional clues for obtaining a definitive diagnosis, especially regarding neoplastic lesions. Cellular arrangements can be classified as acinar, palisade, pavement, honeycomb, papillary, trabecular, storiform, or perivascular pattern (Masserdotti, 2006).

Acinar patterns are recognized when cells are grouped around an empty central area (which may at times be filled with secretory material) (Figure 7.75b). When sampled, cells from normal thyroid tissue exfoliate in an acinar pattern. This pattern can also be found in cytological specimens from a variety of neoplasms of glandular tissues.

Columnar epithelial cells arranged in regular rows have a palisade arrangement. The columnar ciliated epithelial cells from the respiratory tract found in tracheal washes are frequently found in this arrangement. Gastric columnar epithelial cells from gastric wash samples may also align themselves in this fashion.

When flat cells exfoliate as pieces of a mosaic in a monolayer (often referred to as a cobblestone arrangement), the arrangement is called a pavement pattern. Exfoliations of superficial epithelial cells from the surface of skin, eyelids, and the oral cavity often arrange themselves in this pattern.

A honeycomb arrangement is like a pavement arrangement, but consists of cuboidal or columnar glandular cells. Imprints of biopsies from multilayered parenchyma, such as the stomach or intestine often reveal cells in this pattern.

A papillary arrangement occurs when epithelial cells arrange themselves around a stromal axis (that may not always be evident) where the outer cells may show a palisade arrangement. This pattern is often seen in neoplasms derived from tubular epithelium.

Cells that exfoliate in large, elongated 2- to 3-dimensional clusters that exhibit branching have a trabecular cell pattern. This is characteristic of epithelial neoplasms that are supported by fibrous stroma, such as some mammary and hepatic tumors.

When spindle cells are arranged in wavelike bundles, they have a storiform pattern. This is a typical mesenchymal arrangement that can be seen in many malignant mesenchymal tumors (i.e., fibrosarcoma or malignant fibrous histiocytoma).

Cells arranged around single or multiple vascular structures, such as the elongated endothelial elements of capillaries that contain erythrocytes, have a perivascular arrangement. This arrangement can be found in cytology specimens from hemangiosarcomas.

Neoplasia of the Gastrointestinal Tract

The most common epithelial tumors found in the oropharynx of domestic mammals include squamous cell carcinoma and odontogenic neoplasms (including the epulides) (Figure 7.82). The common mesenchymal tumors of the mouth in domestic mammals include fibrosarcoma, chondrosarcoma, osteosarcoma, and malignant melanoma. The common round cell tumors of the mouth and mucous membranes of domestic mammals include mast cell tumors, plasma cell tumors, and lymphoma.

Neoplasia of the stomach is rare in domestic mammals. Cytodiagnosis of a gastric carcinoma can be difficult because of the location of the tumor; however, a cytodiagnosis of a gastric lymphoma is easier because it would be similar to lymphoma in other locations.

Lymphoma is the most common intestinal neoplasm of domestic mammals, especially in the cat, but it can be confused with inflammatory bowel disease based on cytology alone. Intestinal adenocarcinoma can be identified by aggregates of epithelial cells exhibiting features of malignancy. Smooth muscle tumors (leiomyomas or leiomyosarcomas) located in the intestinal submucosa can be identified as mesenchymal cells that exfoliate poorly and have characteristic, long and narrow or "cigar-shaped" nuclei.

Common tumors of the rectum and anal area in domestic mammalian species include perianal gland tumors and apocrine anal sac adenocarcinoma. Cells in perianal gland tumors are described as being hepatoid because cytologically they resemble hepatocytes. The cytology of apocrine anal sac adenocarcinomas generally consists of ruptured cells and free nuclei stripped of their cytoplasm. The few intact cells have a scant rim of basophilic cytoplasm and a large round nucleus with a small but prominent nucleolus. Other tumors of the colon and rectum include adenocarcinoma, lymphoma, and plasma cell tumors.

A variety of neoplastic diseases involving the gastrointestinal tract have been reported in small mammals. Neoplasia involving the gastrointestinal tract can be identified based upon the appearance of cells with features of malignant neoplasia. Adenocarcinomas of the stomach are the most common gastrointestinal neoplasms of ferrets (Williams and Weiss, 2004).

Adenocarcinomas, leiomyomas, and leiomyosarcomas of the stomach and intestines and papillomas of the sacculus rotundus are the most frequent gastrointestinal neoplasms in rabbits (Jenkins, 2004).

Neoplasia of the Respiratory Tract

Neoplasia of the respiratory tract is uncommon in exotic animals; however, when present, neoplasia can often be identified by the presence of cells with features of malignancy in the cytology specimens (Effron et al., 1977). These features have been described above, and an attempt to classify the neoplasm can be made based upon the cytology. Neoplasia of the lungs of animals occurs with either primary or metastatic lesions. Neoplasia of the lungs of small mammals is usually of metastatic origin (Meredith, 2000; Williams and Weiss, 2004).

Cutaneous Neoplasms

Common epithelial tumors of the skin in domestic mammals include squamous cell carcinoma, basal cell tumors, hair follicle tumors, sebaceous adenomas, perianal gland tumors, and apocrine anal sac adenocarcinomas. Distinguishing the different mesenchymal tumors based upon cytology alone is difficult; therefore, a general diagnosis of sarcoma or mesenchymal tumor is made, with the presence of these cells demonstrating features of malignancy. Histopathology, usually with immunohistochemical staining in samples from domestic species, is necessary to arrive at the specific diagnosis. Reliable cytologic criteria that distinguishes neoplastic from reactive spindle cells is lacking; however, computer-based nuclear morphometry on cytologic preparations is a reproducible method that may be able to differentiate cutaneous soft tissue sarcomas from reactive mesenchymal lesions, at least in the dog (Meachem et al., 2012).

Round cell tumors commonly found in the skin of domestic mammals include lymphoma, mast cell tumor, plasma cell tumor, histiocytoma, and transmissible venereal tumors (dogs only). Each of these cell types can easily be differentiated from the others based upon cytology alone. For example, cells in mast cell tumors contain red to purple cytoplasmic granules; cells in transmissible venereal tumors contain multiple, discrete, cytoplasmic vacuoles; cells in histiocytomas exhibit peripheral clearing of the cytoplasm; and plasma cells exhibit a perinuclear clearing in the cytoplasm.

Cutaneous neoplasms are common in many species of exotic animals and can be epithelial, mesenchymal, or vascular in origin (Campbell and Grant, 2010). Spontaneous cutaneous neoplasia is rare in mice, rats, hamsters, chinchillas, and rabbits; however, the skin is the second most common site of primary neoplasia in the gerbil and guinea pig (Collins, 1987; Harkness and Wagner, 1989; Burgmann, 1991; Scott et al., 1995, 2001; Harcourt-Brown, 2002a; Da Costa et al., 2007). Spontaneous cutaneous neoplasia is common in captive African hedgehogs (*Atelerix albiventris*) (Raymond and Garner, 2001).

Papillomas have been reported in ferrets, mice, rats, and rabbits, and usually appear as solitary lesions that can occur anywhere on the skin (Scott et al., 2001). Papillomas of domestic rabbits frequently occur at the mucocutaneous junction of the mouth, eye, or anus and appear as small, friable, cauliflower-shaped tumors that easily bleed. Shope papillomas of wild rabbits appear as multiple hornlike growths, especially on the face and eyelids, which originate from a single site and are caused by an oncogenic papovavirus (Scarff, 2000).

Papillomas of all species of animals are often identified by the gross appearance of a cauliflower or warty lesion; however, other conditions may at times resemble papillomas. Examples of these include chronic inflammatory lesions with fibrous proliferation and other neoplastic lesions. Cytology may be helpful in the differentiation of these conditions. The cytology of the wart-like lesions of squamous papillomas reveals predominately normal mature squamous epithelial cells, a lack of inflammatory cells, or cells with obvious features of neoplasia.

Apocrine gland neoplasms in ferrets typically involve the prepuce, but have also been reported on the tail and in the perianal area. They are highly aggressive in behavior, with frequent local recurrence and metastasis to local tissues and lymph nodes resulting in a median disease-free interval in ferrets with a histological diagnosis of less than two months (Pinches et al., 2008).

Cutaneous lymphoma is infrequently found in small mammals. However, it is a common skin neoplasm of pet rabbits in Europe, but is rarely reported in pet rabbits in North America. These tumors have been classified as diffuse, large B-cell lymphomas with 56% being a centroblastic/centrocytic subtype and 44% being a T-cell-rich B-cell subtype (a rare subtype other than in horses), and there has been no support for a viral etiology (Ritter et al., 2012). Unlike other domestic animals, cutaneous lymphomas in European pet rabbits were highly pleomorphic and frequently contained multinucleated giant cells.

Fibromas and fibrosarcomas are common neoplasms of the integument of exotic small mammals, especially in rodents, where mesenchymal neoplasms are more common than are epithelial neoplasms. Cytologic preparations often reveal a population of individually arranged oval to spindle-shaped cells that exhibit moderate anisocytosis and anisokaryosis. The cytoplasm may stain unevenly basophilic and contain clear, round vacuoles and occasional paranuclear pale areas suggestive of the Golgi apparatus (Johnson et al., 2014). The cells may have one or more cytoplasmic processes with relatively indistinct cytoplasmic borders.

Rabbit (Shope) fibroma virus (Poxviridae) is a tumorigenic, transmissible virus infecting eastern cottontail and European rabbits and is similar to rabbit myxoma virus, and fibroma viruses of hares and squirrels (Dehghanpir et al, 2016). The virus ordinarily produces localized fibromas where cytologic preparations consist of spindle-shaped cells exhibiting moderate anisocytosis and anisokaryosis (Figures 7.86a and 7.86b). The nuclei are large (1–3 times the size of erythrocytes), round to oval, eccentric, and exhibit finely stippled chromatin with multiple nucleoli. The basophilic cytoplasm occasionally contains round to oval eosinophilic inclusions that vary in size (3–5 µm) and shape (Dehghanpir et al., 2016).

Carcinomas or adenocarcinomas are common malignant tumors of mammary epithelium in rodents. Fibroadenomas are a common spontaneous benign mammary tumor in rats.

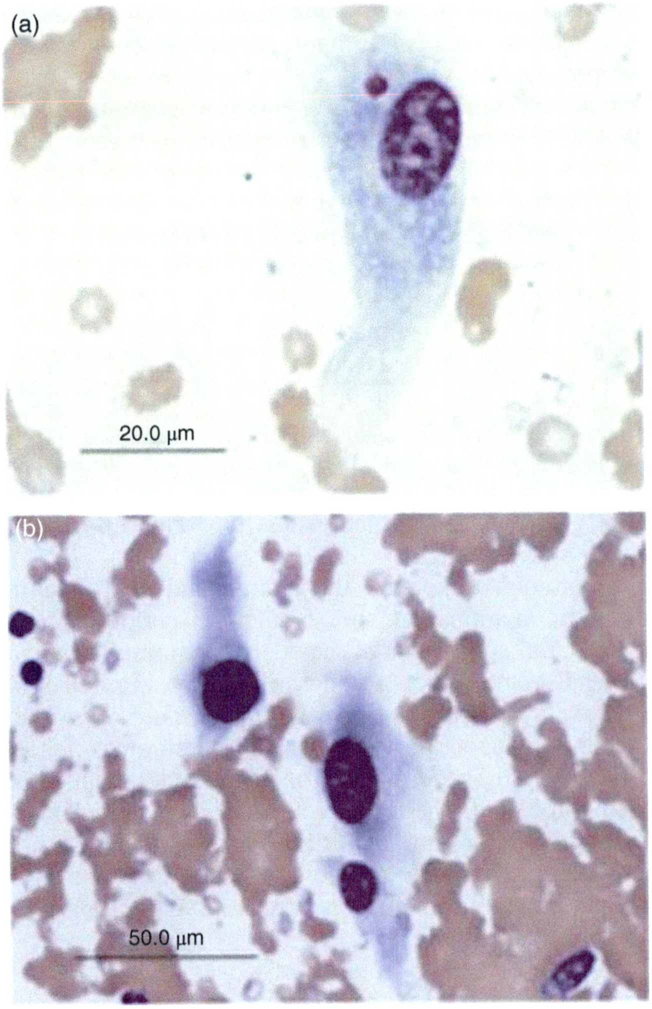

Fig. 7.86. (a) A fine-needle aspirate of a nodule on the muzzle in a rabbit revealed low to moderate numbers of spindle-shaped cells with rare nonkeratinized squamous epithelial cells. The spindle cells exhibited moderate anisocytosis and anisokaryosis. Nuclei were round to oval, eccentric, large (measuring 1.5–3× the diameter of an erythrocyte), and occasionally binucleated with finely stippled chromatin and 1–4 variably sized prominent nucleoli. Aqueous Romanowsky stain (50×). Source: Image from Dehghanpir et al. (2016). (b) The cytoplasm was moderate in amount and moderately basophilic with occasional round to oval eosinophilic inclusions that varied in size (3–5 µm) and shape. The cytologic interpretation was mesenchymal neoplasm with presumptive diagnosis of Shope fibroma. Aqueous Romanowsky Stain (100×). Source: Dehghanpir et al. (2016).

Fine-needle aspiration (FNA) has proved to be a simple, rapid, less invasive, and cost-effective method to differentiate benign from malignant lesions and has been widely used in veterinary medicine (Karim et al., 2008). Mammary tumors of other mammals may differ from those of rodents. For example, malignant epithelial cells from mammary tumors of adult European hedgehogs (often classified as simple tubulopapillary carcinomas) when immunolabeled by antibodies specific for various cytokeratins (CKs) reveal a profile that differs from that shown by mammary epithelial cells of other mammalian species (Döpke et al., 2007).

Mammary adenocarcinoma appears to occur with some frequency in marsupials (e.g., macropods); however, it has not been well described in sugar gliders, a popular pet (Churgin et al., 2015). Cytological preparations reveal cohesive clusters that are polygonal to spindle-shaped with variably distinct cytoplasmic borders, high N:C ratios, and moderately basophilic cytoplasm that contain occasional coarse, blue-gray granules (Keller et al., 2014) (Figure 7.87).

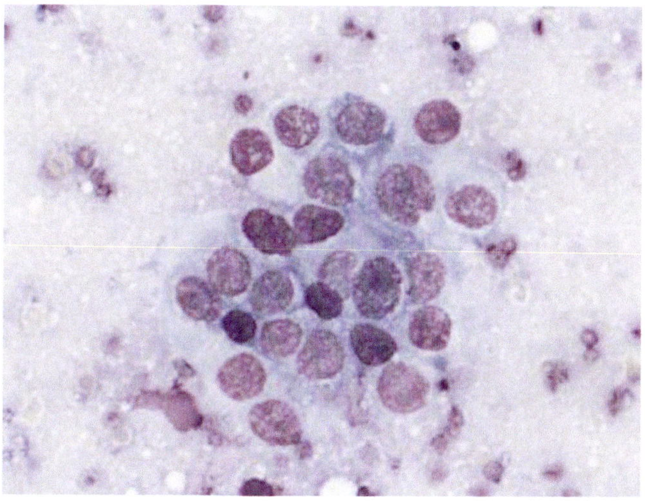

Fig. 7.87. A fine-needle aspirate of a mass protruding from the right aspect of the marsupium of a sugar glider (*Petaurus breviceps*) revealed neoplastic cells exhibiting high nucleus to cytoplasmic (N:C) ratios, anisocytosis, and anisokaryosis. Likely differentials include carcinoma or adenocarcinoma, although an amelanotic melanoma could not be ruled out. Anaplastic mammary adenocarcinoma was determined on histopathology. Modified Wright Stain (50×). Source: Keller et al. (2014).

As in the dog, the use of FNA biopsy of mammary gland tumors in rats is controversial. Although fibroadenomas represented 53% of subcutaneous masses in companion rats and carcinomas represented 12%, cytologic results were inconclusive in 55% of the samples in one study (Vergneau-Grosset et al., 2016). In that study, cytologic results of aspirates of mammary gland carcinomas indicated septic inflammation and those of mammary gland fibroadenomas indicated a hematoma, likely resulting from peripheral blood contamination.

Anal sac neoplasms can be evaluated by fine-needle aspirate cytologic preparations from a perianal mass. When present, bare nuclei throughout the preparation are suggestive of an endocrine/neuroendocrine appearance. Cells arranged in cohesive clusters exhibiting moderate to marked anisocytosis and anisokaryosis with poorly defined cell borders, light blue cytoplasm, round to oval nuclei with finely stippled chromatin and round to irregular, prominent nucleoli are suggestive of an adenocarcinoma (Vilalta et al., 2017b) (Figures 7.88a and 7.88b). A definitive diagnosis of an anal sac neoplasm generally requires histopathologic examination of the tissue and classification into one of three distinct histological patterns (solid, rosette, and tubular or mixtures of these), and the presence of neuroendocrine differentiation in some cases (Suzuki et al., 2013).

Melanocytic tumors, such as melanomas, are mesenchymal neoplasms; however, their cytological appearance can be a mixture of spindle, round, and epithelial-like

(a) (b)

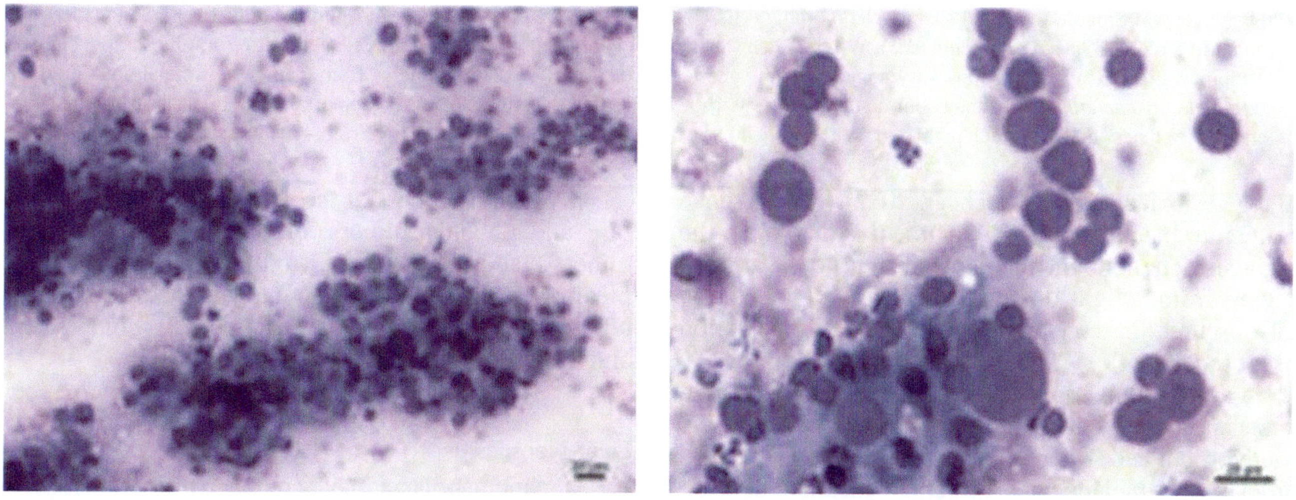

Fig. 7.88. (a) A fine-needle aspirate of a perianal mass from a ferret (*Mustela putorius furo*) revealed cohesive clusters of epithelial cells with poorly defined cell borders, mid-to-light blue cytoplasm, and round to oval nuclei with finely stippled chromatin. The cells have prominent, variably shaped, and sometimes multiple nucleoli. Moderate anisocytosis and anisokaryosis were observed. The cytologic was compatible with anal sac adenocarcinoma. Modified Wright stain (bar = 50 μm). (b) Same sample as in left figure, revealing bare nuclei suggesting a cell population of endocrine/neuroendocrine origin. Modified Wright stain (bar = 50 μm). Source: Vilalta et al. (2017b).

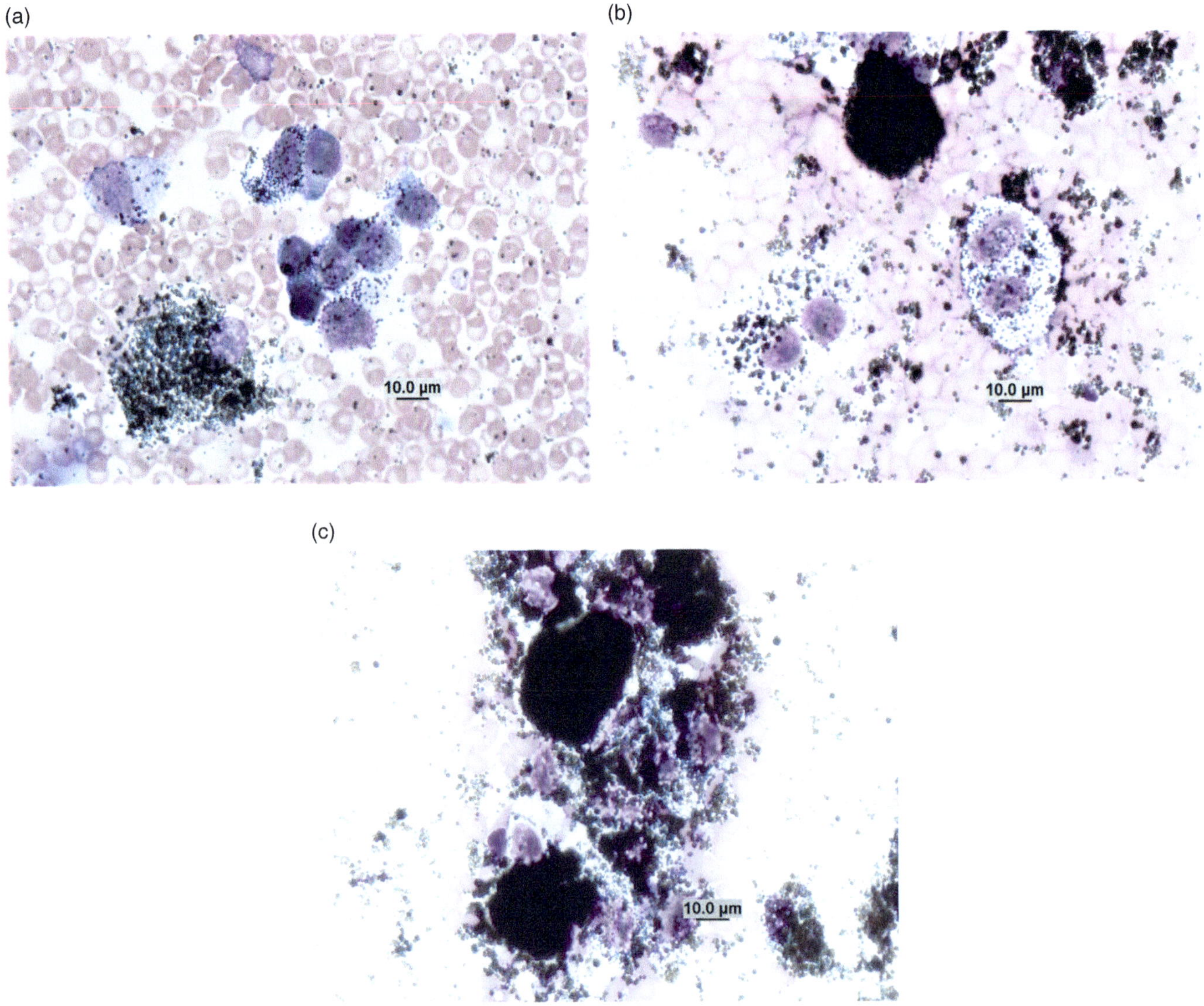

Fig. 7.89. (a) Spindle- to round-shaped pleomorphic cells containing spherical, green-black melanin granules from a cutaneous melanoma in a rabbit (*Oryctolagus cuniculus*), Wright–Giemsa stain. (b) Pleomorphic cells and binucleated cells from the sample cytologic sample as Figure 7.95a containing varying amounts of spherical, green-black melanin granules from a cutaneous melanoma in a rabbit (*Oryctolagus cuniculus*), Wright–Giemsa stain. (c) Cells in a lymph node aspirate (from the same rabbit patient as in Figures 7.95a and 7.95b) that contain so much pigment that it is difficult to examine other cytologic features, Wright–Giemsa stain.

aggregates (Meuten and Meichner, 2022). The presence of green to black cytoplasmic pigment is the key to the diagnosis. The amount of pigment present is variable, ranging from a light dusting to a heavy pigmentation that obscures the cell nucleus. Rarely is pigmentation absent (amelanotic) (Allnoch et al., 2020).

In domestic mammals, most melanomas are benign except when they occur in certain locations such as the mouth or nail bed, where they tend to be malignant. The cytoplasm of melanocytes in benign melanomas typically contains so much pigment that it is difficult to examine other cytologic features. By contrast, the cells in malignant melanomas often have little to no pigment, making it easy to identify the criteria of malignancy (Figures 7.89a–7.89c, 7.90a, 7.90b).

In general, tumors of the external auditory canal are rare, and glandular tumors comprise a minority of these tumors (Jan et al., 2008). Cytologic preparations reveal pleomorphic cells with abundant cytoplasm and variable numbers of vacuoles (Suckow et al., 2002) (Figures 7.55a and 7.55b).

Liver Neoplasms

Hepatic neoplasia may occur as a primary neoplasm of the hepatocytes or bile duct epithelium, or as a secondary neoplasia such as metastatic disease or hepatic lymphoma. Benign neoplasia involving hepatocytes and nodular regeneration cannot be differentiated based on cytology alone because both conditions exhibit

(a) (b)

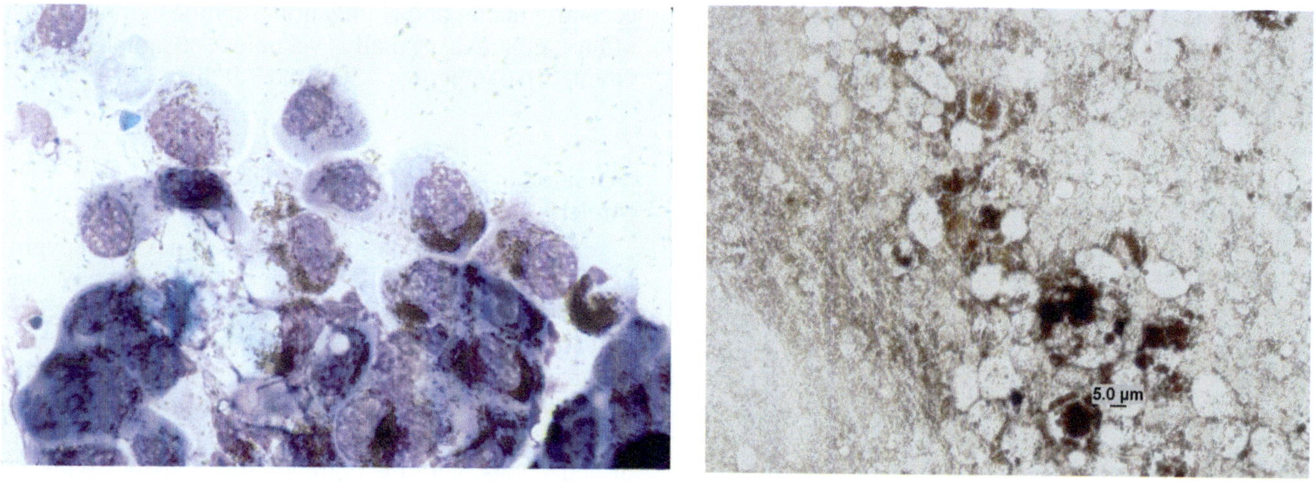

Fig. 7.90. (a) Melanocytes containing variable amounts of rod-shaped, brown-black to black melanin granules in a fine-needle aspiration biopsy from a cutaneous melanoma in a guinea pig (*Cavia porcellus*), Wright–Giemsa stain (100× oil). (b) Imprint of a black cutaneous mass on a rat (*Rattus norvegicus*) diagnosed with a cutaneous melanoma, Wright–Giemsa stain.

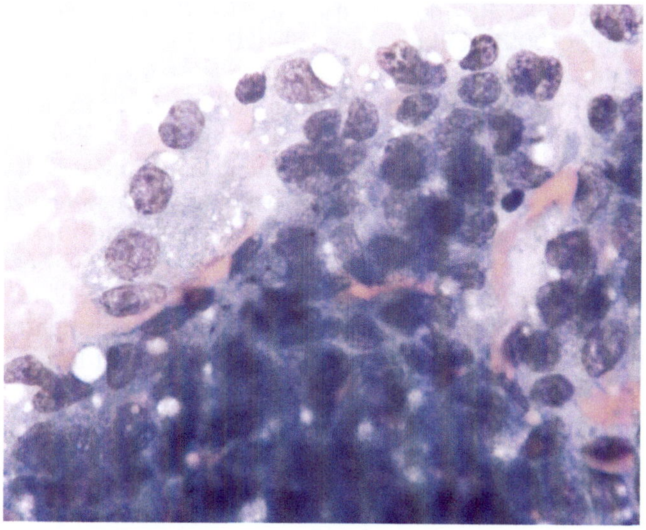

Fig. 7.91. Hepatocytes with moderate anisocytosis and anisokaryosis; some with large nucleoli and vacuolated cytoplasm in an imprint of a liver biopsy with a histologic diagnosis of biliary carcinoma from a ferret (*Mustela putorius furo*). Although the cytology is suspicious for a hepatic neoplasm, hepatocellular carcinomas can be challenging to diagnose based on cytology alone. Wright–Giemsa stain (100× oil).

hepatocytes that appear normal or exhibit mild anisocytosis and anisokaryosis (Figure 7.91). Hepatocellular carcinomas can be challenging to diagnose based on cytology alone. Only hepatocytes with obvious cytologic criteria for malignancy can be used as a cytological basis in the diagnosis of hepatocellular carcinomas. Neoplasia originating from the biliary epithelium (bile duct neoplasia) can also be difficult to identify based upon cytology alone because of the exfoliation of normal-appearing bile duct epithelial cells (Meyer, 2001a). Hepatic neoplasia has been reported in small mammals and lower vertebrates.

Renal Neoplasms

Renal adenomas and adenocarcinomas arise from epithelial cells of the kidney. Adenomas may be difficult to identify based on cytology alone, whereas adenocarcinomas that contain epithelial cells with features of malignant neoplasia may be easier to identify.

Embryonal nephromas (nephroblastomas) arise from pluripotential embryonal renal tissue. The undifferentiated vestigial tissue retains its primitive characteristics and is often described as an adenosarcoma because of the presence of tubular and glandular epithelium and connective tissue. Embryonal nephromas often contain neoplastic cuboidal epithelial cells with much fibrous stroma. The fibrous stroma contains spindle-shaped cells dispersed among large amounts of mucinous material. It may undergo metaplasia to form bone or cartilage. The noncellular background may contain a heavy eosinophilic substance suggestive of a cellular attempt to produce a matrix (e.g., chondroid or osteoid).

Reproductive Tract Neoplasia

Imprint cytology is a simple, inexpensive, diagnostic tool that plays a major role in rapid intraoperative diagnosis of ovarian neoplasms similar to frozen histopathologic sections (Sireesha et al., 2018). Cytopathologic features of ovarian tumors have been well described in domestic animals, especially in the bitch, where the cellular morphology depends on the cell type from which the tumor is derived (Bertazzolo et al., 2004). Papillary adenocarcinomas exhibit papillary structures that are associated with tridimensional cell clusters in acinar or tubular arrangements. Granulosa cell tumors commonly exhibit single pleomorphic (round, oval, polyhedral, or flame shaped) cells arranged in monolayered cell clusters with acinar to tubular patterns. Teratomas are characterized by highly variable cell populations that reflect the multiple different tissue types from which they originate. Ovarian dysgerminomas have been described in cytologic specimens as consisting of large, round neoplastic cells with marked anisocytosis and anisokaryosis; nuclei are oval, with prominent nucleoli and reticular chromatin (Bertazzolo et al., 2004). Mixed dysgerminoma/granulosa cell tumors are described as containing mixed neoplastic cell populations composed of two different morphologic cell types (neoplastic germ cells and granulosa cells) (Bertazzolo et al., 2004).

Neoplasia of Ferrets (*Mustela putorius furo*)

Of neoplasms involving the skin, cutaneous mast cell tumors, basal cell tumors, squamous cell carcinomas, and sebaceous epitheliomas are commonly diagnosed in ferrets of all ages, whereas fibromas, fibrosarcomas, sebaceous gland adenomas, hemangiomas, and benign cystic adenomas are frequently identified in middle-aged to older ferrets (Kelleher, 2001; Hoppman and Barron, 2007; Mitchell and Tully, 2009). Endocrine tumors are the most common neoplasm reported in ferrets, constituting almost 40% of the tumors in one study where pancreatic islet cell tumors comprised 21.7% and adrenocortical tumors comprised 16.7% of tumors (Li et al., 1998). In another study, pancreatic tumors comprised 23.4% and adrenocortical tumors comprised 36.6% of tumors in ferrets (Avallone et al., 2016). The cytology of neuroendocrine lesions reveals a homogenous population of mononuclear cells with eccentric nuclei and abundant basophilic cytoplasm that often contains small vacuoles (Campbell and Grant, 2010) (Figures 7.92a and 7.92b).

Neoplasia of African Pygmy Hedgehogs (*Atelerix albiventris*)

Neoplasms are commonly reported in African pygmy hedgehogs (*Atelerix albiventris*). Approximately one-third of these patients presented to veterinary practices will be for the treatment of neoplasia, with most occurring in females (Hoefer, 1994; Raymond and White, 1999). Neoplasia, both benign and malignant, has been observed with considerable frequency in all organs of hedgehogs, with the common locations involving the integumentary, hemolymphatic, digestive, and endocrine systems, and the most common types of tumors are mammary gland adenocarcinoma, lymphosarcoma, and oral squamous cell carcinoma (Hoefer, 1994; Raymond et al., 1998; Raymond and White, 1999; Raymond and Garner, 2001; Fukuzawa et al., 2004; Díaz -Delgado et al., 2017).

Thyroid follicular adenoma, follicular adenocarcinoma, and C-cell carcinoma have been described in African pygmy hedgehogs (Raymond and Garner, 2001; Miller et al., 2002). Cytologic preparations may reveal clustered epithelial cells (occasionally arranged in acinar formations) with variably distinct cytoplasmic borders and many free nuclei. When intact, these cells are round to polygonal (rarely spindle shaped) with lightly to moderately basophilic cytoplasm and round to oval

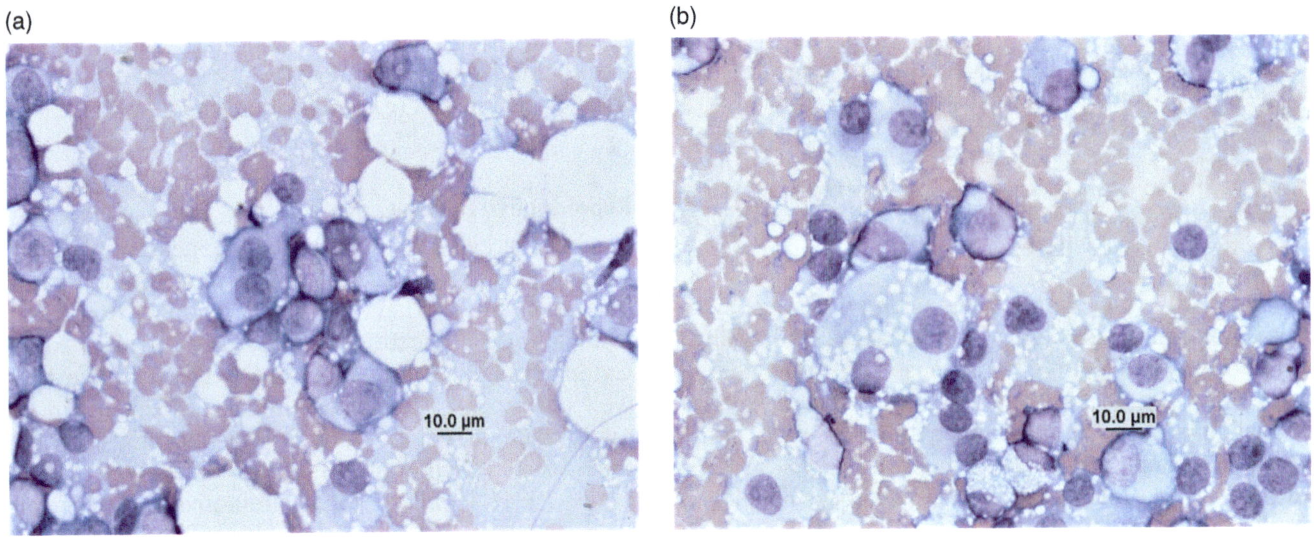

Fig. 7.92. (a), (b) A homogeneous population of mononuclear cells with eccentric nuclei and abundant basophilic cytoplasm that often contain small vacuoles from a fine-needle aspiration biopsy of an adrenal gland adenoma from a ferret (*Mustela putorius furo*), Wright–Giemsa stain.

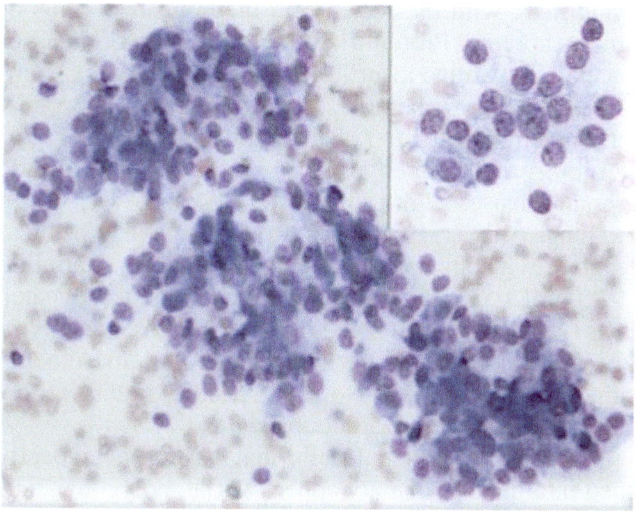

Fig. 7.93. A fine-needle aspiration of a ventral right cervical mass (malignant thyroid tumor) in a hedgehog (*Atelerix albiventris*) revealed clustered epithelial cells with indistinct cytoplasmic borders and many free nuclei. Intact cells were round to polygonal to rarely spindloid. Moderate anisocytosis and anisokaryosis, coarsely stippled chromatin, and one or two prominent nucleoli were observed (inset). These cells were occasionally arranged in acinar formations. Nuclei were round to oval, approximately 1.5 to 3 times the diameter of an erythrocyte, and variably located. Source: LaRue et al. (2016).

nuclei with moderate anisocytosis and anisokaryosis, coarsely stippled chromatin, and nuclei with one or two prominent nucleoli (LaRue et al., 2016) (Figure 7.93).

Neoplasia of Sugar Gliders (*Petaurus breviceps*)

Neoplasia reported in sugar gliders (*Petaurus breviceps*) include cutaneous lymphosarcoma (cutaneous), transitional cell carcinoma (pericloacal), biliary cystadenomas, hepatocellular tumors, mammary gland adenocarcinoma, melanoma, leukemia, leiomyoma of the skin, vascular hamartoma, bronchoalveolar carcinoma, and duodenal adenocarcinoma (Keller et al., 2014; Churgin et al., 2015).

Neoplasia of Chinchillas (*Chinchilla lanigera*)

Neoplasia is rarely reported in chinchillas compared to other exotic pets. For example, squamous cell carcinoma, which is common in other rodents and exotic pets, rarely occurs in chinchillas (Szabo et al., 2019).

Effusions

The peritoneum produces a small amount of lubricating fluid to facilitate organ movement. In normal animals, little if any fluid can be collected from the thoracic and abdominal or coelomic cavity; however, pathological conditions result in the accumulation of fluid. Pleural and peritoneal fluids accumulate in animals as a result of decreased reabsorption or increased production of normal fluid, an inflammatory process, disruption of vessels or viscous structures, or a neoplastic condition (Baker and Lumsden, 2000).

Abdominocentesis may be performed on small mammals to obtain ascitic fluid for evaluation. The procedure begins by surgical preparation of the aspiration site. A 21- to 25-gauge needle is inserted along the ventral midline of the abdomen distal to the umbilicus of mammals. The abdominal cavity of some mammals, such as rabbits and guinea pigs, is large, and the gastrointestinal tract occupies much of the space and lies just under the body wall. Care should be taken not to penetrate the gastrointestinal tract of these animals.

Fluid accumulation disorders are characterized by the location and cytologic characterization of a collected sample, which is important for determining the pathogenesis of an effusion. Normal pleural and peritoneal fluid is colorless, clear, and poorly cellular with the presence of a few mesothelial cells, macrophages, and lymphocytes. Neutrophils/heterophils are rarely found in normal fluid. The pathophysiological process involved with the production of pleural and peritoneal effusions (ascitic fluid) include inflammatory, circulatory, or malignant disorders. These effusions can then be further described as a transudate, modified transudate, exudative effusion, hemorrhagic effusion, chylous effusion, pseudochylous effusion, malignant effusion, or other species-related effusion.

Effusion analysis is a common, routine test in veterinary clinical laboratories that involves both the qualitative and quantitative evaluation of a fluid sample. Body fluid analysis in veterinary and medical laboratories typically includes assessment of physical features (i.e., color, turbid, cloudy, and containing particles), protein quantitation, red blood cell (RBC) count, total nucleated cell count (TNCC), differential cell count, and when indicated, evaluation of lipid content (Hotz et al., 2005). Quantitative protein concentration of body fluids can be obtained by refractometric or rapid chemical methods, such as biuret. Refractometry is the method of choice for determination of protein in peritoneal, pericardial, and pleural fluids (George, 2001). Most American-made refractometers give direct protein readings of 2.5 g/dL (25 g/L) or greater; reliable results for protein concentrations as low as 0.6 g/dL (6 g/L) can be obtained from published conversion tables (George and O'Neill, 2001).

In addition, pathologists routinely evaluate a stained smear of the fluid to assess cell morphology and the presence of organisms. For an accurate cytological evaluation of fluids, it is essential that the sample be fresh. The sample should be refrigerated if it cannot be examined immediately. The microscopic findings together with other qualitative and quantitative results are used to categorize the fluid as a transudate, modified transudate, exudate, chylous effusion, hemorrhagic effusion, or neoplastic effusion. Fluid classification is useful for determine the underlying disease process resulting in the effusion (Hotz et al., 2005).

Transudate

Transudative effusions are fluids that have accumulated in the serous cavities because of oncotic pressure changes and other circulatory disturbances (i.e., increased hydrostatic vascular pressure) or decreased lymphatic drainage (Stockham and Scott, 2008). The primary causes of the formation of transudates in domestic mammals include hypoproteinemia (hypoalbuminemia), overhydration, and lymphatic or venous congestion (Baker and Lumsden, 2000). Cardiac insufficiency, portosystemic shunt, and hepatic cirrhosis and insufficiency are examples of conditions that result in transudate formation.

The term *modified transudate* has been used to describe effusions that do not fit neatly into the transudate or exudate category based on nucleated cell counts and protein concentrations; however, describing an effusion as a modified transudate has limited utility because of the wide variety of potential underlying disorders (Allison, 2022). Transudates can be classified as protein-poor (pure transudates) or protein-rich (modified transudates).

Protein-poor transudates are typically clear and colorless to straw colored grossly and are characterized by low specific gravity (<1.017), low cellularity (<1500 nucleated cells/μL), and low total protein (<2.5 g/dL) (Baker and Lumsden, 2000). Some authors suggest that the cell counts should be less than 3000 cells/mL (Baker and Lumsden, 2000). The nucleated cells found in transudates are primarily made up of macrophages, and occasional mesothelial cells, small lymphocytes, and nondegenerate neutrophils/heterophils. The most common cause of protein-poor transudative effusion is severe hypoalbuminemia caused by protein-losing nephropathy or enteropathy or hepatic insufficiency/failure. Other causes include portal hypertension (presinusoidal or sinusoidal), portosystemic shunt, and early cardiac insufficiency.

Protein-rich transudates are effusions that have also been referred to as modified transudates. They most commonly form secondary to congestive heart failure and portal hypertension (postsinusoidal). Increased hydrostatic pressure causes high-protein fluid to escape vessels in the lungs or liver. Protein-rich transudates may be clear to hazy with an increased total protein concentration (>2.5 g/dL) and low to moderate numbers of nucleated cells (<5000/μL) consisting of mononuclear cells and nondegenerate neutrophils. Mesothelial cells may be reactive. Protein-rich transudates are long-standing transudative effusions that have become "modified" with the increase in the number of cells or protein content. Protein-rich transudates are often associated with cardiac insufficiency, cardiomyopathy, compression of vascular structures from neoplasia, inflammation or torsion of an organ, and the presence of sterile irritants (Shelly, 2001). Increased hydrostatic pressure causes high-protein fluid to escape vessels in the lungs or liver. Protein-rich transudates may be clear to hazy with an increased total protein concentration (>2.5 g/dL) and low to moderate numbers of nucleated cells (<5000/μL) consisting of macrophages, small lymphocytes, nondegenerate neutrophils, and mesothelial cells that may be reactive. The specific gravity is low (1.017–1.025) (Baker and Lunsden, 2000).

Normal mesothelial cells that have been recently shed into the body cavity appear as flat, polygonal cells with thin, homogenous, weakly basophilic cytoplasm and centrally positioned round or oval nuclei and occur singly or in clusters of sheets. Mesothelial cells become reactive when irritation of the serous membranes occurs, or when long-standing effusions are present. Reactive mesothelial cells are cuboidal to round, larger in size, exfoliate singly or in clusters, and contain a moderate amount of basophilic cytoplasm compared to nonreactive cells. The cytoplasm may contain large vacuoles that can push the nucleus to the cell margin, creating a signet ring appearance (Baker and Lumsden, 2000). The nucleus of reactive mesothelial cells tends to be large and round, and often contains coarsely granular chromatin and one to three prominent nucleoli. Many reactive mesothelial cells also have scalloped or villus-like eosinophilic cytoplasmic margins (pink to red fringe). Additional features that might be noted include multinucleation, cytoplasmic vacuolation, anisocytosis, anisokaryosis, and mitotic activity.

Proliferation of mesothelial cells results in the formation of irregular aggregates. These irregular aggregates may exfoliate, appearing in the cytology sample as cellular sheets, balls, or rosettes, which can resemble abnormal cellular clusters seen with some neoplastic disorders (i.e., adenocarcinomas). The uniform appearance of the nuclei in the cell clusters helps to differentiate reactive mesothelial cells from neoplasia.

Macrophages appear as large, variably shaped mononuclear cells containing round, oval, or variably shaped nuclei (the nucleus often appears kidney bean shaped) that may contain fine chromatin and nucleoli. The cytoplasm is granular, abundant, light blue to gray in color, and may contain phagocytic vacuoles and/or foreign material. "Foamy" macrophages that contain small, round cytoplasmic vacuoles may be present as well, and often result from the phagocytosis of lipids derived from cellular degeneration. Macrophages can reproduce as free-floating cells in fluids. An estimated 90% of the mitotic figures seen in mammalian body fluids are reproducing macrophages (Cowell et al., 1999).

Exudative Effusion

Exudative effusions are fluids containing increased protein content and cellularity. Exudative effusions vary in color and turbidity, may have a foul odor, and often clot during sample collection. Fluid samples suggestive of an exudative effusion should be placed into a collection tube containing an anticoagulant (e.g., EDTA) to prevent clotting of the sample. Exudates typically result from inflammatory processes or chemotactic stimulation within the peritoneal cavity that causes increased capillary permeability.

The gross appearance of an exudative effusion varies dependent upon the etiology (i.e., the type of infectious or noninfectious agent), host response, and duration of time. Cloudy, red, or pink samples frequently contain blood, which may indicate intracavitary hemorrhage or contamination during sampling and opaque, tan or beige samples are generally highly cellular, often containing numerous inflammatory cells, which are consistent with an exudate (Allison, 2022).

In general, exudates are characterized by a high cellularity (>5000/μL), protein content (>3.0 g/dL), and specific gravity (>1.025). The cellular contents of exudates are primarily inflammatory cells that vary with etiology, host response, and duration. Mononuclear leukocytes are characteristic of mild irritation to the coelomic cavity and nonseptic conditions. Exudates demonstrating a neutrophilic/heterophilic inflammation suggest an acute inflammatory response. Septic exudates may demonstrate intracellular bacteria and degenerate neutrophils/heterophils. Chronic exudates contain an increased number of macrophages, lymphocytes, and plasma cells (Figures 7.38b, 7.94, and 7.95).

The cytological appearance of the microorganism may provide clues to the etiology of the exudative effusion. For example, a pleural effusion consisting of neutrophilic inflammation with numerous clusters of rod-shaped to serpentine microorganisms that measure between 2 and 3 μmm in length and surrounded by a clear halo have been associated with *Pseudomonas luteola* infection in ferrets (Martínez et al., 2012).

Hemorrhagic Effusion

Traumatic injury, neoplasia, and hemostatic disorders may result in bleeding into the thoracic or peritoneal cavities, resulting in a hemorrhagic effusion. Hemorrhagic effusions present as red, turbid fluid. Peracute or ongoing hemorrhagic effusions may resemble peripheral blood (based on cell counts, leukocyte differentials, and the packed cell volume). Established hemorrhagic effusions contain a variable number of erythrocytes and leukocytes. In general, a packed cell volume (PCV) of the fluid greater than 3% is suggestive of a hemorrhagic effusion (Stockham and Scott, 2008).

Hemorrhagic effusions present as red, turbid fluid. Peracute or ongoing hemorrhagic effusions may resemble peripheral blood (based on cell counts, leukocyte differentials, and the packed cell volume). Established hemorrhagic effusions contain a variable number of erythrocytes and leukocytes.

It is important to differentiate hemorrhagic effusions from peripheral blood contamination of the sample during collection. Observation of the sudden appearance of a red fluid in a clear fluid during sample collection indicates peripheral blood contamination of the sample. The

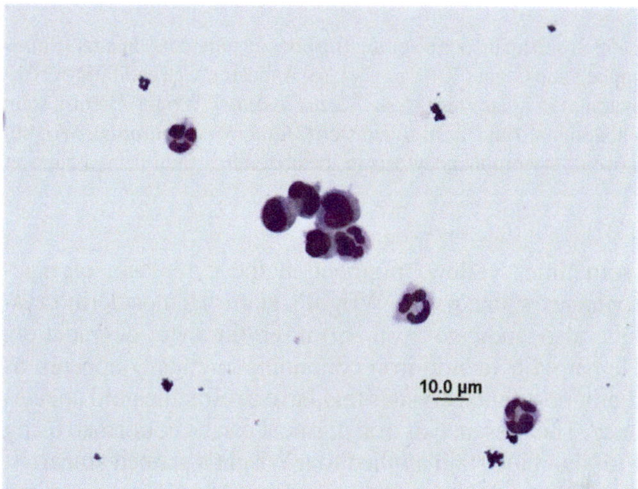

Fig. 7.94. A direct smear of abdominal fluid reveals a mixed cell inflammation with numerous nondegenerate neutrophils indicating an exudative effusion (peritonitis) in a ferret (*Mustela putorius furo*), Wright–Giemsa stain.

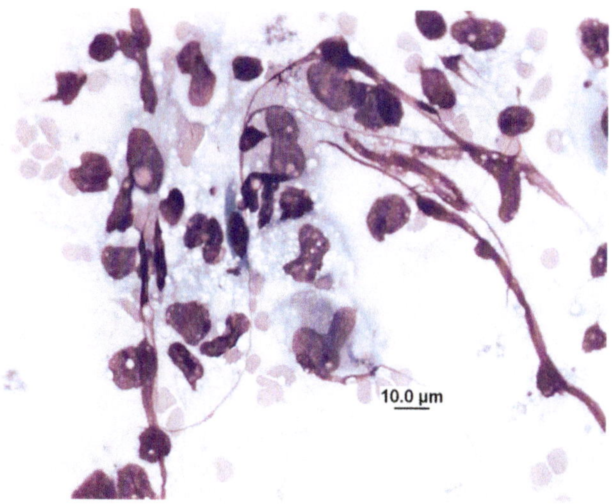

Fig. 7.95. A cytocentrifuge concentrated abdominal fluid sample reveals numerous macrophages indicating an exudative effusion (peritonitis) in a ferret (*Mustela putorius furo*), Wright–Giemsa stain.

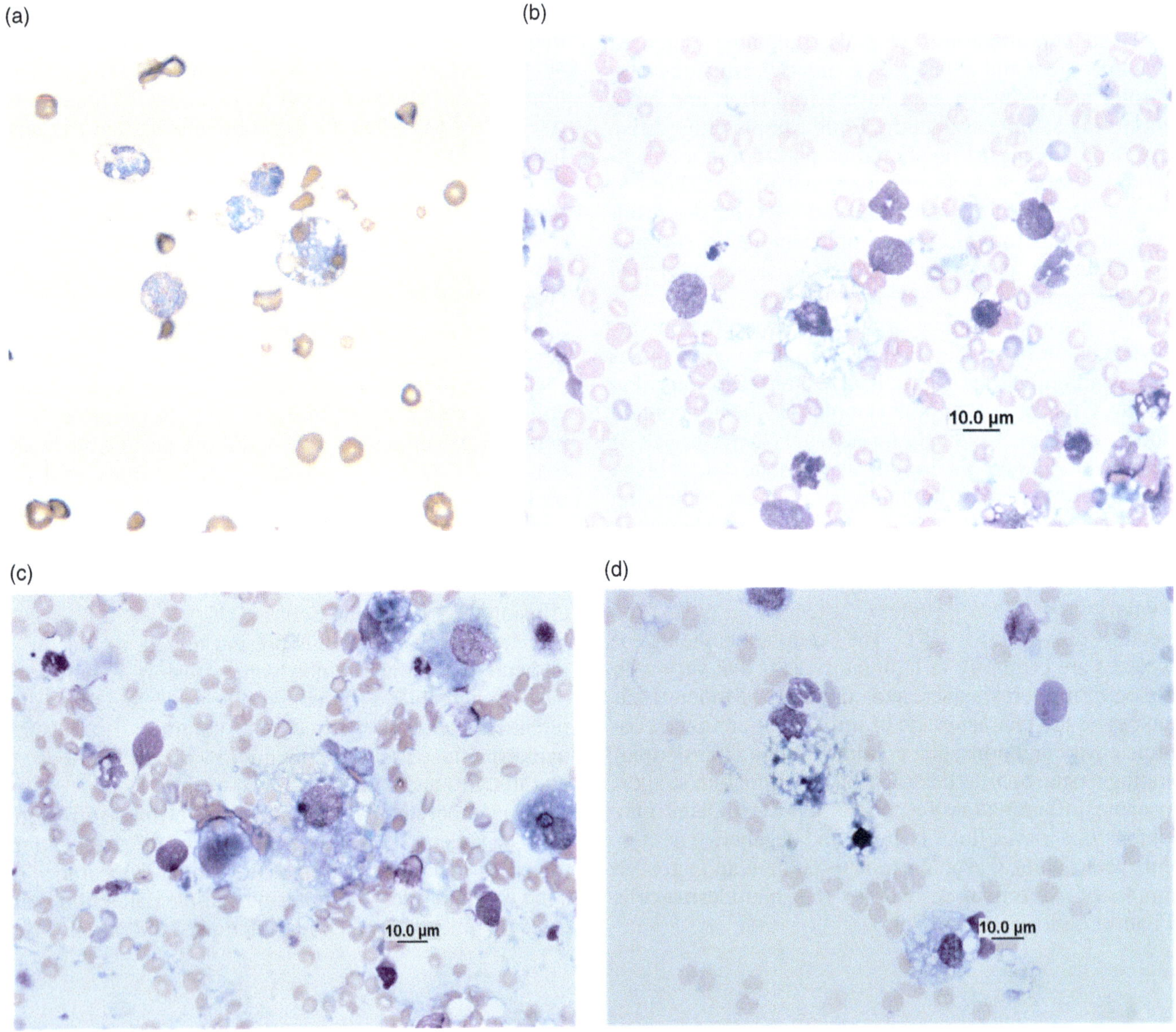

Fig. 7.96. (a) A macrophage exhibiting erythrophagocytosis in a fluid-filled subcutaneous swelling (resolving hematoma) in a rat (*Rattus norvegicus*), Wright–Giemsa stain (100× oil). Source: Image from Campbell and Grant (2010, p. 174). (b) A macrophage exhibiting erythrophagocytosis in a fluid-filled subcutaneous swelling (resolving hematoma) in a hamster (*Mesocricetus auratus*), Wright–Giemsa stain (100× oil). (c) A macrophage exhibiting erythrophagocytosis in the abdominal fluid from a hamster (*Mesocricetus auratus*), Wright–Giemsa (100× oil). (d) A macrophage containing iron pigment indicative of erythrophagocytosis in the abdominal fluid from a hamster (*Mesocricetus auratus*), Wright–Giemsa (100× oil).

presence of platelets is suggestive of peripheral blood contamination because platelets of mammals disappear quickly in hemorrhagic effusions.

Chronic (duration greater than 24 h) and resolving hemorrhagic effusions exhibit varying degrees of erythrophagocytosis (erythrophagia). Erythrophagocytosis is indicated by leukocytic (usually macrophagic) phagocytosis of intact erythrocytes, or macrophages containing remnants of erythrocytes such as red cell fragments and breakdown products, such as hemosiderin and hematoidin (Figures 7.96a–7.96d). The iron-containing pigment hemosiderin appears as a blue-green to black or gray (sometimes yellow) pigment in the cytoplasm of macrophages stained with Wright's stain. Hemosiderin crystals also indicate iron from erythrocyte degradation. Hematoidin (a non-iron-containing pigment) appears as diamond-shaped crystals that have a refractile gold appearance. The presence of iron pigment can be confirmed using Prussian blue stain applied to a Wright's stained smear.

The cytologic appearance of an early hematoma of the skin and subcutis initially resembles that of peripheral blood; early hematomas typically contain fluid that resembles blood without platelets (Hall and McWilliams, 1988). The cytology of established hematomas contains macrophages exhibiting various degrees of erythrophagocytosis (Campbell and Grant, 2010). Early erythrophagocytosis is indicated by macrophages that contain intact erythrocytes. As organization of the hematoma progresses, the hemoglobin from the erythrocytes breaks down within the macrophages, and blue-green to black pigmented intracytoplasmic inclusions called hemosiderin granules appear. Hematoidin crystals, golden rhomboid crystals formed from the iron-poor hemoglobin pigment, may also be found. Hematoidin crystals suggest chronic hemorrhage. Hematomas that have organized into a solid firm mass contain numerous fibroblasts. The gross appearance of this type of hematoma is often confused with a neoplastic condition.

A seroma is an accumulation of poorly cellular fluid under the dermis as a sequela to cutaneous injury. The fluid is typically poorly cellular and appears clear to slightly blood tinged. Cellular concentration may be required in order to evaluate the few cells that are present. The cells are primarily macrophages and occasionally other inflammatory cells.

Hemarthrosis is commonly caused by trauma, but other causes include coagulopathies (for example, hemarthrosis associated with vitamin C deficiency in guinea pigs) and neoplasia. Hemarthrosis, or true hemorrhage into a joint, is indicated by the presence of erythrocytes, erythrophagia, hematoidin crystals, hemosiderin, and lack of platelets. Hemarthrosis must be differentiated from peripheral blood contamination due to a traumatic joint tap.

In true hemarthrosis, the sample is typically noted to be bloody from the very beginning of collection rather than starting out clear, and cytologically, erythrocytes and leukocytes are generally present in numbers proportional to those seen in peripheral blood collected from the patient at the same time as the joint fluid was collected (Meinkoth, 2022). Evidence of erythrophagocytosis (erythrophagia) by leukocytes (primarily macrophages) is supportive of a diagnosis of hemarthrosis. The presence of macrophages with dark pigment representing hemosiderin from hemoglobin metabolism in the cytoplasm is also supportive of true hemarthrosis. With chronic hemarthrosis, xanthochromia, a yellowish discoloration that forms from production of pigments from hemoglobin metabolism, may be noted in the supernatant formed following synovial fluid centrifugation (Meinkoth, 2022). The presence of platelets indicates contamination of the synovial sample. Platelets are typically not present when hemarthrosis is present, because platelets disappear rapidly in a long-standing hemorrhagic lesion.

Chylous Effusions

Cloudy fluid should be centrifuged, and the protein measured on the supernatant. Samples with high concentrations of lipoproteins will demonstrate an increased refractive index that results in an artifactually increased total protein measurement. Samples with a white or milky appearance may contain high concentrations of lipoproteins that are suggestive of chyle, and these samples will continue to appear milky after centrifugation (Allision, 2022).

Chylous effusions form when lymphatic fluid leaks from lymphatic vessels. In domestic mammals, this occurs most often in the pleural cavity. Chylous effusions are composed of chyle, which is a mixture of lymph and chylomicrons (triglycerides). Chylous effusions have a "milky" white to pink-tinged appearance and contain variable cell counts and protein content. In general, chylous effusions are classified as either modified transudates or exudates, depending upon the degree of chronicity (Meadows and MacWilliams, 1994; Shelly, 2001). Samples are often obtained by an ultrasound-guided fine-needle aspirate of abdominal or thoracic fluid (Liptovszky et al., 2017). The definitive diagnosis of chylous effusion is made by gross examination, biochemical analysis, and cytologic examination of the peritoneal fluid.

The most specific diagnostic method to identify chylous effusion is based on the cytologic predominance of lymphocytes and macrophages and by the comparison of cholesterol and by comparing the concentrations of triglyceride and cholesterol in the fluid to serum concentrations in samples taken at the same time (Terrell et al., 2003; Vilalta et al., 2017b). The triglyceride concentration is typically 2 to 3 times greater in the effusion than in the serum, and the cholesterol concentration in the effusion is lower than in the serum (Vilalta et al., 2017b). The triglyceride content of peritoneal fluid above 110 mg/dl is indicative of chylous effusion (Connally, 2003).

Chylous fluid is generally composed of small lymphocytes with lesser numbers of lipid droplets, mesothelial cells, and macrophages (Figures 7.97a and 7.97b). Macrophages often contain numerous fine, clear vacuoles consistent with lipid. Long-standing chylous effusions are associated with a mixed population of small, mature lymphocytes, vacuolated macrophages, and nondegenerate neutrophils. The reason for this is that the small lymphocytes are rapidly replaced by inflammatory cells secondary to the chronic inflammation caused by the irritant effect of the chyle on the serosal surface.

Chylous ascites is the accumulation of triglyceride-rich fluid within the peritoneum related to disruption of the lymphatic network (Cárdenas and Chopra, 2002; Almakdisi et al., 2005; Ludwig et al., 2010; Roh et al., 2014;). In most cases, it is secondary to traumatic injury, obstruction (from benign or malignant causes), or external compression of the lymphatics and can be related to infections, hepatic cirrhosis, or inflammatory diseases (Chassang et al., 2018).

Chylothorax is caused by various disease states adversely effecting lymphatic flow (e.g., caudal vena cava thrombus and rupture of the thoracic duct). When

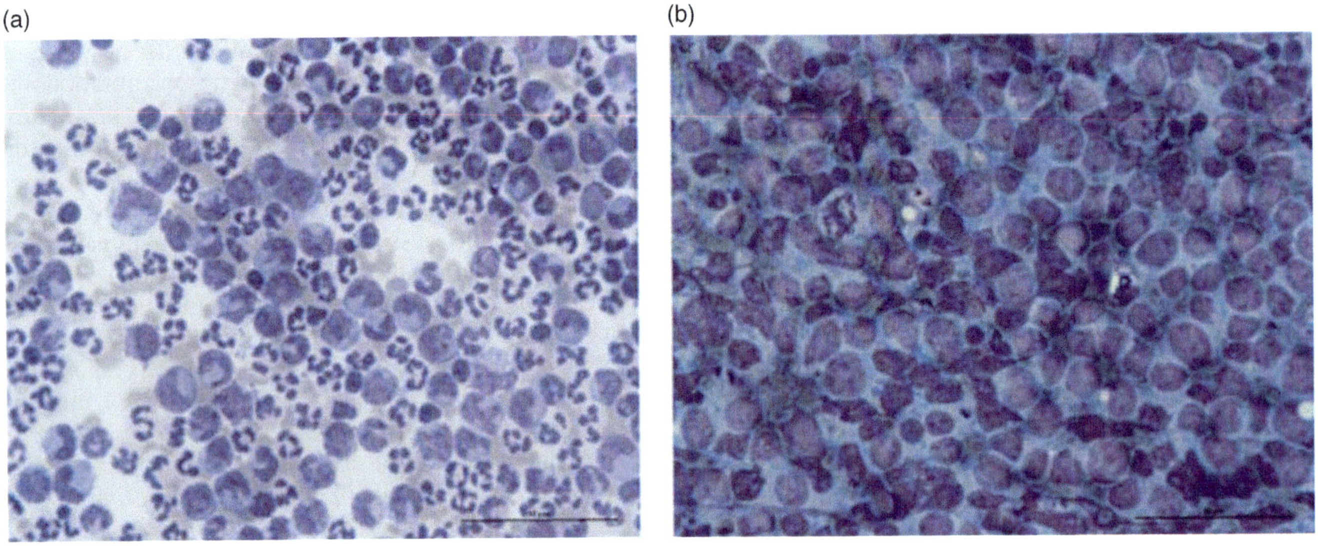

Fig. 7.97. (a) A cytocentrifuged preparation of the abdominal fluid obtained from the ferret (*Mustela putorius furo*) with chylous ascites reveals a mixed population of nondegenerate neutrophils and macrophages that show intermittent foamy cytoplasm. Small lymphocytes are also identified in low numbers. Modified Wright stain (bar = 50 μm). Source: Image from Vilalta et al. (2017a). (b) A smear preparation from a fine-needle biopsy of the abdominal mass collected from the same ferret in Figure 7.103a reveals a mildly pleomorphic population of lymphoid cells with scant, pale blue cytoplasm and occasional vacuoles. Nuclei are round and occasionally indented with coarse chromatin and prominent irregular nucleoli. Aberrant mitotic figures are occasionally seen (black arrow). The cytologic diagnosis was lymphoma. Modified Wright stain; (bar = 50 μm). Source: Image from Vilalta et al. (2017a).

the cause of the chylothorax remains undetermined, it is termed *idiopathic* (Center, 2012). Chylous effusions in the thoracic cavity of mammals are caused by leakage of lymphatic vessels from trauma or obstruction associated with neoplasia, cardiovascular disease, lung torsion, heartworm disease, mediastinal granulomas, and occasionally chronic coughing or vomiting (Waddle and Giger, 1990; Forrester et al., 1991; Fossum, 1993; Shelly, 2001). Conditions associated with chylous effusion in the abdominal cavity include malignant neoplasia, biliary cirrhosis, lymphatic leakage, or obstruction of the thoracic duct (Fossum et al., 1992; Gores et al., 1994, Shelly, 2001). The pathogenesis of chylous ascites associated with liver disease is complicated, but in most cases the ascites is due to liver cirrhosis or portal hypertension, which may cause dilation of, and leakage from, intestinal lymphatic flow (Roh et al., 2014).

Pseudochylous effusions are associated with chronic peritonitis or pleuritis in mammals and differ from true chylous effusions in having a higher cholesterol content (Shelly, 2001). A cholesterol-to-triglyceride ratio less than 1.0 and a triglyceride concentration greater than 100 mg/dL are supportive of a chylous effusion compared to a pseudochylous effusion (Fossum et al., 1986; Waddle and Giger, 1990).

Uroabdomen

Traumatic rupture of the urinary bladder as well as a variety of other disorders involving the urinary tract may result in urine leaking into the peritoneal cavity. In domestic mammals, creatinine (preferred to urea (BUN) because urea diffuses faster from the effusion back into blood) and/or potassium concentrations can be measured in abdominal fluid and compared with serum concentrations to confirm a uroabdomen (Allison, 2022). Generally, a creatinine concentration in the effusion greater than twice that of serum and an abdominal:serum potassium ratio greater that 1.4:1 in samples obtained concurrently confirms a uroabdomen (Schmiedt et al., 2001; Allison, 2022). Although urine is sterile (unless there is a urinary tract infection involved), the chemicals that it contains incite an inflammatory response, which can be variable depending upon the duration of the effusion.

Malignant (Neoplastic) Effusion

An effusion is characterized as malignant or neoplastic if neoplastic cells can be identified in the fluid sample. Although many types of tumors can exfoliate cells into an effusion, round cell tumors (such as lymphoma or mast cell tumor), carcinomas, and mesotheliomas tend to do so more readily than do mesenchymal tumors (sarcomas) (Allison, 2022). Malignant (neoplastic) effusions created by round cell tumors produce individual cells that resemble neoplastic cells that resemble those in other cytologic samples. Large individual cells with rounded cell borders are easily confused with reactive or hyperplastic mesothelial cells. Effusions caused by carcinomas or adenocarcinomas may reveal neoplastic epithelial cells that tend to form cohesive clusters or are found in large sheets. Mesotheliomas produce cells

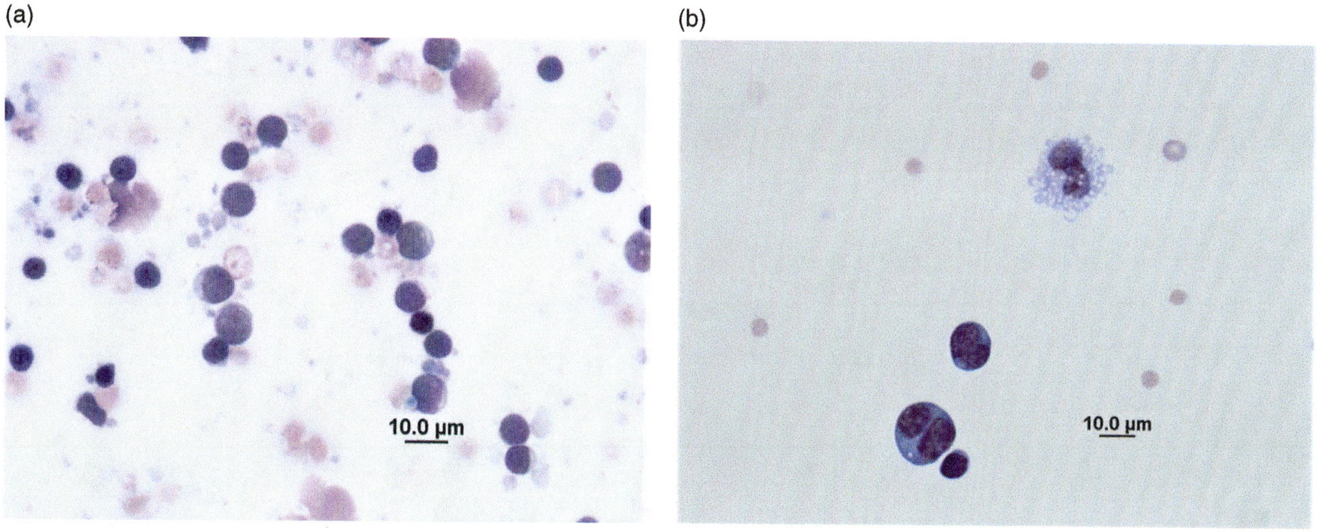

Fig. 7.98. (a) Lymphocytes (an equal mix of large and small) in the thoracic fluid from a ferret (*Mustela putorius furo*) with thoracic lymphoma, Wright–Giemsa stain (100× oil). (b) Immature lymphocytes (binucleated), small mature lymphocytes, and a macrophage in the abdominal fluid of a domestic mouse (*Mus musculus*) with ascites and abdominal lymphoma, Wright–Giemsa stain.

having the same criteria of malignancy as described for carcinomas and are frequently present in large papillary clusters with irregular outlines (Whitaker, 2000). Sarcomas rarely exfoliate sufficient numbers of neoplastic cells into an effusion to allow diagnosis, even hemangiosarcomas (a common sarcoma of the spleen) composed of neoplastic endothelial cells (Allison, 2022). Lack of identifiable neoplastic cells does not exclude neoplasia as the underlying cause of an effusion.

Malignant (neoplastic) effusions often result from blood or lymphatic vessel blockage and can have features of modified transudates, hemorrhagic effusions, or exudates, and may demonstrate cells with features of malignant neoplasia. High-protein transudates can occur and are typically associated with hepatic neoplasms that cause compression of the outflow of the sinusoids. Neoplastic cells may be present in the effusion, and their cytological features may allow the cytologist to classify the malignancy involved (sarcoma, carcinoma, or lymphoid neoplasia) (Figures 7.98a and 7.98b). When undifferentiated malignant cells are present in the peritoneal effusion, determination of cell origin is very difficult. Neoplasia is easiest to recognize when there are large numbers of neoplastic cells with marked criteria of malignancy without the presence of inflammation or hemorrhage. The presence of numerous reactive mesothelial cells may be confounding (Allison, 2022).

Synovial Cyst

Synovial cysts are herniations of synovial membrane associated with degenerative joint disease. Their formation is presumed to be the result of increased intra-articular pressure. Despite the prevalence of degenerative joint disease, synovial cysts are rare.

Synovial cysts are filled with synovial fluid and are found adjacent to joints. The cellularity of the fluid collected from the cysts may be increased and consists primarily of synovial lining cells (synoviocytes) – large, mononuclear cells with eccentric nuclei and abundant, vacuolated cytoplasm that often contains pink-staining granules (Figure 15.112 in Chapter 15). The cells in the highly viscous synovial fluid tend to line up in parallel rows, called "wind rowing of cell," during slide preparation.

Cutaneous Cysts

Cutaneous cysts may originate from underlying tissues. For example, an infraorbital cyst may originate from the secretory epithelium lining the infraorbital sinus. Infraorbital cysts contain a poorly cellular serosanguinous to mucinous fluid with a proteinaceous background (Stiles and Greenacre, 2001).

Mucocele

Normal cytology of the salivary glands is predominated by glandular epithelial cells arranged in clusters and with cytoplasm filled with multiple discrete cytoplasmic vacuoles. The nuclei are round with condensed chromatin. The smaller ductal epithelial cells are less frequently observed. They present as aggregates of round cells with a scant rim of basophilic cytoplasm and a large, round nucleus. The most characteristic feature of salivary gland cytology is the thick, pale, eosinophilic viscous mucin that entraps the cells, causing them to line up in rows or windrows.

Accumulation of saliva in the subcutaneous tissue of mammals results in the formation of a cystic lesion originating from underlying tissues and is referred to as a

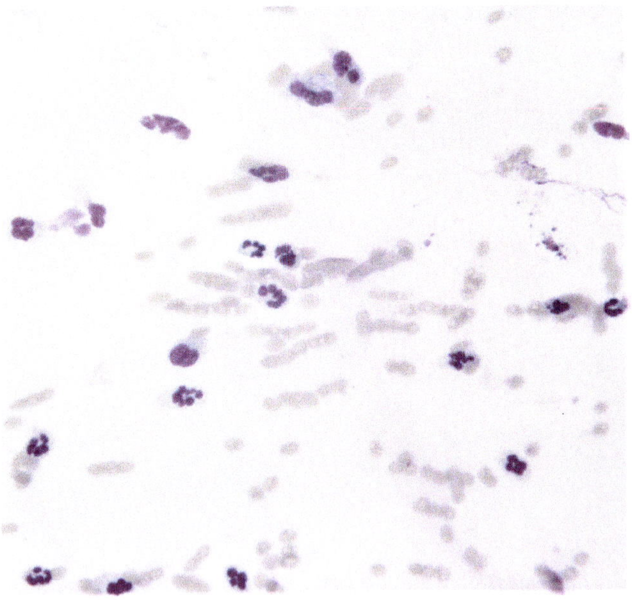

Fig. 7.99. Nondegenerate neutrophils and erythrocytes exhibiting a linear arrangement indicative of a highly viscous fluid in fluid obtained from a fluctuant mass on the head of a ferret (*Mustela putorius furo*) mucocele, Wright–Giemsa stain (500×). Source: Image from Campbell and Grant (2010, p. 171).

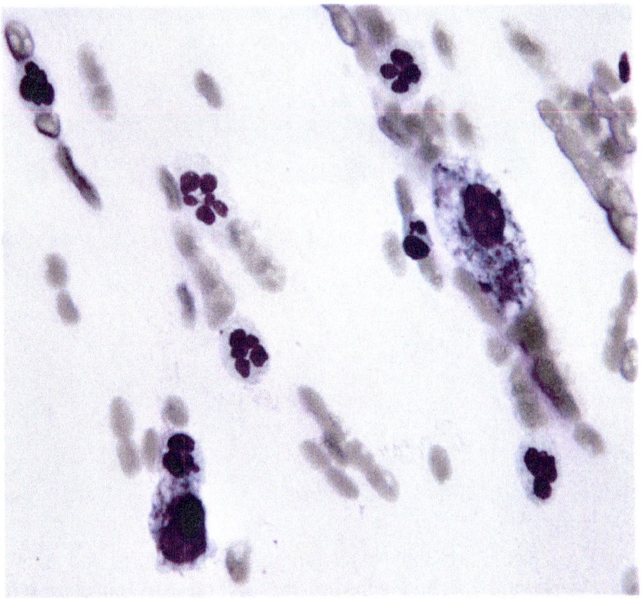

Fig. 7.100. Nondegenerate neutrophils, two macrophages, and erythrocytes exhibiting a linear arrangement indicative of a highly viscous fluid in fluid obtained from a fluctuant mass on the head of a ferret (*Mustela putorius furo*) mucocele, Wright–Giemsa stain (100× oil). Source: Image from Campbell and Grant (2010, p. 171).

mucocele or sialocele. A salivary mucocele is a nonepithelial lined cavity adjacent to the salivary duct. The accumulated saliva results in an inflammatory response, typically consisting primarily of macrophages. Hemorrhage is a common feature of these structures, and hematoidin crystals are often observed. The fluid collected from these lesions tends to be sticky and tenacious, and affects the quality of the cytology slides by reducing cell spreading (Campbell and Grant, 2010). The resulting cytology slides typically have a thick background, and the trapped cells (typically exhibiting "wind rowing") tend to appear as dark pyknotic cells with limited features (Figures 7.99 and 7.100). Other cytological features include an overall uniformly basophilic staining to the specimen owing to the high protein content of the fluid. Amorphous material representing the saliva is present, and erythrophagocytosis and hematoidin crystals may be seen if chronic hemorrhage has occurred. The large highly vacuolated macrophages or salivary gland epithelial cells may be noted as well; the two can be difficult to differentiate on the cytological specimen.

Infectious Agents

Intracellular organisms are those that have been phagocytized and therefore provide evidence of pathogenicity. If only extracellular organisms are seen, contamination or presence of normal flora must be considered (Allison, 2022).

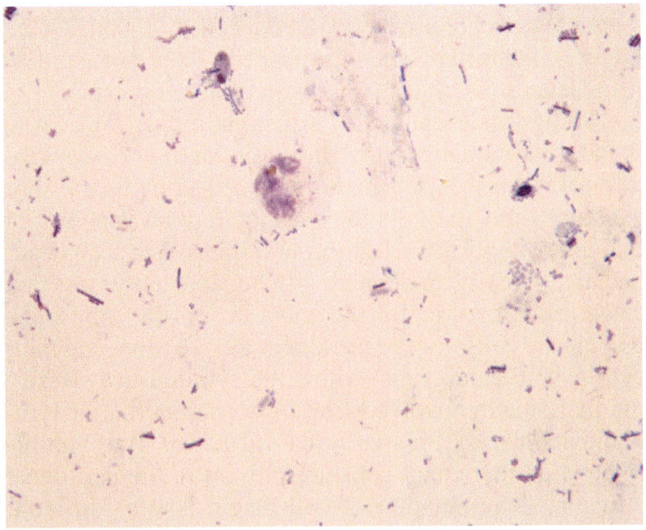

Fig. 7.101. A fecal sample with a degenerate neutrophil and intracellular bacteria that have been phagocytized from a hamster (*Mesocricetus auratus*), Wright–Giemsa stain (100× oil).

Bacteria

Bacteria stain blue with Romanowsky stains; however, phagocytized or dying bacteria may stain poorly. The morphological types of bacteria commonly identified include cocci, rods, filamentous bacteria, and spirochetes. In general, bacterial infections are associated with neutrophilic (suppurative) inflammation (Figures 7.33 and 7.101). However, mixed cell inflammation (pyogranulomatous inflammation) is often associated with filamentous bacterial infections.

Bacterial cocci are blue spheres that occur individually, in small clusters, or in chains. Cocci usually stain gram positive with gram staining.

Bacterial rods may occur individually or in chains. They vary in size. Small bacterial rods typically stain gram negative (i.e., *E. coli*, *Klebsiella* spp., *Pseudomonas* spp.); however, some pleomorphic rods stain gram positive (i.e., *Rhodococcus* spp.) (Allison, 2022). Large bacterial rods may be gram positive (i.e., *Bacillus* spp.) or gram negative (i.e., *Clostridium* spp.). Gram staining may be attempted on cytologic samples; however, the results are not reliable; gram staining is best performed on organisms grown in culture (Allison, 2022).

Filamentous rods (i.e., *Actinomyces* and *Nocardia* spp.) appear as long, slender chains that may have a beaded appearance. These organisms are often difficult to see, especially in the presence of background debris.

Spirochetes are gram-negative, spiral-shaped bacteria. They are often part of the normal oral and gastrointestinal flora of mammals. *Helicobacter* spp. may be found in gastric samples from normal mammals, but they have also been implicated as a cause of gastritis, especially in domestic ferrets.

Mycoplasma (Mycoplasmosis)

See Chapter 15 for a description of the organism.

Clostridium

Bacteria are commonly found in rectal or fecal samples of mammals and are typically represented by a wide variety of morphological types. Neutrophils or heterophils are not normally found in these samples, and when present, suggest an active infection. A monomorphic population of bacteria, *Clostridium*-like bacteria, *Candida*-like yeast, protozoa, parasite ova, and fungal elements also constitute abnormal cytologic findings in the rectal, cloacal, or fecal samples of animals.

Clostridia are anaerobic, spore-forming bacteria that appear as large, rod-shaped bacteria with a clear center and an increased density on one end (the endospore) on cytologic samples. This is often referred to as a "safety pin" or "tennis racquet" appearance (Figures 7.102a and 7.102b). Certain species of *Clostridium* are known to be highly pathogenic in animals. For example, C. *spiroforme* of rabbits causes a severe enterotoxemia owing to the production of an iota-like toxin (Deeb, 2000; Jenkins, 2004).

Sources of clostridial infections can include chronic antibiotic therapy, contaminated food or food containers, soil, or drinking water.

Clostridia can produce disease in one of two ways. Certain species, such as C. *tetani* and C. *botulinum*, produce extremely potent toxins outside the host or in localized areas within the host. Other clostridial species, such as C. *perfringens*, C. *colinum*, C. *septicum*, C. *tertium*,

(a) (b)

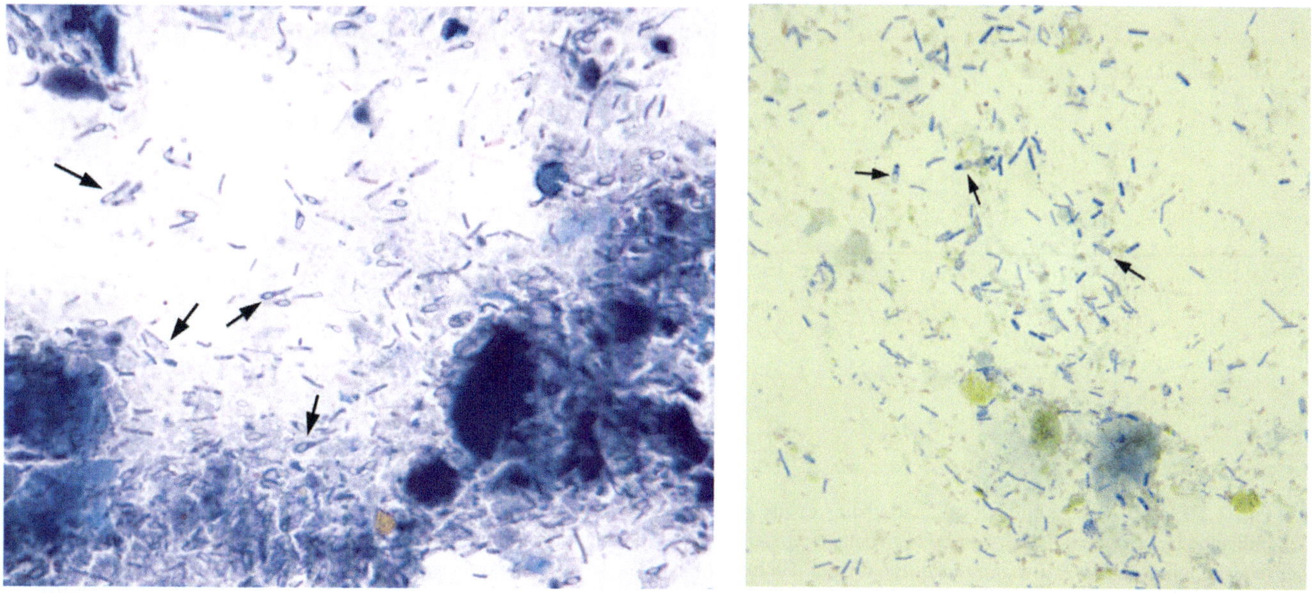

Fig. 7.102. (a) Numerous *Clostridium*-like bacteria (a few indicated by arrows) in a fecal swab cytology from a hedgehog (*Atelerix albiventris*) with diarrhea, Diff–Quik stain (100× oil). (b) A large number of rod-shaped bacteria with a clear center and an increased density on one end (the endospore) resembling "safety pins" or "tennis racquets," indicative of an overgrowth of *Clostridium*-like bacteria (a few indicated by arrows) in the feces of a ferret (*Mustela putorius furo*), Wright–Giemsa stain (100× oil).

and C. *novyi*, are invasive and produce less potent toxins. Invasion of the intestinal tract can result in damage to the gastrointestinal mucosa by direct colonization resulting in a fatal enteritis and enterotoxemia. The fecal cytology of animals exhibiting melena may reveal lysed and intact erythrocytes, neutrophils or heterophils, and a monomorphic population of large bacteria consistent in size and shape with *Clostridium* spp. is indicative of clostridial enteritis or colitis.

Campylobacter

Campylobacter spp. are potentially pathogenic bacteria found on fecal cytology specimens from a variety of animals (Turowski et al., 2014). These small bacteria are often overlooked among the numerous other bacteria found on fecal smears (Figures 7.103a–7.103d). *Campylobacter* spp. have a characteristic "gull wing" appearance created by small chains of the slender, comma-shaped or curved bacilli (Walberg and Loar, 2004).

(a) (b) (c) (d)

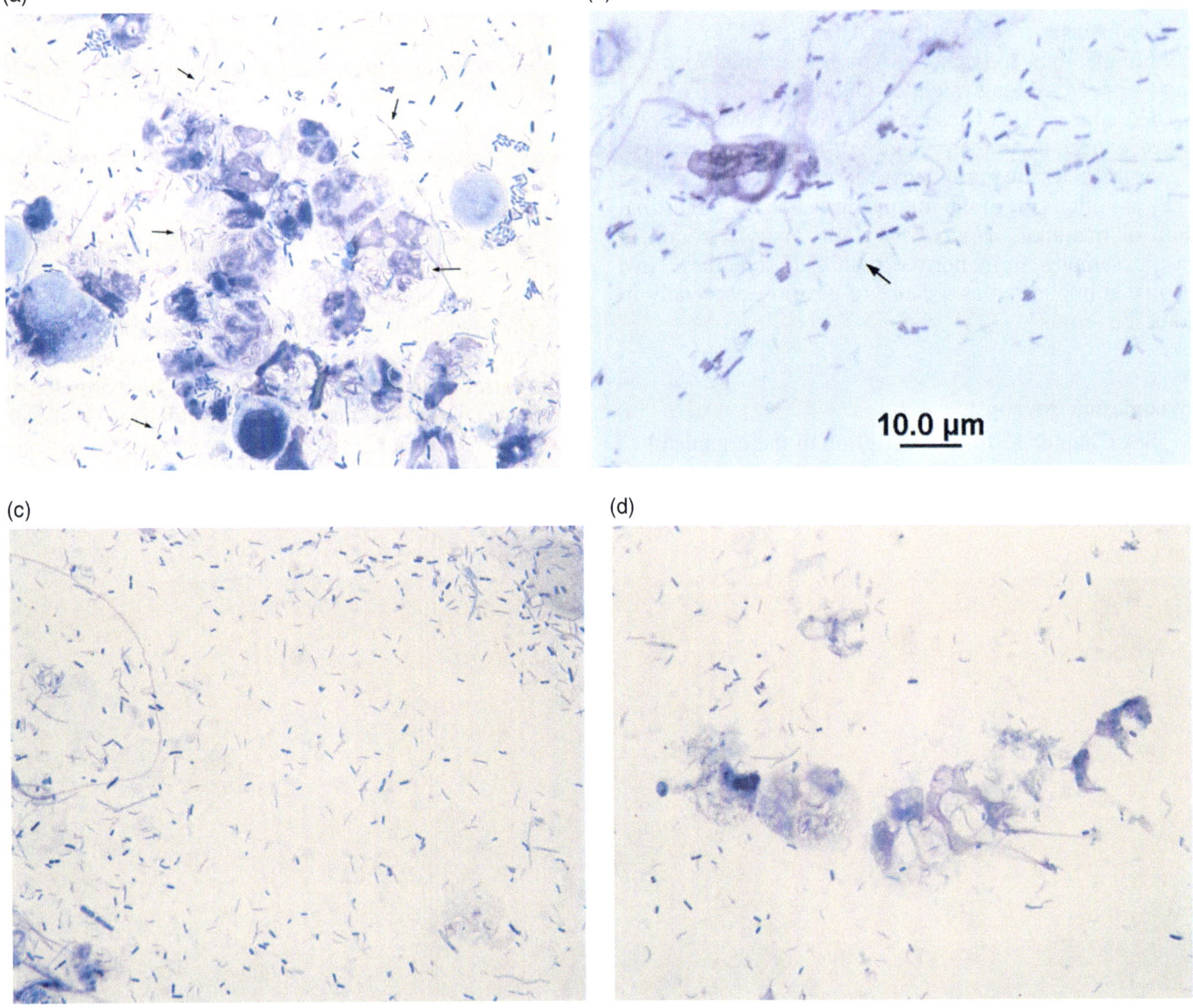

Fig. 7.103. (a) A large number of small chains of the slender, comma-shaped, or curved bacilli with a "gull wing" appearance (a few indicated by arrows) outside of and within degenerate leukocytes indicative of *Campylobacter*-like bacteria causing a septic colitis in the feces of a hamster (*Mesocricetus auratus*), Wright–Giemsa stain (100× oil). (b) Same fecal sample from the hamster (*Mesocricetus auratus*) with colitis as in Figure 7.109a revealing numerous small slender, curved bacilli indicative of *Campylobacter*-like bacteria (represented by an arrow), Wright–Giemsa stain (100× oil). (c) A rectal swab from another hamster (*Mesocricetus auratus*) with colitis revealing numerous, small, curved bacilli indicative of *Campylobacter*-like bacteria, Wright–Giemsa stain (100× oil). (d) A rectal swab from a hamster (*Mesocricetus auratus*) with colitis revealing numerous, small, curved bacilli indicative of *Campylobacter*-like bacteria, some of which are phagocytized in degenerate neutrophils, Wright–Giemsa stain (100× oil).

Spirochetes

Spirochetal infections are occasionally seen in veterinary medicine. The spirochete, *Borrelia burgdorferi*, is the causative agent of arthritis in Lyme disease in dogs; however, the organism is not always found in the cytology of affected joint fluid (Fernandes, 2008).

Helicobacter

Helicobacter (phylum Proteobacteria, class Epsilonprotebacteria, order Campylobacterales, family *Helicobacteraceae*) are a genus of spiral-shaped, gram-negative bacteria that are phylogenetically distinct from bacteria within the phylum Spirochaetes. In mammals, *Helicobacter* have been associated with gastric ulcers, ulcerative colitis, cholangiohepatitis, cellulitis, and bacteremia.

The domestic ferret, *Mustela putorius furo*, is known to be colonized with a gastric helicobacter, *Helicobacter mustelae*, which is associated with gastritis and gastric ulcers. Another member of the Mustelidae family, the Southern sea otter, also harbors a *Helicobacter*, *H. enhydrae* (Shen et al., 2017). The slightly curved bacterial rods stain positive with silver stain. *H. mustelae* and *H. pylori*, the causative agent of peptic ulcers in humans, are urease positive; however, *H. enhydrae* is not.

Chlamydia/Chlamydophila

Many animals are susceptible to chlamydial infections that are responsible for a variety of disease syndromes (i.e. abortion, pneumonia, enteritis, polyarthritis, encephalomyelitis, and conjunctivitis) that depends upon the species of the organism (Strik et al., 2005). Chlamydial conjunctivitis is a common cause of infectious conjunctivitis in guinea pigs. It is caused by members of the order Chlamydiales, which are obligate intracellular bacteria. These organisms have a two-stage development cycle and unique pathogenicity. The intracellular vegetative, reticulate body is the noninfectious form that measures between 0.5 and 1.5 μm in diameter. The smaller infectious, extracellular form called the elementary body measures 0.3 μm. The elementary body is endocytosed into a cytoplasmic inclusion by eukaryotic host cells, within which it replicates by binary fission into a reticulate body. Reticulate bodies, therefore, are large, membrane-bound populations of elementary bodies.

Cytologic diagnosis of chlamydiosis requires identification of reticulate bodies (0.5 to 1.5 μm) or elementary bodies (0.3 μm) on Romanowsky-stained cytologic preparations. Chlamydial conjunctivitis in guinea pigs may reveal moderately cellular preparations consisting of heterophils (neutrophils), small lymphocytes, and oval to polygonal epithelial cells. The cytoplasm of a few epithelial cells may contain clumps of coccoid basophilic organisms measuring 0.3–1.5 μm in diameter that are consistent with the intraepithelial inclusions of chlamydial elementary and reticulate bodies (Strik et al., 2005). Detection of intracytoplasmic inclusions in Romanowsky-stained or Macchiavello (basic fuchsin–citric acid–methylene blue)–stained cytologic preparations do not allow for a definitive diagnosis. Absence of the organisms does not rule out chlamydiosis because they often disappear from tissues by the time a patient presents with clinical disease. Therefore, the most sensitive and reliable method of diagnosis of chlamydiosis is PCR testing (Everett and Andersen, 1999; Everett et al., 1999; Laroucau et al., 2001). Other methods of identifying chlamydial organisms include culture and fluorescent antibody staining of swab specimens (Perez-Martínez and Storz, 1985).

It has been suggested to reclassify the family *Chlamydiaceae* into two genera: *Chlamydia* and *Chlamydophila*. Consequently, the genus *Chlamydia* would include the species *C. trachomatis*, *C. suis*, and *C. muridarum* and the genus *Chlamydophila* would include the species *C. abortus*, *C. caviae*, *C. felis*, *C. pecorum*, *C. pneumoniae*, and *C. psittaci*. Also, three new *Chlamydophila* species derived from *Chlamydia psittaci* would include *C. abortus*, *C. caviae*, and *C. felis* (Everett et al., 1999). Both the old and new nomenclature can be found in the literature, and research continues to sort out these organisms; for example, *Chlamydophila caviae*, the causative agent of chlamydial conjunctivitis in guinea pigs, was formerly known as the GPIC strain of *C. psittaci* and now has five known identical isolates with identical ompA (omp1) sequences (Prain and Pearce, 1989; Zhao et al., 1993).

Mycobacterium

Mycobacterium species are aerobic, non-spore-forming, nonmotile, acid-fast rods. A cytologic specimen that contains macrophagic inflammation and negative-staining, slender rods in the cytoplasm of macrophages is suggestive of *Mycobacterium* spp. infection (Campbell and Grant, 2010) (Figure 7.104). Because *Mycobacteria* spp. do not stain with Romanowsky stains routinely used for cytology specimens, an acid-fast, positive staining of the rods will provide further support for a diagnosis of mycobacteriosis.

Mycobacterium genavense is a non-tuberculous, slow-growing, acid-fast opportunistic bacterium responsible for disseminated diseases in an increasing number of mammalian patients, including chinchillas and ferrets (Lucas et al., 2000; Huynh et al., 2014; Theuss, 2010). The clinical and histopathological features of this bacterial infection are indistinguishable from those caused by members of the *Mycobacterium avium-intracellulare* complex. Mycobacteriosis caused by opportunistic pathogens of the *Mycobacterium avium* complex (four

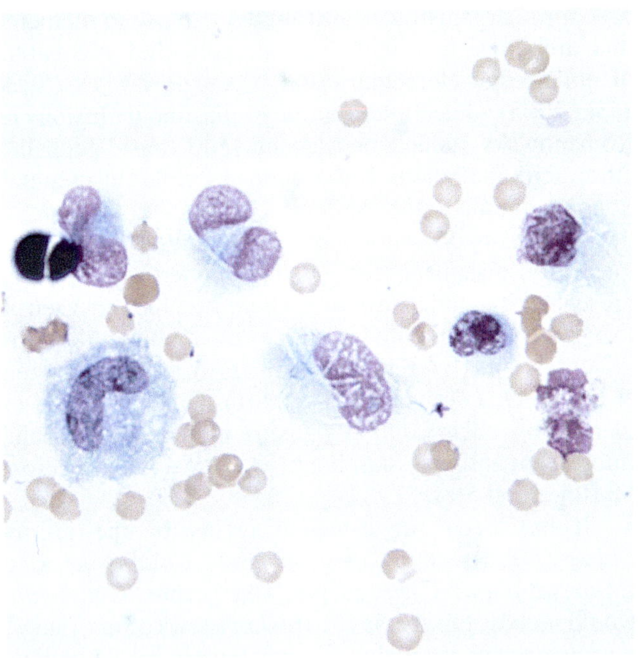

Fig. 7.104. Macrophages in a thinner part of a contact smear of a liver revealing several bacterial filamentous rods that fail to stain (negative staining) with routine cytology stains from a ferret (*Mustela putorius furo*) with a *Mycobacterium goodii* infection. Wright–Giemsa stain (100× oil). Source: Image from Campbell and Grant (2010, p. 184).

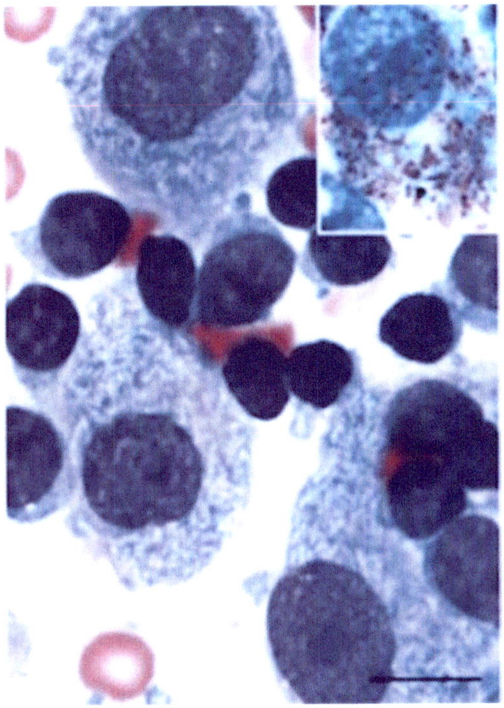

Fig. 7.105. A smear of a pancreaticoduodenal mass in a ferret (*Mustela putorius furo*) with *Mycobacterium genavense* infection, showing macrophages, multinucleate cells, lymphocytes, and myriad intracytoplasmic, negative-staining 2 × 0.5 μm rods. May-Grünwald/Giemsa stain (bar = 20 μm). Inset: Intracellular rods are acid-fast positive. Ziehl–Neelsen stain. Source: Image from Dequéant et al. (2019).

subspecies *avium*, *silvaticum*, *paratuberculosis*, and *hominissuis*) is an important infectious disease that affects a wide range of animals globally. These organisms are ubiquitous in the environment, and ingestion, followed by invasion of the gastrointestinal tract, is the most important route of infection (Bertram et al., 2020a). Spontaneous mycobacteriosis is rare in most exotic pet mammals except for ferrets (Mentre and Bulliot, 2015; Bertram et al., 2020a).

Cytologic preparations stained with MayGrünwald/ Giemsa (MGG) may reveal epithelioid macrophages admixed with small lymphocytes and a few binucleate cells containing myriad intracytoplasmic, 2 × 0.5 μm, negative-staining, bacterial rods (Dequéant et al., 2019) (Figure 7.105). Destaining MGG-stained slides with alcohol and restaining with Ziehl–Neelsen (ZN) stain reveals numerous acid-fast bacilli within macrophages. This technique yields a staining quality comparable to direct acid-fast staining, does not affect cytologic features, and avoids repeat sampling (Dequéant et al., 2019).

Dimorphic Fungi

Dimorphic fungi can cause systemic infections. They exist as yeasts at body temperature, but can form hyphae in the environment, and the morphologies of the yeast forms are distinctive enough to allow for definitive cytologic identification (Allison, 2022).

Candidiasis

Candidiasis is an infection caused by the fungus of the genus *Candida* that can affect many types of animals, especially those with a gastrointestinal dysbiosis or are immunocompromised. Candidiasis is detected by the presence of many oval, thin-walled, narrow-based budding yeast that measure 2–6 μm in diameter (Campbell and Grant, 2010) (Figures 7.106 and 7.107). Candida typically stain deeply basophilic in color with Wright's stain and gram positive with Gram's stain, although occasionally the yeast and hyphae stain poorly. A marked amount of background debris is often present, but few inflammatory cells are typically noted unless mucosal ulceration has occurred. The presence of short, extracellular, septate, acute-angle-branching, fungal-type hyphae (occasionally with globose terminal ends) and round to oval blastospores and germinal tubes indicate tissue invasion by the *Candida* organism.

The approximately 150 species of *Candida* are commensals of animals and normally inhabit the alimentary, upper respiratory, and lower urogenital tracts; however, a small percentage are frequent pathogens of mammals (Duchaussoy et al., 2015). Interruption of normal defense mechanisms is necessary for them to become pathogenic (Kennedy et al., 1987). Complications

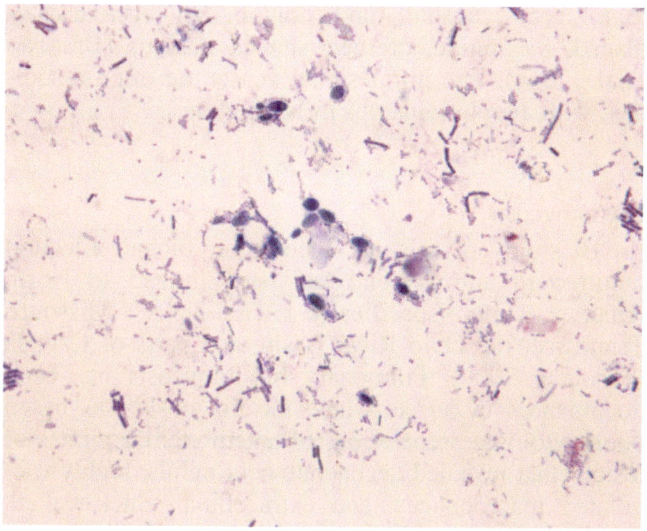

Fig. 7.106. Several budding *Candida*-like yeast in a fecal cytology from a hamster (*Mesocricetus auratus*) with diarrhea, Wright–Giemsa stain (100× oil).

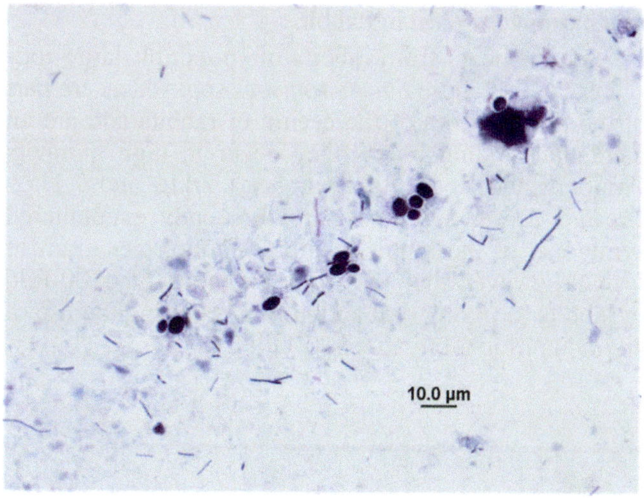

Fig. 7.107. Several budding *Candida*-like yeast in a fecal cytology from a ferret (*Mustela putorius furo*) with diarrhea – note some yeast fail to stain – Wright–Giemsa stain (100× oil).

secondary to local overgrowth and extension due to impairment of the mucosal barrier are the most common causes of invasive mycoses. In rats, it has been shown that *C. albicans* can delay gastrointestinal ulcer healing by releasing cytokines (IL-1beta and TNF-alpha), which perpetuate ongoing inflammation and promote conditions for gastrointestinal wall invasion and adherence (Brzozowski et al., 2005).

Malassezia

Cytology typically reveals broadly budding yeast structures in various stages of budding that stain heterogeneously (Figure 7.108).

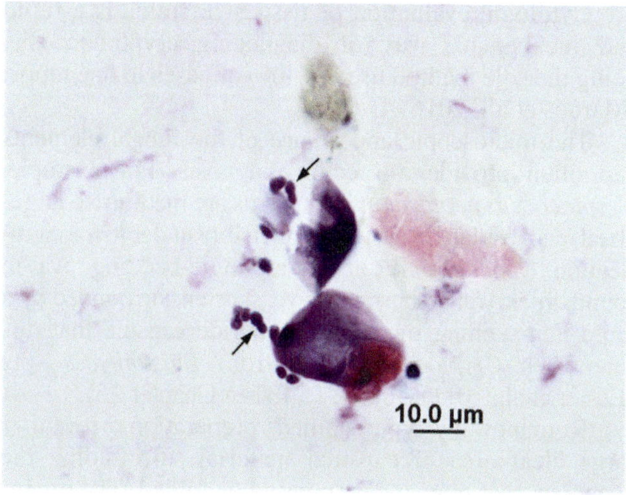

Fig. 7.108. *Malassezia* yeast in an ear swab from a ferret (*Mustela putorius furo*) with otitis media, Wright–Giemsa stain (100× oil).

The hyphal form of this organism used to be called "Malassezia" and the yeast form was called "Pityrosporum"; however, mycologists realize they were the same organism. The genus *Malassezia* includes 17 species comprising the former taxon *M. pachydermatis* and the splitting of *M. furfur* (*sensu lato*) into 6 new lipid-dependent species, *M. furfur* (*sensu stricto*), *M. sympodialis*, *M. globosa*, *M. obtusa*, *M. restricta*, and *M. slooffiae* and the addition of 10 new lipid-dependent species, *M. arulanokei*, *M. brasiliensis*, *M. caprae*, *M. cuniculi*, *M. dermatis*, *M. equina*, *M. japonica*, *M. nana*, *M. psittaci*, and *M. yamatoensis* (Puig et al., 2018). These yeasts adapt to different animal hosts. For example, *M. furfur* has been found on a broad spectrum of animals, including birds held in captivity. *Malassezia* spp. has often been reported to be associated with otitis media and/or chronic pruritic dermatitis in domestic ferrets. Multifocal pustular dermatitis with hyperkeratosis, rather than seborrheic dermatitis, without otitis, can be associated with *Malassezia* overgrowth in domestic ferrets with a concurrent bacterial infection contributing to the pustular reaction, and adrenal diseases may be the underlying primary cause of this condition (Bongiovanni et al., 2017).

Cryptococcus neoformans

Cryptococcosis is an opportunistic, systemic fungal disease with a worldwide distribution that primarily affects the respiratory of mammals. Transmission of *Cryptococcus* spp. is through inhalation of spores, or, less commonly, by contamination of wounds (Nevitt et al., 2013). Infection is typically caused by *Cryptococcus neoformans* var. *gattii* and *C.* n. var. *neoformans* (Martínez-Nevado et al., 2017).

Cytologic evaluation of tissues or fluids is a rapid and inexpensive way of diagnosing cryptococcosis, being the sole method used in 40% of cases in one report (Marcos et al., 2016).

The microscopic appearance of the fungal elements can often provide a specific diagnosis. For example, *Cryptococcus neoformans* organisms are medium to large-sized, encapsulated yeast that are visible under low magnification. *C. neoformans* appear as single-budding, oval to round, thick-walled basophilic yeast often surrounded by a large non-staining mucopolysaccharide capsule that differentiates *Cryptococcus* spp. from *Blastomyces* spp. (Lester et al., 2011) (Figure 15.131 in Chapter 15).

Romanowsky-type stained preparations reveal a large clear area of capsular material surrounding the organism that may appear creased or folded. The organism itself measures 1–7 µm, but with the capsule, the entire mass may measure up to 30 µm (Baker and Lumsden, 2000). The blue to magenta yeasts are often well defined in films with a heavy background substance. India ink and new methylene blue can be used to delineate the yeasts in thinner smears. Other stains such as Gram, periodic acid–Schiff (PAS), and Gomori methenamine silver (GMS) can also be used (Marcos et al., 2016). However, the morphologic details of the cells are often lost when using stains other than Romanowsky-type stains. On the other hand, quick stains, such as Diff–Quik, often make the yeast unrecognizable. In such cases, GMS can be used to confirm the presence of the yeast when ill-defined structures are seen (Marcos et al., 2016). Serum cryptococcal antigen testing can be used to detect the presence of the organism in some cases (Krockenberger et al., 2003). Lack of an inflammatory response is typical, presumably due to the thick capsule that protects the yeast from the host's immune system. Small numbers of neutrophils, foamy macrophages, erythrocytes, and lymphocytes may be found in some specimens. Occasionally, the associated inflammation consists of macrophages and multinucleated giant cells (granulomatous) with low numbers of eosinophils (Allison, 2022).

Histoplasma

Histoplasmosis is an important fungal disease caused by *Histoplasma capsulatum*, a soil-borne, dimorphic fungus found endemic to large areas of temperate and tropical regions of the world. In the United States, most clinical cases occur in warm, moist, and humid regions along the Ohio, Missouri, and Mississippi rivers, with Tennessee considered an area of high endemicity in animals (Greenacre et al., 2019). A diagnosis of histoplasmosis can be made based upon cytologic preparations from a transtracheal wash, bronchiolar lavage, rectal scraping, FNA, or biopsy of affected tissue. The organisms are 3–5 µm in diameter, round to oval, with a thin, clear capsule, and contain an eccentrically placed, basophilic, crescent-shaped nucleus (Brandão et al., 2014). The intralesional yeasts are often associated with a granulomatous inflammation.

Blastomycosis

Blastomycosis is an uncommon fungal infection reported in animals and has been limited to North America, and specifically Mississippi, Missouri, Tennessee, the Ohio River Basin, and parts of Canada (Taboada, 2000). Pulmonary blastomycosis has been documented in ferrets where the diagnosis was based upon cytologic preparations of antemortem aspirates of lesions that revealed degenerate neutrophils, highly vacuolated macrophages, and extracellular, thick-walled, spherical (5–20 µm diameter), deeply basophilic, broad-based budding yeast consistent with *Blastomyces dermatitidis* (Darrow et al., 2014; Le et al., 2019) (Figure 7.109).

Saccharomyces Yeast in Rabbits

Fecal smears from rabbits often exhibit large rod-shaped yeast. These *Saccharomyces* spp. yeasts are part of the normal flora of the cecum of rabbits and are an incidental finding unless they occur in high numbers (Walberg and Loar, 2004) (Figures 7.110 and 7.111). *Saccharomyces* spp. yeast are frequently encountered symbionts of the rabbit cecum (3 million per gram of feces); however, they may increase more than 100-fold in rabbits receiving oral antibiotics, requiring the use of an oral antifungal treatment (Malley, 2000).

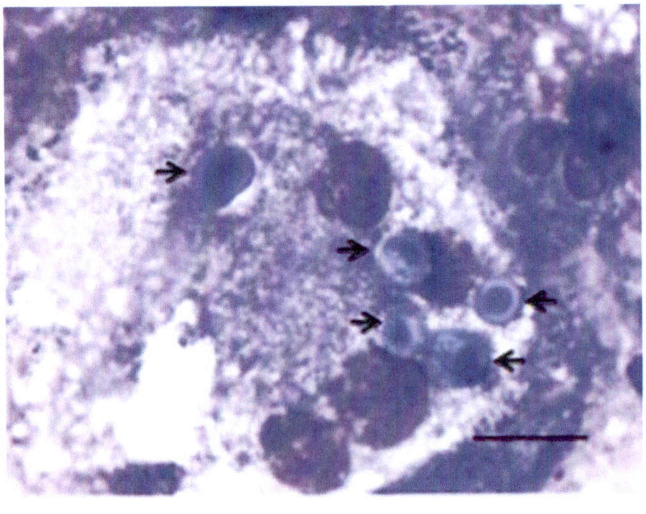

Fig. 7.109. A fine-needle aspirate from the lung of a ferret with blastomycosis reveals that a multinucleated giant cell contains several *Blastomyces dermatitidis* yeast organisms (arrows). Wright–Giemsa stain (bar = 20 µm). Source: Darrow et al. (2014).

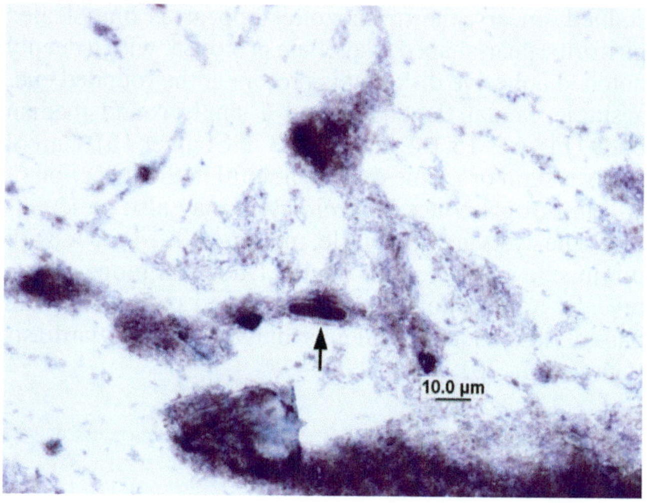

Fig. 7.110. The large *Saccharomyces* spp. yeast (arrow) are part of the normal flora of the cecum and frequently seen in the fecal cytology of rabbits (*Oryctolagus cuniculus*), Wright–Giemsa stain.

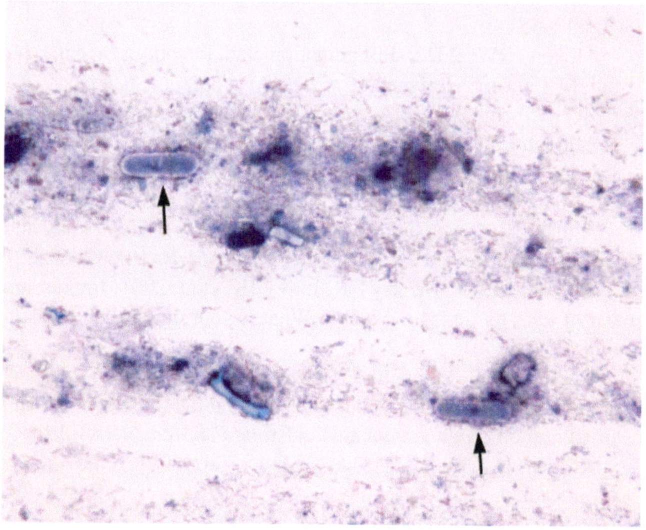

Fig. 7.111. The large *Saccharomyces* spp. yeast (arrows) are part of the normal flora of the cecum and frequently seen in the fecal cytology of rabbits (*Oryctolagus cuniculus*), Diff–Quik stain (100× oil).

Hyphae-Forming Fungi

Many hyphae-forming fungi can cause local or systemic infections in animals whereby fungal hyphae can be seen in cytologic specimens. Depending upon the organism, hyphae can vary in size and shape, be septate or nonseptate, or have pigmentation. Fungal hyphae are often associated with aggregates of macrophages and may not stain well, if at all (Allison, 2022). The histochemical stain GMS can be helpful to highlight fungal hyphae.

Aspergillosis

Aspergillosis is a mycosis that affects a diverse range of animal hosts (Latgé, 1999). Aspergillus spp. are ubiquitous saprophytic fungi found in the soil, in feeds as grains, and in decomposing vegetables (Perdelli et al., 2006). Animals are exposed regularly through the inhalation of hundreds of conidia daily; however, these fungi are considered opportunistic pathogens that may cause either localized sinonasal infections or disseminated infections, including pulmonary involvement in mammals.

Certain species of fungi of the genus *Aspergillus* produce cells around the cleistothecium called Hülle cells. These are thick-walled cells characterized by thin-walled pores and may act as nurse cells. Formation of Hülle cells indicates regression of the aspergillosis organism and may be found following antifungal treatment (Carvalho et al., 2002; Savelieff et al., 2018). See Chapter 15 for a further description of the organism.

Protozoa

Trichomoniasis

Trichomoniasis is a common disease of exotic animals. Trichomonads are best detected on wet-mount smears, where they appear as motile, flagellate protozoa with anterior flagella and an undulating membrane. However, an air-dried sample of the lesion may be obtained when trichomoniasis is not suspected. In such cases, the cytology specimens stained with Romanowsky stains (Wright's or Diff–Quik) often reveal inflammatory cells (heterophilic or mixed cell inflammation), background debris, and trichomonad organisms. The protozoa vary in staining intensity from poorly stained to deeply basophilic, and have an anterior flagellum, undulating membrane, and prominent axostyle (Figure 7.112). The nucleus stains more eosinophilic compared to most cell nuclei, and the axostyle can be identified as an eosinophilic-staining straight line between the nucleus and the opposite pole of the cell. Flagella occur at the nuclear end of the cell, and the undulating membrane occurs along one side. These structures are eosinophilic in color as well.

Cryptosporidiosis

Cryptosporidium is a coccidian protozoal parasite that affects the gastrointestinal and respiratory tracts of fish, reptiles, birds, and mammals (Figures 23.65 and 23.66a, b in Chapter 23). Twenty-six *Cryptosporidium* species are considered valid, and over 40 genotypes or cryptic species have been identified (Ryan et al., 2014). Cryptosporidium infection has been reported in asymptomatic and diarrheic domestic mammals (especially dogs, cats, and horses) and is associated with either

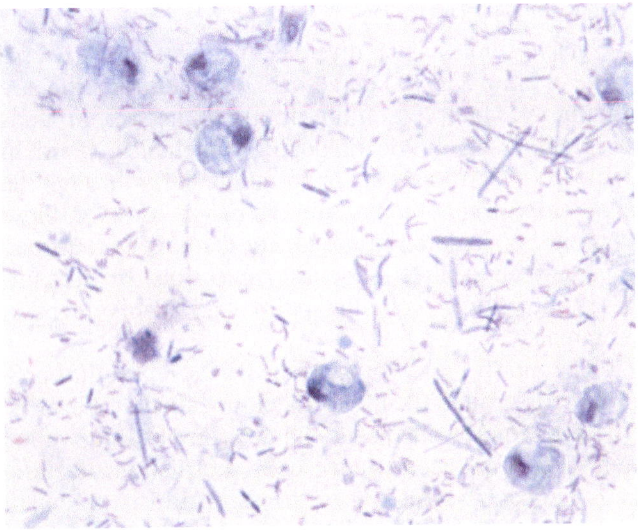

Fig. 7.112. Stained piriform-shaped organisms in the feces that previously was examined as a wet-mount preparation that revealed numerous motile flagellate protozoa with undulating membranes that was supportive of a diagnosis of trichomoniasis in a rat (*Rattus norvegicus*) with diarrhea, Wright–Giemsa stain (100× oil). Source: Image from Campbell and Grant (2010, p. 144).

Cryptosporidium parvum, *C. felis*, *C. canis*, *C. meleagridis*, and *C. muris* with infections being acquired via the fecal-oral route either directly or indirectly (Smith et al., 2009). *Cryptosporidium* also causes diseases in aquatic species, such as wild-ranging and captive aquatic mammals (Borges et al., 2017). Methods for detection of *Cryptosporidium* include Sheather's sugar flotation technique and modified acid-fast staining, as well as molecular biology techniques used to determine the species and genotypes of the organism in clinical specimens and to improve the sensitivity of the detection method (Gu et al., 2016). See Chapter 23 for a further description of the organism.

Giardia

Giardia has a direct life cycle and is transmitted by the orofecal route. Studies have shown that dogs and livestock can substantially contribute to the *Giardia* load in wetlands, and large volumes of wetland effluents can contribute to the contamination of surface waters. (Mashinsky et al., 2009).

Trophozoites of *Giardia* may be found in the feces or on samples obtained from a rectal swab. On wet-mount preparations, *Giardia* trophozoites appear as motile, flat flagellates that are 10–20 μm × 5–15 μm in size with eight pairs of flagella (the one trailing out from the posterior end is the most visible) with a movement typically described as a "falling leaf" motion.

Epifluorescence microscopy can be used to detect the organism in fecal samples (Beck et al., 2011). On stained smears, the trophozoites appear as binucleated piriform (pear-shaped) flagellate protozoa, with a deeply notched adhesive disk that is present at the rounded end, a single caudal flagellum, and a single round median body (Figures 15.142 and 15.143 in Chapter 15). Carbol fuchsin stain or iodine may be helpful in the detection of *Giardia* trophozoites. *Giardia* cysts may also be identified. The cysts are nonmotile, measure 10–14 μm × 8–10 μm in size and have four nuclei. Duodenal biopsies that reveal cytomorphology of pear-shaped organisms with paired flagella and nuclei is diagnostic for giardiasis (Garg et al., 2019).

References

Affolter VK, Moore PF. 2002. Localized and disseminated histiocytic sarcoma of dendritic cell origin in dogs. *Vet Pathol* 39:74–88.

Agarwal K, Pahuja S, Agarwal C, et al. 2007. Fine needle aspiration cytology of gouty tophi with review of literature. *Journal of Cytology* 24(3):142–145.

Allen SW, Prasse KW, Mahaffey EA. 1986. Cytologic differentiation of benign from malignant canine mammary tumors. *Vet Pathol* 23(6):649–55.

Allison, RW. 2022. Inflammation and infectious agents. In: Thrall MA (ed), *Veterinary Hematology, Clinical Chemistry, and Cytology*, 3rd edn. Ames, IA: Wiley-Blackwell, in press.

Allnoch L, Kostlinger S, Steffensen N, et al. 2020. Amelanotic malignant melanoma in a Himalayan rex guinea pig (*Cavia porcellus*). *J Comp Pathol* 181:13–17.

Almakdisi T, Massoud S, Makdisi G. 2005. Lymphomas and chylous ascites: Review of the literature. *Oncologist* 10:632–635.

Al-Rukibat RK, Irizarry AR, Lacey JK, et al. 2001. Impression smear of liver tissue from a rabbit: What is your diagnosis? *Vet Clin Pathol* 30(2):57–61.

Anderson KB, Meinkoth J, Hallman M, et al. 2019. Cytological diagnosis of gastric neuroendocrine carcinoma in a pet Inland bearded dragon (*Pogona vitticeps*). *J Exotic Pet Med* 29:188–193.

Andreasen CB, Jergens AE, Meyer DJ. 2001. Oral cavity, gastrointestinal tract, and associated structures. In: Raskin R, Meyer D (eds), *Atlas of Canine and Feline Cytology*. Philadelphia, PA: WB Saunders.

Arndt TP, Shelly SM. 2014. The liver. In: Valenciano AC, Cowell RL (eds), *Cowell and Tyler's Diagnostic Cytology and Hematology of the Dog and Cat*, 3rd ed. St. Louis, MO: Mosby Elsevier, pp. 317–319.

Avallone G, Forlani A, Tecilla M, et al. 2016. Neoplastic disease in the domestic ferret (*Mustela putorius furo*) in Italy: classification and tissue distribution of 856 cases (2000–2010). *BMC Veterinary Research* 12:1–8.

Avery AC, Avery PR. 2007. Determining the significance of persistent lymphocytosis. *Vet Clin North Am Small Anim Pract* 37:267–282.

Baggiolini M, Hirsch JG, De Duve C. 1969. Resolution of granules from rabbit heterophil leukocytes into distinct populations by zonal sedimentation. *J Cell Biol* 40:529–541.

Baggiolini M, Hirsch JG, De Duve C. 1970. Further biochemical and morphological studies of granule fractions from rabbit heterophil leukocytes. *J Cell Biol* 45:586–597.

Baker R, Lumsden JH. 2000. Cytopathology techniques and interpretation. In: Baker R, Lumsden J (eds), *Color Atlas of the Dog and Cat*. St. Louis: Mosby.

Banks WJ. 1974. Histology and comparative organology. In: Banks, WJ (ed), *Histology and Comparative Organology: A Text Atlas*. Baltimore: Williams and Wilkins.

Barger AM, MacNeill AL. 2016. Liver cytology. In: Taylor and Francis Group (ed), *Small Animal Cytologic Diagnosis*, 1st edn. Boca Raton, FL: CRC Press. pp. 246–247.

Barrios-Arpi LM, Morales-Cauti SM. 2020. Cytomorphological characterization of lymphadenopathies in guinea pigs: study of 31 clinical cases. *J Exotic Pet Med* 32:1–5.

Barton CL. 1987. Cytologic diagnosis of cutaneous neoplasia: an alogorithmic approach. *Compend Cont Ed Pract* 9:20–33.

Bau-Gaudreault L, Grimes CN. 2017. What is your diagnosis? Cystic prostatic lesion in a domestic ferret. *Vet Clin Pathol* 46(2): 367–368.

Beck R, Sprong H, Bata I, et al. 2011. Prevalence and molecular typing of (*Giardia* spp.) in captive mammals at the zoo of Zagreb, Croatia. *Vet Parasitol* 175(1/2):40–46.

Bellows J. 2011. Intraoral cytology. DVM: The News magazine of Veterinary Medicine 42(9):2S–4S.

Bertazzolo W, Dell'Orco M, Bonfanti U, et al. 2004. Cytological features of canine ovarian tumours: a retrospective study of 19 cases. *J Small Anim Pract* 45:539–545

Bertram CA, Klopfleisch R, Muller K. 2019. Fine needle aspirate of an intestine-associated mass in a domestic rabbit (Oryctolagus cuniculus). *J Exotic Pet Med* 31:1–3.

Bertram CA, Barth SA, Glockner B, et al. 2020a. Intestinal *Mycobacterium avium* infection in pet dwarf rabbits (*Oryctolagus cuniculus*). *J Comp Pathol* 180:73–78.

Bertram CA, Garner MM, Reavill D, et al. 2020b. Giant cell sarcomas in domestic rabbits (*Oryctolagus cuniculus*). *Vet Pathol* 57(4):490–496.

Bongiovanni L, Della Salda P, Selleri P, et al. 2017. Multifocal pustular dermatitis associated with Malassezia overgrowth in a ferret. *J Comp Pathol* 156(1):107.

Borges JCG, Lima DD, Da Silva EM, et al. 2017. *Cryptosporidium* spp. and *Giardia* spp., in aquatic mammals in northern and northeastern Brazil. *Dis Aquat Org* 126:25–31.

Budgeon C, Mans C, Chamberlin T, et al. 2014. Diagnosis and surgical treatment of a malignant trichoepithelioma of the ear canal in a pet rabbit (*Oryctolagus cuniculus*). *J Am Vet Med Assoc* 245(2):227–231.

Brandão J, Woods S, Fowlkes N, et al. 2014 Disseminated histoplasmosis (*Histoplasma capsulatum*) in a pet rabbit: case report and review of the literature. *J Vet Diagn Invest* 26(1):158–162.

Brombini GC, Rahal SC, Bergamini BCS, et al. 2017. Brief communication: analysis of synovial fluid of the Capybara's stifle joints. *Vet Clin Pathol* 46(1):179–182.

Brzozowski T, Zwolinska-Weislo M, Konturek PC, et al. 2005. Influence of gastric colonization with *Candida albicans* on ulcer healing in rats: effect of ranitidine, aspirin and probiotic therapy. *Scand J Gastroenterol* 40(3):286–296.

Burgmann PM. 1991. Dermatology of rabbits, rodents, and ferrets. In: Nesbitt G, Ackerman L (eds), *Dermatology for the Small Animal Practitioner*. Trenton, NJ: Veterinary Learning Systems Co.

Burkhard MJ, Valenciano A, Barger A. 2001. Respiratory tract. In: Raskin R, Meyer D (eds), *Atlas of Canine and Feline Cytology*. Philadelphia, PA: WB Saunders.

Campbell LH, Fos GJ, Snyder SB. 1973. Ocular bacteria and mycoplasma of the clinically normal cat. *Feline Pract*. 1:10–12.

Campbell TW.1983. Disorders of the avian crop. *Compend Cont Ed Pract* 5(10):813–824.

Campbell TW. 1995. Avian Hematology and Cytology. In: Ritchie B, Harrison G, Harrison L (eds), *Avian medicine: principles and application*, 2nd edn. Ames: Iowa State University Press.

Campbell TW, Ellis CS. 2007. Avian *and Exotic Animal Hematology and Cytology*, 3rd edn. Ames, IA: Blackwell Publishing.

Campbell TW, Grant KR. 2010. *Clinical Cases in Avian and Exotic Animal Hematology and Cytology*. Ames, IA: Wiley-Blackwell.

Camus MS, Rech RR, Choy FS, et al. 2009. Pathology in practice. *J Am Vet Med Assoc* 235(8):949–951.

Camus MS, Priest HL, Koehler JW, et al. 2016. Cytologic criteria for mast cell tumor grading in dogs with evaluation of clinical outcome. *Vet Pathol* 53(6) 1117–1123.

Cantile C, Youssef S. 2016. Nervous system. In: Maxie MG (ed), *Jubb, Kennedy, and Palmer's Pathology of Domestic Animals*, 6th edn. St. Louis, MO: Elsevier, pp. 250–406.

Cárdenas A, Chopra S. 2002. Chylous ascites. *Am J Gastroenterol* 97:1896–1900.

Carvalho MDF, Baracho MS, Baracho IR. 2002. An investigation of the nuclei of Hülle cells of *Aspergillus nidulans*. *Genet Mol Biol* 25(4).

Cazzini P, Watson VE, Brown HM. 2013. Laboratory Medicine: Yesterday- Today- Tomorrow: the many faces of Mott cells. *Vet Clin Pathol* 42/2:125–126.

Center SA. 2012. Fluid accumulation disorders. In: Willard MD, Tvedten H (eds), *Small Animal Clinical Diagnosis by Laboratory Methods*, 5th edn. St. Louis, MO: Elsevier Saunders. pp. 247–269.

Chassang L, Langlois I, Loos P, et al. 2018. Chylous ascites associated with abdominal trauma and intestinal resection-anastomosis in a pet ferret (*Mustela putorius furo*). *J Am Vet Med Assoc* 252(10):1272–1278.

Chung T-H, Kim H-J, Choi U-S. 2014. Case report: multicentric epitheliotropic T-cell lymphoma in an African hedgehog (*Atelerix albiventris*). *Vet Clin Pathol* 43(4):601–604.

Churgin SM, Deering KM, Wallace R, et al. 2015. Metastatic mammary adenocarcinoma in a Sugar glider (*Petaurus breviceps*). *J Exotic Pet Med* 24:441–445.

Cian F. 2014. Cytology (part 3): Round cell tumours. *Companion Animal (2053–0889)* 19(10):508–511.

Cole JE, Steeil JC, Sarro SJ, et al. 2020. Chordoma of the sacrum of an adult naked mole-rat. *J Vet Diagn Invest* 32(1):132–135.

Collins BR. 1987. Dermatologic disorders of common small nondomestic animals. In: Nesbitt G (ed), *Dermatology*. New York: Churchill Livingstone.

Connally HE. 2003. Cytology and fluid analysis of the acute abdomen. *Clin Tech Small Anim Pract*. 18:39–44.

Conrado FdO, Bruno SF, De Alencar NX. 2013. What is your diagnosis? Scapular mass in a Chinese hamster. *Vet Clin Pathol* 42(4):533–534.

Cowell RL, Tyler RD, Meinkoth JH. 1999. Diagnostic cytology and hematology of the dog and cat. In: Cowell RL, Tyler RD, Meinkoth JH (eds), *Diagnostic Cytology and Hematology of the Dog and Cat, 2nd edn*. St. Louis: Mosby.

Da Costa RMG, Rema A, Payo-Puente P, et al. 2007. Immunohistochemical characterization of a sebaceous gland carcinoma in a gerbil (*Meriones unguiculatus*). *Journal of Comparative Pathology* 137(2–3):130–132.

Darrow BG, Mans C, Drees R, et al. 2014. Pulmonary blastomycosis in a domestic Ferret (*Mustela putorius furo*). *J Exotic Pet Med* 23:158–164.

De Cecco BS, Da Silva TM, Felin DV, et al. 2018. Malignant peripheral nerve sheath tumor in a cat: cytological, histopathological, and immunohistochemical aspects. *Comparative Clinical Pathology* 27(3):803–806.

Deeb B. 2000. Digestive system and disorders. In: Flecknell P (ed), *Manual of Rabbit Medicine and Surgery*. Gloucester: British Small Animal Veterinary Association.

Dehghanpir SD, Canady LK, Wakamatsu N, et al. 2016. What's Your Diagnosis? Subcutaneous nodules on the muzzle of a rabbit. *Vet Clin Pathol* 45(2):383–384.

Delk KW, Carpenter JW, Biller DS. 2013. Diagnostic challenge. *J Exotic Pet Med* 22:409–412.

Dequéant B, Pascal Q, Bilbault H, et al. 2019. Identification of *Mycobacterium genavense* natural infection in a domestic ferret. *J Vet Diagn Invest* 31(1):133–136

Díaz -Delgado J, Pool R, Hoppes S, et al. 2017. Spontaneous multicentric soft tissue sarcoma in a captive African pygmy hedgehog (*Atelerix albiventris*): case report and literature review. *J of Vet Med Sci* 79:889–895.

Di Tommaso M, Rocconi F, Marruchella G, et al. 2015. Invasive pleural malignant mesothelioma with rib destruction and concurrent osteosarcoma in a dog. *Acta Veterinaria Scandinavica* 57:1–5.

Donnelly TM. 1997. Disease problems of small rodents. In: Hillyer E, Quesenberry K (eds), *Ferrets, Rabbits, and Rodents Clinical Medicine and Surgery*. Philadelphia, PA: WB Saunders.

Donnelly TM. 2004. Disease problems of small rodents. In: Quesenberry KE, Carpenter JW (eds), *Ferrets, Rabbits, and Rodents*,2nd edn. St Louis, MO: Elsevier Saunders, pp. 299–315.

Donovan TA, Moore FM, Bertram CA, et al. 2021. Mitotic figures- Normal, atypical, and imposters: a guide to identification. 2021. *Vet Pathol* 58(2) 243–257.

Döpke C, Fehr M, Thiele A, et al. 2007. Morphological and immunohistochemical characterization of spontaneous mammary tumours in European hedgehogs (*Erinaceus europaeus*). *Journal of Comparative Pathology* 137(1):22–29.

Duchaussoy A-C, Rose A, Talbot JJ, et al. 2015. Gastrointestinal granuloma due to *Candida albicans* in an immunocompetent cat. *Medical Mycology Case Reports* 10:14–17.

Dusick A, Young KM, Muir P. 2014. Relationship between automated total nucleated cell count and enumeration of cells on direct smears of canine synovial fluid. *The Veterinary Journal* 202(3): 550–554.

Effron M, Gringer L, Benirschke K. 1977. Nature and rate of neoplasia found in captive wild mammals, birds, and reptiles at necropsy. *J Natl Cancer Inst* 59:185–198.

Everett KDE, Andersen AA. 1999. Identification of nine species of the Chlamydiaceae using PCR-RFLP. *Int J Syst Bacteriol* 49:803–813.

Everett KDE, Hornung LJ, Andersen AA. 1999. Rapid detection of the Chlamydiaceae and other families in the order Chlamydiales: three PCR tests. *J Clin Microbiol.* 37:575–580.

Fernandes PJ. 2008. Synovial fluid analysis. In: Cowell RL, Tyler RD, Meinkoth JH, et al. (eds), *Diagnostic Cytology and Hematology of the Dog and Cat*, 3rd edn. St. Louis: Mosby Elsevier, pp.193–209.

Fisher DJ. 2001. Musculoskeletal system. In: Raskin R, Meyer D (eds), *Atlas of Canine and Feline Cytology*. Philadelphia, PA: WB Saunders.

Forrester SD, Fossum TW, Rogers KS. 1991. Diagnosis and treatment of chylothorax associated with lymphoblastic lymphosarcomas in four cats. *J Am Vet Med* Assoc 198:291–294.

Fossum TW. 1993. Feline chylothorax. *Compend Contin Edu Pract Vet* 15:549–567.

Fossum TW, Jacobs RM, Birchard SJ. 1986. Evaluation of cholesterol and triglyceride concentrations in differentiating chylous and nonchylous pleural effusions in dogs and cats. *J Am Vet Med Assoc* 188:49–51.

Fossum TW, Hay WH, Boothe HW, et al. 1992. Chylous ascites in three dogs. *J Am Vet Med Assoc* 200:70–76

Fox JG, Muthupalani S, Kiupel M, et al. 2014. Neoplastic diseases. In: Fox JG, Marini RP (eds), *Biology and Diseases of the Ferret*, 3rd edn. Ames, IA: Wiley-Blackwell, pp. 587–626.

Fry MM, Viesselmann L, Yao B, et al. 2018. Diagnostic performance of cytology for assessment of hepatic lipid content in dairy cattle. *Journal of Dairy Science* 101(2):1379–1387.

Fukuzawa R, Fukuzawa K, Abe H, et al. 2004. Acinic cell carcinoma in an African pygmy hedgehog (*Atelerix albiventris*). *Vet Clin Pathol* 33:39–42.

Fulmer AK, Mauldin GE. 2007. Canine histiocytic neoplasia: An Overview. *Can Vet J* 48:1041–1050.

Gardhouse SM, Guzman DS-M, Sadar MJ, et al. 2016. Partial gastrectomy for resection of a gastric leiomyoma in a guinea pig (*Cavia porcellus*). *J Am Vet Med Assoc* 249(12):1415–1420.

Garg N, Singh J, Anjum H, et al. 2019. Cytopreparation of duodenal biopsy fixative improves detection rate of giardia in clinically suspected cases. *Cytopathology* 30(3):309–313.

Garma-Aviña A. 2004. Cytology of the normal and abnormal choroid plexi in selected domestic mammals, wildlife species, and man. *J Vet Diagn Invest* 16:283–292.

Garner MM, Ramsell K, Morera N, et al. 2006. Clinicopathologic features of a systemic coronavirus-associated disease resembling feline infectious peritonitis in the domestic ferret (*Mustela putorius*). *Vet Pathol* 45:236–246.

Garner MM. 2007. Cytologic diagnosis of diseases of rabbits, guinea pigs, and rodents. *Vet Clin North Am Exot Anim Pract* 10:25–49.

George JW. 2001. The usefulness and limitations of hand-held refractometers in veterinary laboratory medicine: an historical and technical review. *Vet Clin Pathol* 30:201–210.

George JW, O'Neill SL. 2001. Comparison of refractometer and biuret methods for total protein measurement in body cavity fluids. *Vet Clin Pathol* 30:16–18.

Gibbons PM, Garner MM, Kiupel M. 2012. Morphological and immunohistochemical characterization of spontaneous thyroid gland neoplasms in guinea pigs (*Cavia porcellus*). *Veterinary Pathology* 50(2):334–342.

Goad MEP, Fox JG. 1988. Neoplasia in ferrets. In: Fox JG (ed), *Biology and Diseases of the Ferret*. Philadelphia, PA: Lea & Febiger.

Goldschmidt MH, Goldschmidt KH. 2017. Epithelial and melanocytic tumors of the skin. In: Meuten DJ (ed), *Tumor in domestic animals*, 5th edn. Ames, IA: Wiley- Blackwell, pp. 88–141.

Gores BR, Berg J, Carpenter JL, et al. 1994. Chylous ascites in cats: nine cases (1978–1993). *J Am Vet Med Assoc* 205:1161–1164.

Grandi F, Ferreira I, Rocha RM, et al. 2012. What is your diagnosis? Subcutaneous enlargement near the base of the ear canal in a Sprague-Dawley rat. *Vet Clin Patho*l 41:160–161.

Green L. 1992. Gastrointestinal cytology. In: Atkinson B (ed), *Atlas of Diagnostic Cytopathology*. Philadelphia, PA: WB Saunders.

Greenacre CB. 2004. Spontaneous tumors of small mammals. *Vet Clin North Am Exot Anim Pract* 7:627–651.

Greenacre CB, Dowling M, Nobrega-Lee M. 2019. Diagnosis and treatment of histoplasmosis in a group of four domestic ferrets (*Mustela putorius furo*) and a review of histoplasmosis. *J Exotic Pet Med* 29:194–201.

Grieshaber TL, McKeever PJ, Conroy JD. 1991. Spontaneous cutaneous (erruptive) xanthomatosis in two cats. *J Am Anim Hosp Assoc* 27:509–512.

Gu Y, Wang X, Zhou C, et al. 2016. Investigation on *cryptosporidium* infections in wild animals in a zoo in Anhui Province. *J Zoo Wildl Med* 47(3):846–854.

Gupta A, Gumber S, Schnellbacher R, et al. 2010. Malignant B-cell lymphoma with mott cell differentiation in a ferret (*Mustela putorius furo*). *J Vet Diagn Invest* 22:469–473.

Hall RL, McWilliams PS. 1988. The cytological examination of cutaneous and subcutaneous masses. *Semin Vet Med Surg* 3(2):94–108.

Harcourt-Brown F. 2002a. Skin diseases. In: Harcourt-Brown F (ed), *Textbook of Rabbit Medicine*. Oxford: Butterworth-Heinemann.

Harcourt-Brown F. 2002b. Abscesses. In: Harcourt-Brown F (ed), *Textbook of Rabbit Medicine*. Oxford, UK: Butterworth-Heinemann, pp. 206–223.

Harkness JE, Wagner JR. 1989. The biology and medicine of rabbits and rodents. In: Harkness JE, Wagner JR (eds), *Vol. III, The Biology and Medicine of Rabbits and Rodents*. Philadelphia, PA: Lea & Febiger.

Harr KE, Thielen L, MacNeill AL. 2018. Validation of an immunocytochemical assay for immunophenotyping of lymphoma in guinea pigs (*Cavia porcellus*). *Vet Clin Pathol* 47(4):682–687.

Heatley JJ, Smith AN. 2004. Spontaneous neoplasms of lagomorphs. *Vet Clin North Am Exot Anim Pract* 7:561–577.

Hoefer HL. 1994. Hedgehogs. *Vet Clin North Am Small Anim Pract* 24:113–120.

Hoefer HL, Bell JA. 2004. Gastrointestinal diseases. In: Carpenter J, Quesenberry K (eds), *Ferrets, Rabbits, and Rodents Clinical Medicine and Surgery*, 2nd edn. St. Louis: Saunders Elsevier.

Hoppman E, Barron HW. 2007. Ferret and rabbit dermatology. *J Exot Pet Med* 16:225–237.

Hotz CS, Templeton SJ, Christopher MM. 2005. Comparative analysis of expert and machine-learning methods for classification of body cavity effusions in companion animals. *J Vet Diagn Invest* 17:158–164.

Huynh M, Pingret J-L, Nicolier A. 2014. Disseminated *mycobacterium genavense* infection in a chinchilla (*Chinchilla lanigera*). *J Comp Pathol* 151:122–125.

Jan J-C, Wang C-P, Kwan P-C, et al. 2008. Ceruminous adenocarcinoma with extensive parotid, cervical, and distant metastases, Case report and review of literature. *Arch Otolaryngol Head Neck Surg* 134(6):663–666.

Jenkins JR. 2004. Gastrointestinal disease. In: Carpenter J, Quesenberry K (eds), *Ferrets, Rabbits, Rodents Clinical Medicine and Surgery*. St. Louis: Saunders Elsevier.

Johnson JG, Blair R, Brandão J, et al. 2014. Case report: atypical fibrosarcoma in the skin of a roborovski hamster (*Phodopus roborovskii*). *Vet Clin Pathol* 43(2):281–284.

Kanfer S, Reavill DR. 2013. Cutaneous neoplasia in ferrets, rabbits, and guinea pigs. *Vet Clin Exot Anim* 16:579– 598.

Karim BO, Ali SZ, Landolfi JA, et al. 2008. Cytomorphologic differentiation of benign and malignant mammary tumors in fine needle aspirate specimens from irradiated female Sprague–Dawley rats. *Vet Clin Pathol* 37(2):229–236.

Karim KR, Izawa T, Pervin M, et al. 2017. Cutaneous histiocytic sarcoma with regional lymph node metastasis in a Netherland dwarf rabbit (*Oryctolagus cuniculus*). *J Comp Pathol* 156:169–172.

Kelleher SA. 2001. Skin diseases of ferrets. *Vet Clin North Am Exot Anim Pract* 4:136–140.

Keller KA, Nevarez JG, Rodriguez D, et al. 2014. Diagnosis and treatment of anaplastic mammary adenocarcinoma in a Sugar glider (*Petaurus breviceips*). *J Exotic Pet Med* 23:277–282.

Kennedy MJ, Volz PA, Edwards CA, et al. 1987. Mechanisms of association of *Candida albicans* with intestinal mucosa. J *Med Microbiol* 24(4):333–341

Kern TJ. 1989. Ocular disorders of rabbits, rodents, and ferrets. In: Kirk R, Bonagura J (eds), *Current Veterinary Therapy X*. Philadelphia, PA: WB Saunders.

Kerr PJ, Donnelly TM. 2013. Viral infections of rabbits. *Vet Clin North Am Exot Anim Pract* 16:437–468.

Kondo H, Hara K, Sukegawa A, et al. 2018. Chordoma of the tail in a degu (octodon degus). *J Exotic Pet Med* 27:1–4.

Krimer PM, Haley AC, Harvey SB, et al. 2016. Evaluation of cytospin precision in low cellularity canine cerebrospinal fluid. *J Vet Diagn Invest* 28(2):158–164.

Krockenberger MB, Canfield PJ, Malik R. 2003. *Cryptococcus neoformans* var *gattii* in the koala (*Phascolarctos cinereus*): a review of 43 cases of cryptococcosis. *Med Mycol* 41:225–234.

Kuramochi M, Izawa T, Hori M, et al. 2015. Chordoma of the thoracic vertebrae in a Bengal tiger (panthera tigris tigris). *J Vet Med Sci* 77:893–895.

Laroucau K, Souriau A, Rodolakis A. 2001. Improved sensitivity of PCR for Chlamydophila using pmp genes. *Vet Microbiol* 82:155–164.

LaRue MK, Flesner BK, Higbie CT, et al. 2016. Treatment of a thyroid tumor in an African pygmy hedgehog (*Atelerix albiventris*). *J Exotic Pet Med* 25:226–230.

Latgé JP. 1999. *Aspergillus fumigatus* and aspergillosis. *Clin Microbiol Rev* 12:310–350.

Le K, Beaufrére H, Laniesse D, et al. 2019. Diagnosis and long-term management of blastomycosis in two ferrets (*Mustela putorius furo*). *J Exotic Pet Med* 31:39–44.

Leissinger M, Brandão J, Wakamatsu N, et al. 2013. Case report: Pulmonary histiocytic sarcoma in a rabbit. *Vet Clin Pathol* 42(3):364–367.

Lester S, Malik R, Bartlett K, et al. 2011. Cryptococcosis: update and emergence of *Cryptococcus gattii*. *Vet Clin Pathol* 40:4–17.

Lin T-Y, Hamberg A, Pentecost R, et al. 2010. Mast cell tumors in a llama (*Lama glama*). *J Vet Diagn Invest* 22:808–811.

Lipman NS, Marini RP, Murphy JC, et al. 1993. Estradiol17 beta secreting adrenocortical tumor in a ferret. *J Am Vet Med Assoc* 203:1552–1555.

Liptak JM, Forrest LJ. 2007. Soft tissue sarcomas: Overview and surgical management. In: Withrow SJ, Vail, DM (eds), *Withrow and MacEwen's Small Animal Clinical Oncology*, 4th edn. St. Louis, MO: Elsevier Saunders, p. 435.

Liptovszky M, Kerekes Z, Perge E, et al. 2017. Mediastinal lymphoma and chylothorax in a Striped skunk (*Mephitis mephitis*). *J Zoo Wildl Med* 48(2):598–601.

Li X, Fox JG, Padrid PA. 1998. Neoplastic diseases in ferrets: 584 cases (1968–1998). *J Am Vet Med Assoc* 212:1402–1406.

Long H, di Girolamo N, Selleri P, et al. 2016. Polyostotic lymphoma in a ferret (*Mustela putorius furo*). *J Comp Pathol* 154:341–344.

Lopez GT, Moore AR, Rao S, et al. 2020. Characterization of cells collected from nasolacrimal duct flush samples in healthy rabbits (*Oryctolagus cuniculus*). *J Exotic Pet Med* 35:58–62.

Lowenstine LJ, McManamon R, Terio KA. 2016. Comparative pathology of aging great apes: bonobos, chimpanzees, gorillas, and orangutans. *Vet Pathol* 53(2) 250–276.

Lucas A, Furber H, James G, et al. 2000. *Mycobacterium genavense* infection in two aged ferrets with conjunctival lesions. *Aust Vet J* 78:685–689.

Ludwig LL, Simpson AM, Han E. 2010. Pleural and extrapleural diseases. In: Ettinger SJ, Feldmand EC (eds), *Textbook of Veterinary Internal Medicine*, 3rd edn. St Louis, MO: Saunders Elsevier, pp. 1125–1137.

Malley D. 2000. Handling, restraint, and clinical techniques. In: Flecknell P (ed), *Manual of Rabbit Medicine and Surgery*. Gloucester: British Small Animal Veterinary Association.

Manzocchi S, Venco L, Di Cesare A. 2016. What is your diagnosis? Squash preparation from the lung of a hedgehog. *Vet Clin Pathol* 45(4):715–716.

Marcos R, Malhão F, Santos J, et al. 2016. The cryptic Cryptococcus. *Vet Clin Pathol* 45(4):532–533.

Marshall KL. 2008. Rabbit hematology. *Vet Clin N Am Exot Anim Pract* 11:551–567.

Martínez J, Martorell J, Abarca ML, et al. 2012. Pyogranulomatous pleuropneumonia and mediastinitis in ferrets (*Mustela putorius furo*) associated with *pseudomonas luteola* infection. J Comp Pathol 146:4–10.

Martínez-Nevado E, Alonso-Alegre GE, Martínez MAJ, et al. 2017. Atypical presentation of cryptococcus neoformans in a koala (phascolarctos cinereus): a magnetic resonance imaging and computed tomography study. *J Zoo Wildl Med* 48(1):250–254.

Martorell J, Melero A. 2013. Diagnostic challenge. *J Exotic Pet Med* 22:85–89.

Mashinsky Y, Thompson RA, Koru O, DaSilva A. 2009. Human zoonotic enteropathogens in constructed free-surface flow wetland. *Parasitol Res* 105(2):423–428.

Masserdotti C. 2006. Architectural patterns in cytology: correlation with histology. *Vet Clin Pathol* 35:388–396.

Masserdotti C. 2020. The cytologic features of biliary diseases: A retrospective study. *Vet Clin Pathol* 49:440–450.

Mauldin EA, Peters-Kennedy J. 2016. Integumentary system. In: Maxie MG (ed), Jubb, Kennedy, and Palmer's pathology of domestic animals, 6th edn. Vol. 1. St. Louis, MO: Elsevier, pp. 509–736.

Mayer J, Erdman SE, Fox JG. 2014. Diseases of the hematopoietic system. In: Fox JG, Marini RP (eds), *Biology and Diseases of the Ferret*. Ames: John Wiley & Sons, pp. 311–334.

Meachem MD, Burgess HJ, Davies JL, et al. 2012. Utility of nuclear morphometry in the cytologic evaluation of canine cutaneous soft tissue sarcomas. *J Vet Diagn Invest* 24(3):525–530.

Meadows RL, MacWilliams PS. 1994. Chylous effusions revisited. *Vet Clin Pathol* 23:54–62.

Meinkoth J. 2022. Cytology of synovial fluid. In: Thrall MA (ed), *Veterinary Hematology, Clinical Chemistry, and Cytology*, 3rd edn. Ames, IA: Wiley-Blackwell, in press.

Meinkoth JH, Cowell RH, Tyler RD. 2007. Cell types and criteria of malignancy. In: Cowell RL, Tyler RD, Meinkoth JH, et al. (eds), Diagnostic cytology and hematology of the Dog and Cat. Mosby: Elsevier, pp. 37–46.

Mentre V, Bulliot C. 2015. A retrospective study of 17 cases of mycobacteriosis in domestic ferrets (*Mustela Putorius furo*) between 2005 and 2013. *J Exotic Pet Med* 24:340–349.

Meredith A. 2000. Respiratory system and disorders. In: Lecknell PF (ed), *Manual of Rabbit Medicine and Surgery*. Gloucester: British Small Animal Veterinary Association.

Messick JB. 2014. The lymph nodes. In: Cowell RL, Tyler RD(eds), Diagnostic cytology and hematology of the dog and cat, 4th edn. Saint. Louis, MO: Elsevier, pp. 180–94.

Meuten DJ, Meichner K. 2022. Inflammation and infectious agents. In: Thrall MA (ed), *Veterinary Hematology, Clinical Chemistry, and Cytology*, 3rd edn. Ames, IA: Wiley-Blackwell, in press.

Meyer DJ. 2001a. The liver. In: Raskin R, Meyer D (eds), *Atlas of Canine and Feline Cytology*. Philadelphia, PA: WB Saunders.

Meyer DJ. 2001b. Eyes and adnexa. In: Raskin R, Meyer D (eds), *Atlas of Canine and Feline Cytology*. Philadelphia: WB Saunders.

Meyer DM. 2016. The liver. In: Raskin E, Meyer DJ (eds), *Canine and Feline Cytology: A Color Atlas and Interpretation Guide*, 4th edn. St. Louis, MO: Elsevier, pp. 259–270.

Miller DL, Styer EL, Stobaeus JK, et al. 2002. Thyroid c-cell carcinoma in an African pygmy hedgehog (Atelerix albiventris). *J Zoo Wildl Med* 33:392–396.

Mitchell MA, Tully TN. 2009. *Manual of Exotic Pet Practice*. St. Louis, MO: Elsevier Saunders.

Munasinghe L, Dougherty C, Sridharan S, et al. 2017. What is your diagnosis? a mass on the right tarsus in a rabbit. *Vet Clin Pathol* 46(1):187–18.

Murphy IM. 1988. Exfoliative cytologic examination as an aid in diagnosing ocular diseases in the dog and cat. *Semin Vet Med Surg* 3:10–14.

Nagata K, McHale B, Sladakovic I, et al. 2019. Total body irradiation for the treatment of lymphoma in a guinea pig (*Cavia porcellus*). *J Exotic Pet Med* 28:132–136.

Nasser IA, Fayyad LM, Soudi NM, et al. 1994. Fine needle aspiration cytology in the diagnosis of gouty tophi: the role of diff-quick stain in the evaluation of unexpected lesions. *Acta Cytol* 38:840.

Naylor AD, Morrison LR, Girling SJ. 2018. Mandibular squamous cell carcinoma in a Rock hyrax (Procavia capensis). *J Zoo Wildl Med* 49(2):489–492.

Nevitt BN, Langan JN, Adkesson MJ, et al. 2013. Multifocal *crytococcus neoformans* var. *neoforms*: infection, treatment, and monitoring by serial computed tomography in a Schmidt's red-tailed guenon (*Cercopithecus ascanius schmidti*). *J Zoo Wildl Med* 44(3):728–736.

Nevitt BN, Langan JN, Adkesson MJ, et al. 2014. Diagnosis and treatment of chronic lymphocytic leukemia in a bat-eared fox (*Otocyon megalotis*). *J Am Vet Med Assoc* 245 (12):1391–1395.

Ogihara K, Itoh T, Mizuno Y, et al. 2016. Disseminated histiocytic sarcoma in an African hedgehog (*Atelerix albiventris*). *J Comp Pathol* 155:361–364.

Ogihara K, Suzuki K, Madarame H. 2017. Primary histiocytic sarcoma of the brain in an African hedgehog (*Atelerix albiventris*). *J Comp Pathol* 157:241–245.

Orr H. 2009. Rodents: neoplastic and endocrine disease. In: Keeble E, Meredith A (eds), *BSAVA Manual of Rodents and Ferrets*. Gloucester, UK: BSAVA, pp. 181–192.

Padrid PA, Feldman BF, Funk K, et al. 1991. Cytologic, microbiologic and biochemical analysis of bronchoalveolar lavage fluid obtained from 24 healthy cats. *Am J Vet Res* 52:1300–1307.

Pantanowitz L, Goulart RA, Martínez-Girón R. 2011. Mimics and contaminants. In: L Pantanowitz, P Michelow, WE Khalbuss (eds), *Cytopathology of Infectious Diseases*. New York: Springer, pp. 351– 377.

Patel S, Mahadevappa A, Vimalambike MG. 2016. Fine needle aspiration cytology of papulonodular lesions of skin: a study of 50 cases. *Journal of Clinical & Diagnostic Research*. 10(12):9–13.

Perdelli F, Sartini M, Spagnolo AM, et al. 2006. A problem of hospital hygiene: the presence of aspergilli in hospital wards with different air-conditioning features. *Am J Infect Control* 34(5):264–8.

Perez-Martínez JA, Storz J. 1985. Antigenic diversity of chlamydia psittaci of mammalian origin determined by microimmunofluorescence. *Infect Immun* 50:905–910.

Perman V, Alsaker RD, Riis RC. 1979. Cytology of the dog and cat. In: Perman V, Alsaker RD, Riis RC (eds), *Cytology of the Dog and Cat*. South Bend, IN: American Animal Hospital Association.

Perpiñán D, López C. 2008. Clinical aspects of systemic granulomatous inflammatory syndrome in ferrets (*Mustela putorius furo*). *Vet Rec* 162(6):180–184.

Pinches MDG, Liebenberg G, Stidworthy MF. 2008. What is your diagnosis? preputial mass in a ferret. *Vet Clin Pathol* 37(4):443–446.

Prain CJ, Pearce JH. 1989. Ultrastructural studies on the intracellular fate of *chlamydia psittaci* (strain guinea pig inclusion conjunctivitis) and *chlamydia trachomatis* (strain lymphogranuloma venereum 434): modulation of intracellular events and relationship with endocytic mechanism. *J Gen Microbiol* 135:2107–2123.

Protain HJ, Kutzler MA, Valentine BA. 2009. Assessment of cytologic evaluation of preputial epithelial cells as a diagnostic test for detection of adrenocortical disease in castrated ferrets. *Am J Vet Res* 70(5):619–623.

Pucheu-Haston CM, Brandão J, Jones KL, et al. 2016. Zymbal gland (auditory sebaceous gland) carcinoma presenting as otitis externa in a pet rat (*Rattus norvegicus*). *J Exotic Pet Med* 25:133–138.

Puig L, Bragulat MR, Castellá G, et al. 2018. Phenotypic and genetic diversity of *Malassezia furfur* from domestic and zoo animals. *Medical Mycology* 56:941–949.

Rebar AH, DeNicola DB, Muggenburg BA. 1980. Bronchopulmonary lavage cytology in the dog: normal findings. *Vet Clin North Am (Sm Anim)* 22:1065–1085.

Quereshi MA. 1998. Role of macrophages in avian health and disease. *Poult Sci* 77:978–982.

Raymond JT, Clarke KA, Schafer KA. 1998. Intestinal lymphosarcoma in captive African hedgehogs. *J Wildl Dis* 34:801–806.

Raymond JT, Garner MM. 2001. Spontaneous tumours in captive African hedgehogs (*Atelerix albiventris*): a retrospective study. *J Comp Pathol* 124:128–133.

Raymond JT, White MR. 1999. Necropsy and histopathologic findings in 14 African hedgehogs (*Atelerix albiventris*): a retrospective study. *J Zoo Wildl Med* 30:273–277.

Raskin RE. 1996. Myelopoiesis and myeloproliferative disorders. *Vet Clin North Am Small Anim Pract* 26:1023–1042.

Raskin, 2001a. Skin and subcutaneous tissues. In: Raskin R, Meyer D (eds), *Atlas of Canine and Feline Cytology*. Philadelphia, PA: WB Saunders.

Raskin RE. 2001b. Eyes and adnexa. In: Raskin R, Meyer D (eds), *Atlas of Canine and Feline Cytology*. Philadelphia, PA: WB Saunders.

Raskin, 2001c. General categories of cytologic interpretation. In: Raskin R, Meyer D (eds), *Atlas of Canine and Feline Cytology*. Philadelphia, PA: WB Saunders.

Raskin RE, Meyer DJ. 2016. *Atlas of Canine and Feline Cytology*, 3rd edn. Philadelphia, PA: Saunders, pp. 91–137.

Rebar A. 1978. *Handbook of veterinary cytology*. St. Louis: Ralston Purina.

Reimnitz L, Guzman DS-M, LaDouceur E, et al. 2019. Peripheral nerve sheath tumor in the pelvic limb of a domestic rabbit (*Orycytolagus cuniculus*). *J Exotic Pet Med* 28:137–142.

Reyes-Matute A, Méndez-Bernal S, Ramos-Garduno L-A. 2017. Osteosarcoma in African hedgehogs (Atelerix albiventris): Five cases. *J Zoo Wildl Med* 48(2):453–460.

Ritter JM, von Bomhard W, Wise AG, et al. 2012. Cutaneous lymphomas in European pet rabbits (*Oryctolagus cuniculus*). *Vet Pathol* 49(5): 846–851.

Roh Y-S, Kim E-J, Cho A, et al. 2014. Chylous ascites in a hedgehog (*Atelerix albiventris*). *J Zoo Wildl Med* 45:951–954.

Ryan U, Fayer R, Xiao L. 2014. Cryptosporidium species in humans and animals: current understanding and research needs. *Parasitology* 141:1667–1685.

Sapierzyński R, Czopowicz M, Ostrzeszewicz M. 2017. Factors affecting the diagnostic utility of canine and feline cytological samples. *J Small Anim Pract* 58(2):73–78.

Sautier L, Guillier D, Coste M, et al. 2019. Coccygeal chordoma in a degu: case report and review of the literature. *J Vet Diagn Invest* 31(1) 142–145.

Savelieff MG, Pappalardo L, Azmanis P. 2018. The current status of avian aspergillosis diagnoses: veterinary practice to novel research avenues. Vet Clin Pathol 2018 47(3):342–362.

Scarff DH. 2000. Dermatoses. In: Flecknell P (ed), *Manual of Rabbit Medicine and Surgery*. Gloucester: British Small Animal Veterinary Association

Schmiedt C, Tobias KM, Otto CM. 2001. Evaluation of abdominal fluid: peripheral blood creatinine and potassium ratios for diagnosis of uroperitoneum in dogs. *J Vet Emerg Crit Care* 11(4):275–280.

Scott DW, Miller WH, Griffin CE. 1995. Dermatoses of pet rodents, rabbits, and ferrets. In: Scott DW, Miller WH, Griffin CE (eds), *Muller and Kirk's Small Animal Dermatology*, 5th edn. Philadelphia, PA: WB Saunders

Scott DW, Miller WH, Griffin CE. 2001. Dermatoses of pet rodents, rabbits, and ferrets. In: Scott D, Miller W, Griffin C (eds), *Muller and Kirk's Small Animal Dermatology*, 6th edn. Philadelphia, PA: WB Saunders.

Schaeffer DO, Donnelly TM. 1997. Disease problems of guinea pigs and chinchillas. In: Hillyer E, Quesenberry K (eds), *Ferrets, Rabbits, and Rodents Clinical Medicine and Surgery*. Philadelphia, PA: WB Saunders.

Shelly SM. 2001. Body cavity fluids. In: Raskin R, Meyer D (eds), *Atlas of Canine and Feline Cytology*. Philadelphia, PA: WB Saunders.

Shen Z, Batac F, Mannion A, et al. 2017. Novel urease-negative *Helicobacter* sp. 'H. *enhydrae* sp. nov.' isolated from inflamed gastric tissue of southern sea otters. *Dis Aquat Org* 123:1–11.

Shigemoto J, Muraoka Y, Wise AG, et al. 2014. Two case of systemic coronavirus associated disease resembling feline infectious peritonitis in domestic ferrets in Japan. *J Exotic Pet Med* 23:196–200.

Sireesha A, Triveni B, Parmer S, et al. 2018. Role of Imprint cytology in rapid diagnosis of ovarian neoplasms with histopathology correlation. IAIM 5(11):56–62.

Sirivisoot S, Arya N, Kiupel M, et al. 2021. Disseminated haemophagocytic histiocytic sarcoma in an African pygmy hedgehog (*Atelerix albiventris*). *J Comp Pathol* 182:54–57.

Smith RP, Chalmers RM, Elwin K, et al. 2009. Investigation of the role of companion animals in the zoonotic transmission of cryptosporidiosis. *Zoonoses & Public Health* 56(1):24–33.

Snow S, Higbie C, Tully TN, et al. 2018. Diagnostic challenge: Multiple myeloma in an African hedgehog (Atelerix albiventris) based on necropsy findings. *J Exotic Pet Med* 30:82–84.

Son NV, Chambers JK, Dung LT, et al. 2020. Histological and immunohistochemical features of normal histiocytes and langerhans cells, and histiocytic sarcomas in Four-Toed hedgehogs (*Atelerix albiventris*). *J Comp Pathol* 178:1–8.

Stiles J, Greenacre C. 2001. Infraorbital cyst in a White cockatoo (*Cacatua alba*). *J Avian Med Surg* 15:40–43.

Strik NI, Alleman AR, Wellehan JFX, 2005. What is your diagnosis: conjunctival swab cytology from a guinea pig: it's elementary. *Vet Clin Pathol* 34:169–171.

Stockham SL, Scott MA. 2008. Cavitary effusions. In: Stockham SL, Scott MA (eds), *Fundamentals of Veterinary Clinical Pathology*, 2nd edn. Ames, IA: Blackwell, pp. 831–866.

Suckow MA, Rebelatto MC, Schulman AA, HogenEsch H. 2002. Sebaceous adenocarcinoma of the external auditory canal in a New Zealand white rabbit. *J Comp Path* 127(4):301–303.

Suzuki K, Morita R, Hojo Y, et al. 2013. Immunohistochemical characterization of neuroendocrine differentiation of canine anal sac glandular tumours. *J Comp Pathol* 149:199–207.

Szabo Z, Reavill DR, Kiupel M. 2019. Squamous cell carcinoma in chinchillas: a review of three cases. *J Exotic Pet Med* 28:115–120.

Taboada J. 2000. Systemic mycoses. In: Ettinger SJ, Feldman EC (eds), *Textbook of Veterinary Internal Medicine*, 5th edn. Philadelphia, PA: Elsevier Saunders, pp. 453–476.

Tauziede-Espariat A, Bresson D, Polivka M, et al. 2016. Prognostic and therapeutic markers in chordomas: a study of 287 tumors. *J Neuropathol Exp Neurol* 75:111–120.

Taylor KR, Garner MM, Russell K, et al. 2016. Chordomas at high prevalence in the captive population of the endangered perdido key beach mouse (*Peromyscus polionotus trissyllepsis*). *Vet Pathol* 53(1) 163–169.

Terrell SP, Fontenot DK, Miller MA, et al. 2003. Chylous ascites in a cheetah (Acinonyx jubatus) with venoocclusive liver disease. *J Zoo Wildl Med* 34(4):380–384.

Theuss T. 2010. Disseminated infection with *Mycobacterium genavense* in a grizzled giant squirrel (*Ratufa macroura*) associated with the isolation of an unknown mycobacterium. *J Comp Pathol* 143:195–198.

Turowski EE, Shen Z, Ducore RM, et al. 2014. Isolation of a *campylobacter lanienae*-like bacterium from laboratory chinchillas (*Chinchilla laniger*). *Zoonoses & Public Health* 61(8):571–580.

Tvedten H. 2009. Atypical mitoses: morphology and classification. *Vet Clin Pathol* 38(4):418–420.

Tyler RD, Cowell RL, Meinkoth JH. 1999. Cutaneous and subcutaneous lesions: masses, cysts, ulcers, and fistulous tracts. In: Tyler RD, Cowell RL, Meinkoth JH (eds), *Diagnostic Cytology and Hematology of the Dog and Cat*. St. Louis: Mosby.

Vail DM, Mahler PA, Soergel SA. 1995. Differential cell analysis and phenotypic subtyping of lymphocytes in bronchoalveolar lavage fluid from clinically normal dogs. *Am J Vet Res* 56:282–285.

van der Woerdt A. 2004. Ophthalmologic diseases in small pet mammals. In: Carpenter J, Quesenberry K (eds), *Ferrets, Rabbits, and Rodents Clinical Medicine and Surgery*. St. Louis: Saunders Elsevier.

Vergneau-Grosset C, Keel MK, Goldsmith D, et al. 2016. Description of the prevalence, histologic characteristics, concomitant abnormalities, and outcomes of mammary gland tumors in companion rats (*Rattus norvegicus*): 100 cases (1990–2015). *J Am Vet Med Assoc* 249(10):1170–1179.

Vernau W, Moore PF. 1999. An immunophenotypic study of canine leukemias and preliminary assessment of clonality by polymerase chain reaction. *J Vet Immunol Immunopathol* 69:145–164.

Vilalta L, Meléndez-Lazo A, Doria G, et al. 2016. Clinical, cytological, histological and immunohistochemical features of cutaneous mast cell tumours in ferrets (*Mustela putorius furo*). *J Comp Pathol* 155:346–355.

Vilalta L, Altuzarra R, Molina J, et al. 2017a. Chylous ascites in 2 ferrets. *J Exotic Pet Med* 26:150–155.

Vilalta L, Meléndez-Lazo A, Canturri A, et al. 2017b. Anal sac adenocarcinoma with metastases and hypercalcemia in a ferret (Mustela putorius furo). *J Exotic Pet Med* 26:143–149.

Vujovic S, Henderson S, Presneau N, et al. 2006. Brachyury, a crucial regulator of notochordal development, is a novel biomarker for chordomas. *J Pathol* 209:157–165

Waddle JR, Giger U. 1990. Lipoprotein electrophoresis differentiation of chylous and nonchylous pleural effusions in dogs and cats and its correlation with pleural effusion triglyceride concentration. *Vet Clin Pathol* 19:80–85.

Walberg J, Loar AS. 2004. Cytology and hematology of small mammals. In: Carpenter J, Quesenberry K (eds), *Ferrets, Rabbits, and Rodents Clinical Medicine and Surgery*. St. Louis: Saunders Elsevier.

Weeden, AL, Wamsley, HL. 2015. Dry-mount fecal cytology. In: RE Raskin, D Meyer (eds), *Canine and Feline Cytology*. St. Louis, MI: Elsevier, pp. 525- 526.

Weisbroth SH. 1994. Neoplastic diseases. In: Manning P, Ringler D, Newcomer C (eds), *The Biology of the Laboratory Rabbit*, 2nd edn. New York: Academic Press.

Weiser G. 2012. Interpretation of leukocyte responses in disease. In: Thrall MA, Weiser G, Allison RW (eds),*Veterinary Hematology and Clinical Chemistry*, 2nd edn. Ames, IA: Wiley-Blackwell, pp. 127–139.

Whitaker D. 2000. The cytology of malignant mesothelioma. *Cytopathology* 11(3):139–151.

Williams BH, Weiss CA. 2004. Neoplasia. In: Carpenter J, Quesenberry K (eds), *Ferrets, Rabbits, and Rodents Clinical Medicine and Surgery*, 2nd edn. St. Louis: Saunders Elsevier.

Williams BH, Wyre NR. 2021. Neoplasia in ferrets. In Quesenberry KE, Mans C, Orcutt CJ, Carpeter JW (eds), *Ferrets, Rabbits, and Rodents, Clinical Medicine and Surgery*, 4th edn. St. Louis, MO: Elsevier, pp. 92–108.

Williams ES, Thorne ET, Kwiatkowski DR, et al. 1992. Comparative vaginal cytology of the estrous cycle of black-footed ferrets (*Mustela nigripes*), Siberian polecats (M. *eversmanni*), and domestic ferrets (M. *putorius furo*). *J Vet Diagn Invest* 4:38–44.

Wu D, Henriksen M, Grant K, et al. 2019. Ocular findings and selected ophthalmic diagnostic tests in a group of young commercially available Guinea and Skinny pigs (*Cavia porcellus*). *Veterinary Ophthalmology* 23(2):234–244.

Yildirim F, Gurel A. 2012, Comparison between cytological and histopathological evaluations of canine mammary tumours. *Revue Méd Vét* 163(3):116–122.

Yui T, Ohmachi T, Matsuda K, et al. 2015. Histochemical and immunohistochemical characterization of chordoma in ferrets. *J Vet Med Sci* 77:467–473

Zhao Q, Schachter J, Stephens RS. 1993. Lack of allelic polymorphism for the major outer membrane protein gene of the agent of guinea pig inclusion conjunctivitis. *Infect Immun* 61:3078–3080.

8 Mammalian Cytology: Clinical Case Presentations

Case 1: Hedgehog with Swelling under the Right Forelimb

Signalment

2-year-old female African pygmy hedgehog (*Atelerix albiventris*)

History

Presented with a swelling under the right forelimb.

Physical Examination

Bright, alert, responsive. Body weight of 314 gm. 1-cm round discrete mass present in the tissues of the right axilla.

A fine-needle aspirate of the mass was performed for cytodiagnosis (Figures 8.1a–8.1d).

Interpretive Discussion

The fine-needle aspirate stained with Wright–Giemsa–Romanowsky stain revealed a highly cellular sample containing primarily epithelial cells with distinct cell borders and occurring in adherent groups. Figures 8.1a–8.1d revealed epithelial cells that commonly have eccentric, round to oval nuclei with coarse chromatin, moderate nuclear pleomorphism, and prominent nucleoli that are sometimes large, angular, and multiple. There was a variable N:C ratio among the cells, and binucleated cells were found. The variably stained basophilic cytoplasm contained vacuoles suggestive of the production of a secretory product. Because these epithelial cells exhibited features of malignant neoplasia with secretory vacuoles, a diagnosis of an adenocarcinoma was made.

Summary

The mass was removed under general anesthesia and submitted for histopathology. The subcutaneous axillary mass was confirmed to be a mammary adenocarcinoma and was completely excised. The hedgehog was released without complications.

Case 2: Dumbo Rat with a Mass on Its Face

Signalment

8-month-old intact male Dumbo rat (*Rattus norvegicus*)

History

The rat was presented for a rapidly growing (3 days duration) mass on its face. The rat was adopted four months prior to presentation. He was housed with another male rat and was active and playful with normal appetite and urination/defecation. He did not appear to be bothered by the mass.

Physical Examination

On presentation, the 445-g rat was bright, alert, responsive, playful, and active with appropriate mentation. He had normal ambulation and was in good body condition. His pulse rate was 250 bpm and respiratory rate was 60 bpm.

Exotic Animal Hematology and Cytology, Fifth Edition. Terry W. Campbell and Krystan R. Grant.

Companion website: www.wiley.com/go/campbell/exotic

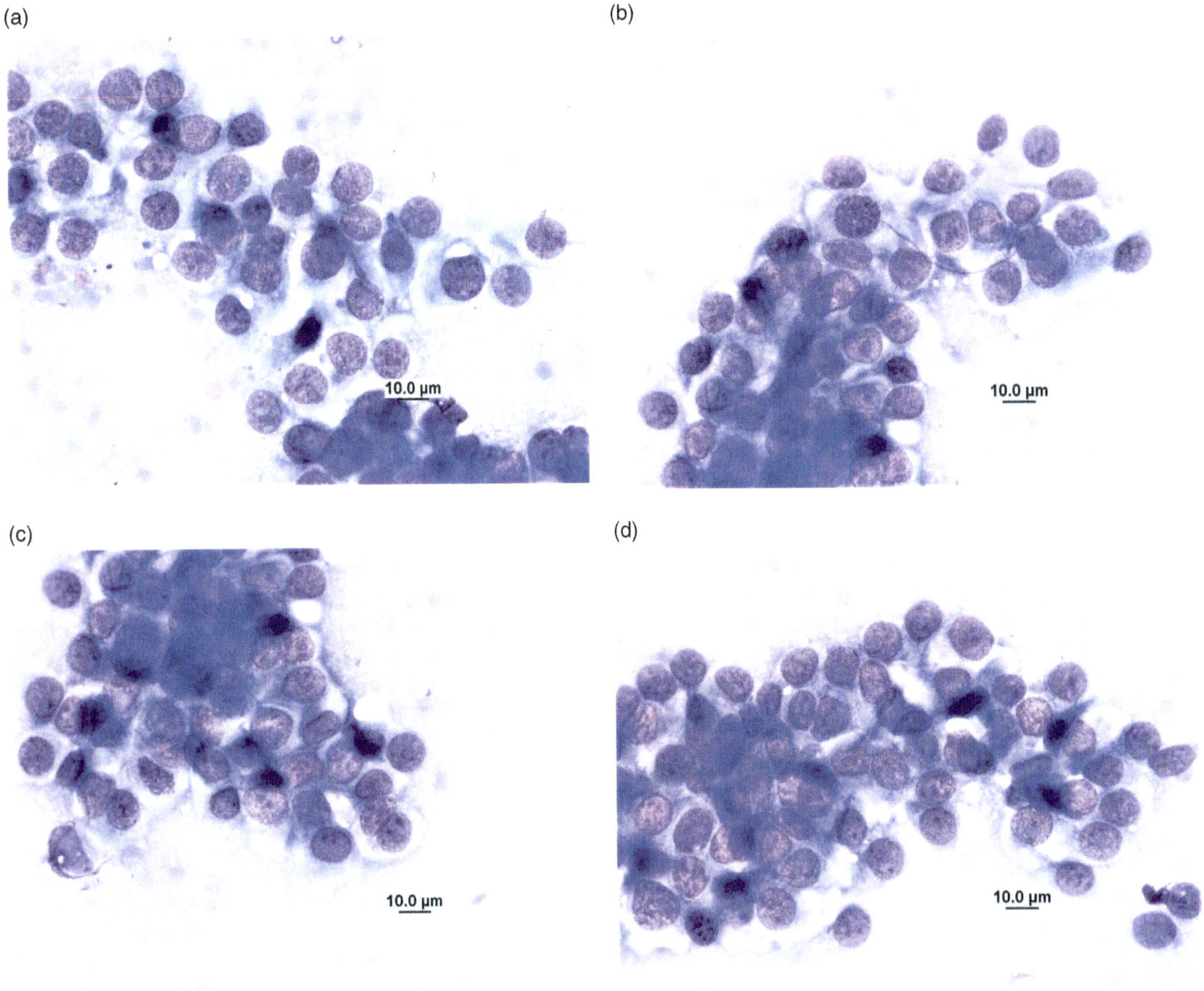

Fig. 8.1. (a)–(d) Cytology of a fine-needle aspirate of the mass (Wright–Giemsa stain, 100× oil).

A 1.5-cm-diameter round firm cutaneous mass was present on the right lateral face, cranial to the ear, caudal to the eye. A dark thick crust with dried bloody discharge covered the mass. Figures 8.2a and 8.2b show the appearance of the mass upon presentation and after the removal of the overlying crust and dried bloody discharge while the rat was under general anesthesia. The mass was cleaned with saline and was found to extend into the ear canal.

A fine-needle aspirate was obtained for cytodiagnosis, and the sample was stained with Wright–Giemsa–Romanowsky stain (Figures 8.3a–8.3c).

Interpretive Discussion

The fine-needle aspirate stained with Wright–Giemsa–Romanowsky stain revealed a highly cellular sample containing epithelial cells with distinct cell borders and occurring in adherent groups. The background contained numerous erythrocytes and occasional degenerate neutrophils. Figures 8.3a–8.3c revealed dense clusters of pale foamy cells with a dense, centrally placed round to oval nucleus. The cells demonstrated moderate anisocytosis and anisokaryosis with mild nuclear pleomorphism and variable N:C ratios. The cells resembled foamy or phagocytic macrophages.

The cytology is indicative of a sebaceous carcinoma with a differential diagnosis of Zymbal gland adenocarcinoma based upon the location of the mass.

Summary

Diagnostic and treatment options for this case included (1) a fine-needle aspiration biopsy with cytology, (2) palliative care with pain medications, anti-inflammatories, and antibiotics if needed, (3) debulking excisional biopsy

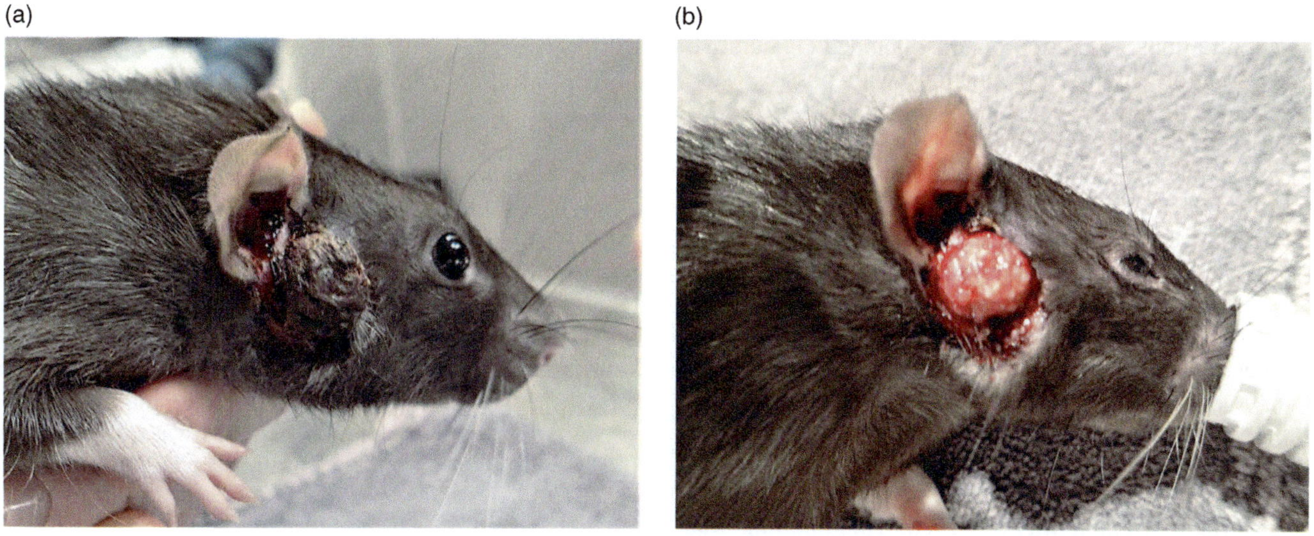

Fig. 8.2. (a) The gross appearance of mass on the rat at presentation during physical examination. (b) With the rat under general anesthesia, gross appearance of mass after removal of overlying crust and discharge.

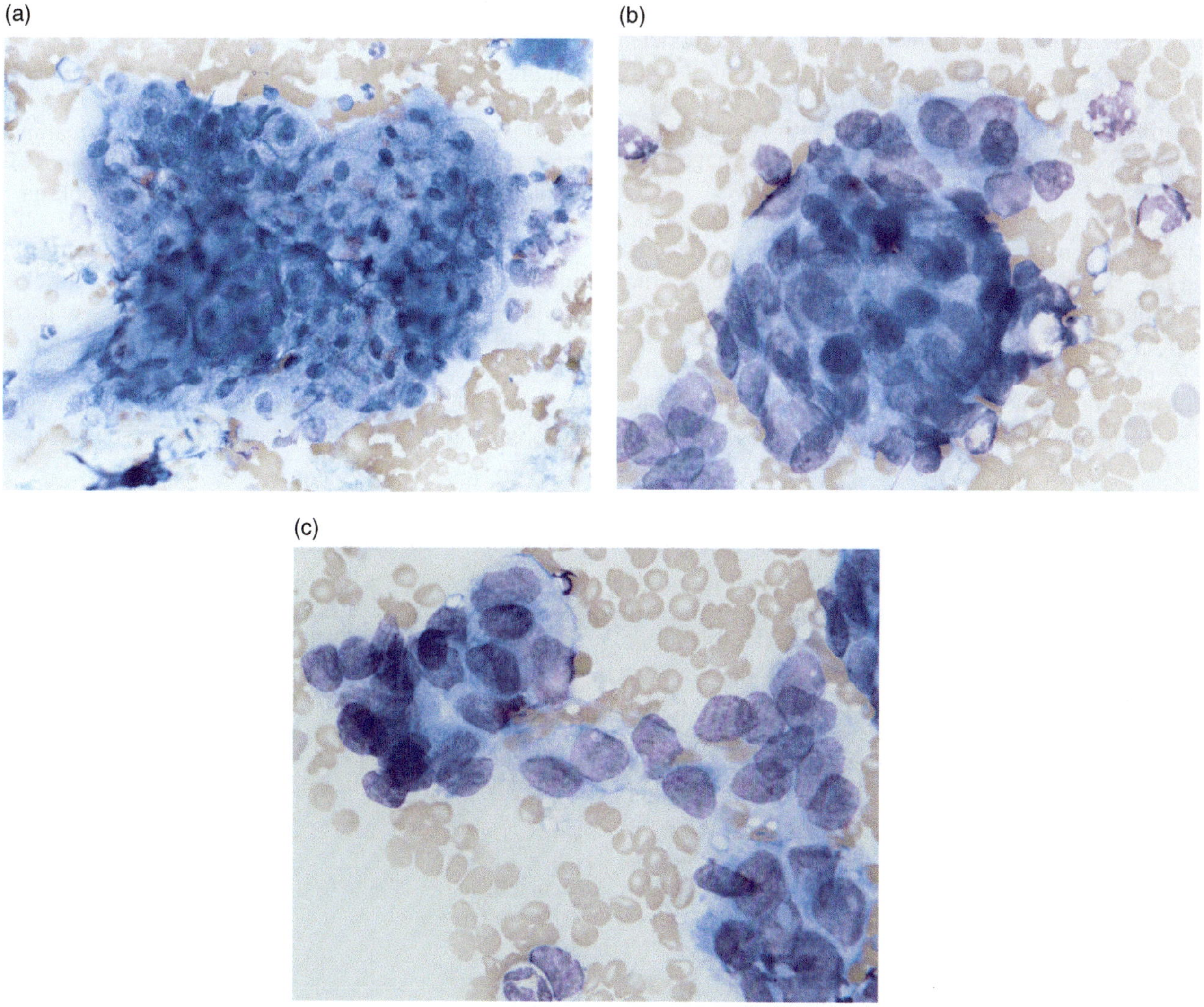

Fig. 8.3. (a)–(c) Aspirate of the mass (Wright–Giemsa stain, 100×, oil).

surgery with histopathology, and (4) different levels of radiation options. Radiation options included (1) curative local radiation (high-level radiation) with possible side effects including pain, vestibular abnormalities, or blindness due to the close proximity to eyes, ears, and brain, (2) three fractions of lower-dose radiation, which is less curative and requires anesthesia for each fraction, and (3) palliative low-dose radiation with once-a-week-fractions following a debulking surgery, which could lead to local cure with less severe side effects. CT planning would be required for the first two radiation options.

The client chose to start with the fine-needle aspiration biopsy and based upon the possibility of a sebaceous carcinoma, a decision to proceed with a debulking surgical procedure with histopathology of the tissue was made. During the mass debulking procedure, entry into the external ear canal was observed. This opening was closed with suture following the removal of the mass.

Histopathologic examination of the mass revealed basaloid cells surrounding cores of cells with sebaceous and squamous differentiation, some containing keratin, and showing moderate anisocytosis. The nuclei were round to ovoid with 1–2 nucleoli, and there was moderate anisokaryosis. A diagnosis of a sebaceous carcinoma was made. The mass was infiltrated diffusely by moderate numbers of neutrophils admixed with lymphocytes and plasma cells. Moderate, multifocal hemorrhage was also noted.

Owing to the proximity of the mass to the ear canal, postoperative neurologic abnormalities consisting of head tilt, circling, and loss of balance were of concern. The patient was fitted with a collar and placed on an antibiotic and nonsteroidal analgesic.

Zymbal glands (auditory sebaceous glands) are small bilateral sebaceous glands located ventral to the orifice of the external ear canal. Zymbal gland tumors arise from acini or ductal epithelium and may be classified as adenomas or adenocarcinomas. Cytologic preparations typically reveal abundant extracellular keratin and small three-dimensional clusters of basaloid round to oval cells with orangeophilic cytoplasm and round to oval monomorphic nuclei with a smooth chromatin in a pale basophilic background. Differential diagnoses included epidermal inclusion cyst, basal cell tumor, Zymbal gland ductular hyperplasia, and Zymbal gland adenoma. Zymbal gland neoplasms are often malignant, locally invasive, and may metastasize to the lungs. Complete mass removal is often impossible due to the aggressive local invasion. Therefore, Zymbal gland neoplasia, like sebaceous carcinoma, has a poor prognosis.

Case 3: Hedgehog with a vaginal mass

Signalment

2-year-old female African pygmy hedgehog (*Atelerix albiventris*)

History

Presented as an emergency for vaginal bleeding and mass protruding from the vagina.

Physical Examination

Bright, alert, responsive. Body weight was 275 g. A 1-cm-diameter round firm ulcerated broad-based mass was intermittently protruding 3 mm from the vagina (Figure 8.4). The mass exhibited areas of vascularity and areas of more normal pink soft tissue. There was blood staining on the fur surrounding the perineal region from a previous hemorrhagic episode from the mass.

A fine-needle aspirate of the mass was obtained and prepared for cytodiagnosis (Figures 8.5a–8.5c).

Interpretive Discussion

The fine-needle aspirate stained with Wright–Giemsa–Romanowsky stain revealed a poorly cellular sample containing pleomorphic mesenchymal cells with indistinct cell borders and a marked number of erythrocytes in the background (Figures 8.5a–8.5c). The cells exhibited a high N:C ratio, often with a scant amount of blue cytoplasm. There was marked anisokaryosis, and the ovoid to elongate nuclei contained coarse chromatin and often multiple nucleoli of varying sizes and shapes. The cytology was consistent with mesenchymal neoplasia.

Summary

A firm swelling surrounding the left elbow associated with a white discoloration of the overlying skin was also discovered on physical examination. With the patient under general anesthesia, an abdominal mass in the area of the uterus could be palpated. The client was

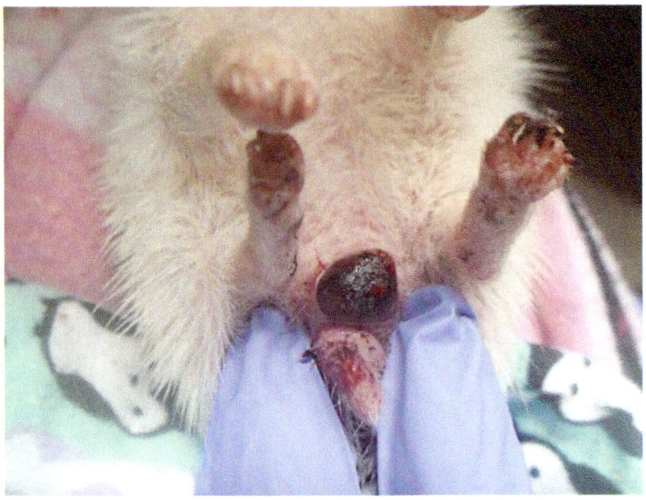

Fig. 8.4. Gross appearance of the vaginal mass on the hedgehog.

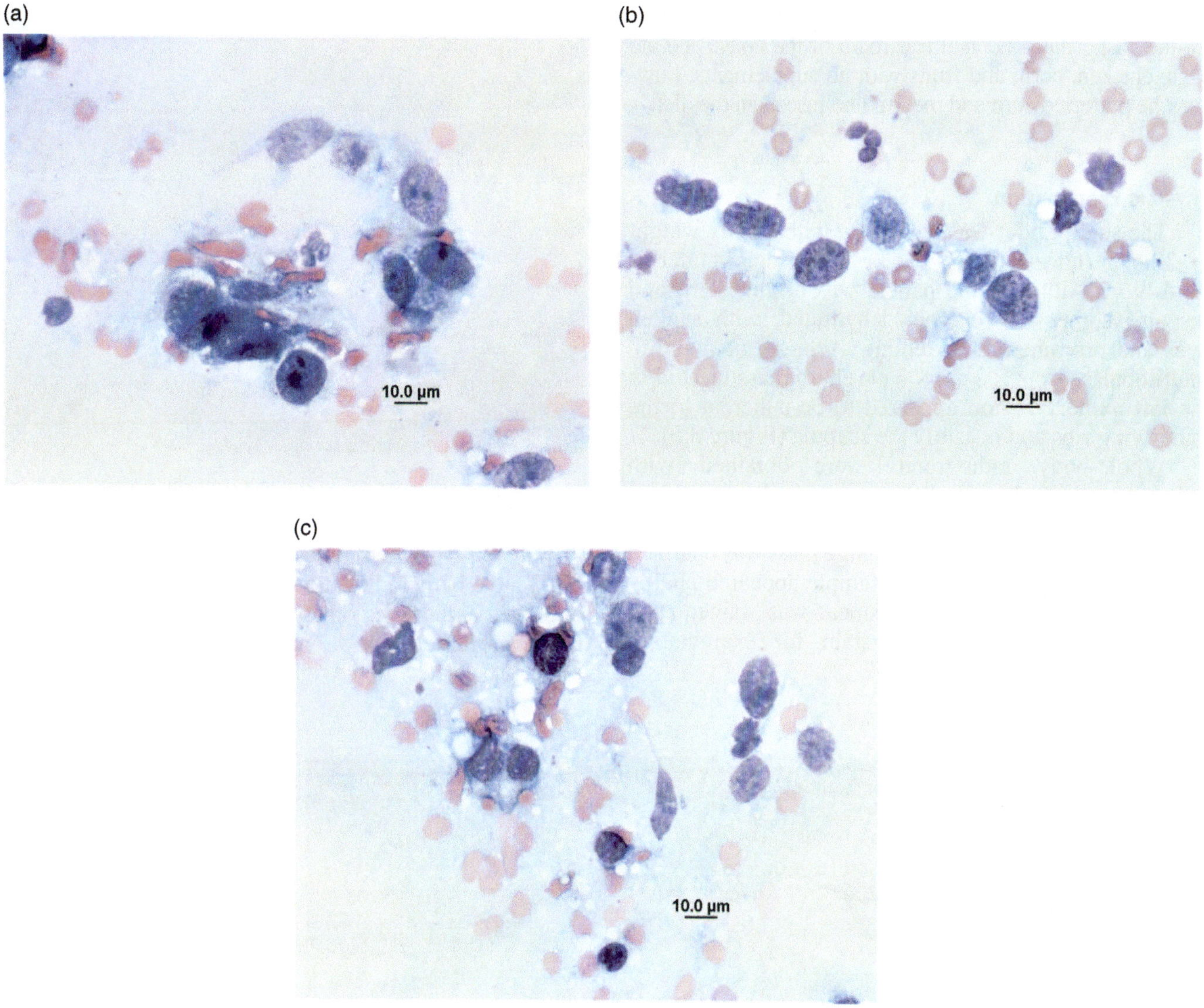

Fig. 8.5. (a)–(c) Cytology of fine-needle aspirate (Wright–Giemsa stain, 100× oil).

offered further diagnostic testing that included a thoracic radiograph to check for metastasis and surgical exploration for possible removal of a uterine mass. The client decided to euthanize the patient, and the body was submitted for necropsy.

Post-mortem findings of a leiomyosarcoma within the vagina and right uterine horn were consistent with clinical suspicion of neoplasia. Findings within the left elbow were consistent with osteosarcoma that likely arose from the cortical bone of the radius. Histopathology revealed the submucosa and myometrium of the vagina and right uterine horn were multifocally expanded and effaced by interlacing bundles and streams of poorly differentiated mesenchymal cells that frequently entrap the normal glandular structures and elevate the overlying endometrium. These neoplastic cells were highly pleomorphic, with varying amounts of eosinophilic cytoplasm with indistinct cells borders. Nuclei were ovoid to elongate, with vesiculate chromatin, 0–2 nucleoli, and displayed marked anisokaryosis. Mitotic index was observed to be 1–2 per single high-powered field (400×). The overlying endometrium was multifocally ulcerated and replaced by large numbers of degenerate neutrophils accompanied by large amounts of hemorrhage and organizing fibrin.

Case 4: Sugar Glider with a Mass in the Left Axilla

Signalment

4-year-old intact male sugar glider (*Petaurus breviceps*)

History

The sugar glider presented as an emergency for severe lethargy and not using his left forelimb. During Thanksgiving, he had a severely lethargic episode that was treated by warming up. He had not been eating or drinking as normal for the past 3 days. He had free roam of the house and ate eggs, chicken, corn, and fruits with no supplements; however, he preferred corn and received no insects in the diet.

Physical Examination

The sugar glider was emaciated with a body weight of 38.6 g (normal for an adult male sugar glider is 90–149 g). Although the patient was bright, alert, and responsive, he was severely dehydrated, with sunken eyes and prominent skin tenting. A large, nonpainful, multilobular (1 cm × 2 cm × 3 cm) hard mass located in the left axillary region appeared to be adherent to the underlying ribs and possibly the scapula (Figure 8.6).

Whole-body radiographs were obtained with the patient under isoflurane general anesthesia (Figures 8.7a–8.7c).

A fine-needle aspirate of the large mass was obtained for cytodiagnosis. Grossly, the sample appeared chalky on the slide (Figure 8.8). The smear was stained with Wright–Giemsa–Romanowsky stain for examination (Figures 8.9a and 8.9b).

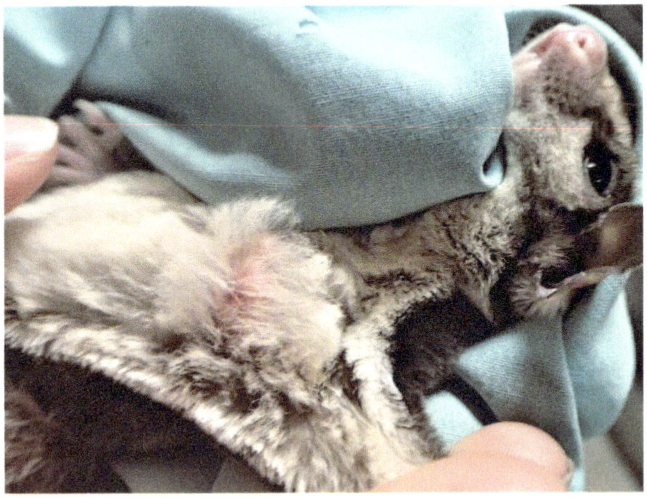

Fig. 8.6. Image of the mass in the left axillary region.

Interpretive Discussion

Whole-body radiographs revealed a mineralized mass in the left axillary region that was associated with the left rib cage, the left elbow, and the left scapula. A smaller mass associated with the right scapula was also identified.

(a)

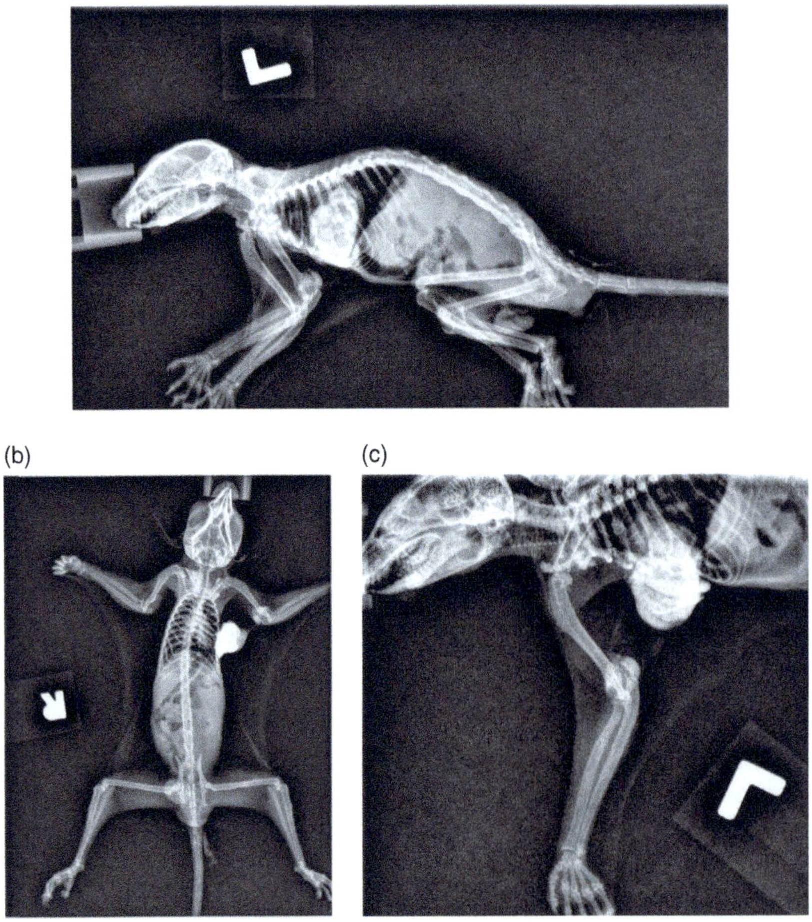

Fig. 8.7. (a) Lateral whole-body radiograph, (b) VD whole-body radiograph, (c) lateral radiograph of thoracic area.

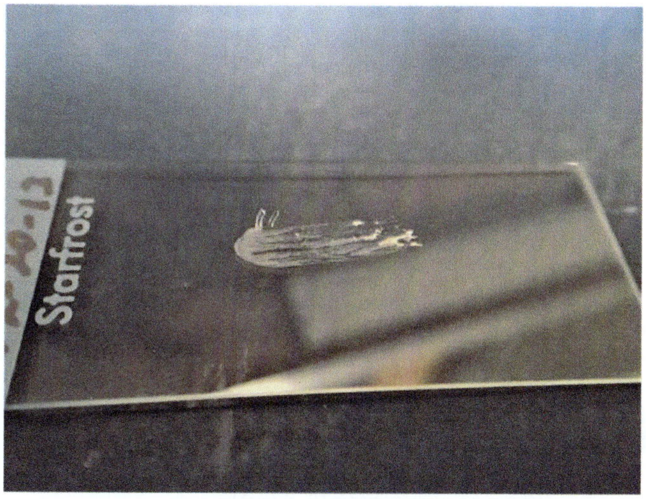

Fig. 8.8. Appearance of aspirated sample.

The cytology revealed numerous refractile crystals of varying shapes and sizes. A few cells presumed to be macrophages and lymphocytes were seen among the crystals. A cytodiagnosis of calcinosis circumscripta was made based upon this finding.

Summary

Recommended treatment for calcinosis circumscripta is complete surgical removal of the lesion; however, in this case, such a procedure would likely have an unfavorable outcome considering the poor health (likely associated with chronic malnutrition) of the patient and the location of the lesion. Therefore, correction of the husbandry and improvement of the overall health was the first order of medical care for this patient.

Case 5: Ferret with an Abdominal Mass

Signalment

11-month-old neutered male ferret (*Mustela putorius furo*)

History

Presented with a two-week history of vomiting and lethargy. The ferret was treated for diarrhea caused by a clostridium infection (based upon fecal cytology) when he was 3 months old.

Physical Examination

On physical examination, the ferret appeared thin (body weight 675 g) and lethargic. A nonpainful, firm abdominal mass was noted on abdominal palpation.

A blood sample was obtained for a blood profile (Tables 8.1 and 8.2). Whole-body radiographs and an abdominal ultrasound examination were performed (Figures 8.10a and 8.10b).

Radiograph images revealed multiple gas-filled loops of small bowel within the right caudal abdomen. There was decreased serosal detail within the mid-ventral abdomen on the lateral view. A poorly defined soft tissue mass effect within the mid-abdomen was seen on both views, causing displacement of the bowel. The stomach was empty. Multiple rounded soft tissue opacities (representing either loops of bowel or mesenteric lymph nodes) were seen on the VD view within the mid-abdomen medial to the head of the spleen. The liver, spleen, kidneys, thorax, and osseous structures appeared normal. The radiograph findings suggested (1) decreased serosal detail could represent peritoneal effusion, such as neoplastic effusion, hemorrhage, or transudate

(a) (b)

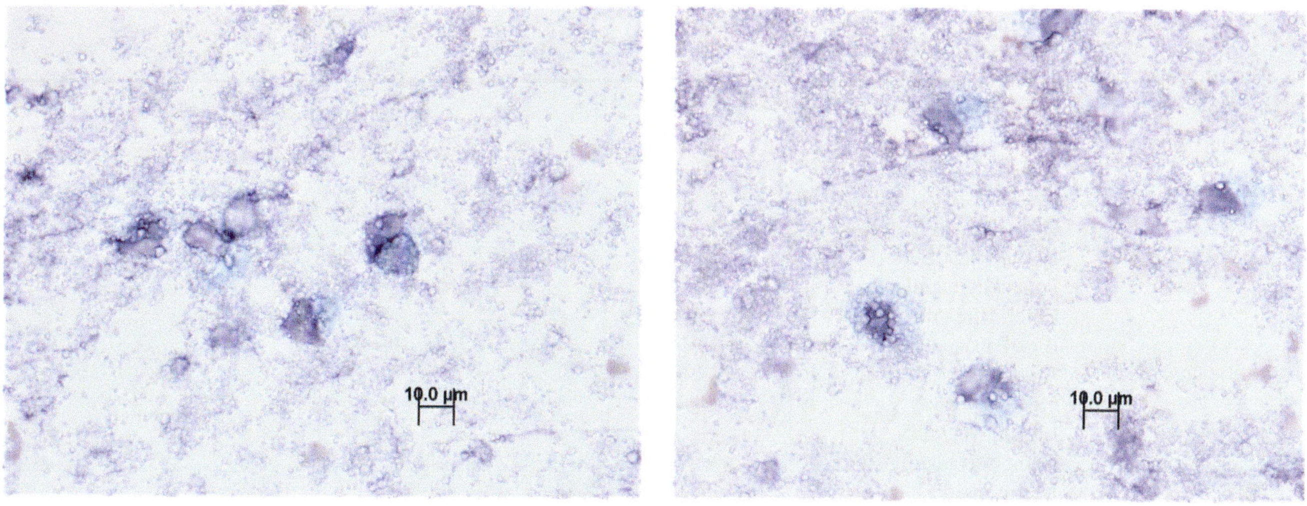

Fig. 8.9. (a), (b) Aspirate of the mass (Wright–Giemsa stain, 100× oil).

Table 8.1. Ferret hematology results (Case 5).

		Reference[a]	Reference[b]	Reference[c]
WBC ×10³/µL	16.9	4.0–9.0	4.4–19.1	7.7–15.4(11.3)
Neutrophils ×10³/µL	11.2	1.5–3.5		—
%	66		11–82	24–78(40)
Lymphocytes ×10³/µL	5.6	0.5–5.0		—
%	33		12–54	28–69(50)
Monocytes ×10³/µL	0.2	0–0.5		—
%	1		0–9	3.4–8.2(6.6)
Eosinophils ×10³/µL	0	0–0.5		—
%	0		0–7	0–7(2)
Basophils ×10³/µL	0	0		—
%	0		0–2	0–2.7(0.7)
Plasma protein g/dL	7.9	5.0–6.5	—	—
RBC × 10⁶/µL	9.6	7.0–11.0	7.3–12.2	—
Hb g/dL	14.1	12–18	16.3–18.2	12.0–16.3(14.3)
PCV %	43	35–53	44–61	36–50(43)
MCV fL	45	47–52	—	—
MCHC g/dL	33	33–55	—	—
RDW	12.8	—	—	—
Platelets 10³/µL	180	—	297–730	—
MPV fL	7.7	—	—	—
Clumped platelets	Present			

[a]Colorado State University reference ranges; [b]Fox (1988); [c]Carpenter (2005, male fitch ferret).

Table 8.2. Ferret plasma biochemical results (Case 5).

		Reference[a]	Reference[b]	Reference[c]
Glucose mg/dL	112	95–140	94–207	63–134(101)
BUN mg/dL	10	10–26	10–45	12–43(28)
Creatinine mg/dL	0.4	0–0.5	0.4–0.9	0.2–0.6(0.4)
Phosphorus mg/dL	5.0	3.0–5.5	4.0–9.1	5.6–8.7(6.5)
Calcium mg/dL	7.9	8.0–9.7	8.0–11.8	8.6–10.5(9.3)
Total protein g/dL	7.1	5.0–6.4	5.1–7.4	5.3–7.2(5.9)
Albumin g/dL	1.1	2.9–4.1	2.6–3.8	3.3–4.1(3.7)
Globulin g/dL	6.0	1.8–3.0	—	2.0–2.9(2.2)
A/G ratio	0.2	1.0–2.2	—	1.3–2.1(1.8)
Cholesterol mg/dL	284	70–200	64–296	—
T. Bilirubin mg/dL	0	0–0.3	<1	—
CK IU/L	84	80–400	—	—
ALP IU/L	14	10–60	9–84	30–120(53)
ALT IU/L	27	80–270	—	82–289(170)
AST IU/L	40	30–75	28–120	—
GGT IU/L	2	1–15	—	5
Sodium mg/dL	140	147–153	137–162	146–160(152)
Potassium mg/dL	3.2	3.3–4.5	4.5–7.7	4.3–5.3(4.9)
Chloride mg/dL	119	114–120	106–125	102–121(115)
Bicarbonate mg/dL	15.6	15–23	—	—
Anion gap	15	14–21	—	—
Calc. osmolality	297	—	—	—
Lipemia mg/dL	5	—	—	—
Hemolysis mg/dL	20	—	—	—
Icterus mg/dL	0	—	—	—

[a]Colorado State University reference ranges; [b]Fox (1988); [c]Carpenter (2005, fitch ferret).

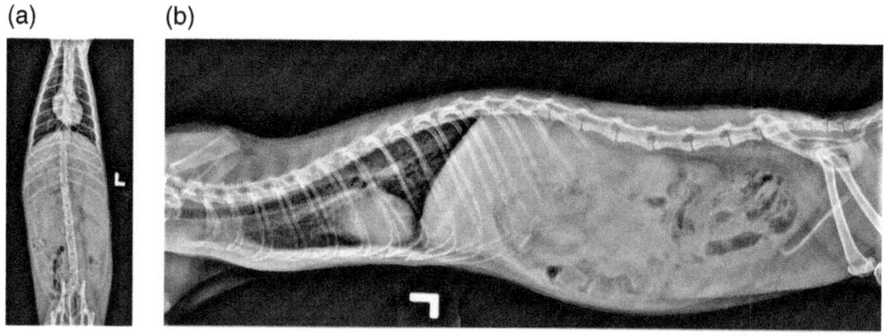

Fig. 8.10. (a) VD whole-body radiograph, (b) lateral whole-body radiograph.

secondary to lymphatic obstruction; (2) soft tissue mass effect in the mid-abdomen could be neoplasia (or abscess or cyst) arising from the spleen, gastrointestinal tract, or mesentery; and (3) gas-filled loops of bowel could be secondary to mechanical or functional ileus.

The abdominal ultrasound detected a large, smoothly marginated, heterogeneous mass with a moderate amount of internal vasculature characterized by Doppler ultrasound within the mid-abdomen between the two kidneys. The mass had multiple hypoechoic areas throughout the parenchyma. The remaining organs of the abdomen were ultrasonographically normal.

The mass in the mid-abdomen, likely of mesenteric origin, was suggestive of severe lymphadenopathy secondary to neoplastic infiltration; however, reactive or granulomatous disease could not be ruled out. Therefore, fine-needle aspirates for cytodiagnosis were performed without immediate complication (Figures 8.11a–8.11d).

Interpretive Discussion

The hemogram indicated a significant leukocytosis and neutrophilia with increased plasma total protein indicative of an inflammatory leukogram.

Significant plasma biochemistry findings indicated a hyperproteinemia and hyperglobulinemia that also supported an inflammatory disease. The hypokalemia was likely associated with anorexia or loss of potassium.

The imprint of the abdominal mass stained with Wright–Giemsa–Romanowsky stain revealed a highly cellular sample with a marked number of mature erythrocytes. The sample consisted of mostly blood as indicated by the presence of numerous platelet microclots. Within this, there were neutrophils that were interpreted to be variously degenerate and increased more than could be accounted for by blood; however, based upon a hemogram indicating a considerable neutrophilia, the sample could be reflective of peripheral blood contamination. There were occasional macrophages. No organisms were seen. The mixture of cells was not specific; however, this pattern is consistent with feline infectious peritonitis lesions. Overall, the cytology indicated suppurative inflammation.

Summary

Based upon the cytology findings, which were compatible with feline infectious peritonitis, the pursuit of a viral etiology was made. However, tests on fresh fecal samples using polymerase chain reaction (PCR) for Aleutian disease virus and ferret enteric coronavirus were negative.

Ten days later, after the ferret was not responding favorably to treatment (famotidine and orbifloxacin), an exploratory surgery was performed where what appeared to be an inoperable effaced lymph node was found. Biopsies of the mass and small intestine were obtained for histopathology.

Histopathology of the mesenteric mass revealed numerous coalescing inflammatory foci composed centrally of large numbers of intact and degenerate neutrophils, admixed with and surrounded by abundant epithelioid macrophages, with a peripheral rim of reactive fibroblasts and fewer lymphocytes and plasma cells. Multifocally admixed with reactive fibroblasts were moderate numbers of small- to medium-caliber blood vessels (neovascularization). Rarely, inflammatory cells surrounded and separated low numbers of mature adipocytes. Peripherally, the inflammatory mass was segmentally lined by villous projections of hyperplastic mesothelial cells. These finding provided a diagnosis of a severe, chronic, diffuse, pyogranulomatous steatitis with villous mesothelial hyperplasia.

Histopathology of the intestinal biopsy indicated a mild to moderate, chronic, diffuse, lymphoplasmacytic, neutrophilic, and eosinophilic enteritis.

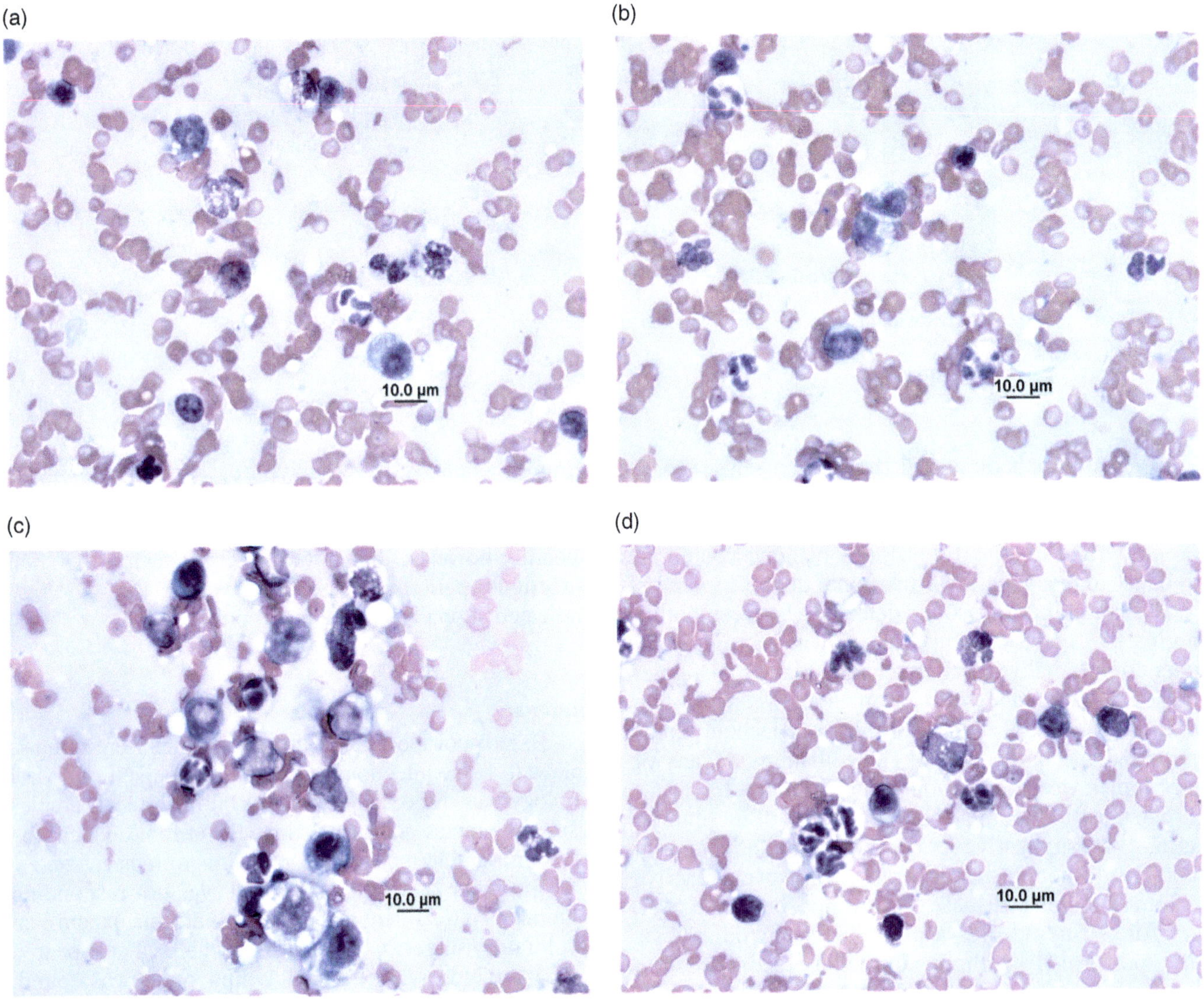

Fig. 8.11. (a)–(d) Aspirate of the mass (Wright–Giemsa stain, 100× oil).

References

Carpenter JW. 2005. *Exotic Animal Formulary*, 3rd edn. St. Louis: Elsevier Saunders, pp. 464–465.

Fox JG. 1988. Normal clinical and biological parameters. In: Fox JG (ed), *Biology and Diseases of the Ferret*. Philadelphia: Lea and Febiger, pp. 159–173.

SECTION II

Avian

9 Blood and Bone Marrow Sample Collection and Preparation in Birds

Blood Sample Collection

Hematology of avian patients consists of a variety of tests and parameters used to evaluate the overall health status of the bird, rule in or rule out disease, evaluate the progression of disease or response to therapy, establish a prognosis, or establish a baseline or database. Consistency in technique when restraining the patient, collecting the blood sample, handling and preparing the blood sample, and processing the blood sample will contribute to the integrity of the sample.

In preparation of blood collection, supplies such as cotton balls, alcohol, needles, syringes, Microtainer® tubes, capillary tubes, and slides should be gathered. The health status of the patient should be determined and the weight obtained during the physical examination. Having a plan in place and determining the priority of diagnostic tests will also contribute to efficient processing and integrity of the blood sample.

Restraint

Blood collection should be performed safely and quickly. Most birds, especially ill birds and small birds (such as finches and canaries), are easily stressed when handled. The stress associated with the capture and restraint of the avian patient, especially those that are ill or those not accustomed to being handled, can further compromise the health of the patient and may affect the hematologic indices.

Blood collection for hematologic evaluation in birds begins with proper restraint. Proper restraint of birds has been previously described in other texts (Ritchie et al. 1997; Wilson, 2001; Girling, 2009) and therefore is not discussed in complete detail here. Many birds can be physically restrained without anesthesia for venipuncture. Cloth towels may be used to restrain most of the common pet psittacine and passerine birds. Birds should be held in an upright position or parallel to the floor; they should not be held upside down, because this may compromise their respiration. Birds must be able to move the keel (sternum) in order to breathe; therefore, excessive restraint around the body should be avoided to prevent asphyxiation. Lastly, the wings and legs should be supported during the process of blood collection to prevent injury to those limbs. Many birds become tractable when the head is covered to reduce vision using a snug-fitting lightweight cloth or hood (i.e., cotton sack or pillowcase-type bag). Birds used for falconry or those in raptor rehabilitation facilities often have properly fitting leather hoods available.

Proper restraint of the avian patient should be safe for both the bird and the handler. Some species of birds are capable of inflicting serious injury to the handler. The talons of raptors and the spurs of Galliformes can injure handlers; therefore, care should be taken to properly and safely restrain the legs of these birds during venipuncture. The beak of many birds can also serve as a weapon; therefore, proper restraint of the head is required to protect the handlers. Large birds, such as ratites, are especially dangerous as their kicks are potentially lethal to the handlers. Communication between the handler(s) and the phlebotomist is also important to ensure the safety of those involved in the procedure.

Blood Volume Collection

Estimates of the total blood volume in birds range from 6 to 12 mL/100 g (approximately 6–12% of body weight), and are variable depending upon the species (Sturkie, 1976). For example, the blood volume of the galah (*Eolophus* [*roseicapillus*] *roseicapilla*) was determined to be 10.66 ± 2.9% of the body weight using the

Exotic Animal Hematology and Cytology, Fifth Edition. Terry W. Campbell and Krystan R. Grant.

Companion website: www.wiley.com/go/campbell/exotic

indocyanine green method (Jaensch and Raidal, 1998). Using 10% as an estimate of the total blood volume, blood samples representing 1% or less of a bird's body weight can usually be withdrawn from a healthy bird without detrimental effects. For example, a healthy 90 g cockatiel (*Nymphicus hollandicus*) or a 30 g budgerigar (*Melopsittacus undulatus*) can easily tolerate the removal of 0.9 and 0.3 mL of blood, respectively. The sample size taken from severely ill birds must be reduced to avoid further compromising the health of the patient. For routine hematologic evaluations in birds, a sample size of 0.2 mL is usually adequate.

Blood Collection Methods

There are a variety of blood collection sites available in birds. The site chosen depends upon the size of the bird, peculiarities of the species, preference of the collector, volume of blood needed, and physical condition of the patient. Blood obtained by venipuncture is used for hematologic studies because venous blood provides the best sample. Capillary blood, such as blood obtained by the clipping of a toenail, is not recommended for hematologic studies. Capillary blood contains abnormal cell distributions, cells, cellular debris, and tissue fluid not found in venous blood, which subsequently interferes with the hematology results. Osteoblasts and osteoclasts in the peripheral blood film have been reported when blood is collected by the toenail clip method owing to the inadvertent biopsy of the third phalanx (Clark and Tvedten, 1999).

A variety of blood collection methods may be used in the avian patient. In general, a short (1.0 inch or less) 27–22-gauge needle attached to a 1- or 3-cc syringe may be used when performing venipuncture on the jugular vein or other large veins in most avian species. A needle with an extension tube, such as a butterfly catheter (Abbott Hospitals, Inc., North Chicago, IL), often aids in the stabilization of the needle during sample collection, which may be useful when collecting blood from some species. Once blood is collected into the syringe, it should be quickly introduced into a collection tube after removal of the needle from the syringe. Remove the tube stopper prior to transfer of the sample to prevent hemolysis and clotting. This method allows the blood sample to be divided into various collection tubes or into other containers, depending on the intended use of the sample.

Blood samples are typically collected into syringes containing no anticoagulant. In certain circumstances, use of a syringe containing anticoagulant may be recommended. However, a disadvantage of this technique is that the amount of blood collected is not always predictable and often results in an inappropriate ratio of anticoagulant and blood. Excessive amount of a liquid anticoagulant could cause dilution of the blood sample and abnormal staining of the cells.

Alternatively, blood can be collected following venipuncture by allowing it to flow through the needle and drip into a microcollection device. An advantage of this method is that collecting blood by allowing it to flow through the needle rather than aspirating into a syringe minimizes hematoma formation. A variety of microcollection devices containing ethylenediaminetetraacetic acid (EDTA) are available for hematologic studies (i.e., Microtainer tubes, Becton-Dickinson, Rutherford, NJ) and may be utilized for this procedure. Microtainer tubes are also available as plain tubes with or without a serum separator or as tubes containing heparin (lithium heparin is preferred) for blood chemistry studies.

Collections Sites

Veins commonly used for venipuncture include the jugular, basilic (cutaneous ulnar, wing or brachial), and medial metatarsal (caudal tibial). Jugular venipuncture can be performed in most species of birds and is the blood collection method of choice for small birds that lack other veins large enough for venipuncture (Law, 1960; Stevens and Ridgeway, 1966; Dein, 1986; Hawkey and Dennett, 1989; Campbell, 1995). Jugular venipuncture allows for a rapid collection time and the ability to easily collect adequate amounts of blood even in small birds, and the tendency for hematoma formation can be minimized with proper attention to technique and hemostasis. The right jugular vein is the site of choice for this procedure because it is typically the larger of the two jugular veins in birds, or may be the only jugular vein present in some species.

Jugular Vein

The jugular vein tends to be highly movable and is surrounded by a large subcutaneous space that predisposes it to hematoma formation during venipuncture. Therefore, the jugular vein must be stabilized before attempting venipuncture. Depending on the size of the bird and whether or not sedation or anesthesia is used, an assistant to hold and restrain the bird may be required. Following adequate restraint, extend the bird's head and neck to allow the jugular vein to fall into the jugular furrow along the lateral side of the neck. Lightly wet the feathers with alcohol to expose the featherless tract (apterium) that overlies the jugular furrow. With a few exceptions (pigeons and doves), the jugular vein is visible through the thin skin on the neck (Figure 9.1). Pressure should be applied to the jugular vein just cranial to the thoracic inlet to occlude and distend the vein, which will facilitate the blood collection process.

Jugular venipuncture should be performed using an appropriate-sized needle and syringe because the large flow rate and the volume of blood present make it difficult to collect blood as it flows from a needle alone

(Figures 9.2a and 9.2b). Introduce the needle into the vein and collect the blood sample by applying only enough negative pressure on the syringe to allow blood to enter the syringe. More vigorous aspiration will cause collapse of the vein, promotes hematoma formation of the vessel, and may cause hemolysis of the sample. Collection of blood with vacuum tubes is not recommended because of the excessive negative pressure that occurs.

Basilic Vein

The basilic (cutaneous ulnar, wing, or brachial) vein is a blood collection site that may be utilized in medium to large birds. This method of blood collection will require an assistant to restrain the bird and to apply pressure to the humeral area to occlude the vein, because proper restraint is crucial in order to prevent wing movement and hematoma formation. Typically, the bird is restrained in dorsal recumbency. One wing is then stretched away from the bird's body, with the elbow almost fully extended. Anesthesia may be required to facilitate restraint because many birds will struggle during this procedure.

The basilic vein crosses the ventral surface of the humeral-radioulnar joint (elbow) directly beneath the skin and is easily visualized by wetting the area lightly with alcohol. Using an appropriate-sized needle, blood can be collected following cannulation of this vein either by aspiration into a syringe or by allowing the blood to drip from the needle hub into a microcollection tube (Figures 9.3a and 9.3b).

To prevent needle movement while aspirating blood into a syringe, the needle can be stabilized by the phlebotomist. This is accomplished by placing the index finger of the free hand alongside the ulna where the basilic vein crosses the elbow. The needle can then be supported as it rests on top of the index finger while it is guided into the vein. If necessary, additional support can be provided by placing the thumb of the free hand on top of the needle (Figure 9.3b). A needle with an extension tube may also minimize needle movement when using a syringe. Hematoma formation is the most common complication associated with this procedure because of movement of the wing or the needle following venipuncture.

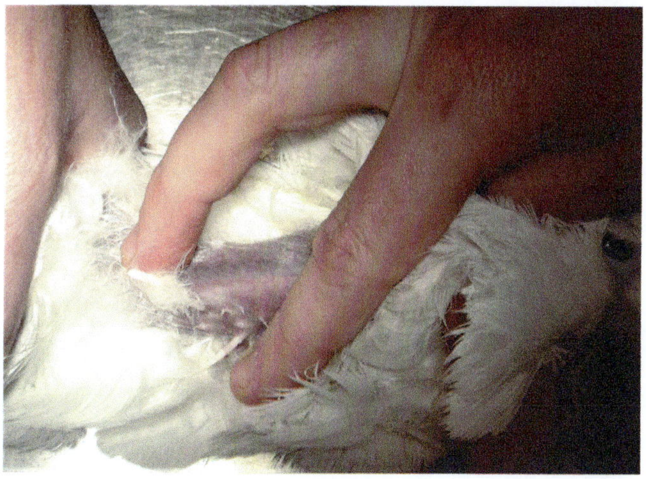

Fig. 9.1. Right jugular vein within the jugular furrow under the apterium of an umbrella cockatoo (*Cacatua alba*).

Medial Metatarsal

Venipuncture of the medial metatarsal (caudal tibial) vein is another common blood collection method in medium to large birds. The medial metatarsal vein is located on the caudomedial aspect of the tibiotarsus just above the tibiotarsus–tarsometatarsal joint and often hides beneath the calcaneal tendon. In order to access this vein, the bird should be restrained in dorsal or lateral recumbency, with the leg extended. Once the leg is

(a) (b)

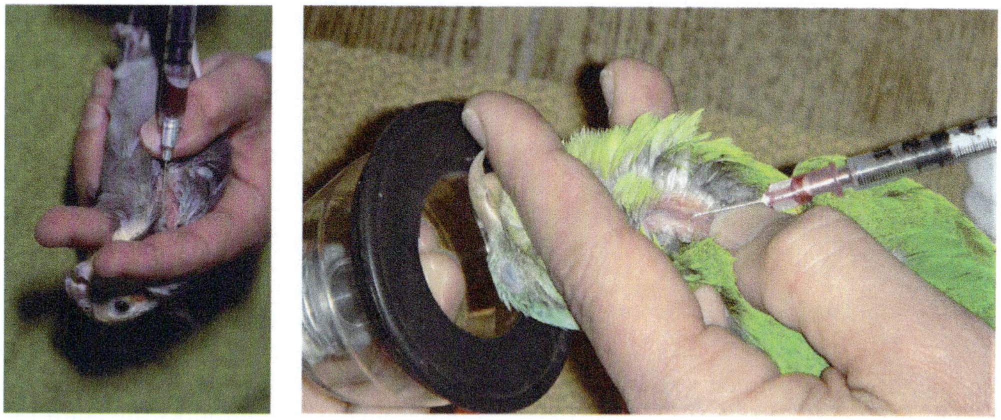

Fig. 9.2. (a) Jugular venipuncture in a cockatiel (*Nymphicus hollandicus*). (b) Jugular venipuncture in a grey-cheeked parakeet (*Brotogeris pyrrhoptera*) while under general anesthesia.

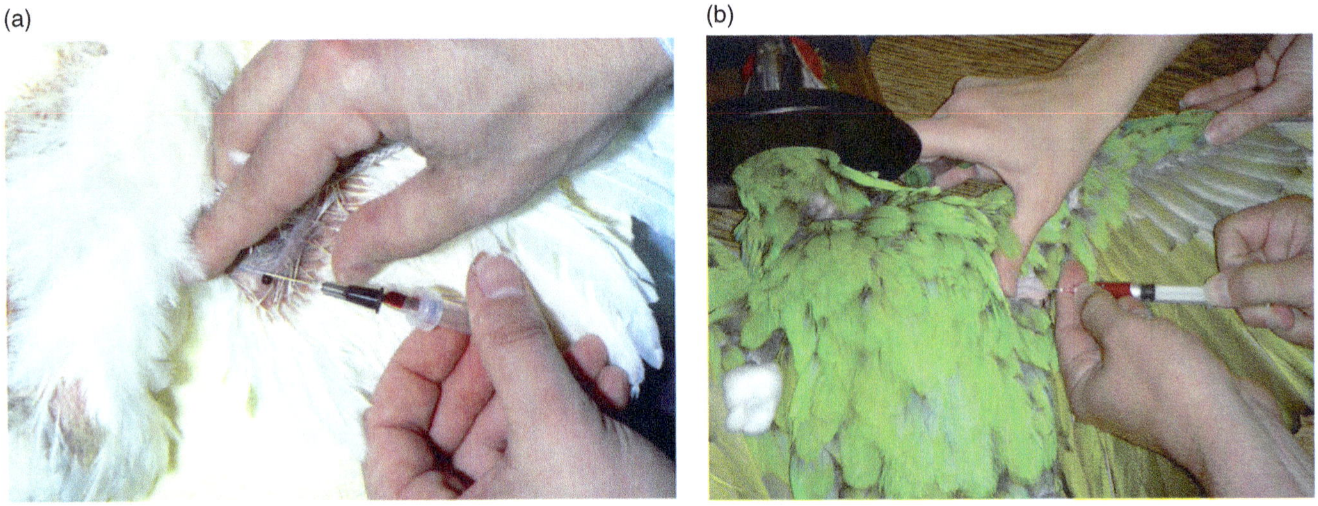

Fig. 9.3. (a) Venipuncture of the basilic vein of a chicken (*Gallus gallus domesticus*). (b) Venipuncture of the basilic vein of a military macaw (*Ara militaris*) under general anesthesia.

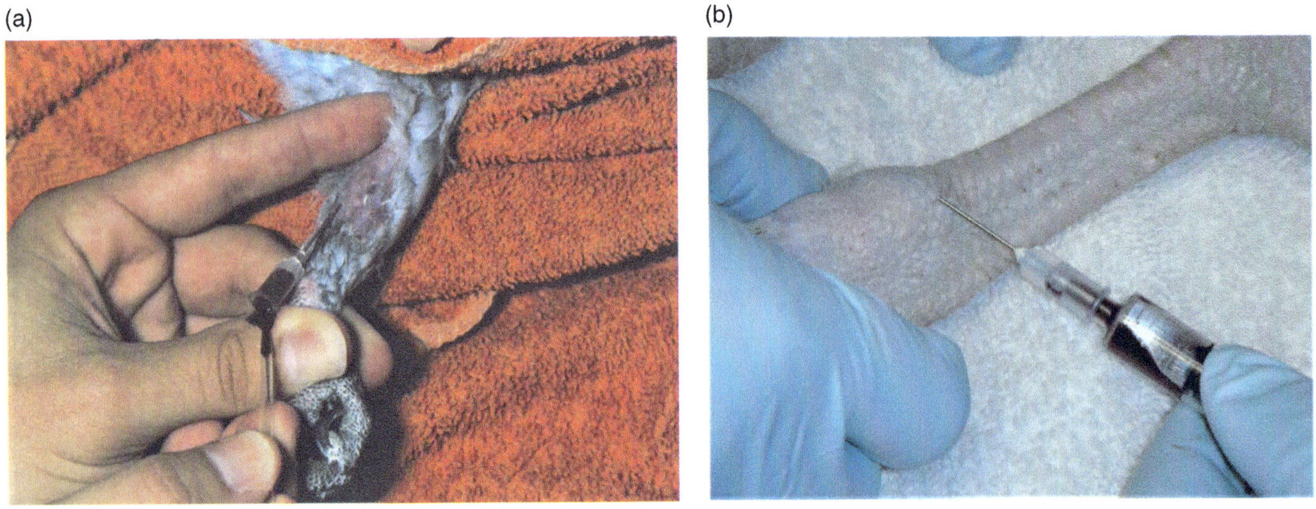

Fig. 9.4. (a) Venipuncture of the medial metatarsal vein of a African gray parrot (*Psittacus erithacus*). (b) Venipuncture of the medial metatarsal vein of a turkey (*Meleagris gallopavo*).

extended and stabilized, a needle is introduced into the medial metatarsal vein at a shallow angle. Blood can be collected by aspiration into a syringe or by allowing blood to drip from the needle hub into a collection tube. Compared to venipuncture of the jugular and basilic veins, hematoma formation is typically minimal following venipuncture at this site because the leg is relatively easy to restrain, and the vein is protected by the surrounding muscles of the leg (Figures 9.4a and 9.4b).

Lancet Wounding

Lancet wounding of vascular structures, such as the basilic vein, medial metatarsal vein, and external thoracic vein, for blood collection should be reserved for very small birds, or when attempts at venipuncture have failed. This method is often used by field researchers collecting small blood samples from small birds. Following alcohol cleansing of the skin overlying the vein, the vessel is punctured through the skin using a lancet (i.e., needle), and the blood is allowed to drip into a microcollection tube.

Cardiac Puncture

Cardiac puncture may be used to collect large volumes of blood (MacArthur, 1944; Andrews, 1950; Utter et al., 1970; Campbell, 1995). This procedure is potentially dangerous and should be reserved for blood sampling from birds used for research or prior to euthanasia. Cardiac puncture may be performed using an anterior or a lateral approach. Restrain the bird in dorsal

(a) (b)

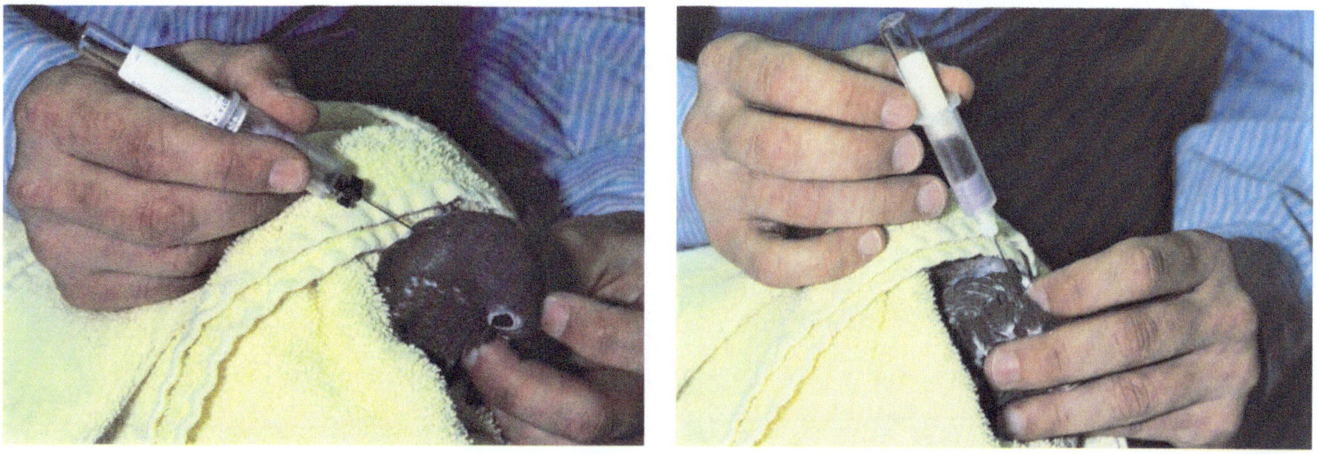

Fig. 9.5. (a) Blood collection from the occipital venous sinus in a pigeon (*Columba livia*) using an evacuated tube with needle and holder. (b) Blood collection from the occipital venous sinus in a pigeon (*Columba livia*) by filling an evacuated tube after penetration of the needle into the sinus.

recumbency for the anterior approach, and approach the heart by inserting a needle along the ventral floor of the thoracic inlet near the V formed by the furculum. Direct the needle toward the dorsal midline and caudal toward the heart. Care must be taken to avoid the ingluvies (crop) in some avian species. Vibration will be felt in the syringe when the needle is placed properly, and the heart is penetrated. The lateral approach is typically used in Galliformes and is performed with the bird held in lateral recumbency. Insert the needle at the fourth intercostal space near the sternum (keel), and angle the needle toward the dorsal midline. There may be some species variability with this approach.

Dorsal Occipital Venous Sinus

The dorsal occipital venous sinus is located at the juncture of the base of the dorsal skull and the first cervical vertebra and may be used to collect large volumes of blood from birds (Vullaume, 1983; Campbell, 1995). Blood collection from the occipital venous sinus requires the use of evacuated glass tubes with appropriate needles and needle holders. Proper restraint is imperative with this technique because of the risk of permanent damage to the brain stem and possible death of the patient. Because of these risks, this method of blood collection should be reserved for birds used in research or prior to euthanasia. Birds should be restrained with the head and neck extended so that the head is positioned in a straight line with the cervical vertebrae. The bird's head is then firmly flexed ventrally. The dorsal occipital venous sinus can then be located by palpation as a depression between the skull and cervical vertebrae. A needle is inserted through the skin at a 30–40° angle to the vertebrae. As soon as the needle penetrates the skin, the rubber stopper of the evacuated tube is perforated gently by the needle in the tube holder, and the needle is advanced until the sinus is reached (Figures 9.5a and 9.5b). Penetration of the sinus results in a rapid flow of blood into the tube.

Toenail

Blood collection using the toenail clip method has been described as a method of sample collection that may be used in some avian species, but is a subject of much debate. When this procedure is performed, blood is collected from a toenail that has been clipped to the bleeding quick after it has been cleaned with alcohol and allowed to dry. Blood is collected into a microcollection tube or microhematocrit tube as it drips from the cut nail. Bleeding is then stopped by applying a hemostatic agent (e.g., silver nitrate or ferrous subsulfate) directly to the nail. Proponents of this method feel that it is quick and easy to perform and causes minimal stress to the bird. Opponents of this method feel that cutting the nail to the bleeding quick is more painful than venipuncture because often birds are temporarily lame following the procedure. The primary disadvantage of this method is that the sample collected from the bleeding nail quick is capillary blood, not venous blood, and often contains cellular debris and cells, such as macrophages, that are not normally found in peripheral blood (Campbell, 1994). For example, osteoblasts and osteoclasts in the peripheral blood film have been reported when blood is collected by the toenail clip method owing to the inadvertent biopsy of the third phalanx (Clark and Tvedten, 1999). In Moluccan cockatoos, *Cacatua moluccensis*, there was agreement in blood samples obtained from the jugular vein and toenail, although there were differences in some parameters like WBC count and hemoglobin (Bennett et al., 2015). Use of the toenail clip method for

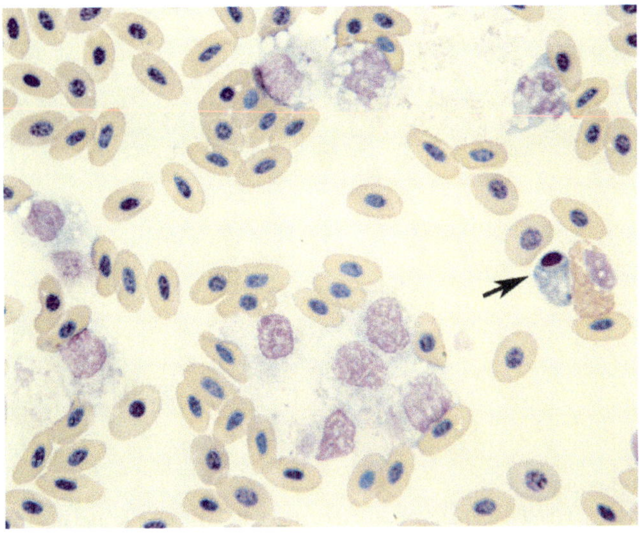

Fig. 9.6. Clumping and vacuolation of cells and cells with pyknotic nuclei (arrow) associated with prolonged exposure (48 h) to EDTA in a blood film from a turkey (*Meleagris gallopavo*). Wright–Giemsa stain, 100× oil.

blood collection in birds should be reserved for very small birds and/or when other methods for blood collection are not feasible (Murray, 1997).

Blood Sample Handling and Preparation

Anticoagulant

Blood samples collected without the use of an anticoagulant require immediate processing for cell counting following collection. If immediate processing is not possible, blood should be transferred immediately from the syringe into tubes containing an anticoagulant. Most avian blood samples are collected into tubes containing an anticoagulant, such as ethylenediaminetetraacetic acid (EDTA), heparin, or sodium citrate. Regardless of the type of anticoagulant used, hematologic testing should be performed as soon as possible after blood collection to avoid artifacts such as increased cell smudging, vacuolization, clumping, or cells with pyknotic nuclei created by prolonged exposure to any anticoagulant (Figure 9.6). Anticoagulant volume should be limited to the smallest amount needed to prevent clot formation. Excessive volume of liquid anticoagulants will dilute the blood sample, resulting in artifactually decreased hematocrit and total cell concentrations. Excess amounts of dry anticoagulants may cause shrinkage of red blood cells, which will affect the hematocrit.

Ethylenediaminetetraacetic Acid (EDTA)

EDTA is the most used anticoagulant. In optimal concentrations, EDTA allows for proper staining of the cells and does not tend to cause clumping of the leukocytes, making it the anticoagulant of choice for hematologic studies (Dein, 1986; Hawkey and Dennett, 1989; Campbell, 1995). However, blood from certain avian groups (crows, jays, ravens, magpies, and some species of ducks, cranes, hornbills, and ratites) may show incomplete anticoagulation or partial hemolysis when collected in EDTA, rendering the blood sample unfit for hematologic studies (Dein, 1986; Hawkey and Dennett, 1989; Walberg, 2001; Cray and Zaias, 2004; Sabino et al., 2010) (Figure 9.7).

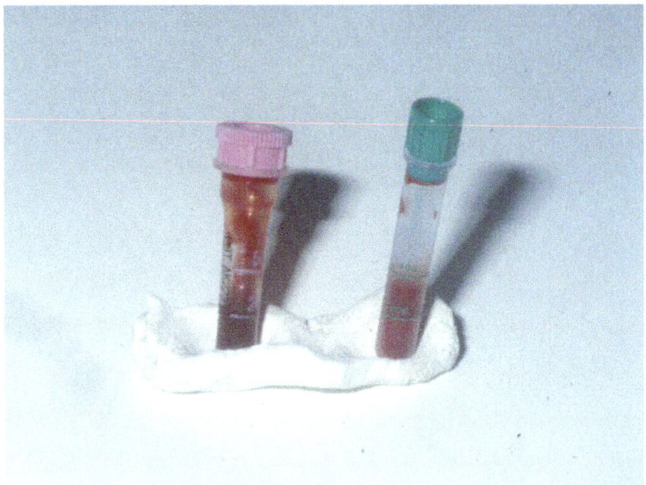

Fig. 9.7. Blood collected from a magpie (*Pica pica*) that has undergone hemolysis when exposed to EDTA (tube on the left), but not in heparin (tube on the right).

Heparin

Heparin prepared at a dilution of 0.2 mL of 1% heparin to 5 mL of blood can substitute for EDTA in situations where the latter cannot be used. Heparin has the advantage of providing anticoagulated blood for hematology and plasma for blood chemistry evaluations. However, heparinized blood may result in improper staining of cells, resulting in erroneous leukocyte counts and poor cellular morphology in stained blood films (Dein, 1986; Jain, 1986; Hawkey and Dennett, 1989; Campbell, 1995). Heparin may also cause clumping of leukocytes and thrombocytes, resulting in inaccurate cell counts (Figures 9.8a and 9.8b). A 3.8% sodium citrate solution used in a ratio of one part citrate solution to nine parts blood is the anticoagulant of choice for coagulation studies.

Whole Blood Preservatives

The use of whole blood preservatives may be useful when there is a delay between blood collection and the determination of the packed cell volume, complete blood cell count, and assessment of hemic cell morphology.

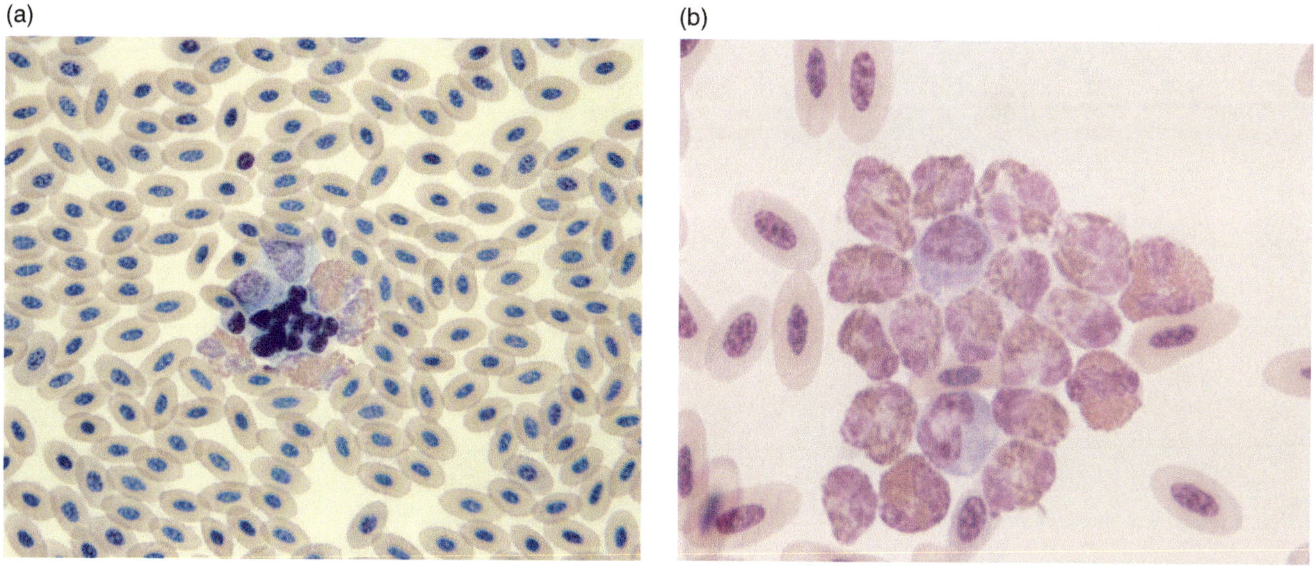

Fig. 9.8. (a) Clumping of leukocytes and thrombocytes in an avian blood film following exposure of the blood to heparin, Wright–Giemsa stain, 1000×. (b) Clumping of leukocytes (heterophils and monocytes) in a red-tailed hawk (*Buteo jamaicensis*) blood film following exposure of the blood to heparin, Wright–Giemsa stain, 1000×.

This is a common situation involving wildlife populations in distant locations. Streck Cell Preservative© (a proprietary proteinaceous stabilizer developed for human flow cytology that has been validated in mammalian species) and formalin (which has been used in fish hematology) can be used is this situation (Arnold et al., 2014; Whitehead et al., 2019; Parlier et al., 2020). Although formalin (200 µL blood combined with 800 µL 10% neutral buffered formalin) is useful for obtaining total white blood cell counts measured by hemocytometer in delayed samples, it results in irregular staining characteristics that prevent an accurate analysis of differential counts and cellular morphology; therefore, use of the Streck Cell Preservative© method is preferred. Both preservatives altered the packed cell volume; however, the values remained constant over time, thus necessitating method-specific reference intervals.

Blood Film Techniques

A stained blood film is an essential part of the hematologic examination because it provides the opportunity to determine the differential leukocyte count and allows assessment of pathologic abnormalities of the various blood cells. A properly made blood film should contain areas with a cellular monolayer that contains evenly distributed individually dispersed cells. Blood films are made using blood with or without an anticoagulant and using a variety of techniques. Avian blood cells are easily ruptured with improper blood film preparation techniques; therefore, it is advisable to use pre-cleaned, bevel-edged microscope slides to minimize cell damage during blood film preparation.

Push-Slide or Two-Slide Wedge Method

The standard or push-slide method commonly used for preparing human and mammalian blood films can be used to create blood films for avian hematology (Schalm et al., 1975; Coles, 1986; Campbell, 1995; Cray and Zaias, 2004; Weiser, 2012). This method involves placement of a drop of blood near one end of a microscope slide that is supported by a solid surface, such as a countertop. The second (pusher or spreader) slide is placed on top of the first slide to form a "wedge" at a 30–45° angle in front of the drop of blood. The pusher slide is backed into the drop of blood and quickly advanced forward in one rapid motion to create the blood film (Figures 9.9a and 9.9b). This method usually provides good cellular distribution and adequate monolayer fields for proper slide evaluation; however, cells are commonly damaged when too much pressure is applied to the pusher slide. To minimize cell damage, a drop of commercially available purified bovine albumin can be applied to a glass microscope slide, followed by an equal amount of blood placed on top of the albumin prior to making the blood film. The albumin should not be allowed to dry before making the blood film.

Alternate Two-Slide Wedge Technique

Another method of blood film preparation using the two-slide wedge technique may aid in minimizing cell damage. Hold the slides rather than allowing one of the slides to rest on a firm surface. The slide on which the blood film will be placed is held in one hand while the pusher slide is held in the other hand. A drop

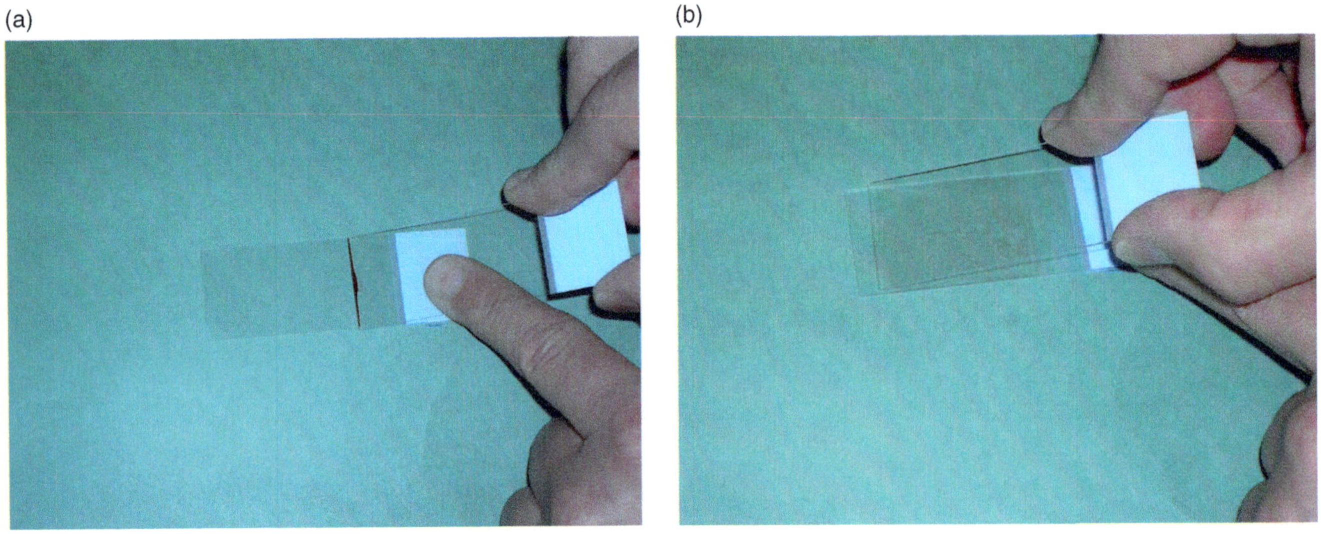

Fig. 9.9. (a) Blood film preparation using the push-slide technique with the slide held on a solid surface and the pusher slide is pulled through the blood droplet. (b) The pusher slide pushed away from the preparer.

of blood is placed near the end of the slide farthest from the person making the blood film, and the pusher slide is immediately placed in front of the drop of blood. The pusher slide is then quickly backed completely through the drop of blood while being held at an angle of approximately 30–45° to the blood film slide. The direction of the pusher slide is immediately reversed toward the opposite end of the blood film slide to make the blood film. The pusher slide, therefore, is brought toward the person making the blood film rather than being pushed away. Most people have better control of the spreader slide when it is being pushed toward them than when it is being pushed away. This step should be performed in one rapid motion that involves a flip of the wrist holding the pusher slide. The advantage of holding the slides rather than allowing the blood film slide to rest on a solid surface is that less downward pressure can be applied to the pusher slide when making the blood film, which results in less cell damage (Figures 9.10a, 9.10b, and 9.10c).

Coverslip Method

Alternatively, blood films can be prepared by using a slide and coverslip, or two coverslips. With proper attention to technique, these methods minimize cellular disruption and maintain good cellular distribution with monolayered areas for examination (Davidson and Henry, 1974; Dein, 1984; Cray and Zaias, 2004; Russell and Heatley, 2020). These methods utilize a coverslip that is pulled across a drop of blood that has been placed on a glass microscope slide or another coverslip. The primary disadvantages of this method include the inability to use an automatic stainer, and the potential for cell rupture (smudge cell formation) and improper cell distribution when improper technique is used.

Stains

Blood cell stains that have been used for staining air-dried avian blood films for hematologic examination include Wright, Wright–Giemsa, Wright–Leishman, and May Grünwald–Giemsa staining methods. Wright's stain or Wright–Giemsa modified stains are the most common stains used in the microscopic evaluation of cells in avian blood films. Quick stains or modified Wright's stains (i.e., Diff–Quik, Dade Diagnostics, Aguada, Puerto Rico, or Hemacolor, Miles Laboratories, Inc., Elkhart, IN) can also be used to stain avian blood films. These stains are convenient and are the most commonly used stains in veterinary practice settings. The use of automatic slide stainers simplifies the staining procedure and provides a means for consistency and high-quality staining of blood films. Automatic stainers remove much of the staining variation that occurs with the hand-staining methods.

Laboratory Submission

When submitting blood samples to a diagnostic laboratory, it is helpful to submit fresh blood films, stained and unstained, along with appropriately filled Microtainer tubes of the blood. Understanding the requirements of submission will help ensure appropriate sample preparation. Helpful information to include with the blood samples and slides are the date and time of

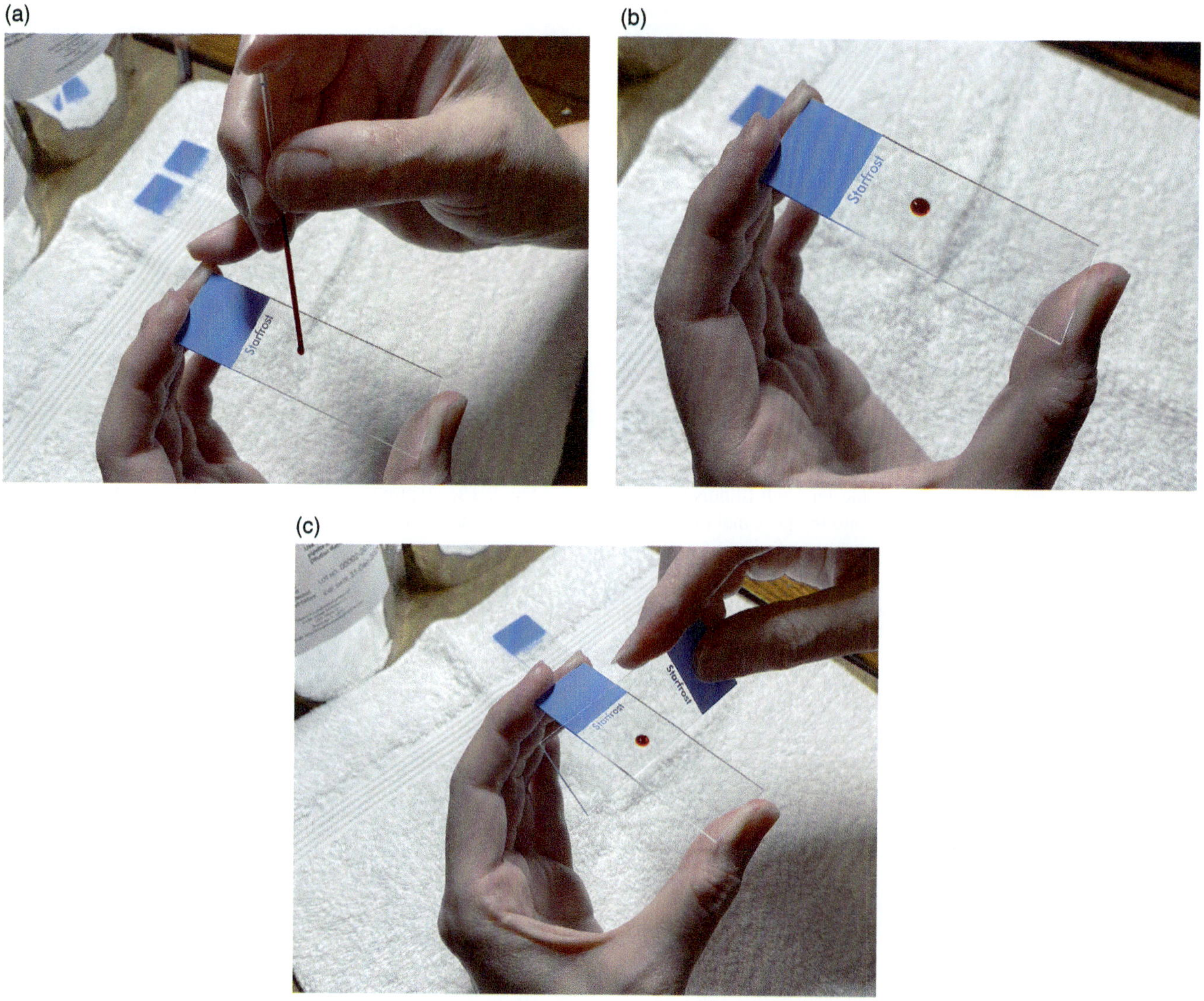

Fig. 9.10. (a) Blood film preparation using the push-slide technique with the slide held in one hand and the pusher slide pushed toward the preparer – using a microhematocrit tube to place the drop of blood onto the slide. (b) Blood film preparation using the push-slide technique with the slide held in one hand and the pusher slide pushed toward the preparer – the blood film is made as soon as the drop of blood is applied to the slide. (c) Blood film preparation using the push-slide technique with the slide held in one hand and the pusher slide pushed toward the preparer.

blood collection, date and time of slide preparation, blood sample condition for the blood film (with/without anticoagulant, anticoagulant type, estimated ratio of anticoagulant and blood), and the stain used if applicable (and/or whether or not the slide was fixed).

Bone Marrow Collection

Bone marrow aspiration may be used to collect bone marrow samples for cytologic evaluation in most avian species. Sites commonly used for bone marrow collection in birds include the proximal tibiotarsus, sternum (keel), and most of the long bones. Marrow cannot be collected from the pneumatic bones (such as the humerus of most birds and femur of raptors). A general anesthetic is usually not required but is recommended to prevent pain and stress to the patient, and to limit patient movement. When necessary, large birds may be manually restrained, and a local anesthetic can be used. Use of an analgesic agent may provide comfort following the procedure.

Collection Sites for Marrow Aspiration

Proximal Tibiotarsus

The most used site for bone marrow collection in birds is the proximal tibiotarsus because the procedure is relatively simple (Van der Heyden, 1987; Campbell, 1995). The medial or cranial aspect of the

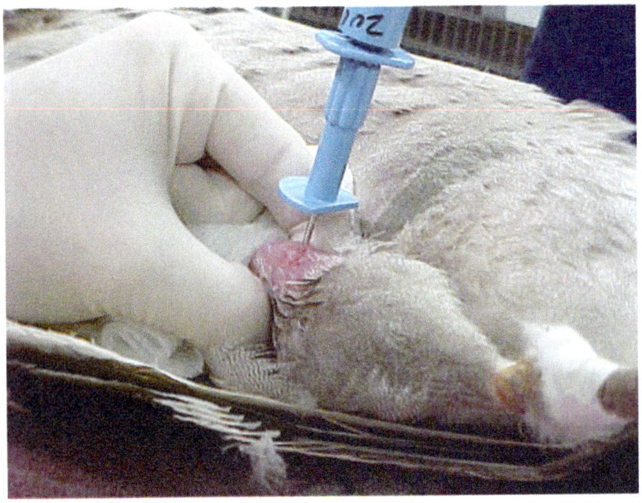

Fig. 9.11. Placement of a disposable Jamshidi Illinois Sternal/Illiac bone marrow biopsy needle into the proximal tibiotarsus of a mallard (*Anas platyrhynchos*).

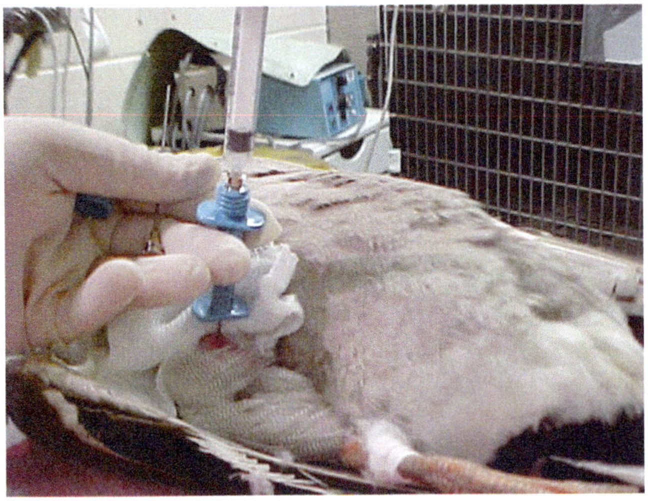

Fig. 9.13. Aspiration of the marrow sample from the proximal tibiotarsus of a mallard (*Anas platyrhynchos*) into the biopsy needle.

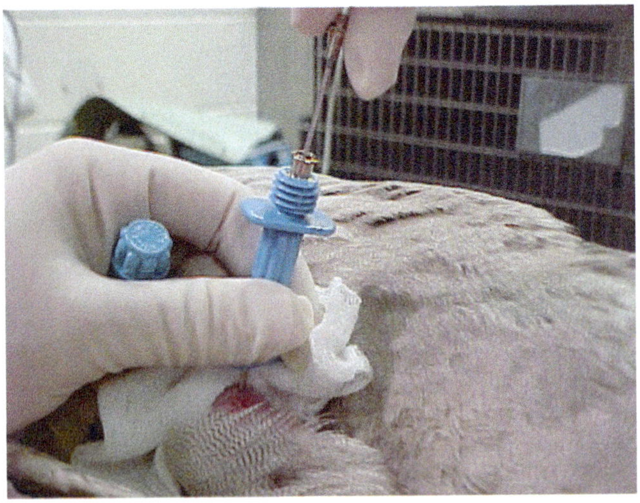

Fig. 9.12. Removal of the stylet of the bone marrow biopsy needle after placement in the proximal tibiotarsus of a mallard (*Anas platyrhynchos*).

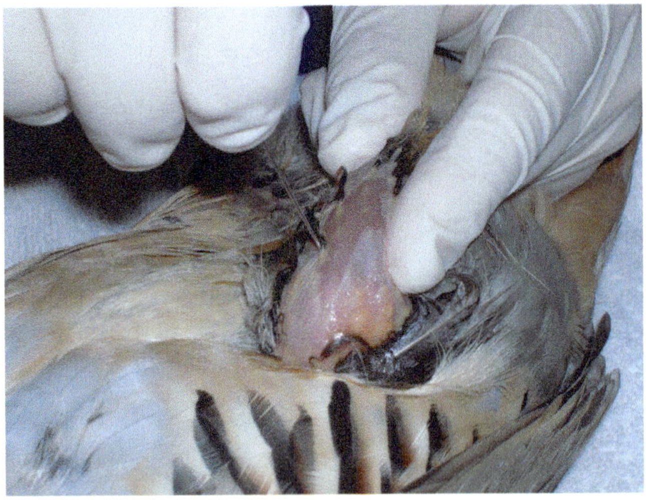

Fig. 9.14. Placement of a disposable spinal needle used as a bone marrow biopsy needle in the proximal tibiotarsus of a chukar partridge (*Alectoris chukar*).

proximal tibiotarsus just below the femoral-tibiotarsal joint is a suitable location for aspiration because of the minimal amount of soft tissue overlying the bone in this area. The site should be prepared as for surgery, a local anesthetic is applied, and a small skin incision is made using a scalpel blade to facilitate passage of the needle through the skin. The needle with a stylet is placed against the bone at a perpendicular angle and is then advanced through the cortex and into the marrow cavity using gentle pressure and rotary movements. The hand not used for manipulating the needle is used to stabilize the tibiotarsus (Figures 9.11–9.17).

Once the needle is positioned into the marrow cavity, the stylet is removed and a 6–12 mL syringe is attached to the hub of the needle (Figures 9.12 and 9.16). Marrow is aspirated into the lumen of the needle by applying negative pressure to the syringe (Figures 9.13 and 9.17). Excessive or prolonged negative pressure should be avoided to minimize blood contamination of the marrow sample. Unlike bone marrow collection from most domestic mammals, an avian marrow sample will be found within the lumen of the biopsy needle; marrow should not appear in the syringe due to the small marrow volume in most birds. Very large birds may be the exception.

When aspiration has been completed, the needle and syringe are removed from the tibiotarsus, making sure negative pressure is not being applied to the syringe to prevent the sample from aspirating into the syringe. The needle is removed from the syringe, and the syringe is

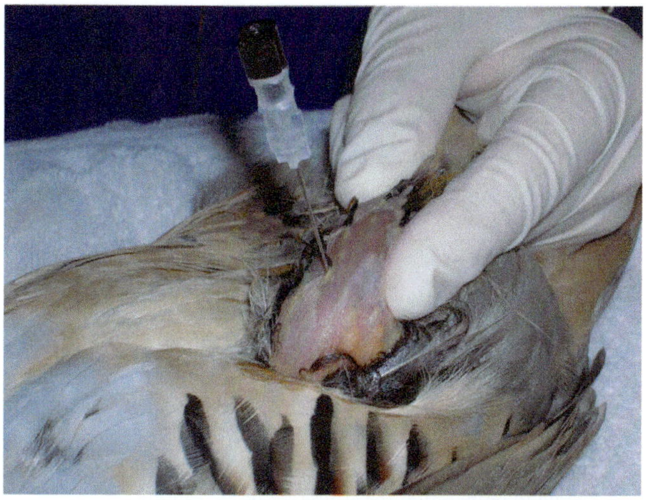

Fig. 9.15. Proper placement of a spinal needle in the proximal tibiotarsus for obtaining a bone marrow sample from a chukar partridge (*Alectoris chukar*).

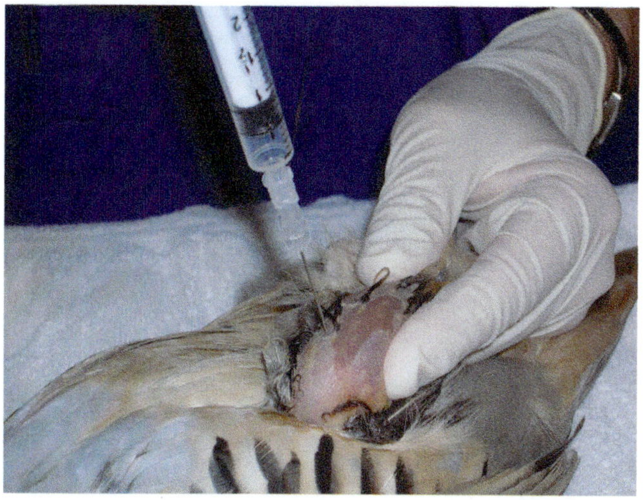

Fig. 9.17. Aspiration of the marrow sample into the lumen of a spinal needle used to obtain a bone marrow sample from the proximal tibiotarsus from a chukar partridge (*Alectoris chukar*).

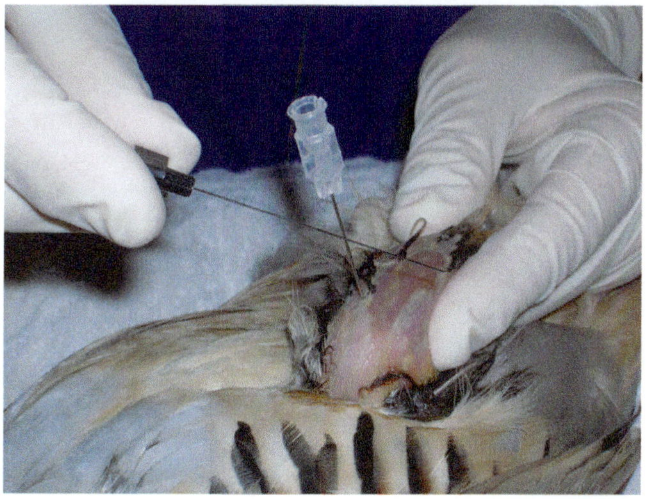

Fig. 9.16. Removal of the stylet from a spinal needle used to obtain a bone marrow sample from the proximal tibiotarsus of a chukar partridge (*Alectoris chukar*).

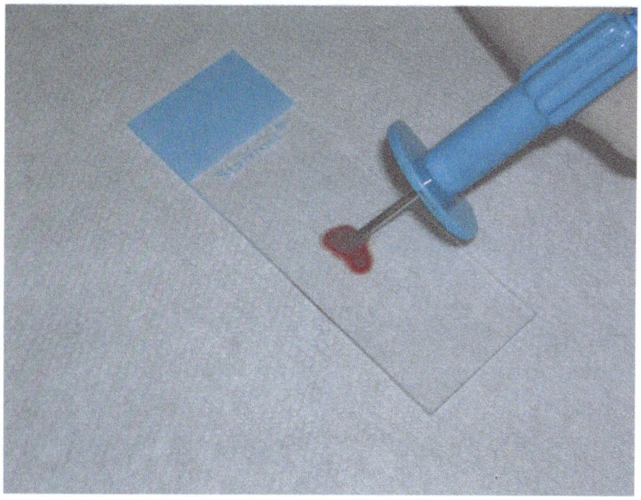

Fig. 9.18. Placement of the marrow sample from within the biopsy needle onto a microscope slide.

filled with air to force the marrow from the needle lumen onto a glass microscope slide (Figure 9.18). A second glass microscope slide is placed on top of the marrow sample, and the marrow is allowed to spread between the two slides as they are pulled apart (Figure 9.19).

Sternum (Keel)

The sternum (keel) is sometimes used as a site for bone marrow collection in some birds, such as Galliformes. A sample is typically collected from the widest part of the sternal ridge. Following surgical preparation and local anesthesia, a biopsy needle is introduced in the same manner described for the proximal tibiotarsus (Figures 9.20–9.23).

Preparation of the Bone Marrow Sample

Aspirated Bone Marrow

Drops of aspirated bone marrow are placed on glass microscope slides that are tilted to allow excess blood to run off. Slides are prepared using a squash prep technique with the remaining bone marrow spicules and stained with routine stains for hematology (Schwartz et al., 2019).

Marrow Core Biopsy

Marrow core biopsies for histologic evaluation can be obtained from birds using a technique similar to marrow aspiration. The biopsy needle is placed in the bone

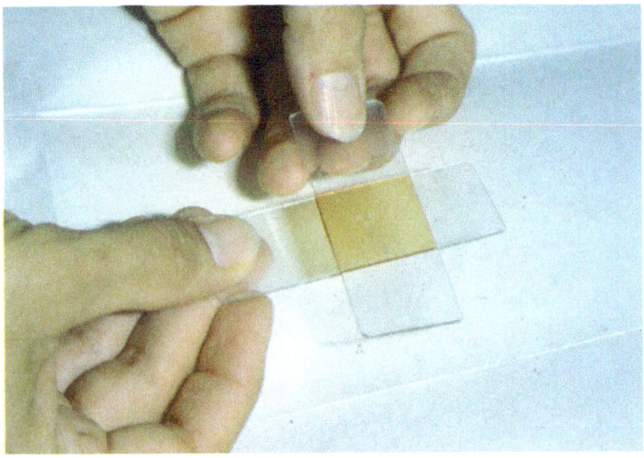

Fig. 9.19. Preparation of the bone marrow aspiration biopsy sample for cytologic evaluation.

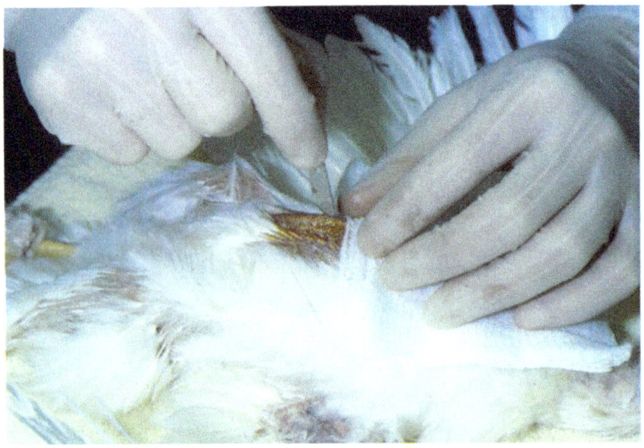

Fig. 9.20. Making a small skin incision over the keel of a chicken (*Gallus gallus domesticus*) in preparation for obtaining a bone marrow sample.

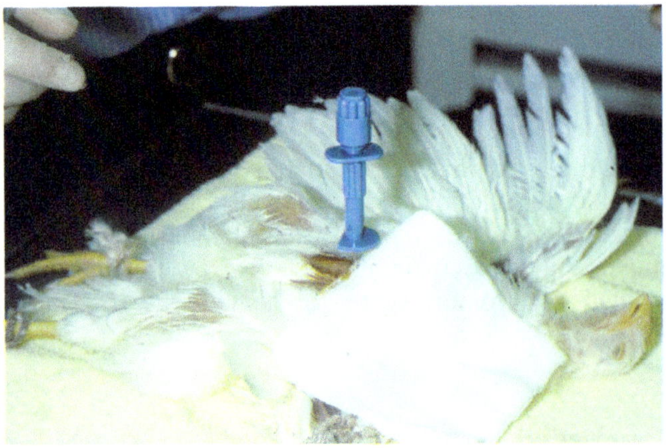

Fig. 9.21. Placement of a disposable Jamshidi Illinois Sternal/Iliac bone marrow needle into the marrow space of the keel of a of a chicken (*Gallus gallus domesticus*).

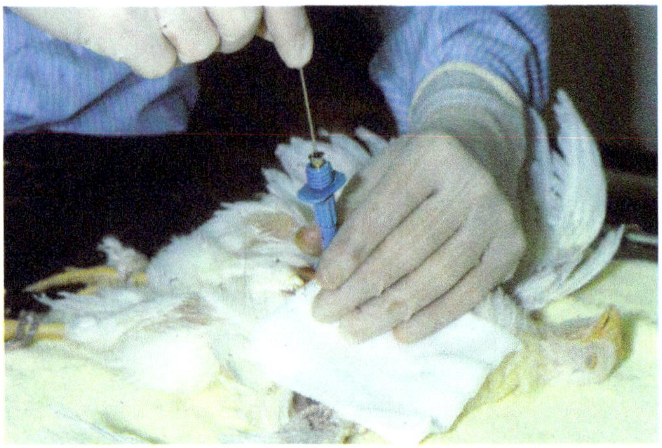

Fig. 9.22. Removal of the stylet from the bone marrow biopsy needle in preparation for aspiration of the sample.

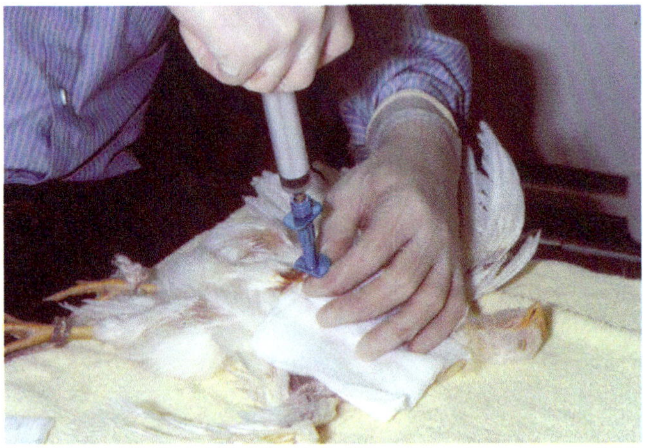

Fig. 9.23. The marrow sample being aspirated into the lumen of the biopsy needle that is placed within the keel of a chicken (*Gallus gallus domesticus*).

as previously described, but once the bone marrow biopsy needle is introduced into the marrow space, the stylet is removed, and the needle is advanced deeper into the marrow cavity toward the opposite cortex. When the opposite cortex has been reached, the needle is twisted and redirected slightly to detach the marrow plug within the lumen of the needle. The needle is then withdrawn from the marrow cavity as gentle negative pressure is applied to the syringe in order to hold the marrow plug inside the lumen of the needle.

The marrow core sample is removed from the needle by reinserting the stylet (usually beginning at the tip of the needle) to push the sample out of the needle. Imprint films can be made from the core sample for cytologic evaluation before the sample is placed in 10% neutral buffered formalin. A sample holder (e.g., tissue cassette for small biopsies intended for histology) is often required to maintain the marrow core while it is being fixed in the formalin solution.

References

Andrews FX. 1950. Simplified heart puncture in poultry diagnosis. *J Am Vet Med Assoc* 16:38–39.

Arnold JE, Matsche MA, Rosemary K. 2014. Preserving whole blood in formalin extends the specimen stability period for manual cell counts for fish. *Vet Clin Pathol* 43(4):613–620.

Bennett TD, Lejnieks DV, Koepke H, et al. 2015. Comparison of hematologic and biochemical test results in blood samples obtained by jugular venipuncture versus nail clip in moluccan cockatoos (*Cacatua moluccensis*). *J Avian Med Surg* 29(4):303–312.

Campbell TW. 1994. Hematology. In: Ritchie B, Harrison G, Harrison L (eds), *Avian Medicine: Principles and Application.* Lake Worth, FL: Wingers Publishing.

Campbell TW. 1995. *Avian Hematology and Cytology*, 2nd edn. Ames, IA: Iowa State University Press.

Clark P, Tvedten HW. 1999. Peripheral blood from a young lorikeet, what is your diagnosis? *Vet Clin Pathol* 28:71–74.

Coles EH. 1986. *Veterinary Clinical Pathology*, 4th edn. Philadelphia, PA: WB Saunders.

Cray C, Zaias J. 2004. Laboratory procedures. *Vet Clin North Am (Exotic Anim Pract): Exotic Pet Manag Tech* 7:487–518.

Davidson I, Henry JB. 1974. *Todd-Sanford Clinical Diagnosis by Laboratory Methods*, 15th edn. Philadelphia, PA: WB Saunders.

Dein FJ. 1984. *Laboratory Manual of Avian Hematology.* East Northport, NY: Association of Avian Veterinarians.

Dein FJ. 1986. *Hematology.* In: Harrison G, Harrison L (eds), *Clinical Avian Medicine and Surgery.* Philadelphia, PA: WB Saunders.

Girling S. 2009. Avian anesthesia. In: Welsh L (ed), *Anaesthesia for Veterinary Nurses*, 2nd edn. Ames, IA: Wiley-Blackwell.

Hawkey CM, Dennett TB. 1989. *A Colour Atlas of Comparative Veterinary Haematology.* London: Wolfe Medical Publications, Ltd.

Jaensch SM, Raidal SR. 1998. Blood volume determination in galahs (*Eolophus roseicapillus*) by indocyanine green clearance. *J Avian Med Surg* 12(1):21–24.

Jain NC. 1986. Veterinary hematology. In: Jain NC (ed), *Schalm's Veterinary Hematology*, 4th edn. Philadelphia, PA: Lea & Febiger.

Law GRJ. 1960. Blood samples from the jugular vein of turkeys. *Poult Sci* 39:1450–1452.

MacArthur FN. 1944. An improved method of obtaining blood from the chicken heart. *Poultry Sci* 23:542–544.

Murray MJ. 1997. Diagnostic techniques in avian medicine. *Semin Avian Exotic Pet Med* 6:48.

Parlier MR, Moore R, Molter CM, Marrow JC. 2020. Evaluation of cell preservatives on the integrity of Attwater's prairie chicken (*Tympanuchus cupido attwater*) whole blood samples over time. *J Zoo Wildl Med* 51(1):116–122.

Ritchie BW, Harrison GJ, Harrison LR. 1997. *Avian Medicine: Principles and Application.* Lake Worth, FL: Wingers Publishing.

Russell KE, Heatley JJ. 2020. Introduction. In: Heatley JJ, Russell KE, (eds), *Exotic Animal Laboratory Diagnosis.* Hoboken, NJ: Wiley-Blackwell, pp. 1–15.

Sabino AJ, Trevelin SC, Ciarlini PC. 2010. Comparison of the effect of ethylenediaminetetraacetic acid (EDTA) and heparin on erythrocytes of ostriches (*Struthio camelus* L.). *Revista Ceres*, *57*(3), 338–342. https://dx.doi.org/10.1590/S0034–737X 2010000300008

Schalm OW, Jain NC, Carroll EJ. 1975. *Veterinary Hematology, Vol. 3.* Philadelphia, PA: Lea & Febiger.

Schwartz D, Guzman DS-M, Beaufrere H, et al. 2019. Morphologic and quantitative evaluation of bone marrow aspirates from Hispaniolan Amazon parrots (*Amazona ventralis*). *Vet Clin Pathol* 2019 48(4):645–651.

Stevens RWC, Ridgeway GJ. 1966. A technique for bleeding chickens from the jugular vein. *Poult Sci* 45:204–205.

Sturkie PD. 1976. Blood: physical characteristics, formed elements, hemoglobin, and coagulation. In: Sturkie PD (ed), *Avian Physiology.* New York: Springer-Verlag.

Utter JM, LeFebure EA, Greenlaw J. 1970. A technique for sampling blood from small passerines. *Auk* 88:169–170.

Van der Heyden N. 1987. Avian hematology. In: Keever M (ed), *Care and Rehabilitation of Injured Owls.* Lincoln, ON: Rannie.

Vullaume A. 1983. A new technique for taking blood samples from ducks and geese. *Avian Pathol* 12:389–391.

Walberg J. 2001. White blood cell counting techniques in birds. *Semin Avian Exotic Pet Med* 10:72–76.

Weiser G. 2012. Laboratory technology for veterinary medicine. In: Thrall M, Weiser G, Allison RW, Campbell TW, (eds), *Veterinary Hematology and Clinical Chemistry*, 2nd edn. Ames, IA: Wiley-Blackwell, pp. 3– 33.

Whitehead MC, Vanetten CL, Zheng Y, Lewbart GA. 2019. Hematological parameters in largemouth bass (*Micropterus salmoides*) with formalin-preservation: comparison between wild tournament-caught and captive-raised fish. *PeerJ* DOI 10.7717/peerj.6669

Wilson L. 2001. Psittacine restraint in the examination room. In: Rupley A (ed).*Vet Clin North Am (Exotic Anim Pract): Avian Pet Medicine.* Philadelphia, PA: WB Saunders.

10 Hematologic Techniques for Quantitative Assessment in Birds

The in-house veterinary laboratory evaluation of the blood sample of birds involves the same routine procedures used in mammalian hematology, with a few modifications. As in mammalian hematology, hematologic evaluation of avian blood samples begins after the sample is prepared with preferred stains and solutions using a centrifuge, microhematocrit tube, refractometer, hemacytometer, and slides. The systematic approach to evaluating the avian hemogram involves an assessment of cell and plasma parameters, morphologic features of the cells, and intra- and extracellular parasites. This chapter focuses on obtaining the sample parameter counts or concentrations, with some interpretation of the avian hemogram. Chapter 11 will continue with procedures on the avian hemogram with a focus on evaluating the blood film by identifying the morphologic features of the cells and parasites as well as the interpretation of findings.

Erythrocyte and Plasma Parameters

The basic primary avian hematologic procedures include a packed cell volume (PCV) by centrifugation (or hematocrit (HCT) by calculation), a plasma total protein estimation by refractometry, determination of hemoglobin concentration by spectrophotometry or hemoglobinometer, erythrocyte concentration using Natt and Herrick's solution dilution and a hemacytometer, and a stained blood film evaluation. Appendix B, Table B.5 provides guidelines for evaluating avian erythrocytes.

PCV

The PCV provides the percentage of whole blood that is composed of erythrocytes. Determination of the PCV via the microhematocrit method is the most commonly used method for evaluating the red cell mass of birds. The total erythrocyte count (TRBC) or erythrocyte concentration value, described later in the chapter, is commonly reported as well, but it is not as useful for clinical interpretation and generally parallels the PCV and hemoglobin concentration (Weiser, 2012). The TRBC may be useful in calculating red cell indices or for calculating the HCT when instrument determinations are used.

Preparation of the microhematocrit tube with the blood sample can be done as described for mammals (Weiser, 2012). It is determined using the standard manual technique that employs microhematocrit tubes, tube sealant, a microhematocrit centrifuge (12 000 *g* for 5 min), and a tube-reading card or device. The three distinct layers observed in the spun microhematocrit tube of mammals are also present in blood samples from birds. The plasma column is located at the top of the tube, and the packed erythrocytes are located at the bottom. The buffy coat appears as a small white band located just above the erythrocyte column, and consists of leukocytes and thrombocytes. The buffy coat typically increases in size when the leukocyte concentration increases.

A smear of the buffy coat can be prepared by breaking the spun microhematocrit tube at the plasma–buffy coat interface using a diamond pen (or other tool) to cleanly break the tube. The buffy coat is deposited onto a glass microscope slide, and a cytologic sample is prepared using a technique similar to the preparation of a bone marrow aspiration sample and stained with a Romanowsky used for the examination of a blood film. The buffy coat smear is examined to study the presence of atypical blood cells and hemoparasites. It should be noted that the buffy coat is slightly variable in avian hematology and differs from that of mammals. In mammals, the position of cells

Exotic Animal Hematology and Cytology, Fifth Edition. Terry W. Campbell and Krystan R. Grant.

Companion website: www.wiley.com/go/campbell/exotic

in the buffy coat layer is related to cell densities, with heavier cells (granulocytes) in the bottom layer and lighter cells (platelets) at the top, with younger erythrocytes positioned below the granulocytes; however, in birds, there is extensive mixing of the cells (lymphocytes and thrombocytes; heterophils and erythrocytes), and immature erythrocytes are found above the granulocytes (Pinto et al., 2018). Because heterophils can be found admixed with erythrocytes inside the buffy coat, the use of the height of the buffy coat layer as a rough indicator of leukocyte number is not warranted in lower vertebrates (especially in reptiles).

Much as in mammals, the PCV of birds is affected by the number and size of the erythrocytes, as well as changes in the plasma volume that do not affect the total cell mass. These changes include increased plasma volume (hemodilution), decreased plasma volume (hemoconcentration), improper blood sampling (hemodilution), and epinephrine administration and hypothermia, which may result in hemoconcentration. The normal PCV of many species of birds ranges between 35% and 55% (see Appendix B for the PCV ranges of selected species). Therefore, a PCV less than 35% is suggestive of anemia, and a PCV greater than 55% suggests dehydration or erythrocytosis (polycythemia). Anemia and erythrocytosis are described in more detail in Chapter 11.

Hemoglobin

There are generally two methods of determining the total hemoglobin concentration for birds: the cyanmethemoglobin method (using alkaline Drabkin's solution), which estimates hemoglobin from methemoglobin with a spectrophotometer, or by using a hemoglobinometer, which estimates hemoglobin from azide-methemoglobin (Clark et al., 2008; Velguth et al., 2010; Gustavsson, 2015; Samour, 2016). The standard cyanmethemoglobin method used to obtain the total hemoglobin concentration for birds is similar to that used for mammals, with one modification: the cyanmethemoglobin reagent–blood mixture has to be centrifuged prior to analysis. The free nuclei from lysed erythrocytes are removed before obtaining the optical density value, in order to avoid overestimating the hemoglobin concentration. Using a hemoglobinometer, such as the HemoCue® (HemoCue America, Brea, CA), allows the blood to be mixed with a dry reagent within a cuvette prior to insertion into the device, which reads the sample with a built-in photometer. The use of the HemoCue system has been validated for some avian species, but the obtained values may need to be corrected (Harter et al., 2015; Gustavsson, 2015).

It should be noted that a proportional relationship exists between hemoglobin (Hgb) concentration from a hemoglobinometer and PCV in avian blood samples. A simplified relationship of Hgb (g/dL) = 0.30 × PCV provides a reasonable estimate of Hgb concentration from the PCV of birds from the orders Anseriformes, Columbiformes, Falconiformes, Galliformes, Passeriformes, Psittaciformes, Sphenisciformes, and Strigiformes, but a separate relationship of Hgb = 0.217 × PCV + 6.69 might be warranted for the order Phoenicopteriformes (Velguth et al., 2010).

Avian hemoglobin has four iron-containing heme subunits, as with mammalian hemoglobin, but the protein moieties (i.e., globulins) are different (Dieterien-Lievre, 1988). In avian erythrocytes, the phosphate compounds influencing the affinity of hemoglobin for oxygen also differ from those in mammals. The hemoglobin of mature birds contains myo-inositol pentaphosphate, not 2,3-diphosglycerate as in mammals. Inositol pentaphosphate causes hemoglobin to have a lower affinity for oxygen, and it shifts the oxygen dissociation curve to the right of the mammalian curve. Therefore, avian tissues can extract oxygen more readily from hemoglobin than from mammalian tissues. Birds that fly at high altitudes during migration, like the bar-headed goose, have a higher affinity to oxygen, which shifts the oxygen dissociation curve to the left, compared to other birds, like ducks and chickens (Scanes, 2014).

The hemoglobin concentration in birds may be used to further assess or confirm their physiologic condition with respect to their ability to fulfill their oxygen need. In conjunction with PCV, hemoglobin concentration can offer a similar assessment from a biochemical perspective as opposed to a cytological one (Minias, 2015).

Total Erythrocyte Concentration

The total erythrocyte concentration in birds can be determined using the same automated or manual methods used for the determination of total erythrocyte counts in mammalian blood. Electronic impedance cell counters provide a rapid, reliable method for obtaining total red blood cell concentrations. Erythrocyte counts with electronic cell counters are slightly inflated by the inclusion of leukocytes and thrombocytes in the count; however, these additional cells are not significant in most samples as they make up approximately 0.1% of the peripheral blood cell population. Alternatives for automated counting include flow cytometry and image processing using thresholding methodology (Beaufrere et al., 2013; Samour, 2016; Autaiem et al., 2019; Meechart et al., 2019; Ochoa et al., 2019). Image processing is used to detect the number of cells from the image or the nuclei of the erythrocytes. Red blood cell counting is used as a basic health screening protocol in the broiler industry, and this method of counting is more practical from an economic perspective compared to cytometry (Meechart et al., 2019; Autaiem et al., 2019).

Previously, the two manual methods for obtaining total red blood cell counts in birds were the erythrocyte Unopette (Unopette, Becton-Dickinson, Rutherford, NJ) method used in mammalian hematology and Natt and Herrick's method, which involves the preparation of Natt and Herrick's solution to be used as a stain and diluent (Natt and Herrick, 1952) (see Appendix A). In 2009, the erythrocyte Unopette system was discontinued, but a similar kit is available for manual red cell counts in mammals (Erythro-pette™, Exotic Animal Solutions, Inc. Hueytown, AL, USA), which has been used for counting avian red blood cells (Ferreyra et al., 2015). Natt and Herrick's solution is commercially available as a stain (Vetlab Supply, Palmetto Bay, FL) or within a kit (Natt-Pette™, Exotic Animal Solutions, Inc. Rockledge, FL, USA; Natt-Herricks-TIC®, Bioanalytic GmbH, Germany).

Obtaining manual red cell counts using Natt and Herrick's method involves making a 1:200 dilution of the blood using Natt and Herrick's solution and red blood cell diluting pipettes. Alternatively, use of commercially prepared Natt and Herrick's solution kits provides an easy method for obtaining accurate dilutions for the total erythrocyte determination, because dilutions are made using a provided capillary tube and not a diluting pipette. After mixing, the diluted blood is discharged into a hemacytometer counting chamber (Figure 10.1), and the cells are allowed to settle for 5 min, to the ruled surface, before counting (Figure 10.2). Erythrocytes located in the four corner squares and central square within the large center square of the Neubauer-ruled hemacytometer chamber are counted using any of the manual methods (Figures 10.3a and 10.3b). Using the 40× objective, the cells can be identified for counting (Figure 10.4). Cells on the borders of the squares should be counted on the top and left, but not on the bottom and right borders to avoid redundancy. Both sides of the hemacytometer should be counted separately. If the count totals from each side are within 10% of each other, then the total red blood cell count can be calculated. The number obtained from either side, or an average of the two sides, is multiplied by 10 000 to calculate the total red blood cell count per cubic millimeter (mm^3) or microliter (µL) of blood:

$$(\text{Average count from both sides of chamber}) \times 10\ 000 = \text{RBC/mm}^3$$

This method, as with all manual counting methods, may have an inherent error of 10%; however, it is commonly used in clinical practice.

The TRBC of birds can also be determined using the modified Dacie's solution (Dacie and Lewis, 1968; Samour, 2016). The method is equivalent to using Natt and Herrick's method with the manual red blood cell diluting pipettes.

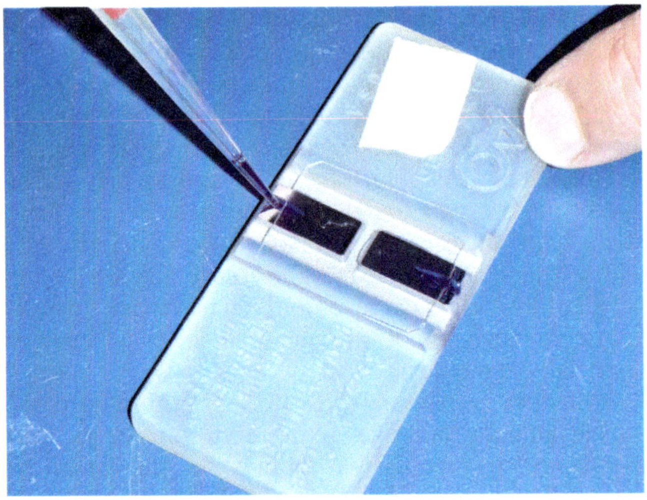

Fig. 10.1. This image shows the diluted blood with Natt and Herrick's solution being discharged into a Neubauer hemacytometer.

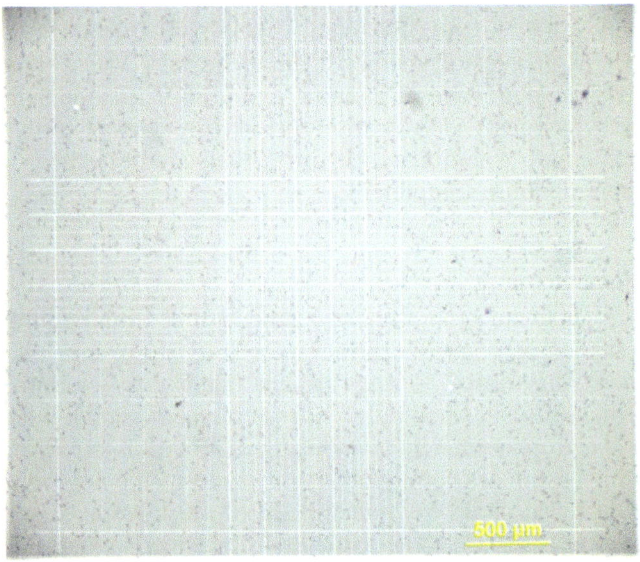

Fig. 10.2. This image shows the counting chamber on one side of the Neubauer-ruled hemacytometer.

Erythrocyte Indices

After the primary hematologic parameters (PCV, erythrocyte count, and hemoglobin concentration) have been determined, the erythrocyte indices can be calculated. These include the mean cell volume (MCV) or mean erythrocyte volume (MEV), mean cell hemoglobin (MCH) or mean erythrocyte hemoglobin (MEH), and mean cell hemoglobin concentration (MCHC) or mean erythrocyte hemoglobin concentration (MEHC). The MCV is an index of the red cell volume and is calculated similarly to mammalian MCV (Samour, 2016):

$$\text{MCV(fL)} = (\text{PCV}(\%) \times 10)/\text{TRBC}$$

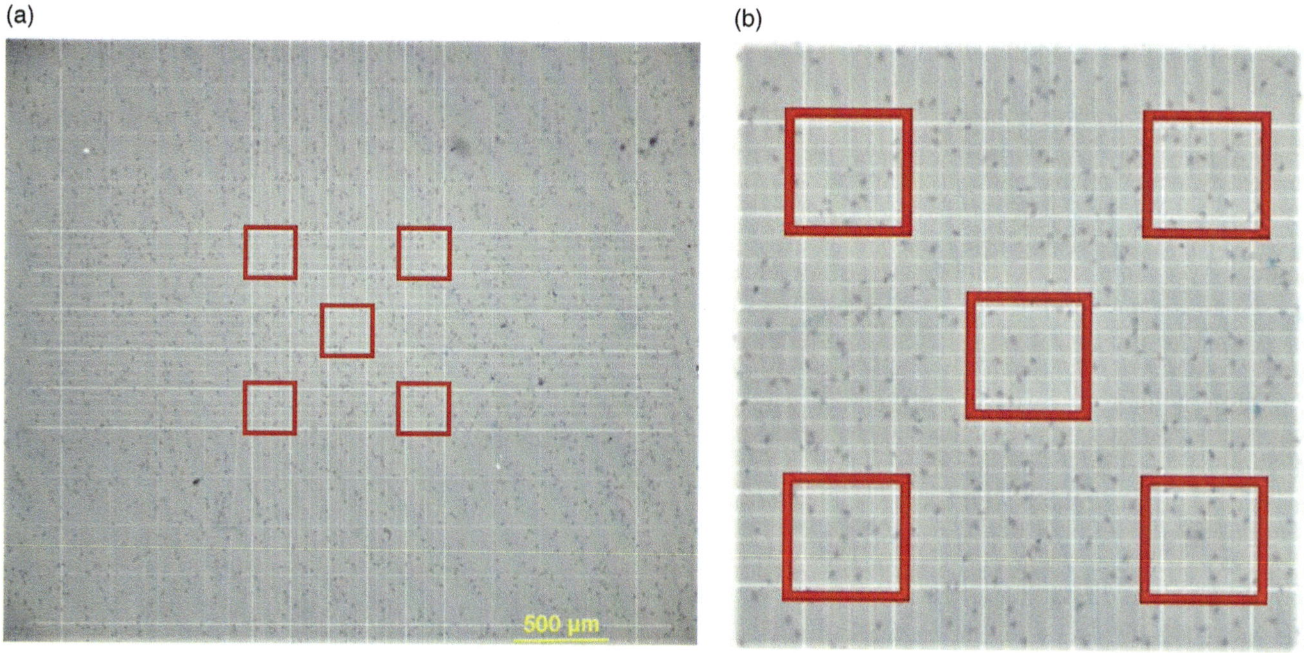

Fig. 10.3. (a) This image identifies the four corners and center square within the large center square of the counting chamber of the Neubauer-ruled hemacytometer. These are the small squares in which the erythrocytes are counted manually. (b) This is a close-up view of the five squares.

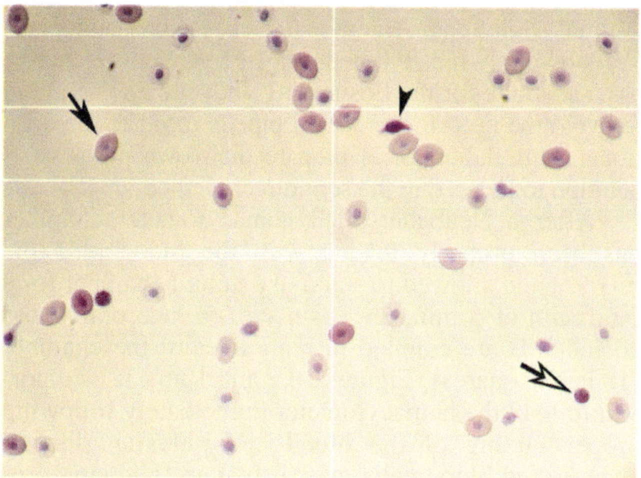

Fig. 10.4. The appearance of cells in a Neubauer-ruled hemacytometer using the Natt-Pette™ system (40×). The solid arrow is pointing to an erythrocyte. The open arrow is pointing to a granulocyte. The arrowhead is pointing to a thrombocyte.

The MCH is an index of hemoglobin content in an average red blood cell and is calculated similarly to mammalian MCH, although it is not commonly used (Weise, 2012). In avian studies, it may help with interpretation when used with other parameters for interpretation (Kloskowski et al., 2017).

MCH (pg) = (Hb (g/dL) × 10)/TRBC

The MCHC is an index denoting the proportion of hemoglobin present in an average erythrocyte and is calculated (Weiser, 2012) as follows:

MCHC (g/dL) = (Hgb (g/dL) × 100)/PCV (%)

Erythrocyte parameters for selected bird species can be found in Appendix B, Table B.5.

Published MCV values for birds generally range between 90 and 210 fL (femtoliters, μm^3), and MCHC values typically range between 20 and 40 g/dL (Hawkins et al., 2018). Although published references are available for the erythrocyte indices of birds, the assessment of abnormal values has not been properly evaluated in these species.

Plasma Appearance and Protein

The color and clarity of the plasma column above the packed erythrocytes should be noted. Normal plasma is typically colorless; however, in some avian species (granivorous birds), it may appear to have a yellow color owing to the presence of diet-related carotene pigments. Clinical icterus is rare because the primary bile pigment of many lower vertebrate species is biliverdin (which is green), not bilirubin (which is yellow). These animals lack the biliverdin reductase enzyme needed to reduce biliverdin to bilirubin. Under rare circumstances, icterus can occur in some avian species (i.e., *Ara* spp.). In these cases, the source of bilirubin is likely associated with posthepatic reduction of biliverdin to bilirubin.

Green plasma is suggestive of biliverdinemia (excess biliverdin bile pigment in blood), and typically is indicative of a poor prognosis for survival. Biliverdinemia may be an indication of hepatic failure or renal failure because the kidney is normally very efficient at clearing bile pigments from the blood. Currently, there are no commercial biochemical tests available to confirm the presence of biliverdin.

Lipemia may be noted in some samples and is most commonly associated with postprandial conditions. It is often not possible to obtain a true fasting blood sample from many avian patients owing to their digestive physiology associated with the presence of a crop (ingluvies). In some cases, lipemic samples may reflect disorders involving lipid metabolism.

Hemolysis may occur and usually results from lysis of erythrocytes during blood collection or sample handling. Intravascular hemolysis may also cause hemolysis of the sample in some instances. If the PCV is normal, then the presence of the hemolysis is probably associated with artifactual lysis of erythrocytes.

Plasma protein concentration is typically determined using handheld refractometers, which have been the standard instruments for determining protein concentration in plasma and body cavity fluid samples since the 1960s (George and O'Neill, 2001). Some authors report good correlation between protein estimation by refractometry and biuret protein in avian samples, but others have not (Morgan et al., 1975; Green et al., 1982; Lumeij and deBruijne, 1985; Andreasen et al., 1989; Lumeij and Maclean, 1996). The major discrepancies between the biuret and refractometric results in these reports may be due to differences in the brand of refractometers used in the study, changes in the alteration of the chemical composition of the biuret reagent, use of different standards, or changes in reaction conditions (George and O'Neill, 2001). Sample-related causes of error in protein determination by refractometric methods include increased nonprotein solids, such as cholesterol, urea, lipoproteins, and glucose (George and O'Neill, 2001). These compounds can increase the refractometric protein measurements by 0.5–1.0 g/dL (5–10 g/L) (George and O'Neill, 2001).

Leukocyte Parameters

Leukocyte counts may be obtained using manual or automated methods. However, significant differences may occur between the manual absolute and relative microscopic leukocyte differential count and the automated absolute and relative leukocyte count techniques (Post et al., 2003). Manual methods for the determination of a leukocyte differential exhibit greater variability compared to automated methods (Russo et al., 1986).

The presence of nucleated erythrocytes and thrombocytes in the blood of lower vertebrates presents a challenge when attempting to apply the automated counting methods used for obtaining mammalian white blood cell counts. The fact that these animals have an erythrocyte that is similar in size to many of the leukocytes, small lymphocytes, and thrombocytes presents an additional challenge. Automated methods tend to yield a higher percentage of monocytes and lower percentage of basophils compared to manual methods when using avian blood; however, there appears to be no difference between the mean percentage of heterophils and lymphocytes. This makes automated methods suitable for determination of heterophil/lymphocyte (H/L) ratios in birds.

Direct and semidirect manual methods for obtaining absolute (total) leukocyte concentrations in animals with nucleated erythrocytes and thrombocytes have been developed.

Semidirect Method for Manual Leukocyte Concentration

A commonly used semidirect method involves the staining of heterophils and eosinophils using phloxine B (a specific stain for mammalian eosinophils) as the diluent. The procedure was simplified utilizing the Eosinophil Unopette 5877 System (Becton-Dickinson, Rutherford, NJ), which was developed for determining total eosinophil concentrations in mammalian blood, but it was discontinued in 2007 (Costello, 1970). When it was available, the avian blood sample was diluted 1:32 with the phloxine B solution in the Unopette vial using the 25 μL pipette provided. The Eopette Test Kit (Exotic Animal Solutions, Hueytown, AL) and Leukopet™ (Vetlab Supply Inc., Palmetto Bay, FL) are now available as a substitute for the Eosinophil Unopette 5877 System to avoid the need for a manual pipette to make the dilutions. Some laboratories prepare their own phloxine B solution to be used in the semidirect method.

After a Neubauer-ruled hemacytometer chamber has been properly loaded with the blood–phloxine mixture and allowed to stand in a humid chamber for a minimum of 5 min, the eosin-stained heterophils and eosinophils are counted in both sides of the chamber (18 large squares) (Figures 10.5 and 10.6). It is important to load the hemacytometer immediately following proper mixing of the blood and phloxine diluent, because red blood cells may also stain following prolonged exposure. Next, the total leukocyte concentration (TWBC/mm^3) is calculated after completing a leukocyte differential to obtain the percent heterophils and eosinophils on the stained blood film using the following equation:

$$\mathrm{WBC/mm^3} = \frac{\left(\text{Total count in both sides of hemacytometer}\right)\times 1.1\times 16\times 100}{\%\ \text{Heterophils} + \%\ \text{Eosinophils from differential}}$$

For example, if the total number of eosin-stained cells counted in the nine large squares on both sides of a Neubauer-ruled hemacytometer chamber (total of 18 squares) is 73, and the differential leukocyte count revealed 16% heterophils and 2% eosinophils, then

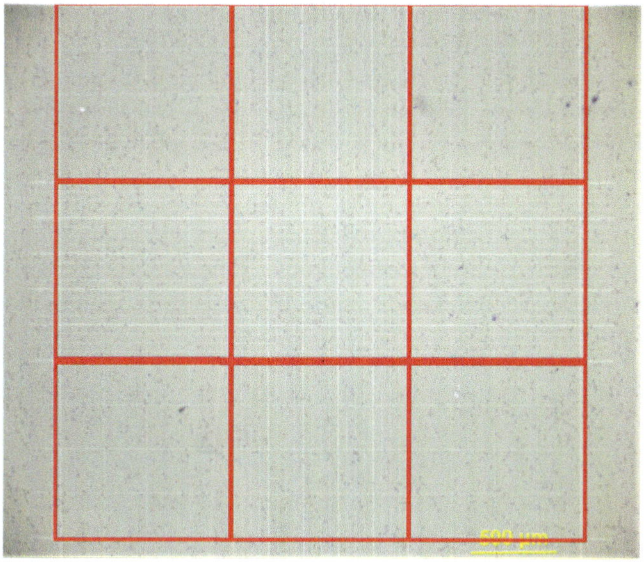

Fig. 10.5. This image identifies the nine large squares of the counting chamber of the Neubauer-ruled hemacytometer. These are the nine squares in which the leukocytes are counted manually.

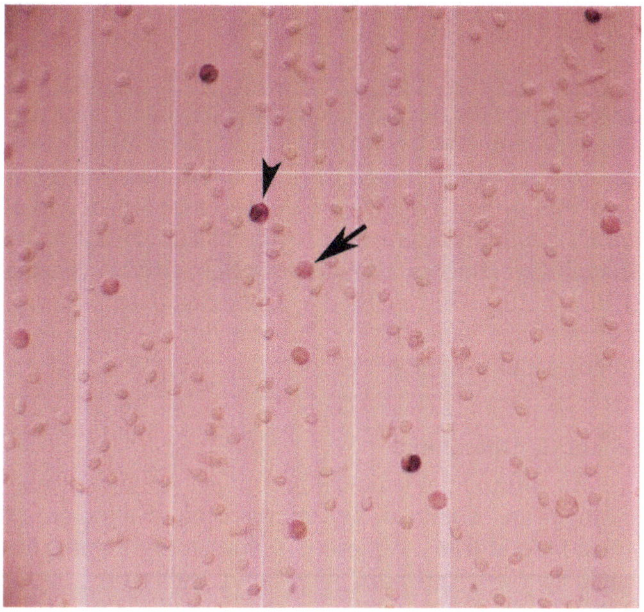

Fig. 10.6. The appearance of cells in a Neubauer-ruled hemacytometer using the Eopette system (40×). The solid arrow is pointing to a heterophil. The arrowhead is pointing to an eosinophil.

using the above formula, the TWBC/mm^3 is calculated to be 7,138/mm^3 when rounded to the nearest whole number.

The phloxine B semidirect method is relatively easy to perform and has been shown to be more precise for hemacytometer counting than Natt and Herrick's method (see next section) (Dein et al., 1994). A disadvantage of this method is that the determination of the total leukocyte count depends on an accurate leukocyte differential (in particular, the number of heterophils and eosinophils present), and the count often becomes less accurate when the mononuclear leukocytes exceed the granulocytes.

Direct Methods for Manual Leukocyte Concentration

Natt and Herrick's Solution

A direct method of obtaining total leukocyte concentrations in avian blood is to make a 1:200 dilution with Natt and Herrick's solution (see Appendix A) using a standard red blood cell diluting pipette. An alternative method would be to add 20 µL of blood to 4 mL of Natt and Herrick's solution. Use of commercially prepared Natt and Herrick's solution kits (Natt-Pette™, Exotic Animal Solutions, Rockledge, FL; Natt-Herricks-TIC®, Bioanalytic GmbH, Germany) provides easy methods of obtaining accurate dilutions for the total leukocyte determination because dilutions are made using a provided capillary tube and not a diluting pipette (Carisch et al., 2019). The leukocytes in the sample will stain dark blue (Figure 10.4). The total leukocyte concentration is obtained by counting all the leukocytes (dark blue cells) in the nine large squares on both sides of the ruled area of the Neubauer-ruled hemacytometer chamber (Figure 10.5). If they are within 10% of each other, the average count of both sides is used in the following equation:

$$\text{TWBC/mm}^3 = (\text{total cells in nine large squares} + 10\%) \times 200$$

The advantage of using this method is that a total erythrocyte and thrombocyte count can also be obtained using the same charged hemacytometer. A disadvantage is that it is often difficult to differentiate thrombocytes from small lymphocytes, thus creating errors in the counts. It has been recommended that staining the blood sample for 60 min in Natt and Herrick's solution improves the differentiation between small lymphocytes and thrombocytes (Robertson and Maxwell, 1990). An alternative approach to the problem of differentiating lymphocytes and thrombocytes using this method is to include thrombocytes in the leukocyte differential and subtract the absolute thrombocyte count from the total count to obtain the total leukocyte count. A lab in Zurich, Switzerland, performed a study comparing their total leukocyte results between the standard Natt-Herrick's method and the Natt-Herricks-TIC® (Carisch et al., 2019). They found that the Natt-Herricks-TIC® showed acceptable precision and good agreement with the standard method. Their method, in an effort to reduce counting errors likely introduced from the difficulty in differentiating lymphocytes and thrombocytes, is to only count granulocytes in either counting method. To include lymphocytes and monocytes in the total leukocyte count, the uncorrected leukocyte count (including only granulocytes) is multiplied by 100 and divided by the sum of the percentages of heterophils, eosinophils, and basophils that were determined in the leukocyte differential (Carisch et al., 2019).

Toluidine Blue Solution

A second direct method for obtaining a total leukocyte count involves diluting the anticoagulated blood sample 1:100 with 0.01% toluidine blue in phosphate-buffered saline before charging a Neubauer-ruled hemacytometer (Zinkle, 1986; Joseph et al., 1989). Toluidine blue will stain leukocytes blue, erythrocytes pale orange, and thrombocytes pale blue.

All blue cells equal to or larger than the width of an erythrocyte are counted in the nine large squares on one side of the Neubauer-ruled hemacytometer. The total leukocyte count is then calculated using the following equation:

$$\text{TWBC/mm}^3 = \left[\left(\text{total cells in nine large squares}\right) \times 10 \times 100\right]/9$$

or to simplify the math,

$$\text{TWBC/mm}^3 = \left(\text{total cells in nine large squares} + 10\%\right) \times 100$$

Counting only the cells that are equal to or larger than the width of erythrocytes should rule out thrombocytes, which tend to be smaller than the width of erythrocytes. Small lymphocytes tend to be equal to or larger than the width of the erythrocytes. Immature erythrocytes may be distinguished from small lymphocytes by their round to irregular shape, round centrally positioned nucleus with dark irregularly clumped chromatin, and moderate volume of basophilic hyaline cytoplasm. When a large number of immature erythrocytes are present in the blood sample, a corrected total leukocyte concentration can be obtained using the following formula:

$$\text{Corrected TWBC/mm}^3 = (\text{TWBC} \times 100)/(100 + \text{number of immature RBCs per 100 leukocytes})$$

When using counting methods that require the use of a hemacytometer, the difference between the counts obtained from each chamber should not exceed 10%, to ensure accuracy between the two sides. If a discrepancy greater than 10% occurs, the procedure should be repeated. To date, no comparisons have been made between the toluidine blue method and the other methods of obtaining avian leukocyte counts; however, the results should be similar to Natt and Herrick's method.

Leukocyte Estimation from Blood Film

Crude estimation of cell numbers from blood films is an inappropriate method for obtaining a routine total leukocyte count in birds. Estimated leukocyte counts should be used only when quantitative counts (i.e., phloxine, Natt and Herrick's, or toluidine blue methods) are unavailable, or may be used as a means of detecting submission or laboratory error (e.g., if the number of leukocytes observed in a blood film appear to be less than that reported from a quantitative count) (Weiss, 1984). Crude estimation of the leukocyte concentration in a well-prepared blood film is made by obtaining the average number of leukocytes in five 1000× (oil-immersion) monolayer fields and using the following equation:

$$\text{Estimated TWBC/mm}^3 = \left(\text{average WBCs per 5 fields/1000}\right) \times 3\,500\,000$$

Typically, the average number of erythrocytes in five 1000× (oil-immersion) monolayer fields is 1000. The approximated number of erythrocytes per cubic millimeter in birds with normal PCV is 3 500 000. If the PCV is outside the normal range (35–55%), then the estimated count should be corrected for the PCV, using this equation:

$$\text{Corrected estimated TWBC/mm}^3 = (\text{estimated WBC} \times \text{observed PCV})/\text{normal PCV } (45\%)$$

An estimated total WBC count can be obtained by counting leukocytes in 10 monolayer fields at 400× magnification and dividing by 10 to calculate an average number per-high-power field count, and that average is multiplied by 2000 to calculate an estimated total WBC count in units of cells/μL. (That value can be divided by 1000 to convert to cells $\times 10^9$/L) (Kanda et al., 2020). This method is considered to be more accurate than using 1000× (oil-immersion) magnification to count the cells.

Leukocyte Differential

The differential leukocyte count and leukocyte morphology are obtained by microscopic evaluation of stained blood films. A variety of hematologic stains are available (see Appendix A). Rapid stains (i.e., Diff–Quik, Dade Diagnostics, Aguada, Puerto Rico) or Hemacolor (Miles Laboratories, Inc., Elkhart, IN) have a shorter staining time, but do not always provide adequate differentiation between the various leukocytes. Additionally, heterophil granules tend to coalesce more with rapid stains, especially those of reptiles and some species of birds, making evaluation of these cells difficult (Muro et al., 1998). Stains such as Wright's and May–Grünwald–Giemsa stains are more time consuming, but provide better differentiation of the leukocytes, thrombocytes, and immature erythrocytes (Alleman et al., 1992; Muro et al., 1998).

The leukocyte differential is performed during the microscopic evaluation of Romanowsky-stained blood films. Blood samples collected into heparin make it necessary to prepare the blood films immediately following sample collection in order to decrease the incidence of cell clumping. Whenever possible, preparing blood films using blood containing no anticoagulant is preferred. The differential leukocyte count is performed by counting a minimum of 100 leukocytes in a monocellular area in the blood film. The cells counted are those consecutively encountered as one moves from one counting field to the next. The cells are classified as heterophils (Figure 11.15), eosinophils (Figure 11.19), basophils (Figure 11.21), lymphocytes (Figure 11.10), and monocytes (Figure 11.14). The number of each cell type becomes a fraction of the total or a percentage of the leukocyte population. Absolute numbers of each cell type are obtained by multiplying the total leukocyte concentration by the percentage of that type of leukocyte from the differential count.

Thrombocyte Parameters

The concentrations of thrombocytes in the blood of lower vertebrates vary. The best-studied thrombocyte concentrations have been in birds, where the numbers range between 20 000 and 30 000 per cubic millimeter of blood, or 10 and 15 thrombocytes per 1000 erythrocytes in most avian species (Fox and Solomon, 1981; Campbell, 1995). The actual thrombocyte concentration is difficult to determine because thrombocytes tend to clump; therefore, thrombocyte concentration is often reported as normal, increased, or decreased, based upon estimates from peripheral blood films.

Blood films may be used to assess thrombocyte numbers. Approximately 1–5 thrombocytes can be seen in a monolayer 1000× (oil-immersion) field in a blood film from a normal bird, unless the thrombocytes clump excessively during preparation.

The absolute thrombocyte concentration can be obtained using the same hemacytometer used for obtaining total leukocyte and erythrocyte counts with Natt and Herrick's method. The number of thrombocytes counted in the central large square on both sides of the Neubauer-ruled hemacytometer is multiplied by 1000 to obtain the number of thrombocytes per microliter of blood (Figure 10.7).

Thrombocytopenia is suggested by thrombocyte numbers less than one per monolayer 1000× field. Thrombocytosis is suggested by numbers greater than five in an average monolayer 1000× field.

Quantitative Evaluation of Bone Marrow Aspirates

Stained bone marrow aspirates are examined for cellularity and quality where the monolayer of hematopoietic cells is ideal. A 500-cell differential count (1000-cell

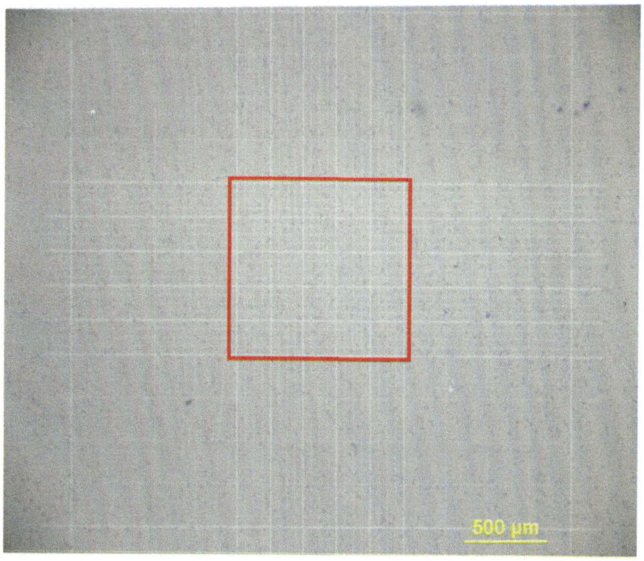

Fig. 10.7. This image identifies the large center square of the counting chamber of the Neubauer-ruled hemacytometer. This is the large square in which the thrombocytes are counted manually.

differential is more precise) is considered adequate for bone marrow assessment (Schwartz et al., 2019).

References

Alleman AR, Jacobson ER, Raskin RE. 1992. Morphologic and cytochemical characteristics of blood cells from the desert tortoise (*Gopherus agassizii*). *Am J Vet Res* 53:1645–1651.

Andreasen CB, Latimer KS, Kircher IM, et al. 1989. Determination of chicken and turkey plasma and serum protein concentration by refractometry and the biuret method. *Avian Dis* 33:93–96.

Autaiem T, Auethavekiat S, Sa-ing V, et al. 2019. A novel Iterative method for automatic avian red blood cell counting. *BMEiCON-2019*.

Beaufrere H, Ammersback M, Tully TN. 2013. Complete blood cell count in psittaciformes by using high-throughput image cytometry: a pilot study. *J Avian Med Surg* 27(3):211–217.

Campbell TW. 1995. *Avian Hematology and Cytology*, 2nd edn. Ames, IA: Iowa State University Press.

Costello RT. 1970. A unopette for eosinophil counts. *Am J Clin Pathol* 54:249.

Carisch L, Stirn M, Hatt JM, et al. 2019. White blood cell count in birds: evaluation of a commercially available method. *BMC Vet Res* 15:93 DOI: 10.1186/s12917-0191834-8.

Clark TD, Eliason EJ, Sandblom E, et al. 2008. Calibration of a hand-held haemoglobin analyser for use on fish blood. *J Fish Biol* 73(10):2587–2595.

Dacie JV, Lewis K. 1968. *Practical Hematology*, 4th edn. London: Churchill Livingstone.

Dein FJ, Wilson BA, Fischer MT. 1994. Avian leucocyte counting using the hemocytometer. *J Zoo Wildl Med* 25:432–437.

Dieterien-Lievre F. 1988. Birds. In: Rawley AF, Ratcliffe NA (eds), *Vertebrate Blood Cells*. Cambridge, UK: Cambridge University Press, pp. 257–336.

Ferreyra H, Beldomenico PM, Marchese K, et al. 2015. Lead exposure affects health indices in free-ranging ducks in Argentina. *Exotoxicology* DOI: 10.1007/s10646-015-1419-7.

Fox AJ, Solomon JB. 1981. Chicken non-lymphoid leukocytes. In: Rose L, Payne L, Freeman M (eds), *Avian Immunology*. Edinburgh: Poultry Science Ltd.

George JW, O'Neill SL. 2001. Comparison of refractometer and biuret methods for total protein measurement in body cavity fluids. *Vet Clin Pathol* 30:16–18.

Green SA, Jenkins SJ, Clark PA. 1982. A comparison of chemical and electrophoretic methods of serum protein determination in clinically normal domestic animals of various ages. *Cornell Vet* 72:416–426.

Gustavsson F. 2015. Validation study: HemoCue Hb 201+ as a tool in comparative physiological field studies on avian blood. Linköpings, Sweden: universitet SE-581 83.

Hawkins MG, Sanchez-Migallon Guzman D, Beaufrere H, et al. 2018. Birds. In: Carpenter JW (ed), *Exotic Animal Formulary*, 5th edn. St. Louis, MO: Elsevier.

Joseph V, Wagner D, Stouli J, et al. 1989. Toluidine blue stain for avian WBC count. *J Assoc Avian Vet* 3:191, 229.

Kanda I, Robertson J, Meinkoth J, et al. 2020. Complete blood cell count and white blood cell counting method comparison in 49-day-old Bobwhite quail (*Colinus virginianus*). *J Avian Med Surg* 34(2):132–141.

Kloskowski J, Kaczanowska E, Krogulec J, et al. 2017. Hematological indicators of habitat quality: erythrocyte parameters reflect greater parental effort of red-necked Grebes under ecological trap conditions. *Condor Ornithol Appl* 119:239–250.

Lumeij JT, deBruijne JJ. 1985. Evaluation of refractometric method for the determination of total protein in avian plasma or serum. *Avian Pathol* 14:441–444.

Lumeij JT, Maclean B. 1996. Total protein determination in pigeon plasma and serum: comparison of refractometric methods with biuret method. *J Avian Med Surg* 10:150–152.

Meechart K, Auethavekiat S, Sa-ing V. 2019. An automatic detection for avian blood cell based on adaptive thresholding algorithm. *BMEiCON-2019*.

Minias P. 2015. The use of haemoglobin concentrations to assess physiologic condition in birds: a review. *Conserv Physiol* 3(1):cov007. DOI: 10.1093/conphys/cov007

Morgan GW, Thaxton P, Edens FW. 1975. Estimation of protein content in the plasma of young chickens by a refractometric method. *Poult Sci* 54:1312–1214.

Muro J, Cuenca R, Pastor J, et al. 1998. Effects of lithium heparin and tripotassium EDTA on hematologic values of Hermann's tortoises (*Testudo hermanni*). *J Zoo Wildl Med* 29:40–44.

Natt MP, Herrick CA. 1952. A new blood diluent for counting erythrocytes and leucocytes of the chicken. *Poult Sci* 31:735–738.

Ochoa D, Redondo T, Moreno-Rueda G. 2019. Mizutama: a quick, easy, and accurate method for counting erythrocytes. *Physiol Biochem Zool* 92(2):206–210.

Pinto FF, Lopes C, Marcos R. 2018. Unraveling avian and reptilian hematology: an optical and electron microscopic study of the buffy coat. *Vet Clin Pathol* 47(3):407–414.

Post J, Rebel JMJ, Ter Huurne AAHM. 2003. Automated blood cell count: a sensitive and reliable method to study corticosterone related stress in broilers. *Poultry Sci* 82:591–595.

Robertson GW, Maxwell MH. 1990. Modified staining techniques for avian blood cells. *Br Poultry Sci* 31:881–886.

Russo EA, McEntee L, Applegate I, et al. 1986. Comparison of two methods for determination of white blood cell counts in macaws. *J Am Vet Med Assoc* 189:1013–1016.

Samour J. 2016. Clinical and laboratory diagnostic examination. In: Samour J (ed), *Avian Medicine*, 3rd edn. St. Louis, MO: Elsevier.

Scanes CG. 2014. Blood. In: Scanes CG (ed), *Sturkie's Avian Physiology*. Philadelphia, PA: Elsevier.

Schwartz D, Guzman DS-M, Beaufrere H, et al. 2019. Morphologic and quantitative evaluation of bone marrow aspirates from Hispaniolan Amazon parrots (*Amazona ventralis*). *Vet Clin Pathol* 2019 48(4):645–651.

Velguth KE, Payton ME, Hoover JP. 2010. Relationship of hemoglobin concentration to packed cell volume in avian blood samples. *J Avian Med Surg* 24(2):115–121.

Weiss DJ. 1984. Uniform evaluation and semiquantitative reporting of hematologic data in veterinary laboratories. *Vet Clin Pathol* 13(2):27–31.

Weiser G. 2012. Laboratory technology for veterinary medicine. In: Thrall M, Weiser G, Allison RW, et al. (eds), *Veterinary Hematology and Clinical Chemistry*, 2nd edn. Ames, IA: Wiley-Blackwell, pp. 3–33.

Zinkle JG. 1986. Avian hematology. In: Jain C (ed), *Schalm's Veterinary Hematology*. Philadelphia, PA: Lea & Febiger.

11 Evaluation and Interpretation of Peripheral Blood of Birds

Evaluation and interpretation of avian blood cell morphology and counts are used to rule in or rule out disease, monitor response to therapy, establish a prognosis, or develop a database. In general, the basic hematological principles of domestic mammalian hematology apply to avian hematology with a few differences and modifications. The major differences between mammalian and avian hematology include the presence of nucleated erythrocytes, thrombocytes, and heterophil granulocytes in the peripheral blood of birds. The modified procedures are labor intensive, and the reliability of the results depends on the experience and expertise of the individual performing the analysis.

The normal reference intervals of any avian hematologic parameter have a broad range owing to the influence of various intrinsic and extrinsic factors. Avian hematological values are subject to extensive variability resulting from different environment and management practices, which can affect physiological responses (Fourie and Hattingh, 1980). Normal hematologic reference intervals vary between the avian species as well. The different avian species as well as the different collection and preparation methods from which blood samples are submitted to veterinary laboratories create a significant logistical challenge for the development of clinically relevant reference intervals. Those factors, along with the differences in analytical methods, introduce additional variability in results. Thus, published reference intervals should be used only as guidelines. When monitoring trends in individuals, it is important to maintain consistency with materials and techniques.

This chapter continues with the procedures of assessing the avian hemogram with blood film evaluation. The information gathered from the blood film, coupled with the results from cell counts and red blood cell indices, allows for complete evaluation of the avian hemogram.

Representative hemic cells found in avian blood films can be found in Appendix C.

Avian Erythrocytes

Morphology and Color

Evaluation of avian erythrocyte morphology involves observation of the cells in a monolayer 1000× field in which approximately half the erythrocytes touch one another. In general, such fields represent approximately 200 erythrocytes in most species of birds. Monolayer fields may be difficult to achieve, however, in some situations, such as in severely anemic birds where the films are too thin or in poorly prepared blood films (films are made too thick or thin). Avian erythrocytes should be evaluated based on size, shape, color, nuclear morphology and position, and presence of cellular inclusions.

Erythrocyte Size

Mature avian erythrocytes generally are larger than mammalian erythrocytes, but smaller than reptilian and amphibian erythrocytes. Avian erythrocytes vary in size depending on the species, but they generally range between 10.7 × 6.1 and 15.8 × 10.2 µm (Sturkie and Griminger, 1986). Erythrocytes of adult Coturnix quail, for example, measure 11.06 ± 0.70 µm in length and 6.80 ± 0.67 µm in width in males and 11.40 ± 0.63 µm in length and 6.73 ± 0.45 µm in width in females (Tadjalli et al., 2003). Mature avian erythrocytes are elliptical and

Exotic Animal Hematology and Cytology, Fifth Edition. Terry W. Campbell and Krystan R. Grant.

Companion website: www.wiley.com/go/campbell/exotic

have an elliptical, centrally positioned nucleus. Nuclear chromatin is uniformly clumped and becomes increasingly condensed with age.

Erythrocyte Shape

Variations in the normal erythrocyte morphology occur in blood films from normal healthy birds as well as those with medical disorders. Careful examination of erythrocyte morphology may reveal significant clues in the detection of disorders affecting avian erythrocytes. It is important to note, however, that the presence of atypical erythrocytes in a blood film may sometimes be associated with poor technique in blood film preparation. Disruption and/or smudging of avian erythrocytes are common artifacts of slide preparation. Severely ruptured cells result in the presence of purple, amorphous, nuclear material in the blood film. A semiquantitative scale can be used to estimate the number of abnormal erythrocytes based on the average number per monolayer 1000× field (Appendix B, Table B.4) (Bessis, 1977; Rebar et al., 1981; Weiss, 1984).

Changes in Morphology

In most species of birds, erythrocyte shape is relatively uniform; however, the shape of the red blood cells may be somewhat variable. Therefore, atypical erythrocytes may vary in both size and shape. Changes that typically occur in the size of avian erythrocytes include microcytosis, macrocytosis, and anisocytosis (unequal in size). The presence of macrocytes or microcytes should also be noted during assessment of the blood film. The degree of variation in the size of erythrocytes (anisocytosis) can be scored from 1+ to 4+ based on the number of variable-sized erythrocytes in a monolayer field (Appendix B, Table B.4) (Weiss, 1984). A significant change in the mean size of the erythrocyte is reflected in the mean corpuscular volume (MCV). A slight variation in the size of erythrocytes (1+ anisocytosis) is normal for birds. A greater degree of anisocytosis, however, usually is observed in birds with a regenerative anemia and is associated with polychromasia. Erythrocyte subpopulations have been reported in ducks, in which larger erythrocytes (MCV, 308 fL/cell) most likely represent those most recently released from the hematopoietic tissue, and smaller cells (MCV, 128 fL/cell) most likely represent the older, aging cells (Herbert et al., 1989). Microcytic, hypochromic, nonregenerative anemia is often associated with chronic inflammatory diseases in birds, especially those with an infectious etiology (Tell et al., 2004). The degree of poikilocytosis (abnormally shaped) can also be estimated using the scale outlined in Appendix B, Table B.4.

Likewise, minor deviations from the normal shape of avian erythrocytes (1+ poikilocytosis) are considered to be normal in the peripheral blood of birds, but marked poikilocytosis may indicate erythrocytic dysgenesis. For example, round erythrocytes with oval nuclei occasionally are found in the blood films of anemic birds and suggest a dysmaturation of the cell cytoplasm and nucleus, which may be a result of accelerated erythropoiesis.

Erythrocyte Color

In Wright-stained blood films, the nucleus stains purple, whereas the cytoplasm stains orange-pink with a uniform texture (Figures 11.1a–11.1c). Variations in erythrocyte color include hypochromasia and polychromasia.

Hypochromasia

Hypochromatic erythrocytes are abnormally pale in color compared with mature erythrocytes, and they have an area of cytoplasmic pallor that is greater than half the cytoplasmic volume (Figures 11.2a–11.2c). They may also have cytoplasmic vacuoles and round, pyknotic nuclei. Hypochromatic erythrocytes frequently appear in blood films from birds with nutritional deficiencies that lead to iron deficiency, lead toxicosis, and chronic inflammatory diseases presumably related to iron sequestration as part of the bird's defense against infectious agents. In such cases, hypochromatic cells are often observed in blood films before the red cell indices (mean corpuscular hemoglobin concentration (MCHC) and mean corpuscular hemoglobin (MCH)) suggest hypochromasia (Hawkey and Dennett, 1989; Lloyd, 1992). A significant hypochromasia is reflected as a decrease in the MCHC and MCH values. The degree of hypochromasia can be estimated using the scale presented in Appendix B, Table B.4. The presence of many hypochromatic erythrocytes (i.e., 2+ hypochromasia or greater) indicates an erythrocyte disorder such as iron deficiency.

Chronic lead toxicosis may also be associated with an inappropriate release of normal-appearing immature erythrocytes into the peripheral blood of nonanemic birds (Figure 11.3). When this condition occurs, the blood film reveals small, senescent, mature erythrocytes with pyknotic nuclei and immature erythrocytes (usually late polychromatic rubricytes) without the presence of normal mature erythrocytes. This hematologic response resembles the inappropriate release of nucleated erythrocytes in the blood of nonanemic dogs affected by chronic lead poisoning. Basophilic stippling in the cytoplasm of erythrocytes may be seen with lead poisoning in birds, but is rare. Stippled basophilia is more commonly associated with erythrocyte regeneration and hypochromic anemia in birds.

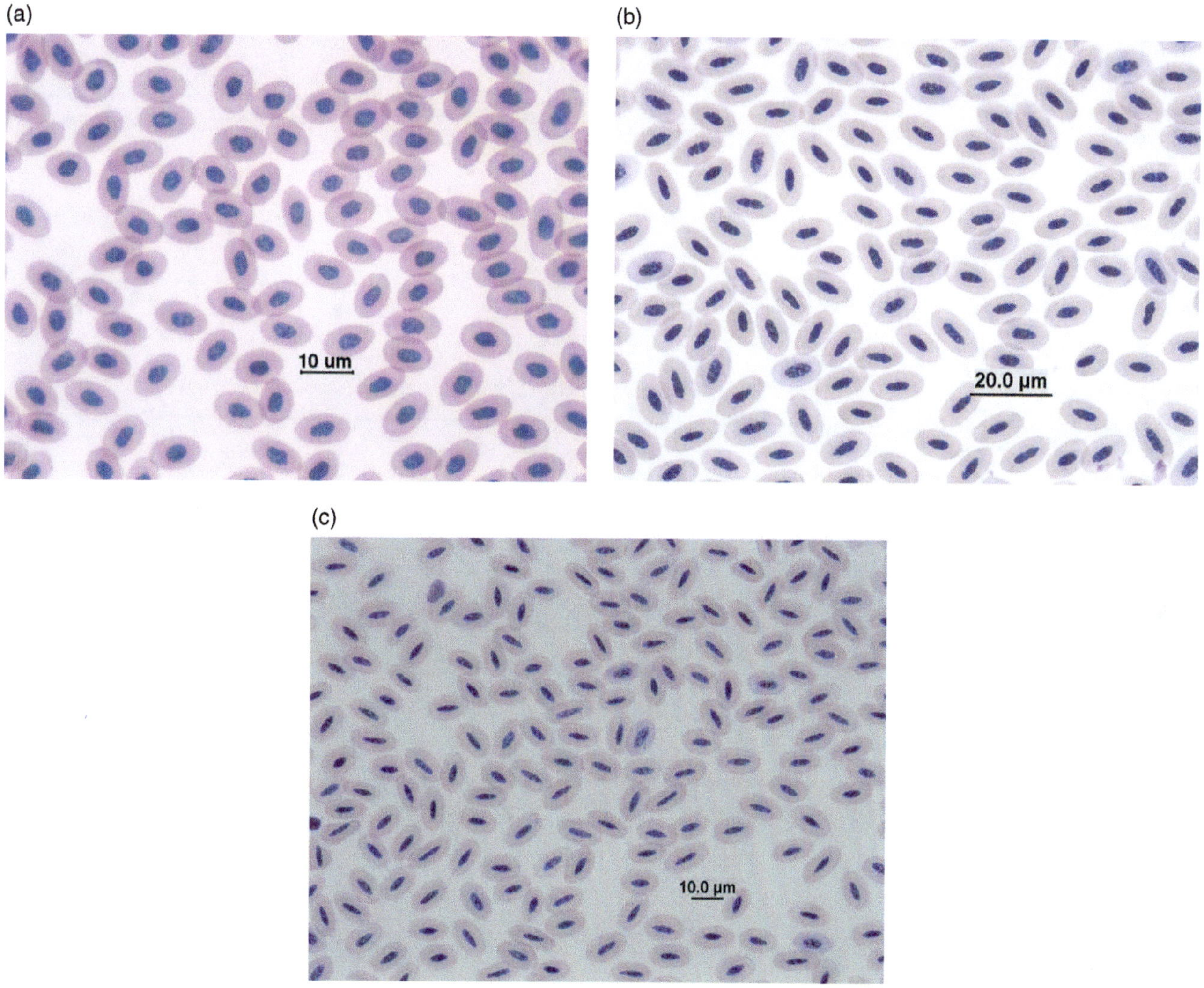

Fig. 11.1. (a) Normal erythrocytes in the blood film of a domestic chicken (*Gallus gallus domesticus*), Wright–Giemsa stain. (b) Normal erythrocytes in the blood film of an eclectus parrot (*Eclectus roratus*), Wright–Giemsa stain. (c) Normal erythrocytes in the blood film of a bald eagle (*Haliaeetus leucocephalus*).

Polychromasia

Polychromatophilic erythrocytes are similar in size to mature erythrocytes and appear as reticulocytes when stained with vital stains, such as new methylene blue. The cytoplasm appears weakly basophilic, and the nucleus is less condensed than the nucleus of mature erythrocytes (Figures 11.4a and 11.4b). The degree of polychromasia can be graded according to the guideline presented in Appendix B, Table B.4. Polychromatophilic erythrocytes occur in low numbers (usually <5% of erythrocytes) in the peripheral blood of most normal birds.

Reticulocytes

Reticulocytes are the penultimate cell in the erythrocyte maturation series, and their presence in the peripheral blood of normal birds suggests that the final stages of red cell maturation occur in circulating blood. Reticulocytes tend to be smaller in size and less elongated compared to the mature erythrocyte. For example, reticulocytes of adult Coturnix quail measure 9.80 ± 0.77 µm in length and 8.23 ± 0.72 µm in width in males, and 9.80 ± 0.77 µm in length and 7.73 ± 0.70 µm in width in females (Sturkie and Griminger, 1986). Determination of the reticulocyte concentration can be made by staining erythrocytes with a vital stain such as new methylene blue. Reticulocytes have a distinct ring of aggregated reticular material that encircles the nucleus (Figures 11.5a and 11.5b) (Lucas and Jamroz, 1961; Hawkey and Dennett, 1989). As the cells mature, the amount of aggregated reticular material decreases, and it becomes more dispersed throughout the cytoplasm. With further maturation, the reticular material becomes nonaggregated, thereby resembling the "punctate" reticulocytes of felids. Most mature avian erythrocytes

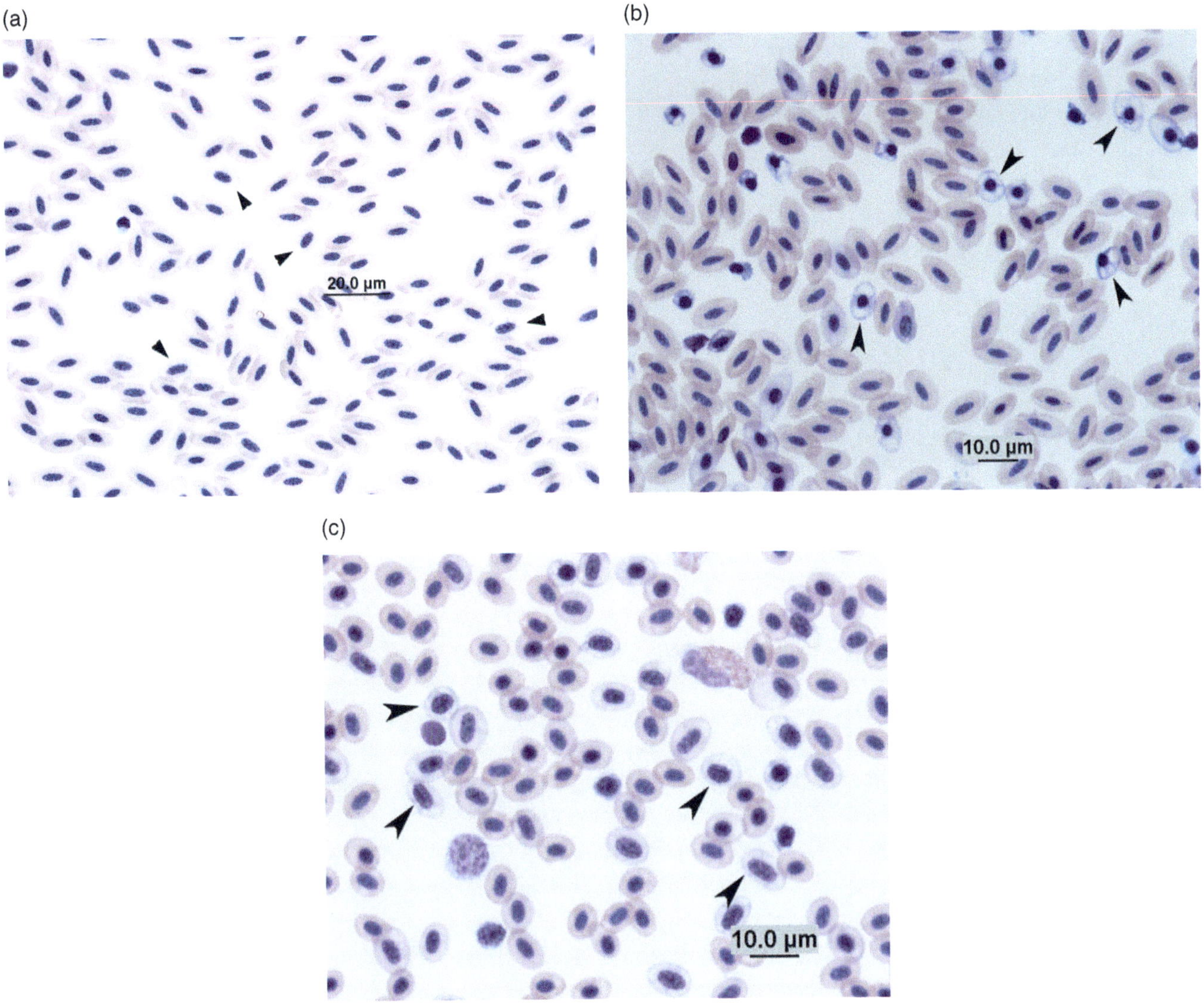

Fig. 11.2. (a) Hypochromatic erythrocytes (arrowheads) in the blood film of an eclectus parrot (*Eclectus roratus*), Wright–Giemsa stain. (b) Hypochromatic erythrocytes (arrowheads) in the blood film of a peregrine falcon (*Falco peregrinus*), Wright–Giemsa stain. (c) Hypochromatic erythrocytes (arrowheads) in the blood film of a blue-throated macaw (*Ara glaucogularis*), Wright–Giemsa stain.

contain a varying amount of aggregate or punctate reticulum. Reticulocytes that reflect the current erythrocyte regenerative response, however, are those with a distinct ring of aggregated reticulum that encircles the red cell nucleus. (Hawkey and Dennett, 1989; Campbell and Ellis, 2007). Significantly high numbers of these cells would represent a regenerative response to anemia.

Other Erythrocyte Features

Nucleus

The nucleus may vary in its location within the erythrocyte, and may contain indentions, protrusions, or constrictions. Nuclear morphologic variations have been identified in a wide range of avian species (Clark, 2015). Micronuclei and nuclear budding are potential indices of environmental genotoxic exposure (Wolf and Luepke, 1997; Wolf et al., 2002; Gómez-Meda et al., 2006). Chromophobic streaking suggestive of chromatolysis or achromic bands indicating nuclear fracture with displacement of the fragments may also be present (Lucas and Jamroz, 1961). Mitotic activity is occasionally noted in blood films and is suggestive of a marked regenerative response or erythrocytic dyscrasia. Binucleated erythrocytes rarely occur in blood films of normal birds; however, the presence of large numbers of binucleated erythrocytes plus other features of red blood cell dyscrasia is suggestive of neoplastic, viral, or genetic disease (Romagnano, 1994). Anucleated erythrocytes (erythroplastids) or the presence of cytoplasmic fragments are occasionally noted in small proportions in normal avian blood films (Figure 11.6) (Clark and Raidal, 2014). The degree of erythroplastid presence can be graded according to the guideline outlined in Appendix B, Table B.4.

Perinuclear rings are common artifacts of improper slide preparation (e.g., exposure to solvent or formalin fumes, or excessively slow drying of the slide) and represent nuclear shrinkage. Clear, irregular, refractile spaces in the cytoplasm may also occur when blood films are allowed to dry too slowly (Figure 11.7). This artifact, a form of erythrocyte crenation, should not be confused with avian blood parasites, such as gametocytes of *Hemoproteus* and *Plasmodium*.

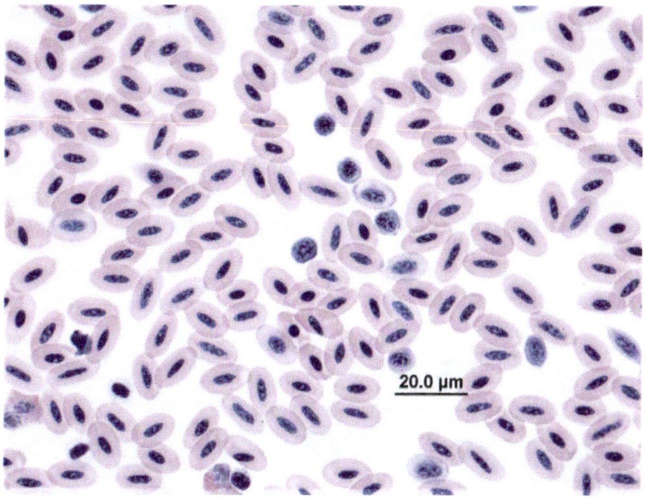

Fig. 11.3. Increased numbers of immature erythrocytes (early and mid-polychromatic rubricytes) without an appropriate increase in polychromasia in the blood film of a turkey vulture (*Cathartes aura*) with lead poisoning, Wright–Giemsa stain.

Cytoplasm

Variations may occasionally be noted in the cytoplasm of erythrocytes. Punctate basophilia is characterized by the appearance of punctate aggregations of small, irregular, basophilic-staining granules throughout the cytoplasm of erythrocytes in Wright's-stained blood films and is most likely associated with degenerative changes in ribosomal ribonucleic acid (RNA). This change is typically indicative of a response to anemia or, rarely, lead poisoning, which is similar to the significance of these changes in mammalian hematology. Basophilic stippling can occur during the preparation and staining of the blood film. Blood films made using fresh blood without an anticoagulant or blood films made from EDTA-anticoagulated blood that undergo rapid drying provide the best films for demonstration of basophilic stippling (George and Duncan, 1981). This change is less apparent when alcohol fixation of blood is used.

Heinz Bodies

Heinz bodies have been reported rarely in birds and are the result of hemoglobin denaturation (oxidized hemoglobin) (Maxwell, 1981a). Heinz bodies appear as refractile inclusions in the cytoplasm of the erythrocytes in unstained blood films. In blood films stained with Wright's stain, Heinz bodies appear as round to irregular inclusions of densely stained hemoglobin, and in blood films stained with new methylene blue, they appear as round to irregularly shaped, pale blue cytoplasmic inclusions.

(a) (b)

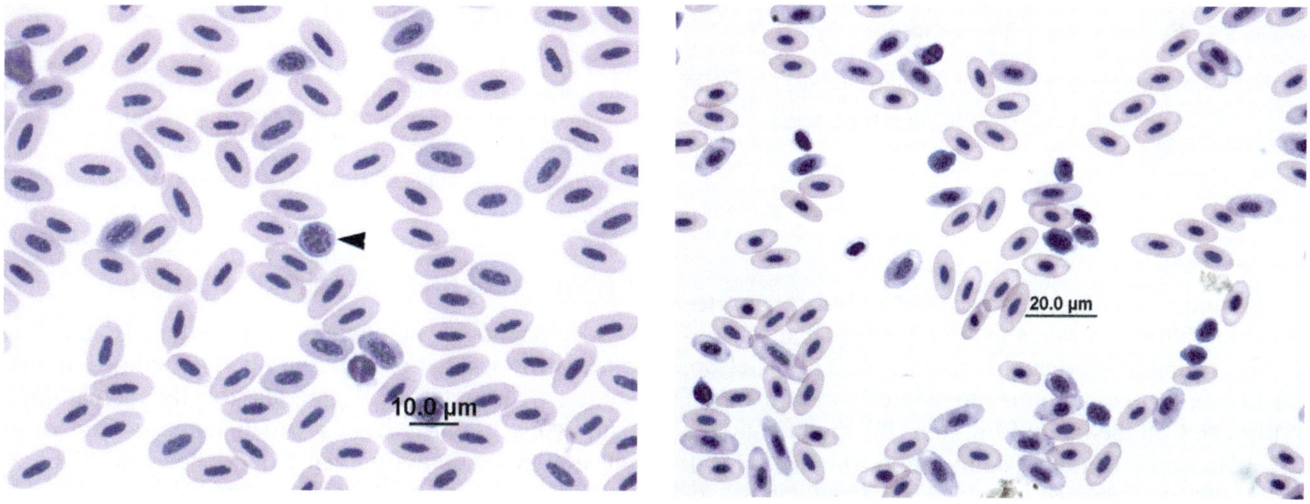

Fig. 11.4. (a) Increased polychromatophilic erythrocytes and a rubricyte, a mid-polychromatic rubricyte (arrowhead), in the blood film of a conure (*Aratinga solstitialis*), Wright–Giemsa stain. (b) Increased polychromatophilic erythrocytes in the blood film of a red-tailed hawk (*Buteo jamaicensis*), Wright–Giemsa stain.

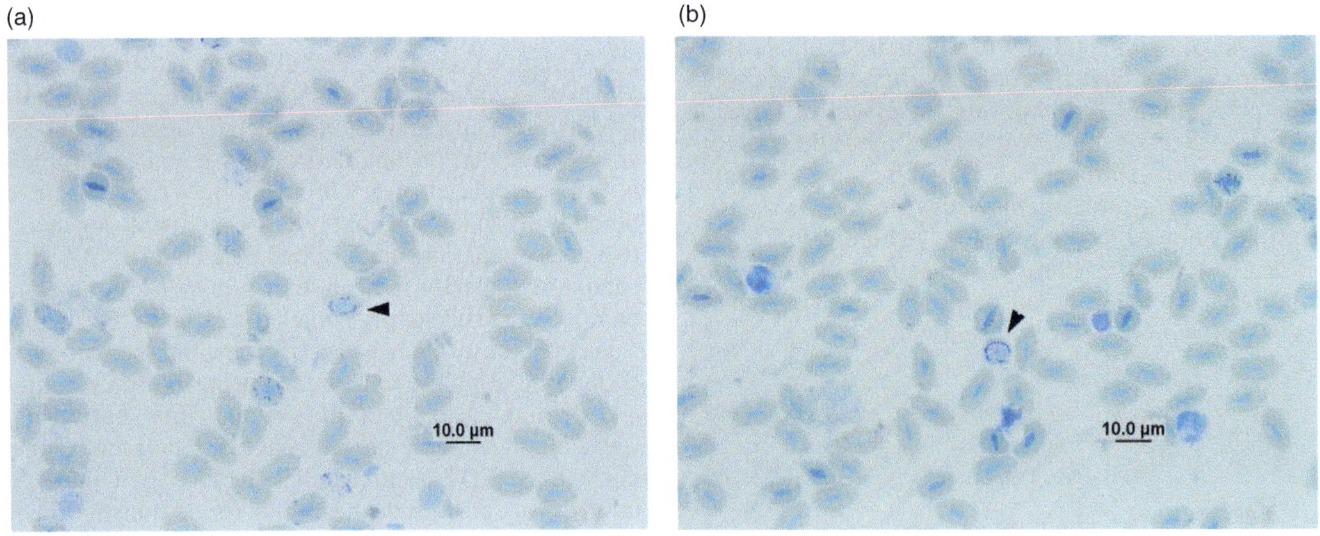

Fig. 11.5. (a) Reticulocyte with a distinct ring of aggregated reticular material (arrowhead) that encircles the erythrocyte nucleus in the blood film of an African gray parrot (*Psittacus erithacus*), new methylene blue stain. (b) A round immature erythrocyte with a distinct ring of aggregated reticular material that encircles the cell nucleus (arrowhead) in the blood film of an African gray parrot (*Psittacus erithacus*), new methylene blue stain.

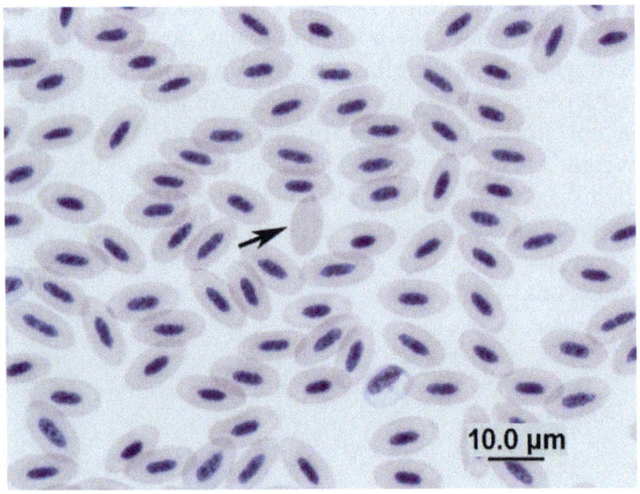

Fig. 11.6. Anucleated erythrocyte (erythroplastids) (arrow) in the blood film of a conure (*Aratinga solstitialis*), Wright–Giemsa stain.

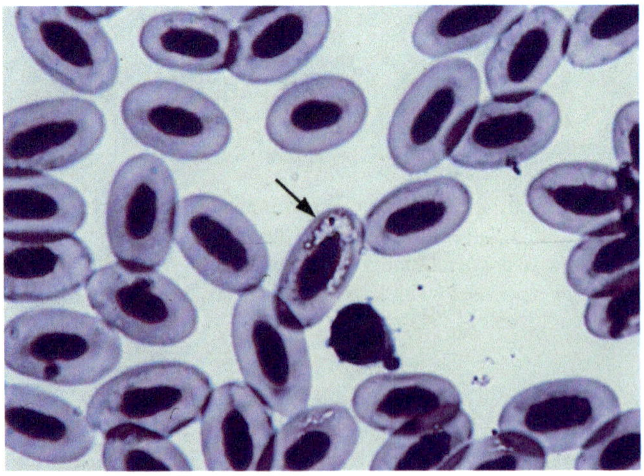

Fig. 11.7. Clear irregular, refractile spaces in the cytoplasm (arrow) may occur when blood films are allowed to dry too slowly. This artifact, a form of erythrocyte crenation, should not be confused with avian blood parasites, such as gametocytes of *Hemoproteus* and *Plasmodium*, Wright–Giemsa stain (100× oil).

Agglutination

Agglutination of erythrocytes and erythrophagocytosis in blood films are rare abnormal findings that are suggestive of immune-mediated disease (Figures 11.8a, 11.8b, and 11.8c). Agglutination is represented by clumping of erythrocytes on the blood film. Red cell agglutination is best observed on low magnification (Figure 11.8a). Erythrophagocytosis is identified by phagocytosis of whole red blood cells or iron pigment from hemoglobin degradation in the cytoplasm of leukocytes, typically monocytes.

Factors Affecting the Avian Erythrogram

Hematologic parameters are frequently used as indices for assessing health and body condition in bird studies. The reference intervals for the hematologic parameters of birds have a broad range owing to the physiologic and environmental influences on the blood cells. The hematologic parameters of birds can fluctuate with sex, age, time of day, season, nutritional status, and hydration. Seasonal variations, age, and species have been shown to affect the erythrocyte parameters, such as

(a) (b) (c)

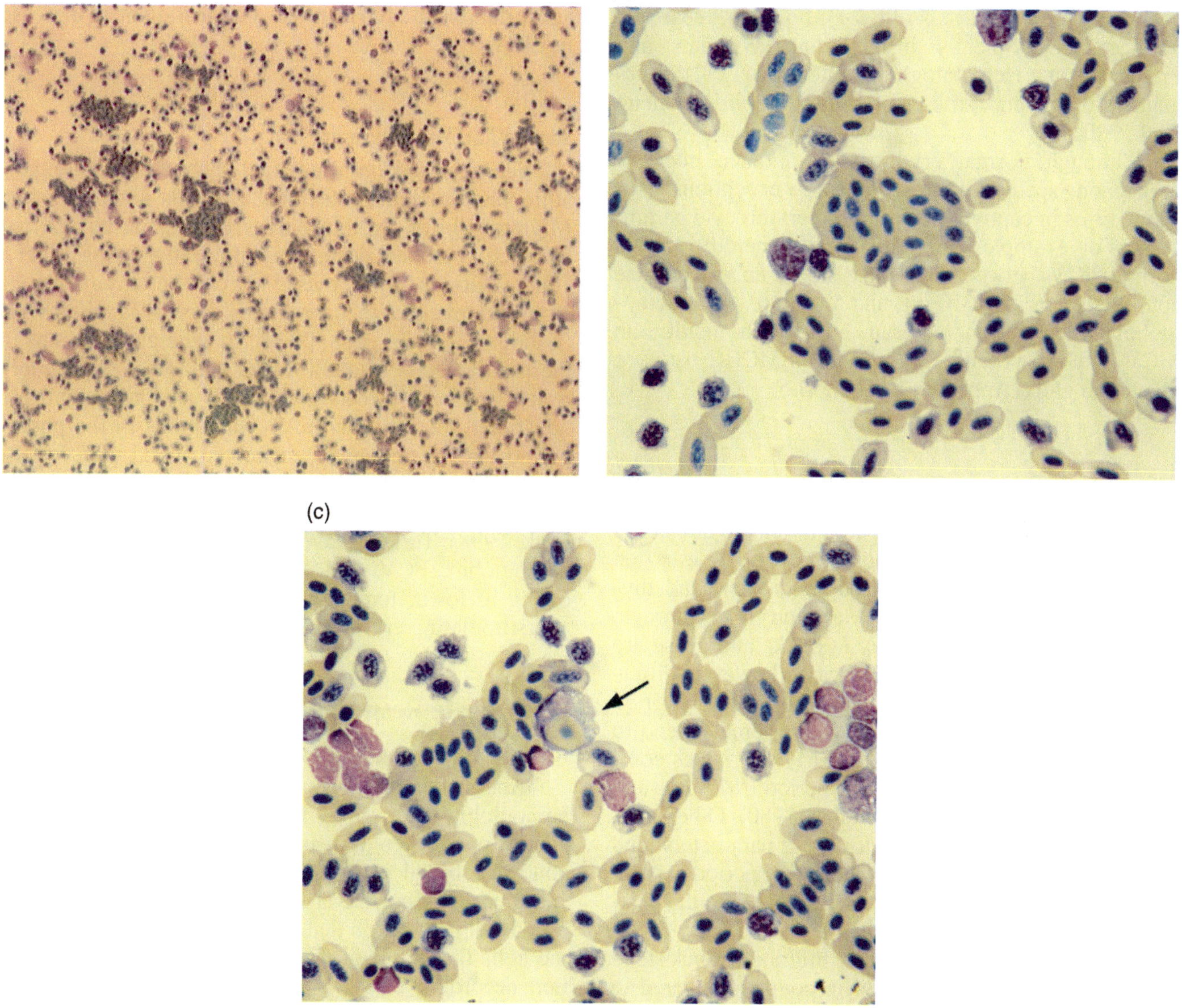

Fig. 11.8. (a) Erythrocyte agglutination in the blood film of an eclectus parrot (*Eclectus roratus*), Wright–Giemsa stain (10×). (b) Erythrocyte agglutination in the blood film of an eclectus parrot (*Eclectus roratus*), Wright–Giemsa stain (10× oil). (c) Erythrocyte agglutination and erythrophagocytosis (arrow) in the blood film of an eclectus parrot (*Eclectus roratus*), Wright–Giemsa stain (100× oil).

packed cell volume (PCV), total erythrocyte count (TRBC), hemoglobin concentration (Hb), MCHC, and MCV of normal birds, especially wildlife (Williams and Trainer, 1971; Kocan and Pitts, 1976; Shave and Howard, 1976; Mulley, 1979; Mulley, 1980; Rehder et al., 1982; Morton, 1994; Harper and Lowe, 1998; Bearhop et al., 1999; Hauptmanova et al., 2006; Schmidt et al., 2007). The hematocrit has been used as a method of determining nutritional status in wild birds. In some studies, decreased hematocrit (reflecting anemia) caused by reduced erythropoiesis has been reported during periods of nutritional stress in wild birds, although the reliability of hematocrit values as a condition index has been questioned (Dawson and Bortolotti, 1997).

Species

Significant differences occur between species of birds in regard to the red blood cell parameters. For example, mallard ducks (*Anas platyrhynchos*), a dabbling duck, have higher average PCV and TRBC values in the winter and pre-nesting period compared to diving ducks (*Aythya* spp. and *Oxyura jamaicensis*) (Shave and Howard, 1976). The same study demonstrated that diving ducks, on the other hand, have higher MCV values during the winter and pre-nesting period compared to mallards. In general, ducks tend to have higher TRBC values than geese, but geese have higher MCV and Hb than ducks during the winter (Shave and Howard, 1976). Total erythrocyte counts tend to be slightly higher for

Snow geese (*Chen caerulescens*) compared to Canada geese (*Branta canadensis interior*); however, these differences are clinically insignificant (Williams and Trainer, 1971). Hematologic parameters may also fluctuate with genetic strains of domestic birds (Cheng et al., 2001).

Although normal erythrocyte reference intervals vary among species of birds, with a few exceptions, psittacine birds in captivity have similar erythrocyte parameters. For example, psittacine birds generally have a normal PCV between 35% and 55%; an erythrocyte count between $2.4 \times 10^6/\mu L$ and $5.0 \times 10^6/\mu L$; a hemoglobin concentration between 11 and 16 mg/dL; an MCV between 90 and 235 fL; and an MCHC between 20 and 40 g/dL (Appendix B, Table B.5).

Sex

Generally, the total erythrocyte counts and PCV tend to be higher in male compared to female birds. The reason for this may be a hormonal effect: estrogen depresses erythropoiesis, whereas androgens and thyroxin stimulate erythropoiesis. Variations in erythrocyte parameters associated with sex in ducks and geese are generally not statistically significant; however, differences between males and females have been reported and reflect a seasonal variation, where females tend to have higher PCV, Hb, TRBC, and MCHC values compared to males in the pre-nesting period (Williams and Trainer, 1971; Mulley, 1979; Mulley, 1980). Other studies have shown that averages for these parameters tend to be higher in the winter and pre-nesting period in adult ducks and geese regardless of sex compared to the post-nesting period and fall (Williams and Trainer, 1971; Shave and Howard, 1976). During migration, ducks tend to have slightly lower erythrocyte counts compared to wintering ducks, and post-nesting MCV averages for these birds tend to be higher in the winter or pre-nesting periods (Kocan and Pitts, 1976; Shave and Howard, 1976). These changes also occur in captive ducks that are not able to migrate.

Age

Age can cause variation in the normal hemogram of healthy birds. For example, 4- to 10-week-old ducklings exhibit a lower PCV and slightly higher protein concentration compared to adult ducks (Kocan and Pitts, 1976). Other studies showed significantly lower PCV, Hb, and TRBC in select Strigiformes chicks compared to juveniles and adults, and in ducklings compared to adults (Montolio et al., 2017; Bhattacherjee et al., 2018). This difference is likely associated with the high metabolic rate of young rapidly growing ducks that are consuming diets higher in protein and carbohydrates. In general, the total erythrocyte count, PCV, and MCV increase with age. In cases where Hb does not appear to be affected by age, a decline in MCHC is likely a function of an increase in MCV.

Season and Environment

Seasonal and environmental changes affect temperature, photoperiods, nutritional demands, and hormones. Migratory birds exhibit increased hematocrits and red blood cell numbers during migration, suggesting either a compensation for increased aerobic requirements or oxygen demand of the larger body mass of fattened birds (Landys-Ciannelli et al., 2002). In general, variations in these parameters in adult ducks and geese most likely reflect seasonal effects associated with hormonal and nutritional changes caused by alterations in the photoperiod and migration. Chicken red blood cell counts, and hematocrit values have also been found to be greater during dark periods versus light periods (Zhou et al., 1998). Turkeys have also shown to have increased hemoglobin, PCV, and TRBC during winter months owing to lower temperatures and increased metabolic rate stimulating erythropoiesis (Gattani et al., 2016).

Erythrocyte Response to Disease

Anemia in Birds

Anemia is the reduction in the total mass of hemoglobin-bearing erythrocytes, resulting in a deficiency of oxygen transport. Anemias result from an abnormal blood cell loss that cannot be compensated sufficiently by normal erythropoiesis or from decreased blood cell production that fails to adequately replace the red cells that are naturally lost. Anemias can be classified according to their pathophysiology as hemolytic (increased red cell destruction), hemorrhagic (blood loss), or hypoplastic (decreased red cell production or depression of hematopoiesis). Appendix B, Table B.5 provides guidelines for evaluating avian erythrocytes.

Birds, like mammals, respond to blood loss and blood destruction by increasing erythropoietin production, which stimulates erythropoiesis. Avian erythropoietin (a glycoprotein produced by the kidney) acts directly on the bone marrow to increase erythrocyte production. Avian erythropoietin does not stimulate mammalian erythropoiesis, however, and mammalian erythropoietin has no effect on avian hematopoiesis (Sturkie and Griminger, 1986).

Birds appear to develop anemia due to the lack of erythropoiesis (depression anemia) more quickly than mammals. This may be due in part to the relatively short avian erythrocyte half-life. The erythrocyte life span varies with the species of bird, but is generally shorter in comparison to mammals (Sturkie, 1976; Campbell and Dein, 1984). For example, the erythrocyte life span of

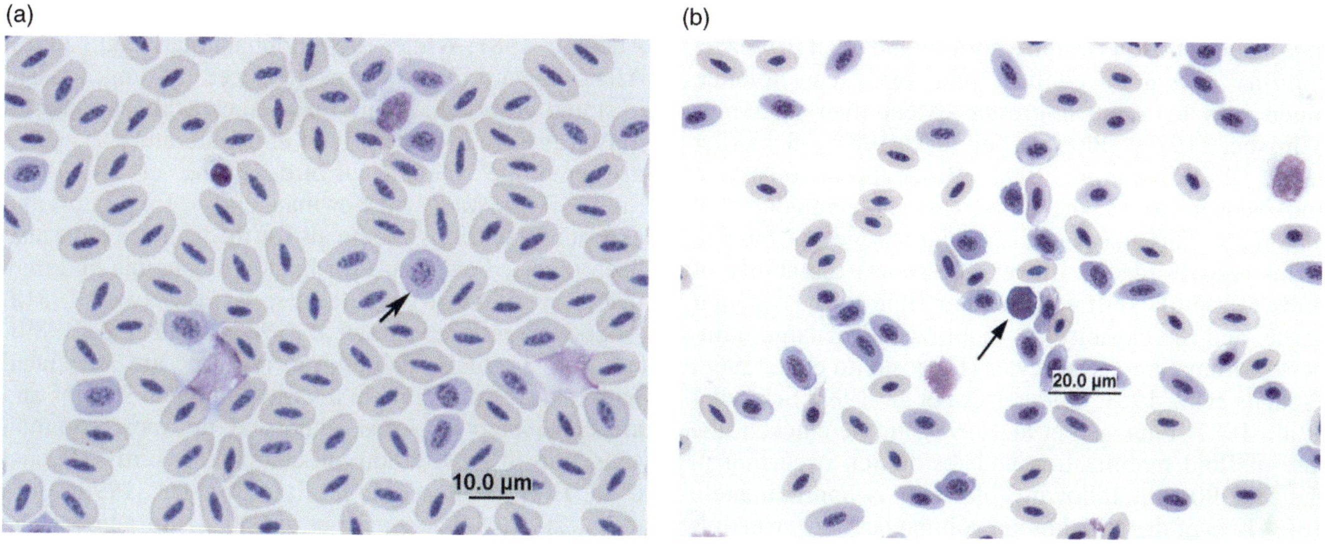

Fig. 11.9. (a) Immature erythrocytes, rubricytes (arrow), and increased polychromasia in the blood film of a wrinkled hornbill (*Aceros corrugatus*), Wright–Giemsa stain. (b) A basophilic rubricyte (arrow) and increased polychromasia in the blood film of a ferruginous hawk (*Buteo regalis*), Wright–Giemsa stain.

chickens is 35 days; ducks, 42 days; pigeons, 48 days; and quail, 34 days (Sturkie, 1976; Scanes, 2014). In general, avian erythrocytes in peripheral circulation have a half-life of 28–45 days (King and McLelland, 1984).

The PCV is the quickest and most practical method for evaluating the red cell mass of birds. Much as in mammals, the PCV of birds is affected by the number and size of the erythrocytes, as well as changes in the plasma volume that do not affect the total cell mass. These changes include increased plasma volume (hemodilution), decreased plasma volume (hemoconcentration), improper blood sampling (hemodilution), and epinephrine administration and hypothermia, which may result in hemoconcentration.

Since the normal PCV of many species of birds ranges between 35% and 55%, a PCV less than 35% is suggestive of anemia and a PCV greater than 55% suggests dehydration or erythrocytosis (polycythemia). Dehydration can be differentiated from erythrocytosis by using the total serum protein. Increased total protein indicates dehydration, and normal or low total protein supports erythrocytosis.

The presence and degree of erythrocyte polychromasia and reticulocytosis may be used as an indication of erythrogenesis. Polychromatic erythrocytes are expected to make up 5% or less of the total erythrocyte population in the blood of normal birds. Anemic birds with greater than 10% polychromasia (3+ and 4+ polychromasia) are exhibiting an appropriate regenerative response to their anemia, whereas those with a smaller response are not.

The number of reticulocytes present in the blood film may also be an indication of a bird's current response to anemia; however, absolute reticulocyte counts are rarely performed in avian hematology. Reticulocyte counts can be used in conjunction with assessment of the degree of polychromasia to determine the bird's current erythropoietic response.

Other evidence of active erythropoiesis is the presence of binucleate immature erythrocytes and an increase in the number of normal immature erythrocytes in the peripheral blood. The presence of immature erythrocytes (i.e., rubricytes) in the peripheral blood films of anemic birds, in addition to the presence of increased polychromasia, indicates a marked erythrocyte response (Figures 11.4a, 11.4b, 11.9a, and 11.9b). In nonanemic birds, however, these cells would be indicative of abnormal erythropoiesis. The presence of immature erythrocytes may also suggest early release from the hematopoietic tissue following anoxic insult or toxicity (i.e., lead poisoning) (Figure 11.3).

Hemorrhagic Anemia

The most common causes of hemorrhagic anemia in birds include traumatic injury, blood-sucking parasites, coagulopathies, ulcerated neoplasms, and hemorrhagic lesions of internal organs such as gastric ulceration or rupture of the liver or spleen. Heavy infestation with blood-sucking ectoparasites, such as ticks or mites (i.e., *Dermanyssus* mites) or gastrointestinal parasites, such as coccidia, can lead to severe anemia due to blood loss in birds (Szabo et al., 2002). Coagulopathies are usually acquired and are often associated with toxicities such as aflatoxicosis or coumarin poisoning, or with severe liver diseases such as papovavirus infections (Jacobson et al., 1984; Wainright et al., 1987; Lothrop et al., 1988; Gaskin, 1989; James et al., 1998).

Humane studies performed in pigeons (*Columba livia*), domestic fowl (*Gallus gallus*), and quail (*Coturnix coturnix japonica*) confirm that birds can tolerate blood loss to a much greater extent than mammals (Christie, 1979; Ploucha et al., 1981; Schindler et al., 1987; Bos et al., 1990). Birds appear to survive and recover from acute blood loss more rapidly than mammals. This may be due to the absence of mechanisms responsible for irreversible shock, the ability of birds to rapidly shift extracellular fluid to the vascular space, and the capacity for mobilization of large numbers of immature erythrocytes (Djojosugito et al., 1968; Ploucha et al., 1981; Gildersleeve et al., 1985; Schindler et al., 1987; Finnegan et al., 1997). In the chicken, the rate of fluid mobilization and restoration occurring in the first 90 min following bleeding is approximately 13%–17% of the initial blood volume per hour, which is twice that of the dog (Herbert et al., 1989). Diving and flying birds are more resistant to blood loss than nondiving birds such as Galliformes.

Hemolytic Anemia

Normally, a small percentage of damaged or senescent red blood cells is continually removed from circulation by the macrophages of the spleen and other hemopoietic tissues, and the iron contained within it is recycled. With hemolytic anemia, the destruction rate is higher than normal, the rate of erythrocyte production is increased to compensate, and immature erythrocyte stages are commonly found in the circulating blood. There are few reports of hemolytic anemia in birds, although systemic or hematogenous bacterial infection (septicemia), infectious disease, hemoparasites, and toxicities have all been associated with cases of avian hemolytic anemia (Assoku et al., 1970; Weiden and Blaese, 1971; Woerpel and Rosskopf, 1982; Leighton et al., 1983; Atkinson and Van Ripper, 1991; Powers, 2000). Hemolytic anemia is considered a responsive anemia, because it is associated with increased numbers of polychromatic erythrocytes, and is often associated with a subsequent increase in the hematocrit following successful treatment.

Salmonellosis or spirochetosis may cause bacterial septicemias that result in severe hemolytic anemia, and a regenerative anemia caused by chronic inflammation and hemolysis due to oxidation-associated increased red blood cell membrane fragility has been reported in birds with pansteatitis (Assoku et al., 1970; Wong et al., 1999). Most avian blood parasites have the potential to cause an anemia in the host; however, the two parasites most frequently associated with hemolytic anemia are *Plasmodium* and *Aegyptianella*.

Toxicosis is a frequent cause of hemolytic anemia in birds. Toxins that have been associated with hemolytic anemia in birds include aflatoxins, certain plant toxins, chemicals used in medical treatments, heavy metals, and petroleum products (Leighton et al., 1983; Fry and Addiego, 1987; White, 1990; Sobhakumari et al., 2018). Aflatoxins are fungal toxins produced by fungi present in stored grains, and plant toxins such as those found in mustards have been described in the literature as causes of hemolytic anemia in birds (Tung et al., 1975; Smith, 1980; Wade and Newman, 2004). Treatments and exposure to various chemicals for medical use have also been reported as causes for hemolytic anemia and may involve an immune-mediated response (Maxwell, 1981a; Abdo et al., 1983; Clark et al., 1988; Datta et al., 1989).

Heavy metals such as lead and zinc are associated with hemolytic anemia in a variety of avian species and are considered by some authors as the most common cause of this condition in companion birds (Droual et al., 1991; Ochiai et al., 1993; Marks et al., 1999; Jones et al., 2002; Sobhakumari et al., 2018). In general, the anemia caused by heavy metal poisoning is typically mild to moderate, with evidence of regeneration (Woerpel and Rosskopf, 1982; Campbell, 1995; Katavolos et al., 2007; Campbell and Grant, 2010).

Birds affected by lead poisoning may have diverse forms of poikilocytosis present in the hemogram. Erythrocyte morphological changes suggestive of heavy metal toxicosis in birds included prominent hypochromasia (including D cells: hypochromatic cells with ballooning or large clear areas in the cytoplasm), cytoplasmic stippling, poikilocytosis (dacryocytes, fusiform cells, distorted cells), and decreased size of polychromatic erythrocytes (Guthrie et al., 2020). Anemia results from damaged and defective erythrocytes that are removed in the spleen, liver, and kidney, producing hemosiderosis in those tissues (DeFrancisco et al., 2003). Severe zinc toxicosis can lead to faulty hematopoiesis and shortened erythrocyte life span due to alterations in copper and iron metabolism (Pimental et al., 1992). However, unlike dogs, zinc-poisoned birds generally do not exhibit a hemolytic crisis or morphologic changes in red blood cells (Romagnano et al., 1995). A regenerative anemia associated with reticulocytosis, increased numbers of immature erythrocytes, and abnormal red blood cell morphology, such as binucleated erythrocytes and increased poikilocytosis, has been reported in birds with experimental zinc intoxication (Levengood et al., 2000).

Hemolytic anemia and Heinz body anemia occur in marine birds associated with oil pollution or exposure to petroleum products and is characterized by low red cell indices and numerous immature erythrocytes (Leighton, 1985; Yamato et al., 1996). This anemia is caused by multiple factors and may be associated with or exacerbated by a variety of captivity-associated stressors and the age of the affected birds (Newman et al., 1999).

Heinz bodies may be associated with hemolytic anemia in birds. Heinz bodies represent oxidative damage to erythrocytes. The presence of these bodies in the red blood cell causes the cell membrane to change from pliable to rigid, which impedes passage of the cells through the microcirculation of the spleen. This in turn results in intravascular hemolysis or erythrophagocytosis by the reticuloendothelial system. Avian Heinz bodies resemble those seen in mammals except that they are considerably smaller (less than 2 μm in length), lack the classic button appearance (are oval or irregularly shaped), and occupy both the nucleoplasm and the cytoplasm (light blue inclusions found throughout the cytoplasm) (Simpson, 1971; Harr et al., 2017). In a variety of mammalian species, Heinz-body-associated hemolysis has occurred following the ingestion of onions (Valli, 1993). Anemia associated with onion ingestion is rare in birds; however, the toxic compounds in onions do damage the red blood cell membrane in birds as well (Crespo and Chin, 2004).

Hemolysis with agglutination of erythrocytes in blood films is a rare, abnormal finding that is suggestive of immune-mediated disease (Hawkey and Dennett, 1989; Jones et al., 2002; Campbell and Grant, 2010). Immune-mediated hemolytic anemia is rarely reported in birds other than poultry, and may be primary or secondary. Secondary causes of hemolytic anemia in birds may include drugs, infectious agents that stimulate an immune response to the remove erythrocytes from circulation, or other factors such as neoplasia. Some drugs bind to erythrocytes, causing an antibody response to the drug–erythrocyte antigen combination. Immune complexes subsequently form that adhere to erythrocyte membranes, or combine with an erythrocyte component, exposing its haptenic determinant (Schwartz et al., 2000). Some infectious agents induce antibodies that cross-react with erythrocyte epitopes. Neoplasia, especially the lymphoproliferative disorders, can also induce immune-mediated hemolytic anemia (Schwartz et al., 2000).

The clinical presentation of immune-mediated anemia in birds would include a strongly regenerative anemia with the presence of small, round erythrocytes (presumed to be spherocytes), and biliverdinuria resulting from extravascular hemolysis. This type of anemia would be expected to respond quickly to immunosuppressive treatment with corticosteroids. Other hematologic evidence of immune-mediated anemia might include a marked reticulocytosis, erythroid hyperplasia in the bone marrow, extramedullary erythropoiesis, and erythrophagocytosis. A definitive diagnosis would be based on a positive direct or indirect Coombs test (Assoku et al., 1970; Schwartz et al., 2000). Polyclonal antibody to chicken IgY does cross-react with parrot IgY; therefore, the chicken reagent could be used in either the direct or indirect Coombs tests to detect bound antierythrocytic antibodies in the cases of immune-mediated anemia in psittacines (Phalen et al., 1995).

Hemochromatosis has been associated with severe anemia with a marked regenerative response (4+ polychromasia and the presence of immature erythrocytes as early as prorubricytes) in one report in a psittacine bird (Rupiper and Read, 1996; Woerpel et al., 1992). It is possible that the hemochromatosis may have altered erythrocyte maturation as a result of defective iron uptake.

Nonregenerative (Depression) Anemia

Poorly regenerative or nonregenerative anemia is likely caused by an inflammatory or infectious disease combined with a catabolic state and the stress of captivity in many avian patients. Nonregenerative, normocytic, normochromic anemia is indicative of decreased erythropoiesis (depression anemia), which can develop rapidly in birds affected by inflammatory diseases, especially those involving infectious agents. The degree of polychromasia or reticulocytosis is poor to absent in birds with this type of anemia. Disorders frequently associated with depression anemia in birds include tuberculosis, aspergillosis, chlamydiosis, chronic hepatic or renal disease, hypothyroidism, neoplasia, and other chronic inflammatory diseases (Lothrop et al., 1988; Newell et al., 1991; Helmer et al., 2000). Nonregenerative anemia can also be associated with parasites, such as *Baylisascaris procyonis* infections (Wolf et al., 2007). Treatment with myelosuppressive medication for neoplastic lesions can also lead to depression anemia (Kisseberth and MacEwen, 1996). Chronic inflammation is often associated with a marked nonregenerative anemia, leukocytosis, and heterophilia (Kolmstetter et al., 1995a).

A macrocytic, normochromic anemia occurs in birds affected by food restriction or folic acid deficiency (Maxwell et al., 1991). Folic acid deficiency causes defective DNA synthesis, resulting in erythrocyte nuclear maturation that is out of step with hemoglobinization of the cytoplasm (Jain, 1993). Food restriction anemia is also associated with leukopenia, thrombocytopenia, abnormal erythrocyte shapes (marked poikilocytosis), and hypersegmentation of granulocytes (Maxwell et al., 1991). A dietary deficiency in vitamin B_{12} and folate was suspected to be responsible for an anemia (PCV 16%) with slight polychromasia (poor regenerative response) and folded and dacrocyte-like erythrocytes in a macaw with no abnormalities in the leukogram and thrombocyte count (Gupta et al., 2011).

Avian Erythrocytosis

Erythrocytosis (polycythemia) is rarely reported in birds and is probably caused by the same conditions associated with polycythemia in mammals (Taylor, 1987; Campbell and Grant, 2010, Fernandes et al., 2014). Primary erythrocytosis is a myeloproliferative disorder resulting in an absolute erythrocytosis, which is rarely

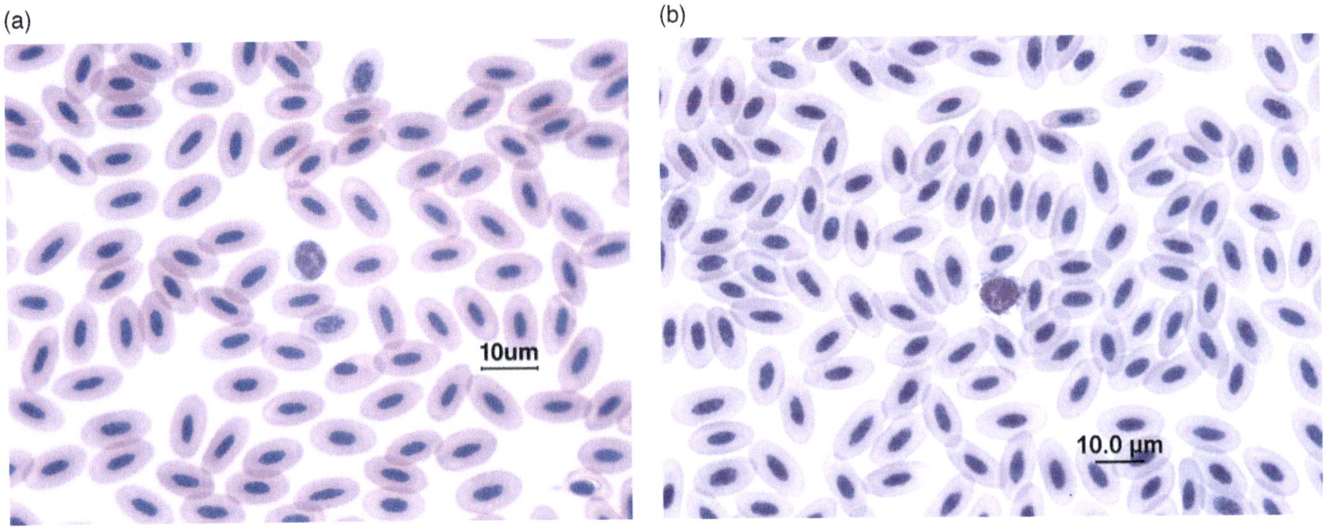

Fig. 11.10. (a) Lymphocyte in the blood film of a ring-necked parakeet (*Psittacula krameri*), Wright–Giemsa stain. (b) Lymphocyte in the blood film of a yellow-headed amazon (*Amazona oratrix*), Wright–Giemsa stain.

reported in birds. Most reported cases of an absolute erythrocytosis (PCV usually greater than 70%) in birds are secondary and are associated with chronic pulmonary disease. For example, a hornbill (*Aceros corrugatus*) with chronic erythrocytosis for two years was diagnosed with severe heart disease secondary to a pulmonary carcinoma which resulted in hypoxia (Romano et al., 2020). Other rule-outs to consider for erythrocytosis include cardiac insufficiency, increased erythropoietin associated with renal disease, or the presence of a relative erythrocytosis associated with dehydration. The last rule-out is likely responsible for most avian cases of erythrocytosis. A hemoconcentration phenomenon in chickens with a relative erythrocytosis was reported in one study during experimental aflatoxicosis (Fernandez et al., 1995). However, in another study, the hemoconcentration, a relative polycythemia, was seen in young chicks, but not adults (Lanza et al., 1980).

Erythrocytic neoplasia may occur in birds and is typified by the presence of numerous immature erythrocytes, especially rubriblasts, and abnormal-appearing immature erythrocytes in the peripheral blood. Erythroblastosis in poultry with avian leukosis complex is an example of this condition.

Avian Leukocytes

Accurate interpretation of leukocyte counts, especially when determined by semidirect methods, is dependent upon accurate identification and differentiation of leukocytes in the blood film. Leukopoiesis in normal birds is like that of mammals, in that leukocytes are released into the peripheral circulation only when they are mature. Leukocytes in bird blood include lymphocytes, monocytes, and granulocytes. The granulocytes are further classified as heterophils, eosinophils, and basophils.

Lymphocytes

Avian lymphocytes resemble mammalian lymphocytes. They are typically identified as round cells that often show cytoplasmic irregularity as they mold around adjacent erythrocytes in the blood film (Figures 11.10a and 11.10b). Avian lymphocytes must be differentiated from other cells in the peripheral blood that resemble them (Figures 11.11a–11.11e). Lymphocytes have a round, occasionally slightly indented, centrally, or slightly eccentrically positioned nucleus. The nuclear chromatin is heavily clumped or reticulated in mature lymphocytes. The cytoplasm is typically scant, giving lymphocytes a high nucleus to cytoplasm ratio (N:C); typically appears homogenous and weakly basophilic (pale blue); and lacks vacuoles or granules. Occasionally, lymphocytes may contain distinct azurophilic granules or irregular cytoplasmic projections (Figures 11.11a and 11.11c).

Differentiating Small Lymphocytes from Thrombocytes

Cytoplasmic features are important when differentiating small lymphocytes from thrombocytes. Thrombocytes have a cytoplasm that is clear and colorless, and often appears vacuolated with a few distinct specific granules. (Figures 11.11a–11.11e). Lymphocytes tend to be round, but may often mold around adjacent cells, whereas thrombocytes tend to cluster (Figure 11.11e).

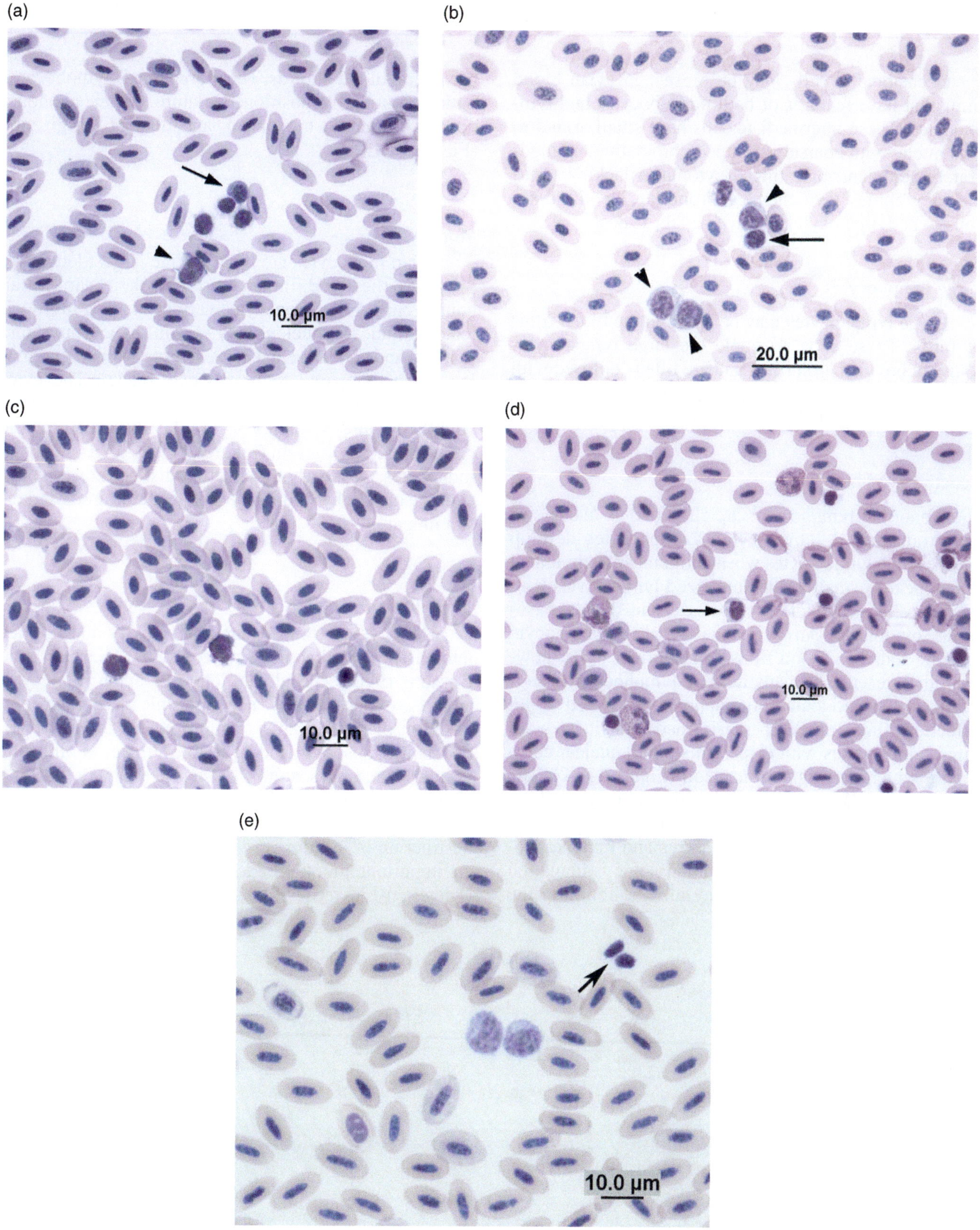

Fig. 11.11. (a) Immature erythrocyte—early polychromatic rubricyte (arrow), lymphocyte (arrowhead), and thrombocytes in the blood film of a conure (*Aratinga solstitialis*), Wright–Giemsa stain. (b) Large lymphocytes (arrowheads), medium lymphocyte (arrow), and thrombocyte in the blood film of a domestic chicken (*Gallus gallus domesticus*), Wright–Giemsa stain. (c) Lymphocyte with irregular cytoplasmic projections in the blood film of a yellow-headed amazon (*Amazona oratrix*), Wright–Giemsa stain. (d) Lymphocyte with azurophilic cytoplasmic granules (arrow) and thrombocyte in the blood film of a barred owl (*Strix varia*), Wright–Giemsa stain. (e) Two large lymphocytes (center) and two thrombocytes (arrow) in the blood film of a domestic duck (*Anas platyrhynchos domesticus*), Wright–Giemsa stain.

Occasionally, cells may be present in avian blood films that have features of both thrombocytes and lymphocytes. These intermediate cells have small, round to oval nuclei with coarsely clumped chromatin, and moderately abundant, blue-tinged cytoplasm lacking vacuoles or granules. Cytochemical properties identify these cells to be lymphocytes (Swayne et al., 1986).

Large Lymphocytes

Large lymphocytes may be noted in the blood films of birds. These cells resemble the large lymphocytes found in bovine blood films and are often confused with monocytes due to their size, large cytoplasmic volume, and pale staining nuclei (Figure 11.11b).

Reactive Lymphocytes

Abnormal lymphocytes are classified as reactive or blast-transformed lymphocytes. Lymphocytes develop into reactive lymphocytes when antigenically stimulated and appear as small to medium-sized lymphocytes with heavily clumped nuclear chromatin and deeply basophilic cytoplasm. An occasional reactive lymphocyte may be found in blood films from normal birds; however, the presence of many reactive lymphocytes is suggestive of antigenic stimulation associated with infectious diseases. Blast-transformed lymphocytes are large lymphocytes with dispersed smooth nuclear chromatin, which may contain nucleoli (Figure 11.12). The cytoplasm of these cells is basophilic and may exhibit a prominent clear perinuclear halo or Golgi zone. These lymphocytes have anaplastic features and may be neoplastic or may result from immunologic stimulation (Weiss, 1984). Plasma cells may also be found in the peripheral blood of birds. These are large B lymphocytes with eccentrically positioned mature nuclei, abundant deeply basophilic cytoplasm, and distinct Golgi zone (Figure 11.13).

Monocytes

Avian monocytes are typically the largest leukocyte present in the blood film and resemble their mammalian counterpart. Avian monocytes vary in shape from round to amoeboid. The nucleus may vary in shape from round to lobed and is relatively pale with less chromatin clumping when compared to lymphocyte nuclei. The cytoplasm is abundant, blue-gray in color, and may appear slightly opaque. Vacuoles or fine dust-like eosinophilic granules may be present (Figures 11.14a–11.14c). Avian monocytes frequently exhibit two distinct zones in the cytoplasm: a light-staining perinuclear area and a darker-staining area.

Macrophages

Monocytes exhibit phagocytic activity and migrate into tissues to become macrophages (Harmon and Blisson, 1990). The ultrastructure of avian monocytes and macrophages reveals a cytoplasmic membrane composed of blebs or filaments, a prominent Golgi apparatus, many ribosomes, and a variable number of pinocytic vesicles and lysosomes (Dieterien-Lievre, 1988). Monocytes and macrophages possess biologically active chemicals involved in inflammation mediation and the destruction of invading organisms. Monocytes also play an important immunologic role in antigen processing (Dieterien-Lievre, 1988).

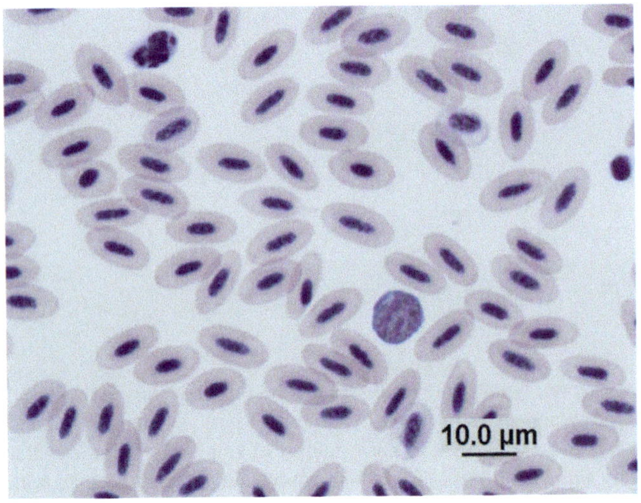

Fig. 11.12. Large reactive lymphocyte in the blood film of a conure (*Aratinga solstitialis*), Wright–Giemsa stain.

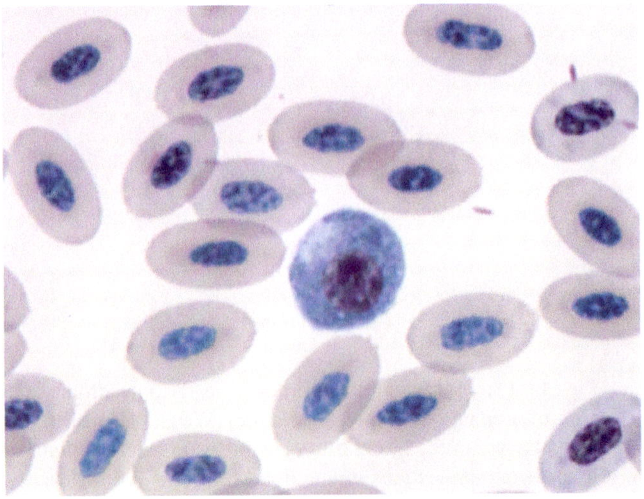

Fig. 11.13. Plasma cell in the blood film of a yellow-headed amazon (*Amazona oratrix*), Wright–Giemsa stain (100× oil).

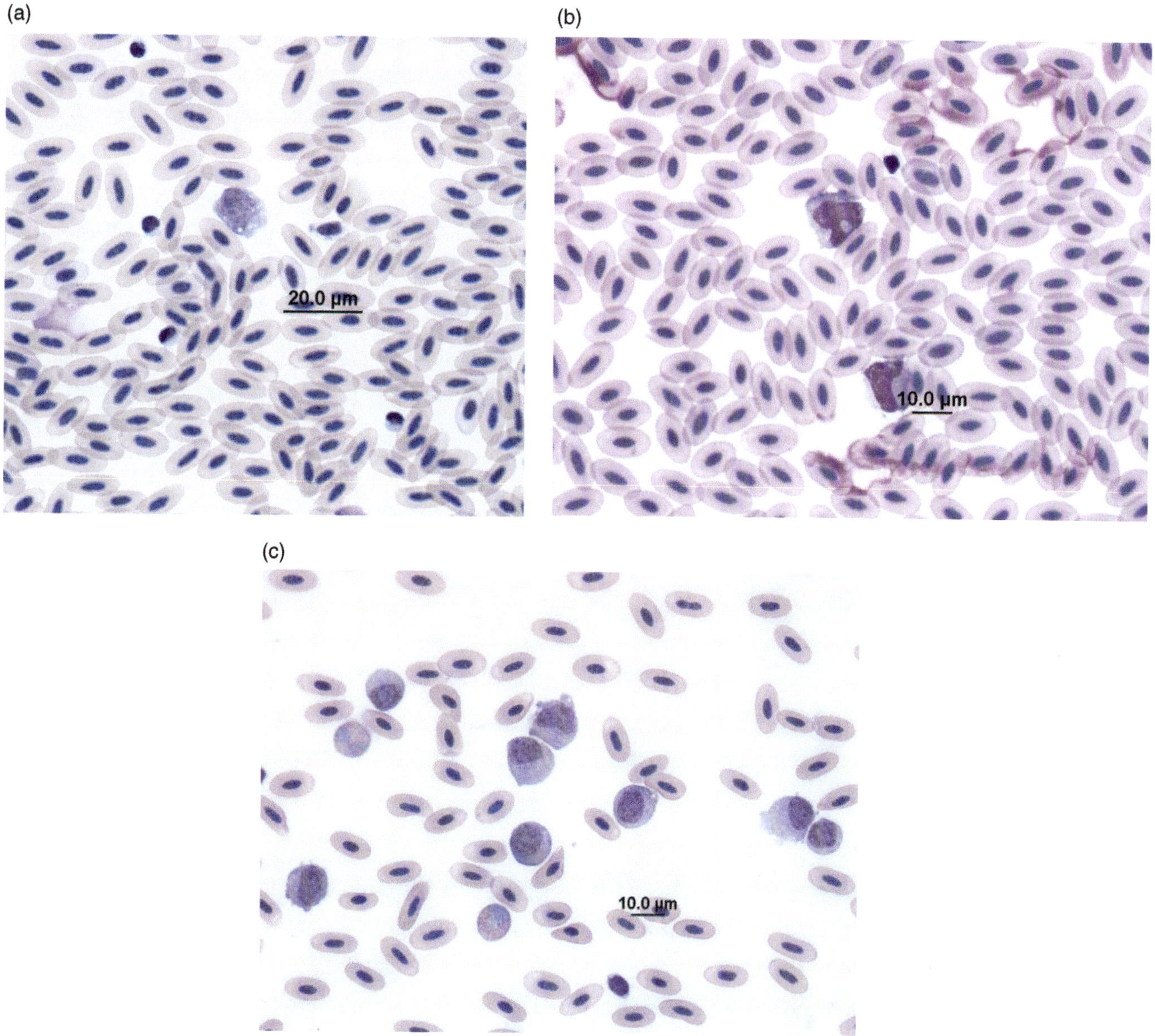

Fig. 11.14. (a) Monocyte in the blood film of an eclectus parrot (*Eclectus roratus*), Wright–Giemsa stain. (b) Monocytes in the blood film of a red-tailed hawk (*Buteo jamaicensis*), Wright–Giemsa stain. (c) Monocytosis in the blood film of a gannet (*Morus* sp.), Wright–Giemsa stain.

Heterophils

The heterophil is functionally equivalent to the mammalian neutrophil and is the most abundant granulocyte of many avian species. The ultrastructure of the avian heterophil has been described by several electron microscopy studies (Campbell, 1967; Wood, 1967; Enbergs and Kriesten, 1968; Dhingra et al., 1969; Maxwell and Trejo, 1970; Ericsson and Nair, 1973; Maxwell, 1973; Nair, 1973; Yamada et al., 1973; Enbergs, 1975; Lewis et al., 1979). In general, heterophils tend to be round, although their shape may be distorted, and have a mean diameter of 8.8 µm. Peripheral pseudopodia and/or lobopodia may occasionally be noted morphologically. Heterophil size tends to be uniform for each species of bird, although slight species variations may be noted morphologically (Maxwell, 1973). Laboratory technique in preparation of the blood film may also be a factor in heterophil size variability (Roberts and Maxwell, 1993).

The nucleus of the mature heterophil is lobed (two to three lobes), with coarse, clumped, purple-staining chromatin. The nucleus is often partially hidden by the cytoplasmic granules.

The cytoplasm of normal mature heterophils appears colorless and contains granules that stain an eosinophilic color (dark orange to brown red) with Romanowsky stains (Figures 11.15a–11.15d). The granules can be affected by the staining process, and may appear atypical

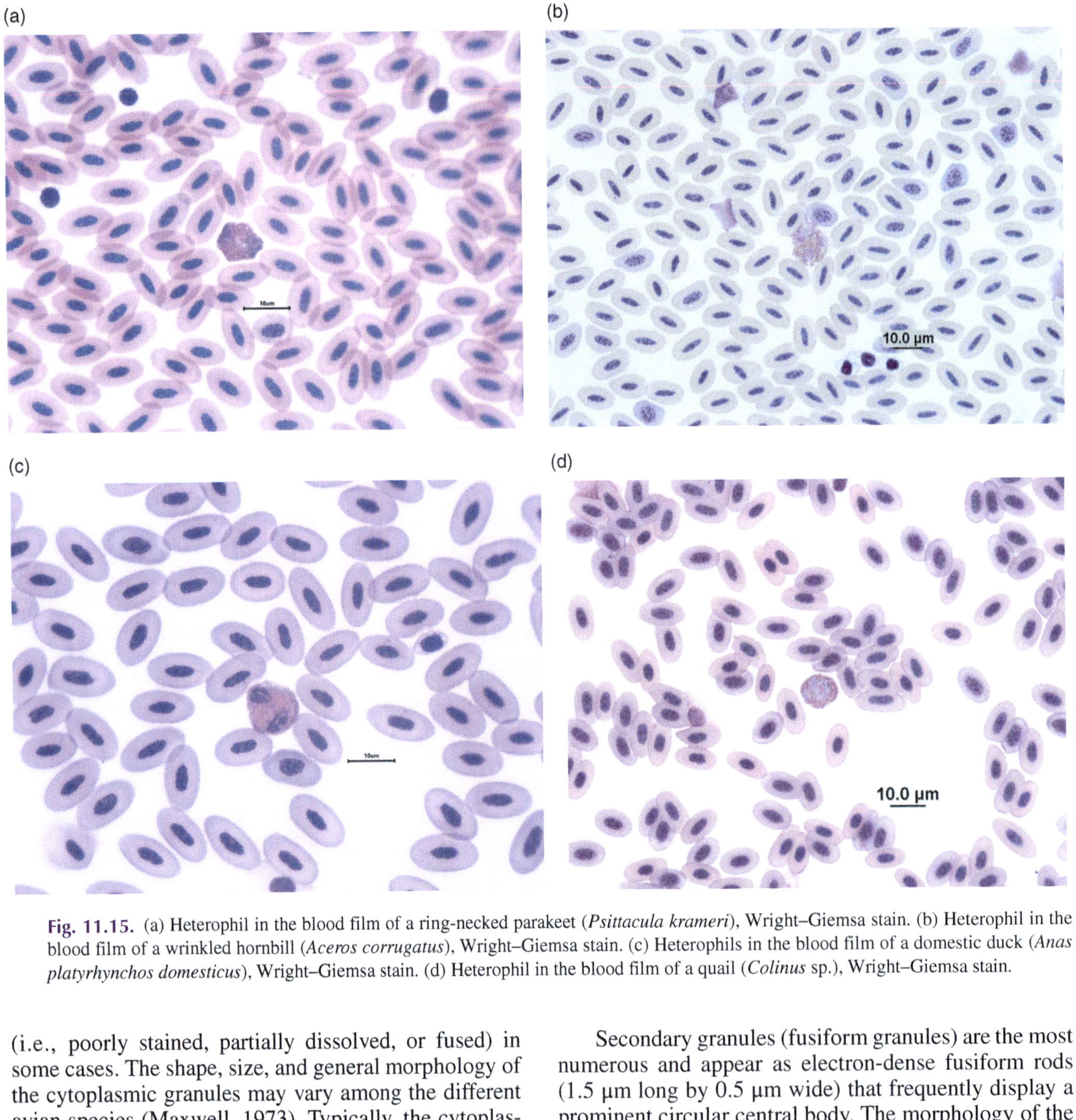

Fig. 11.15. (a) Heterophil in the blood film of a ring-necked parakeet (*Psittacula krameri*), Wright–Giemsa stain. (b) Heterophil in the blood film of a wrinkled hornbill (*Aceros corrugatus*), Wright–Giemsa stain. (c) Heterophils in the blood film of a domestic duck (*Anas platyrhynchos domesticus*), Wright–Giemsa stain. (d) Heterophil in the blood film of a quail (*Colinus* sp.), Wright–Giemsa stain.

(i.e., poorly stained, partially dissolved, or fused) in some cases. The shape, size, and general morphology of the cytoplasmic granules may vary among the different avian species (Maxwell, 1973). Typically, the cytoplasmic granules appear elongate (rod or spiculate shaped), but may appear oval to round as well. Ultrastructural studies of avian heterophils reveal primary, secondary, and tertiary granules (Dieterien-Lievre, 1988). Small- and medium-sized granules may be seen ultrastructurally in avian heterophils as well and probably represent maturation stages of the cytoplasmic granules (Dieterien-Lievre, 1988). Functionally, the cytoplasmic granules contain lysosomal and nonlysosomal enzymes used for bactericidal activity (Brune and Spitznagel, 1973; Pinneall and Spitznagel, 1975; Daimon and Caxton-Martins, 1977; Hodges, 1977).

Secondary granules (fusiform granules) are the most numerous and appear as electron-dense fusiform rods (1.5 µm long by 0.5 µm wide) that frequently display a prominent circular central body. The morphology of the central body can be variable depending on the avian species, but often appears circular. These central bodies are electron dense and contain a less dense granular matrix that may be proteinaceous in nature. The density of the granular matrix is similar in density to the crystalline interna present in eosinophil granules of certain birds (Maxwell and Siller, 1972; Maxwell, 1979; Hayat, 1989; Egami and Sasso, 1991).

Other granules are smaller (0.5 µm diameter), less dense, and contain eccentric inclusions composed of loose filamentous material. These granules can be identified in the heterophils of most avian species (Maxwell and Robertson, 1998). Tertiary granules are very small comparatively (0.1 μm) and have a dense core separated from a membranous envelope of an electron-lucent area.

Heterophils are highly phagocytic, have considerable bactericidal activity, and actively participate in inflammatory lesions (Topp and Carlson, 1972a, 1972b). Studies indicate that the bactericidal activity of the avian heterophil is primarily mediated through nonoxidative mechanisms that rely on oxygen-independent mechanisms, lysozyme, and cationic proteins (i.e., acid hydrolases and cathepsin) to destroy microorganisms (Dri et al., 1978; Harmon, 1998). Other studies using a more sensitive detection system have demonstrated oxidative responses (Desmidt et al., 1996). For example, chicken heterophils lack alkaline phosphatase, catalase, and myeloperoxidase needed for oxygen-dependent killing of microorganisms, but do consume oxygen and produce oxygen radicals and hydrogen peroxide, albeit to a lesser extent than mammalian neutrophils (Dri et al., 1978; Andreasen and Latimer, 1990; Brooks et al., 1996). As previously stated, unlike mammalian neutrophils, avian heterophils are devoid of myeloperoxidase (Kelenyi and Nemeth, 1969a, 1969b; Brune and Spitznagel, 1973; Pinneall and Spitznagel, 1975; Rausch and Moore, 1975; Daimon and Caxton-Martins, 1977; Breton-Gorius et al., 1978; Andreasen and Latimer, 1990; Egami and Sasso, 1991). Despite this, avian heterophils are still capable of phagocytosis. Avian heterophils phagocytize and destroy microorganisms using oxygen-dependent and oxygen-independent mechanisms. The cytoplasmic granules contain hydrolytic bactericidal lysosomal and nonlysosomal enzymes that can perform in the phagocytic role (Brune and Spitznagel, 1973; Pinneall and Spitznagel, 1975; Daimon and Caxton-Martins, 1977; Hodges, 1977). These enzymes include acid phosphatase, arylsulfatase, b-glucuronidase, phosphorylase, uridine diphosphate glucose–glycogen glycosyltransferase, neutral and acid a-glucosidases, acid tri-metaphosphatase, and lysozyme (Osculati, 1970; Topp and Carlson, 1972a, 1972b; Ericsson and Nair, 1973; Nair, 1973; Rausch and Moore, 1975; Fujimori et al., 1979; Maxwell, 1984). Although cytochemical staining is useful in differentiating mammalian blood cells, it is not as useful for differentiating avian blood cells where there is considerable staining heterogeneity. For example, Periodic Acid-Schiff (PAS) staining is used to differentiate granulocytic and megakaryocytic precursors in mammals; however, it is not useful in avian cytochemical studies (Salakij et al., 2019).

Heterophils appear to play a crucial role in controlling bacterial invasion and subsequent pathogenesis of bacterial infections in birds, and heterophils have also been shown to participate in viral and parasitic infections (Rose et al., 1979; Penigrahy et al., 1986; Janes et al., 1994; Lam et al., 1996). In the presence of certain bacterial pathogens (*Salmonella* species and *Escherichia coli*), heterophils appear to be more effective than macrophages in the absence of antibody-assisted bacterial phagocytosis and killing (Stabler et al., 1994; Kogut et al., 1995; Ziprin, 1997; Maxwell and Robertson, 1998). In the early phase of bacterial infections, heterophils mobilize within a few hours; a decrease in the number of circulating heterophils in the peripheral blood may be noted early in the course of infection (Tellez et al., 1993).

Abnormal-Appearing Heterophils

Abnormal-appearing heterophils in blood films include both immature and toxic heterophils. Immature heterophils have increased cytoplasmic basophilia, non-segmented nuclei, and immature cytoplasmic granules when compared to normal mature heterophils (Figure 11.16).

The immature heterophils most frequently encountered in the blood are myelocytes and metamyelocytes (Figure 11.17). Heterophil myelocytes are larger than mature heterophils and have a round to oval non-segmented nucleus, blue cytoplasm, and contain rod-shaped granules, which occupy less than one-half the cytoplasmic volume. Heterophil metamyelocytes resemble myelocytes, except that the nucleus is indented and the rod-shaped granules occupy more than one-half the cytoplasmic volume.

Band heterophils resemble mature heterophils except that the nucleus is not lobed. The nucleus of the band cell has smooth parallel sides and is frequently horseshoe shaped. It is often difficult to recognize a band cell, because the nucleus is frequently hidden by the cytoplasmic granules. Therefore, a true assessment of the concentration of band cells in blood films of birds

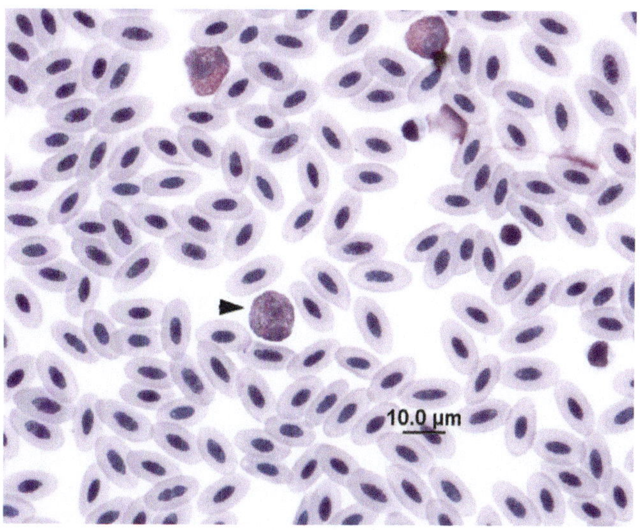

Fig. 11.16. Immature heterophil (arrowhead) in the blood film of a yellow-headed amazon (*Amazona oratrix*), Wright–Giemsa stain.

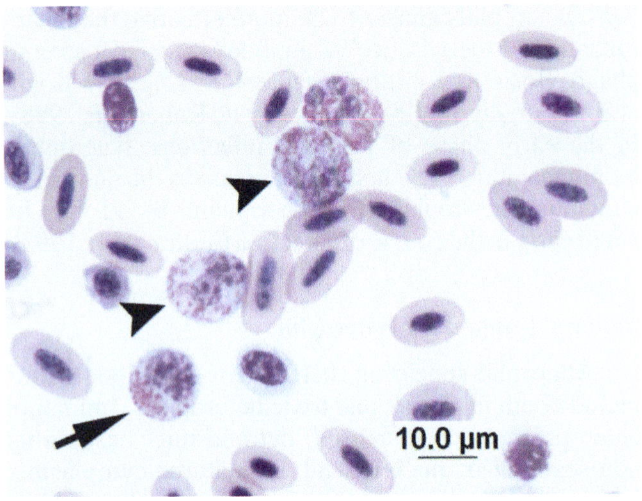

Fig. 11.17. Immature heterophils. A myelocyte (arrow) and two metamyelocytes (arrowheads) in the blood film of a ferruginous hawk (*Buteo regalis*), Wright–Giemsa stain. The heterophil at the top of the image is mature, as indicated by the rod-shaped granules filling the cytoplasm and segmented nucleus.

requires the use of a nuclear stain, such as hematoxin, which stains only the nucleus and not the cytoplasmic granules. The presence of band cells indicates an early release of heterophils into the peripheral circulation.

Immature heterophils are rarely found in the blood film of normal birds. When present, they represent a left shift indicating an increased demand for heterophils owing to an inflammatory stimulus and can be associated with either a heterophilia or heteropenia.

Toxic Change

In response to severe systemic illness, avian heterophils exhibit toxic changes similar to those seen in mammalian neutrophils (Schalm et al., 1975; Coles, 1986; Campbell, 1995; Campbell and Grant, 2010). Toxic changes are subjectively quantified as to the number of toxic cells and severity of toxicity present, as in mammalian hematology (Weiss, 1984). When present, toxic heterophils represent a severe inflammatory response regardless of the leukocyte count. The heterophil toxic changes associated with inflammatory responses are probably the cause of the same toxic changes present in human and mammalian neutrophils. Originally, in human medicine, the "toxic changes in neutrophils" were thought to be caused by an alteration of cell morphology and function in association with toxemia (Zieve et al., 1966). It is now believed that the cells have normal function and that the morphologic changes are attributable to altered bone marrow production (Weiser, 2012). The bone marrow responds to an inflammatory stimulus by accelerating the rate of heterophil production, resulting in the presence of heterophils that may have increased amounts of organelles that are present during early development.

The principal manifestation of toxic change is cytoplasmic basophilia, which is attributable to a larger-than-normal complement of ribosomes. Other manifestations accompanying cytoplasmic basophilia include cytoplasmic vacuolization, abnormal granulation (degranulation, granules that appears deeply basophilic, or granules that appear to coalesce into large round granules), retention of primary granules, decreased number of definitive granules, and degeneration of the cell nucleus (Figures 11.18a–11.18f).

The degree of heterophil toxic change can be rated subjectively on a scale of 1+ to 4+. A 1+ degree of toxicity is assigned when the heterophils exhibit an increase in cytoplasmic basophilia. A 2+ degree of toxicity is assigned when the cells demonstrate deeper cytoplasmic basophilia and partial degranulation. Heterophils with a 3+ degree of toxicity have dark cytoplasmic basophilia, moderate degranulation, abnormal granules, and cytoplasmic vacuolization. Heterophils with a 4+ degree of toxicity exhibit deep cytoplasmic basophilia, moderate to marked degranulation with the presence of abnormal granules, cytoplasmic vacuolization, and karyorrhexis or karyolysis. The number of toxic heterophils is graded as few (5–10%), moderate (11–30%), and marked (greater than 30%) (Table 11.1).

Eosinophils

Most avian eosinophils are similar in size to the heterophil, although species variation does exist (Hawkey and Dennett, 1989). The mean diameter of most avian eosinophils is 7.9 μm. Comparatively, the mean diameter of the heterophil is 8.8 μm (Maxwell, 1984). The nucleus of the eosinophil is lobed and usually stains darker than the nucleus of a heterophil, and the cytoplasm stains clear blue in contrast to the colorless cytoplasm of normal mature heterophils (Figures 11.19a–11.19f). Granules are present in the cytoplasm and are strongly eosinophilic in appearance. The granules are typically round in shape, although the granules of some avian species may be described as oval or elongate. Eosinophil granules tend to stain more intensely compared to the granules of the heterophil and may vary in appearance when Romanowsky stain is used; may appear colorless; may stain pale blue; or may appear large, swollen, and round (Figures 11.20a and 11.20b).

The cytoplasmic granules of avian eosinophils lack the central refractile body noted in many avian heterophils. Ultrastructural studies of the avian eosinophils reveal the presence of large spherical primary granules and mature rod-shaped specific granules. The larger primary granules are most likely precursors to the smaller specific granules. The specific granules appear to be similar to those present in mammalian eosinophils and contain

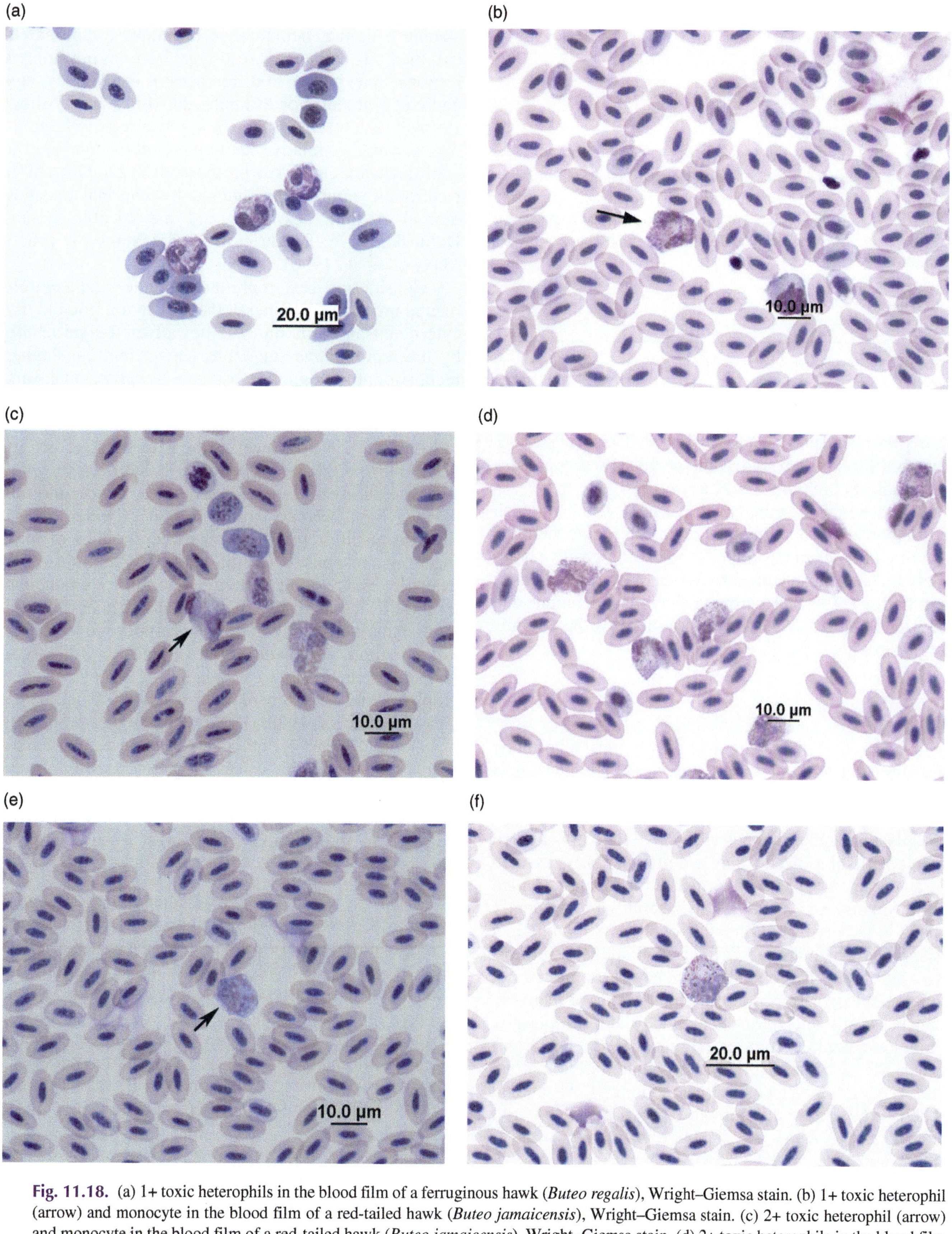

Fig. 11.18. (a) 1+ toxic heterophils in the blood film of a ferruginous hawk (*Buteo regalis*), Wright–Giemsa stain. (b) 1+ toxic heterophil (arrow) and monocyte in the blood film of a red-tailed hawk (*Buteo jamaicensis*), Wright–Giemsa stain. (c) 2+ toxic heterophil (arrow) and monocyte in the blood film of a red-tailed hawk (*Buteo jamaicensis*), Wright–Giemsa stain. (d) 2+ toxic heterophils in the blood film of a great horned owl (*Bubo virginianus*), Wright–Giemsa stain. (e) 3+ toxic heterophil (arrow) in the blood film of a conure (*Aratinga solstitialis*), Wright–Giemsa stain. (f) 3+ toxic heterophil in the blood film of an eclectus parrot (*Eclectus roratus*), Wright–Giemsa stain.

Table 11.1. Summary of heterophil toxicity scale and grade.

Toxicity Scale	
1+	Increased cytoplasmic basophilia
2+	Deeper cytoplasmic basophilia and partial degranulation
3+	Dark cytoplasmic basophilia, moderate degranulation, abnormal granules, cytoplasmic vacuolization
4+	Deep cytoplasmic basophilia, moderate to marked degranulation with presence of abnormal granules, cytoplasmic vacuolization, karyorrhexis or karyolysis
Grade*	
Few	5–10%
Moderate	11–30%
Marked	>30%

*Based on the number of cells exhibiting toxicity per [×1000] monolayer field.

high concentrations of arginine and enzymes such as peroxidase, acid phosphatase, and arylsulfatase (Dieterien-Lievre, 1988). In some birds, the specific granules possess a crystalline core (Dieterien-Lievre, 1988).

Cytochemical stains may be used to distinguish eosinophils from heterophils. For example, cytochemical staining of chicken eosinophils indicates a positive reactivity for acid phosphatase and Sudan black B (Andreasen and Latimer, 1990). A peroxidase staining technique can be used to differentiate peroxidase-negative heterophils from peroxidase-positive eosinophils.

Basophils

Avian basophils contain deeply metachromatic granules that often obscure the nucleus. The nucleus is usually nonlobed, causing avian basophils to resemble mammalian mast cells (Figures 11.21a and 11.21b). The cytoplasmic granules of basophils are frequently affected by alcohol-solubilized stains and may partially dissolve or coalesce and appear abnormal in blood films stained with Romanowsky stains. Avian basophils are frequently found in the peripheral blood, in contrast to mammalian basophils, which are rarely found in blood films of normal animals. The function of avian basophils is not known, but is presumed to be similar to that of mammalian basophils and mast cells, since their cytoplasmic granules contain histamine (Hodges, 1974; Dieterien-Lievre, 1988). They participate in acute, inflammatory, and type IV hypersensitivity reactions (Carlson and Allen, 1969; Fox and Solomon, 1981).

Normal Variation to the Leukogram of Birds

Changes in the avian leukogram, when comparing to individual baseline results or to reference intervals, may be from a physiologic and/or pathologic response. When comparing results to documented reference intervals, variation may also exist due to differences in sample handling, hematologic techniques, and analytical methods. Changes resulting from a physiologic response may be due to differences in species, sex, age, and environment. For example, ducklings and goslings younger than 60 days of age have lower relative lymphocyte and higher relative heterophil counts compared to adult ducks and geese (Fairbrother and O'Loughlin, 1990). Heterophil numbers are altered by seasonal changes, diurnal rhythm, sex, age, and diet (Dobinsky and Dobinska, 1976; Reddy et al., 1981; Maxwell, 1981b; Maxwell et al., 1990).

Considering sex, reproductive state, and environmental influence, in general, the leukogram (total leukocyte count and H:L ratio) is not affected significantly by the reproductive state (pre–egg laying, egg laying, incubation, molting, and post–egg laying) of ducks and geese and there is no significant difference between sexes (Williams and Trainer, 1971; Fairbrother and O'Loughlin, 1990). However, the percentage of heterophils in the peripheral blood of ducks has been shown to decrease during and immediately following the molting of the flight feathers (remige molt) (Driver, 1981). Significant differences occur between species of birds regarding responses to inflammatory stimulus. For example, birds with a normal heterophil to lymphocyte ratio (H:L) less than 1.0, such as many species of waterfowl, exhibit an initial leukogram response to stress and inflammation, with leukopenia associated with a lymphopenia followed up to 12 h later by leukocytosis, heterophilia, and lymphopenia (Davidson and Flack, 1981; Gross and Siegel, 1983). Birds with a higher proportion of heterophils than lymphocytes in their normal leukograms tend to exhibit a less dramatic response in the stress leukogram.

Leukocyte Response to Disease

The general causes of leukocytosis in birds include inflammation, which may be associated with infectious or noninfectious etiologies; toxicities; hemorrhage into a body cavity; rapidly growing neoplasms; and leukemia. The leukocyte differential aids in the assessment of a leukocytosis. The type of leukocytes present and the morphology of the cells are often a useful diagnostic tool when assessing the avian patient and establishing rule-out lists and treatment protocols and may serve as a prognostic indicator as well. Appendix B, Table B.6 provides guidelines for evaluating avian leukocytes.

Inflammatory Leukogram

The presence of an inflammatory leukogram is an indicator of the presence of a severe illness or condition, such as the presence of a gastrointestinal foreign body, severe infection, toxicity, traumatic injury, or neoplasia.

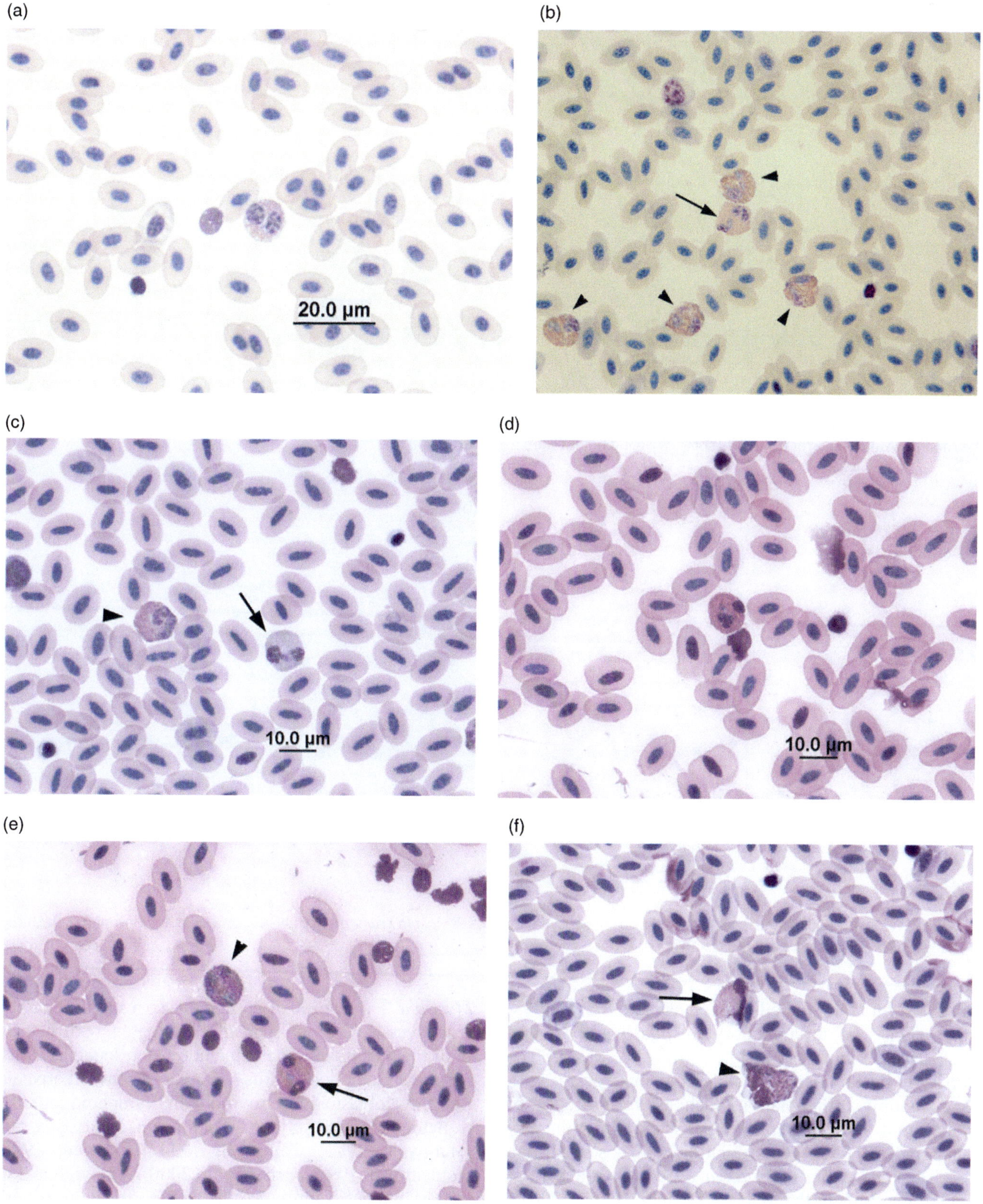

Fig. 11.19. (a) Eosinophil in the blood film of a domestic chicken (*Gallus gallus domesticus*), Wright–Giemsa stain. (b) Eosinophil (arrow) and heterophils (arrowheads) in the blood film of a red-tailed hawk (*Buteo jamaicensis*), Wright–Giemsa stain (100× oil). (c) Eosinophil (arrow) and heterophil (arrowhead) in the blood film of a barred owl (*Strix varia*), Wright–Giemsa stain. (d) Eosinophil in the blood film of a golden eagle (*Aquila chrysaetos*), Wright–Giemsa stain. (e) Eosinophil (arrow) and heterophil (arrowhead) in the blood film of a golden eagle (*Aquila chrysaetos*), Wright–Giemsa stain. (f) Eosinophil (arrow) and a 1+ toxic heterophil (arrowhead) in the blood film of a red-tailed hawk (*Buteo jamaicensis*), Wright–Giemsa stain.

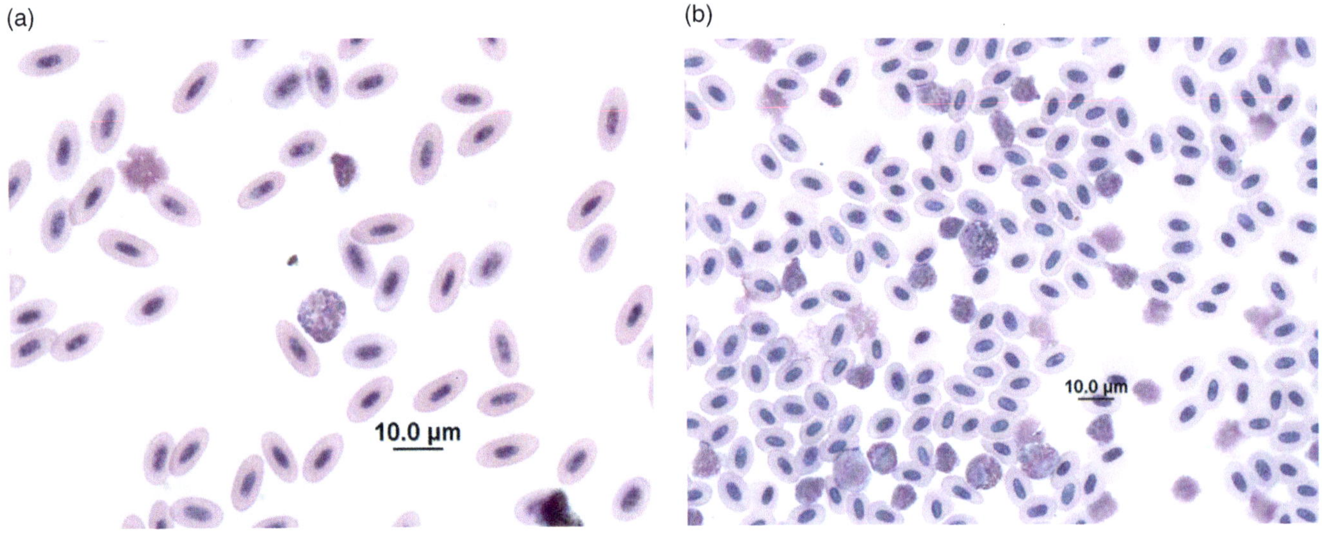

Fig. 11.20. An eosinophil with blue staining cytoplasmic granules in the blood film of an (a) African gray parrot (*Psittacus erithacus*) and (b) Amazon parrot (*Amazona* spp.), Wright–Giemsa stain.

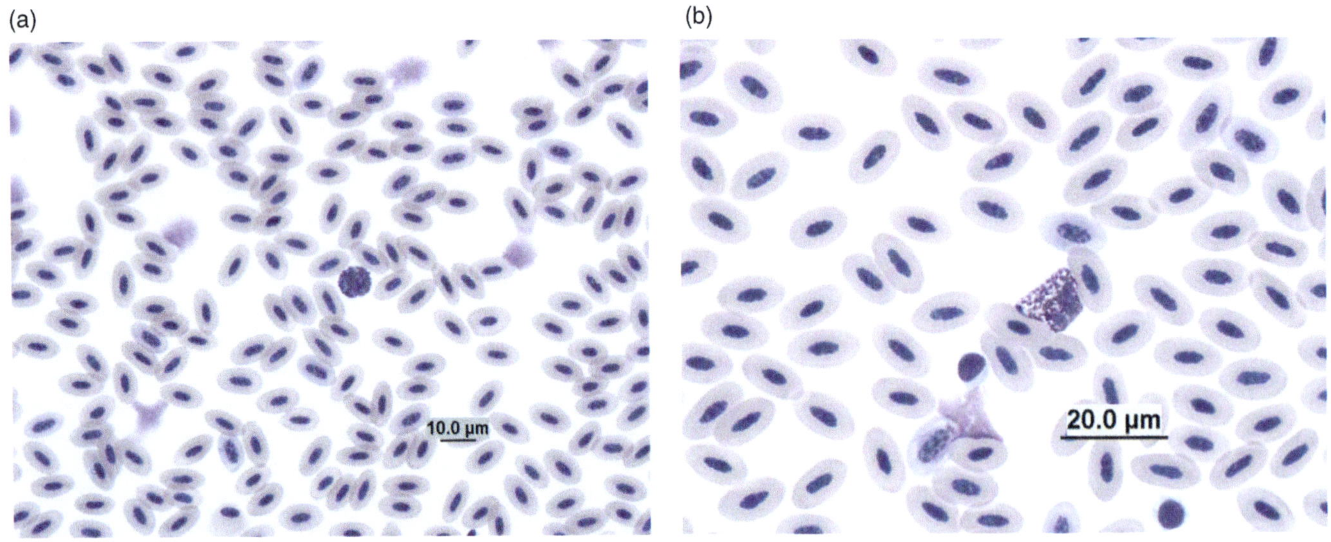

Fig. 11.21. (a) Basophil in the blood film of a ring-necked parakeet (*Psittacula krameri*), Wright–Giemsa stain. (b) Basophil in the blood film of an eclectus parrot (*Eclectus roratus*), Wright–Giemsa stain.

Intracoelomic foreign bodies, such as radio transmitters, may elicit an inflammatory response (Korschgen et al., 1996; Schultz et al., 1998; Mulcahy et al., 2007). Persistent inflammatory leukograms may occur with long-standing inflammation, such as the presence of granulomas. For example, a persistent inflammatory leukogram of three years duration was observed in a peach-fronted conure (*Aratinga aurea*) with a barium granuloma within the trachea (Latney et al., 2007). Inflammatory leukograms have been reported in ducklings fed mycotoxins (Chowdhury et al., 2005). A marked leukocytosis and heterophilia are often associated with diseases produced by common avian pathogens, such as *Chlamydia*, *Aspergillus*, *Salmonella*, and *Mycobacterium*. Viral diseases can also result in a marked leukocytosis, but not typically associated with heterophilic leukocytosis. These include avian leukosis virus, reticuloendotheliosis virus, Marek's disease (herpesvirus), myeloblastosis (retrovirus), and lymphoid leukosis (reticuloendotheliosis virus and avian leukosis virus) (Halliwell, 1971; Campbell, 1994; Coleman, 1995; Heidenreich, 1997; Forbes et al., 2000). Although leukocytosis and heterophilia have been reported in birds with avian bornavirus infections, the experimental results were inconsistent; therefore, leukocyte changes are likely related to stress or the existence of secondary infections (Högemann et.al., 2017). A marked leukocytosis can also be associated with noninfectious etiologies, such as trauma, neoplasia, and toxicities (such as mycotoxins, aflatoxicosis, and microcystin toxicosis) (Campbell, 1994; Chowdhury et al., 2005; McCain et al., 2020).

Although the nature of the immune response to bacterial infections in birds has not yet been fully elucidated, nonlymphoid cells, such as macrophages and heterophils, play a crucial role in immunity to bacteria (Kogut et al., 1995; Barrow, 1996; Harmon, 1998; Quereshi, 1998). Therefore, increases in the numbers of heterophils and monocytes in the peripheral blood would be expected with bacterial infections. The degree of the inflammatory response present in the blood may be associated with the location of the bacterial infection. For example, psittacine birds with varying degrees and causes of sinusitis often exhibit normal complete blood cell counts or have only a mild inflammatory leukogram, perhaps because the lesions remained a focal one (Pye et al., 2000).

An inflammatory leukogram characterized by heterophilia and/or monocytosis is often associated with infections with *Chlamydia* or mycotic infections, such as aspergillosis (Johns et al., 2009). The presence of toxic or immature heterophils indicates severe inflammation and a poor prognosis for survival.

An inflammatory leukogram characterized by heterophilia, lymphopenia, and monocytosis may be associated with neoplastic diseases such as squamous cell carcinoma, papillomatosis, and other neoplasms in birds (Helmer et al., 2000; Jones et al., 2001; Gibbons et al., 2002; Campbell and Grant, 2010). Bacterial or fungal infections within the lesions may be responsible for this; however, tissue necrosis and granulocyte breakdown can also stimulate the inflammatory response. A hematopoietic factor capable of promoting a leukocytosis may also be produced by some tumors and could be a factor in the presence of the inflammatory leukogram (Ogilvie, 1996). For example, the hemogram of a peach-fronted conure (*Aratinga aurea*) with internal papillomatosis, intrahepatic cholangiocarcinoma, and gastrointestinal adenocarcinoma revealed toxic heterophils, a left shift of the heterophils, and lymphopenia (Gibbons et al., 2002). Chronic mucosa irritation of the gastrointestinal tract due to the presence of the internal papillomatosis could have served as the source of the inflammatory leukogram (Sunber et al., 1986).

Common hematologic abnormalities associated with avian mycobacteriosis include mild to moderate nonregenerative anemia, marked to severe leukocytosis, heterophilia, lymphopenia, monocytosis, eosinophilia, and immature heterophils (Gibbons and Sakas, 1997; Tell et al., 2004; Steinmetz et al., 2006; Heatley et al., 2007; Mans and Guzman, 2007; Hannon et al., 2012). Thrombocytosis has also been reported in birds with mycobacteriosis (Tell et al., 2004). Laboratory findings can be variable and reflect the stage of the disease, presence of concurrent illness, and species differences. Initial hematologic results may be normal in some individuals. In such cases, repeat and serial complete blood cell counts may be useful in the diagnosis of mycobacteriosis. A leukocytosis with a moderate to marked monocytosis, with or without heterophilia, is supportive of possible mycobacteriosis (Bale et al., 2020). High leukocyte counts are typically seen in birds with advanced mycobacteriosis (Sutherland et al., 2018). When present, immature heterophils indicate a poor prognosis.

Heterophilia

Leukocytosis and heterophilia can be associated with localized or systemic infections caused by a veritable spectrum of infectious agents (i.e., bacteria, fungi, *Chlamydia*, viruses, *Mycoplasma*, and parasites) and noninfectious etiologies (i.e., traumatic injury, toxicities, stress). For example, leukocytosis has been associated with hepatic trematode infestations (Kuiken and Danesik, 1999), and a marked leukocytosis and heterophilia can be associated with organophosphate toxicity (Heatley and Jowett, 2000). Experimental and natural zinc intoxication has been associated with heterophilia and lymphopenia in birds as well (Woerpel and Rosskopf, 1982; VanSant, 1991; Romagnano et al., 1995; Marks et al., 1999; Levengood et al., 2000). This leukocytosis appears to be related to the zinc-mediated toxemia, gastrointestinal inflammation, stress, and a subsequent reduced resistance to pathogens. The hemogram of birds with active West Nile virus infections often reveal a mild to moderate leukocytosis with mature heterophilia, but this response is not persistent (D'Agostino and Isaza, 2004). A marked to severe leukocytosis and heterophilia have been described in vultures with *Mycoplasma*-associated polyarthritis and tenosynovitis (Van Wettere et al., 2012). Experimental and natural infections with *Mycoplasma gallisepticum* in finches reveal an increase in both heterophils and monocytes with peak response at 7 to 14 days that corresponded to the development of conjunctivitis (Davis et al., 2004; Bale et al., 2020).

When leukocytosis is associated with inflammation, a heterophilia is usually present. During the early inflammatory phase, heterophils can respond to chemotactic agents within 30 min and demonstrate sensitive and selective phagocytosing properties. The magnitude of the heterophilia is dependent upon the etiology and severity of the inflammation. The greater the degree of heterophilia, the greater the severity of the inflammation.

Marked heterophilias are not necessarily protective against disseminated infection (Kolmstetter et al., 1995b; Tully et al., 1995, Bale et al., 2020). Assessment of cell morphology is an important tool in determining the prognosis of a sick bird with a leukocytosis and heterophilia. The appearance of toxic changes in the heterophils is associated with a sudden worsening in the control of an infectious process, regardless of the value of the total leukocyte count (Bienzle et al., 1997; Whittington and Williams, 2000; Wilson et al., 2001; Campbell and Grant, 2010). Toxic heterophils are frequently associated with severe systemic illness such as septicemia, viremia, chlamydiosis, mycotic infections, and severe tissue necrosis (Campbell, 1995; Wissman, 1995; Fudge, 1997; Tully et al., 2000). The degree of heterophil toxicity usually indicates the severity of the bird's condition, and the presence of a marked number of 4+ toxic heterophils indicates a grave prognosis.

The lymphocyte is the most numerous leukocyte present in circulation in most clinically healthy domestic birds of various species (e.g., Anseriformes), and the heterophil is the second most numerous cell type. These birds typically respond to acute inflammation with heterophilia (Latimer et al., 1988). Initially, these species may show leukopenia, but later (i.e., up to 12 h) demonstrate the typical leukocytosis, heterophilia, and lymphopenia (Davidson and Flack, 1981; Gross and Siegel, 1983). Other avian species (psittacines, ratites, raptors) have a higher proportion of heterophils than lymphocytes in circulation, and typically demonstrate a less dramatic change in the stress leukogram (Hawkey and Dennett, 1989; Maxwell and Robertson, 1998). An H/L ratio of less than 1.0 may be normal for some avian species, such as those that are more lymphocytic, whereas it is indicative of stress in other species. Greater responses are seen in species with normal H/L ratios of 3.0:1.0 versus those with ratios of 0.5:1.0.

Immature heterophils are rarely present in the peripheral blood of normal birds. Much like mammals, their presence usually is a result of excessive peripheral utilization of mature heterophils with depletion of the mature storage pool in the hematopoietic tissue, indicating a severe inflammatory response, especially when associated with leukopenia (Tangredi, 1981; Echols et al., 2000). Marked increases in immature heterophil concentration may also result from granulocytic leukemia, a rare condition in birds.

Heterophilia of Excitement and Stress in Birds

A slight to moderate leukocytosis may occur in response to environmental stress (stress leukogram) (McFarlane and Curtis, 1989). The mechanisms mediating these cellular changes are poorly defined in birds, but appear to be associated with changes in endogenous corticosteroid levels (Gross and Siegel, 1983; Gross, 1989; Dohms and Metz, 1991; Gibbons and Horton, 2000). Corticosteroid levels change rapidly during stress; however, absolute leukocyte numbers change more slowly (30 min to 20 h) in response to stress, and are less variable, but more enduring (Maxwell, 1993; Vleck et al., 2000). Blood samples ideally should be collected quickly with minimal stress to the patient to avoid leukogram changes associated with handling. When working with wild birds, blood should be collected immediately after capture.

Absolute heterophil numbers may also increase during mildly to moderately stressful conditions as a response to endogenous corticosteroid release (Gray et al., 1989; Post et al., 2003). Transport-related stress (including transport to veterinary hospitals) can alter the total and differential white blood cell counts of birds, resulting in leukocytosis, heterophilia, and lymphopenia (Mitchell et al., 1992; Speer and Kass, 1995; Parga et al., 2001; Campbell and Grant, 2010). Short transport times are not as likely to be a factor in the development of a stress leukogram (Parga et al., 2001).

An absolute leukocytosis may also occur when exogenous glucocorticoids are administered to birds. A moderate mature heterophilia and lymphopenia accompany a stress leukogram. The stimulus for heterophil recruitment or mobilization arises from bone marrow interactions with the hypothalamic-pituitary-adrenal cortical axis (Maxwell and Robertson, 1998).

An absolute leukocytosis with a moderate mature heterophilia and lymphopenia are typically the hallmarks of a stress leukogram (Gross and Siegel, 1983; Gross, 1989; McFarlane and Curtis, 1989). Stressors elevate the number of heterophils and depress the number of lymphocytes (Gross and Siegel, 1983; Gross, 1989; McFarlane and Curtis, 1989). Consequently, the heterophil/lymphocyte ratio (H/L ratio) can be used to detect the presence of physiologic stress in many avian patients (Maxwell and Robertson, 1998). For example, in chickens, the H/L ratio has proved to be a valuable tool in stress-related research (Davison et al., 1983; Gross and Siegel, 1983). Since the early 1980s, elevations in corticosterone and H/L ratios have been recognized as responses to stress in birds (Davison et al., 1983; Gross and Siegel, 1983).

Corticosterone levels may be a more sensitive indicator of short-term stressors, whereas the H/L ratio may be a more persistent indicator of stress associated with injury, reproductive cycles, and seasonal changes. Leukocyte changes in response to environmental stress are less variable but more enduring than corticosterone responses, suggesting that leukocyte changes are more reliable indicators of stress (McFarlane and Curtis, 1989). The mechanisms mediating these cellular changes are poorly defined in birds, but appear to be associated with changes in corticosteroids (Gross and Siegel, 1983; Gross, 1989; Dohms and Metz, 1991).

The H/L ratio has been shown to be a reliable indicator of stress associated with injury, reproductive cycles, and seasonal changes in birds in both captive and field situations (Ots et al., 1998; Moreno et al., 2002). The H/L ratio appears to be the most accurate indicator of stress because it is less variable than the number of heterophils or lymphocytes alone (Gross and Siegel, 1983; Mitchell et al., 1992; Maxwell, 1993). The H/L ratio has also been used as a measurement of body condition (Hanauska-Brown et al., 2003). In free-living birds, H/L ratios may be more useful than a single measure of plasma corticosterone in assessing response to chronic stressors like injury or crowded conditions in the breeding colony, and H/L ratios have been shown to be a valuable tool to measure stress in passerine birds and to evaluate management practices for critically endangered passerines (Vleck et al., 2000; Groombridge et al., 2004). In two species of gulls, the H/L ratio was approximately 0.6 in normal individuals, compared to 2.9 in birds that were oiled, emaciated, injured, or infected with endoparasites (Averbeck, 1992). In the poultry industry, H/L reference values of 0.20, 0.50, and 0.80 are characteristic of low, optimal, and high degrees of stress, respectively (Gross and Siegel, 1983).

There are limitations to the accuracy of the H/L ratio as an indicator of stress in birds, however. The H/L ratio may vary with conditions that affect heterophil and lymphocyte numbers, such as age and inflammatory disease (Janes et al., 1994; Branton et al., 1997). There may also be species variation in the hemic response to corticosteroids and stress, which would in turn affect the magnitude of the leukocytosis (Bhattacharyya and Sarkar, 1968). In some extreme circumstances, a bird may even exhibit a heteropenia and basophilia (Maxwell and Robertson, 1998).

Leukopenia in Birds

Leukopenia is associated with either consumption of peripheral leukocytes or decreased production. In many species of birds, an absolute heteropenia is the cause of a leukopenia. Leukopenias associated with heteropenias can occur with severe bacterial infections or certain viral diseases (e.g., Pacheco's parrot disease) (Olson, 1965; Rosskopf et al., 1981; Lopes et al., 2007; Owen et al, 2013). Severe leukopenia is commonly associated with parrots infected with psittacine circovirus, where peracute infections can present with leukopenia, anemia, and pancytopenia (Schoemaker et al., 2000). Hematologic changes associated with togavirus infections, such as eastern equine encephalomyelitis virus, across host–pathogen systems are not consistent. Although total leukocyte counts may not be predictive of a viral response, a decrease in lymphocytes, monocytes, and heterophils can be a significant indication of an eastern equine encephalomyelitis virus infection in some birds (Owen et al, 2013).

Leukopenia and heteropenia with the presence of immature heterophils suggests exhaustion of the mature heterophil storage pool because of excessive peripheral demand for heterophils, as seen with severe inflammation. A degenerative response is reflected by leukopenia, heteropenia, immature heterophils, and toxic heterophils. Degenerative responses and depletion are differentiated by the presence of toxic heterophils or by following the decreasing leukocyte count with serial leukograms. In general, a degenerative response in the leukogram of a bird indicates a poor prognosis for survival. As discussed earlier, leukopenia and lymphopenia can occur as an early corticosteroid-induced leukogram response in some species of birds (Davidson and Flack, 1981). Leukopenia and lymphopenia may also suggest a viral etiology, although such causes have been poorly documented in birds (Schoemaker et al., 2000).

Leukopenia associated with heteropenia, marked anemia, and thrombocytopenia suggests stem cell injury to the bone marrow, which can be associated with certain neoplastic conditions (Marshall et al., 2004). A rapid leukopenia that resolved with discontinuation of therapy with tamoxifen, a nonsteroidal agent with potent antiestrogenic properties, was observed in budgerigars (*Melopsittacus undulatus*) being treated to prevent egg production (Lupu, 2000).

Heteropenia

Heteropenia results from a decreased survival of mature heterophils or decreased or ineffective production. Heteropenia is seen with acute inflammatory disease or in diseases with marked severity because heterophils are being consumed at a faster rate than they are being produced and released to peripheral circulation. A heteropenia with a left shift and toxic changes is indicative of an acute inflammatory response associated with excessive peripheral utilization of heterophils.

An absolute heteropenia in conjunction with immature heterophilia and heterophil toxicity indicates either an overwhelming demand for heterophils in the periphery due to bacterial sepsis or viral disease, a reduced production of heterophils in the bone marrow, or ineffective granulopoiesis due to a maturation arrest. This type of leukogram carries a poor prognosis (Bienzle et al., 1997; Ferrell and Tell, 2001). Bone marrow evaluation may be helpful to rule out these conditions.

Immune-mediated heteropenia, should it occur in birds, would result in a profound heteropenia in the peripheral blood and depletion of the maturation pool in the bone marrow. Injury to the stem cells in the bone marrow can occur with chemicals, drugs, or infectious agents, such as viral agents, that affect rapidly dividing cells, resulting in a profound heteropenia. Stem cell injury would first appear as a profound heteropenia followed by a thrombocytopenia and eventually a nonregenerative anemia.

A heteropenia with a left shift, no anemia, and adequate thrombocytes is indicative of an acute inflammatory response with exhaustion of the mature heterophil storage pool owing to excessive peripheral utilization of heterophils (Olson, 1965; Rosskopf et al., 1981).

A heteropenia with no left shift, no anemia, and adequate thrombocytes is indicative of an acute viral infection or acute marrow injury. For example, severe heteropenia has been associated with experimental infections with the herpesvirus that causes Pacheco's disease in psittacine birds (Godwin et al., 1982). A heteropenia associated with a nonregenerative anemia and possibly a thrombocytopenia is indicative of a chronic marrow injury. Fenbendazole toxicity in birds causes bone marrow toxicosis in Columbiformes, Psittaciformes, painted storks, vultures, and marabou storks that results in transient leukopenia, severe heteropenia, and anemia as the result of a compromise to cellular division that impacts rapidly dividing cells (Short et al., 1988; Pedersoli et al., 1989; Taylor et al., 1993; Stalis et al., 1995; Papendick et al., 1998; Rivera et al., 2000; Howard et al., 2002; Weber et al., 2002; Bonar et al., 2003).

Lymphopenia

Lymphopenia is usually indicative of corticosteroid excess. Leukopenia associated with lymphopenia can occur as an early corticosteroid-induced leukogram response in some species of birds (Bale et al., 2020). Lymphopenia may suggest a viral disease, although such cases have been poorly documented in birds (Davidson and Flack, 1981). Immunosuppressive drugs other than corticosteroids, such as chemotherapeutic agents, may also cause lymphopenia. A lymphopenia with numerous atypical large lymphocytes containing scalloped cytoplasmic margins has been documented in birds with lymphosarcoma (Heatley et al., 1999).

Lymphocytosis in Birds

A marked leukocytosis with lymphocytosis is suggestive of lymphocytic leukemia (Counihan et al., 2020). Chronic lymphocytic leukemia in birds is characterized by extremely high total leukocyte counts (e.g.,100 000/µL or greater), with lymphocytes representing greater than 80% of the white blood cell differential. Review of the blood smears is crucial for distinguishing the lymphocytes as neoplastic where the cells typically appear as intermediate to large lymphocytes with round to indented nuclei, finely stippled chromatin, and occasional nucleoli; mitotic figures are occasionally present (Keeney et al., 2021). Immunocytochemical staining of blood films in a bearded dragon with B-cell leukemia was reported to be negative for CD3 and positive for CD79a (Gavazza et al., 2019). Immature lymphocytes are not always present and may be represented by normal-appearing small to medium (intermediate) mature lymphocytes (Cummings et al., 2020). Lymphocytes with scalloped cytoplasmic margins may be present in varying numbers. Bone marrow samples from patients with chronic lymphocytic leukemia typically reflect the peripheral blood findings.

Monocytosis in Birds

Monocytosis can be seen with acute and chronic inflammation and occurs with an increased demand for monocytes (Figure 11.22). Monocytosis in avian patients is typically associated with infectious and inflammatory diseases, especially those associated with granulomatous inflammation. Other causes of monocytosis may include hemic reaction to a foreign body, and certain nutritional deficiencies, such as zinc deficiency (Wight et al., 1980; Adamcak et al., 2000; Maldonado and Larson, 2004).

Anemia and leukocytosis with increases in monocyte, heterophil, and basophil numbers are a common hematologic feature of chronic inflammation in birds (Hawkey et al., 1984; Hawkey et al., 1985; D'Aloia et al., 1994). Early in the inflammatory process, an initial leukocytosis and heterophilia generally occur; however, some infectious agents may elicit acute monocytosis. For example, acute *Mycoplasma* infections can result in heterophilia, lymphopenia, monocytosis, and eosinophilia (Branton et al., 1997). Anemia and monocytosis then develop as the inflammation become chronic (Graham et al., 2004). Organisms such as *Mycobacterium*, *Chlamydia*, and fungi such as *Aspergillus* typically cause granulomatous inflammation in birds and are often associated with monocytosis. A profound nonregenerative anemia and severe monocytosis can occur with chronic clostridial infections (Hess et al., 1998; Campbell and Grant, 2010).

Neoplasia may cause monocytosis in some birds (Campbell and Grant, 2010). Quail exposed experimentally

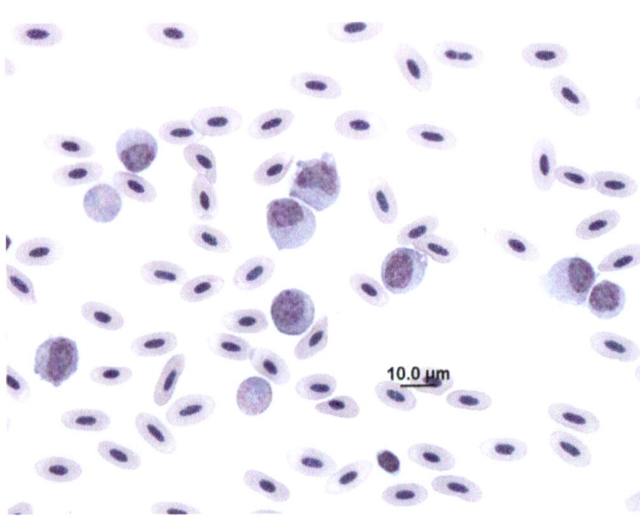

Fig. 11.22. A blood film showing monocytosis in a gannet (*Morus* spp.) Wright–Giemsa stain.

to Rous sarcoma virus developed leukocytosis as tumor growth developed. The leukocyte counts returned to normal in birds that showed regression of the tumors; however, those with progression of tumor growth continued to exhibit leukocytosis with heterophilia, monocytosis, and lymphopenia (Janes et al., 1994).

Eosinophilia and Eosinopenia in Birds

Eosinophilia is difficult to interpret in birds because the exact function of the avian eosinophil is unknown. Even though this avian granulocyte was given the name "eosinophil," avian eosinophils may behave differently from mammalian eosinophils. Regardless of the limited information available about the function of the avian eosinophil, peripheral eosinophilia in birds can be loosely interpreted as a response to internal or external parasitism or exposure to foreign antigen (hypersensitivity response) (Latas et al., 2020). It has been noted, however, that parasitic infections may not elicit a peripheral eosinophilia in birds (Armstrong et al., 1989; Kwiecien et al., 1993; Suedmeyer et al., 1996).

Avian eosinophils may serve as modulators of inflammation in delayed hypersensitivity responses, differing in this respect from mammalian eosinophils (Chad and Eyre, 1978; Maxwell, 1987). Eosinophilias associated with gastrointestinal nematode infestations have been reported in birds, although experiments utilizing parasite antigens have failed to induce peripheral eosinophilia (Maxwell, 1980; Work et al., 2004). Peripheral eosinophilias have also been reported in birds with acute *Mycoplasma* infections (Branton et al., 1997).

Eosinopenia may be difficult to document in birds. If present, it would be expected to be associated with a stress response or glucocorticosteroid administration. Eosinopenia, as with lymphopenia, observed with infectious agents may be a relative mean proportion associated with an increase in other types of cells, such as heterophils and monocytes (Bale et al., 2020).

Avian Thrombocytes

Avian thrombocytes are nucleated cells that are the second most numerous cell (after erythrocytes) found in the blood. Thrombocytes are typically small, round to oval cells (smaller than erythrocytes) with a round to oval nucleus that contains densely clumped chromatin. The nucleus is more rounded than an erythrocyte nucleus, and thrombocytes tend to have a high N:C ratio.

The appearance of the cytoplasm is an important feature used to differentiate thrombocytes from small, mature lymphocytes (Figures 11.11a, 11.11b, 11.11e, and 11.23). The cytoplasm of normal mature thrombocytes is colorless to pale gray and may be reticulated in

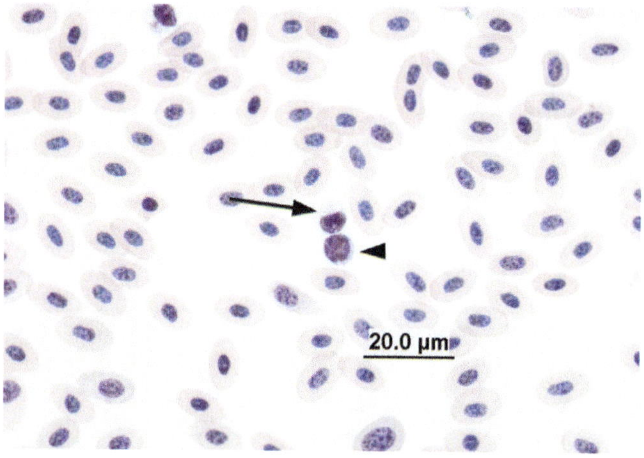

Fig. 11.23. A thrombocyte (arrow) and lymphocyte (arrowhead) in the blood film of a domestic chicken (*Gallus gallus domesticus*), Wright–Giemsa stain.

appearance (Figure 11.23). Ultrastructurally, the cytoplasm resembles that of mammalian platelets, and cytoplasmic vacuolation can occur in activated or phagocytic thrombocytes (Fox and Solomon, 1981; Du Plessis and van Wilpe, 2009). Occasionally, immature thrombocytes may be found on the blood film. Mid-immature thrombocytes are usually round cells with a round nucleus, moderately granular chromatic pattern, and moderately blue cytoplasm (Figure 11.24a). As maturation progresses, the cell and nuclei become more elliptical and may develop cytoplasmic vacuoles and granules (Figure 11.24b).

Thrombocytes frequently contain one or more distinct eosinophilic (specific) granules located in one area of the cytoplasm. These granules frequently appear as aggregates of many small granules when viewed through an electron microscope and contain primarily 5-hydroxytryptamine. The granules are an unlikely source of thromboplastin (Sturkie, 1976).

The primary function of the thrombocyte is in hemostasis. Avian thrombocytes function in much the same manner as mammalian platelets, although in a slower manner; therefore, they secrete thromboplastin, which polymerizes fibrinogen in the formation of clots in blood coagulation (Sweeny and Carlson, 1968; Scanes, 2014). Because thrombocytes participate in the hemostatic process, they tend to clump or form aggregates in blood films. Activated thrombocytes occurring in aggregates may have indistinct cellular outlines and cytoplasmic pseudopodia and may demonstrate degranulation of specific granules, cellular degeneration, and nuclear pyknosis. The life span of thrombocytes in vitro appears to be only a few hours (Lam, 1997).

The primary role of the thrombocyte in hemostasis is the formation of the initial hemostatic plug via adhesion and aggregation. The secondary hemostatic plug develops via the coagulation cascade following injury to a blood vessel wall. Although there is evidence of an

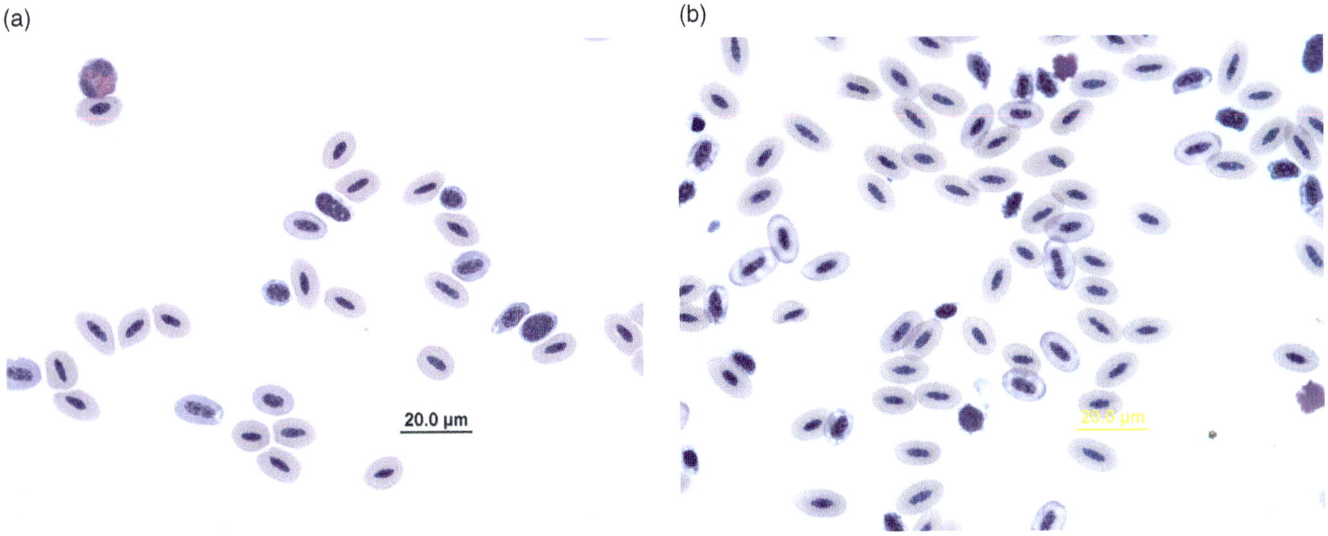

Fig. 11.24. (a) Mid-stage immature thrombocytes (center) and (b) late-stage immature thrombocytes (center) in the blood film of an eclectus parrot (*Eclectus roratus*), Wright–Giemsa stain.

intrinsic clotting mechanism in some species of birds, coagulation of avian blood appears to be dependent upon the extrinsic clotting system, which involves the release of tissue thromboplastin (factor III) (Sturkie and Griminger, 1986). The majority of clotting factors involved in avian blood coagulation are similar to those of mammals.

The extrinsic and common pathways can be evaluated using a one-step prothrombin time (OSPT) test. Avian brain thromboplastin is required for avian prothrombin time testing because commercially available rabbit brain thromboplastin and other mammalian reagents give unreliable results in birds. Studies suggest that the source of thromboplastin should be from the brain of the same species of bird as the patient for prothrombin time determinations (Campbell and Coles, 1986; Sturkie and Griminger, 1986). The normal prothrombin time for most birds is 13 s or less (Campbell and Coles, 1986). Increased prothrombin time is produced by a defect in the intrinsic and common pathway of coagulation and is caused by a deficiency of factors V, VII, X, fibrinogen, and prothrombin (factor II) (Jain, 1986). Increased prothrombin times in affected birds can be related to the presence and the severity of hepatic lesions (Fernandez et al., 1995; Raju and Devegowda, 2000).

Avian thrombocytes may play a role in innate immunity because they are capable of phagocytosis and may participate in removing foreign materials from the blood (Grecchi et al., 1980). Theoretically, even though thrombocytes are less phagocytic than heterophils, avian thrombocytes may act as a nonspecific "scavenging" phagocyte, capable of clearing a wide range of foreign objects, including bacteria (Wigley et al., 1999). Therefore, thrombocytes may play a role in fighting bacterial infection, although the mechanisms by which thrombocytes interact with, adhere to, or respond to bacteria are largely unknown. Light and electron microscopy has demonstrated that thrombocytes contain lysosomal vesicles and are actively phagocytic in vitro for vital dyes and gram-positive bacteria (Carlson et al., 1968; Sweeny and Carlson, 1968).

Others have demonstrated that avian thrombocytes can phagocytose bacteria other than gram-positive bacteria, and oxidative burst activity has been demonstrated in avian thrombocytes after phagocytosis of bacteria (Wigley et al., 1999). In some studies, oxygen radicals were detected in thrombocytes after activation by binding the monoclonal antibody 11C3 that targets the avian homologue of the platelet integrin GPIIb-IIIa (Corbel et al., 1995). Further studies on how thrombocytes interact with other cells and the role of complement and Fc receptors in phagocytosis and antimicrobial activity are needed to determine the specific roles of thrombocytes in avian immunity.

Normal Variation in the Thrombogram of Birds

Thrombocyte concentrations are influenced by environmental factors, seasonal changes, and physiologic factors. For example, a decrease in thrombocyte concentration has been demonstrated in female ducks during the incubation, molting, and post-reproductive periods compared to other periods (Fairbrother and O'Loughlin, 1990). Age also influences the thrombocyte count. Young ducklings and goslings tend to have lower thrombocyte concentrations compared to adult birds of the same species. The number of thrombocytes in the peripheral blood begins to increase at 5 days of age and reaches adult concentrations by 18 days of age (Fairbrother and O'Loughlin, 1990).

Thrombocytopenia

Thrombocytopenia is usually the result of decreased bone marrow production or excessive peripheral utilization or destruction and may be associated with severe septicemia and possibly diffuse intravascular coagulation (DIC). Thrombocytopenia has also been noted with viral infections, experimentally induced malaria infection, and intravenous administration of cellulose microparticles (Scanes, 2014). The presence of immature thrombocytes in an eclectus parrot (*Eclectus roratus*) were presumed to be a result of accelerated maturation. The parrot experienced a hemorrhagic episode that likely led to thrombocytopenia (Campbell and Grant, 2010).

Thrombocytosis

Thrombocytosis associated with large thrombocytes has been reported in birds with chronic inflammation, which may be related to the thrombocyte's phagocytic role in inflammatory disease (D'Aloia et al., 1994). Increased thrombocyte numbers were noted after lipopolysaccharide challenge, and some pesticides appear to increase thrombocyte concentrations (Scanes, 2014).

Avian Blood Parasites

Apicomplexan protozoan parasites of the genera *Hemoproteus*, *Plasmodium*, and *Leukocytozoon* and microfilaria of filarial nematodes are commonly found in avian blood films. Microfilarial nematodes are typically found between the cells. *Hemoproteus*, *Plasmodium*, and *Leukocytozoon* produce merozoites that invade erythrocytes, and their gametocytes are found within the erythrocyte. Most of the species of *Hemoproteus* and *Leukocytozoon* that infect birds are host specific. Many species of *Plasmodium* can infect a wide range of hosts (Peirce et al., 2004).

In general, the presence of blood parasites in wild birds has no effect on the health of the bird, although combined infections with *Hemoproteus* and *Leukocytozoon* can produce a fatal anemia in young raptors (Michot et al., 1995; Evans and Otter, 1998). Birds may be infected with a single blood parasite or may have mixed infections based on the examination of stained blood films. Wild birds may also have high parasite prevalence with low parasitemia (Granthon and Williams, 2017). Transmission of the hemoparasites of wild birds to captive birds may result in fatal infections in the more susceptible hosts (García-del-Río et al., 2020).

Populations of certain free-ranging species of birds in various parts of the world appear to be free of blood parasites, whereas birds in other areas often have multiple infections (Gilardi et al., 1995; Merino et al., 1997; Pung et al., 1997; Rooney et al., 2001; Holmstad et al., 2003; Valkiunas et al., 2003; Remple, 2004; Mijares et al., 2012). Avian hemosporidian parasites can vary in their degree of host specificity and even have a broad host range, likely relying on a key host species (Hellgren et al., 2011). Free-living birds may exhibit seasonal variation in the degree of parasitemia. For example, one study of accipiter hawks demonstrated a spring recrudescence of latent blood parasite infections (Phalen et al., 1995). In another study, waterfowl exhibited higher parasitemias in the fall compared to the summer (DeJong and Muzzall, 2000).

The age and effects of captivity may affect the occurrence of blood parasites in birds. For example, *Hemoproteus* and *Leukocytozoon* were more commonly found in birds held in captivity for longer than 365 days, and *Leukocytozoon* was found more commonly in adults and juveniles than in nestlings (Ziman et al., 2004)

Identification of avian blood parasites can usually be made using stains commonly used for evaluation of blood cells. Films made from fresh blood, without the addition of an anticoagulant, provide samples with fewer artifacts affecting the parasite. A method of using the buffy coat to evaluate parasites in avian blood samples in the field has also been described by evaluating the capillary tube with low magnification, placing the buffy coat sample on a slide as a wet mount, and as a stained sample. The evaluation of this method resulted with various sensitivities, specificities, and agreement when comparing to evaluation using standard blood films depending on the parasite (Chagas et al., 2020).

Hemoproteus

Protozoan blood parasites of the genus *Hemoproteus* are common in many species of wild birds, but the pathogenicity is usually low (Boal et al., 1998a; Blanco et al., 2001). Parasitized birds rarely show serious disease problems; however, clinical disease can occur in certain avian species, such as pigeons, quail, nestling birds, and birds suffering from diseases that may result in immunodeficiency. For example, in one study, *Hemoproteus lophortyx* parasitemia in bobwhite quail was associated with anemia and a mortality rate over 20% (Cardona et al., 2002). *Hemoproteus noctuae*, *H. syria*, and *H. tinnunculi* have been identified in the blood of healthy raptors, most commonly in Strigiformes (Kocan et al., 1977; Apanius and Kirkpatrick, 1988; Joseph, 1999).

Hemoproteus is transmitted by blood-sucking insect vectors such as the hippoboscid flies and midges of the genus Culicoides. The insect host ingests *Hemoproteus* gametocytes when feeding on an infected host. The gametocytes then undergo a series of developmental stages to become sporozoites within the salivary glands of the insect vector. The sporozoites are then injected into a new avian host when the insect feeds again.

Once the sporozoites have entered a new avian host, they enter the vascular endothelial cells of various tissues

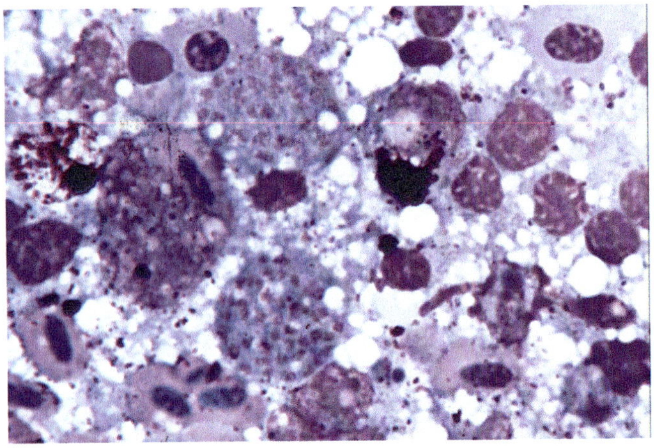

Fig. 11.25. *Hemoproteus* schizonts in a splenic imprint from an American kestrel (*Falco sparverius*), Wright–Giemsa stain (100× oil).

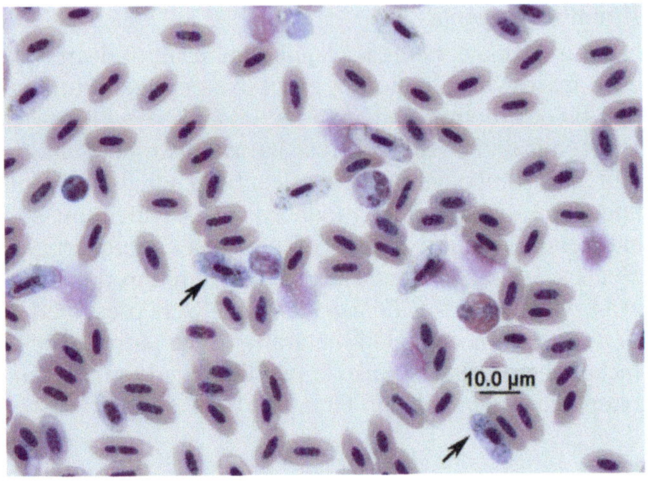

Fig. 11.26. *Hemoproteus* macrogametocyte (arrow) within an erythrocyte in the blood film of a flicker (*Colaptes auratus*), Wright–Giemsa stain.

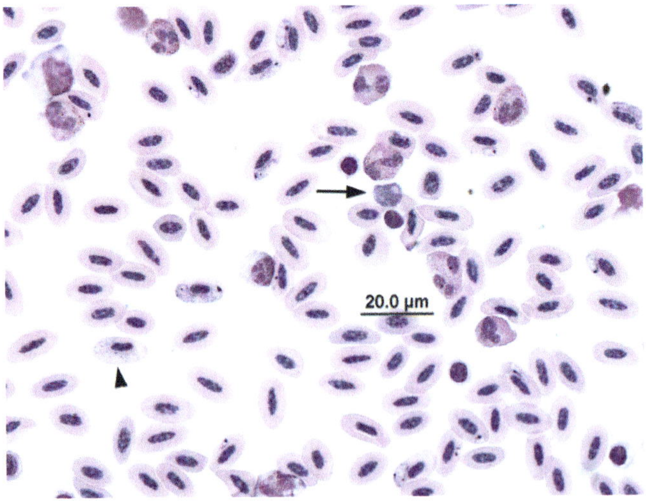

Fig. 11.27. Extracellular *Hemoproteus* macrogametocyte (arrow) and intracellular microgametocyte (arrowhead) in the blood film of a great horned owl (*Bubo virginianus*), Wright–Giemsa stain.

(primarily, lung, liver, bone marrow, and spleen) and undergo schizogony. *Hemoproteus* schizonts are occasionally found in cytologic or histologic samples of infected tissue and appear as large, round cysts that contain numerous multinucleated bodies that produce numerous merozoites (Figure 11.25). Merozoites escape into the blood stream when the endothelial cell ruptures. The merozoites then enter erythrocytes and become gametocytes, which are ingested by insect hosts to complete the cycle.

The clinical signs associated with *Hemoproteus* parasitemia include hemolytic anemia, anorexia, and lethargy. Hemolytic anemia is probably a sequela to lysis of the fragile parasitized erythrocyte as it passes through the fine trabecular network of the spleen. Hepatomegaly and splenomegaly may be observed on radiographs or during a postmortem evaluation.

Hematologic changes associated with *Hemoproteus* infection may include leukocytosis and anemia. For example, in one study, elevated numbers of lymphocytes, heterophils, basophils, eosinophils, and monocytes, as well as decrease in PCV, were associated with the erythrocytic phase of experimental infections of captive juvenile blue jays (Garvin et al., 2003).

Hemoproteus only appears in the peripheral blood of birds in the gametocyte stage. The appearance of the gametocyte varies and may range from small, developing ring forms to the elongated, crescent-shaped, mature gametocytes that partially encircle the erythrocyte nucleus to form the characteristic "halter-shape" (Soulsby, 1982) (Figures 11.26 and 11.27). Mature gametocytes typically occupy greater than one-half of the cytoplasmic volume of the host erythrocyte and cause minimal displacement of the host cell nucleus; the nucleus is never pushed to the cell margin. *Hemoproteus* gametocytes contain refractile, yellow to brown to black pigment granules representing iron pigment deposited as a result of hemoglobin utilization. Erythrocytes parasitized by *Hemoproteus* are larger-than-normal erythrocytes, which likely causes the cells to become fragile. Polymerase chain reaction (PCR) analysis for *Hemoproteus* can be used to detect low parasitemia (Fallon et al., 2003; Fallon and Ricklefs, 2008).

Occasionally, extraerythrocytic macrogametes and microgametes can be found in blood films, especially those made from the blood collected several hours prior to preparing the film (Campbell and Grant, 2010). Extraerythrocytic macrogametes are round and resemble the gametocytes normally seen within the erythrocyte (Figures 11.27 and 11.28). Microgametes are small, spindle-shaped structures scattered throughout the blood film (Figure 11.29). Macrogametocytes typically stain

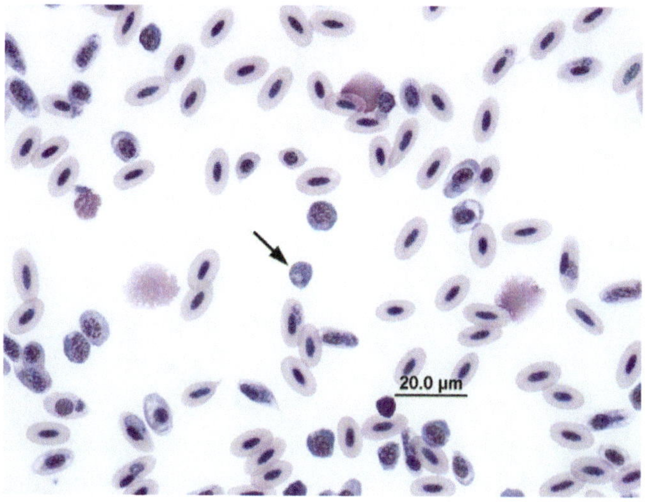

Fig. 11.28. Extracellular *Hemoproteus* macrogametocyte (arrow) in the blood film of an American kestrel (*Falco sparverius*), Wright–Giemsa stain.

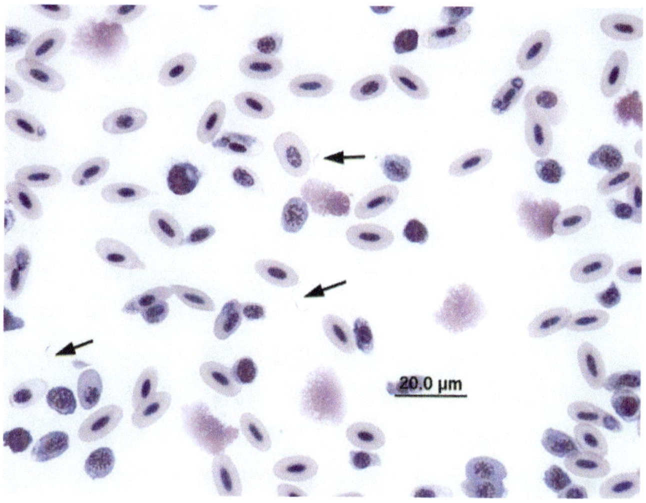

Fig. 11.29. Extracellular *Hemoproteus* microgametocytes (arrows) in the blood film of an American kestrel (*Falco sparverius*), Wright–Giemsa stain.

dark blue with Romanowsky stains and have iron pigment dispersed throughout the cytoplasm of the parasite. Microgametocytes typically stain pale blue to pink, and the iron pigment appears as an aggregated spherical mass. Typically, these forms are found in the midgut of the insect host following a blood meal, but can appear in blood films when erythrocytes begin to deteriorate as the blood sample ages.

A banana-shaped ookinete, the zygote formed by the union of a macrogametocyte and a microgametocyte, may also be found in the blood film (Figure 11.30). Macrogametocytes, microgametocytes, and ookinetes are rarely found in the peripheral blood films of animals, and when this occurs, it is likely associated with a substantial delay between blood collection and preparation of the blood film. It is difficult to determine if the ookinete is from the *Hemoproteus* or another parasite, *Plasmodium*. A delay between blood collection and blood film preparation also creates an increased number of smudge cells on the blood film.

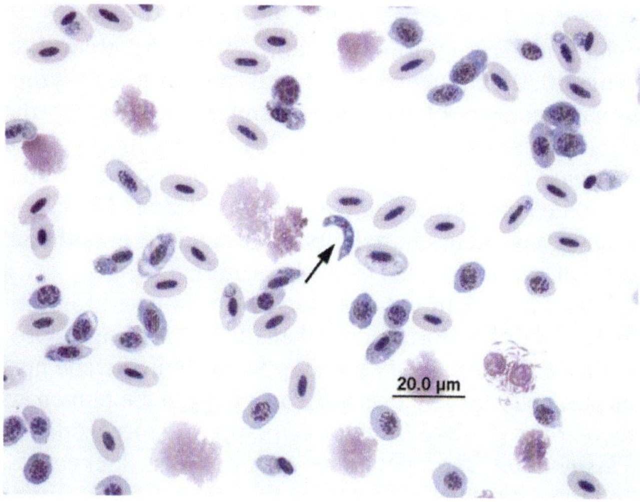

Fig. 11.30. An extracellular ookinete (arrow) in the blood film of an American kestrel (*Falco sparverius*), Wright–Giemsa stain.

Table 11.2. Semiquantitative evaluation of parasitemia.

Grade*	
0	No parasites observed
1	<1 parasite observed
2	1–5 parasites observed
3	6–10 parasites observed
4	>10 parasites observed

*Based on the number of gametocytes per [×400] monolayer field.

The degree of parasitemia can be graded semiquantitatively based on the number of gametocytes per field when viewed under 400× magnification (Cardona et al., 2002). A score of 0 is assigned if no parasites are observed; a 1, with less than 1 parasite; a 2, if 1–5 parasites; a 3, if 6–10 parasites; and a 4, if more than 10 parasites (Table 11.2). The degree of parasitemia associated with *Hemoproteus* can be used as an index to assess the recovery of birds (especially raptors) from traumatic injuries or diseases. For example, an injured raptor may present with marked *Hemoproteus* parasitemia, with greater than 15% of the erythrocytes affected. As the bird recovers from its injuries, the parasitemia decreases dramatically. It is presumed that this represents the improved immune status of the bird.

Plasmodium

Parasites of the genus *Plasmodium* can be pathogenic and are responsible for malaria. Certain species of birds, such as canaries, penguins, ducks, pigeons, raptors, and domestic poultry, are highly susceptible to avian malaria (Grilo et al., 2016, Spottiswoode et al., 2020). Other species of birds appear to be asymptomatic carriers of the parasite and do not develop the clinical disease (Castro et al., 2011). The life cycle of *Plasmodium* is like that of *Hemoproteus* except that Culicine mosquitoes serve as the intermediate hosts, and schizogony occurs in red blood cells and the endothelial cells of various organs (Soulsby, 1982).

The organism is transmitted from infected to uninfected birds by mosquitoes when, during feeding, sporozoites from the salivary glands of a mosquito invade host tissues and reproduce as schizonts to produce numerous merozoites. Unlike *Hemoproteus* spp., the merozoites of *Plasmodium* spp. penetrate erythrocytes, leukocytes, and thrombocytes and become ring-shaped trophozoites that mature into schizonts or infectious gametocytes (Bensch et al., 2000). The schizonts rupture, killing the infected cells and releasing merozoites to infect more blood cells. Blood smear examination is a definitive diagnostic method because the intermediate forms of *Plasmodium* spp. (trophozoites, schizonts, and gametocytes) can be seen in the cells. In both *Plasmodium* spp. and *Hemoproteus* spp., refractile yellow-to-brown-pigmented granules are observed because schizonts ingest and metabolize hemoglobin, resulting in refractile granule formation.

Outbreaks of avian malaria occur sporadically in endemic areas, especially during seasons associated with increases in the mosquito population. Clinical signs associated with avian malaria include anemia, anorexia, lethargy, and acute death. Hemoglobinuria or biliverdinuria may also occur, and splenomegaly and hepatomegaly are often seen on postmortem examination. The hemogram often reveals hemolytic anemia, leukocytosis, and lymphocytosis. *Plasmodium relictum* has been associated with fatal hemolytic anemia in many species of birds, especially raptors (Joseph, 1999).

Detection of *Plasmodium* is based on the presence of the organism in blood films. Key features used to differentiate *Plasmodium* from *Hemoproteus* are the presence of schizogony in the peripheral blood, parasite stages within thrombocytes and leukocytes, and gametocytes that cause marked displacement of the erythrocyte nucleus. Identification of the *Plasmodium* species is dependent upon the location and appearance of the schizonts, the number of merozoites present within the schizonts, and gametocytes (Soulsby, 1982). PCR analysis for *Plasmodium* can be used to detect low parasitemia (Fallon et al., 2003; Fallon and Ricklefs, 2008).

Unlike *Hemoproteus*, developmental stages of *Plasmodium* such as the gametocytes, schizonts, and trophozoites can be found within erythrocytes, thrombocytes, and leukocytes (Figures 11.31–11.34). *Plasmodium* gametocytes contain refractile, yellow to brown iron pigment granules that tend to be scattered. Macrogametocytes

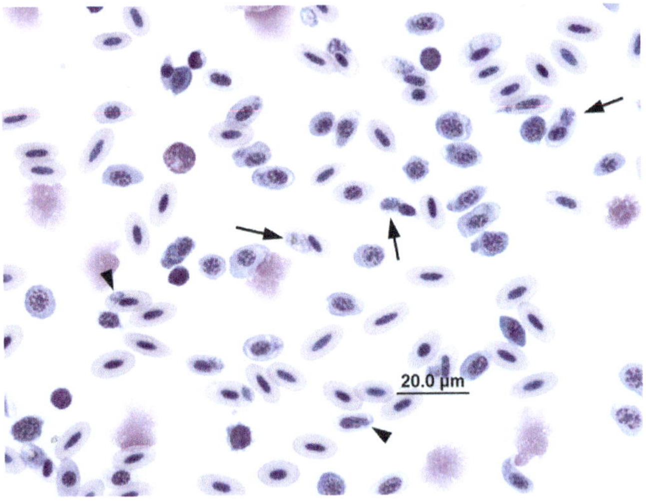

Fig. 11.31. *Plasmodium* gametocytes (arrows) and trophozoites (arrowheads) within an erythrocyte in the blood film of an American kestrel (*Falco sparverius*), Wright–Giemsa stain.

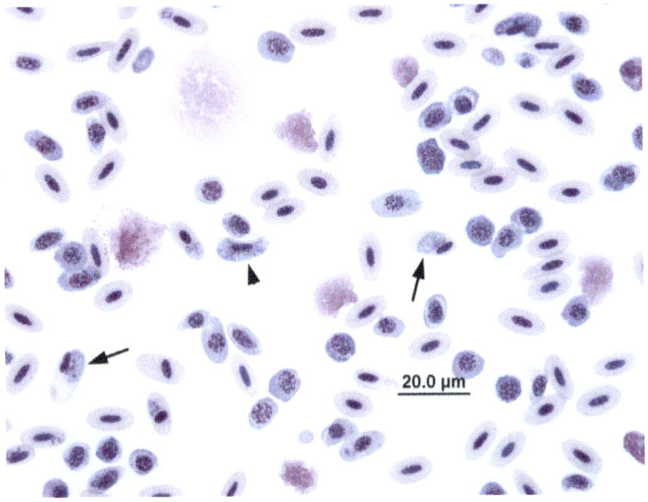

Fig. 11.32. *Plasmodium* macrogametocytes (arrows) and a *Hemoproteus* macrogametocyte (arrowhead) within an erythrocyte in the blood film of an American kestrel (*Falco sparverius*), Wright–Giemsa stain.

and microgametocytes may be present; macrogametocytes stain deeper blue than microgametocytes. The gametocytes of certain *Plasmodium* species are round to irregular in shape and cause marked displacement of the nucleus of the host cell. Other species of *Plasmodium* have elongated gametocytes that do not displace the host cell nucleus.

Schizonts appear as round to oval inclusions containing several deeply staining merozoites (Figure 11.34). Schizonts with developing merozoites exhibit clusters of merozoites that appear fused, whereas mature merozoites appear as distinct bodies that are separate from each other. *Plasmodium* trophozoites appear as small, round

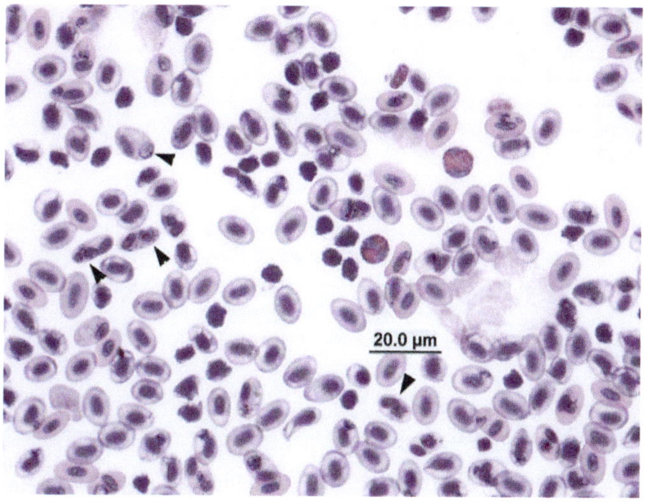

Fig. 11.33. *Plasmodium* gametocytes (arrowheads) within erythrocytes in the blood film of a skua (*Stercorarius* sp.), Wright–Giemsa stain.

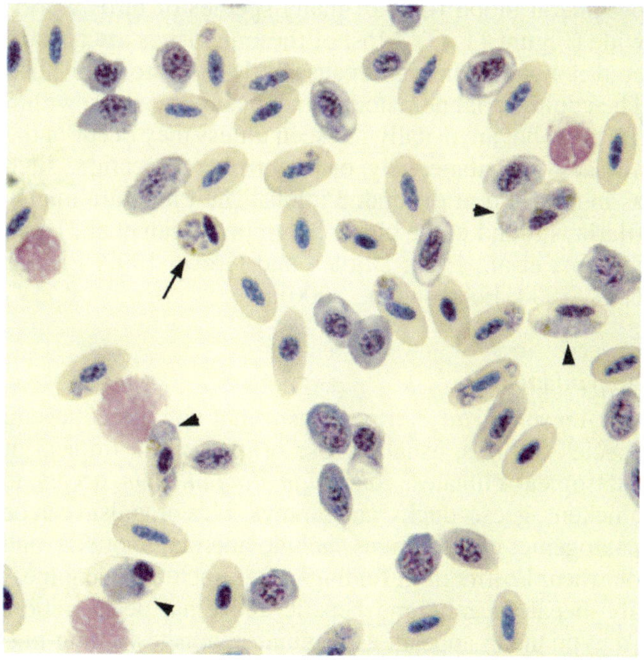

Fig. 11.34. *Plasmodium* gametocytes (arrowheads), schizont (arrow), and trophozoites within an erythrocyte in the blood film of an American kestrel (*Falco sparverius*), Wright–Giemsa stain (100× oil).

to oval amoeboid forms that contain a large vacuole, which pushes the parasite nucleus to one edge, giving the trophozoites a "signet-ring" appearance.

Leukocytozoon

Leukocytozoon is a protozoan parasite commonly found in the blood of wild birds. The name *Leukocytozoon* is derived from the belief that leukocytes serve as the host cell for this parasite. Despite this distinction, some parasitologists believe that immature erythrocytes serve as the host cell for *Leukocytozoon* (Soulsby, 1982). This parasite occurs worldwide and can be identified by the presence of large, dark-staining macrogametocytes or light-staining microgametocytes within erythrocytes in the peripheral blood. The pathogenicity of *Leukocytozoon* is usually low; however, certain species can be highly pathogenic for some birds. (Hunter et al., 1997; Boal et al., 1998a; Raidal and Jaensch, 2000).

The life cycle of *Leukocytozoon* includes the passing of sporozoites from the salivary glands of the insect vector (usually the blackfly, family Simuliidae) into the blood of susceptible species of birds (Gardiner et al., 1988). The sporozoites then invade the endothelial and parenchymal cells of various tissues, such as the reticuloendothelial system, liver, heart, and kidney, where schizogony occurs (Bennett and Pierce, 1992).

Primary schizogony typically occurs in the liver. When the schizonts mature, they release thousands of merozoites, which then initiate a second generation of schizonts in the liver and in phagocytic cells throughout the body. The schizonts in phagocytic cells become very large and are called megaschizonts. The megaschizonts release millions of merozoites that can either initiate schizogony elsewhere or enter circulating erythrocytes (or perhaps leukocytes), where they develop into macrogametes or microgametes.

The macrogametocyte appears as a parasite inclusion that occupies 77% of the area of the host cell–parasite complex (Bennett and Pierce, 1992). Microgametocytes are similar in morphology, but are usually 5–10% smaller (Bennett and Pierce, 1992). The remainder of the life cycle occurs in the insect vector following ingestion of blood containing the gametes (Gardiner et al., 1988)

Most *Leukocytozoon* infections in birds are subclinical; however, fatal infections can occur, especially in immature birds (Macwhirter, 1994; Joseph, 1999; Stuht et al., 1999). The clinical signs associated with this parasite include anemia, anorexia, and lethargy (Dresser, 1967; Siccardi et al., 1971; Miller et al., 1983; Fite, 1987). Clinical laboratory evaluation may reveal a hemolytic anemia, leukocytosis, and elevated serum enzymes, such as aspartate aminotransferase or alanine aminotransferase, suggesting hepatocellular necrosis. Postmortem findings may include splenomegaly and hepatomegaly with hepatic necrosis.

As with *Hemoproteus*, only gametocytes of *Leukocytozoon* occur in the peripheral blood. *Leukocytozoon* gametocytes are different from the gametocytes *Hemoproteus* and *Plasmodium* in that they do not contain the refractile iron pigment granules. Typically, the large gametocytes of most *Leukocytozoon* species grossly distort the infected host cell, causing the cell to become elongated and distended and making the identification of the cell difficult (Figures 11.35

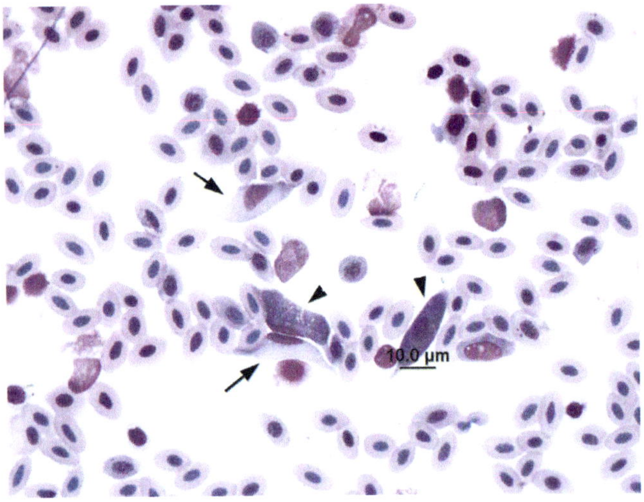

Fig. 11.35. *Leukocytozoon* gametocytes: dark macrogametocytes (arrowheads) and lighter microgametocytes (arrows) within an erythrocyte in the blood film of a red-tailed hawk (*Buteo jamaicensis*), Wright–Giemsa stain.

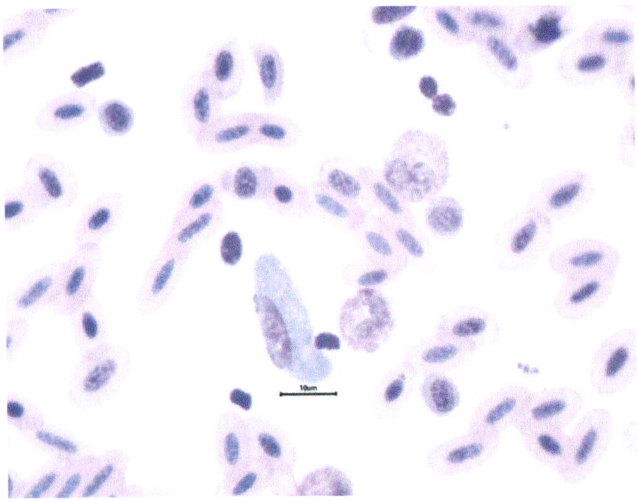

Fig. 11.36. *Leukocytozoon* microgametocytes within an erythrocyte in the blood film of a red-tailed hawk (*Buteo regalis*), Wright–Giemsa stain.

and 11.36). Parasitized cells appear to have two nuclei: a dark-staining host cell nucleus that lies along the cell membrane and a pale-pink-staining parasite nucleus that lies adjacent to the host cell nucleus. Appearance of the gametes in the peripheral blood can vary depending upon the species of *Leukocytozoon* present. For example, gametocytes of *Leukocytozoon sakharoffi*, the *Leukocytozoon* parasite of birds in the family Corvidae (crows, jays, and magpies), are round, and the host cell nucleus covers nearly 80% of the periphery of the parasite.

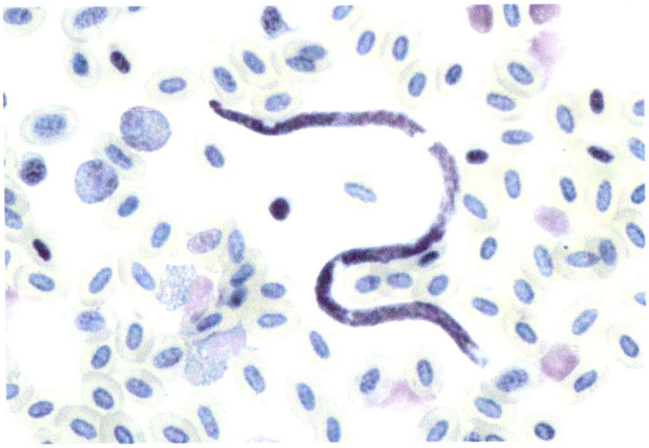

Fig. 11.37. Microfilaria in the blood film of a Moluccan cockatoo (*Cacatua moluccensis*), Wright–Giemsa stain (100× oil).

Microfilaria

Microfilariae are commonly found in the stained peripheral blood films of many species of birds worldwide (Figure 11.37). Most of these parasites are considered nonpathogenic and cause little harm to their host. The adult filarial nematodes may occur anywhere within the body but are usually not seen unless they occur in the air sacs, subcutaneously, or in peripheral locations such as in the fluid of distended joints. The immature microfilaria is found in the blood or lymph (Allen et al., 1985; Dharma et al., 1985; Doolen and Greve, 1992; Pizarro et al., 1994, Echols et al., 2000).

Aegyptianella

Aegyptianella is a piroplasm that can affect several species of birds, usually those originating in tropical or subtropical climates. *Aegyptianella pullorum* occurs in chickens, geese, ducks, and turkeys. This organism can be pathogenic; clinical signs include anemia, anorexia, and diarrhea. Postmortem findings often include splenomegaly, hepatomegaly, and hepatic and renal degeneration. Aegyptianella appears as a minute parasite lacking pigment granules located within erythrocytes in blood films (Figure 11.38). Three forms can occur (Soulsby, 1982). The first form is called the initial body and appears as a small (<1 µm), round, basophilic intracytoplasmic, anaplasma-like inclusion. The second form resembles *Babesia* in that it appears as a round to piriform-shaped inclusion with pale blue cytoplasm and a chromatin body at one pole. The third form presents as a larger (2–4 µm) round to elliptical inclusion within the cell.

Isosporosis or Atoxoplasmosis

Isospora (formerly *Atoxoplasma*) is a polyphyletic clade with two distinct monophyletic groups: those infecting mammals and those infecting birds (Landolfi,

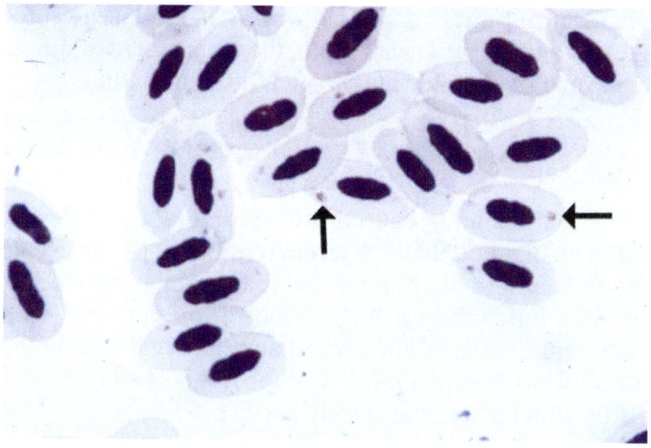

Fig. 11.38. Erythrocytes with intracytoplasmic *Aegyptianella* inclusions (arrows) in the blood film of a parrot (*Ara* sp.), Wright–Giemsa stain (100× oil).

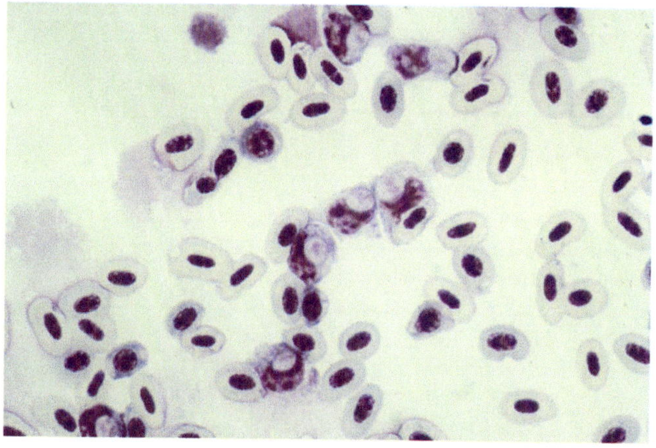

Fig. 11.39. Lymphocytes containing intracytoplasmic *Atoxoplasma* inclusions in the buffy-coat preparation of a black-throated laughing-thrush (*Garrulax chinensis*), Wright–Giemsa stain (100× oil).

et al., 2020). Systemic isosporosis (formerly atoxoplasmosis) is a protozoal infection that causes death in passerine nestlings. *Isospora serini* (formerly *Atoxoplasma serini* and *Lankesterella garnhami*) can be highly pathogenic, especially to canaries (Dorresteine et al., 1985; Flammer, 1987). The asexual phase of this parasite occurs in tissues and circulating mononuclear leukocytes, especially lymphocytes, where it is detected on a stained blood film. Transmission occurs via the oral–fecal route when susceptible birds are exposed to sporulated oocysts present in the feces of infected birds. A sexual phase of development then occurs in the intestinal tract of the infected individual, which results in the passage of sporulated oocysts in the excreted feces of that individual bird (Levine, 1982). An asexual phase of development occurs in body tissues such as the spleen, liver, and intestinal lamina propria and in circulating mononuclear leukocytes such as lymphocytes and monocytes.

Clinical signs of isosporosis may vary. Infected birds may be asymptomatic, may exhibit weight loss, or may be found dead without having previously exhibited any signs of illness. Infected adult birds are usually asymptomatic, but shed fecal oocysts that are ingested by their nestlings. Isosporosis has been implicated in the deaths of birds, especially Bali mynahs (*Leucopsar rothschildi*) raised in captivity (Greiner et al., 1995). Young, fledgling-age birds are the group most affected, where mortality can approach 80%.

Isosporosis is identified by the presence of the characteristic sporozoites within lymphocytes in peripheral blood films or in cytology imprints of organs (especially the liver, spleen, and lungs), where numerous parasite-laden lymphocytes can be found. Antemortem diagnosis of *Isospora* (*Atoxoplasma*) in peripheral blood can be improved by preparing a buffy-coat film to concentrate the leukocytes for examination.

A buffy-coat smear is prepared by filling a microhematocrit tube with blood from an EDTA tube that contains the blood sample. The microhematocrit tube is centrifuged in the same manner as during the preparation of a microhematocrit in order to concentrate the buffy coat. After centrifugation, the tube is broken at the cell–plasma interface to obtain the concentrated cells located in the buffy-coat area. The sample containing the concentrated cells is applied to two or three microscope slides and spread as blood films.

Affected lymphocytes contain small (3–5 µm), pale, round to oval eosinophilic intracytoplasmic inclusions or sporozoites in Romanowsky-stained preparations (Figure 11.39). Some lymphocytes may contain multiple organisms. Sporozoites may occasionally be identified in the cytoplasm of monocytes or macrophages as well. The sporozoites do not contain pigment granules, are made up of an outer pale zone surrounding a red granular area, and indent the host lymphocyte nucleus, resulting in a characteristic crescent shape (Levine, 1982).

Trypanosomes

Trypanosomes (*Trypanosoma* spp.) are occasionally found in the peripheral blood of wild birds, especially passerines, Galliformes, waterfowl, and pigeons. Transmission occurs via biting insects, such as mosquitoes, hippoboscid flies, blackflies, or mites. Trypanosomes have an undulating membrane, a slender tapering posterior end, a short anteriorly directed flagellum, and closely resemble those found in mammals (Figure 11.40). Trypanosomes are usually considered to be an incidental finding and are not typically pathogenic.

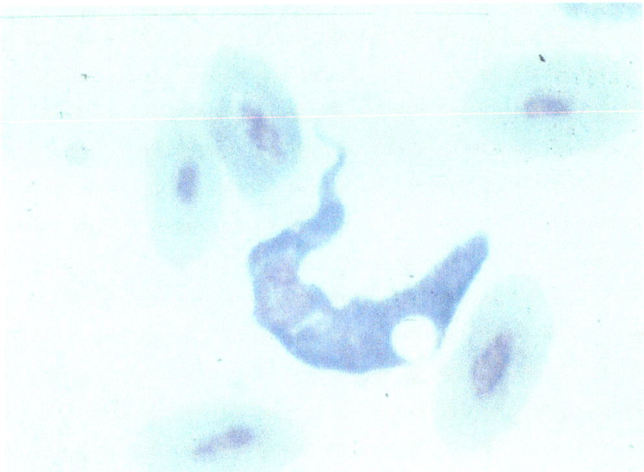

Fig. 11.40. A trypanosome (*Trypanosoma* spp.) in an avian blood film, Wright–Giemsa stain (100× oil).

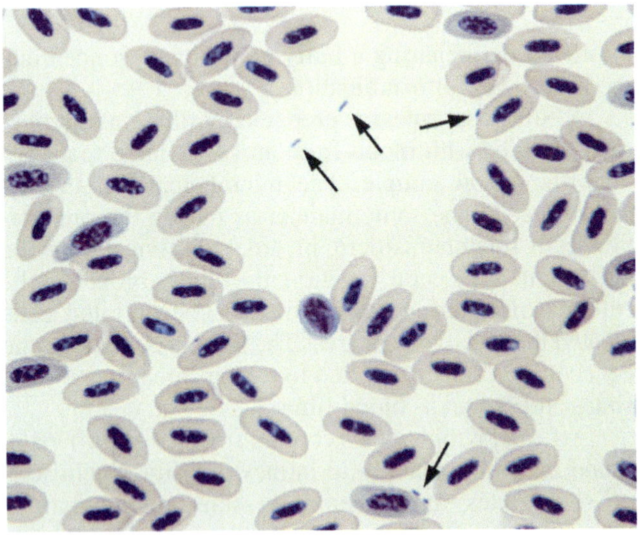

Fig. 11.41. Bacteria (arrows) in the blood film of a budgerigar (*Melopsittacus undulatus*), Wright–Giemsa stain (100× oil).

Borrelia anserina

Borrelia anserina is the causative agent of avian spirochetosis, which can affect several species of birds, especially Galliformes and waterfowl. Transmission occurs via arthropod vectors, such as ticks and mites. Studies have identified Argasid tick prevalence in poultry farms as a widespread concern throughout the world (Aslam et al., 2015; Ouchene et al., 2020). Clinical signs of avian spirochetosis include lethargy, anemia, and weakness. Postmortem findings often include splenomegaly and hepatomegaly. Birds recovering from the disease exhibit a regenerative anemia. *Borrelia* organisms may be found free in the plasma of affected birds and appears as a loosely spiraled spirochete that tapers into fine filaments. In acute stages of the disease, the organism is spiral shaped; however, as the disease progresses and the bird nears death, the organism may appear abnormal or clumped and is often difficult to find.

Bacteremia

Fowl cholera, caused by *Pasteurella multocida*, often results in a fatal bacteremia in birds. Because cats are the carriers of *P. multocida*, bacteremias may occur in birds following cat bites. Blood from the birds with bacteremias reveals numerous bacterial organisms in the blood film (Figure 11.41) (Campbell and Grant, 2010). Birds with bacteremias rarely survive.

References

Abdo KM, Timmons PR, Graham DG, Abou-Donia MB. 1983. Heinz body production and hematological changes in the hen after administration of a single oral dose of n-butyl mercaptan and n-butyl disulfide. *Fundam Appl Toxicol* 3:69–74.

Adamcak A, Hess LR, Quesenberry KE. 2000. Intestinal string foreign body in an adult umbrella cockatoo (*Cacatua alba*). *J Avian Med Surg* 14(4):257–263.

Allen JL, Kollias GV, Greiner EC, Boyce W. 1985. Subcutaneous filariasis (*Pelecitus* sp.) in a yellow-collard macaw (*Ara auricollis*). *Avian Dis* 29:891–894.

Andreasen CB, Latimer KS. 1990. Cytochemical staining characteristics of chicken heterophils and eosinophils. *Vet Clin Pathol* 19:51–54.

Apanius V, Kirkpatrick CE. 1988. Preliminary report of *Haemoproteus tinnunculi* in a breeding population of American kestrels. *J Wildl Dis* 24:150.

Armstrong DL, Montali RJ, Doster AR, Kazacos KR. 1989. Cerebrospinal nematodiasis in macaws due to *Baylisascaris procyanis*. *J Zoo Wildl Med* 20:254–359.

Aslam B, Hussain I, Azhoor MA, Mahmood MS, Rasool MH. 2015. Prevalence of *Borrelia anserine* in *Argas* Ticks. *Pakistan J Zool* 47(4):1125–1131.

Assoku R, Pehale W, Buxton A. 1970. An immunological basis for the anemia of acute *Salmonella gallinarium* infection of chickens. I. Hematological changes and their association with in vivo modification of the erythrocytes. *Clin Exp Immunol* 7:865–874.

Atkinson CT, VanRipper C. 1991. Pathogenicity and epizootiology of avian haematozoa: *Plasmodium*, *Leucocytozoon*, and *Haemoproteus*. In: Loye J, Zuk M (eds), *Bird–Parasite Interactions*. New York: Oxford University Press.

Averbeck C. 1992. Haematology and blood chemistry of healthy and clinically abnormal great black-backed gulls (*Larus marinus*) and herring gulls (*Larus argentatus*). *Avian Pathol* 21:215–223.

Bale NM, Leon AE, Hawley DM. 2020. Differential house finch leukocyte profiles during experimental infection with *Mycoplasma gallisepticum* isolates of varying virulence. *Avian Pathol* 49(4):342–354.

Barrow PA. 1996. Immunity to salmonella and other bacteria. In: Davison T, Morris T, Payne L (eds), *Poultry Immunology*. Abingdon, UK: Carfax Publishing Company.

Bearhop S, Griffiths R, Orr K, Furness RW. 1999. Mean corpuscular volume (MCV) as a measure of condition in birds. *Ecol Lett* 2:352–356.

Bennett GF, Pierce MA. 1992. Leucocytozoids of seven old world passeriform families. *J Nat Hist* 26:693–707.

Bensch S, Stjernman M, Hasselquist D, et al. 2000. Host specificity in avian blood parasites: a study of *Plasmodium* and *Haemoproteus* mitochondrial DNA amplified from birds. *Proc R Soc Lond B* 267:1583–1589.

Bessis M. 1977. *Blood Smears Reinterpreted.* Berlin, Heidelberg: Springer-Verlag.

Bhattacherjee A, Acharya CP, Rana N, Mallik BK, Mohanty PK. 2018. Haematological and morphometrical analysis of blood cells of Khaki Campbell duck (*Ana platyrhynchos*) in different age groups with respect to sexual dimorphism. *Comp Clin Pathol* 27:1465–1472.

Bhattacharyya TK, Sarkar AK. 1968. Avian leucocytic responses induced by stress and corticoid inhibitors. *Ind J Exp Biol* 6:26–28.

Bienzle D, Pare JA, Smith DA. 1997. Leukocyte changes in diseased non-domestic birds. *Vet Clin Pathol* 26:76–84.

Blanco G, Rodrigues-Estrella R, Merino S, Bertellotti J. 2001. Effects of spatial and host variables on hematozoa in white-crowned sparrows wintering in California. *J Wildl Dis* 37:786–790.

Boal CW, Hudelson KS, Mannan RW, Estabrook TS. 1998a. Hematology and hematozoa of adult and nestling copper's hawks in Arizona. *J Raptor Res* 32:281–285.

Bonar CJ, Lewandowski AH, Schaul J. 2003. Suspected fenbendazole toxicosis in 2 vulture species (*Gyps africanus, Torgos tracheliotus*) and marabou storks (*Leptoptilos crumeniferus*). *J Avian Med Surg* 17:16–19.

Bos JH, Todd B, Tell LA, et al. 1990. Treatment of anemic birds with iron dextran therapy: homologous and heterologous transfusions. In: Proceedings of the Association of Avian Veterinarians, Phoenix, AZ, September 10–15, 1990.

Branton SL, May JD, Lott BD, Maslin WR. 1997. Various blood parameters in commercial hens acutely and chronically infected with *Mycoplasma gallisepticum* and *Mycoplasma synoviae*. *Avian Dis* 41(3):540–547.

Breton-Gorius J, Coquin Y, Guichard J. 1978. Cytochemical distinction between azurophils and catalase-containing granules in leukocytes. I. Studies in developing neutrophils and monocytes from patients with myeloperoxidase deficiency: comparison with peroxidase-deficient chicken heterophils. *Lab Invest* 38:21–31.

Brooks RL, Bounous DI, Andreasen CB. 1996. Functional comparison of avian heterophils with human and canine neutrophils. *Comp Haemat Inter* 6:153–159.

Brune K, Spitznagel JK. 1973. Peroxidaseless chicken leukocytes: isolation and characterization of anti-bacterial granules. *J Infect Dis* 127:84–94.

Campbell F. 1967. Fine structure of the bone marrow of the chicken and pigeon. *J Morphol* 123:405–440.

Campbell TW. 1994. Hematology. In: Ritchie BW, Harrison GJ, Harrison LR (eds), *Avian Medicine: Principles and Application.* Lake Worth, FL: Wingers Publishing, Inc., pp. 176–198.

Campbell TW. 1995. *Avian Hematology and Cytology*, 2nd edn. Ames, IA: Iowa State University Press.

Campbell TW, Coles EH. 1986. Avian clinical pathology. In: Coles EH (ed), *Veterinary Clinical Pathology*, 4th edn. Philadelphia, PA: WB Saunders Co.

Campbell TW, Dein FJ. 1984. Avian hematology, the basics. *Vet Clin North Am (Small Anim Pract)* 14:223–248.

Campbell TW, Ellis CK. 2007. *Avian and Exotic Animal Hematology and Cytology*, 3rd edn. Ames, IA: Blackwell Publishing.

Campbell TW, Grant KR. 2010. *Clinical Cases in Avian and Exotic Animal Hematology and Cytology.* Ames, IA: Wiley-Blackwell.

Cardona CJ, Ihejirika A, McClellan L. 2002. *Haemoproteus lophortyx* infection in Bobwhite quail. *Avian Dis* 46:249–255.

Carlson HC, Allen JR. 1969. The acute inflammatory reaction in chicken skin: blood cellular response. *Avian Dis* 14:817–833.

Carlson HC, Sweeny PR, Tokaryk JM. 1968. Demonstration of phagocytic and trephocytic activities of chicken thrombocytes by microscopy and vital staining techniques. *Avian Dis* 12:700–715.

Castro I, Howe L, Tompkins DM, Barraclough RK, Slaney D. 2011. Presence and seasonal prevalence of *Plasmodium* spp. in a rare endemic New Zealand passerine (Tieke or Saddleback, *Philesturnus carunculatus*). *J Wildl Dis* 47(4):860–867.

Chad N, Eyre P. 1978. Immunological release of histamine and SRS in domestic fowl. *Can J Comp Med* 42:519–524.

Chagas CRF, Binkiene R, Ilgunas M, Iezhova T., Valkiunas G. 2020. The buffy coat method: a tool for detection of blood parasites without staining procedures. *Parasites Vectors* 13(104): https://doi.org/10.1186/s13071-020-3984-8.

Cheng HW, Eicher SD, Chen Y, Singleton P, Muirt WM. 2001. Effect of genetic selection for group productivity and longevity on immunological and hematological parameters of chickens. *Poult Sci* 80:1079–1086.

Counihan KL, Tuomi PA, Hollmén TE. 2020. Differential progression of lymphoma in two captive Steller's eiders (*Polysticta stelleri*). *J Avian Med Surg* 34(3):302–305.

Chowdhury SR, Smith TK, Boermans HJ, et al. 2005. Effects of feeding blends of grains naturally contaminated with *Fusarium* mycotoxins on performance, metabolism, hematology, and immunocompetence of ducklings. *Poult Sci* 84:1179–1185.

Christie G. 1979. Hematological and biochemical findings in an experimentally produced hemolytic anemia in eight-week-old brown leghorn cockerels. *Br Vet J* 135:279–285.

Clark MW, Gildersleeve RP, Thaxton JP, et al. 1988. Hematological effects of ethyl methanesulfonate, paraquat and phenylhydrazine in Japanese quail. *Comp Biochem Physiol C Toxicol Pharmacol* 89:15–30.

Clark P. 2015. Assessment of avian erythrocytes that exhibit variant nuclear morphology. *Comp Clin Pathol* 24:485–490.

Clark P, Raidal SR. 2014. Evaluation of the erythroplastid component of avian blood. *Comp Clin Pathol* 23:1117–1123.

Coleman CW. 1995. Lymphoid neoplasia in pet birds: a review. *J Avian Med Surg* 9:3–7.

Coles EH. 1986. *Veterinary Clinical Pathology*, 4th edn. Philadelphia, PA: WB Saunders Co.

Corbel C, Lacoste-Eleaume AS, Bleux C, et al. 1995. Platelet intergrin GPIIb-IIIa homologue identified on chicken thromboytes. In: Davison T, Bumstead N, Kaiser P (eds), *Advances in Avian Immunology Research.* Abingdon, UK: Carfax Publishing Company.

Crespo R, Chin RP. 2004. Effect of feeding green onions (*Allium ascalonicum*) to White Chinese geese (*Threskiornis spinicollis*). *J Vet Diagn Invest* 16:321–325.

Cummings CO, Tully TN, Stöhr AC, et al. 2020. What Is Your Diagnosis? *J Avian Med Surg* 34(4):403–408.

D'Agostino JJ, Isaza R. 2004. Clinical signs and results of specific diagnostic testing among captive birds housed at zoological institutions and infected with West Nile virus. *J Am Vet Med Assoc* 224:1640–1643.

Daimon T, Caxton-Martins A. 1977. Electron microscopic and enzyme cytochemical studies on granules of mature chicken granular leucocytes. *J Anat* 123:553–562.

D'Aloia M-A, Samour JH, Howlett JC, Bailey TA, Naldo J. 1994. Haemopathological responses to chronic inflammation in the houbara bustard (*Chlamydotis undulata macqueenii*). *Comp Haematol Int* 4:203–206.

Datta K, Soni JL, Awadhiya RP, Datta IC. 1989. Erythrophagocytosis in phenylhydrazine induced acute anemia in chickens. *Res Vet Sci* 47:136–137.

Davidson TF, Flack IH. 1981. Changes in the peripheral blood leucocyte populations following an injection of corticotropin in the immature chicken. *Res Vet Sci* 30:79–82

Davis, AK, Cook, KC, Altizer, S. 2004. Leukocyte profiles in wild house finches with and without mycoplasmal conjunctivitis, a recently emerged bacterial disease. *EcoHealth* 1:362–373.

Davison TF, Rowell JG, Rea J. 1983. Effects of dietary corticosterone on peripheral blood lymphocytes and granulocyte populations in immature domestic fowl. *Res Vet Sci* 34:236–239.

Dawson RD, Bortolotti GR. 1997. Are avian hematocrits indicative of condition? American kestrels as a model. *J Wildl Manag* 61:1297–1306.

DeFrancisco N, Ruiz Troya JD, Aguera EI. 2003. Lead and lead toxicity in domestic and free living birds. *Avian Pathol* 32:3–13.

DeJong RJ, Muzzall PM. 2000. Hematozoa of waterfowl of Michigan. *J Wildl Dis* 36:767–773.

Desmidt M, Van Nerom A, Haesbrouck F, et al. 1996. Oxygenation activity of chicken blood phagocytes as measured by luminol- and lucigenin-dependent chemiluminescence. *Vet Immunol Immunopathol* 53:303–311.

Dharma DN, Purnomo PD, Arsana IB. 1985. Filariasis and microfilariasis in parrots in the eastern islands of Indonesia. *Avian Dis* 29:881–885.

Dhingra LD, Parrish WB, Venzke WG. 1969. Electron microscopy of granular leucocytes of chicken (*Gallus domesticus*). *Am J Vet Res* 30:637–642.

Dieterien-Lievre F. 1988. Birds. In: Rawley AF, Ratcliffe NA (eds), *Vertebrate Blood Cells*. Cambridge, UK: Cambridge University Press, pp. 257–336.

Djojosugito AM, Folkow B, Kovach AGB. 1968. The mechanisms behind rapid blood volume restoration after hemorrhage in birds. *Acta Physiol Scand* 74:114–122.

Dobinsky O. and Dobinska E. 1976. Season changes in the blood picture of adult pheasants. *Zentralblatt Veterinaire Medizin* 23:609–615.

Dohms JE, Metz A. 1991. Stress-mechanisms of immunosuppression. *Vet Immunol Immunopathol* 30:89–109.

Doolen MD, Greve, JH. 1992. Pet bird medicine: case report—description of a microfilaria from an Umbrella Cockatoo (*Cacatua alba*) and an unsuccessful attempt to infect mosquitoes (*Culex pipiens pipiens*). *Avian Dis* 36:484–487.

Dorresteine GM, vand de Hage MN, Zwart P. 1985. Diseases of passerines, especially canaries and finches. *Proc Assoc Avian Vet*, pp. 53–70.

Dresser SS. 1967. Schizogony and gametogony of *Leucocytozoon simondi* and associated reactions in the avian host. *J Protozool* 14:224—254.

Dri P, Bisiacchi B, Cramer R, Bellavite P, De Nicola G, Patriarca P. 1978. Oxidative metabolism of chicken polymorphonuclear leucocytes during phagocytosis. *Mol Cell Biochem* 22:159–166.

Driver EA. 1981. Haematological and blood chemical values of mallard, *Anas platyrhynchos platyrhynchos*, drakes before, during, and after remige molt. *J Wildl Dis* 17:413–421.

Droual R, Meteyer CU, Galey FD. 1991. Zinc toxicosis due to ingestion of a penny in a grey-headed chachalaca (*Ortalis cinereiceps*). *Avian Dis* 35:1007–1011.

Du Plessis L, Van Wilpe E. 2009. Thrombocyte morphology and morphometric observations in two vulture species. *Vet Clin Pathol* 38(3):316–320.

Echols MS, Craig TM, Speer BL. 2000. Heartworm (*Paronchocerca ciconarum*) infection in 2 saddle-billed storks (*Ephippiorhynchus senegalensis*). *J Avian Med Surg* 14(1): 42–47.

Egami MI, Sasso WS. 1991. Topochemistry of blood cells of the *Gallus domesticus* (Aves, Galliforme). *Rev Braz Biol* 51:211–214.

Enbergs H. 1975. *Die Feinstruktur der Leukozyten des Hausgeflugels, Die Feinstruktur der Leukozyten des Hausgeflugels*. Berlin: Verlag Paul Parry.

Enbergs H, Kriesten K. 1968. Die weissen Blutzellen de Haushuhns in elektronenmikroskopischen Bild. *Deutsche Tierartliche Wochschrift* 75:271–274.

Ericsson JLE, Nair MK. 1973. Electron microscopic demonstration of acid phosphatase activity in the developing and mature heterophils of the chicken. *Histochemie* 37:97–105.

Evans M, Otter A. 1998. Fatal combined infection with *Haemoproteus noctuae* and *Leucocytozoon ziemanni* in juvenile snowy owls (*Nyctea scandiaca*). *Vet Rec*143(3):72–76.

Fairbrother A, O'Loughlin D. 1990. Differential white blood cell values of the mallard (*Anas platyrhynchos*) across different ages and reproductive states. *J Wildl Dis* 29:78–82.

Fallon SM, Ricklefs RE. 2008. Parasitemia in PCR-detected *Plasmodium* and *Haemoproteus* infections in birds. *J Avian Biol* 39:514–522.

Fallon SM, Ricklefs RE, Swanson BL, Bermingham E. 2003. Detecting avian malaria: an improved polymerase chain reaction diagnostic. *J Parasitol* 89:1044–1047.

Fernandez A, Verde MT, Gomez J, et al. 1995. Changes in the prothrombin time, haematology and serum proteins during experimental aflatoxicosis in hens and broiler chickens. *Res Vet Sci* 58:119–122.

Fernandes AF, Fenton H, Martinson S, Desmarchelier M, Ferrell ST. 2014. Absolute polycythemia in a Bald eagle (*Haliaeetus leucocephalus*). *J Zoo Wildl Med* 45(4):958–960.

Ferrell ST, Tell LA. 2001. *Clostridium terium* infection in a rainbow lorikeet (*Trichoglossus haematodus haematodus*) with enteritis. *J Avian Med Surg* 14(3):204–208.

Finnegan MV, Daniel JB, Ramsay EC. 1997. Evaluation of whole blood transfusions in domestic pigeons (*Columba livia*). *J Avian Med Surg* 11(1):7–14.

Fite RW. 1984. Diagnosis and control of Leucocytozoonosis in captive water fowl. *Proceedings of the First International Conference of Zoological and Avian Medicine*, pp. 193–198.

Flammer K 1987. Clinical aspects of atoxoplasmosis in canaries. *Proceedings of the First International Conference of Zoological and Avian Medicine*, pp. 33–35.

Forbes NA, Cooper JE, Higgins RJ. 2000. Neoplasms of birds of prey. In: Lumeij JT (ed), *Raptor Biomedicine III*. Lake Worth, FL: Zoological Education Network, Inc., pp. 127–145.

Fourie F. Le R. Hattingh J. 1980. Variability in bird haematology. *Comp Biochem Physiol* 65a:147–150.

Fox AJ, Solomon JB. 1981. Chicken non-lymphoid leukocytes. In: Rose L, Payne L, Freeman M (eds), *Avian Immunology*. Edinburgh: Poultry Science Ltd.

Fry DM, Addiego L. 1987. Hemolytic anemia complicates the cleaning of oiled seabirds. *Wildl J* 10:3–6.

Fudge AM. 1997. What is your diagnosis? *J Avian Med Surg* 11(4):279–281.

Fujimori K, Yamada M, Imai K. 1979. Distribution of neutral and acid glucosidases of granule fractions from chicken heterophil leucocytes. *Cell Mol Biol* 23:391–402.

García-del-Río M, Sancho R, Martínez J, Merino S. 2020. Blood parasite infections in Strigiformes and Psittaciformes species in captivity with a new record of potential fatal blood parasite transmission to parrots. *J Zoo Wildl Med* 51(4):799–813.

Gardiner CH, Fayer R, Dubey JP. 1988. An atlas of protozoan parasites in animal tissues. In: *U.S. Department of Agriculture, Agriculture Handbook*. Washington, DC: U.S. Government Printing Office.

Garvin MC, Homer BL, Greiner EC. 2003. Pathogenicity of *Haemoproteus danilewskyi*, Kruse, 1890 in blue jays (*Cyanocitta cristata*). *J Wildl Dis* 39:161–169.

Gaskin JM. 1989. Psittacine viral diseases: a perspective. *J Zoo Wildl Med* 20:249–264.

Gattani A, Pathak A, Kumar A, Mishra V, Bhatia JS. 2016. Influence of season and sex on hemato-biochemical traits in adult turkeys under arid tropical environment. *Veterinary World* 9(5):530–534.

Gavazza A, Galosi L, Croce V, et al. 2019. A case of lymphocytic leukemia in a bearded dragon (*Pogona vitticeps*) and a review of literature. *Acta Vet (Beogr)* 69:360–368.

George JW, Duncan JR. 1981. Effect of sample preparation on basophilic stippling in bovine blood smears. *Vet Clin Pathol* 10:37–39.

Gibbons PM, Horton S. 2000. What is your diagnosis? *J Avian Med Surg* 14(1):60–64.

Gibbons PM, Sakas PS. 1997. What is your diagnosis? *J Avian Med Surg* 11(4):282–285.

Gibbons PM, Busch MD, Tell LA, et al. 2002. Internal papillomatosis with intrahepatic cholangiocarcinoma and gastrointestinal adenocarcinoma in a peach-fronted conure (*Aratinga aurea*). *Avian Dis* 46:1062–1069.

Gilardi KVK, Lowenstine L, Gilardi JD, Munn CA. 1995. A survey for selected viral, chlamydial, and parasitic diseases in wild Dusky-headed parakeets (*Aratinga-weddellii*) and Tui parakeets (*Brotogeris-sanctitihomae*) in Peru. *J Wildl Dis* 31(4).

Gildersleeve RP, Galvin M, Thaxton JP, McRee DI. 1985. Hematological response of Japanese quail to acute hemorrhagic stress. *Comp Biochem Physiol* 81A (2):403–409.

Godwin JS, Jacobson ER, Gaskin JM. 1982. Effects of Pacheco's parrot disease virus on hematologic and blood chemistry values of Quaker parrots (*Myopsitta monachus*). *J Zoo Anim Med* 113:127–132.

G6mez-Meda BC, Zamora-Perez AL, Luna-Aguirre J, et al. 2006. Nuclear abnormalities in erythrocytes of parrots (*Aratinga canicularis*) related to genotoxic damage. *Avian Pathol* 35(3):206–210.

Graham JE, Tell LA, Lamm MG, Lowenstine L. 2004. Megacloaca in a Moluccan cockatoo (*Cacatua mouccensis*). *J Avian Med Surg* 18(1):41–49.

Granthon C, Williams DA. 2017. Avian malaria, body condition, and blood parameters in four species of songbirds. *Wilson J Ornithol* 129(3):492–508.

Gray HG, Paradis TJ, Chang PW. 1989. Physiological effects of adrenocorticotropic hormones and hydrocortisone in laying hens. *Poult Sci* 68:1710–1713.

Grecchi R, Saliba AM, Mariano M. 1980. Morphological changes, surface receptors and phagocytic potential of fowl mononuclear phagocytes and thrombocytes in vivo and in vitro. *J Pathol* 130:23–31.

Greiner EC, Norton TM, Latimer KS. 1995. Atoxoplasmosis—an impediment to the Bali mynah (*Leucopsar rothschilli*) species survival plan. In: *Proceedings of the Joint Conference AAZV/WDA/AAWV*.

Grilo ML, Vanstreels RET, Wallace R, et al. 2016. Malaria in penguins – current perceptions. *Avian Pathol* 45(4):393–407.

Groombridge JJ, Massey JG, Bruch JC, et al. 2004. Evaluating stress in a Hawaiian honeycreeper, *Paroreomyza montana*, following translocation. *J Field Ornithol* 75:183–187.

Gross WB. 1989. Factors affecting chicken thrombocyte morphology and the relationship with heterophil: lymphocytre ratios. *Br Poult Sci* 30:919–925.

Gross WB, Siegel HS. 1983. Evaluation of the heterophil/lymphocyte ratio as a measure of stress in chickens. *Avian Dis* 27:972–979.

Gupta A, Tully TN, Beaufre're H, et al. 2011. What is your diagnosis? Bone marrow aspirate from a hyacinth macaw (*Anodorhynchus hyacinthinus*). *Vet Clin Pathol* 40(4):565–566.

Guthrie AL, Jayson SL, Strike TB, et al. 2020. Diagnosis and treatment of heavy metal toxicosis in six Waldrapp ibis (*Geronticus eremita*). *J Avian Med Surg* 34(4):371–380.

Halliwell WH. 1971. Lesions of Marek's disease in a great horned owl. *Avian Dis* 15:49–55.

Hanauska-Brown LA, Duffy AM, Roloff GJ. 2003. Blood chemistry, cytology, and body condition in adult northern goshawks (*Accipiter gentilis*). *J Raptor Res* 37:299–306.

Hannon DE, Bemis DA, Garner MM. 2012. *Mycobacterium marinum* infection in a blue-fronted Amazon parrot (*Amazona aestiva*). *J Avian Med Surg* 26(4):239–247.

Harmon BG. 1998. Avian heterophils in inflammation and disease resistance. *Poult Sci* 77:972–977.

Harmon BG, Blisson JR. 1990. Disassociation of bacterial and fungistatic activities from the oxidative burst of avian macrophages. *Am J Vet Res* 51:71–75.

Harper EJ, Lowe B. 1998. Hematology values in a colony of budgerigars (*Melopsittacus undulatus*) and changes associated with aging. *J Nutr* 28:2639S–2640S.

Harr KE, Cunningham FL, Pritsos CA, et al. 2017. Weathered MC252 crude oil-induced anemia and abnormal erythroid morphology in double-crested cormorants (*Phalacrocorax auritus*) with light microscopic and ultrastructural description of Heinz bodies. *Ecotox Environ Safe* 146:29–39.

Hauptmanova K, Maly M, Literak I. 2006. Changes of haematological parameters in common pheasant throughout the year. *Vet Med* 51:29034.

Hawkey CM, Dennett TB. 1989. *A Colour Atlas of Comparative Veterinary Haematology*. London: Wolfe Medical Publications, Ltd.

Hawkey CM, Hart MG, Samour JH, et al. 1984. Haematological findings in healthy and sick captive rosy flamingos (*Phoenicopterus ruber ruber*). *Avian Pathol* 13:163–172.

Hawkey CM, Samour JH, Henderson GM, et al. 1985. Haematological findings in captive Gentoo penguins (*Pygoscelis papua*) with bumblefoot. *Avian Pathol* 14:251–156.

Hayat MA. 1989. Principles and techniques of electron microscopy: biological applications. In: Hayat M (ed), *Principles and Techniques of Electron Microscopy: Biological Applications*, 3rd edn. London: Macmillan Press Ltd.

Heatley JJ, Jowett PLH. 2000. What is your diagnosis? *J Avian Med Surg* 14(4):283–284.

Heatley JJ, Williams J, Mitchell MA, et al. 1999. What is your diagnosis? *J Avian Med Surg* 13(2):138–142.

Heatley JJ, Mitchell MM, Cho DY, Williams DL, Tulley TN. 2007. Disseminated mycobacteriosis in a bald eagle (*Haliaeetus leucocephalus*). *J Avian Med Surg* 21:201–209.

Heidenreich M. 1997. Infectious diseases. In: Heidenreich M (ed), *Birds of Prey: Medicine and Management*. Osney Mead, Oxford: Blackwell Science, pp. 103–129.

Hellgren O, Križanauskienė A, Hasselquist D, Bensch S. 2011. Low haemosporidian diversity and one key-host species in bird malaria community on a mid-Atlantic island (SÃO Miguel, Azores). *J Wildl Dis* 47(4):849–859.

Helmer PJ, Carpenter JW, Hoskinson JJ. 2000. What is your diagnosis? *J Avian Med Surg* 14(3):200–203.

Herbert R, Nanney J, Spano JS, Pedersoli WM, Krista LM. 1989. Erythrocyte distribution in ducks. *Am J Vet Res* 50:958–960.

Hess L, Bartick T, Hoefer H. 1998. *Clostridium tertium* infection in a Moluccan cockatoo (*Cacatua moluccensis*) with megacolon. *J Avian Med Surg* 12(1):30–35.

Hodges RD. 1974. *The Histology of the Fowl*. London: Academic Press.

Hodges RD. 1977. Normal avian (poultry) haematology. In: Archer R, Jeffcott L (eds), *Comparative Clinical Haematology*. London: Blackwell Scientific Publications.

Högemann C, Richterb R, Korbel R, Rinder M. 2017. Plasma protein, haematologic and blood chemistry changes in African grey parrots (*Psittacus erithacus*) experimentally infected with bornavirus. *Avian Pathol* 46(5):556–570.

Holmstad PR, Anwar A, Iezhova T, Skorping A. 2003. Standard sampling techniques underestimate prevalence of avian hematozoa in willow ptarmigan (*Lagopus lagopus*). *J Wildl Dis* 39:354–358.

Howard LL, Papendick R, Stalis IH, et al. 2002. Fenbendazole and albendazole toxicity in pigeons and doves. *J Avian Med Surg* 16:203–210.

Hunter DB, Rohner C, Currie DC. 1997. Mortality in fledgling great horned owls from black fly hematophaga and leucocytozoonosis. *J Wildl Dis* 33(3):486–491.

Jacobson ER, Hines SA, Quesenberry K, et al. 1984. Epornitic of papova-like virus-associated disease in a psittacine nursery. *J Am Vet Med Assoc* 185:1337–1341.

Jain NC. 1986. *Schalm's Veterinary Hematology*, 4th edn. Philadelphia, PA: Lea & Febiger.

Jain NC. 1993. *Essentials of Veterinary Hematology*. Philadelphia, PA: Lea & Febiger.

James SB, Raphael BL, Cook RA. 1998. Brodifacoum toxicity and treatment in a white-winged wood duck (*Cairnina scutulata*). *J Zoo Wildl Med* 29(3):324–327.

Janes ME, Bower RK, Anthony NB. 1994. The leukocyte response of Japanese quail to Rous sarcoma virus-induced tumors. *Avian Dis* 38:610–615.

Johns JL, Luff JA, Shooshtari MP, Zehnder AM, Borjesson DL. 2009. What is your diagnosis? Blood smear from an injured red-tailed hawk. *Vet Clin Pathol* 38(2):247–252.

Jones JS, Thomas JS, Bahr A, Phalen DN. 2002. Presumed immune-mediated hemolytic anemia in a blue-crowned conure (*Aratinga acuticaudata*). *J Avian Med Surg* 16:223–229.

Jones MP, Orosz SE, Richman LK, et al. 2001. Pulmonary carcinoma with metastases in a Moluccan cockatoo (*Cacatua moluccensis*). *J Avian Med Surg* 15(2):107–113.

Joseph V. 1999. Raptor hematology and chemistry evaluation. *Vet Clin North Am (Exotic Anim Pract): Clin Pathol Sample Collect* 2(3):689–699.

Katavolos P, Staempfli S, Sears W, et al. 2007. The effect of lead poisoning on hematologic and biochemical values in trumpeter swans and Canada geese. *Vet Clin Pathol* 36:341–347.

Keeney CMH, Intile JL, Sims CS, Harrison TM. 2021. Lymphoid leukemia in five bearded dragons (*Pogona vitticeps*). *J Am Vet Med Assoc* 258(7):748–757.

Kelenyi G, Nemeth A. 1969a. Comparative histochemistry and electron microscopy of the eosinophil leucocytes of vertebrates. *Acta Biol Acad Sci Hung* 20:405–422.

Kelenyi G, Nemeth A. 1969b. Comparative studies on eosinophils. *Acta Biol Hung* 20:405–417.

King AS, McLelland J. 1984. Integument. In: King AS, McLelland J (eds), *Birds: Their Structure and Function*, 2nd edn. London: Bailliere Tindall.

Kisseberth WC, MacEwen EG. 1996. Complications of cancer and its treatment. In: Withrow S, MacEwen E (eds), *Small Animal Clinical Oncology*. Philadelphia, PA: WB Saunders.

Kocan AA, Snelling J, Greiner EC. 1977. Some infectious and parasitic diseases in Oklahoma raptors. *J Wildl Dis* 13:304.

Kocan RM, Pitts SM. 1976. Blood values of the Canvasback duck by age, sex, and season. *J Wildl Dis* 12:341–345.

Kogut MH, McGruder ED, Hargis BM, Corrier DE, DeLoach JR. 1995. in vivo activation of heterophil function in chickens following injection with *Salmonella enteritidis*-immune lymphokine. *J Leukoc Biol* 57:56–62.

Kolmstetter CM, Carpenter JW, Morrisey J, Ball R. 1995a. What is your diagnosis? *J Avian Med Surg* 9:50–56.

Kolmstetter CM, Carpenter JW, Ernst S. 1995b. What is your diagnosis? *J Avian Med Surg* 9(3):195–197.

Korschgen CE, Kenow KP, Gendron-Fitzpatrick A, et al. 1996. Implanting intra-abdominal radiotransmitters with external whip antennas in ducks. *J Wildl Manag* 60:132–137.

Kuiken T, Danesik KL. 1999. Hematology and serum chemistry of captive juvenile double-crested cormorants (*Phalacrocorax auritus*). *Can Vet J* 40:493–496.

Kwiecien JM, Smith DA, Key DW, et al. 1993. Encephalitis attributed to larval migration of *Baylisascaris* sp. in emus. *Can Vet J* 34:176–178.

Lam KM. 1997. Activation, adhesion, migration and death of chicken thrombocytes. *Comp Haematol Int* 1:81–87.

Lam KM, Kabbur MB, Eiserich JP. 1996. Newcastle disease virus-induced functional impairments and biochemical changes in chicken heterophils. *Vet Immunol Immunopathol* 53:13–327.

Landolfi JA, Adkesson MJ, Ahmed N, et al. 2020. Systemic isosporosis (formerly atoxoplasmosis), is a protozoal infection that causes death in nestling and fledgling passerine birds affecting ex situ breeding and reintroduction programs. *J Zoo Wildl Med* 51(2):391–397.

Landys-Ciannelli MM, Haerdawei JJ, Piersma T. 2002. Blood parameter changes during stopover in a long-distance migratory shorebird, the bar-tailed godwit *Limosa lapponica taymyrensis*. *J Avian Biol* 33:451–455.

Lanza GM, Washburn KW, Wyatt RD. 1980. Variation with age in response of broilers to aflatoxin. *Poult Sci* 59:282–288.

Latas P, Auchland LD, Teel PD, Hamer SA. 2020. *Argas (Persicargas) giganteus* soft tick infection with *Rickettsia hoogstraali* and replapsing fever *Borrelia* on wild avian species of the desert southwest. *USA: J Wildl Dis* 56(1):113–125.

Latimer KS, Tang KN, Goodwin MA, et al. 1988. Leukocyte changes associated with acute inflammation in chickens. *Avian Dis* 32:760–772.

Latney L, Guzman DS-M, Tully TN, et al. 2007. What is your diagnosis? *J Avian Med Surg* 21:77–79.

Leighton FA. 1985. Morphological lesions in red blood cells from herring gulls and Atlantic puffins ingesting Prudhoe Bay crude oil. *Vet Pathol* 23:393–402.

Leighton FA, Peakall DB, Butler RG. 1983. Heinz-body hemolytic anemia from the ingestion of crude oil: primary toxic effect in marine birds. *Science* 220:871–873.

Levengood JM, Sanderson GC, Anderson WL, et al. 2000. Influence of diet on the hematology and serum biochemistry of zincintoxicated mallards. *J Wildl Dis* 36:111–123.

Levine ND. 1982. The genus Atoxoplasma (Protozoa, Apicomplexa). *J Parasitol* 68:719–723.

Lewis JH, Hasiba U, Spero JA. 1979. Comparative hematology: studies on class Aves, domestic turkey (*Meleagris gallopavo*). *Comp Biochem Physiol* 62A:735–745.

Lloyd M. 1992. Heavy metal ingestion: medical management and gastroscopic foreign body removal. *J Assoc Avian Vet* 6:25–26.

Lopes H, Redig P, Glaser A, Armien A, Wünschmann A. 2007. Clinical findings, lesions, and viral antigen distribution in great gray owls (*Strix nebulosa*) and barred owls (*Strix varia*) with spontaneous West Nile virus infection. *Avian Dis* 51(1):140–145.

Lothrop C, Harrison G, Schultz D, Utteridge T. 1988. Miscellaneous diseases. In: Harrison G, Harrison L (eds), *Clinical Avian Medicine and Surgery*. Philadelphia, PA: WB Saunders Co.

Lucas AJ, Jamroz C. 1961. *Atlas of Avian Hematology*. United States Department of Agriculture Monograph 25. Washington, DC: U.S. Government Printing Office.

Lupu CA. 2000. Evaluation of side effects of tamoxifen in buderigars (*Melopsittacus undulatus*). *J Avian Med Surg* 14(4): 237–242.

Macwhirter P. 1994. Passeriformes. In: Ritchie B, Harrison G, Harrison L (eds), *Avian Medicine: Principles and Application*. Lake Worth, FL: Wingers.

Maldonado N, Larson K. 2004. What is your diagnosis? *J Avian Med Surg* 18(2):112–115.

Mans C, Guzman DS-M. 2007. What is your diagnosis? *J Avian Med Surg* 21:235–238.

Marks S, Williams J, Tulley TN, Ryan KA. 1999. What is your diagnosis? *J Avian Med Surg* 13(4):294–297.

Marshall K, Daniel G, Patton C, Greenacre C. 2004. Humeral air sac mucinous adenocarcinoma in a salmon-crested cockatoo (*Cacatua moluccensis*). *J Avian Med Surg* 18(3):167–174.

Maxwell MH. 1973. Comparison of heterophil and basophil ultrastructure in six species of domestic bird. *J Anat* 115:187–202.

Maxwell MH. 1979. The ultrastructure of the eosinophil granules of the black-necked crowned crane. *J Anat* 128:53–63.

Maxwell MH. 1980. Attempted induction of an avian eosinophilia using various agents. *Res Vet Sci* 29:293–297.

Maxwell MH. 1981a. The production of a "Heinz body" anaemia in the domestic fowl after oral ingestion of dimethyl disulphate: a haematological and ultrastructural study. *Res Vet Sci* 30:233–238.

Maxwell MH. 1981b. Leucocyte diurnal rhythms in normal and pinealectomized juvenile female fowls. *Res Vet Sci* 31:113–115.

Maxwell MH. 1984. The distribution and localisation of acid trimetaphosphatase in developing heterophils and eosinophils in the bone marrow of the fowl and the duck. *Cell Tissue Res* 235:171–176.

Maxwell MH. 1987. The avian eosinophil—a review. *World's Poult Sci* 43:190–207.

Maxwell MH. 1993. Avian blood leucocyte responses to stress. *World's Poult Sci* 49:34–43.

Maxwell MH, Robertson GW. 1998. The avian heterophil leucocyte: a review. *World's Poult Sci* 54:155–178.

Maxwell MH, Robertson GW, Spence S, McCorquodale CC. 1990. Comparison of haematological values in restricted and ad libitum-fed domestic fowls. II White blood cells and thrombocytes. *Br Poult Sci* 31:399–405.

Maxwell MH, Siller WG. 1972. The ultrastructural characteristics of the eosinophil granules in six species of domestic bird. *J Anat* 112:289–303.

Maxwell MH, Trejo R. 1970. The ultrastructure of white blood cells and thrombocytes of the domestic fowl. *Br Vet J* 126:583–592.

Maxwell MH, Robertson GW, Anderson IA, Dick LA, Lynch M. 1991. Haematology and histology of seven-week old broilers after early food restriction. *Res Vet Sci* 50:290–297.

McCain S, Sim RR, Howerth EW, et al. 2020. Myonecrosis and death due to presumed microcystin toxicosis in American white pelicans (*Pelecanus erythrorhynchos*). *J Zoo Wildl Med* 51(2):407–415.

McFarlane JM, Curtis SE. 1989. Multiple concurrent stressors in chicks: effects on plasma corticosterone and the heterophil/lymphocyte ratio. *Poult Sci* 68:522–527.

Merino S, Potti J, Fargallo JA. 1997. Blood parasites of passerine birds from central Spain. *J Wildl Dis* 33(3):638–641.

Michot TC, Garvin MC, Weidner EH. 1995. Survey for blood parasites in redheads (*Aythya americana*) wintering at the Chandeleur Islands, Louisiana. *J Wildl Dis* 31(1):90–92.

Mijares A, Rosales R, Silva-Iturriza A. 2012. Hemosporidian parasites in forest birds from Venezuela: genetic lineage analyses. *Avian Dis* 56:583–588.

Miller RE, et al. 1983. *Leucocytozoon simondi* infection in European and American eiders. *JAVMA* 183:1241–1244.

Mitchell MA, Kettlewell PJ, Maxwell MH. 1992. Indicators of physiological stress in broiler chickens during road transportation. *Anim Welfare* 1:91–103.

Montolio SA, Lopez RM, Cray C, et al. 2017. Hematologic reference intervals and age effect in European Strigiformes. *Vet Clin Pathol* 46(3):483–495.

Moreno J, Merino S, Martinez J, Sanz JJ, Arriero E. 2002. Heterophil/lymphocyte ratios and heat-shock protein levels are related to growth in nestling birds. *Ecoscience* 9:434–439.

Morton ML. 1994. Hematocrits in montane sparrows in relation to reproductive schedule. *Condor* 96:119–126.

Mulcahy DM, Burek KA, Esler D. 2007. Inflammatory reaction to fabric collars from percutaneous antennas attached to intracoelomic radio transmitters implanted in Harlequin ducks (*Histrionicus histrionicus*). *J Avian Med Surg* 21(1):13–21.

Mulley RC. 1979. Haematology and blood chemistry of the black duck (*Anas supercilliosa*). *J Wildl Dis* 15:473–441.

Mulley RC. 1980. Haematology of the wood duck, *Chenonetta jubata*. *J Wildl Dis* 16:271–273.

Nair MK. 1973. The early inflammatory reaction in the fowl—a light microscopical, ultrastructural and autoradiographic study. *Acta B Vet Scand (Suppl)* 42:1–103

Newell SM, McMillan MC, Moore FM. 1991. Diagnosis and treatment of lymphocytic leukemia and malignant lymphoma in a Pekin duck (*Anas platyrhynchas domesticus*). *J Assoc Avian Vet* 5:83–86.

Newman SH, Mazet JK, Ziccardi MH, et al. 1999. Haematological changes and anaemia associated with captivity and petroleum exposure in seabirds. *Comp Haematol Int* 9:60–67.

Ochiai K, Jin K, Goryo M, et al. 1993. Pathomorphologic findings of lead poisoning in white-fronted geese (*Anser albifrons*). *Vet Pathol* 30:522–528.

Ogilvie GK. 1996. Paraneoplastic syndromes. In: Withrow S, MacEwen E (eds), *Small Animal Clinical Oncology*. Philadelphia, PA: WB Saunders.

Olson C. 1965. Avian hematology. In: Biester H, Swarte L (eds), *Diseases of Poultry*, 5th edn. Ames, IA: Iowa State University Press.

Osculati E. 1970. Fine structural localization of acid phosphatase and arylsulfatase in the chick heterophil leucocytes. *Z Zellforsch Mikrosk Anat* 109:398–406.

Ots I, Murumagi A, Horak P. 1998. Haematological health state indices of reproducing great tits: methodology and sources of natural variation. *Funct Ecol* 12:700–707.

Ouchene N, Nebbak A, Ouchene-Khelifi NA, et al. 2020. Molecular detection of avian spirochete *Borrelia anserine* in *Argas persicus* ticks in Algeria. *Comp Immunol Microbiol Infect Dis* 68:101408.

Owen JC, Cornelius EA, Arsnoe DA, Garvin MC. 2013. Leukocyte response to Eastern Equine Encephalomyelitis virus in a wild passerine bird. *Avian Dis* 57:744–749.

Papendick R, Stalis I, Harvey C, et al. 1998. Suspected fenbendazole toxicity in birds. In: *Proceedings of the Annual Conference of the American Association of Zoo Veteterinarians*, Omaha, NE, October 17–22, pp. 144–146.

Parga ML, Pendl H, Forbes NA. 2001. The effect of transport on hematologic parameters in trained and untrained Harris's hawks (*Parabuteo unicinctus*) and Peregrine falcons (*Falco peregrinus*). *J Avian Med Surg* 15:162–169.

Pedersoli WM, Spano JS, Krista LM, et al. 1989. Effects of fenbendazole administration on hematology, clinical chemistries and selected hormones in the white Pekin duck. *J Vet Pharmacol Ther* 12:200–208.

Peirce MA, Lederer R, Adlard RD, O'Donoghue PJ. 2004. Pathology associated with endogenous development of haematozoa in birds from southeast Queensland. *Avian Pathol* 33:445–450.

Penigrahy B, Rowe LD, Corrier DE. 1986. Haematological values and changes in blood chemistry in chickens with infectious bursal disease. *Res Vet Sci* 40:86–88.

Phalen DN, Taylor C, Phalen SW, et al. 1995. Hemograms and hematozoa of sharp-shinned (*Accipiter striatus*) and Coopers-hawks (*Accipiter cooperii*) captured during spring migration in Northern New York. *J Wildl Dis* 31(2):216–222.

Pimental JL, Greger JL, Cook ME, Stahl JL. 1992. Iron metabolism in chicks fed various levels of zinc and copper. *J Nutr Biochem* 3:140–145.

Pinneall R, Spitznagel JK. 1975. Chicken neutrophils: oxidative metabolism in phagocytic cells devoid of myeloperoxidase. *Proc Natl Acad Sci USA* 72:5012–5015.

Pizarro M, Villegas P, Rodriguez A, Rowland GN. 1994. Filariasis (*Pelecitus* sp.) in the cervical subcutaneous tissue of a pigeon with trichomoniasis. *Avian Dis* 38:385–389.

Ploucha JM, Scott JB, Ringer RK. 1981. Vascular and hematologic effects of hemorrhage in the chicken. *Am J Physiol* 240:H9–H17.

Post J, Rebel JMJ, TerHuurne AAHM. 2003. Automated blood cell count: a sensitive and reliable method to study corticosteronerelated stress in broilers. *Poult Sci* 82:591–595.

Powers LV. 2000. Diseases of the avian spleen. *J Am Vet Med Assoc* 22:925–933.

Pung OJ, Maxwell NE, Greiner WC, Robinette ER, Thul JE. 1997. *Haemoproteus greineri* in wood ducks from the Atlantic flyway. *J Wildl Dis* 33:355–358.

Pye GW, Bennet RA, Newell SM, et al. 2000. Magnetic resonance imaging in psittacine birds with chronic sinusitis. *J Avian Med Surg* 14(4):243–256.

Quereshi MA. 1998. Role of macrophages in avian health and disease. *Poult Sci* 77:978–982.

Raidal SR, Jaensch SM. 2000. Central nervous disease and blindness in Nankeen kestrels (*Falco cenchroides*) due to a novel *Leucocytozoon*-like infection. *Avian Pathol* 29:51–56.

Raju MVLN, Devegowda G. 2000. Influence of esterifiedglucomannan on performance and organ morphology, serum biochemistry, and haematology in broilers exposed to individual and combined mycotoxicosis (aflatoxin, ochratoxin, and T-2 toxin). *Br Poult Sci* 41:640–650.

Rausch PG, Moore TG. 1975. Granule enzymes of polymorphonuclear neutrophils: a phylogenetic comparison. *Blood* 46: 913–919.

Rebar AH, Lewis HB, DeNicola DB. 1981. Red cell fragmentation in the dog: an editorial review. *Vet Pathol* 18:415–426.

Reddy VR, Mohiuddin SM, Ramana PV. 1981. Red cell fragmentation in the dog: an editorial review. *Vet Pathol* 18:415–426.

Rehder NB, Lague DM, Mackay C. 1982. Variation in selected hematological parameters of captive red-tailed hawks. *J Wildl Dis* 18:105–109.

Remple JD. 2004. Intracellular hematozoa of raptors: a review and update. *J Avian Med Surg* 18(2):75–88.

Rivera S, Mc Clearen J, Reavill D. 2000. Suspected fenbendazole toxicity in pigeons (*Columba livia*). In: *Proceedings of the Annual Conference of the Association of Avian Veteterinarians*, Portland, OR, August 30–September 1, pp. 207–209.

Roberts GW, Maxwell MH. 1993. Importance of optimal mixtures of EDTA anticoagulant: blood for the preparation of well-stained avian blood smears. *Br Poultry Sci* 34:615–617.

Romagnano A. 1994. Binucleate erythrocytes and erythrocytic dysplasia in a cockatiel. In: *Proceedings of the Annual Conference of the Association of Avian Veterinarians*, Reno, NV, September 28–30.

Romagnano A, Grindem CB, Degernes LA, Mautino M. 1995. Treatment of a hyacinth macaw with zinc toxicity. *J Avian Med Surg* 9(3):185–189.

Romano J, Campbell TW, Grant KR, Montgomery C, Han S. 2020. Absolute Erythrocytosis in a Sunda Wrinkled Hornbill (*Aceros corrugatus*). *J Avian Med Surg* 34(2):192–197.

Rooney MB, Burkhard MJ, Greiner EC, et al. 2001. Intestinal and blood parasites in Amazon parrots destined for relocation in Guatemala. *J Zoo Wildl Med* 32:71–73.

Rose ME, Hesketh P, Ogilvie GM. 1979. Peripheral blood leucocyte response to coccidial infection: a comparison of the response in rats and chickens and its correlation with resistance to reinfection. *Immunology* 36:71–79.

Rosskopf WJ, Woerpel RW, Howard EB, Holshuh HJ. 1981. Chronic endocrine disorder associated with inclusion body hepatitis in a sulfur-crested cockatoo. *J Am Vet Med Assoc* 179:1273–1276.

Rupiper DJ, Read DH. 1996. Hemochromatosis in a hawkheaded parrot (*Deroptyus accipitrinus*). *J Avian Med Surg* 10:24–27.

Salakij C, Pornpanom P, Salakij J, Jakthong P. 2019. Quantitative and qualitative characteristics of blood cells in black-shouldered, Brahminy, and black kites. *Vet Clin Pathol* 2019 48(1):19–30.

Scanes CG. 2014. Blood. In: Scanes CG (ed), *Sturkie's Avian Physiology*. Philadelphia, PA: Elsevier.

Schalm OW, Jain NC, Carroll EJ. 1975. *Veterinary Hematology*, Vol. 3. Philadelphia, PA: Lea & Febiger.

Schmidt EMDS, Paulillo AC, Dittrich RL, et al. 2007. The effect of age on hematological and serum biochemical values in juvenile ring-necked pheasants (*Phasianus colchicus*). *Int J Poult Sci* 6:459–461.

Schindler SL, Gildersleeve RP, Thaxton JP, McRee DI. 1987. Hematological response of hemorrhaged Japanese quail after blood volume replacement with saline. *Comp Biochem Physiol A* 87:933.

Schoemaker NJ, Dorrestein GM, Latimer KS, et al. 2000. Severe leukopenia and liver necrosis in young African grey parrots (*Psittacus erithacus erithacus*) infected with psittacine circovirus. *Avian Dis* 44(2):470–478.

Schultz JH, Burmudez AJ, Tomlinson JL, et al. 1998. Effects of implanted radiotransmitters on captive mourning doves. *J Wildl Manag* 62:1451–1460.

Schwartz RS, Berkmand EM, Silberstein LE. 2000. Autoimmune hemolytic anemias. In: Hoffman R, Benz E, Shattil S, et al. (eds), *Hematology: Basic Principles and Practices*. Philadelphia, PA: Churchill Livingstone.

Shave HJ, Howard V. 1976. A hematologic survey of captive waterfowl. *J Wildl Dis* 12:195–201.

Short CR, Barker SA, Hsieh LC, et al. 1988. The elimination of fenbendazole and its metabolites in the chicken, turkey and duck. *J Vet Pharmacol Ther* 11:204–209.

Siccardi FJ, Rutherford HO, Derieux WT. 1971. Pathology and prevention of Leucocytozoon smithi infection of turkeys. *JAVMA* 158:1902.

Simpson CF. 1971. The ultrastructure of Heinz bodies in horse, dog, and turkey erythrocytes. *Cornell Vet* 61:228–238.

Smith RH. 1980. Kale poisoning: the brassica anemia factor. *Vet Rec* 107:12–15.

Sobhakumari A, Poppenga RH, Tawde S. 2018. Avian Toxicology. In: Gupta RC (ed), *Veterinary Toxicology*. Philadelphia, PA: Elsevier.

Soulsby EJL. 1982. Helminths, arthropods, and protozoa of domesticated animals. In: Soulsby EJL (ed), *Helminths, Arthropods, and Protozoa of Domesticated Animals*, 7th edn. Philadelphia, PA: Lea and Febiger.

Speer BL, Kass PH. 1995. The influence of travel on hematologic parameters in hyacinth macaws. In: *Proceedings of the Annual Conference of the Association of Avian Veterinarians*, Philadelphia, PA, August 28–September 1.

Spottiswoode N, Bartlett SL, Conley KJ, et al. 2020. Analysis of plasmodium lineages identified in captive penguins (*Sphenisciformes* spp.), eiders (*Somateria* spp.), and Inca terns (*Larosterna inca*) in a North American zoological collection. *J Zoo Wildl Med* 51(1):140–149.

Stabler JG, McCormick TW, Powell KC, Kogut MH. 1994. Avian heterophils and monocytes: phagocytic and bactericidal activities against *Salmonella enteritidis*. *Vet Microbiol* 38:293–305.

Stalis IH, Allen JL, Sutherland-Smith M. 1995. Possible albendazole toxicity in birds. In: *Proceedings of the Annual Conference of the American Association of Zoo Veterinarians*, East Lancing, MI, August 13–17, pp. 216–217.

Steinmetz HW, Rutz C, Hoop RK, et al. 2006. Possible human–avian transmission of *Mycobacterium tuberculosis* in a green-winged macaw (*Ara chloroptera*). *Avian Dis* 50(4):641–645.

Stuht JN, Bowerman WW, Best DA. 1999. Leucocytozoonosis in nestling bald eagles in Michigan and Minnesota. *J Wildl Dis* 35:608–612.

Sturkie PD. 1976. Blood: physical characteristics, formed elements, hemoglobin, and coagulation. In: Sturkie PD (ed), *Avian Physiology*. New York: Springer.

Sturkie PD, Griminger P. 1986. Body fluids: blood. In: Sturkie PD (ed), *Avian Physiology*, 4th edn. New York: Springer, pp. 102–129.

Suedmeyer WK, Bermudez A, Kazacos KR. 1996. Cerebellar nematodiasis in an emu (*Dromaius novaehollandiae*). *J Zoo Wildl Med* 27:544–549.

Sunber JP, Junge RE, Obanion MK, et al. 1986. Cloacal papillomas in psittacines. *Am J Vet Res* 47:928–932.

Sutherland M, Courtman N, Sacks P, Macwhirter P. 2018. Severe leukemoid response associated with *Mycobacterium genavense* infection in a pet Budgerigar (*Melopsittacus undulatus*). *J Exotic Pet Med* 27:11–16.

Swayne DE, Stockman SL, Johnson GS. 1986. Cytochemical properties of chicken blood cells resembling both thrombocytes and lymphocytes. *Vet Clin Pathol* 15:17–24.

Sweeny PR, Carlson HC. 1968. Electron microscopy and histochemical demonstration of lysosomal structures in chicken thrombocytes. *Avian Dis* 12:636–644.

Szabo K, Szalmas A, Liker A, Barta Z. 2002. Effects of haematophagous mites on nestling house sparrows (*Passer domesticus*). *Acta Parasitol* 47(4):318–322.

Tadjalli M, Nazifi S, Eemanparvar A. (2003). Normal cellular morphology of the blood of Japanese quail (*Coturnix coturnix japonica*). *Comp Clin Pathol* 12:102–105.

Tangredi BP. 1981. Heterophilia and left shift with fatal diseases in four psittacine birds. *J Zoo Anim Med* 12:13–16.

Taylor M. 1987. Polycythemia in the blue and gold macaw— a case report of three cases. In: *Proceedings of the First International Conference on Zoological and Avian Medicine*, Turtle Bay, HI, September 6–11.

Taylor SM, Kenny J, Houston A, Hewitt SA. 1993. Efficacy, pharmacokinetics, and effects on egg-laying and hatchability of two dose rates of in-feed fenbendazole for the treatment of *Capillaria* species infections in chickens. *Vet Rec* 133:519–521.

Tell LA, Ferrell ST, Gibbons PM. 2004. Avian mycobacteriosis in free-living raptors in California: 6 cases (1997–2001). *J Avian Med Surg* 18(1):30–40.

Tellez GI, Kogut MH, Hargis BM. 1993. Immunoprophylaxis of *Salmonella enteritidis* infection by lymphokines in Leghorn chicks. *Avian Dis* 37:1062–1070.

Topp RC, Carlson HC. 1972a. Studies on avian heterophils. II: histochemistry. *Avian Dis* 16:369–373.

Topp RC, Carlson HC. 1972b. Studies on avian heterophils. III: phagocytic properties. *Avian Dis* 16:374–380.

Tully TN, Morris JM, Pechman RD, Taylor HW. 1995. What is your diagnosis? *J Avian Med Surg* 9:57–58.

Tully TN, Williams J, McLaughlin LD, Snider TG. 2000. What is your diagnosis? *J Avian Med Surg* 14(4):279–281.

Tung HT, Cook FW, Wyatt RD, Hamilton PB. 1975. The anemia caused by aflatoxin. *Poult Sci* 54(6):1962–1969.

Valkiunas G, Salaman P, Iezhoava TA. 2003. Paucity of hematozoa in Columbian birds. *J Wildl Dis* 39:445–448.

Valli VEO. 1993. The hematopoietic system. In: Jubb K, Kennedy P, Palmer N (eds), *Pathology of Domestic Animals*, 4th edn. San Diego, CA: Academic Press.

VanSant F. 1991. Zinc toxicosis in a hyacinth macaw. In: *Proceedings of the Association of Avian Veterinarians*, Chicago, IL, September 23–28.

Van Wettere AJ, Ley DH, Scott DE, Buckanoff HD, Degernes LA. 2012. *Mycoplasma corogypsi*-associated polyarthritis and tenosynovitis in black vultures (*Coragyps atratus*). *Vet Pathol* 50(2):291–298.

Vleck CM, Vertalino N, Vleck D, Blucher TL. 2000. Stress, corticosterone, and heterophil to lymphocyte ratios in free-living Adelie penguins. *Condor* 102:392–400.

Wade LL, Newman SJ. 2004. Hemoglobinuric nephrosis and hepatosplenic erythrophagocytosis in a dusky-headed conure

(*Aratinga weddelli*) after ingestion of garlic (*Allium sativum*). *J Avian Med Surg* 18(3):155–161.

Wainright PO, Pritchard NC, Fletcher OJ. 1987. Identification of viruses from Amazon parrots with a hemorrhagic syndrome and a chronic respiratory disease. In: *First International Conference on Zoological and Avian Medicine*, Turtle Bay, HI, September 6–11.

Weber MA, Terrell SP, Neiffer DL, Miller MA, Mangold BJ. 2002. Bone marrow hypoplasia and intestinal crypt cell necrosis associated with fenbendazole administration in five painted storks. *J Am Vet Med Assoc* 221:417–419.

Weiden PL, Blaese RM. 1971. Hemolytic anemia in agammaglobulinemic chickens: a model of autoimmune disease in immune deficiency. *J Immunol* 107:1004–1013.

Weiser G. 2012. Interpretation of leukocyte responses in disease. In: Thrall M, Weiser G, Allison RW, Campbell T, (eds), *Veterinary Hematology and Clinical Chemistry*. Ames, IA: Wiley-Blackwell, pp. 127– 139.

Weiss DJ. 1984. Uniform evaluation and semiquantitative reporting of hematologic data in veterinary laboratories. *Vet Clin Pathol* 13(2):27–31.

White J. 1990. Protocol for the rehabilitation of oil-affected waterbirds. In: *Proceedings of the Association of Avian Veterinarians*, Phoenix, AZ, September 10–15.

Whittington A, Williams J. 2000. What is your diagnosis? *J Avian Med Surg* 14(3):205–207.

Wight PAL, Dewar WA, Mackenzie GM. 1980. Monocytosis in experimental zinc deficiency of domestic birds. *Avian Pathol* 9:61–66.

Wigley P, Hulme SD, Barrow PA. 1999. Phagocytic and oxidative burst activity of chicken thrombocytes to *Salmonella*, *Escherichia coli* and other bacteria. *Avian Pathol* 28:567–572.

Williams JI, Trainer DO. 1971. A hematological study of Snow, Blue, and Canada geese. *J Wildl Dis* 7:258–264.

Wilson H, Brown CA, Greenacre CB, et al. 2001. Suspected sodium hypochlorite toxicosis in a group of psittacine birds. *J Avian Med Surg* 15(3):209–215.

Wissman MA. 1995. What is your diagnosis? *J Avian Med Surg* 9(2):147–148.

Woerpel RW, Rosskopf WJ. 1982. Heavy-metal intoxication in cage birds—Part I. *Comp Cont Ed Pract* 4:729–740.

Woerpel RW, Rosskopf WJ, Fudge A, Reavill DR. 1992. Iron storage disease (hemochromatosis) in a citron-crested cockatoo and other psittacine species. In: *Proceedings of the Annual Conference of the Association of Avian Veterinarians*, New Orleans, LA, September 1–5.

Wolf KN, Lock B, Carpenter, JW, Garner MM. 2007. *Baylisascaris procyonis* infection in a Molluccan cockatoo (*Cacatua moluccensis*). *J Avian Med Surg* 21:220–225.

Wolf T, Luepke NP. 1997. Formation of micronuclei in incubated hen's eggs as a measure of genotoxicity. *Mutat Res* 394:163–175.

Wolf T, Niehaus-Rolf C, Luepke NP. 2002. Some new methodological aspects of the hen's egg test for micronucleus induction (HET-MN). *Mutat Res* 514:59–76.

Wong E, Mikaelian I, Desnoyers M, Fitzgerald G. 1999. Pansteatitis in a free-ranging red-tailed hawk (*Buteo jamaicensis*). *J Zoo Wildl Med* 30:584–586.

Wood EM. 1967. *The Fine Structure of the Chick Bone Marrow*. PhD thesis, University of Harvard, Harvard, MA.

Work TM, Meteyer CU, Cole RA. 2004. Mortality in Laysan ducks (*Anas laysanensis*) by emaciation complicated by *Echinuria uncinata* on Laysan Island, Hawaii, 1993. *J Wildl Dis* 40:110–114.

Yamada J, Yamashita T, Misu M. 1973. Fine structures in the blood cells of Japanese quails (*Coturnix coturnix japonica*). 1. Heterophils and eosinophils. *Research Bulletin of Obihiro Zootechnical University* 7:1–22.

Yamato O, Goto I, Meade Y. 1996. Hemolytic anemia in wild seaducks caused by marine oil pollution. *J Wildl Dis* 32:381–384.

Zhou WT, Fujita M, Yamamoto S. 1998. Effects of food and water withdrawal and high temperature exposure on diurnal variation in blood viscosity of broiler chickens. *Br Poult Sci* 39:156–160.

Zieve PD, Haghshenass M, Blanks M, Krevans JR. 1966. Vacuolization of the neutrophil: an aid to the diagnosis of septicemia. *Arch Intern Med* 118:356–357.

Ziman M, Colagross-Schouten A, Griffey S, Stedman B. 2004. *Haemoproteus* spp. and *Leukocytozoon* spp. in a captive raptor population. *J Wildl Dis* 40(1):137–140.

Ziprin RL. 1997. Heterophil response to intraperitoneal challenge with invasion deficient *Salmonella enteritidis* and *Salmonella*immune lymphokines. *Avian Dis* 41:438–441.

12 Evaluation of Avian Bone Marrow

Avian Hematopoiesis

The bone marrow is the primary site for erythropoiesis, granulopoiesis, and thrombopoiesis in late embryonic development and post-hatch birds (Campbell, 1967; Fox and Solomon, 1981; Kaczanowska et al., 1987; Schepelmann, 1990). Hematopoiesis begins in the yolk sac, and as the embryo develops, hematopoietic sites appear in organs, such as the liver and spleen, with the activity predominating in the bone marrow of the post-hatch bird (Bienzle and Smith, 1999).

Erythropoiesis occurs primarily in the central skeleton of pigeon hatchlings, but after two weeks this activity is transferred to the axial skeleton, where by six months of age, one-third of the erythropoietic activity is found in the femurs (Schepelmann, 1990). During embryonic development, granulocyte stem cells colonize to create foci of granulopoiesis in the spleen, kidney, lungs, thymus, gonad, pancreas, and other tissues, including the bone marrow (Lucas and Jamroz, 1961; Jones, 1973; Del Cacho et al., 1991). Therefore, compared to mammals, granulopoiesis in mature birds is more diffuse and found in a variety of tissues. In some adult birds, such as chickens, the hematopoietic activity of the bone marrow is primarily associated with erythropoiesis and possibly thrombopoiesis; only a small percentage appears to be reserved for granulopoiesis and lymphocyte maturation (Glick and Rose, 1976).

Avian bone marrow may be used to evaluate patients for disorders of blood cells because it is the most readily available source of hematopoietic tissue in birds. Cytological evaluation of the bone marrow is indicated in avian patients with nonregenerative anemia, heteropenia, and other unexplained alterations involving the cellular elements in circulating blood.

Avian Erythropoiesis

Avian erythropoietin, a glycoprotein that differs structurally from mammalian erythropoietin, is necessary for the multiplication and differentiation of precursor stem cells committed to the erythroid series (Rosse and Waldmann, 1961; Sturkie, 1976). Avian erythropoiesis occurs within the lumen of vascular sinusoids in the bone marrow (Campbell, 1967; Sturkie, 1976; Fox and Solomon, 1981; Dieterien-Lievre, 1988). These sinuses are lined by elongated endothelial cells, which are associated with the most immature cells of the erythroid series. Erythropoietin is present in the blood of anemic birds; the kidney is the site of its production.

The stages of normal avian erythrocyte maturation appear to be like those of mammals (Campbell, 1967; Campbell and Coles, 1986; Jain, 1993; Campbell, 1995; Tadjalli et al., 1997; Tadjalli et al., 2002). The terminology used for the different stages of erythrocyte maturation varies in the literature; however, in general, there are seven recognizable stages involved in red blood cell development based upon Romanowsky stains (Lucas and Jamroz, 1961; Fox and Solomon, 1981; Hawkey and Dennett, 1989; Campbell, 1995; Schwartz et al., 2019). The stages include rubriblasts (proerythroblasts), prorubricytes (basophilic erythroblasts), basophilic rubricytes (early polychromatic erythroblasts), early polychromatic rubricytes (late polychromatic erythroblasts), late polychromatic rubricytes (orthochromic erythroblasts), polychromatic erythrocytes, and mature erythrocytes (Figure 12.1).

In general, as erythroid cells mature, the nuclear size decreases, the chromatin becomes increasingly condensed, the nuclear shape changes from round to ellipsoid, the amount of cytoplasm increases, the hemoglobin concentration increases (resulting in increasing eosinophilia), and

Exotic Animal Hematology and Cytology, Fifth Edition. Terry W. Campbell and Krystan R. Grant.

Companion website: www.wiley.com/go/campbell/exotic

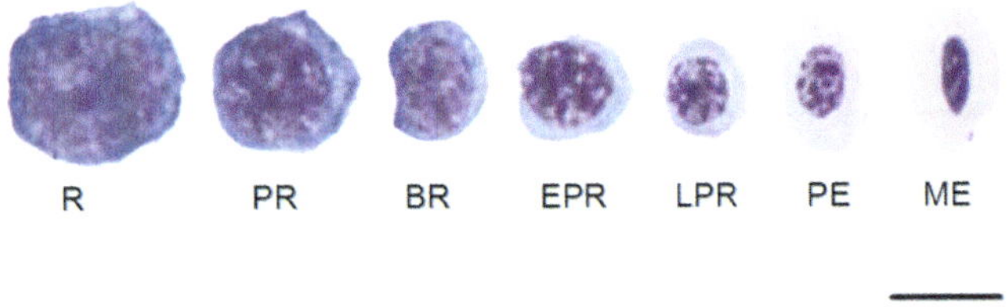

Fig. 12.1. Maturation sequence of the avian erythrocyte from a bone marrow aspirate of a conure (*Aratinga solstitialis*). Rubriblasts (R), prorubricyte (PR), basophilic rubricyte (BR), early polychromatic rubricyte (EPR), late polychromatic rubricyte (LPR), polychromatic erythrocyte (PE), and mature erythrocyte (ME). Bar = 10 μm. Wright–Giemsa.

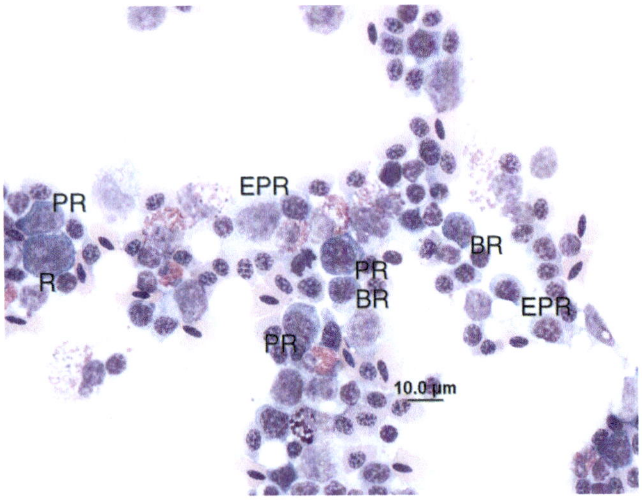

Fig. 12.2. A rubriblast (R), prorubricytes (PR), basophilic rubricytes (BR), and early polychromatic rubricytes (EPR) in the bone marrow aspirate of a conure (*Aratinga solstitialis*). Wright–Giemsa.

the cell shape changes from round to ellipsoid. Unlike mammalian erythrocytes, avian erythrocytes normally retain their nucleus.

Rubriblasts (proerythroblasts) are the cells that represent the first stage of erythrocyte development and appear as large, round, deeply basophilic cells with a large, round central nucleus, resulting in a high nucleus to cytoplasmic ratio (N:C) (Figures 12.1–12.6). The nuclear chromatin is typically coarsely granular, and large prominent nucleoli or nucleolar rings are present. The cytoplasm is deeply basophilic with clear spaces most likely representing mitochondria.

The prorubricyte (basophilic erythroblasts) is the second stage of development and resembles the rubriblast in that the N:C ratio is high, and the large nucleus is usually surrounded by a narrow rim of blue cytoplasm. This cell may be differentiated from the rubriblast because it lacks the mitochondrial spaces of the rubriblast, lacks the prominent nucleoli, and the basophilic cytoplasm often contains spots of reddish material

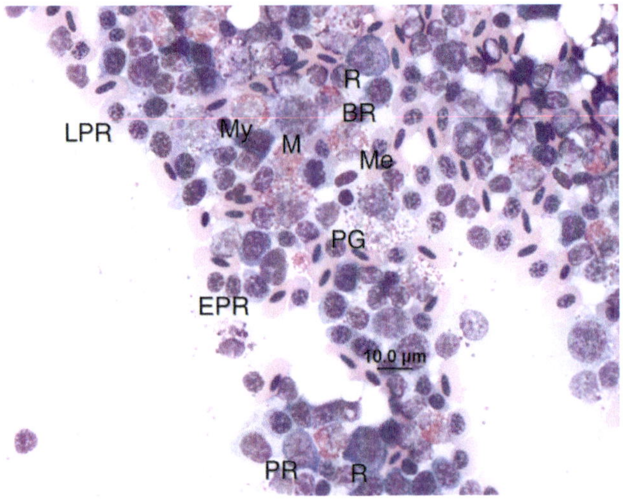

Fig. 12.3. Rubriblasts (R), prorubricyte (PR), basophilic rubricyte (BR), early polychromatic rubricyte (EPR), late polychromatic rubricyte (LPR), myeloblast (M), progranulocyte (PG), myelocyte (My), and metamyelocyte (Me) in the bone marrow aspirate of a conure (*Aratinga solstitialis*). Wright–Giemsa.

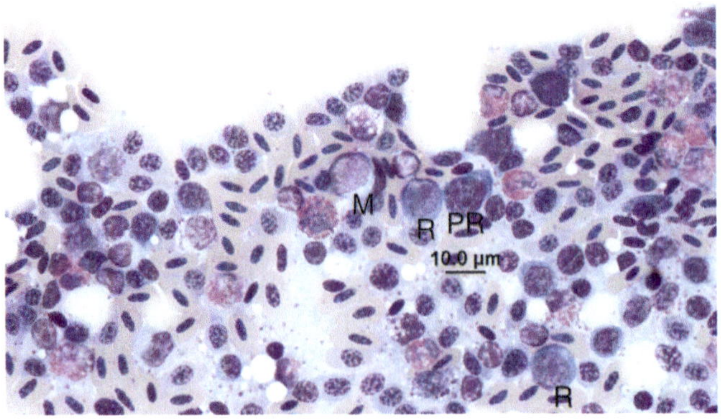

Fig. 12.4. Rubriblasts (R), prorubricyte (PR), and myeloblast (M) in the bone marrow aspirate of a conure (*Aratinga solstitialis*). Wright–Giemsa.

suggestive of the beginning of hemoglobin development (Figures 12.1–12.5, 12.7–12.10).

Rubricytes are round cells that are smaller than both the rubriblasts and prorubricytes. These cells are divided into three stages based primarily upon the appearance of the cytoplasm. The basophilic rubricyte (early polychromatic erythroblasts) represents the earliest rubricyte stage. This cell is characterized by a homogenous basophilic cytoplasm and a round nucleus with clumped chromatin (Figures 12.1–12.3, 12.5, 12.7–12.9). The next stage of development is the early polychromatophilic rubricyte (late polychromatic erythroblasts).

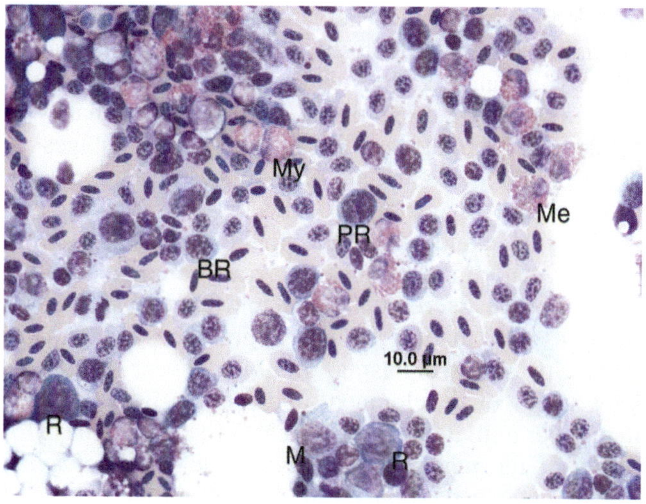

Fig. 12.5. Rubriblasts (R), prorubricyte (PR), basophilic rubricyte (BR), myeloblast (M), myelocyte (My), and metamyelocyte (Me) in the bone marrow aspirate of a conure (*Aratinga solstitialis*). Wright–Giemsa.

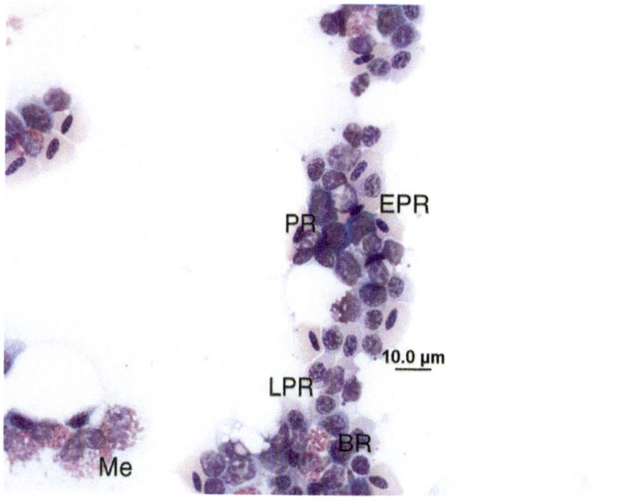

Fig. 12.7. Prorubricyte (PR), basophilic rubricyte (BR), early polychromatic rubricyte (EPR), late polychromatic rubricyte (LPR), and metamyelocyte (Me) in the bone marrow aspirate of a conure (*Aratinga solstitialis*). Wright–Giemsa.

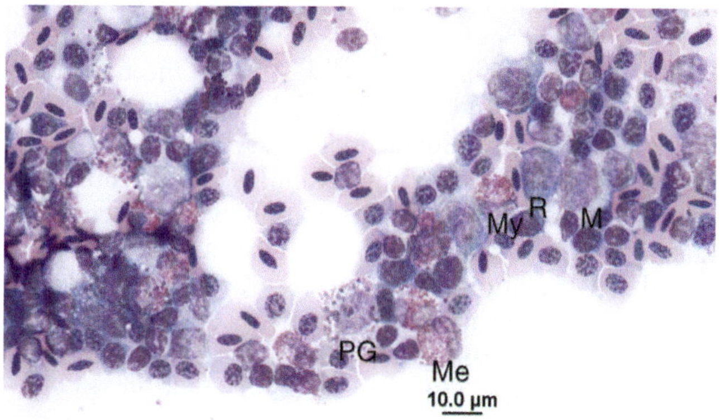

Fig. 12.6. Rubriblast (R), myeloblast (M), progranulocyte (PG), myelocyte (My), and metamyelocyte (Me) in the bone marrow aspirate of a conure (*Aratinga solstitialis*). Wright–Giemsa.

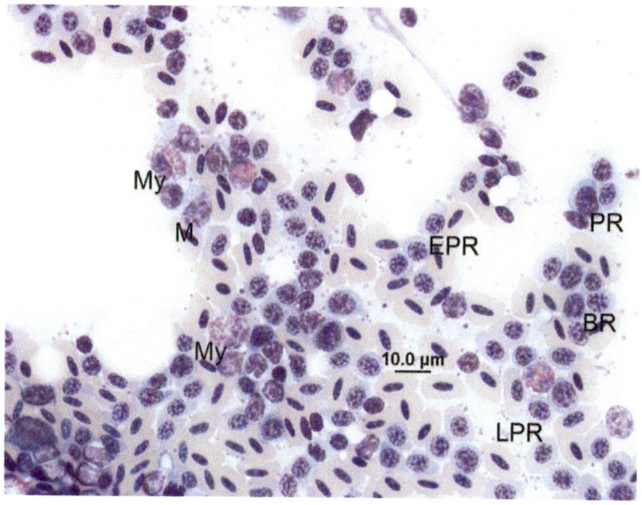

Fig. 12.8. Prorubricyte (PR), basophilic rubricyte (BR), early polychromatic rubricyte (EPR), late polychromatic rubricyte (LPR), myeloblast (M), and myelocytes (My) in the bone marrow aspirate of a conure (*Aratinga solstitialis*). Wright–Giemsa.

This cell is smaller than the basophilic rubricyte and has a lower N:C ratio compared to the more immature erythroblastic cells. The nucleus may vary from round to slightly ellipsoid, the nuclear chromatin is irregularly clumped, and the cytoplasm is gray in color owing to increased hemoglobin production (Figures 12.1–12.3, 12.6–12.10). The final rubricyte stage is the late polychromatophilic rubricyte (orthochromic erythroblasts), which appears as an ellipsoid cell with eosinophilic (eosinophilic gray to weakly eosinophilic) cytoplasm (Figures 12.1, 12.3, 12.7, and 12.8).

Cells in the final stages of erythrocyte development include the polychromatophilic erythrocyte and mature erythrocyte. These cells are found in the peripheral blood of normal birds. The mature erythrocyte has a flattened, ellipsoid shape. The nuclear chromatin is condensed and considered to be transcriptionally inactive.

The primary function of the erythrocyte is to transport hemoglobin, which carries oxygen to the tissues. Although the major function of the avian erythrocyte is to transport oxygen, it may also participate in some immune responses (Passantino, et al., 2007).

The predominance of erythroid cells in avian bone marrow samples results in a granulocyte to erythrocyte (G:E) ratio of less than 1.0 (Schwartz et al., 2019).

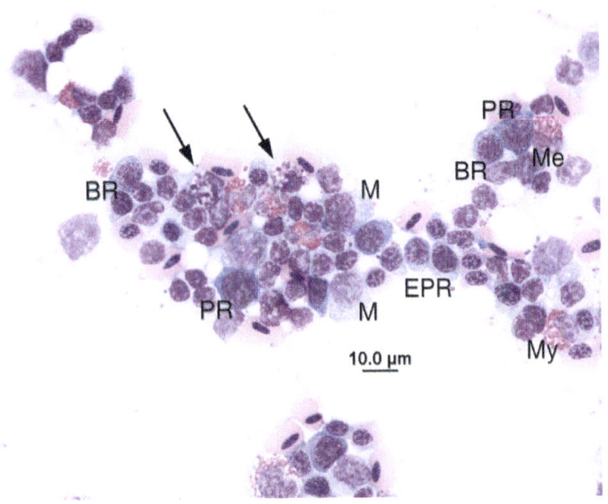

Fig. 12.9. Prorubricytes (PR), basophilic rubricytes (BR), early polychromatic rubricyte (EPR), myeloblasts (M), myelocyte (My), and metamyelocyte (Me) in the bone marrow aspirate of a conure (*Aratinga solstitialis*). The arrows point to basophils. Wright–Giemsa.

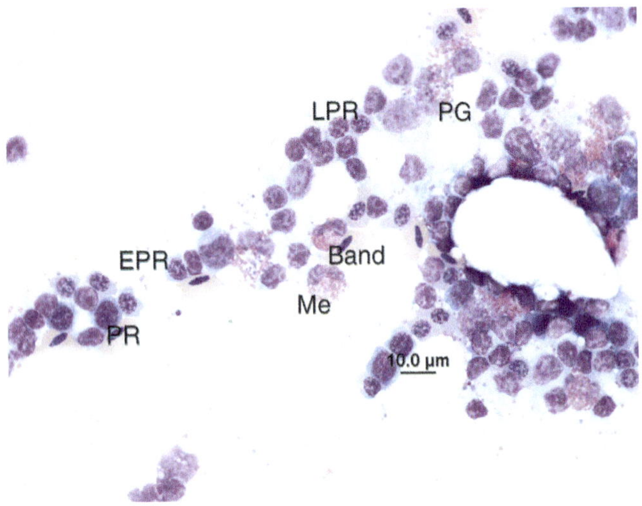

Fig. 12.10. Prorubricyte (PR), early polychromatic rubricyte (EPR), late polychromatic rubricyte (LPR), progranulocyte (PG), metamyelocyte (Me), and band cell in the bone marrow aspirate of a conure (*Aratinga solstitialis*). Wright–Giemsa.

Avian Granulopoiesis

Avian granulocytes appear to develop in a manner similar to those of mammals, although the location of cell origin is different. For example, avian heterophils are derived from stem cells present in the extravascular spaces of the bone marrow, in contrast to mammalian neutrophils, which develop within the vascular spaces (Campbell, 1967: Wood, 1967). Avian heterophils can also be derived from extramedullary hematopoiesis (Lawn, 1979; Olah and Glick, 1984; Randall and Reece, 1996).

The study of avian hematopoiesis lags research in mammalian hematopoiesis because the maturation stages of avian granulocytes have been described based only upon their morphologic appearance, primarily in chicken bone marrow. The developmental stages of avian granulocytes include myeloblasts (granuloblasts), progranulocytes (promyelocytes), myelocytes, metamyelocytes, band cells, and mature granulocytes, in order of maturation. In general, avian granulocytes show a progressive decrease in size and cytoplasmic basophilia as they mature, similar to granulocytes of mammals. Specific cytoplasmic granules appear during the later stages of development and progressively increase in number until a full complement is reached in the cytoplasm of the mature granulocyte. The nuclei of avian granulocytes are initially rounded and progress toward segmentation, and the nuclear chromatin becomes increasingly condensed with maturity. Basophils are the exception because the nucleus of the avian basophil does not segment with maturation.

Avian myeloblasts (granuloblasts) are large round cells with high N:C ratio (Figures 12.3–12.6, 12.8, and 12.9). The cytoplasm of the myeloblast stains a lighter blue than that of rubriblasts, and the nucleus is typically round and contains delicate reticular (fine) chromatin and prominent nucleoli. Myeloblasts do not contain specific cytoplasmic granules and possibly represent a stage common to all granulocytes (heterophils, eosinophils, and basophils). Myeloblasts are frequently found in association with other developing granulocytes, especially in imprints of bone marrow core biopsies.

Avian progranulocytes (promyelocytes) are large cells with light blue cytoplasm and slightly eccentric nuclei (Figures 12.3, 12.6, and 12.10). The N:C ratio of the progranulocyte is less than that of the myeloblast, owing to a larger cytoplasmic volume. The margins of the progranulocyte nucleus may be indistinct, the nuclear chromatin often has a delicate reticular pattern, and nucleoli are absent. Progranulocytes contain primary granules that vary in appearance among the different types of granulocytes.

Heterophil progranulocytes contain primary granules that vary in color and shape. The granules often appear as orange spheres (primary granules) and rings, or deeply basophilic spheres and rings. Eosinophil progranulocytes contain only orange, brightly staining, primary granules and appear to lack the deeply basophilic granules and rings found in heterophilic progranulocytes. Basophil progranulocytes contain basophilic granules and rings. Basophil progranulocytes may be differentiated from heterophil progranulocytes containing basophilic spheres and rings by the size and appearance of the granules. Basophil progranulocytes typically contain fewer ring forms, and the granules appear smaller than the granules present in the immature cells of the heterophil series.

Myelocytes are smaller than myeloblasts and progranulocytes and contain the secondary or specific granules of the mature granulocytes, making identification of this cell somewhat simple (Figures 12.3, 12.5, 12.6, 12.8, and 12.9). The nucleus of myelocytes is round to oval and appears more condensed when compared to the nuclei of myeloblasts and progranulocytes. Heterophil myelocytes typically appear as round cells containing light blue cytoplasm and a mixture of eosinophilic rod-shaped specific granules and primary granules and rings, which occupy less than one-half the cytoplasmic volume. Eosinophil myelocytes lack the deeply basophilic granules and rings occasionally found in early heterophil myelocytes. Basophil myelocytes contain basophilic specific granules, which may have a slightly eosinophilic tinge. Smaller primary granules may also be present and are deep violet in color. The granules occupy less than one-half the cytoplasmic volume of the cell.

Metamyelocytes are slightly smaller than myelocytes, have nuclei that are slightly indented, and possess specific cytoplasmic granules that occupy greater than one-half the cytoplasmic volume (Figures 12.3, 12.5, 12.6, 12.7, 12.9, and 12.10). Heterophil and basophil metamyelocytes have fewer primary granules than the myelocyte and progranulocyte stage cells.

Band cells resemble mature granulocytes, but may be differentiated from mature granulocytes based on the appearance of the nucleus. The nucleus of the band cell appears as a curved or coiled band as compared to the segmented nucleus of the mature granulocyte (Figure 12.10). The nucleus of granulocytes is often obscured by the specific granules present in the cytoplasm of the cell, which may make identification of band cells difficult. Specific nuclear stains, such as hematoxylin, are usually required to determine the concentration of band cells. An exception to this is the band stage of the basophil. The band stage of basophils is not apparent regardless of the staining technique, because mature basophils do not have a segmented nucleus. Mature granulocytes are generally the most abundant cell of each granulocytic cell line in the bone marrow of normal birds.

Mature heterophils have lobed nuclei, colorless cytoplasm and, in general, rod-shaped granules that stain eosinophilic (some species may have round to oval granules). The elliptical cytoplasmic granules often have a distinct refractile central body that appears refractile, which aids in the cell identification in some species.

Heterophils participate in the inflammatory response. The heterophilic response to infection is like that of the mammalian neutrophil: migration to the sites of infection to phagocytize and kill pathogenic microorganisms (Vegad and Katyar, 1995). Avian heterophils contain both lysosomal and nonlysosomal enzymes (Maxwell and Robertson, 1998). Unlike mammalian neutrophils, avian heterophils are devoid of myeloperoxidase and depend primarily on nonoxidative mechanisms, lysozyme, and acid phosphatase for antimicrobial activity (Andreasen and Latimer, 1990). Avian heterophils participate in antibody-dependent cellular cytotoxicity, possess Toll-like receptors, and use extracellular traps to kill antigens (Kogut, et al., 2005; Chuammitri, et al., 2009). The large primary heterophil granules that contain defensins (antimicrobial proteins, previously known as lysosomal cationic proteins) and lysozyme are first detectable in the promyelocyte stage (Wakenell, 2010).

Mature avian eosinophils are similar in size and appearance to mature heterophils. They tend to have round, eosinophilic granules that have tinctorial qualities that differ from those of the heterophil granule on the same stained bone marrow preparation or blood film. The cytoplasm of the eosinophil stains pale blue with Romanowsky stains compared to the colorless cytoplasm of the mature heterophil. Some species of birds may have rod-shaped eosinophilic granules in their eosinophils (e.g., individuals in the families of Anatidae, Tinamidae, Falconidae) (Claver and Quagliab, 2009). The cytoplasmic granules of the eosinophils in other species may stain blue with Romanowsky stains. Crystalline cores similar to those found in mammalian eosinophils have been described in specific granules of eosinophils in some avian species (i.e., such as ducks and geese), but not in others (Maxwell and Siller, 1972). Cytochemical studies have shown that avian eosinophils stain positive for peroxidase and acid phosphatase activity and Sudan black B, whereas the heterophils do not (Andreasen and Latimer, 1990; Bounous and Stedman, 2000). Hydrolytic enzymes, such as acid phosphatase and arylsulfatase have also been detected in avian eosinophilic granules, indicating lysosomal activity. Although the exact functions of the avian eosinophil are poorly understood, peripheral eosinophilias can be associated with the administration of foreign antigens and often with alimentary tract parasitism (Montali, 1988; Latimer and Bienzle, 2000).

Mature avian basophils have nonlobed, round nuclei and violet to reddish purple cytoplasmic granules, thus resembling mammalian mast cells (Figure 12.9). The granules are much smaller than those of the eosinophil. Although the exact function of the avian basophils in not known, it appears to play a role in the early inflammatory response and immediate hypersensitivity reactions; however, it differs from mammalian basophils by not playing a role in delayed hypersensitivity reactions (Maxwell and Robertson, 1995; Bounous and Stedman, 2000; Koutsos, et al., 2007). Peripheral basophilias have also been associated with severe stress responses in birds (Maxwell, 1993).

Avian Thrombopoiesis

Avian thrombocytes are derived from mononuclear precursors in the bone marrow, unlike mammalian platelets, which are cytoplasmic fragments of large, multinucleated megakaryocytes. The avian thrombocyte series consists of thromboblasts, immature thrombocytes, and mature thrombocytes. Thromboblasts appear as small, round to oval cells that resemble rubriblasts, and contain round nuclei with fine to punctate nuclear chromatin, and one or more nucleoli (Figure 12.11). Cytoplasmic blebs may be present on the cell margins.

Immature thrombocytes may be divided into three groups: early, mid-, and late-immature thrombocytes based upon their degree of maturity. Early immature thrombocytes are intermediate in size between thromboblasts and the more mature stages (Figure 12.12) and appear as round to oval cells containing more abundant cytoplasm than the thromboblast. The cytoplasm is basophilic in color and may contain vacuoles, and the nuclear chromatin is aggregated into irregular clumps. Mid-immature thrombocytes appear as slightly elongate or irregular cells with pale blue cytoplasm (Figure 12.13). Cytoplasmic specific granules and vacuoles are occasionally seen at this stage of development, and the nucleus contains heavy chromatin clumping. Late-immature thrombocytes are oval and slightly smaller than the mid-immature stage (Figure 12.14). The cytoplasm stains pale blue with vaguely defined clear areas. Specific granules are frequently seen at one pole of the cell. The nucleus is oval with densely packed chromatin. The mature thrombocyte is the definitive cell in the thrombocyte series.

Mature avian thrombocytes are round to slightly oval cells with a centrally positioned oval to round nucleus that resemble the larger erythrocytes; however, lacking in hemoglobin, the cytoplasm stains light blue or colorless with Romanowsky stains. The cytoplasm of these cells is often vacuolated with a few red granules at one pole of the cell. In the chicken, monoclonal antibodies can be used to differentiate thrombocytes

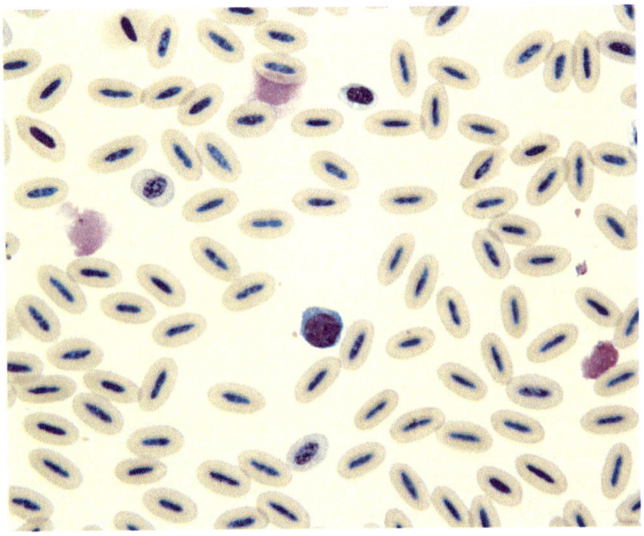

Fig. 12.11. A bone marrow aspiration biopsy from a duck (*Anas platyrhynchos domestica*) reveals a thromboblast. Wright–Giemsa stain (50× oil).

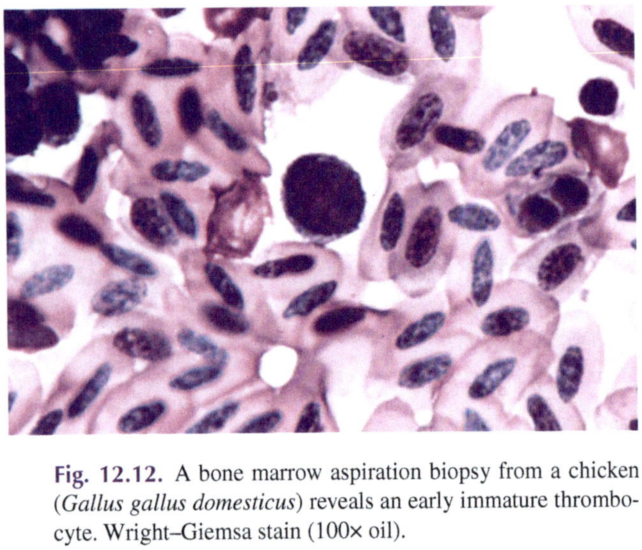

Fig. 12.12. A bone marrow aspiration biopsy from a chicken (*Gallus gallus domesticus*) reveals an early immature thrombocyte. Wright–Giemsa stain (100× oil).

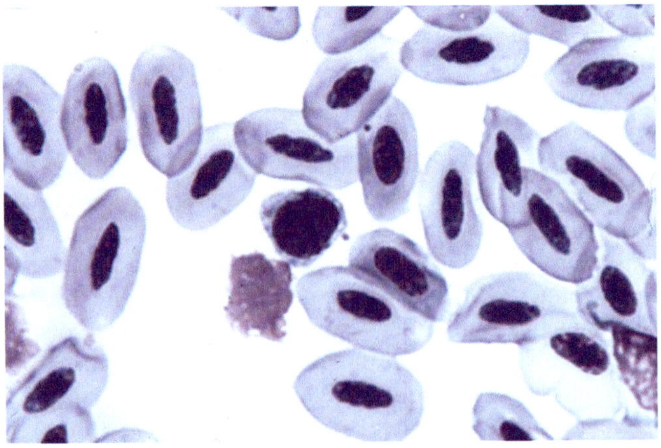

Fig. 12.13. A bone marrow aspiration biopsy from a chicken (*Gallus gallus domesticus*) reveals a mid-immature thrombocyte. Wright–Giemsa stain (100× oil).

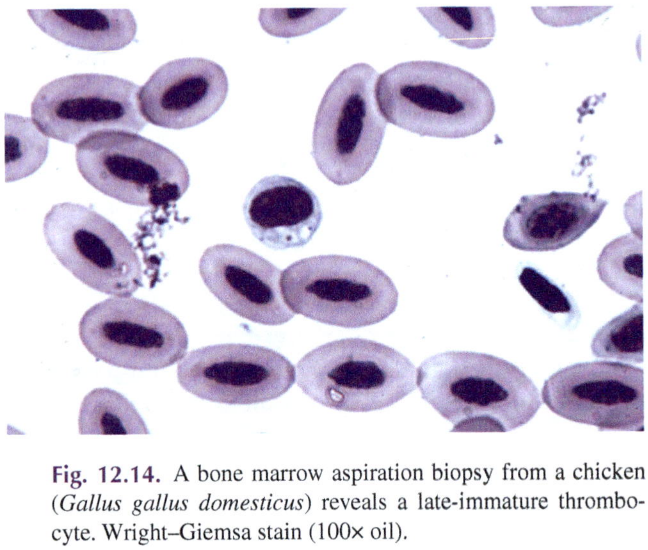

Fig. 12.14. A bone marrow aspiration biopsy from a chicken (*Gallus gallus domesticus*) reveals a late-immature thrombocyte. Wright–Giemsa stain (100× oil).

from other cells types, such as lymphocytes (Horiuchi, et al., 2004).

Avian thrombocytes are the functional equivalent of mammalian platelets. As with mammalian platelets, bird thrombocytes aggregate in a site of vascular injury and form a hemostatic plug (Edmonds, 1968). Like mammalian platelets, activated avian thrombocytes have fibrinogen receptors that facilitate thrombocyte aggregation (Bounous and Stedman, 2000). Avian thrombocytes have acidophilic cytoplasmic granules, stain positive with periodic acid-Schiff (PAS) and Grimelius, and produce little thromboplastin (Wakenell, 2010). Additionally, thrombocytes may have phagocytic abilities and probably have some function in nonspecific immunity (Meseguer, et al., 2002).

Other Cells Present in Avian Bone Marrow

Monocytopoiesis is poorly defined in birds. It is possible that granulocytic precursor cells may be like or identical to monocytic precursor cells (Fox and Solomon, 1981). Monocytes originating in hematopoietic tissue become the monocytes and macrophages found in blood and body tissues, respectively. A variety of tissues, notably bone marrow, embryonic yolk sac, and spleen, can produce macrophage colonies (Fox and Solomon, 1981).

Mature avian monocytes are the largest cells in the blood film and resemble their mammalian counterpart. They are typically round with an abundant blue-gray cytoplasm that may contain fine pink granules and a kidney-shaped nucleus, although the nuclear shape varies considerably.

Avian monocytes function like mammalian monocytes; therefore, they are capable of phagocytosis, oxidative burst activity, and microbial killing. Avian monocytes are phagocytic cells and part of the monocyte–macrophage system that constitutes the replacement pool for tissue macrophages for cellular immunity (Latimer and Bienzle, 2000). Macrophages within the bone marrow usually contain iron pigment within the cytoplasm since they are involved with iron metabolism during hemoglobin synthesis and catabolism. Iron may appear as gray to black granulation or as golden crystalline material.

Aggregates of lymphocytes are found within the bone marrow of birds, although major sites of lymphopoiesis in adult birds are in the spleen, liver, intestines, and cecal tonsils (Dieterien-Lievre, 1988). Avian lymphocytes were used in the initial immunology studies, where they were classified as either B- or T-lymphocytes depending upon their lineages. B-lymphocytes differentiate in the bursa of Fabricius, and T-lymphocytes differentiate in the thymus. Avian lymphocytes classified as B-lymphocytes have immunoglobulin receptors for antigens and therefore provide humoral immunity, and T-lymphocytes are involved in cell-mediated immunity (Dieterien-Lievre, 1988). The two cell types cannot usually be differentiated by morphology alone.

Immature avian lymphocytes are larger than mature lymphocytes and are classified as lymphoblasts or prolymphocytes, based upon morphology. Lymphoblasts have relatively abundant deeply basophilic cytoplasm and contain large nuclei with fine chromatin and one or more prominent nucleoli. Prolymphocytes resemble lymphoblasts, but the nuclear chromatin is coarser, and nucleoli are not present. Mature lymphocytes are smaller than immature lymphocytes and contain scant light blue cytoplasm. The nucleus contains coarse chromatin that is typically clumped.

Mature avian lymphocytes are classified as small, medium, or large based upon size. They tend to be round, but can be irregular as they mold around adjacent cells or distort during slide preparation. Lymphocytes have round nuclei (although nuclear indentations frequently occur), and the cytoplasm stains weakly basophilic with Romanowsky stains. The cytoplasmic volume is scant in small, mature lymphocytes.

Avian osteoblasts may be found in the bone marrow and resemble those of mammals. Osteoblasts appear as large polygonal to fusiform cells with indistinct cytoplasmic margins. The cytoplasm is abundant and basophilic, with a foamy appearance, and a distinct, clear Golgi apparatus is present. The nucleus appears round to oval, is eccentrically located in the cell, and often possesses one or more distinct nucleoli. The nuclear chromatin is reticular to coarsely granular chromatin.

Osteoclasts are large, multinucleated giant cells with an ameboid shape. The cytoplasm is weakly basophilic and vacuolated, and red cytoplasmic granules may be present. The nucleus is round to oval and often contains prominent nucleoli.

Avian Hematopoietic Tissue other than Bone Marrow

Avian Bursa of Fabricius

The sole source of B-lymphocytes in the adult bird is self-regenerating aggregates of B-lymphocytes that originated in the bursa of Fabricius and then subsequently spread to the spleen, liver, intestines, and cecal tonsils. The bursa of pre- and post-hatched birds is a sac-like lymphoid nodule found in the dorsa wall of the proctodeum of the cloaca. During development, the bursa contains numerous deeply basophilic lymphoid precursor cells, which reach a maximum number in the 13–15-day embryo (Dieterien-Lievre, 1988). The number of lymphoid precursors then declines as lymphoid differentiation progresses. The lymphoid precursor cells may originate from an external source, such as the yolk sac or bone marrow, and seeding of the bursa with lymphoid precursor cells appears to occur in the 7–14-day embryo, depending upon the species. The bursa reaches its maximum growth around four weeks post hatch and gradually undergoes involution over a two- to three-month period. Based on research using domestic chicken and quail embryos, lymphoid cells first appear in the developing bursa in the 13–15-day embryo (Dieterien-Lievre, 1988). Granulopoiesis also occurs in the developing bursa of the 12–13-day chick embryo, but disappears at hatching or just prior to hatching.

Avian Thymus

Avian T-lymphocytes are the predominant lymphoid cell of the spleen and peripheral blood of post-hatched birds. T-cells originate in the thymus and then spread to spleen, liver, intestines, and cecal tonsils. Lymphoid precursors originating from the yolk sac or bone marrow begin to colonize the thymus during the first four to eight days of development, depending upon the species (Dieterien-Lievre, 1988). The influx of lymphoid precursors appears to last 24–36 h and ends abruptly. Colonization of the thymus by the precursor cells is followed by a four- to five-day refractory period before another influx occurs. This cyclic colonization of the thymus by precursor cells consists of two to three colonization periods that may extend into the post-hatchling period depending upon the species. This is in contrast to the colonization of the bursa, which occurs during a distinct single episode in the embryo before hatching. T-lymphocytes acquire their T antigen during a 24-h period of development around the time of the second wave of colonization between days 12 and 15 of embryonic life.

Avian Spleen

During embryonic development, the spleen participates in erythropoiesis and granulocytopoiesis. Granulopoiesis becomes more predominant as the embryo matures; however, at hatching the granulocytes begin to disappear, and by three days are replaced by lymphocytes. In mature birds, T- and B-lymphocytes appear in different locations within the white pulp of the spleen (Dieterien-Lievre, 1988). The central arteries of the white pulp are surrounded by a periarteriolar lymphoid sheath made up of densely packed T-lymphocytes. Capillaries branching at right angles from the central arteries are surrounded by periellipsoid lymphoid tissue consisting of B-lymphocytes. B-lymphocytes are also found within the germinal centers located within the periarteriolar lymphoid sheath.

References

Andreasen CB, Latimer KS. 1990. Cytochemical characteristics of chicken heterophils and eosinophils. *Vet Clin Pathol* 19:51–54.

Bienzle D, Smith DA. 1999. Heterophilic leucocytosis and granulocytic hyperplasia associated with infection in a cockatoo. *Comp Haemat Inter* 9:193–197.

Bounous DI, Stedman NL. 2000. Normal avian hematology. In: Feldman BF, Zinkl JG, Jain NC (eds), *Schalm's Veterinary Hematology*, 5th edn. Philadelphia, PA: Lippincott Williams & Wilkins, pp. 1145–1154.

Campbell F. 1967. Fine structure of the bone marrow of the chicken and pigeon. *J Morph* 123:405–440.

Campbell TW, 1995. *Avian Hematology and Cytology*, 2nd edn. Ames: Iowa State University Press.

Campbell TW, Coles EH. 1986. Avian clinical pathology. In: Coles EH (ed), *Veterinary Clinical Pathology*, 4th edn. Philadelphia, PA: WB Saunders Co.

Chuammitri P, Ostojic J, Andreasen CB, et al. 2009. Chicken heterophil extracellular traps (HETs): novel defense mechanism of chicken heterophils. *Vet Immunol Immunopathol* 129:126–131.

Claver JA, Quagliab AIE. 2009. Comparative morphology, development, and function of blood cells in nonmammalian vertebrates. *J Exotic Pet Med* 18(2):87–97.

Del Cacho E, Gallego M, Bascuas JA. 1991. Granulopoiesis in the pineal gland of chickens. *Am J Vet Res* 52:449–452.

Dieterien-Lievre F. 1988. Birds. In: Rawley A, Ratcliffe N (eds), *Vertebrate Blood Cells*. Cambridge: Cambridge University Press.

Edmonds RH. 1968. Electron microscope studies on the hemostatic process in bird embryos I: the initial plug. *J Ultrastruct Res* 24:295–310.

Fox AJ, Solomon JB. 1981. Chicken non-lymphoid leukocytes. In: Rose L, Payne L, Freeman M (eds), *Avian Immunology*. Edinburgh: Poultry Science Ltd.

Glick and Rose, 1976. Cellular composition of the bone marrow in the chicken. I. Identification of cells. *Anat Rec* 185:235–246.

Hawkey CM, Dennett TB. 1989. *A Colour Atlas of Comparative Veterinary Haematology*. London: Wolfe Medical Publications, Ltd.

Horiuchi H, Tanaka K, Shigeta A, et al. 2004. A monoclonal antibody against chicken thrombocytes reacts with the cells of thrombocyte lineage. *J Vet Med Sci* 66:243–250.

Jain NC. 1993. *Essentials of Veterinary Hematology*. Philadelphia, PA: Lea & Febiger.

Jones AW. 1973. Granulopoiesis in the embryonic chick lung: a histologic study. *Poult Sci* 52:1600–1603.

Kaczanowska E, Gromysz-Kalkowska K, Szubartowska E. 1987. Changes in the blood and the bone marrow picture of the pharaoh quail (*Coturnix coturnix* pharaoh) chicks as a manifestation of adaptation to postembryonal life. *Comp Biochem Physiol* 87A:497–501.

Koutsos EA, Garcia Lopez JC, Klasing KC. 2007. Maternal and dietary carotenoids interactively affect cutaneous basophil responses in growing chickens (*Gallus gallus domesticus*). *Comp Biochem Physiol B*. 147:87– 92.

Kogut MH, Iqbal M, He H, et al. 2005. Expression and function of Toll-like receptors in chicken heterophils. *Dev Comp Immunol* 29:791– 807.

Latimer KS, Bienzle D. 2000. Determination and interpretation of the avian leukogram. In: Feldman BF, Zinkl JG, Jain NC (eds), *Schalm's Veterinary Hematology*. Philadelphia, PA: Lippincott Williams & Wilkins, pp. 417– 432.

Lawn AM. 1979. Haemopoietic cells in peripheral nerves of S. P.F chickens. *Avian Pathol* 8:477–481.

Lucas AJ, Jamroz C. 1961. *Atlas of Avian Hematology*, United States Department of Agriculture Monograph #25. Washington, DC: U.S. Government Printing Office.

Maxwell MH. 1993. Avian blood leukocyte response to stress. *World Poult Sci J*. 49:34–43.

Maxwell MH, Robertson GW. 1995. The avian basophilic leukocyte: a review. *World Poult Sci J.* 51:307–325.

Maxwell MH, Robertson GW. 1998. The avian heterophil leukocyte: a review. *World Poult Sci* 54:155–178.

Maxwell MH, Siller WG. 1972. The ultrastructural characteristics of the eosinophil granules in six species of domestic birds. *J Anat* 112:289–303.

Meseguer J, Esteban MA, Rodriquez A. 2002. Are thrombocytes and platelets true phagocytes? *Microsc Res Tech* 57:491– 497.

Montali RJ. 1988. Comparative pathology of inflammation in the higher vertebrates (reptiles, birds and mammals). *J Comp Pathol* 99:1–20.

Olah I, Glick B. 1984. Meckel's diverticulum. 1. Extramedullary myelopoiesis in the yolk sac of hatched chickens (*Gallus domesticus*). *Anat Rec* 208:243–252.

Passantino L, Massaro MA, Jirillo F, et al. 2007. Antigenically activated avian erythrocytes release cytokine-like factors: a conserved phylogenetic function discovered in fish. *Immunopharmacol Immunotoxicol* 29:141–152.

Randall CJ, Reece RL. 1996. Colour atlas of avian histopathology. In: Randall CJ, Reece RL (eds), *Colour Atlas of Avian Histopathology*. London: Mosby-Wolfe.

Rosse WF, Waldmann TA. 1961. Factors controlling erythropoiesis in birds. *Blood* 27:654–661.

Schepelmann K. 1990. Erythropoietic bone marrow in the pigeon: development of its distribution and volume during growth and pneumatization of bones. *J Morphol* 203:21–34.

Schwartz D, Guzman DS-M, Beaufrere H, et al. 2019. Morphologic and quantitative evaluation of bone marrow aspirates from Hispaniolan Amazon parrots (*Amazona ventralis*). *Vet Clin Pathol* 2019 48(4):645–651.

Sturkie PD. 1976. Blood: physical characteristics, formed elements, hemoglobin, and coagulation. In: Sturkie PD (ed), *Avian Physiology*. New York: Springer-Verlag.

Tadjalli M, Nazifi S, Hadipoor MM. 2002. Normal haematopoiesis, cellular components and M/E ratio in the bone marrow of the black-headed gull (*Larus ridibundus*). *Comp Clin Pathol* 11:217–222.

Tadjalli M, Nazifi S, Saeedi M. 1997. Morphological study and determination of M/E ratio of the haematopoietic cells of the duck. *Comp Haemat Inter* 1:117–121.

Vegad JL, Katyar AK. 1995. The acute inflammatory response in the chicken. *Vet Bull* 65:309–409.

Wakenell PS. 2010. Hematology of chickens and turkeys. In: Weiss DJ, Wardrop KJ (eds), *Schalm's Veterinary Hematology*, 6th edn. Ames, IA: Wiley-Blackwell, pp. 958– 967.

Wood EM. 1967. The fine structure of the chick bone marrow. *PhD, Anatomy*. University of Harvard: Harvard, Massachusetts.

13 Avian Hematology and Clinical Chemistry: Clinical Case Presentations

Case 1: Cockatoo with Lethargy and Anorexia

Signalment

10-year-old female umbrella cockatoo (*Cacatua alba*)

History

The cockatoo presented for acute onset of lethargy and not eating well for one day. She resides at a public aquarium and is typically housed in a large cage in the tropical, rainforest habitat area. She is offered a variety of foods in her diet including pellets, fresh fruits, fresh vegetables, pasta, legumes, and occasional seeds or nuts for training treats. It was also reported that she has been snuggling more and laid one egg one month prior to presentation and has been picking her feathers in the region above her coelom. Also, one year ago, she experienced a similar episode where she gained weight over a 3-week period and then laid an egg. She cycled again and gained weight following the egg laying, but no egg was found; she then lost weight (she weighed 560 g).

Physical Examination

Upon physical examination, the 585-g cockatoo was quiet, alert, and responsive. There was evident feather destruction on the anterior coelomic region, and her coelom was slightly distended. She was observed overnight, and it was noted that she did not eat much but was somewhat brighter the following morning. Initial diagnostics included a complete blood count (CBC), biochemical profile, and radiographs.

The cockatoo was placed under general anesthesia (isoflurane via face mask) (Figure 13.1) to obtain a blood sample via jugular venipuncture (Tables 13.1 and 13.2 and Figures 13.2a and 13.2b) and whole-body radiographs (Figures 13.3a and 13.3b). A second radiographic study using contrast in the gastrointestinal tract was performed 2 h and 40 min later with contrast administered 40 min prior to imaging (Figures 13.4a and 13.4b).

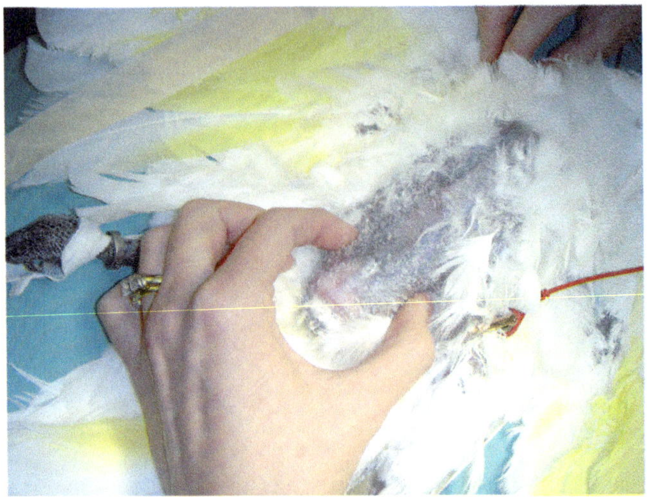

Fig. 13.1. Umbrella cockatoo under general anesthesia for blood collection and radiographs. Apparent feather destruction along chest and coelom, and palpation of coelomic distention.

Exotic Animal Hematology and Cytology, Fifth Edition. Terry W. Campbell and Krystan R. Grant.

Companion website: www.wiley.com/go/campbell/exotic

Table 13.1. Cockatoo hematology results (Case 1).

		Reference[a]	Decision level[b]
PCV (%)	42.0	40–55	35–55
Leukocytes			
WBC (×10³/µL)	23.8	5–13	5.0–20.0
Heterophils (×10³/µL)	21.4	4.68–7.49	2.1–10.0
(%)	90	45–72	—
Lymphocytes (×10³/µL)	1.4	2.08–5.20	1.7–10.0
(%)	6	20–50	—
Monocytes (×10³/µL)	0.5	0–0.2	0–0.7
(%)	2	0–2	—
Eosinophils (×10³/µL)	0.2	0–0.2	0–0.4
(%)	1	0–2	—
Basophils (×10³/µL)	0.2	0–0.1	0–0.4
(%)	1	0–1	—
Thrombocytes			
Adequate thrombocytes	Exist		1–5/1000× field
Plasma protein (refractometry)			
(g/dL)	5.2		3–5
Notes			
Pathologist	Aggregated polychromatophilic erythrocytes		
Technician	Moderate polychromasia		

[a]Carpenter (2018).
[b]Decision levels used by authors when reference values are unavailable.

Table 13.2. Cockatoo plasma biochemical results (Case 1).

		Reference[a]	Decision level[b]
Glucose (mg/dL)	223	214–302	200–500
BUN (mg/dL)	2	3–5.1	
Phosphorus (mg/dL)	8.2	2.5–5.5	5–7
Calcium (mg/dL)	26.9	8.3–10.8	8–11
Uric acid (mg/dL)	3.8	2.9–11.0	<15
Total protein (biuret) (g/dl)	3.9	3.0–5.0	2.5–4.0
Albumin (g/dL)	1.4	1.11–2.28	
Globulin (g/dL)	2.5	—	
Cholesterol (mg/dL)	157	135–355	
Creatine kinase (IU/L)	387	106–305	<500
Aspartate aminotransferase (IU/L)	139	117–314	<275
Sodium (mEq/L)	146	130–155	130–160
Potassium (mEq/L)	3.8	2.5–4.5	2.0–4.0
Chloride (mEq/L)	119	—	

[a]Carpenter (2018).
[b]Decision levels used by authors when reference values are unavailable.

Interpretive Discussion

The hemogram revealed a packed cell volume on the low end of the range compared to the reference values published for umbrella cockatoos. The leukogram revealed a significant leukocytosis with heterophilia and relative lymphopenia. There was also moderate polychromasia. These findings support a stress leukogram; however, a mild inflammatory leukogram and anemia were also considered.

Figure 13.2a shows three heterophils supporting the heterophilia indicated from the leukogram. The erythrocytes reveal a slight increase in polychromasia. Figure 13.2b shows the erythrocytes exhibiting a slight increase in polychromasia.

The plasma biochemical profile revealed a hypercalcemia, which can be expected during reproductive cycling as calcium is mobilized from the bones for use in shell formation. The calcium level here is consistent with

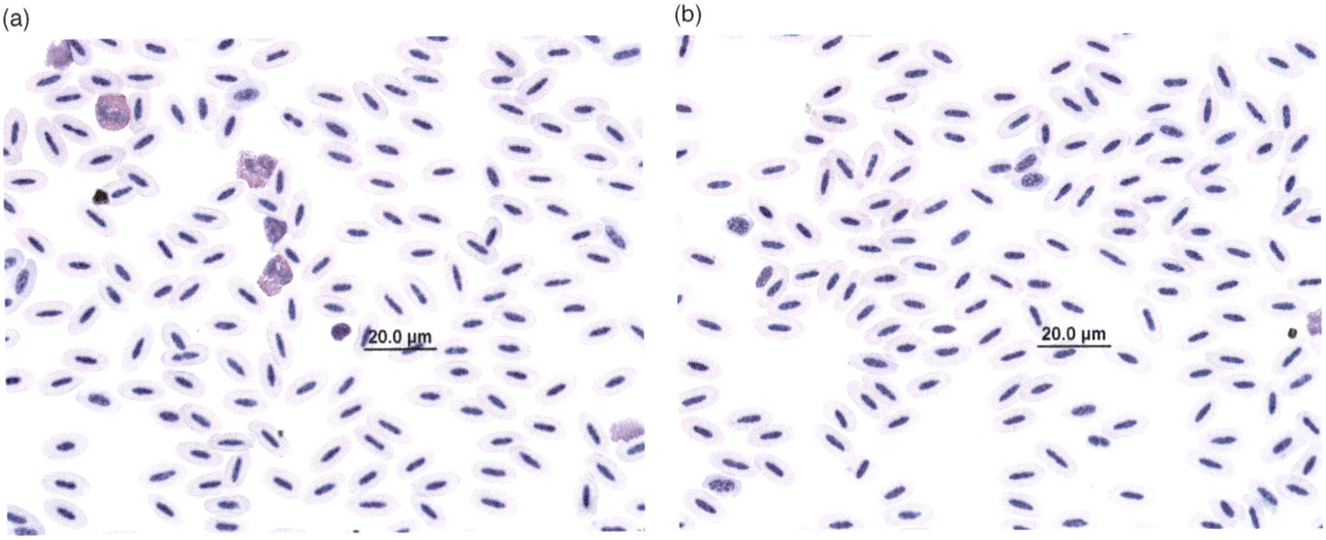

Fig. 13.2. (a), (b) Blood films (Wright–Giemsa stain, 100× oil).

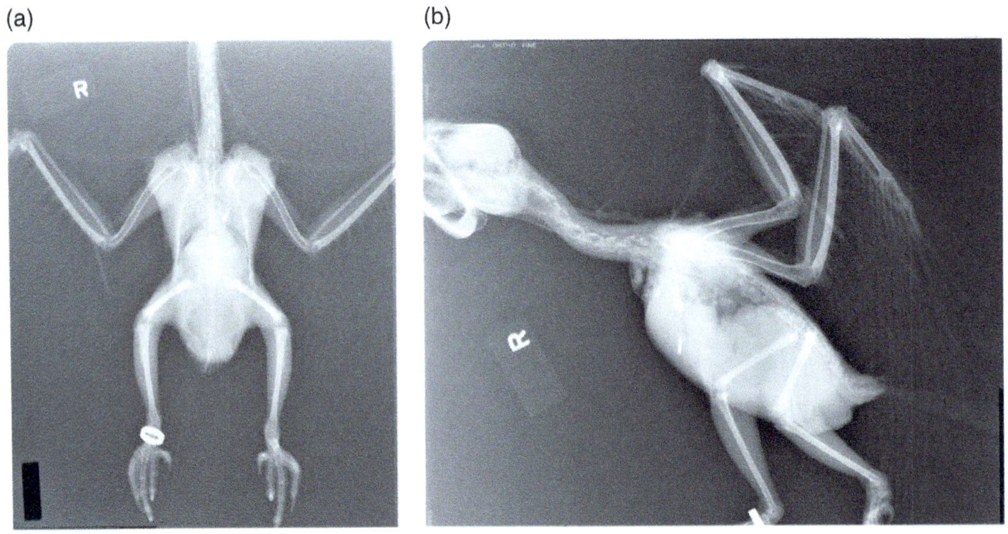

Fig. 13.3. (a) The whole-body ventral-dorsal radiograph, (b) the whole-body lateral radiograph.

a laying bird. Birds experiencing chronic egg laying may also deplete calcium and exhibit hypocalcemia.

Radiographic images (Figures 13.3a and 13.3b) revealed an ill-defined, multilobulated, opaque, soft-tissue mass effect located in the caudodorsal celomic cavity. This mass was compressing the caudal celomic air sacs and was partially superimposed over the ventriculus. On the ventrodorsal (VD) projection, this mass effect was silhouetted with the liver. In the appendicular skeleton, a marked, diffuse, increased intramedullary opacity was located in both radii, ulnae, femurs, and tibias. Incidentally, radiopaque food material within the crop was superimposed over the clavicular air sac. The caudodorsal celomic mass effect may originate from the reproductive tract, kidney, or small intestines. The polyostotic hyperostosis was consistent with hyperestrogenism associated with egg production.

Radiographic images (Figures 13.4a and 13.4b) revealed positive contrast identified within the crop, proventriculus, ventriculus, and multiple small intestinal segments. The gastrointestinal tract was displaced cranially. The large, ill-defined mass effect was located in the caudal celomic cavity and was not associated with the intestinal tract. The caudal celomic mass effect was suspected to be inflammation or a neoplastic mass within the reproductive tract or, less likely, of renal origin.

(a) (b)

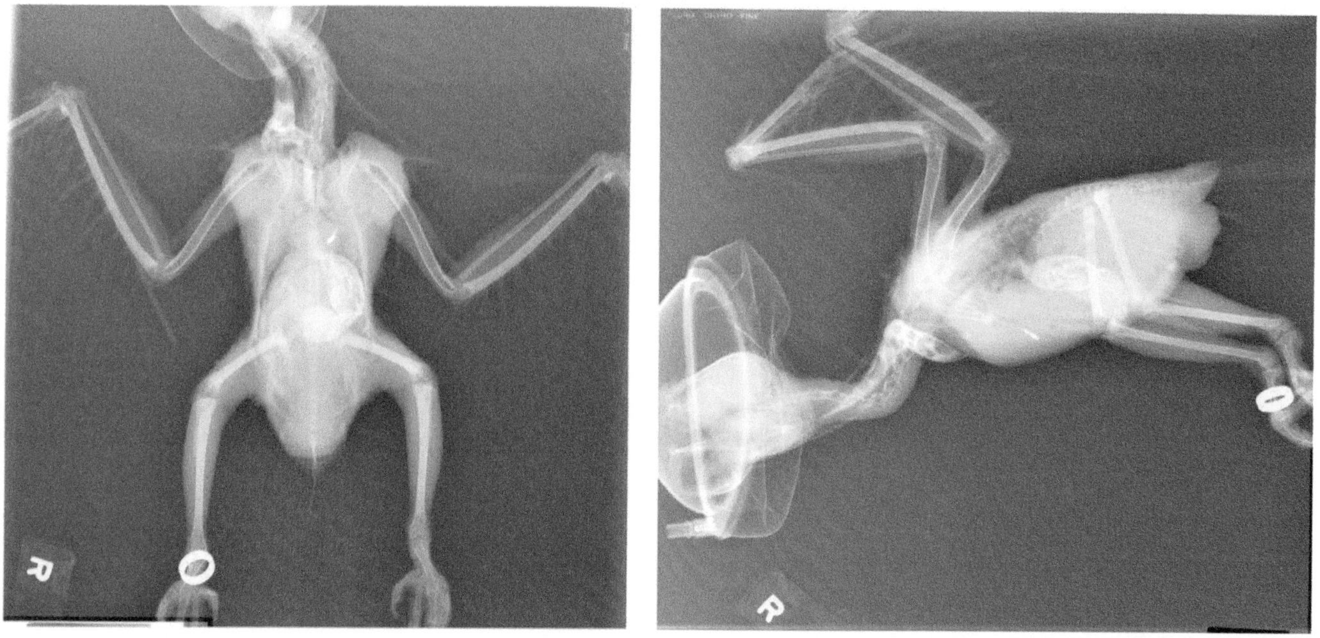

Fig. 13.4. (a) The whole-body ventral-dorsal radiograph with barium contrast in gastrointestinal tract, (b) the lateral radiograph with barium contrast in gastrointestinal tract.

Summary

Due to the cockatoo's recent reproductive activity along with the increased white cell count, a possible salpingitis was suspected, and a salpingohysterectomy was performed. The bird was placed under general anesthesia in preparation for surgery. An incision was made along her ventral midline, and a fully formed egg was found in the distal oviduct. The egg was removed from the oviduct, and the salpingohysterectomy was completed to prevent future egg production. She returned two weeks later for suture removal and was reportedly doing well.

The mass effect on the radiographs was the non-mineralized egg likely in the isthmus of the oviduct. During the time between the last radiograph and surgery, the egg calcified and was located in the distal oviduct, likely in the uterus. The interval between subsequent oviposition in a psittacine with normal reproductive activity is about 48 h (Scagnelli and Tully, 2017).

Egg binding, or dystocia, is a common reproductive disorder in captive psittacine birds. This case represented abnormal reproductive cycling, which often leads to dystocia, the more common clinical presentation.

Case 2: Swainson's Hawk with Head Trauma

Signalment

Adult Swainson's hawk (*Buteo swainsoni*)

History

The hawk presented to a raptor rehabilitation facility after being found sitting in the southbound lane of a local highway, presumably hit by a car.

Physical Examination

Upon physical examination, the 895-g hawk was in good body condition, subdued, and only minimally responsive. There was apparent head trauma evidenced by the blood in the oral cavity, the left eye held closed, and the right eye slow to respond to stimuli. The right wing drooped, and upon palpation, it was discovered that the right clavicle was fractured proximal to the keel. Initial treatment included pain medications for three days, subcutaneous fluids, figure 8 bandage on the right wing with a body band, and supplemental oxygen. Initially, the bird was not eating on its own, so it was tease-fed one-half ounce of mouse and one ounce of mouse was dropped in the enclosure every day until it ate on its own (this occurred five days after presentation). Nine days after presentation, the bird developed green urates. A blood sample was collected for a CBC (Table 13.3 and Figures 13.5a–13.5f), blood lead concentration, and a West Nile Virus (WNV) antibody titer. The lead test result was less than 3.3 ug/dL (considered within normal limits); however, the WNV titer was high and considered positive.

Table 13.3. Swainson's hawk hematology results (Case 3).

	Day 1	Day 7	Reference[a] (*Buteo jamaicensis*)
PCV(%)	34.0	50.0	37.2 ± 4.6
Leukocytes			
WBC (×10³/μL)	38.8	25.3	19.29 ± 7.51
Heterophils (×10³/μL)	20.6	15.2	10.81 ± 4.82
(%)	53	60	—
Lymphocytes (×10³/μL)	4.3	7.1	5.16 ± 2.98
(%)	11	28	—
Monocytes (×10³/μL)	12.4	1.0	1.47 ± 1.24
(%)	32	4	—
Eosinophils (×10³/μL)	1.6	1.0	1.96 ± 1.69
(%)	4	4	—
Basophils (×10³/μL)	0	1.0	0.06 ± 0.19
(%)	0	4	—
Thrombocytes			
*Adequate Thrombocytes	Exist	Exist	
Plasma protein (refractometry)			
(g/dL)	5.2	6.1	3.41 ± 0.65
Notes			
Pathologist	—		
Technician	Many RBC precursor cells in all stages of development. *Hemoproteus* occupies about 30% of the RBCs	Rare *Hemoproteus* observed	

[a]Black (2018).

Interpretive Discussion

The CBC results showed a leukocytosis with heterophilia, severe monocytosis, mild anemia with approximately 30% of erythrocytes with *Hemoproteus*, and immature red blood cells. Figures 13.5a–13.5f revealed a marked degree of polychromasia, indicating that the bird has a regenerative anemia. The images show *Hemoproteus* sp. and *Plasmodium* sp. gametocytes with the erythrocytes, indicating a mixed infection of blood parasites and a possible contributing cause to the anemia (hemorrhage likely contributed to the anemia initially, but this blood sample was collected 10 days after initial presentation to the rehabilitation facility). Figure 13.5a shows several immature erythrocytes along with several mature erythrocytes with mature *Plasmodium* gametocytes and *Hemoproteus* trophozoites and microgametocytes. Figure 13.5b shows the polychromasia from immature erythrocytes, *Plasmodium* gametocytes, one heterophil, one basophil, and two thrombocytes. Figure 13.5c shows immature erythrocytes, different stages of *Hemoproteus* trophozoites and gametocytes, two heterophils, and two monocytes. Figure 13.5d reveals the presence of *Leukocytozoon* microgametocyte. Figure 13.5e shows several heterophils and a mitotic figure among several immature erythrocytes and mature erythrocytes with intracellular protozoa. Figure 13.5f reveals immature erythrocytes, several mature erythrocytes with mature gametocytes from protozoa *Plasmodium* sp., three heterophils, and one monocyte.

Summary

Due to the leukocytosis and WNV titer results, the bird was treated with Nuflor® (SC × 10 days), subcutaneous fluids every other day, and lysine (PO × 7 days). Eleven days after presentation, the bird maintained its body weight on three ounces of mice daily, and the figure 8 bandage and body bandage were removed as the wing was held in a normal position. Seventeen days after initial presentation, the urates appeared normal, and the bird gained weight (993 g), and blood was collected to reevaluate the CBC (Figures 13.6a–13.6d). Overall, the hemogram improved: leukocytosis (depending on what reference interval used) was still present with heterophilia. The anemia had resolved, and hemoparasites were rarely found. Figure 13.6a shows a basophil and two thrombocytes. Figure 13.6b shows two heterophils, one eosinophil, and one monocyte. Figure 13.6c shows one heterophil and one eosinophil. Figure 13.6d shows two heterophils and one monocyte. Another notable finding on the blood film was pyknotic cells (Figures 13.7a and 13.7b). Figure 13.7a shows a pyknotic heterophil and eosinophil and two normal het-

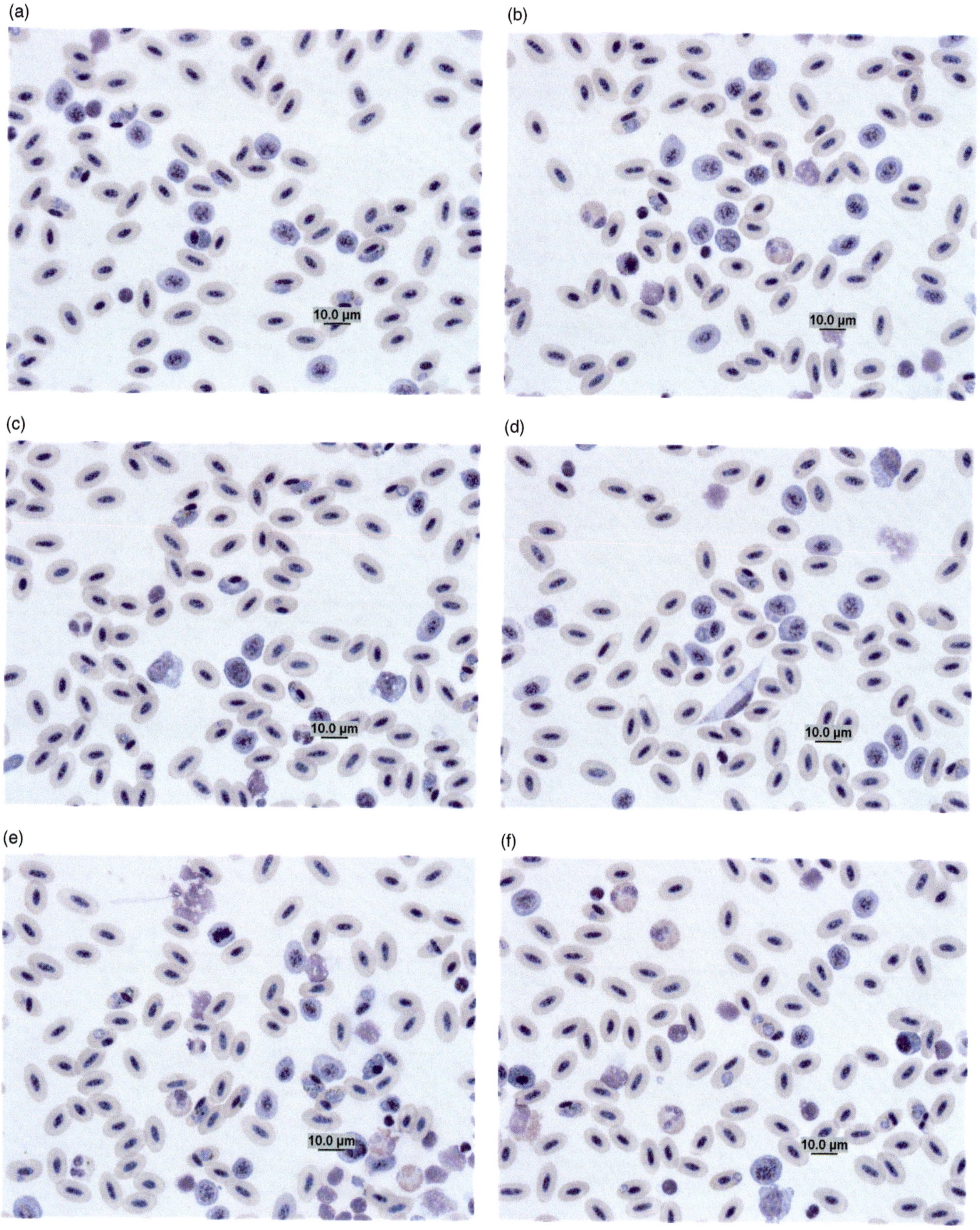

Fig. 13.5. (a)–(f) Blood film (Wright–Giemsa stain, 100× oil).

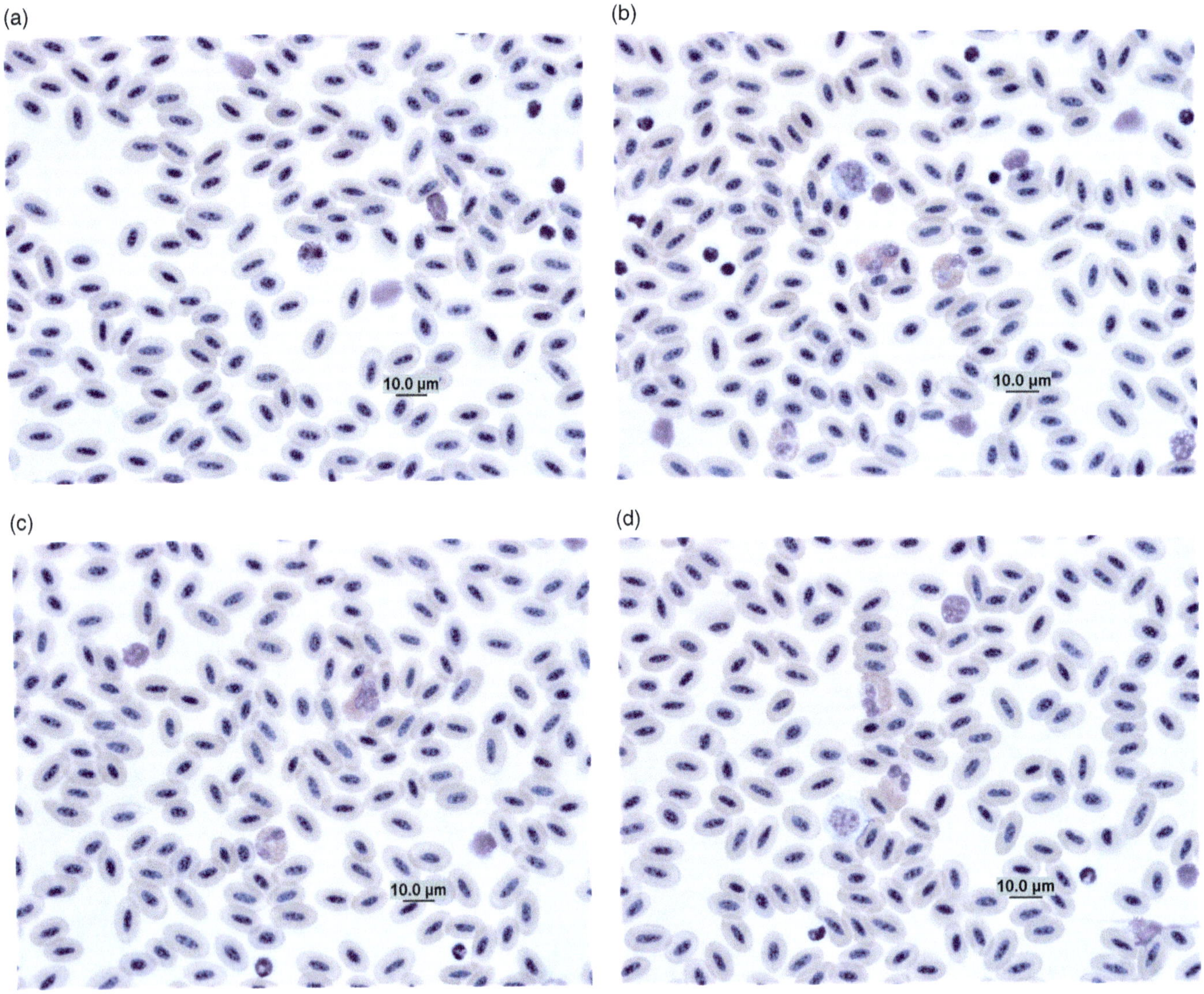

Fig. 13.6. (a)–(d) Blood film (Wright–Giemsa stain, 100× oil).

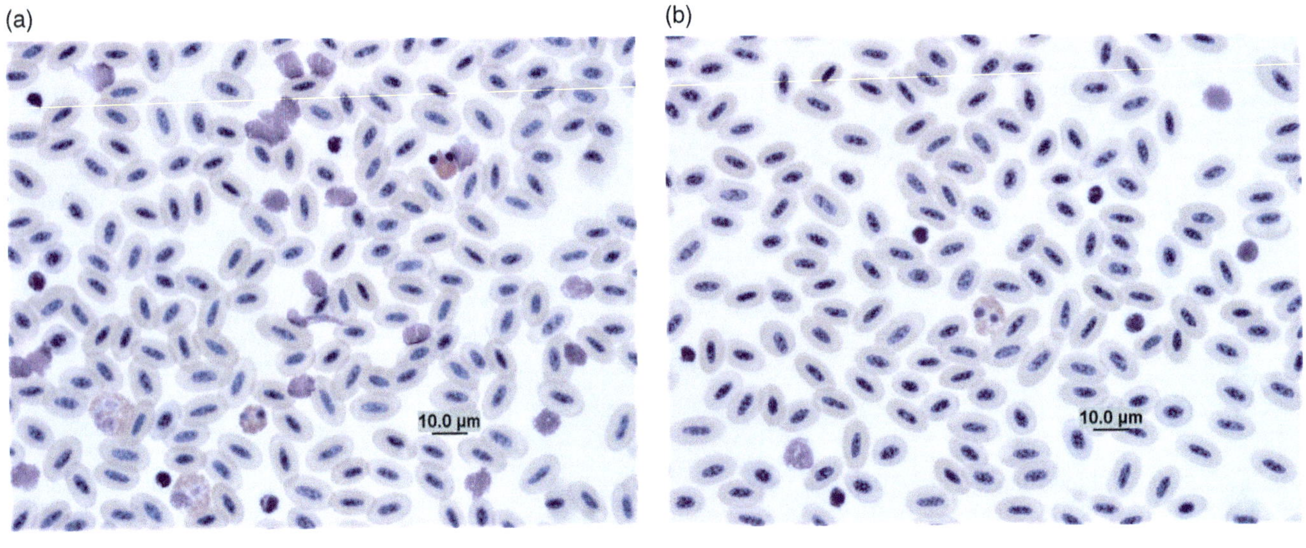

Fig. 13.7. (a), (b) Blood film (Wright–Giemsa stain, 100× oil).

erophils. Figure 13.7b shows a heterophil with a pyknotic nucleus. Overall, the majority of erythrocytes were mature, supporting the resolution of the regenerative anemia.

Once the wings were symmetrical with a good range of motion, the hawk was moved to a recovery enclosure for pre-conditioning exercise. Approximately one month after initial presentation, the bird weighed 1028 g and was moved to a flight enclosure for final flight conditioning, where it resided for three days until it was successfully released back into the wild.

Case 3: Pionus Parrot with Weight Loss, Exercise Intolerance, and Sneezing

Signalment

2-year-old intact male blue-headed Pionus parrot (*Pionus menstruus*)

History

The parrot presented for a previously worked-up respiratory disease evident by sneezing, decreased appetite, chronic weight loss, and exercise intolerance. Three months prior to presentation, he was seen at another veterinary clinic, where diagnostic results included a severely elevated white blood cell count of 93 000/μL (with toxic heterophils) and negative test results for aspergillosis and chlamydiosis. Despite the negative results, he was placed on doxycycline for treatment of chlamydiosis, which appeared to improve his clinical signs. The parrot was referred for a possible exploratory laparoscopy to further evaluate the air sacs.

Additional history included a diet of a variety of pellets and seeds, and the parrot was obtained by a breeder one year prior to presentation.

Physical Examination

On physical examination, the 225-g bird was bright, alert, and responsive with a normal body condition. He had normal inspiratory and expiratory effort, and his vital signs were within normal limits. The parrot was placed under general anesthesia (isoflurane via face mask), and a blood sample via jugular venipuncture (Tables 13.4 and 13.5 and Figures 13.8a–13.8d) and whole-body radiographs (Figures 13.9a and 13.9b) were obtained.

Interpretive Discussion

The hemogram revealed a marked leukocytosis with heterophilia, monocytosis, and eosinophilia. The blood film image in Figure 13.8a is representative of the red blood cells seen throughout the film. The amount of polychromasia seen in the erythrocytes in Figures 13.8a–13.8d is expected for birds. The blood film image in Figure 13.8b shows two normal-appearing heterophils, two normal-appearing monocytes, and a thrombocyte. The blood film image in Figure 13.8c shows two normal-appearing lymphocytes. The blood film image in Figure 13.8d shows a reactive lymphocyte indicated by prominent, smooth nuclear chromatin and a perinuclear Golgi zone. There were no significant concerns with the plasma biochemistry profile.

Radiographic images (Figures 13.9a and 13.9b) reveal that the caudal air sacs are hyperinflated, with the left being more affected than the right. The hepatic silhouette is enlarged, extending beyond the coxofemoral joints. A small amount of mineral opaque material is present within the ventriculus. There is an ill-defined, lobular, soft-tissue opacity in the cranial mid-celomic cavity, best seen on the lateral view. This lobulated mass has a gas lucency passing through it. The radiographic conclusions were consistent with an air sacculitis and enlarged hepatic silhouette that could be related to hepatomegaly secondary to infectious or infiltrative disease. Given these findings, along with the results from the bloodwork and information from the history, chlamydia and aspergillosis were the primary rule-outs. Other differential

Table 13.4. Pionus parrot hematology results (Case 3).

	Visit 1	Visit 10	Reference[a]
PCV (%)	54.0	50.0	44–54
Leukocytes			
WBC (×10³/μL)	29.3	85.7	5–13
Heterophils (×10³/μL)	20.5	72.0	0.48–7.10
(%)	70	84	55–74
Lymphocytes (×10³/μL)	5.6	7.7	1.82–6.72
(%)	19	9	19–70
Monocytes (×10³/μL)	1.8	4.3	0–0.10
(%)	6	5	0–1
Eosinophils (×10³/μL)	1.2	1.7	0–0.10
(%)	4	2	0–1
Basophils (×10³/μL)	0.3	0	0–0.10
(%)	1	0	0–1
Thrombocytes			
Adequate thrombocytes	Exist	Exist	
Plasma protein (refractometry)			
(g/dL)	4.2	4.8	
Notes			
Pathologist	—		
Technician	Visit 10: Slight toxic heterophils		

[a]Carpenter (2018).

Table 13.5. Pionus parrot plasma biochemical results (Case 3).

	Visit 1	Reference[a]	Decision level[b]
Glucose (mg/dL)	252	228–312	200–500
BUN (mg/dL)	<3	3.0–5.4	
Phosphorus (mg/dL)	2.8	2.9–6.6	5–7
Calcium (mg/dL)	8.2	7.8–10.8	8–11
Uric acid (mg/dL)	3.5	2.0–7.9	<15
Total protein (biuret) (g/dL)	3.3	3.6–5.2	2.5–4.0
Albumin (g/dL)	1.2	—	
Globulin (g/dL)	2.1	—	
Cholesterol (mg/dL)	220	130–295	
Creatine kinase (IU/L)	369	169–354	<500
Aspartate aminotransferase (IU/L)	290	140–359	<275
Sodium (mEq/L)	148	145–155	130–160
Potassium (mEq/L)	3.0	3.5–4.6	2.0–4.0
Chloride (mEq/L)	111	—	

[a]Carpenter (2018).
[b]Decision levels used by authors when reference values are unavailable.

(a) (b) (c) (d)

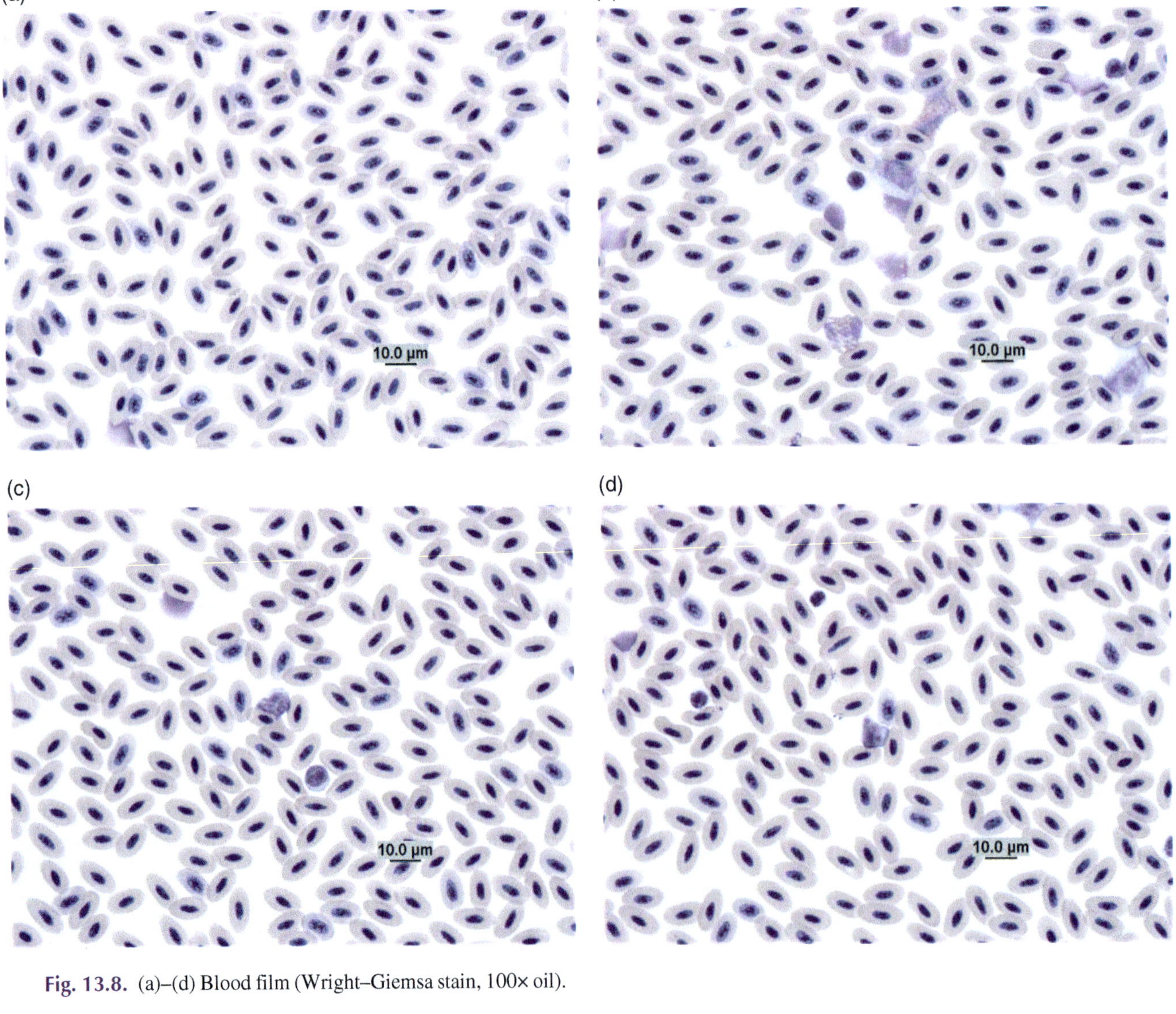

Fig. 13.8. (a)–(d) Blood film (Wright–Giemsa stain, 100× oil).

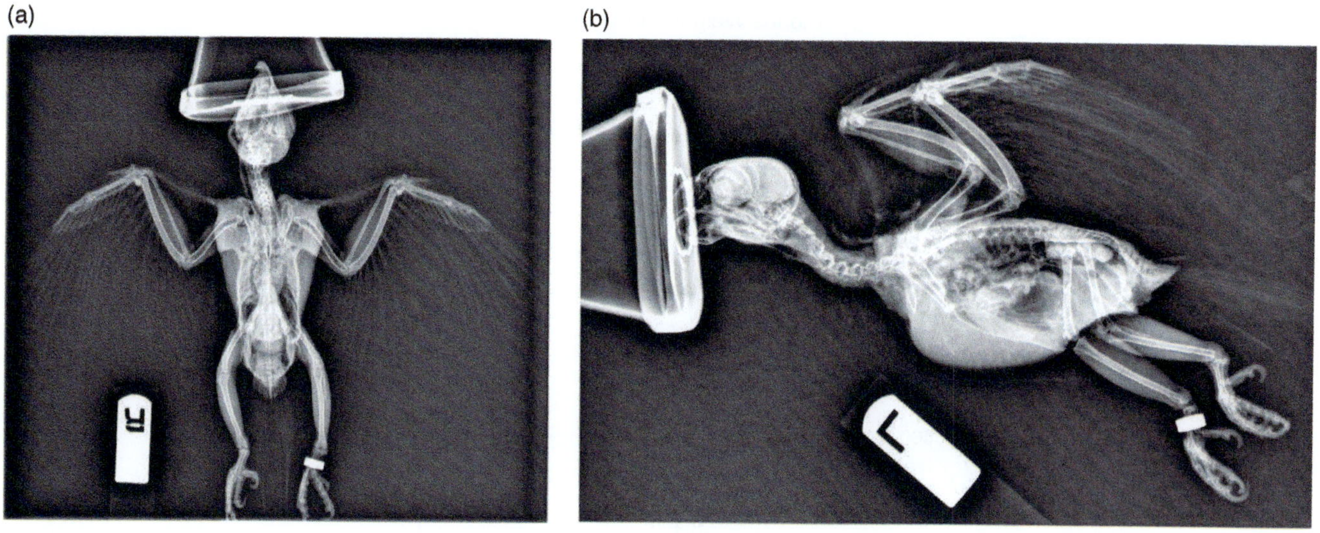

Fig. 13.9. (a) The whole-body ventral-dorsal radiograph, (b) the whole-body lateral radiograph.

diagnoses that often exhibit a severe leukocytosis are mycobacteriosis and neoplasia.

Summary

Given the diagnostic findings and response to doxycycline treatment, a presumptive diagnosis of chlamydiosis was made. The client was instructed to continue the doxycycline treatment for six more weeks. The exploratory laparoscopy was not performed because the parrot had been improving, and there was some concern that the procedure would further compromise his condition. Furthermore, microbial cultures would be compromised by the current antibiotic treatment. It was also suggested that the clients purchase a small home nebulizer to provide topical treatment.

The parrot returned nine days later for a CBC recheck that revealed the same moderate leukocytosis (30 300/μL). At that time, the heterophilia (26 900/μL) persisted; however, the monocyte (600/μL) and lymphocyte (2700/μL) numbers had decreased. The plasma biochemical profile revealed no significant findings. The parrot was discharged, and the client was instructed to continue the current treatment plan.

Four months later, the parrot returned due to continued weight loss (weight down to 187 g) and increased exercise intolerance. The CBC revealed a leukocytosis (48 600/μL) with heterophilia (39 900/μL) and monocytosis (1900/μL). The continued medical expenses were financially draining the clients; therefore, they elected to relinquish the bird to one of the authors (KG).

The treatment approach moving forward included a diet change and medical treatment. The diet was changed to a variety of cooked and fresh foods such as scrambled egg, berries, banana, grapes, sweet potato, green pepper, quinoa, brown rice, whole grain toast, pasta, carrots, beans, peas; pellets; and occasional seed and nuts for treats. The medical treatment regimen was changed to treat systemically and topically for a suspected aspergillosis. A homemade nebulizer was built with a small storage container, acorn nebulizer with the mouthpiece covered, and compressor to deliver topical treatment (Figure 13.10). The treatment was dictated by a combination of the CBC results (9 tests over 15 months), evaluation of the blood film (signs of toxic heterophils), body weight (tracked daily), and overall behavior. A combination of antifungal medications was used: itraconazole (5 mg/kg by mouth once daily), clotrimazole 1% (25 drops in acorn nebulizer for 20 min), or Amphotericin B (5 mg/mL using 0.5 mL with 2.5 mL saline in acorn nebulizer for

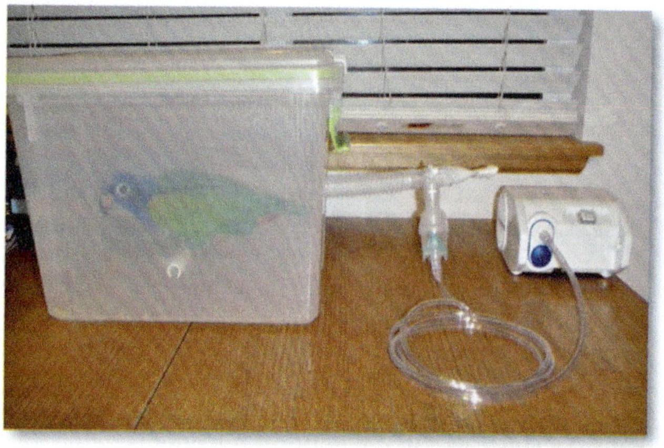

Fig. 13.10. The parrot in a homemade nebulizer receiving topical antifungal treatment. The mouthpiece is covered to divert the mist into the storage container. A half-inch PVC pipe was screwed into the storage container for a perch.

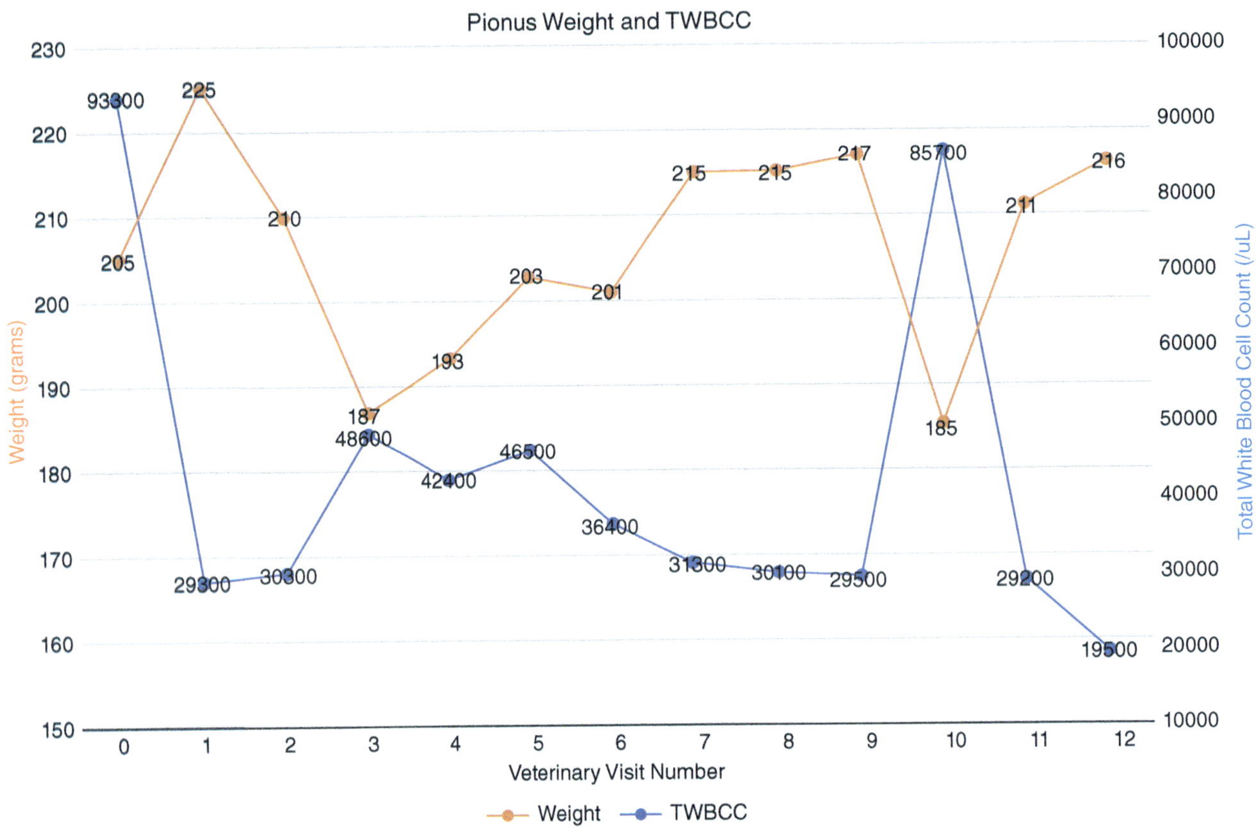

Fig. 13.11. Summary of total white blood cell counts and weight over 22 months. Visit 0 was obtained by the referring veterinarian. Visits 1–3 were obtained by original owner. Visit 3 was the visit during which the bird was relinquished. Visits 4–12 represent results during systemic and topical antifungal treatment regimen. Visits 3–6 were weekly rechecking, visits 7–9 were monthly rechecks, visit 10 was 3 months later, visit 11 was 4 months later, and visit 12 was 5 months later.

20 min). The total white blood cell counts from the CBCs and weights, along with notes regarding changes in the household and treatments given, were tracked from the last visit to the referring veterinarian (visit 0) through 15 months after being relinquished (Figure 13.11). The CBCs and blood films were evaluated once weekly for three weeks (visits 4–6) following the visit the bird was relinquished (visit 3), followed by monthly rechecks for three months (visits 7–9), then three months later (visit 10), four months later (visit 11), and five months later (visit 12). The treatment regimen during the 15 months was as follows: Itraconazole (3 months on/3 months off for the entire 15 months), Clotrimazole (3 months, then 3 months off nebulization), and Amphotericin B (2 months on/1 month off/4 months on, then 2 months off nebulization). There were two periods were the parrot's weight fell below 200 g: the first time at visit 10 and the second time between visits 11 and 12. During both periods, the parrot had been transferred to a relative's house for pet sitting while the owner was out of town, and the decreased weight and leukocytosis (evaluated only during the first episode, visit 10) were attributed to the change in environment prompting relapse of the respiratory condition. Both episodes were treated as described above, and the parrot appeared to recover.

The only visit during which the blood film suggested a leukocytosis with a heterophilia and changes in cell morphology was during visit 10 (Figures 13.12a and 13.12b). The hemogram also revealed the most severe leukocytosis during the 15-month period (Table 13.5). The blood film in Figure 13.12a revealed 13 heterophils, 1 lymphocyte, and 1 monocyte. Figure 13.12b revealed 3 heterophils, 1 monocyte, and 3 lymphocytes. The heterophils exhibit slight toxicity evident by the cytoplasmic basophilia and degranulation.

After visit 12, quantitative assessment included body weights only. Approximately one year later, the parrot experienced one respiratory episode that occurred when a nearby forest wildfire lasted over several weeks. The parrot was treated during this time systemically with itraconazole for one month and topically via nebulizer with Amphotericin B once daily for two weeks. The parrot recovered and remained apparently healthy.

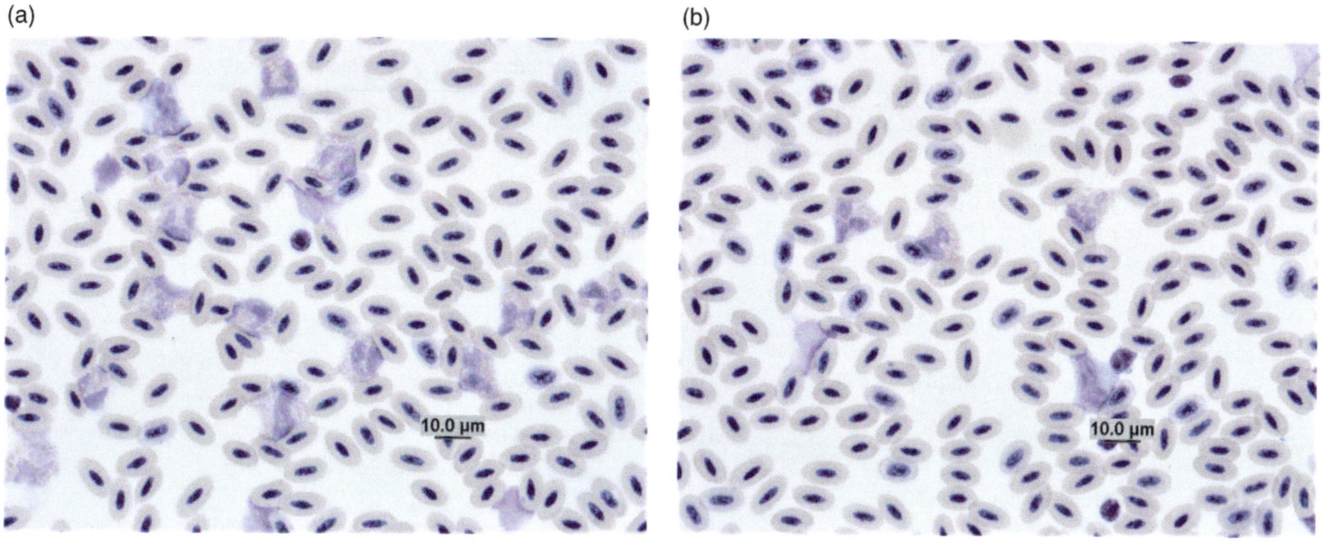

Fig. 13.12. (a), (b) Visit 10 blood film (Wright–Giemsa stain, 100× oil).

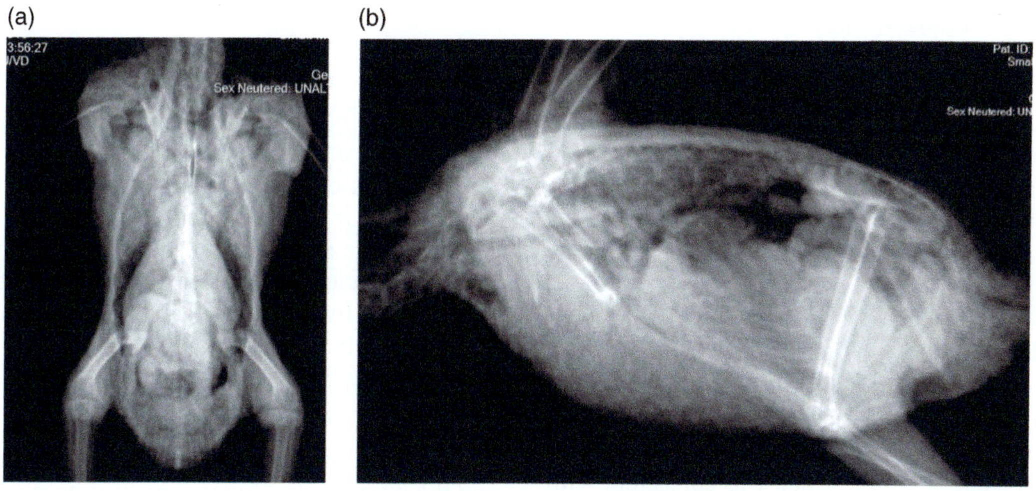

Fig. 13.13. (a) The whole-body ventral-dorsal radiograph (from referring veterinarian), (b) the whole-body lateral radiograph from (from referring veterinarian).

Case 4: Conure with Lethargy and Anorexia

Signalment

7-year-old sun conure (*Aratinga solstitialis*)

History

The conure presented to the hospital for lethargy and anorexia, and was reluctant to open its eyes. The owner mentioned that this seemed like a sudden onset of signs and only noticed a change in behavior beginning the day before presentation, which prompted them to take the bird to an emergency hospital. The radiographs obtained from the emergency hospital (Figures 13.13a and 13.13b) revealed an enlarged cardiohepatic silhouette.

Physical Examination

Upon physical examination, the 110-g bird was lethargic and had decreased pectoral muscle mass, indicating an underconditioned body score. A blood sample was collected for CBC (Table 13.6 and Figures 13.14a–13.14f) and a biochemistry profile (Table 13.7). Contrast radiographs

Table 13.6. Conure hematology results (Case 4).

		Reference[a]	Decision level[b]
PCV (%)	36.0	42–54	35–55
Leukocytes			
WBC (×10³/µL)	1.1	5–13	5.0–20.0
Heterophils (×10³/µL)	0.2	4.22–6.91	2.1–10.0
(%)	18	44–72	—
Lymphocytes (×10³/µL)	0.6	2.11–4.89	1.7–10.0
(%)	60	22–51	—
Monocytes (×10³/µL)	0.2	0–0.09	0–0.7
(%)	16	0–1	—
Eosinophils (×10³/µL)	0.02	0–0.09	0–0.4
(%)	2	0–1	—
Basophils (×10³/µL)	0.04	0–0.09	0–0.4
(%)	4	0–1	—
Thrombocytes			
Adequate thrombocytes	Exist		1–5/1000× field
Plasma protein (refractometry)			
(g/dL)	2.8		3–5
Notes			
Pathologist	Aggregated polychromatophilic erythrocytes		
Technician	Moderate polychromasia		

[a]Carpenter (2018).
[b]Decision levels used by authors when reference values are unavailable.

were also obtained to assess the cause of the enlarged cardiohepatic silhouette on the accompanying radiographs from the referring veterinarian (Figures 13.15a and 13.15b).

Interpretive Discussion

The plasma biochemistry profile revealed a slightly low protein and elevated creatine kinase (CK) and aspartate aminotransferase (AST). The elevated CK was likely due to muscle wasting, which was consistent with the bird's underconditioned appearance on physical examination. An elevated AST is often elevated in coordination with CK and muscle breakdown, but may also be an indication of hepatocellular damage. The CBC revealed mild anemia, hypoproteinemia, and pancytopenia with toxic heterophils. Figure 13.14a revealed a basophil. Figure 13.14b revealed an erythroplastid (anucleated erythrocyte). Figure 13.14c shows hypochromasia and lymphocytes. Figure 13.14d revealed a pyknotic cell (left) and a reactive large lymphocyte. Figures 13.14e and 13.14f each show an example of a toxic heterophil.

Radiographs were taken after the bird was given barium to outline the intestinal tract (Figures 13.15a and 13.15b). Both images revealed that the ingluvies (crop), proventriculus, ventriculus, and small intestines had barium within the lumen. These structures appeared normal and were not pathologically distended. There was mild widening of the cardiohepatic silhouette. The remaining osseous and soft-tissue structures seen on the radiographs appeared normal.

Given the results of the bloodwork and radiographs, it was suspected that the bird had an infectious disease affecting the liver, such as Pacheco's disease, chlamydiosis, or bacterial septicemia.

Summary

Further diagnostics were offered but were declined, and the owner opted to take the bird home with antibiotics. Subcutaneous fluids (4 mL) were given, and the bird was sent home with doxycycline (25 mg/kg PO BID × 14 days) and enrofloxacin (20 mg/kg PO q24h × 14 days). The bird did not return, and therefore follow-up was lost.

Case 5: Hawk with Dehydration and Emaciation

Signalment

Adult, female ferruginous hawk (*Buteo regalis*)

History

This hawk was suspected to be a second-year bird. It was found at the end of the winter season and admitted to the raptor rehabilitation center for being in poor

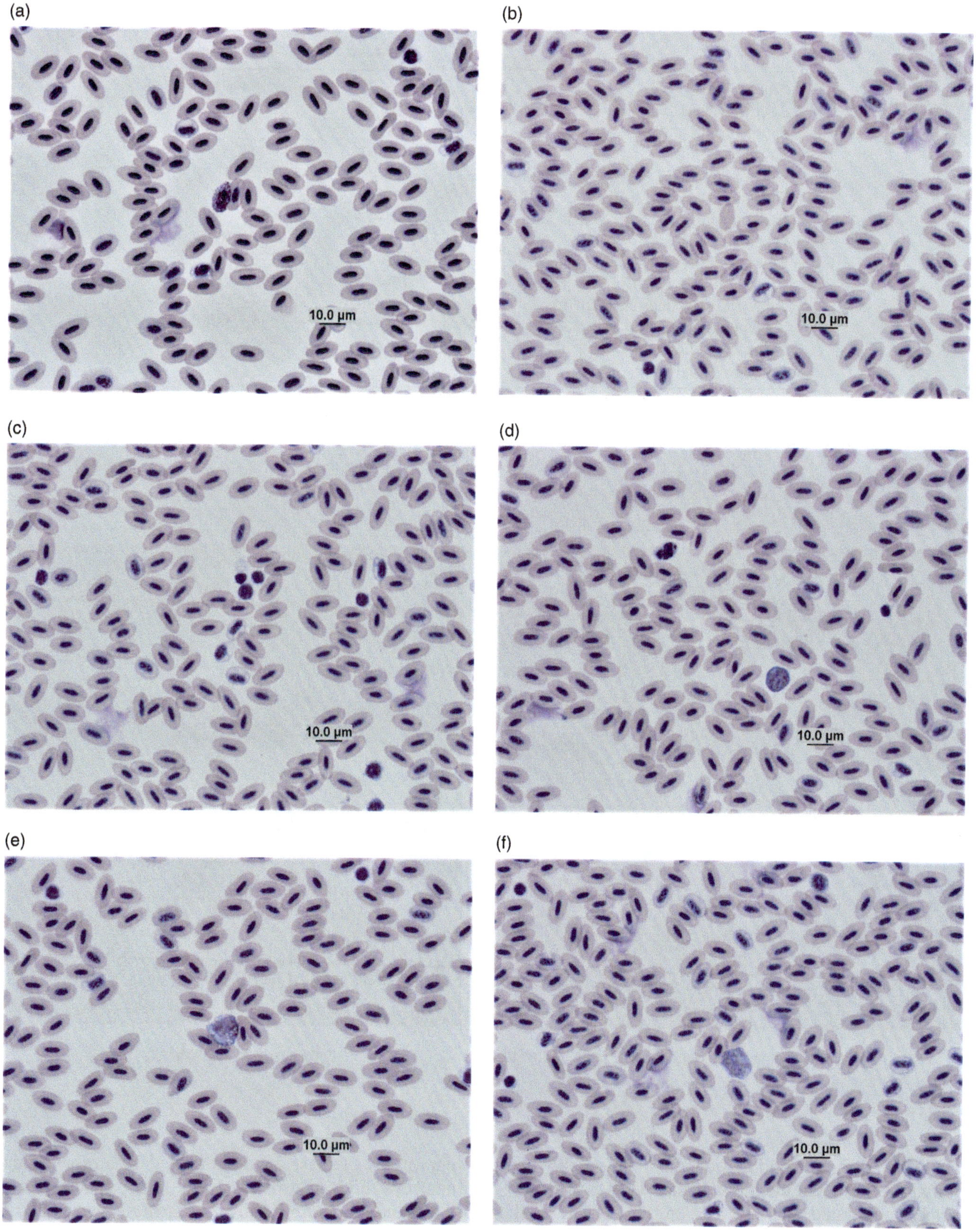

Fig. 13.14. (a)–(f) Blood film (Wright–Giemsa stain, 100× oil).

Table 13.7. Conure plasma biochemical results (Case 4).

		Reference[a]	Decision level[b]
Glucose (mg/dL)	201	217–323	200–500
BUN (mg/dL)	9	2.5–5.4	
Phosphorus (mg/dL)	5.8	2–10	5–7
Calcium (mg/dL)	7.9	7.9–10.8	8–11
Uric acid (mg/dL)	2.6	3.0–11.4	<15
Total protein (biuret) (g/dL)	2.2	2.8–4.6	2.5–4.0
Albumin (g/dL)	0.8	1.01–1.94	
Globulin (g/dL)	1.4	—	
Cholesterol (mg/dL)	84	120–400	
Creatine kinase (IU/L)	1413	154–355	<500
Aspartate aminotransferase (IU/L)	405	178–307	<275
Sodium (mEq/L)	157	135–149	130–160
Potassium (mEq/L)	2.0	3.4–5	2.0–4.0
Chloride (mEq/L)	111	—	

[a]Carpenter (2018).
[b]Decision levels used by authors when reference values are unavailable.

(a) (b)

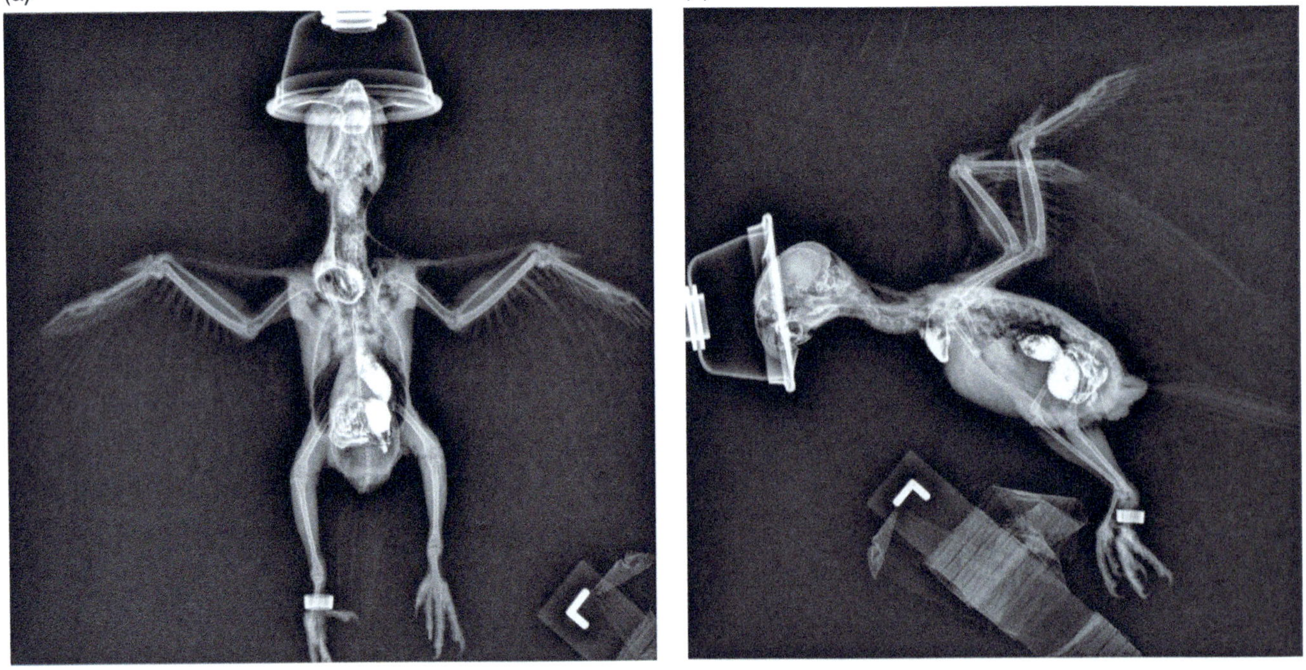

Fig. 13.15. (a) The whole-body ventral-dorsal radiograph with contrast, (b) the whole-body lateral radiograph with contrast.

condition. During the admission examination, the rehabilitation staff noted the bird weighed 1201 g, was emaciated, dehydrated, had bruising on the left side of the cere near the commissure of the mouth, had small feather lice, had a healed keel fracture, and the tissue around the vent was gray with scabs. They treated the bird with subcutaneous fluids, antibiotics, lysine, and provided a heat disc in the enclosure. Over the course of a week and a half, the treatment was continued with the addition of tube feeding Carnivore Care (Oxbow Animal Health,

Table 13.8. Ferruginous hawk hematology results (Case 5).

		Reference[a] (*Buteo jamaicensis*)	Decision level[b]
PCV (%)	25.0	31–43	35–55
Leukocytes			
WBC (×10³/µL)	154.0	19.1–33.4	5.0–20.0
Myelocytes (×10³/µL)	4.6	—	—
(%)	3	—	—
Metamyelocytes (×10³/µL)	4.6	—	—
(%)	3	—	—
Band (×10³/µL)	12.3	—	—
(%)	8	—	—
Heterophils (×10³/µL)	103.2	—	2.1–10.0
(%)	67	35 ± 11	—
Lymphocytes (×10³/µL)	6.2	—	1.7–10.0
(%)	4	44 ± 9	—
Monocytes (×10³/µL)	18.5	—	0–0.7
(%)	12	6 ± 3	—
Eosinophils (×10³/µL)	4.6	—	0–0.4
(%)	3	13 ± 4	—
Basophils (×10³/µL)	0	—	0–0.4
(%)	0	Rare	—
Thrombocytes			
Adequate thrombocytes	Exist		1–5/1000× field
Plasma protein (refractometry)			
(g/dL)	7.7		—
Notes			
Pathologist			
Technician			

[a]Carpenter (2018).
[b]Decision levels used by authors when reference values are unavailable.

Omaha, NE) and an antifungal medication, but the bird did not show much improvement and was not able to gain weight.

Physical Examination

Upon physical exam, the 1184-g bird had a poor body condition (1/10) and was emaciated. The bird had lesions consistent with frost bite, and a healed keel fracture was palpated approximately one inch from the cranial aspect. A blood sample was evaluated on CBC (Table 13.8 and Figures 13.16a–13.16d).

Interpretive Discussion

The CBC (Table 13.8) revealed a severe leukocytosis with a severe heterophilia with a left shift (myelocytes, metamyelocytes, and band heterophils) and monocytosis. Figure 13.16a revealed a *Leukocytozoon* macrogametocyte in the center of the image, one mature heterophil, one band heterophil, two metamyelocytes, one myelocyte, two monocytes, and polychromasia. Figure 13.16b revealed one myelocyte, four metamyelocytes, two band heterophils, one toxic heterophil, and polychromasia. Figure 13.16c revealed two myelocytes, one metamyelocyte, one band heterophil, two mature heterophils, four toxic heterophils, one monocyte, and polychromasia. Figure 13.16d revealed two monocytes, three myelocytes, one band heterophil, one mature heterophil, four toxic heterophils, and polychromasia.

Summary

The severity of the leukocytosis and accelerated production of heterophils indicate a severe inflammatory leukogram, which is likely infectious. White cell counts this high are commonly caused by fungal infections, such as aspergillosis, or bacterial infections, such as chlamydiosis or mycobacteriosis. The bird was euthanized and necropsy revealed respiratory aspergillosis and coelomitis.

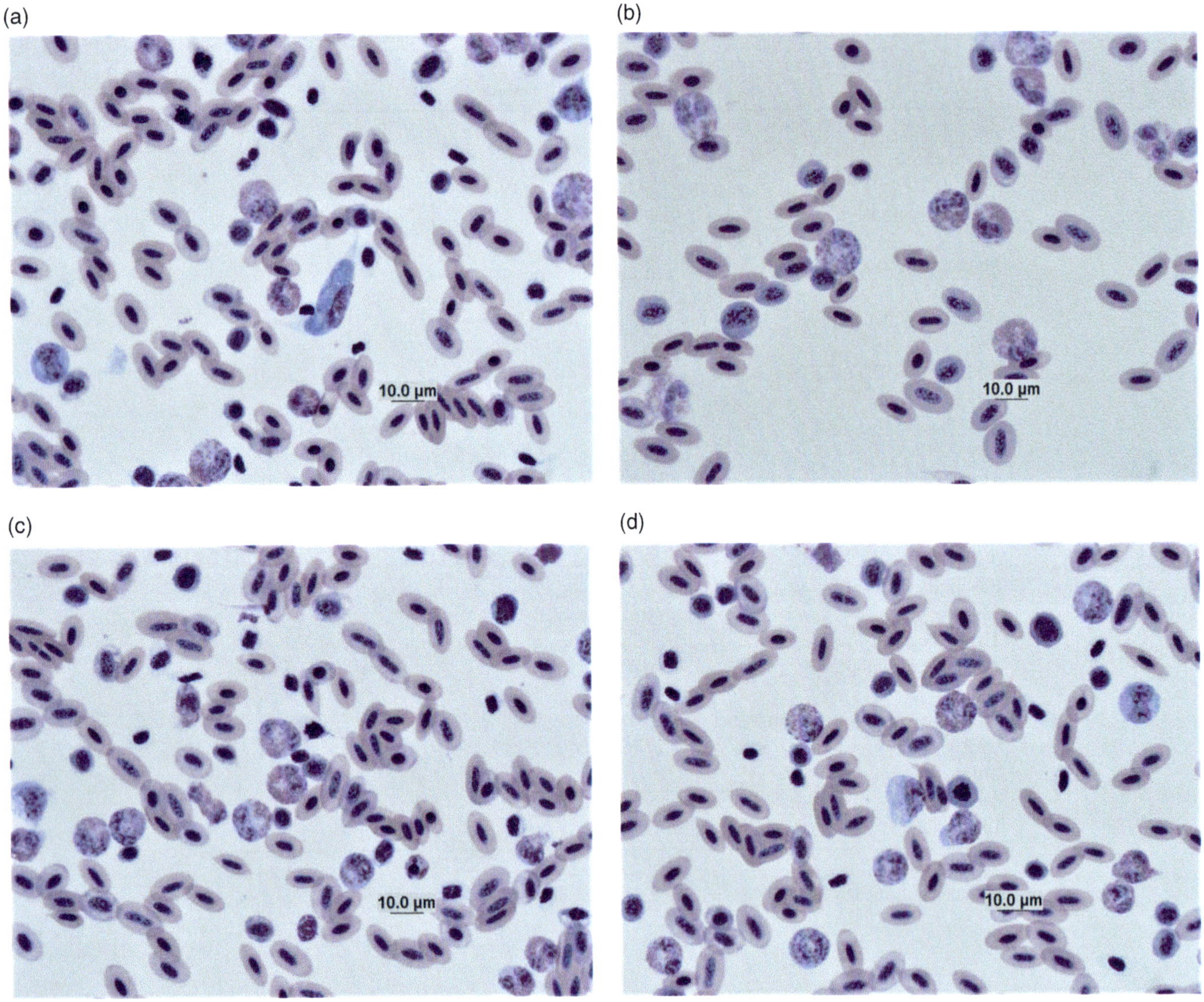

Fig. 13.16. (a)–(d) Blood film (Wright–Giemsa stain 100× oil).

References

Black PA, McRuer DL, Horne LA. 2018. Hematologic parameters in raptor species in a rehabilitation setting before release. *J Avian Med Surg* 25(3):192–198.

Carpenter JW. (ed) 2018. *Exotic Animal Formulary*, 5th edn. St. Louis: Elsevier Saunders, p. 287.

Scagnelli AM, Tully TN. 2017. Reproductive disorders in parrots. In: Jekl V (ed),*Vet Clin North Am (Exotic Anim Pract): Reproductive Medicine*. Philadelphia, PA: Elsevier.

14 Sample Collection for Avian Cytodiagnosis

Review of cytology sampling and evaluation techniques for mammals in Chapter 6 will be helpful in collection and evaluation of samples obtained from avian patients.

Alimentary Tract

Examination of the oral cavity during the routine physical examination of avian patients may reveal excessive mucus, plaques, nodules, or ulcers (Figures 14.1a–14.1c). The differential diagnosis of these lesions includes candidiasis, trichomoniasis, bacterial abscessation, and squamous cell hyperplasia due to hypovitaminosis A. Caseous lesions in the oropharynx of birds have been associated with trichomoniasis, hypovitaminosis A, capillariasis, candidiasis, and bacterial infections (Samour et al., 1995; Heindenreich, 1995; Boydell and Forbes, 1996; Samour, 1999; Samour, 2000).

Cytological examination of smears made from a swab or scraping of the lesion will often prove the presumptive or definitive diagnosis. A swab of the exfoliated cells from an oral lesion can be rolled onto a clean slide for microscopic examination; however, not all masses exfoliate well. For example, rubbing a swab over an encapsulated mass usually will not yield a diagnostic/cellular sample (Bellows, 2011). Masses found in the oral cavity can be aspirated or excised to obtain a cytological sample.

Cytological samples of the esophagus are indicated whenever lesions are detected by palpation or by endoscopy. A cytologic sample can be obtained by a touch imprint of a biopsy sample or a brush cytologic preparation. A sample can also be obtained by passing a sterile cotton swab through the oral cavity into the esophageal lumen. An oral speculum should be used in animals capable of biting and breaking the swab.

Cytologic evaluation of the crop (ingluvies) content of birds is indicated by clinical signs of vomiting, frequent regurgitation other than normal courtship behavior, delayed crop emptying, and other crop disorders. A crop aspirate can be obtained by inserting a sterile, soft plastic or rubber feeding tube into the mouth and esophagus and directing the end into the crop. The tube should pass freely and not be forced into the crop. The procedure should be stopped if any resistance is encountered, to avoid puncture of the esophageal or crop walls. The bird's head and neck should be extended during the procedure to straighten the esophagus and minimize puncture of the thin esophageal wall. Palpation of the tube as it passes through the esophagus or a visual check of the tube path in the mouth can be made to ensure proper tube placement. The crop content is gently aspirated into the sterile syringe attached to the free end of the tube. Excessive negative pressure should be avoided to prevent ischemic lesions, which may result if the tube opening lies against the crop mucosa. A crop wash can be obtained by infusing a small amount (10–15 mL/kg body weight) of sterile isotonic saline into the crop and aspirating the fluid for cytologic evaluation.

Cytologic evaluation of the stomach and intestines is complicated by the presence of many bacteria and much cell debris. Samples are obtained by gastric washes, endoscopy, or exploratory surgery.

Evaluation of the cloacal cytology is indicated whenever inflammation of the cloaca, cloacal prolapse, or cloacal masses is found during the physical examination of a bird. Cloacal cytology and microbiology are often a part of the routine physical examination of pet birds. Cloacal samples from birds are easily obtained by inserting a sterile, saline-moistened, cotton-tipped swab into the cloaca; feathers surrounding the vent must not

Exotic Animal Hematology and Cytology, Fifth Edition. Terry W. Campbell and Krystan R. Grant.

Companion website: www.wiley.com/go/campbell/exotic

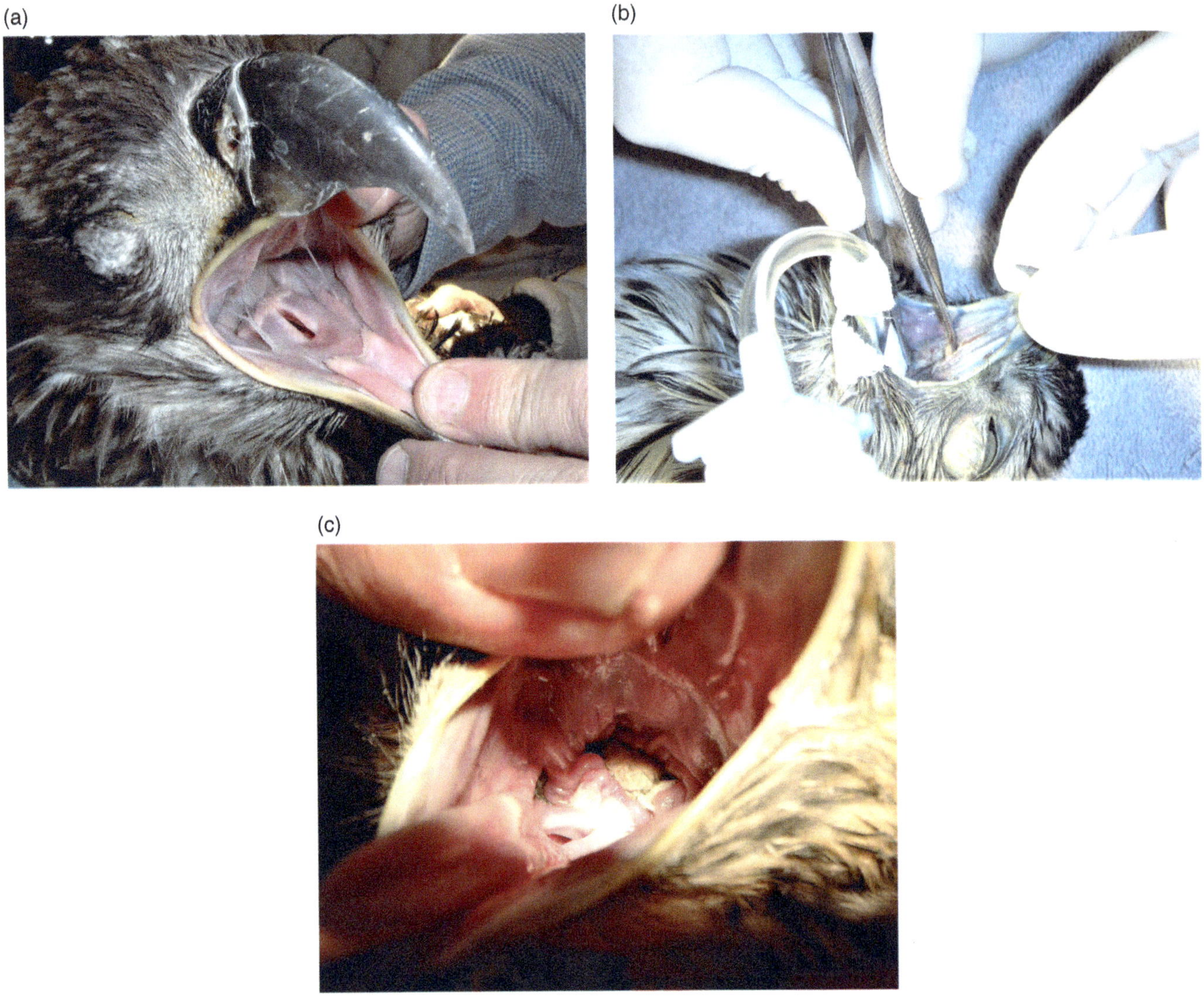

Fig. 14.1. (a) Examination of the mouth of a golden eagle (*Aquila chrysaetos*) shows the position of the rima glottis in the oral cavity, and therefore cytologic material obtained in this area may originate from the respiratory tract. (b) A northern goshawk (*Accipiter gentilis*) with trichomoniasis identified by cytodiagnosis from a sample obtained from the oral cavity. (c) A Swainson's hawk (*Buteo swainsoni*) with an abscess involving the esophagus and ingluvies identified by cytodiagnosis from a sample obtained through the oral cavity.

be touched (Figure 14.2). Fine-needle aspiration biopsy of solid masses or contact films made from excised masses often provides useful cytological samples.

Respiratory Tract

The nasal and infraorbital sinuses of birds and reptiles are lined with nonkeratinized squamous epithelium (Banks, 1974). As in mammals, this also transitions into ciliated pseudostratified columnar epithelium with goblet cells. Pseudostratified columnar epithelium consists of ciliated columnar cells extending from the basement membrane to the lumen, goblet cells, and reserve cells. Reserve cells are small, polygonal cells adjacent to the basement membrane. The glottis is the opening into the trachea of birds and reptiles and is situated at the base of the tongue in most species. The trachea is lined by ciliated pseudostratified columnar epithelium with goblet cells. The syrinx is located at or near the junction of the trachea and bronchi. Its mucosa consists of either bistratified squamous or columnar epithelium (Banks, 1974).

A choanal swab is used as a sampling technique for a screening procedure as part of a wellness examination or in the cytologic diagnosis of upper respiratory disease in birds. The mouth of birds with powerful biting capability is held open using an oral speculum or two gauze loops. A cotton-tip applicator is used to swab the

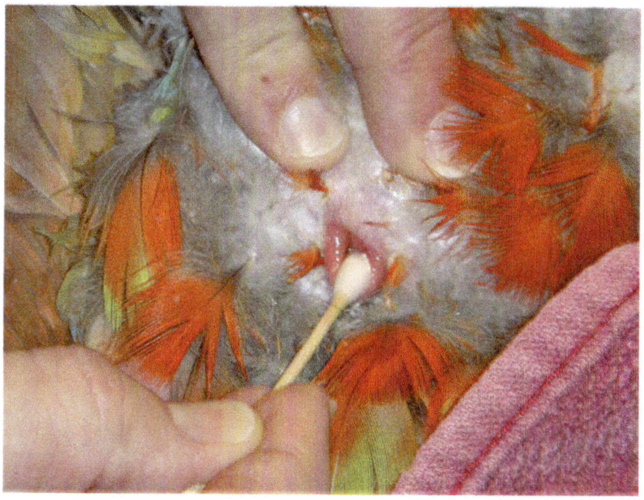

Fig. 14.2. Collection of a cytology sample from the cloaca using a cotton-tipped swab.

nasopharynx dorsal to the choanal slit taking care as to not touch other areas of the oral cavity. The swab is rolled onto a glass slide. Often, cells from the oral cavity contaminate the sample.

A nasal or sinus flush technique is a modification of the choanal swab method. This method is best performed with the bird anesthetized. A cotton swab is placed into the choanal to collect the cytologic sample as sterile saline is flushed into each of the nares (Graham, 1994). The hub of the flushing syringe is placed firmly against the nares to flush the nasal passages.

Because of the likelihood of contamination of the sample from the oral cavity using the choanal swab or nasal flush methods, endoscopy-guided sampling of the choanal slit and internasal septum is a better technique. This allows direct visualization and sampling of lesions using either a rigid or flexible endoscope (Murray and Taylor, 1998).

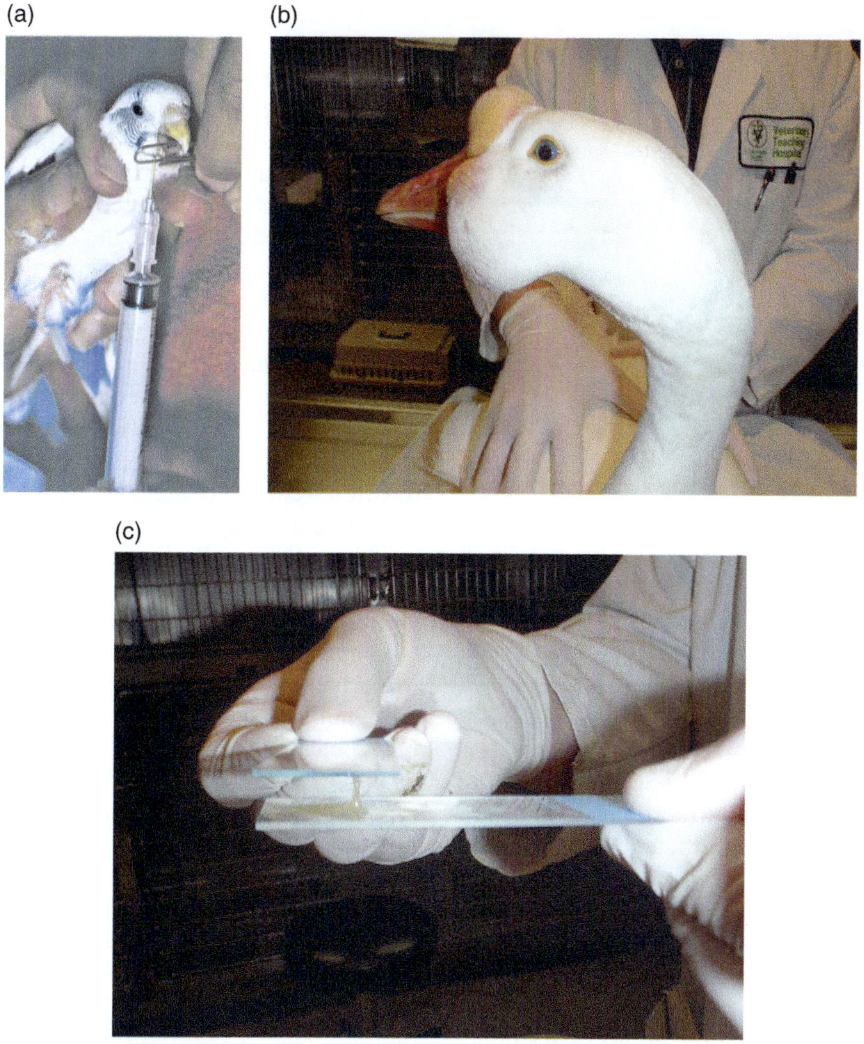

Fig. 14.3. (a) Performing a sinus aspirate from a budgerigar (*Melopsittacus undulatus*). (b) Chinese crested goose (*Anser cygnoid*) with sinusitis. (c) Viscous fluid obtained from the sinus of the Chinese crested goose (*Anser cygnoid*) in Figure 14.3b. See Chapter 6 for sample preparation of viscous fluids.

(a) (b)

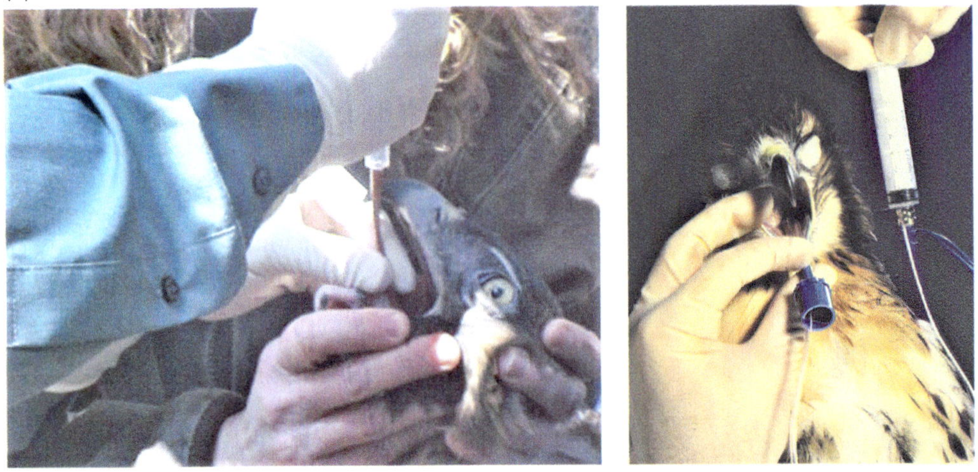

Fig. 14.4. (a) Obtaining a tracheal wash sample from a golden eagle (*Aquila chrysaetos*) by directly passing the collection tube into the trachea. (b) Obtaining a tracheal wash sample from a red-tailed hawk (*Buteo jamaicensis*) by passing the collection tube through an endotracheal tube and into the trachea.

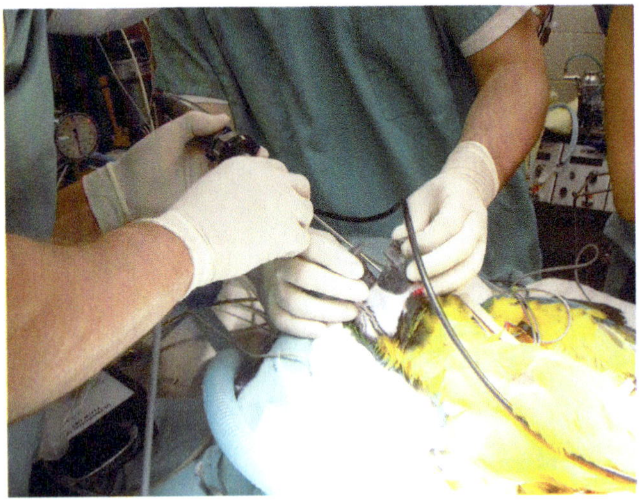

Fig. 14.5. Cytologic samples can be collected during direct examination of the trachea of an anesthetized bird using a small rigid endoscope.

Sinus aspiration of birds with sinusitis allows sampling of the sinus content with a minimal amount of surface contamination; this is especially important for microbial culturing (Figures 14.3a–14.3c). One method of sinus aspiration samples the infraorbital (paranasal) sinus in an area midway between the eye and external nares. The bird's head is held firmly, and proper limb and body restraint is applied. A needle (e.g., 22 gauge) with a syringe attached is inserted at the commissure of the mouth and directed vertically to a point midway between the eye and external nares passing under the zygomatic (or jugal) bone (Figure 14.3a). This bone crosses diagonally from the lower corner of the upper beak to the ear. An oral speculum can be used to hold the mouth open to provide a larger lateral surface at the aspiration site, thus facilitating the passage of the needle under the zygomatic bone. The needle should be held parallel to the skin. Peripheral blood contamination of the sample may occur if the surrounding muscle mass is penetrated. Also, misdirection of the needle caudally may cause penetration of the ocular orbit. This method of sinus aspiration applies primarily to psittacine birds.

A second method samples the sinus immediately ventral to the eye. Two approaches can be used. One is to approach the sinus at a perpendicular angle, entering the sinus directly. The second approach is to enter the sinus from a rostral direction by inserting the needle just caudal to the commissure of the mouth. The needle is directed ventral to the zygomatic arch, ending in the sinus under the eye.

Once the needle is inserted into a sinus, the sinus content can be aspirated into the needle lumen by syringe. Sinusitis leading to periorbital swelling is common in companion birds (Karpinski and Clubb, 1986; Millichamp, 1991). The left and right infraorbital sinuses communicate in some avian species (e.g., psittacine birds) but may not in others (e.g., passerine birds). For example, a single aspirate from one side of a parrot will represent the sinus material on both sides, whereas a bilateral sinusitis in a canary may require bilateral aspirations. See Chapter 6 for sample preparation of viscous fluids (Figure 14.3c).

A tracheal wash is indicated in birds with clinical signs of respiratory disease (e.g., exercise intolerance, persistent coughing, a change in the voice, or dyspnea); radiographic or endoscopic evidence of lower respiratory disease; or detection of tracheal lesions by transillumination of the trachea. Respiratory tract infections in birds (e.g., aspergillosis) are often diagnosed from tracheal wash samples when radiographic evaluation has failed to demonstrate the lesion.

The procedure for tracheal wash sampling of birds may require general anesthesia; however, many properly restrained unanesthetized birds tolerate the procedure because of the ease of access through the rima glottis. The advantage of an unanesthetized bird is its ability to cough following the procedure to aid in the clearing of the airways of any remaining fluid. An appropriately sized, sterile, soft plastic or rubber tube or catheter is passed through the glottis into the trachea (Figures 14.4a and 14.4b). An oral speculum should be used on unanesthetized psittacine birds that can bite off the tube. Sterile, non-bacteriostatic saline is infused into the trachea after the tube has been passed as far as possible (near the syrinx at the thoracic inlet) and then quickly aspirated back into the tube. Excessive fluid infusion should be avoided. A saline volume of 1.0–2.0 mL /kg body weight is generally a safe amount for birds. The procedure using an endotracheal tube in the anesthetized bird as described for mammals can be used in larger birds. Care should be taken in avoiding contamination of the sample with material from the oropharynx. A sterile cotton swab passed down the trachea can also be used to obtain samples of the cranial part of the trachea for cytology or culture. It should be noted that in some birds the tracheal bifurcation lies close to the glottis; therefore, a sample obtained from the healthy side of a unilateral tracheobronchitis would yield false-negative cytologic results.

Direct examination of the trachea of larger birds by endoscopy is performed using either a small, rigid or flexible endoscope (Taylor, 1997; Murray and Taylor, 1998). The neck is fully extended during the procedure to allow easy passage of the endoscope and to prevent perforation of the trachea (Figure 14.5). Endoscopy allows for direct visualization of the trachea and syrinx. Cytologic samples of lesions are obtained either from contact smears from a biopsy or using the brush technique. Available equipment limits the use of bronchoalveolar lavage and bronchial brush biopsy using a fiber-optic bronchoscope in small mammals and lower vertebrate species.

Endoscopy can be used for direct visualization of the lungs and air sacs of birds. The caudal part of the lung and caudal thoracic and abdominal air sacs are visualized using a single endoscopic approach (Taylor, 1997; Murray and Taylor, 1998). The approach can be either from the right or left flank depending upon the location of the lesion based on radiographic findings. Endoscopy allows for direct visualization and sampling of lung and air sac lesions (Figures 14.6a–14.6d). Samples can be obtained for cytological examination (Figures 14.6c–14.6e)

Air sac lavage as a diagnostic tool in birds can be obtained by infusing saline into the trachea and collecting the sample from the air sacs (Fulton et al., 1990; DeRosa et al., 1992). Because cells that line the respiratory tract vary depending upon location, the cells obtained from the air sacs using the tracheal wash method contain cells that do not originate in the air sacs. Endoscopic-directed air sac lavage allows for site-specific sample collection of cytologic samples of the avian air sacs (Crespo et al., 1998). An air sac wash is performed with the anesthetized bird in right or left lateral recumbency. The skin in the area caudal to the last rib, ventral to the synsacrum, and cranial to the femur is aseptically prepared. A small skin incision is made just below the synsacrum, caudal to the last rib, and cranial to the thigh muscle (iliotibialis cranialis muscle). Small hemostats are used to bluntly dissect through the abdominal muscles and puncture the underlying air sacs. A rigid laparoscope or sterile otoscope cone is used to examine the caudal thoracic and abdominal air sacs, caudal aspect of the lung, and internal organs. Samples are collected from the observed lesions using biopsy instruments or a sterile swab passed through an otoscope cone. Sterile physiologic saline is infused through the biopsy channel of a laparoscope or the cone of an otoscope using sterile tubing. After infusion of saline into the air sacs, the bird is rotated with the cranial aspect of the body and the head elevated to keep the wash sample in the air sacs and prevent the saline from entering the lungs. The saline is aspirated quickly and prepared for cytologic examination and culture. Air sac washes from healthy birds have low cellularity and require centrifugation to concentrate the cells. In one study, optimal cell morphology was achieved when the sample was centrifuged at a speed of 1000 rpm (89.4 × gravity) and prepared less than an hour from the time of collection (Crespo et al., 1998). The addition of protein (bovine serum) helped preserve cell quality.

Lymphoid Tissue of Lower Vertebrates

Most species of the lower vertebrates do not possess lymph nodes; however, solitary lymphoid aggregates may occur. For example, in birds, lymphoid aggregates occur as nodules in the walls of the digestive tract, abdominal organs, serous membranes, and skin (e.g., combs of Galliforme birds). Cecal tonsils, which are well-developed lymphoid tissue, occur in the proximal portion of the cecum of some birds. The bursa of Fabricius is a blind sac that opens on the dorsal wall of the proctodeum. The lymph nodules of the avian bursa of Fabricius form follicular-like structures. The spleen is one of the largest single masses of lymphoid tissue in the body of lower vertebrates. Also, many lymphoid aggregates occur throughout the liver.

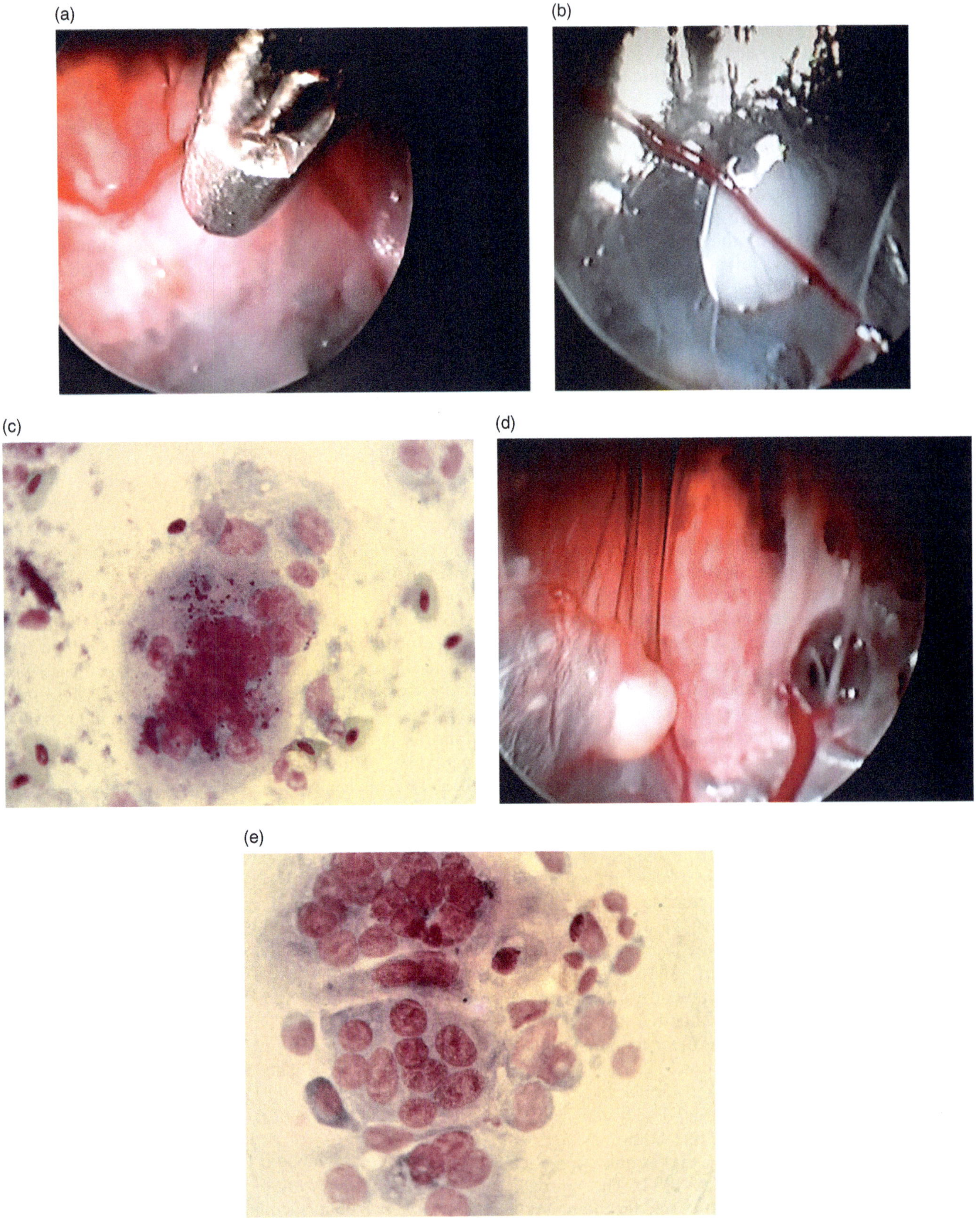

Fig. 14.6. (a) Endoscopy allows for direct visualization and sampling of lung and air sac lesions in birds. (b) An air sac lesion in a thick-billed parrot (*Rhynchopsitta pachyrhyncha*) as viewed through an endoscopic procedure. (c) Multinucleated giant cell in an imprint of a biopsy obtained from the air sac lesion in Figure 14.6b in a thick-billed parrot (*Rhynchopsitta pachyrhyncha*) during an endoscopic procedure. (d) An air sac granuloma in a Timneh African gray parrot (*Psittacus erithacus timneh*) as viewed through an endoscopic procedure. (e) Multinucleated giant cells, macrophages, and plasma cells in an imprint of a biopsy obtained from the air sac lesion in Figure 1.6d in a Timneh African gray parrot (*Psittacus erithacus timneh*) during an endoscopic procedure.

(a) (b)

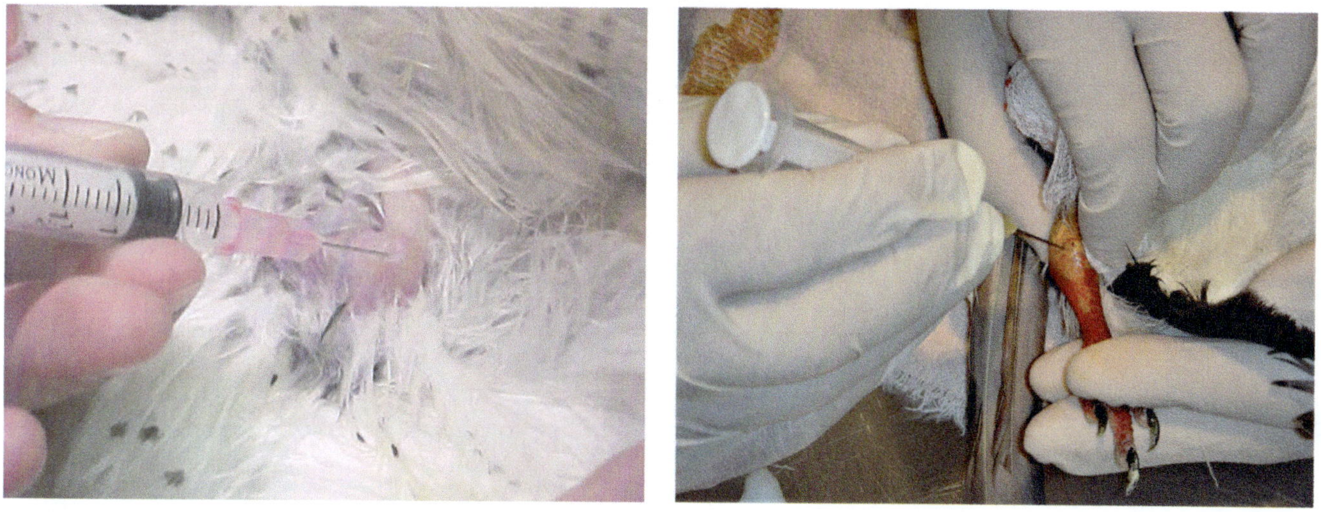

Fig. 14.7. (a) Aspiration of a bone cyst involving the elbow joint of a barn owl (*Tyto alba*). (b) Aspiration of a swollen tarsal joint in a pigeon (*Columbia livia*).

Conjunctiva and Cornea

Cytologic samples of the conjunctiva of birds can be obtained using the same procedures as those used in domestic mammal medicine. Corneal cytology is indicated in superficial erosions and in progressive ulceration associated with infiltrations of inflammatory cells. To obtain a sample for cytology, a topical anesthetic is instilled (1 or 2 drops) and after 60 s the sample is taken by gentle scraping or use of an ophthalmic swab (Bayón et al., 2007). It is important to remember that a topical anesthetic can cause systemic toxicity and even general anesthesia in the avian patient.

Synovial Fluid

Normally, the joints of birds contain a fluid volume that is too small for sampling or proper evaluation; however, fluid distension of a joint may occur with certain arthropathies, allowing for collection of enough synovial fluid for evaluation. To collect synovial fluid, the skin over the joint at the sampling site is prepared using aseptic techniques as one would use for surgery. A 22-gauge (or smaller) needle and syringe (usually a 3-cc syringe) is used to aspirate the synovial fluid sample (Figures 14.7a and 14.7b). Identification of the best site for needle insertion is made by palpation and flexion of the joint. The needle is inserted through the joint capsule, and fluid is withdrawn into the syringe once the joint cavity has been entered. Negative pressure in the syringe should be removed by releasing the plunger prior to removal of the needle from the joint. The sample is then used to prepare direct films using glass microscope slides for microscopic evaluation and fluid analysis if enough sample is obtained as described in Chapter 6.

Coelomic Fluid

Celiocentesis (aspiration of fluid from the coelomic cavity) may be performed on avian patients with fluid accumulation of the coelomic cavity to obtain a sample for cytologic examination. The procedure begins by surgical preparation of the aspiration site. A 21- to 25- gauge needle is inserted immediately distal to the point of the sternum (keel bone). The needle point is directed to the right side of the coelomic cavity to avoid puncture of the ventriculus (gizzard), which lies immediately to the left of the ventral midline, and fluid is aspirated into the sterile syringe (Figures 14.8a–14.8c). Use of extension tubing will help stabilize the needle during the aspiration process when a large volume of fluid is encountered.

A peritoneal wash in birds can be attempted by infusing sterile saline into the peritoneal space of the coelomic cavity and aspirating the fluid. This procedure can be difficult to perform in birds because it is difficult to avoid the abdominal air sacs in a normal bird.

For "Preparation for Cytologic Examination" and "Sample Preparation and Evaluation," see Chapter 6.

(a) (b) (c)

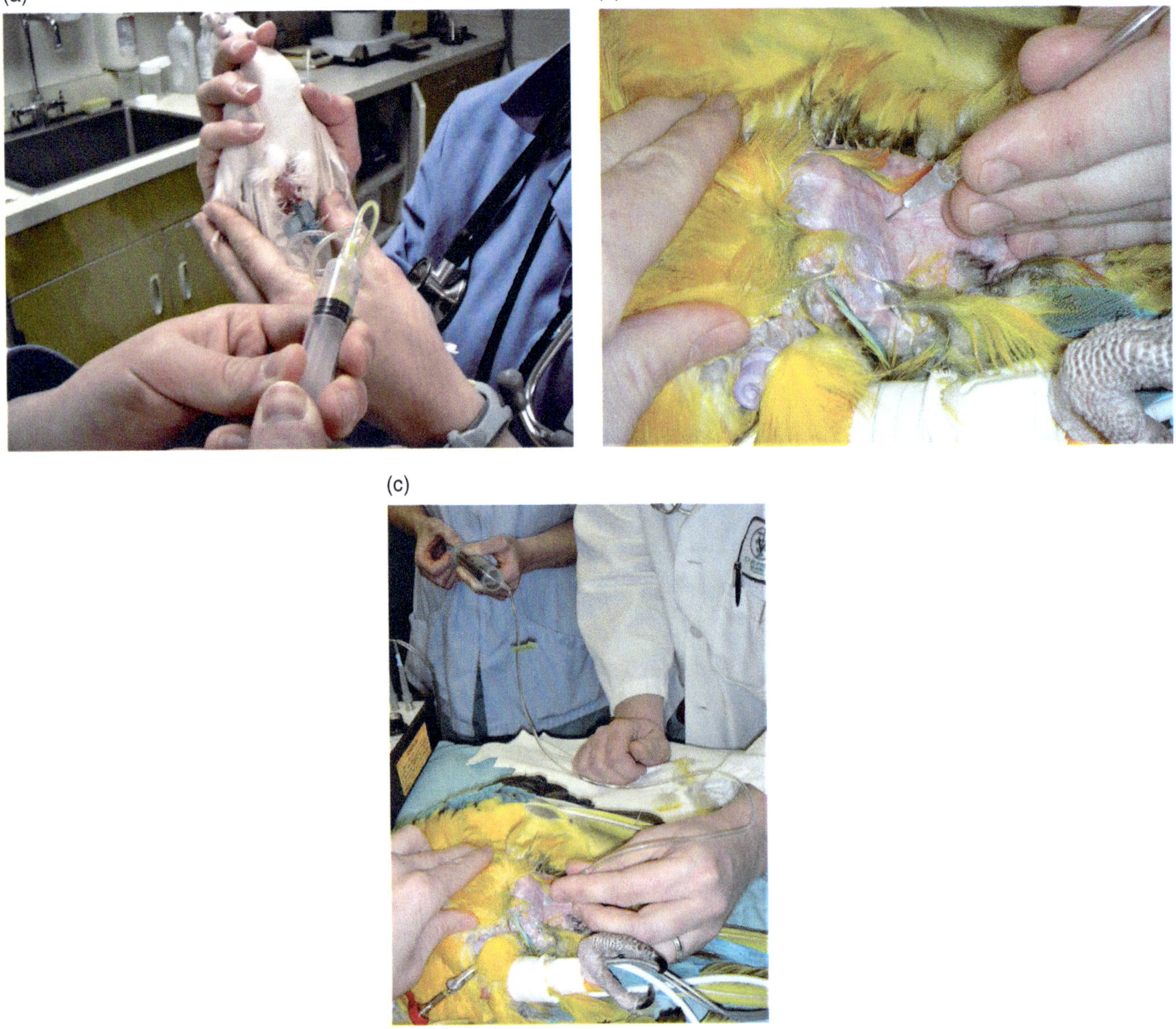

Fig. 14.8. (a) Aspiration of fluid from the coelomic cavity of a budgerigar (*Melopsittacus undulatus*). (b) Placement of a needle in preparation for the aspiration of fluid from the coelomic cavity of a blue and gold macaw (*Ara ararauna*). (c) Aspiration of fluid from the coelomic cavity of a blue and gold macaw (*Ara ararauna*).

References

Banks WJ. 1974. *Histology and Comparative Organology*. In: Banks W (ed), *Histology and Comparative Organology: A Text Atlas*. Baltimore, MD: Williams and Wilkins.

Bayón A, Almela RM, Talavera J. 2007. Avian ophthalmology. *EJCAP* 17(3):1–13.

Bellows J. 2011. Intraoral cytology. *DVM: The Newsmagazine of Veterinary Medicine* 42(9):2S–4S.

Boydell IP, Forbes NA. 1996. *Diseases of the head (including the eye)*. In: Beynon P, Forbes N, Harcourt-Brown N (eds), *Manual of Raptors, Pigeons, and Waterfowl*. Cheltenham, UK: British Small Animal Veterinary Association Ltd.

Crespo R, Stirtzinger T, Hunter DB. 1998. Evaluation of different procedures for processing avian air sac lavage fluid. *Avian Diseases* 42:20–27.

DeRosa M, Ficken MD, Barnes HJ. 1992. Acute airsacculitis in untreated and cyclophosphamide-pretreated broiler chickens inoculated with *Escherichia coli* or *Escherichia coli* cell-free culture filtrate. *Vet Pathol* 29:68–78.

Fulton RM, Reed WM, DeNicola DB. 1990. Light microscopic and ultrastructural characterization of cells recovered by respiratory-tract lavage of 2- and 6- week-old chickens. *Avian Diseases* 34:87–98.

Graham A. 1994. Nasal flushes for diagnosis and treatment. In: *Proceedings Association of Avian Veterinarians*. Reno.

Heindenreich M. 1995. *Birds of Prey: Medicine and Management.* In: Heindenreich M (ed), *Birds of Prey: Medicine and Management.* Munich: Blackwell Science.

Karpinski LG, Clubb SL. 1986. *Clinical aspects of ophthalmology in caged birds.* In: Kirk R (ed), *Current Veterinary Therapy IX* Philadelphia, PA: WB Saunders.

Millichamp NJ. 1991. Exotic animal ophthalmology. In: Gelatt K (ed), *Veterinary Ophthalmology*, 2 nd edn. Philadelphia, PA: Lea & Febiger.

Murray MJ, Taylor M. 1998. Endoscopic collection of diagnostic specimens from the respiratory system. In: *Proceedings Association Avian Veterinarians.* St. Paul, MN.

Samour JH, Bailey TA, Cooper JE. 1995. Trichomoniasis in birds of prey (Falconiformes) in Bahrain. *Vet Rec* 136:358–362.

Samour JH. 1999. Supraorbital trichomoniasis infection in two Saker falcons (*Falco cherrug*). *Vet Rec* 146:139–140.

Samour JH. 2000. *Pseudomonas aeruginosa* stomatitis as a sequel to trichomoniasis in captive Saker falcons (*Falco cherrug*). *J Avian Med Surg* 14:113–117.

Taylor M. 1997. Endoscopic diagnosis of avian respiratory tract disease. *Semin Avian Exotic Pet Med* 4:187–194.

15 Avian Cytodiagnosis

Normal Avian Cytology

Digestive Tract

The oral cavity is lined with cornified squamous epithelium, and the esophagus and ingluvies (crop) with noncornified stratified squamous epithelium. Normal exfoliation of the superficial cells of the epithelium lining the upper alimentary tract reveals normal, mature squamous epithelial cells (superficial and intermediate epithelial cells). These cells resemble those found in mammals (Figures 15.1 and 15.2). These cells often exfoliate singly, are angular, polygonal in shape, contain a condensed pyknotic nucleus, and demonstrate varying degrees of cornification. Cells that are highly cornified typically possess angular or folded cytoplasmic margins and are typically anucleated. Intermediate squamous epithelial cells are common in normal esophageal and crop specimens. Intermediate squamous epithelial cells often occur in sheets and are oval to polygonal in shape, have a low N:C ratio, and possess an oval, centrally located vesicular nucleus with a finely granular chromatin. These cells typically do not have folded cytoplasmic margins and resemble those found in mammals (Figure 15.3). Basal cells may be seen in normal cytology samples if traumatic exfoliation occurs during sample collection. Basal cells are cells that are normally found adjacent to the basement membrane and are smaller in size than intermediate cells. These cells are typically round and contain a deeply basophilic cytoplasm, eccentric nuclei, and high N:C ratio.

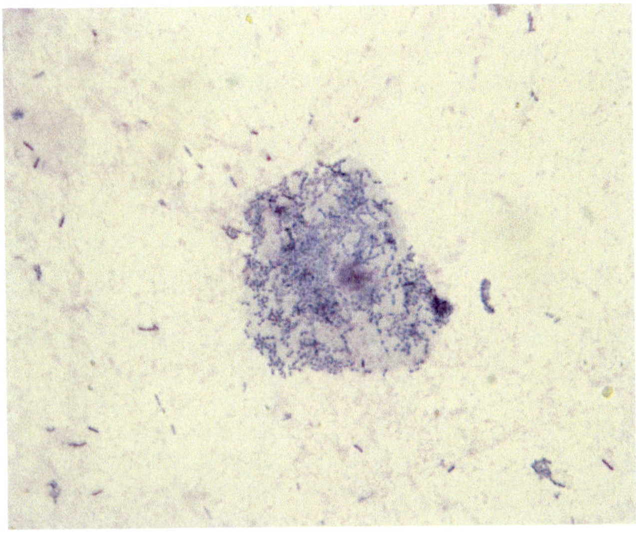

Fig. 15.1. Mature squamous epithelial cells, Wright–Giemsa stain (100× oil).

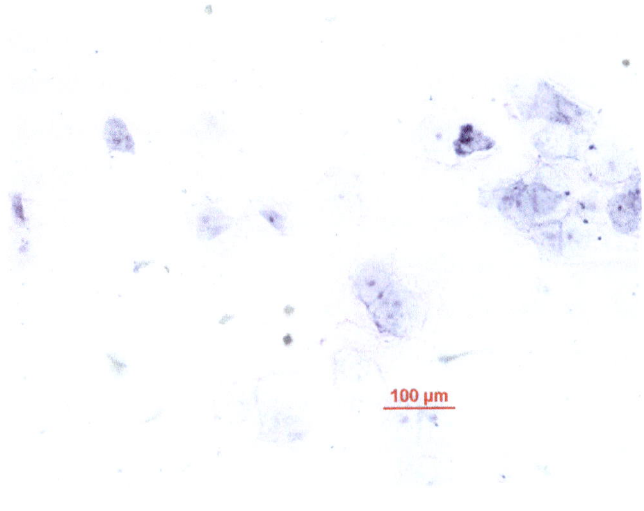

Fig. 15.2. Mature squamous epithelial cells from a crop aspirate of an African gray parrot (*Psittacus erithacus*), Wright–Giemsa stain.

Exotic Animal Hematology and Cytology, Fifth Edition. Terry W. Campbell and Krystan R. Grant.

Companion website: www.wiley.com/go/campbell/exotic

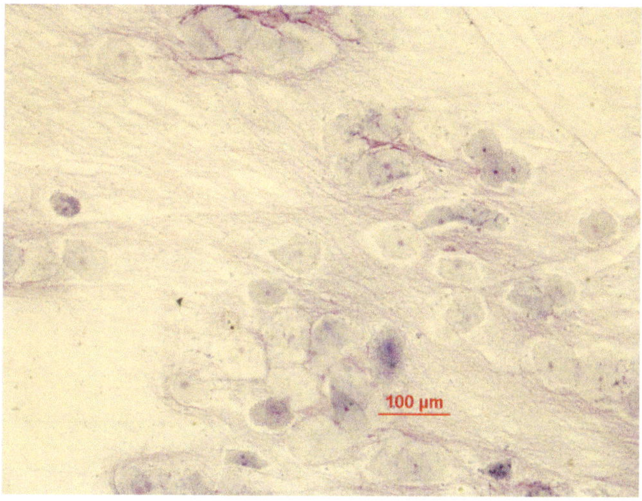

Fig. 15.3. Intermediate squamous epithelial cells from a crop aspirate of an African gray parrot (*Psittacus erithacus*), Wright–Giemsa stain.

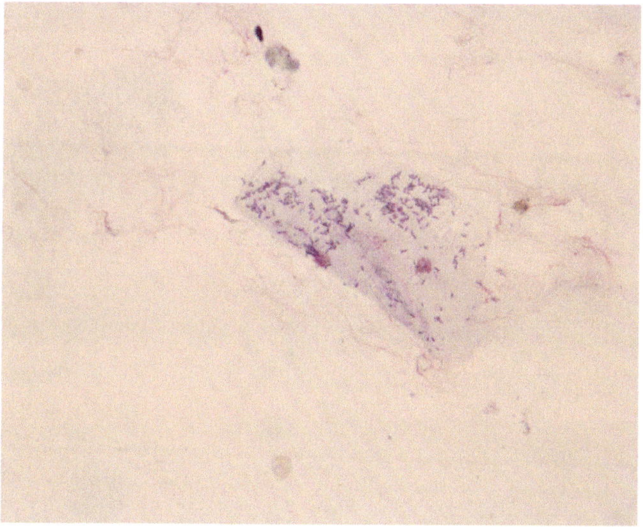

Fig. 15.4. Mature squamous epithelial cells with folded cytoplasmic margins from the oral cavity of an African gray parrot (*Psittacus erithacus*), Wright–Giemsa stain (100× oil).

Several extracellular bacteria represented by a variety of morphological types are often associated with squamous epithelial cells in normal cytological samples from the upper alimentary tract (Figures 15.4 and 15.5). Additionally, a moderate amount of background debris and foreign material (e.g., plant fibers and other material entering the mouth) is often present in samples obtained from the alimentary tract of animals. *Alysiella filiformis* is a normal bacterial inhabitant of the avian upper alimentary tract and should not be confused with infectious agents, such as fungi (Figures 15.6a and 15.6b). The organism occurs as pairs of unicellular bacteria arranged in unbranched, ribbonlike filaments and is related to *Simonsiella* spp., a rounded rectangular bacterium with

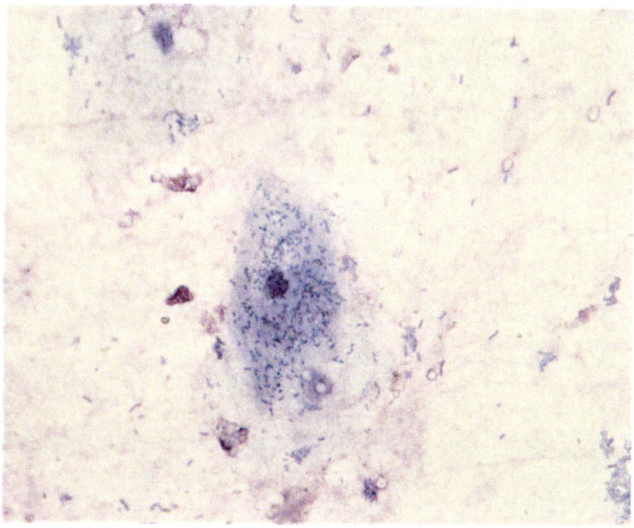

Fig. 15.5. Mature squamous epithelial cells with associated extracellular bacteria from a crop aspirate of an African gray parrot (*Psittacus erithacus*), Wright–Giemsa stain (100× oil).

cross-striations found in oropharyngeal samples of canids. Avian alimentary tract cytology samples may also contain amorphous or calcium carbonate crystals that may have originated from the diet (e.g., cuttlebone or grit), and urate crystals may be seen in samples obtained from coprophagous birds (Figure 15.7a). However, as with any cytologic specimen, contamination of the sample with starch or talc crystals from an examination glove may be found on the slide (Figure 15.7b). Rarely, Candida-like yeast may be present in normal samples from the avian upper alimentary tract.

The mucosa of the stomach is lined with columnar epithelial cells containing moderate amounts of lightly basophilic or eosinophilic cytoplasm, and oval to round nuclei with dispersed chromatin. Columnar epithelial cells tend to exfoliate in clusters of uniform-appearing cells.

The avian cloaca consists of three compartments: the coprodeum (the distal opening of the intestinal tract), the urodeum (the distal opening of the urinary and reproductive tracts), and the proctodeum (the common opening of the coprodeum and urodeum, which terminates at the vent). In birds, the cloacal bursa also opens into the proctodeum.

The cloaca is lined by simple columnar epithelium and lymphoid tissue, and the vent is lined by cornified, stratified squamous epithelium. If cells are present, there is a predominance of epithelial cells. Most of the epithelial cells from normal cloacal tissue appear as noncornified squamous (intermediate squamous epithelial cells) or columnar epithelial cells with a centrally or eccentrically positioned vesicular nucleus (Figure 15.3). Basal epithelial cells may be seen on films obtained by traumatic exfoliation. A variable quantity of bacteria made up of a wide variety of morphologic types, rare Candida-like yeast, and

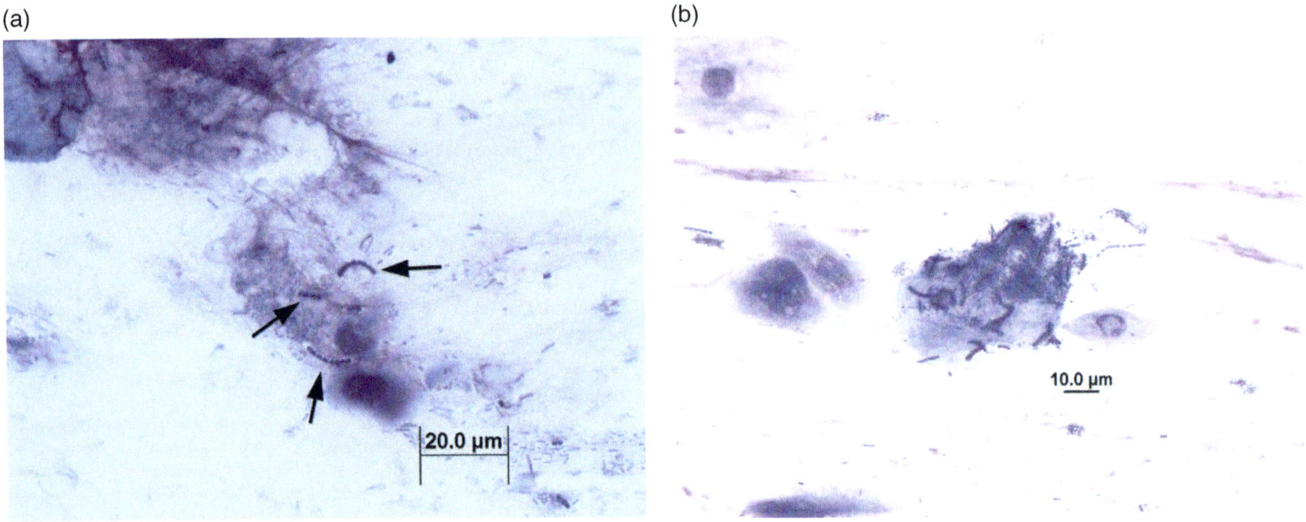

Fig. 15.6. (a) Mature squamous epithelial cell with associated extracellular *Alysiella filiformis* (arrows) from the oral cavity of a yellow-naped Amazon parrot (*Amazona auropalliata*), Wright–Giemsa stain. (b) Mature squamous epithelial cell with associated extracellular *Alysiella filiformis* from the oral cavity of a gentoo penguin (*Pygoscelis papua*), Wright–Giemsa stain.

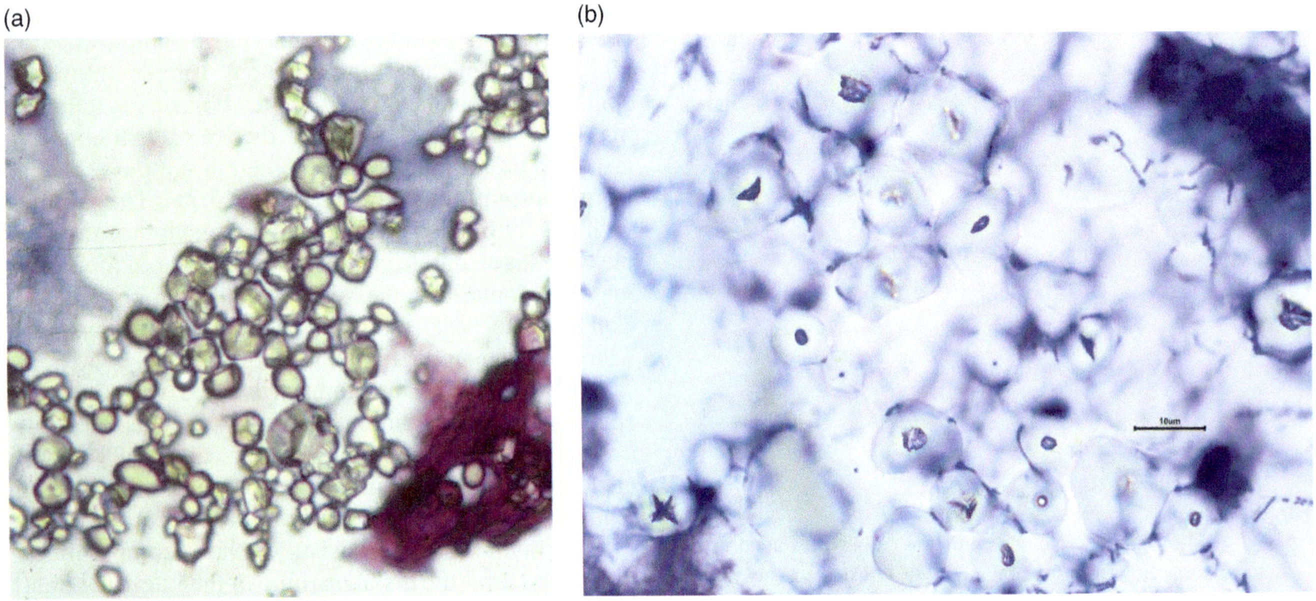

Fig. 15.7. (a) Crystals likely from the diet in a crop aspirate from a cockatiel (*Nymphicus hollandicus*), Wright–Giemsa stain (100× oil). (b) Crystals in a crop aspirate from a cockatiel (*Nymphicus hollandicus*) with a different appearance from those in Figure 15.7a are starch or talc crystal from an examination glove, Wright–Giemsa stain.

background debris are also present on normal specimens (Evans et al., 2014). Urate crystals are commonly seen in normal cloacal and fecal samples as well (Figures 15.8 and 15.9).

The normal gastrointestinal flora of healthy captive psittacine birds is composed predominately of gram-positive bacteria (Summa and Guzman, 2017). Overall, agreement between Gram stain and culture is fair, with a tendency for culture to underestimate the true diversity of bacterial flora (Evans et al., 2014). Because gram-negative bacteria do frequently occur, fecal Gram stains may be of higher value than culture as screening tests for health assessment in captive psittacines (Summa and Guzman, 2017). Fecal culture should be performed whenever abnormal Gram stains are obtained or the avian patient exhibits clinical signs of gastrointestinal disease.

Respiratory Tract

The nasal and infraorbital sinuses of birds are lined with nonkeratinized squamous epithelium that transitions into ciliated pseudostratified columnar epithelium

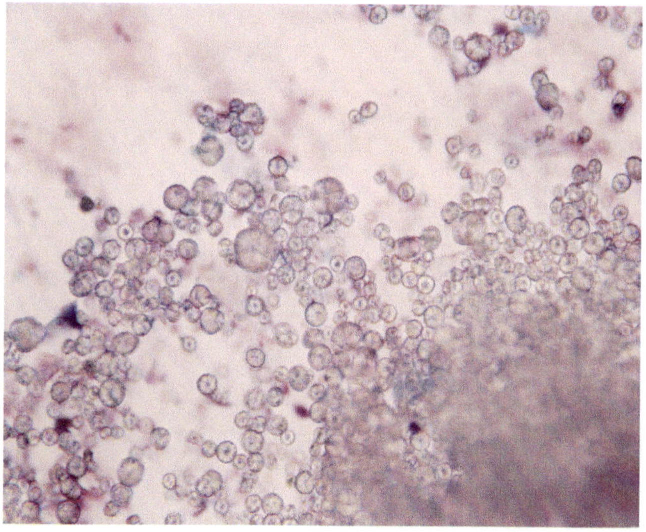

Fig. 15.8. Round urate crystals with a wagon-wheel-like appearance from the urinary tract of a bird. The crystals are frequently found in cloacal and fecal cytology specimens, Diff–Quik stain (100× oil).

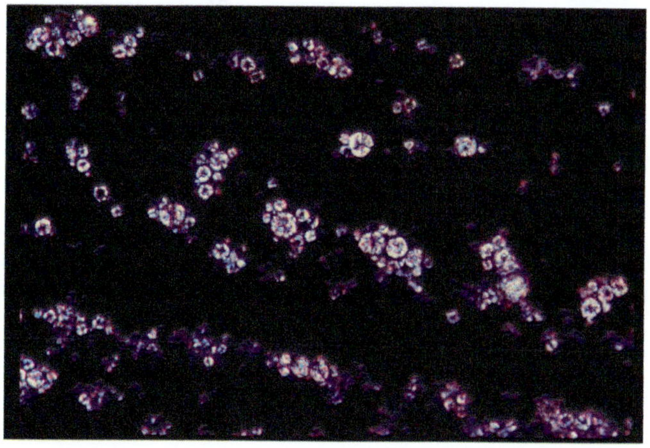

Fig. 15.9. Round urate crystals with a wagon wheel-like appearance from the urinary tract of a bird. These crystals are birefringent under polarized light, Diff–Quik stain (100× oil).

with goblet cells caudally, much as described for mammals (Banks, 1974). The glottis is the opening into the trachea of birds and reptiles and is situated at the base of the tongue in most species.

The trachea of birds is also lined by ciliated pseudostratified columnar epithelium with goblet cells, and extends from the glottis to the syrinx, which is located at or near the junction of the trachea and bronchi. The trachea of some birds, such as penguins, bifurcates a short distance in the cervical region; therefore, a tracheal wash sample usually results in the sampling of only one side. The mucosa of the syrinx consists of either bistratified squamous or columnar epithelium (Banks, 1974).

Samples collected from the respiratory system of normal healthy animals tend to be poorly cellular; however, when present, normal respiratory cells typically include ciliated epithelial cells, round to cuboidal epithelial cells, and macrophages. The normal respiratory epithelial cells and goblet cells of birds resemble those found in mammalian samples. Other cells that may occur less frequently in normal respiratory tract samples include heterophils, lymphocytes, eosinophils (rarely and depending upon the species), and goblet cells (Rebar et al., 1980; Padrid et al., 1991; Vail et al., 1995; Baker and Lumsden, 2000).

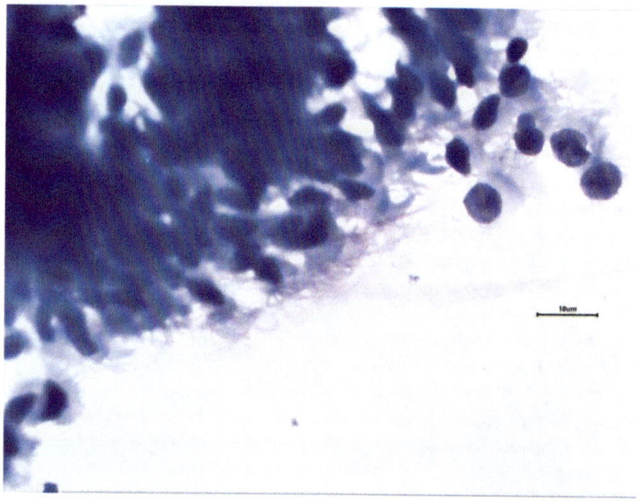

Fig. 15.10. Ciliated respiratory epithelial cells in a tracheal wash from an American kestrel (*Falco sparverius*), Wright–Giemsa stain.

Squamous epithelial cells may also be observed routinely as contaminants in tracheal wash fluids because these cells readily exfoliate from the oral mucosa onto the catheter or bronchoscope. These cells are large cells with abundant blue-gray cytoplasm and a central pyknotic nucleus, and often have adherent bacteria (Figures 15.2, 15.4, and 15.5). Some epithelial cells may be keratinized and have abundant hyalinized, basophilic cytoplasm with angular borders. Small, occasionally pyknotic or karyorrhectic nuclei are usually seen. Avian tracheal wash samples may contain squamous epithelial cells that may be of oral cavity origin or may originate from the lining of the syrinx. Round to cuboidal epithelial cells typically represent bronchiolar epithelial cells and contain a moderate amount of basophilic cytoplasm and a round, centrally positioned nucleus, and typically exfoliate individually or in sheets. The macrophages present in samples collected from the respiratory tract are typically large, highly vacuolated cells that may contain phagocytized material.

Ciliated respiratory epithelial cells are derived from the trachea and bronchi, and tend to exfoliate singly or in clusters. These cells may vary in size and shape, but generally appear as elongated columnar cells with a round to oval nucleus at one pole of the cell, and an abundant basophilic, often granular cytoplasm (Figures 15.10–15.12). Prominent eosinophilic cilia are present at the large end of the cell. The nucleus contains finely

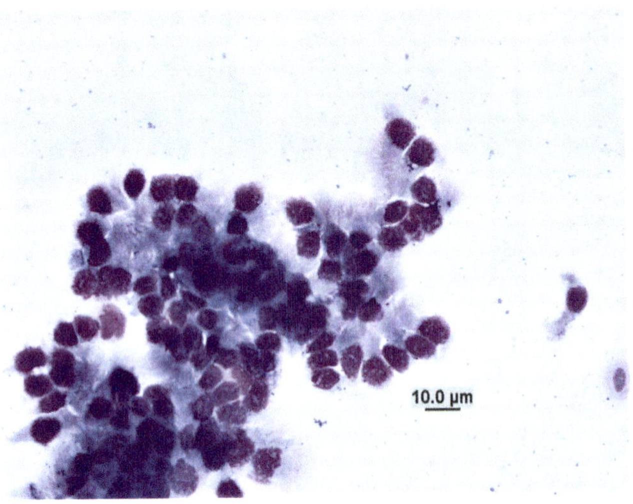

Fig. 15.11. Ciliated respiratory epithelial cells in a tracheal wash from a macaw (*Ara ararauna*), Wright–Giemsa stain. (100× oil).

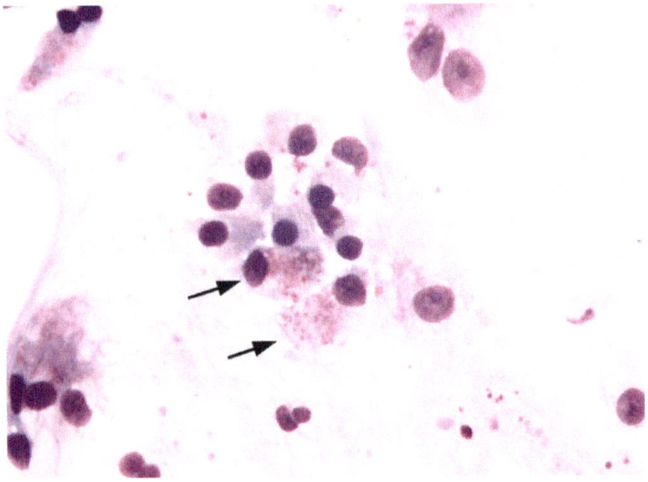

Fig. 15.13. Goblet cells (arrows) in a tracheal wash from a golden eagle (*Aquila chrysaetos*), Wright–Giemsa stain (100× oil).

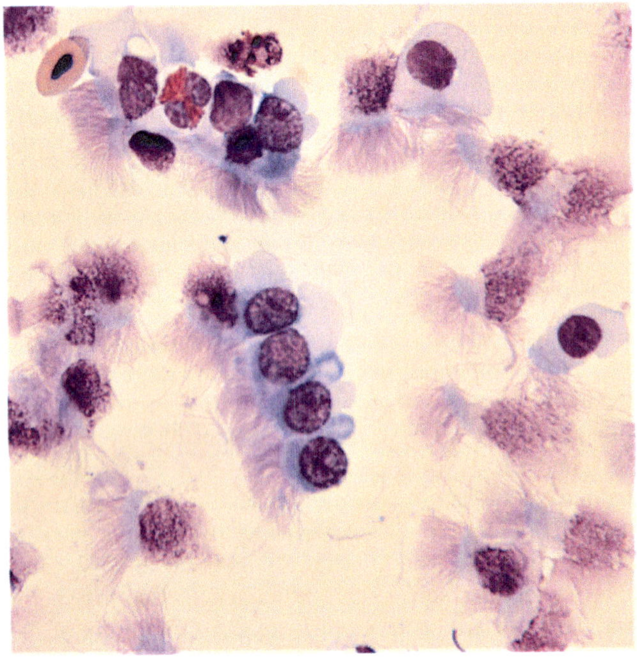

Fig. 15.12. Ciliated respiratory epithelial cells in a tracheal wash from a duck (*Anas platyrhynchos domestica*), Wright–Giemsa stain (100× oil). Source: Image from Campbell and Grant (2010, p. 77).

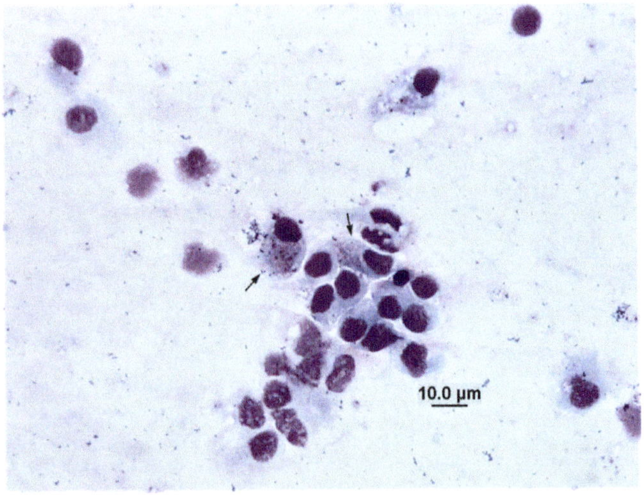

Fig. 15.14. Goblet cells (arrows) in a tracheal wash from a blue and gold macaw (*Ara ararauna*), Wright–Giemsa stain.

granular chromatin with prominent nucleoli and lies on the small pole of the cell opposite the cilia.

Goblet cells exfoliate singly or in clusters and appear as columnar cells that resemble ciliated respiratory epithelial cells, but lack the cilia (Figures 15.13 and 15.14). The cytoplasm is abundant and contains vacuoles and round, uniform eosinophilic granules that frequently distend the cytoplasmic borders. The nucleus is large, round to oval, and basilar in location within the cell. Goblet cells secret mucin, which often appears in the background of air-dried smears stained with Romanowsky stains as amorphous ribbons of lightly basophilic or eosinophilic material. Mucus often entraps cells, making them difficult to identify. Spiral casts of basophilic mucus, called Curschmann's spirals, are seen in association with excessive mucus production (Baker and Lumsden, 2000).

Air sac washes from healthy birds typically have low cellularity and require centrifugation to concentrate the cells. In one study, optimal cell morphology was achieved when the sample was centrifuged at a speed of 1000 rpm (89.4 × gravity) and prepared less than an hour from the time of collection (Crespo et al., 1998). The addition of protein (bovine serum) helped preserve cell quality.

Skin

The skin is composed of the epidermis and dermis. The epidermis is composed of a basal layer, intermediate layer, and a transitional layer (stratum corneum) that is composed of cornified cells that contain keratin (Lucas and Stettenheim, 1972; King and McLelland, 1984). Avian skin is typically thinner than mammalian skin, attaches to muscles at various sites, and contains feather follicles, feathers, and very few glands. It has been suggested that the lipid production of the keratinocytes in the skin of birds makes the entire skin an oil-producing holocrine gland (Cooper and Harrison, 1997).

Normal cytology of skin samples contains the cellular elements of the epidermis and possibly the dermis. Normal mature squamous epithelial cells (keratinocytes) are either anucleate or have a single, small, condensed oval nucleus, with abundant glassy, turquoise cytoplasm, consistent with keratinization when stained with Romanowsky-type stains. Low numbers of bacteria, predominately coccoid, are often found in close association with keratinocytes.

A variable amount of debris and extracellular bacteria (represented by a variety of morphological types) are often present as well. The debris often includes fragments of adnexal structures, such as feathers and variable-sized basophilic structures that resemble yeast (Figures 15.15a and 15.15b). These round to oval, 2–5 micron, deeply basophilic structures have irregular borders, and homogenous staining characteristics represent feather dust (Rosenthal et al., 2004; Schlein et al., 2019). Often, smaller and larger feather dust structures that are adjacent to each other resemble budding yeast or appear similar in size and shape to *Malassezia* yeast organisms (Preziosi et al., 2006; Schlein et al., 2019). However, unlike budding yeast, these structures lack the narrow- or broad-based connection. Feather dust structures result from the degradation of powder down feathers that cover the skin and feathers of birds. Feather dust structures stain positive with multicytokeratin (AE1/AE3) and Masson's trichrome staining indicative of keratinaceous origin (Schlein et al., 2019). Although powder down feathers are rich in lipid, they do not stain positively with the lipid stain Oil Red O (Menon and Menon, 2000; Schlein et al., 2019).

Eye

The conjunctival mucosa is composed of pseudostratified columnar epithelium with numerous goblet cells (Banks, 1974). The portion of the conjunctiva that lines the fornix (the junction of the upper and lower conjunctiva) is lined with stratified cuboidal epithelium. The portion of the conjunctiva (bulbar conjunctiva) that is continuous with the corneal epithelium consists of stratified nonkeratinized epithelium.

The normal cytology of a conjunctival scraping or brush specimen consists of epithelial cells and goblet cells. The background may contain variable amounts of mucus, which appears as strands of lightly basophilic amorphous material. Conjunctival scraping samples often contain cornified squamous epithelial cells derived from the margins of the eyelids (Figure 15.16). The conjunctival epithelial cells present in the sample appear uniformly polygonal, and often contain basophilic

(a)

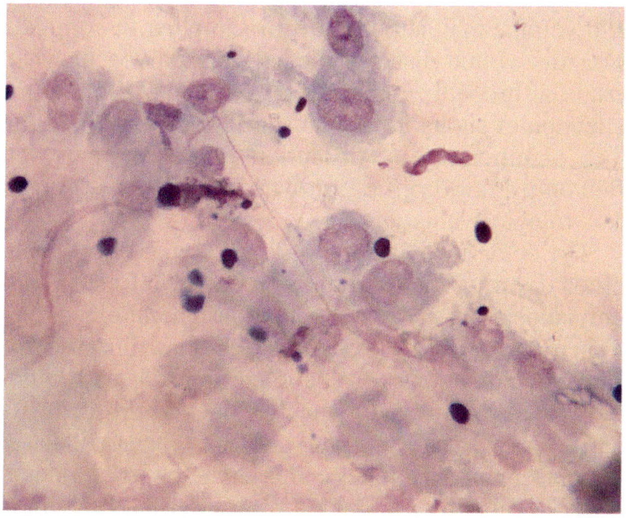

(b)

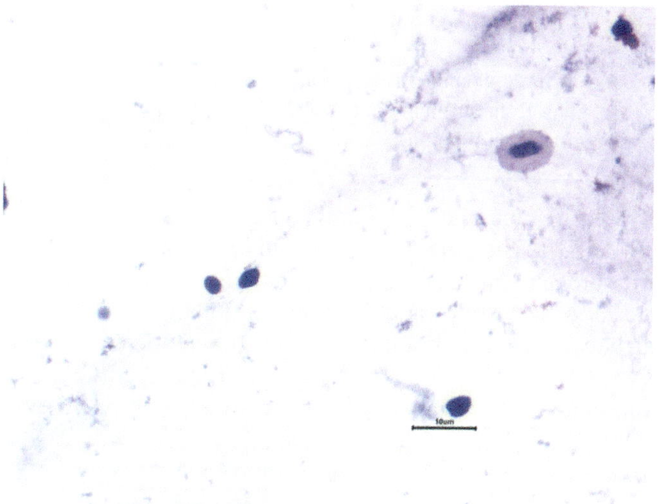

Fig. 15.15. (a) Epithelial cells and fragments of adnexal structures, variable-sized basophilic structures (feather dust) that resemble yeast, in a feather pulp imprint from a blue-fronted Amazon parrot (*Amazona aestiva*), Wright–Giemsa stain (100× oil). (b) Variable-sized basophilic structures (feather dust) that resemble yeast, in a feather pulp imprint from an eclectus parrot (*Eclectus roratus*), Wright–Giemsa stain.

Fig. 15.16. Cornified squamous epithelial cells likely from the margins of the eyelid in a conjunctival scraping derived from a black-neck stilt (*Himantopus mexicanus*), Wright–Giemsa stain (100× oil).

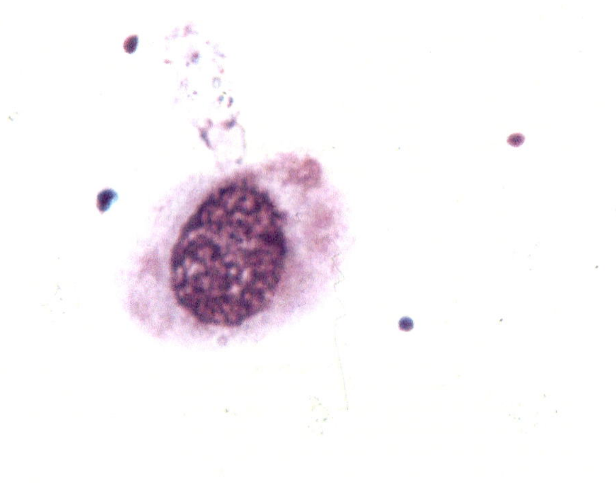

Fig. 15.17. Conjunctival epithelial cell in the conjunctival scraping from an umbrella cockatoo (*Cacatua alba*), Wright–Giemsa stain (100× oil).

cytoplasm and large, round nuclei (Figures 15.17 and 15.18). The goblet cells typically exfoliate singly or in aggregates and contain abundant foamy cytoplasm and large secretory vacuoles. Some goblet cells contain purple cytoplasmic granules. The nuclei are located next to the cell margin. The most frequent flora present in the conjunctival sac in psittacines includes gram-positive bacteria (*Staphylococcus epidermidis*, *Staphylococcus aureus*, β-hemolytic *Streptococcus* and *Corynebacterium* sp.); gram-negative bacteria are rare and only reported to be isolated from 1% of samples (Bayón et al., 2007).

The nictitating membrane of birds is covered by nonkeratinized stratified squamous epithelium on the palpebral and bulbar surfaces. Variable quantities of lymphoid aggregates are found on the bulbar surface. Because of these lymphoid aggregates, numerous plasma cells are often found within the gland of the nictitating membrane of birds (McLelland, 1991).

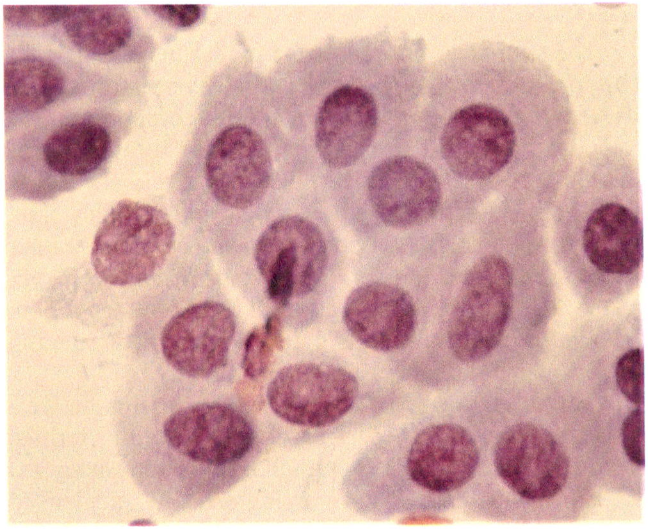

Fig. 15.18. Conjunctival epithelial cell in the conjunctival scraping from an emu (*Dromaius novaehollandiae*), Wright–Giemsa stain (100× oil).

Joint Fluid

Cytologic examination of the synovial fluid is the most valuable part of the diagnostic process involved in the determination of joint disease in birds. When possible, a complete synovial fluid analysis should include assessment of appearance (color and turbidity), protein content, viscosity, a mucin clot test and a nucleated cell count, differential, and cell morphology (Fisher, 2001). Under normal conditions, the joints of birds contain a fluid volume that is too small for sampling or complete evaluation. Fluid distension of a joint may occur when certain arthropathies are present, which will allow for collection of enough synovial fluid for evaluation. Even when significant joint distention is present, however, often only a few drops of synovial fluid can be collected for cytologic evaluation.

The color and character of the synovial fluid should be noted during the aspiration procedure. If blood suddenly appears in the sample, then peripheral blood contamination has likely occurred, which will cause the sample to clot, making evaluation difficult. It also dilutes the sample, making cytological evaluation difficult. If a significant volume of synovial fluid has been collected, then placement of samples contaminated with blood into an EDTA tube to prevent clotting is advised, keeping in mind that EDTA interferes with mucin clot tests and cultures.

Normal synovial fluid is clear or straw-colored and is viscous. A simple viscosity test can be performed on the synovial fluid sample by placing a drop of fresh fluid onto a clean glass slide. The sample is then touched with a finger or wooden applicator stick, and the length of the strand formed as the fluid is lifted from the surface of the slide is measured (Figure 15.19). The viscosity of the fluid is considered reduced if the strand breaks before reaching 2 cm in length from the slide surface. Synovial fluid with poor viscosity indicates a decreased hyaluronic acid content or dilution of the fluid with an effusion, as seen in inflammatory disease.

A mucin clot test is a semiquantitative assessment of the mucin quality or the amount of polymerized hyaluronic acid in the synovial sample. One or two drops of the joint fluid are added to four to eight drops of 2% acetic acid, and the mixture is allowed to stand for 1 min (Fisher, 2001). A firm, thick, homogenous clot will form if there is a normal hyaluronic acid concentration in the sample (Figure 15.20). If the test is performed on a microscope slide, the clot should remain attached to the slide when the slide is inverted. Synovial fluid with reduced hyaluronic acid concentration will not form a clot. The test is typically scored as good, fair, or poor, with normal synovial fluid receiving a good score.

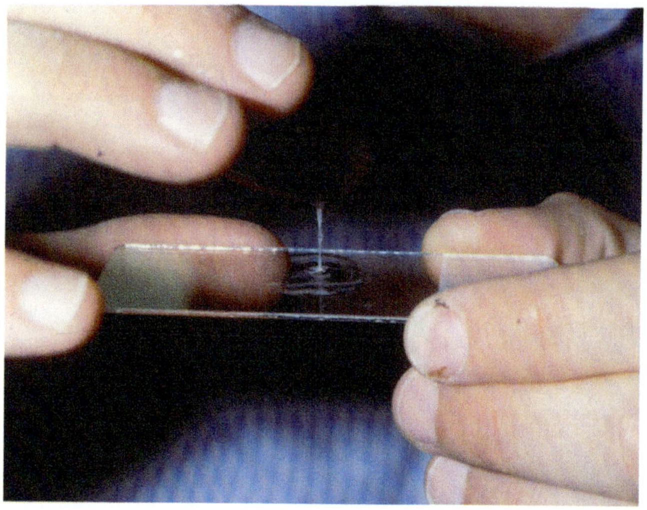

Fig. 15.19. A simple viscosity test.

The protein content of synovial fluid is measured by refractometry. Normal synovial fluid has a low protein concentration (2.5 g/dL). Protein content increases with inflammatory joint disease.

A cell count may be performed on synovial fluid using the same hemacytometer counting method performed with peripheral blood if enough sample volume can be collected. Because synovial fluid often turns into a gel at room temperature (this is called thixotropism), obtaining an accurate cell count can be difficult (Walberg and Loar, 2004). Hyaluronidase can be added to the synovial fluid to reduce the fluid viscosity and prevent clotting to provide a more accurate cell count (Fisher, 2001). If only a small sample volume is obtained, then an estimated cell count can be performed on a synovial fluid film. Fluid from normal joints is poorly cellular and contains less than three cells per high-power field depending upon the thickness of the smear.

Synovial joints are composed of articular cartilage and an articular capsule, which is composed of a fibrous layer and a synovial membrane. The synovial membrane is composed of flat cells that produce the synovial fluid that lubricates the joint. Normal synovial fluid is poorly cellular and contains primarily small and large mononuclear cells (macrophages and synovial lining cells), and granulocytes (neutrophils or heterophils) on a granular background with Wright's stain. Synovial lining cells (synoviocytes) are large mononuclear cells with eccentric nuclei and abundant vacuolated cytoplasm that often contains pink-staining granules (Figures 15.21a and 15.21b). The granulocytes account for less than 10% of the cell differential in normal synovial fluid. The amount of granular background material indicates the amount of mucin present in the fluid. Cells in highly viscous synovial fluid tend to line up in parallel rows (this is called "wind rowing of cell") when the cytological slide is prepared (Walberg and Loar, 2004).

Fig. 15.20. A normal mucin clot test.

(a) (b)

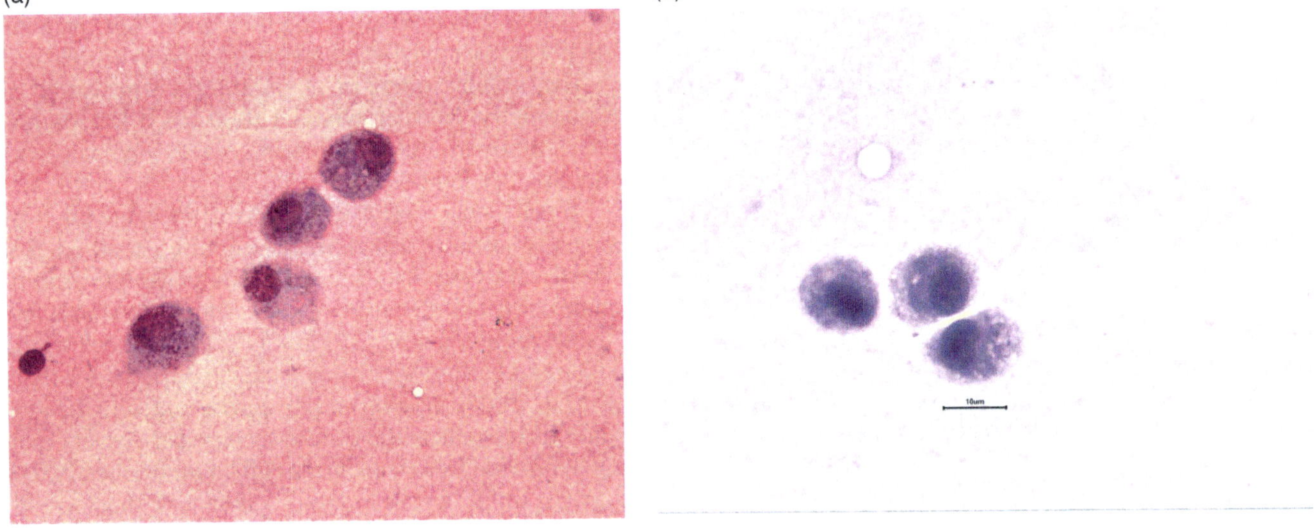

Fig. 15.21. (a) Synoviocytes exhibiting a relatively linear cell arrangement (wind rowing) and the heavy eosinophilic granular background of normal mucin content in the normal avian joint fluid, Wright–Giemsa stain (100× oil). (b) Synoviocytes exhibiting a relatively linear cell arrangement (wind rowing) and the heavy eosinophilic granular background of normal mucin content in the normal joint fluid from a burrowing owl (*Athene cunicularia*), Wright–Giemsa stain.

Lymphoid Tissue

Most species of the lower vertebrates do not possess lymph nodes; however, solitary lymphoid aggregates may occur. For example, in birds, lymphoid aggregates occur as nodules in the walls of the digestive tract, abdominal organs, serous membranes, and skin (e.g., the combs of Galliformes). Well-developed aggregates of lymphoid tissue called cecal tonsils occur in the proximal portion of the cecum of some birds. The bursa of Fabricius is a blind sac that opens on the dorsal wall of the proctodeum of the pre-hatched and immediately post-hatched chick. The spleen is one of the largest single masses of lymphoid tissue in the body, and significant lymphoid aggregates also occur throughout the liver of many of the lower vertebrates, such as birds.

The cytology of normal lymphoid tissue of birds reveals a predominance of small, mature lymphocytes and resembles the normal lymphoid cytology of mammals (Figure 15.22). The small, mature lymphocytes have condensed nuclei with heavy chromatin clumping and scant amount of pale blue to colorless cytoplasm. Other cells such as medium lymphocytes, large lymphocytes (i.e., prolymphocytes and lymphoblasts), plasma cells, macrophages, and heterophils may be present as well and represent less than 10% of the cell population of normal lymphoid tissue.

Immature lymphocytes, such as prolymphocytes, and lymphoblasts are larger than mature lymphocytes. Prolymphocytes have smooth nuclear chromatin and an abundant pale blue cytoplasm. Lymphoblasts are larger than prolymphocytes and have a vesicular nucleus with multiple prominent nucleoli and an abundant basophilic (dark blue) cytoplasm. Prolymphocytes and lymphoblasts are rarely seen in normal lymphoid tissue.

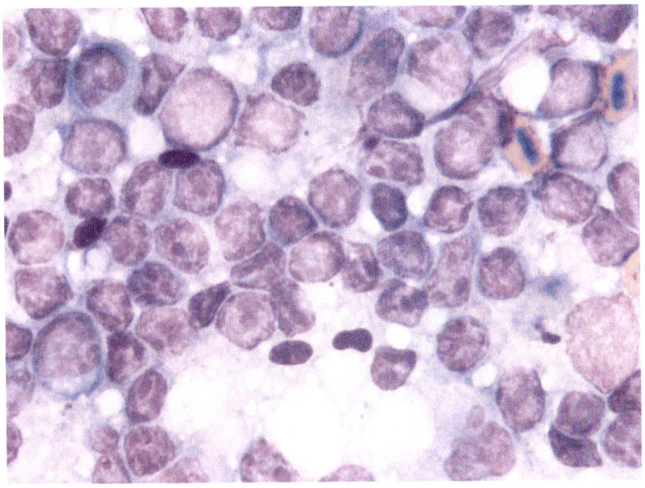

Fig. 15.22. Normal splenic cytology showing a predominance of small, mature lymphocytes in the splenic imprint from a cockatiel (*Nymphicus hollandicus*), Wright–Giemsa stain (100× oil).

Splenic cytology may be helpful in the diagnosis of infectious diseases such as chlamydiosis and some parasitic diseases such as hemic parasites, where developmental stages of blood parasites (such as *Hemoproteus*, *Leukocytozoon*, *Plasmodium*, and *Atoxoplasma*) may be found in splenic samples in some cases (Figure 15.23).

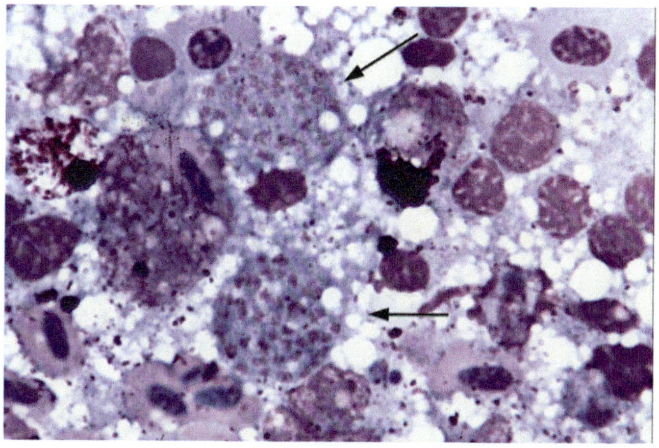

Fig. 15.23. *Hemoproteus* schizonts (arrows) in the splenic imprint from a kestrel (*Falco sparverius*), Wright–Giemsa stain (100× oil).

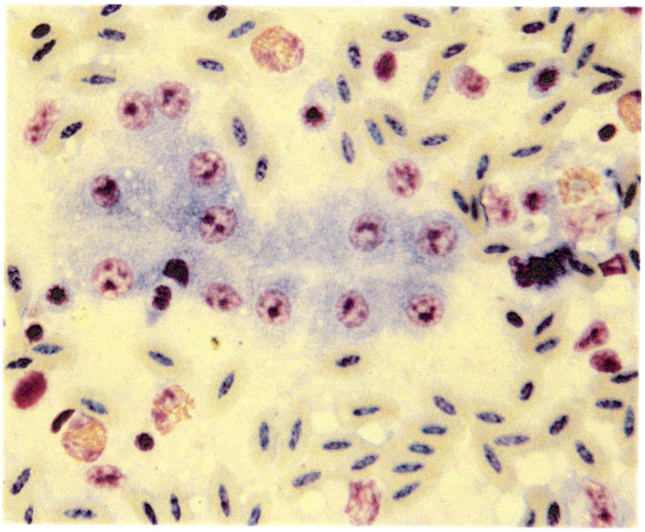

Fig. 15.24. Normal hepatocytes in a liver imprint from an umbrella cockatoo (*Cacatua alba*), Wright–Giemsa stain (100× oil).

Liver

The normal liver provides highly cellular samples that contain hepatocytes and variable amounts of hemic cells from peripheral blood contamination of the sample. Hepatocytes are large (25–30 μm), slightly oval to polygonal cells with distinct cell margins that occur singly or in sheets and clusters (Figures 15.24 and 15.25). The cytoplasm is abundant and lightly basophilic, and fine eosinophilic granulation may be seen occasionally with Wright's stain. The nuclei are round to oval, uniform in appearance, and are slightly eccentric in location within the cells. The nuclei contain coarse chromatin and one or two prominent nucleoli. Binucleation is occasionally seen. Hepatocytes are easily damaged, resulting in numerous free nuclei scattered throughout the smear

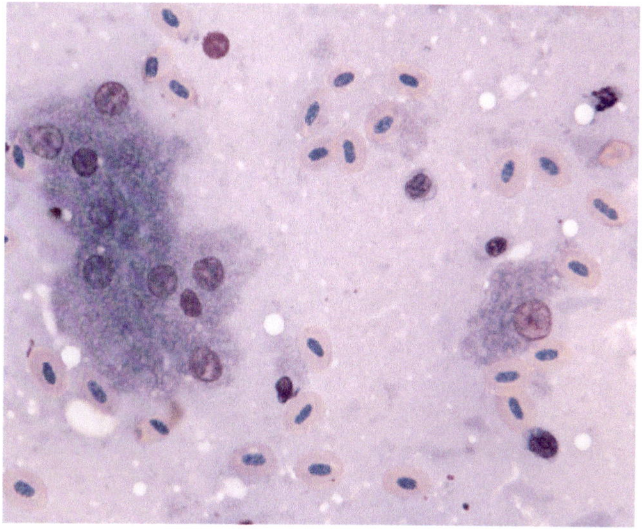

Fig. 15.25. Normal hepatocytes in a liver imprint from a cockatiel (*Nymphicus hollandicus*), Wright–Giemsa stain (100× oil).

and a background that resembles the cytoplasm of intact hepatocytes. Degenerative hepatocytes may be seen with hepatic disease or postmortem autolysis.

Biliary epithelial cells, lymphocytes, plasma cells, macrophages, and spindle-shaped cells are occasionally seen in normal smears. Blue-green bile pigment may occasionally be identified among the cells as well. Biliary epithelial cells are present as clusters of uniform-appearing small, round cells with round nuclei, dense granular to homogenous chromatin, and a scant amount of poorly staining cytoplasm. The macrophages present within the cytology sample often contain iron pigment (hemosiderin), indicating hemoglobin catabolism. Excessive iron pigment within many macrophages may be associated with hemolytic anemias or iron storage secondary to chronic inflammatory disorders.

Normal hepatic hematopoiesis is occasionally seen in hepatic tissue samples of lower vertebrates, such as birds. The cytology of hematopoietic activity is indicated by the presence of a mixed population of hemic cells exhibiting various developmental stages of the cell lines.

Developing stages of parasites, such as schizogony of blood parasites (e.g., *Hemoproteus* and *Leukocytozoon*), sporozoites of *Atoxoplasma*, microfilaria of filarial nematodes, and trematode ova, can occasionally be found in hepatic imprints from birds.

Kidney

Renal tubular epithelial cells exfoliate in clusters or as individual cells and appear as round to columnar cells with abundant basophilic cytoplasm that may contain vacuoles (Figures 15.26a–15.26c). The nuclei of normal renal tubular epithelial cells are uniform in appearance

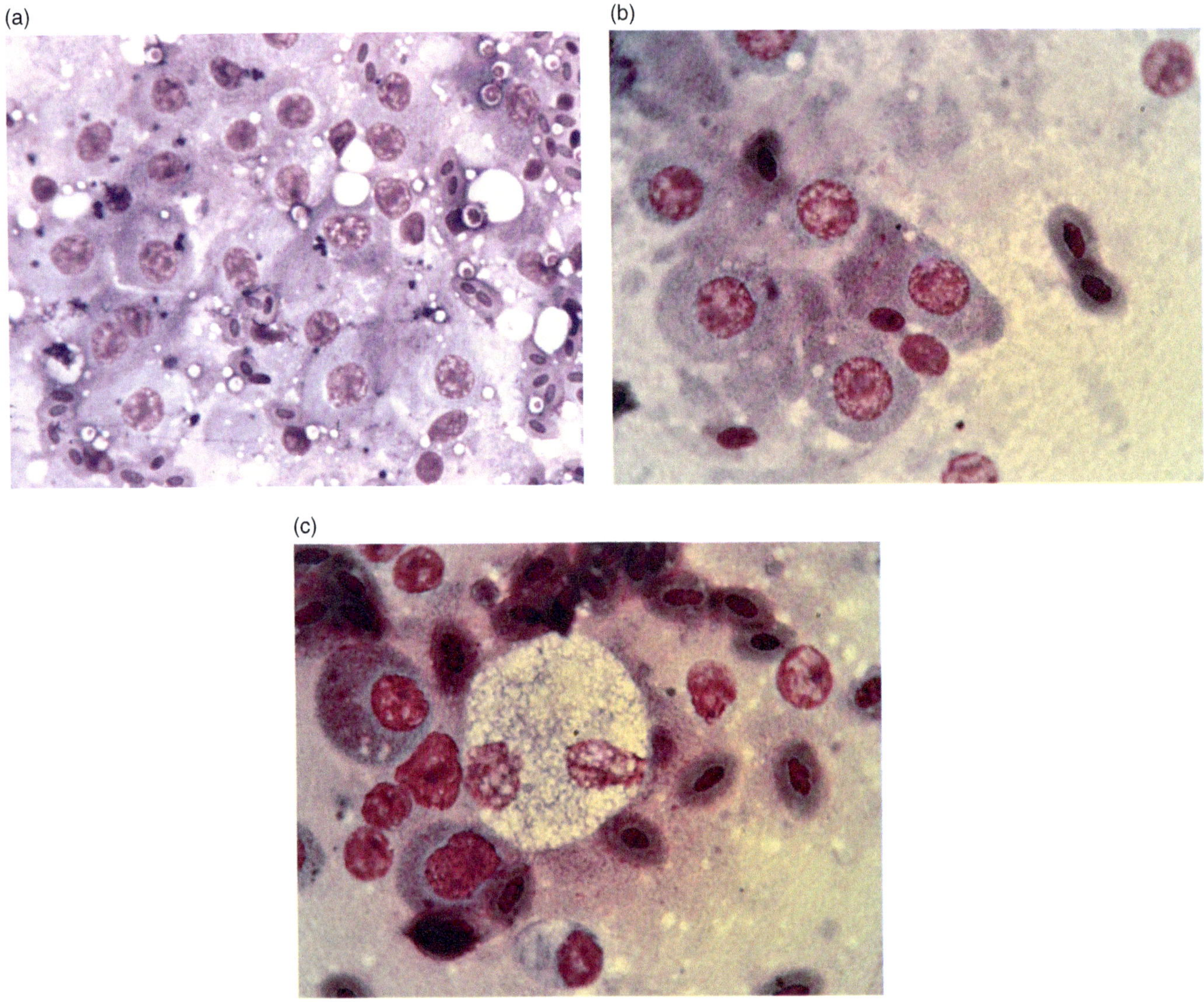

Fig. 15.26. (a) Normal renal epithelial cells in a kidney imprint from a cockatiel (*Nymphicus hollandicus*), Wright–Giemsa stain (100× oil). (b) Renal epithelial cells in an imprint from a kidney biopsy obtained by an endoscopic procedure from a thick-billed parrot (*Rhynchopsitta pachyrhyncha*), Wright–Giemsa stain (100× oil). (c) Renal epithelial cells including a vacuolated, binucleated epithelial cell in an imprint from a kidney biopsy obtained by an endoscopic procedure from a thick-billed parrot (*Rhynchopsitta pachyrhyncha*), Wright–Giemsa stain (100× oil).

and appear round and slightly eccentric. Normal renal cytology samples from birds commonly contain round sodium and potassium urate crystals.

Reproductive Tract

Cytologic examination of testicular biopsy samples from psittacine birds is a reliable method for evaluation of the reproductive status of these male birds (Hänse et al., 2013). Cytologic preparations of natural ejaculates from a golden eagle in cytologic preparations reveal heterogeneous sperm morphology within and among ejaculates, with the most common abnormal morphology being a rounded head with a triangular acrosome (Villaverde-Morcillo et al., 2015). In the same study, a "stinger-shaped" acrosome was also commonly observed, but was deemed normal based on intactness.

Inflammation

Heterophilic Inflammation of Birds

Inflammation occurs whenever chemotactic factors for inflammatory cells are released. The most common causes are microbes and their toxins, physical and chemical trauma, death of cells from circulatory insufficiency, and immune reactions. The rate of the inflammatory response is temperature dependent in poikilotherms such as reptiles, amphibians, and fish, whereas the rate of response in endotherms, such as mammals and birds, is more consistent and predictable.

The inflammatory process begins with the acute phase. Acute inflammation is initiated by the action of vasoactive amines and cell breakdown products released by the damaged tissue on the microcirculation of the affected tissue. These chemicals and products cause capillary dilatation, increased blood flow into the area, and increased lumen diameter of the capillaries, which allows the large serum proteins (such as fibrinogen and immunoglobulins normally confined within circulation) to exude into the tissues. Leukocytes actively migrate into the affected tissue. The degree of the leukocyte migration depends on the stimulus, which is particularly marked in certain bacterial infections. The cells that leave the blood include heterophils, monocytes, lymphocytes, and thrombocytes.

Heterophils are typically the first cells to arrive at the scene, where they destroy ingested organisms. Chemicals released from dying heterophils causes lysis of surrounding tissues and recruitment of other heterophils to form an abscess (a focal accumulation of heterophils, tissue fluids, fibrin, and necrotic tissue). Monocytes in circulation in conjunction with local tissue macrophages (which have multiplied at the site of inflammation) appear quickly and begin to phagocytize tissue debris and infectious agents as the inflammation becomes established. Monocytes and macrophages, stimulated by the cell-mediated immune response, join the heterophils to create a mixed cell inflammation, the most common cellular inflammatory response seen in birds. They can develop into epithelioid and multinucleated giant cells. As the inflammatory process continues and becomes chronic, granulomas may develop as the macrophages form layers that resemble epithelium, and this is the reason for the term *epithelioid cells*. As the lesion matures, fibroblasts proliferate and begin to lay down collagen. These proliferating fibroblasts appear large compared to the small, densely staining fibroblasts of normal fibrous tissue. Lymphocytes appear within the stroma and participate in the cell-mediated immune response. Fusion of macrophages into giant cells occurs in association with material that is not readily digested by macrophages. Therefore, the results of acute inflammation may be complete resolution, development of an exudative or necrotic lesion with continuation of the inflammatory response, or progression to chronic inflammation.

Heterophilic inflammation of birds is represented by a predominance of heterophils (greater than 80% of the inflammatory cells) in the cytologic sample (Figures 15.27 and 15.28). Heterophil granules in cytological specimens tend to lose their normal rod-shaped appearance and appear either more rounded or degranulated (Campbell and Grant, 2010).

Heterophilic inflammation is classified by the presence or absence of degeneration of these granulocytes.

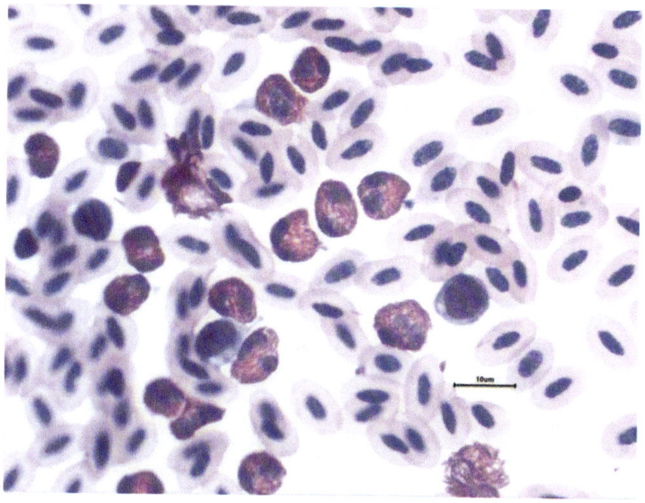

Fig. 15.27. Heterophilic inflammation in an aspirate from the foot of a golden eagle (*Aquila chrysaetos*) with pododermatitis, Wright–Giemsa stain.

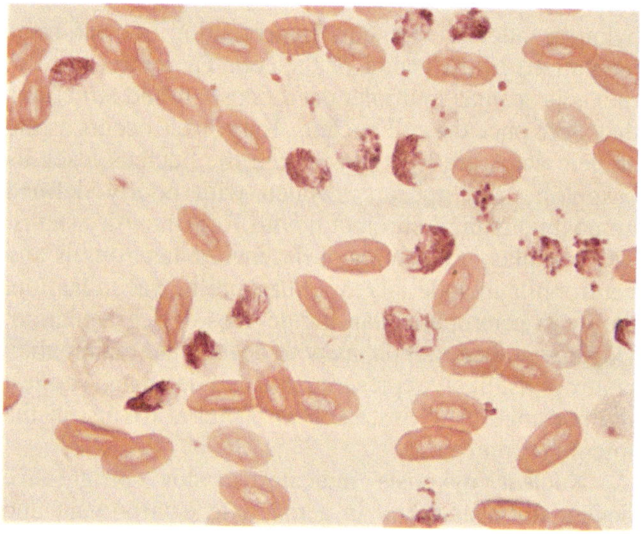

Fig. 15.28. Heterophilic inflammation in an emu (*Dromaius novaehollandiae*), Diff–Quik stain (note the nuclei of all of the cells failed to stain) (100× oil).

Degenerate heterophils have similar characteristics to degenerate mammalian neutrophils. Infectious agents produce toxins and induce cytokine activation, resulting in cell chemotaxis and degenerative changes in the heterophils. Some aerobic bacteria and fungi cause degenerative cell changes, whereas many anaerobic bacteria and mycoplasmas initiate chemotaxis, but do not affect the morphology of the heterophils. The nuclear features of degenerate heterophils include swelling, karyorrhexis, and karyolysis (Figure 15.29). A nucleus that appears larger than normal is considered to be swollen. Karyorrhexis or rupture of the nuclear membrane and fragmentation of the nuclear chromatin indicates the end stage of cell death and is represented by multiple

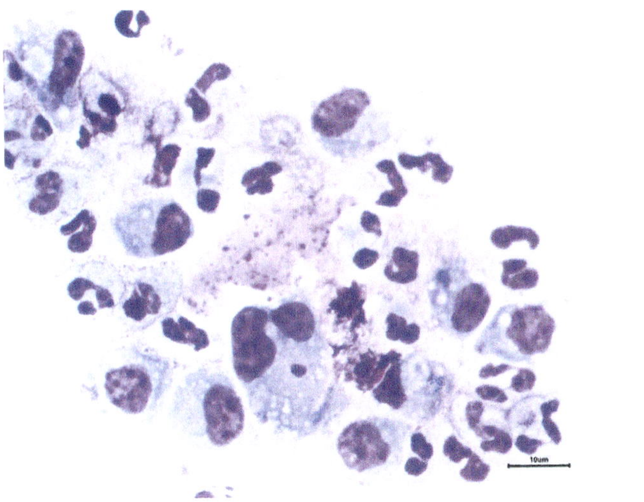

Fig. 15.29. Degenerate heterophils in an aspirate from the foot of a great horned owl (*Bubo virginianus*) with pododermatitis, Wright–Giemsa stain.

pyknotic nuclear segments (representing nuclear fragmentation) in the center of the cell. Therefore, karyorrhexis is seen as multiple, dark, dense, round structures that were once the cell nucleus. Karyolysis occurs as the nucleic acids are hydrolyzed, and the nucleus loses its basophilia and appears swollen with poorly defined homogenous pink chromatin with Romanowsky stains. The cytoplasmic features of degenerate heterophils and neutrophils include increased basophilia, vacuolization, and with heterophils, varying degrees of degranulation. Degenerate heterophils, as with degenerate mammalian neutrophils, likely represent rapid cell death and suggest the presence of toxins, such as bacterial toxins, in the microenvironment.

Nuclear pyknosis indicates a slow progressive degeneration of a cell in a nontoxic environment and may represent the natural aging of the cell. Pyknosis is characterized by nuclear shrinkage, causing the chromatin to become dense and deeply basophilic. Pyknotic nuclei appear as a single round mass with an intact nuclear membrane, or if involving cells with lobed nuclei, such as heterophils, there will be multiple small, round masses.

Heterophilic inflammation usually indicates an acute phase of the inflammatory response in birds. The acute inflammatory response of birds begins with inflammatory cells migrating and adhering to endothelial cells in the venules near the site of the invading agent, whether it is infectious or noninfectious (Klasing, 1991). Heterophils appear in large numbers in dilated blood vessels in the area of inflammation within 30 min of injections of noninfectious and infectious agents (Carlson and Allen, 1969; Nair, 1973). Basophils also appear within hours of injury (Maxwell and Robertson, 1995). Avian thrombocytes also participate in the early inflammatory response, where they actively engage in phagocytosis of foreign materials and bacteria (Awadhiya et al., 1980, 1981; Maxwell and Robertson, 1998). When heterophils arrive at the site of inflammation, they become activated, leading to phagocytosis of the invading agent. The ingested agent initiates a cascade of cellular events, from the release of granule-derived hydrolytic enzymes, oxygen free radicals, and other chemotactic factors to the general disintegration of the cell. This cellular degeneration is a characteristic feature of inflammation with loose, intact granules, and their remnants are accompanied by a gradual increase in phagocytic macrophage activity (Maxwell and Robertson, 1998). Following continued accumulation in the tissues, degranulating heterophils become unrecognizable and necrotic within the center of the lesion. In about seven days, with macrophage involvement, the characteristic heterophilic granuloma develops (Montali, 1988). Apparently, the necrotic center of heterophilic inflammatory lesions produces necrotoxins that are chemotactic to macrophages, and a granuloma quickly develops. Therefore, granuloma formation in birds and reptiles may be in response to necrotic tissue rather than an infectious organism. Giant cell formation is a common occurrence in avian inflammatory lesions because the necrotic tissue stimulates a foreign-body-like reaction. Thus, unlike mammalian giant cell formation, the presence of giant cells in avian inflammatory lesions does not necessarily suggest chronicity.

Heterophilic inflammation in birds is associated with a suppurative inflammatory process that is often associated with infectious agents, especially when these leukocytes are degenerate. Close examination of the heterophils for infectious agents should be made when this type of inflammation is present. Septic lesions caused by pathogenic bacteria are often responsible for heterophilic inflammation; however, fungal agents may also cause heterophilic granulomas associated with degenerate and nondegenerate heterophils. Heterophilic inflammation can also be associated with noninfectious agents, such as foreign material.

Septic Inflammation

Septic inflammation is indicated by the presence of intracellular bacteria (Figure 15.30). Bacteria that have been phagocytized by leukocytes often appear within vacuoles called phagosomes, which are membrane-bound vesicles formed by invagination of the cell membrane. Most bacteria stain blue with Romanowsky stains.

Mixed Cell Inflammation

When there is an influx of macrophages and lymphocytes into the inflammatory lesion, a mixed cell inflammation (pyogranulomatous) is created (Figures 15.29,

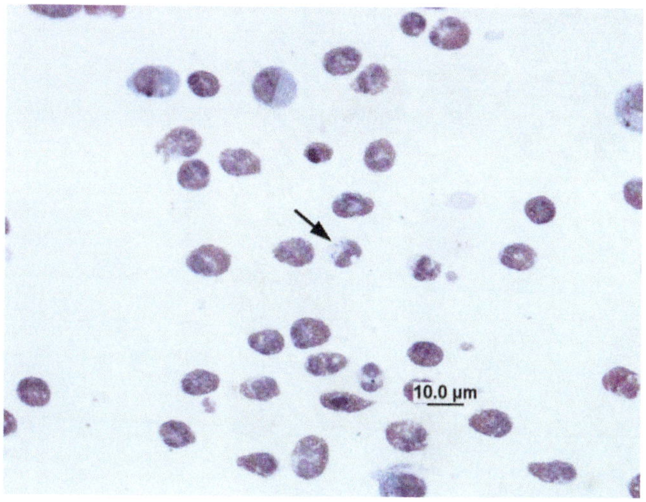

Fig. 15.30. Septic inflammation (arrow) in a green-cheeked conure (*Pyrrhura molinae*), Wright–Giemsa stain.

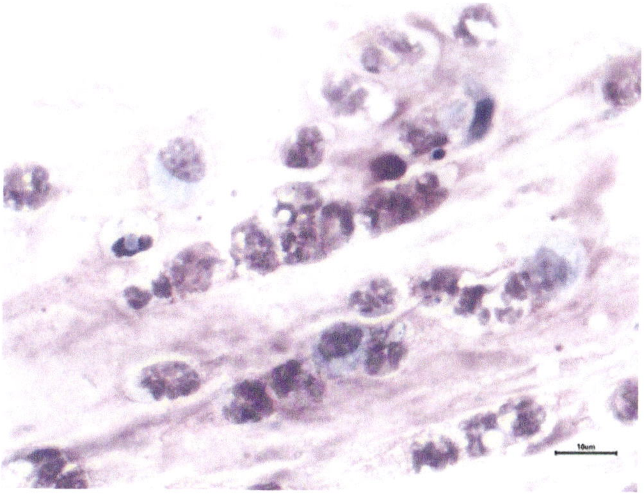

Fig. 15.31. Mixed cell inflammation in a sinus aspirate from a cockatiel (*Nymphicus hollandicus*), Wright–Giemsa stain.

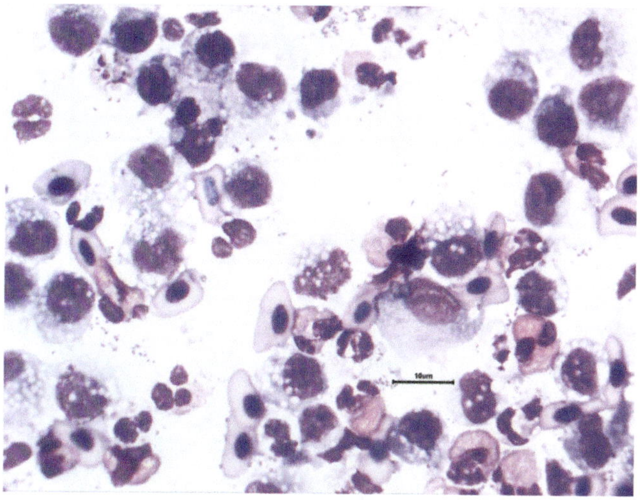

Fig. 15.32. Mixed cell inflammation from an aspirate of an abscess in a red-tailed hawk (*Buteo jamaicensis*), Wright–Giemsa stain.

15.31, and 15.32). A pyogranulomatous response consists of a mixture of heterophils, epithelioid macrophages, and multinucleated giant cells. A mixed cell inflammation indicates an established, active inflammatory lesion (originally known as chronic active inflammation). Mixed cell inflammation is typically represented by a predominance of heterophils (greater than 50% of the inflammatory cells) with an increased number of mononuclear leukocytes. Heterophils in mixed cell inflammatory lesions are usually normal and nondegenerate in appearance. Lymphocytes and plasma cells are often associated with acute heterophilic granulomas, whereas the presence of epithelioid cells (macrophages that contain no vacuoles or phagocytized material) and connective tissue cells (i.e., fibroblasts) suggests chronic granulomas. Frequently, the epithelial and mesenchymal cells adjacent to inflammatory lesions proliferate, resulting in the presence of these cell type demonstrating features of tissue hyperplasia. This type of inflammatory response is commonly observed with a variety of infectious (i.e., bacterial and fungal) and noninfectious (i.e., traumatic and foreign body) etiologies.

Chronic inflammatory lesions, such as bacterial abscesses, may contain a large amount of noncellular, amorphous debris in the center of the lesion. Material obtained from this area will be poorly cellular, and the few cells that are present are often degenerate and difficult to evaluate. Active lesions will reveal an inflammatory response if the sample is obtained from the margin of the lesion. Septic lesions may reveal bacterial phagocytosis in heterophils or macrophages (Campbell and Grant, 2010). Fibroblasts proliferate in mature lesions to lay down collagen (Campbell and Ellis, 2007).

Lymphocytic and plasmacytic infiltration is indicated by increased numbers of lymphocytes and plasma cells in the cellular response. Conditions that are often associated with this type of cellular response include early viral infections, immune-mediated disorders, and chronic inflammation. Infection with *Mycoplasma* spp. is often associated with lymphoplasmacytic inflammation (Nunoya et al., 1997). The lymphocyte population is composed of small and intermediate-sized mature lymphocytes and plasma cells. Plasma cells are large, round to oval lymphocytes with an abundant, deeply basophilic cytoplasm. The nucleus is eccentrically located and appears mature. A prominent Golgi apparatus is found adjacent to the nucleus. Plasma cells distended by round, clear to light blue structures (Russell bodies) are often referred to as Mott cells (Cazzini et al., 2013). The nucleus of the plasma cell is round and contains dense, coarse chromatin and no nucleoli.

Avian Mott cells are heterogeneous group of atypical plasmacytes recognized microscopically by endoplasmic

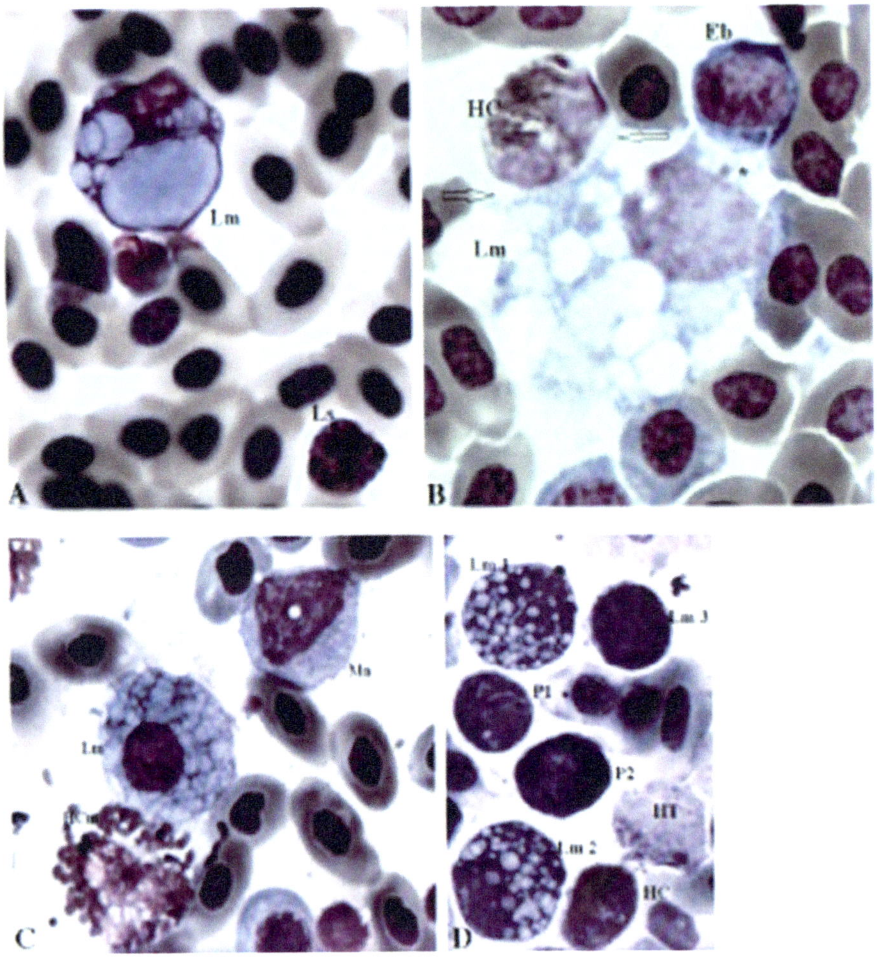

Fig. 15.33. Large and unusual avian Mott cells of blood and bone marrow. (A). Lm is a Mott cell with distended cisternae in blood of an 18-week-old hen. (B). Lm is a bone marrow type from a lame 6-week-old broiler chick, bordered by a classic heterophil (HC). (C). Lm is a bone marrow type from a lame 6-week-old broiler chick and a monocyte (Mn) with a Dutcher body (invaginations of immunoglobulin filled cytoplasm). (D). Lm1 and Lm2 are large bone marrow types; Lm3 is a medium-sized lymphocyte, P1 and P2 are typical plasmacytes from a lame 6-week-old duck. A bacterium has attached to Lm 1 (asterisk), and two others are at either side of P1. A classic heterophil (HC) and a degraded typical heterophil (HT) are in the same field. Sources: Images from Cotter and Bakst (2017).

reticulum distensions known as Russell bodies associated with a retained secretory product (antibody) (Cotter and Bakst, 2017). They are observed in a broad spectrum of immunopathology, sometimes involving hypergammaglobulinemia. Atypical granulocytes and leukocytes frequently accompany Mott cells (Figures 15.33 and 15.34). More information on these cells exists in non-avian species, where they are associated with autoimmunity, leukemia, multiple myeloma, chronic infections, and uveitis (Cotter and Bakst, 2017).

Because of the rapid influx of macrophages (within a few hours) and lymphocytes into inflammatory lesions, mixed cell inflammation (pyogranulomatous) is the most common type of inflammation seen in birds. Mixed cell inflammation is typically represented by a predominance of heterophils (greater than 50% of the inflammatory cells) with an increased number of mononuclear leukocytes. Heterophils in mixed cell inflammatory lesions are usually normal and nondegenerate in appearance. Lymphocytes and plasma cells are often associated with acute heterophilic granulomas, whereas the presence of epithelioid cells (macrophages that contain no vacuoles or phagocytized material) and connective tissue cells (i.e., fibroblasts) suggest chronic granulomas. Heterophilic and mixed cell inflammation are associated with a variety of infectious (i.e., bacterial and fungal) and noninfectious (i.e., traumatic and foreign body) etiologies in birds.

Macrophagic Inflammation

Macrophages are important in antigen presentation, production and secretion of cytokines, phagocytosis, and bacterial killing by the production of reactive

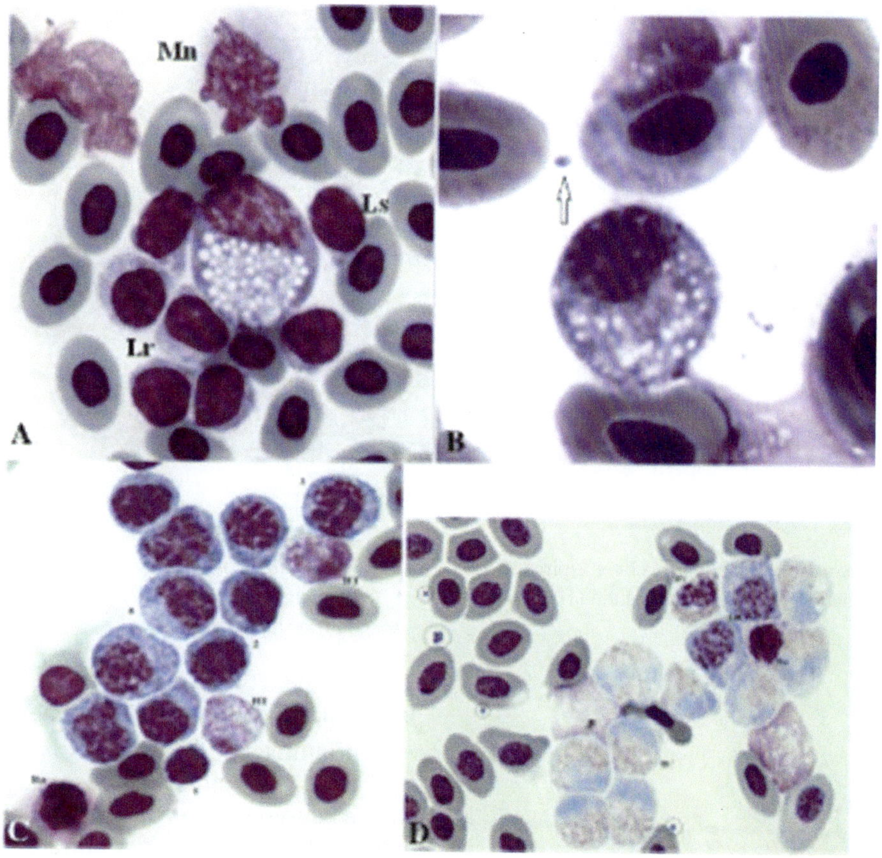

Fig. 15.34. Avian Mott cells with unusual morphology, and reactive clusters. (A). A nest containing a large Mott cell surrounded by small lymphocytes ranging from resting (N/C ~ 1) to reactive types (N/C ~ 0.7) was in the blood of a 77-week-old hen. (B). A Mott cell with cytoplasmic vacuoles varying in size and color was in the blood of a 6-week-old duckling. The arrow locates a solitary encapsulated bacterium. (C). Plasma cells in the blood film of a 32-week-old hen ranging in size from Ls (1) to Lm (2) and larger lymphoid cells (Lm 3, Lm 4) that appear to be developing into Mott cells. Heterophils and a basophil (Ba) are also present. (D). The blood film of a 32-week-old hen reveals a marked number of heterophils and reactive lymphocytes or plasma cells (Lm). Sources: Images from Cotter and Bakst (2017).

oxygen radicals and nitrogen intermediates (Quereshi, 1998). Macrophagic (histiocytic or granulomatous) inflammation consists primarily of macrophages with multinucleated giant cells and lesser numbers of other inflammatory cells. This type of inflammatory response does not always exfoliate well and may be of low cellularity. Macrophagic inflammation may have a different pathogenesis than heterophilic and mixed cell inflammation in birds and is indicated by a predominance of macrophages (greater than 50% of the inflammatory cells) in the cytological sample (Figures 15.35 and 15.36). Large, activated macrophages resembling epithelial cells (epithelioid macrophages) that later develop into multinucleated giant cells, apparently responding to necrotic tissue, are a feature of this type of inflammation (Campbell and Grant, 2010) (Figures 14.6c, 14.6e, and 15.37). Epithelioid cells often appear as clusters of macrophages with blue-gray to pink cytoplasm, and distinct cytoplasmic margins (Burkhard et al., 2001).

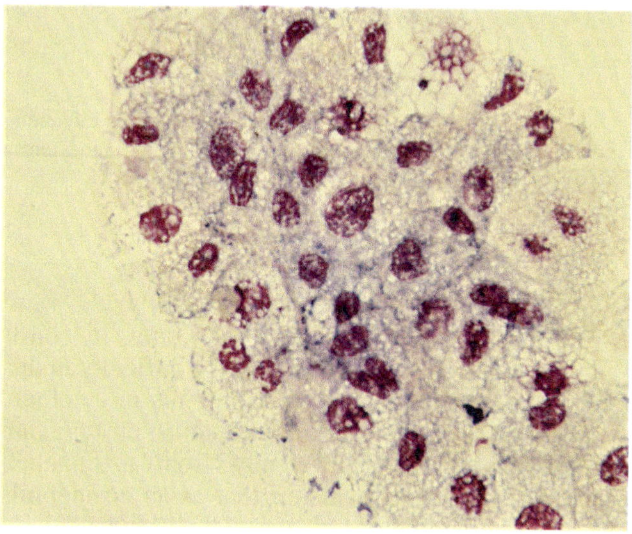

Fig. 15.35. Macrophagic inflammation in a tracheal wash from a golden eagle (*Aquila chrysaetos*), Wright–Giemsa stain (100× oil).

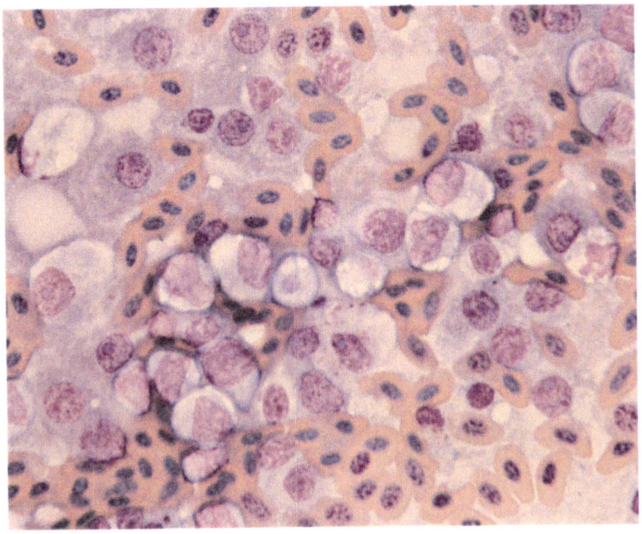

Fig. 15.36. Macrophagic inflammation in a liver aspirate from a chukar (*Alectoris chukar*), Wright–Giemsa stain (100× oil).

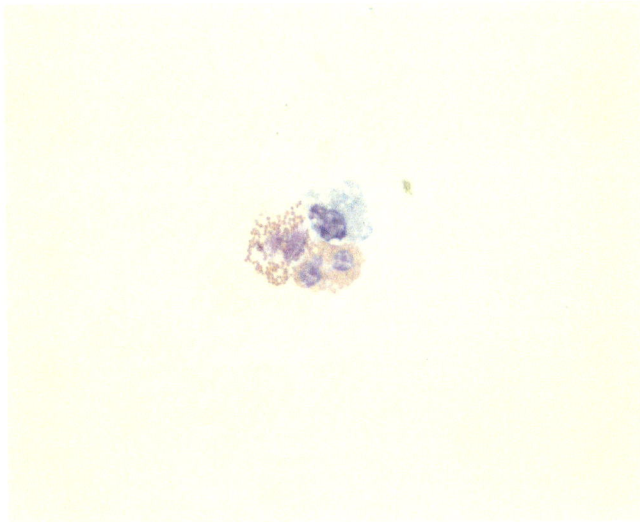

Fig. 15.38. Eosinophils in a tracheal wash from a seasonally coughing bald eagle (*Haliaeetus leucocephalus*), Wright–Giemsa stain (100× oil).

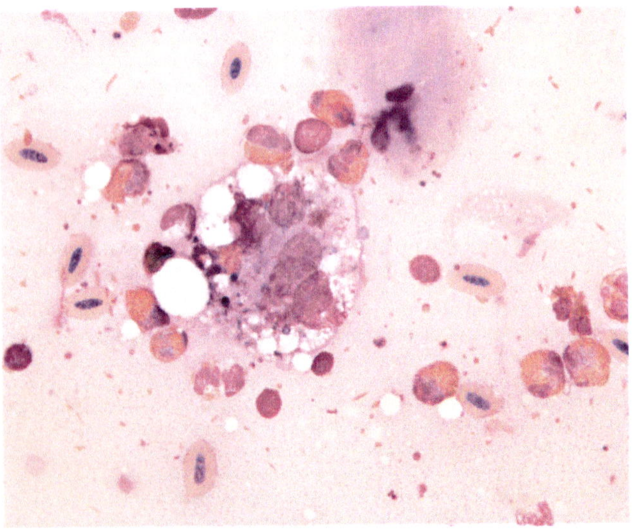

Fig. 15.37. Multinucleated giant cell as part of the inflammatory response in a gyrfalcon (*Falco rusticolus*), Wright–Giemsa stain (100× oil).

Eosinophilic Inflammation

Eosinophilic inflammation is rare in birds (Figure 15.38). This may be due to the difficulty in differentiating eosinophils from heterophils in cytologic samples using routine cytologic stains or to avian eosinophils behaving differently from mammalian eosinophils. There is evidence that avian eosinophils do not act as modulators of immediate hypersensitivity reactions as they do in mammals, but they may participate in delayed hypersensitivity reactions (Chad and Eyre, 1978; Maxwell, 1987).

Inflammatory Lesions of the Alimentary Tract

Inflammatory lesions involving the upper alimentary tract (i.e., stomatitis, esophagitis, and ingluvitis) can be caused by traumatic injury, foreign bodies, chemical irritation (e.g., silver nitrate used for hemostasis when trimming beaks of birds) and infectious agents (Campbell, 1983; Campbell, 1995). The cytology reveals an increased number of inflammatory cells and a variable number of squamous epithelial cells. An increased amount of background debris and lightly basophilic proteinaceous material may be present as well. As with mammalian cytology, basal cells are present in inflammatory lesions when ulceration of the epithelium occurs (Green, 1992). Septic lesions reveal inflammatory cells (heterophilic or mixed cell inflammation) containing intracytoplasmic bacteria (either primary or secondary pathogens) and may contain degenerate heterophils.

Oropharyngeal capillariasis, a common condition in raptors, is often associated with localized tissue inflammation and damage (Royal and Jochems, 2018). Adult capillarids associated with upper alimentary capillariasis live in the esophageal or oropharyngeal mucosa of infected birds and can migrate throughout the oropharynx and into the submucosa. Associated inflammation, ulceration, and secondary bacterial infections may result in the formation of fibrinonecrotic plaques. Capillarid eggs (59 by 28 μm) on slides of cytologic preparations are ovoid, with golden-brown smooth walls, offset bipolar plugs, and pink to tan granular internal structures (Royal and Jochems, 2018).

Chronic inflammatory lesions may reveal many epithelial cells with a high N:C ratio, multiple prominent nucleoli, and abnormal chromatin patterns. These cells represent a reactive epithelial response to the inflammation and should not be confused with a neoplastic condition. In such cases, it is important to correlate the clinical and the cytological findings to arrive at a reasonable interpretation of the cellular response. When deeply ulcerated lesions or chronic inflammatory lesions are present, fibroblasts may be present in the cytology specimen. Fibroblasts appear as spindle-shaped cells with single, oval to elongated nuclei (occasional multinucleation occurs during rapid proliferation).

Caseous lesions in the oropharynx of birds can be associated with bacterial infection, trichomoniasis, hypovitaminosis A, capillariasis, candidiasis, and viral infections (Cooper, 1978; Heidenreich, 1997; Boydell and Forbes, 1996).

Ingluvitis (inflammation of the avian crop) is a common disorder of companion birds. Clinical signs of this disorder include delayed emptying time of the ingluvies, regurgitation, and weight loss. Birds with a peracute bacterial ingluvitis ("sour crop") or candidiasis are typically nestlings being hand-raised. The disorder is characterized by an acidic crop fluid (normal crop pH is 4.5–6.7) with a foul-smelling fermenting odor. Cytological samples of this condition contain few inflammatory cells and many bacteria represented by one morphological type, which is considered abnormal and indicates a need for bacterial culture. This may represent an acute bacterial infection where inflammatory cells have not had time to respond, or the inflammatory response has been overwhelmed. A predominance of gram-negative bacilli presents in a smear from the upper alimentary tract, such as the crop, of noncarnivorous birds should be considered abnormal, whereas they are commonly present in carnivorous birds.

Septic lesions of the ingluvies (septic ingluvitis) reveal inflammatory cells (heterophilic or mixed cell inflammation) exhibiting bacterial phagocytosis (Figure 15.39). The heterophils may appear degenerate.

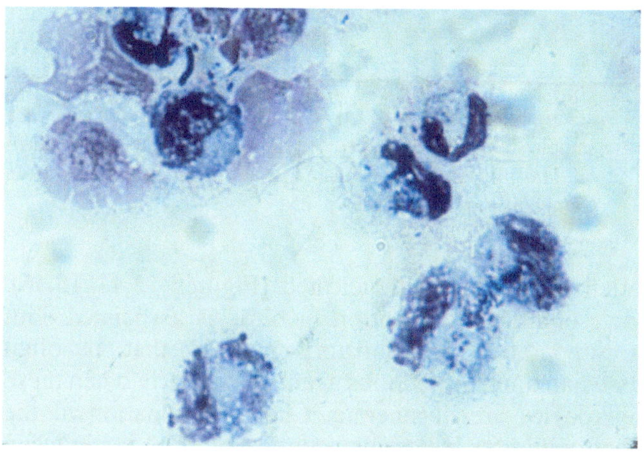

Fig. 15.39. Several degenerate heterophils exhibiting bacterial phagocytosis in a crop aspirate from an Amazon parrot (*Amazona* spp.) with septic ingluvitis, Diff-Quik stain (100× oil).

Gastritis and enteritis are indicated by the presence of inflammatory cells along with bacteria and cell debris. Acute inflammatory lesions exhibit primarily heterophils. A mixed cell inflammation indicates an established lesion. Chronic gastritis and enteritis are indicated by the presence of lymphocytic or lymphoplasmacytic inflammation. Cytologic diagnosis of mycotic infections, such as candidiasis and zygomycete fungi, of the proventriculus and ventriculus of birds is made by identification of fungal elements (narrowly based budding yeast and hyphae) in a gastric wash specimen (Anderson, 1993; Graham, 1994).

Cloacal diseases that have been reported in birds include papillomatous disease and other neoplasms, cloacitis (bacterial, fungal, and parasitic), prolapse (of the cloaca, phallus, oviduct, or rectum), cloacolithiasis, stricture, traumatic injury, and atony (Gill and Helmer, 2020). Inflammatory cells found on cloacal and fecal swab samples from birds are considered abnormal and reflect an inflammatory lesion involving the cloaca, lower intestinal tract, urinary tract, or reproductive tract. Ulcerative lesions may reveal basal epithelial cells and numerous erythrocytes with the inflammatory cells. Granulomatous lesions are typified by numerous macrophages with occasional multinucleated giant cells, plasma cells, and heterophils. Septic inflammation is indicated by leukocytic phagocytosis of bacteria.

Streptococcus species are common inhabitants of the intestinal tract and mucous membranes with a potential for opportunistic infections. Enteric disorders and immunosuppression are major predisposing factors for streptococcosis in avian species, and the species of *Streptococcus* commonly encountered include *S. dysgalactiae*, *S. equi* subsp. zooepidemicus, *S. gallolyticus*, *S. pluranimalium*, and *S. suis* (Crispo et al., 2018).

Inflammation of the Respiratory Tract

The cytology of sinusitis is represented by an increase in inflammatory cells in the sinus aspirate smear. The number and type of inflammatory cells depend on the nature of the infectious agent, severity of the inflammation, and duration of the disease. A moderate to marked amount of background debris, and the causative agent, either primary or secondary, may be present as well. Septic sinusitis is indicated by the presence of a relatively monomorphic population of bacteria, and intracytoplasmic bacteria within leukocytes (typically heterophils) (Figure 15.40). Bacterial sinusitis may not reveal the microorganisms on the cytology specimen; however, a positive culture would support the diagnosis. The presence of bacterial cocci that tend to form chains is suggestive of a *Streptococcus* sinusitis (Figure 15.41).

Chronic irritation or inflammation affecting the respiratory tract leads to cellular hyperplasia, which results

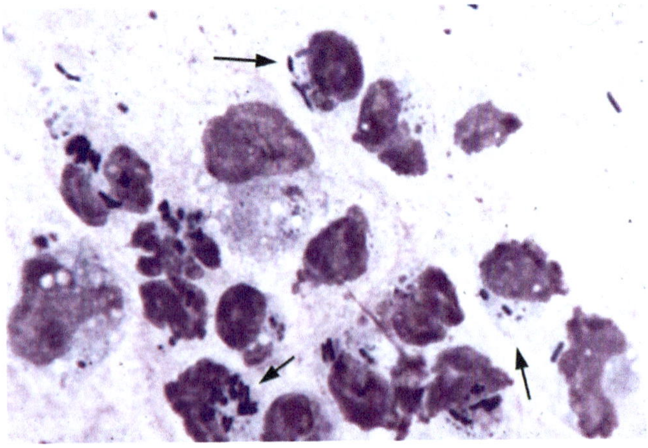

Fig. 15.40. Degenerate heterophils exhibiting bacterial phagocytosis (arrow) and macrophages in a sinus aspirate from an Amazon parrot (*Amazona* spp.) with septic sinusitis, Wright–Giemsa stain (100× oil).

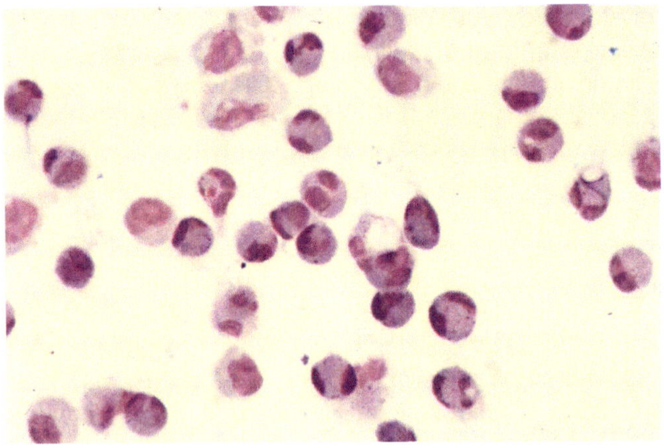

Fig. 15.42. Heterophilic inflammation with nondegenerate heterophils indicative of an acute tracheitis in a tracheal wash sample from a green-winged macaw (*Ara chloropterus*) suffering from smoke inhalation, Diff–Quik stain (100× oil).

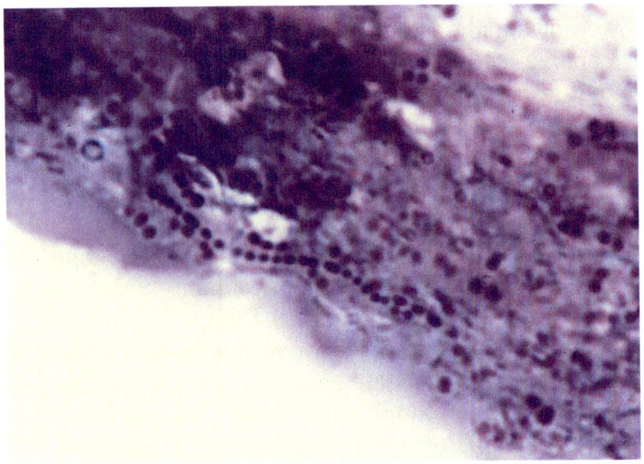

Fig. 15.41. A predominance of bacterial cocci that tend to form chains is characteristic of *Streptococcus* spp. bacteria in a sinus aspirate that was positive for a beta hemolytic *Streptococcus* in an African gray parrot (*Psittacus erithacus*), Diff–Quik stain (100× oil).

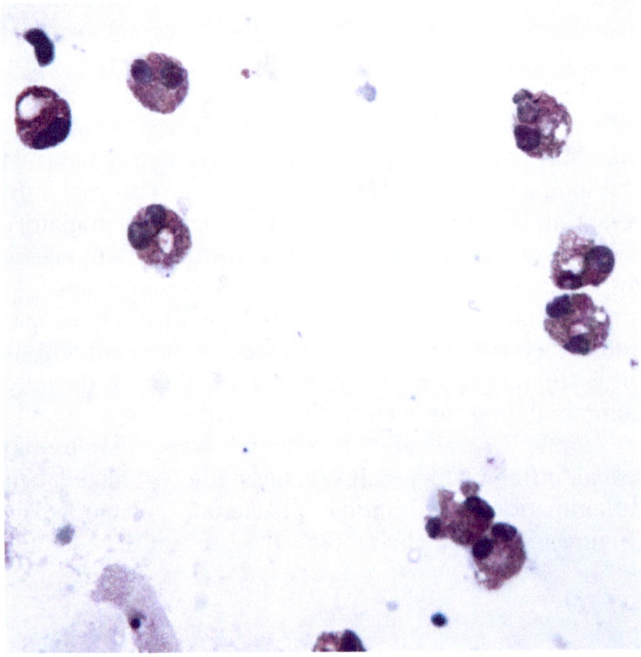

Fig. 15.43. Heterophilic inflammation with nondegenerate heterophils indicative of an acute tracheitis in a tracheal wash sample from yellow-naped Amazon parrot (*Amazona auropalliata*), Wright–Giemsa stain (100× oil). Source: Image from Campbell and Grant (2010, p. 251).

in numerous clusters and sheets of epithelial cells in the cytologic sample. These epithelial cells contain features of tissue hyperplasia, which include increased nuclear-to-cytoplasmic ratios, increased cytoplasmic basophilia, and mild nuclear anisocytosis. Increased numbers of normal mitotic figures may also be seen.

Tracheal wash samples of birds that exhibit many heterophils and macrophages, increased numbers of goblet cells, and increased mucin in the background indicate a tracheobronchitis or pneumonia. Heterophils are more predominant in acute lesions (Figures 15.42 and 15.43). When chronic inflammation is present, increased numbers of macrophages, lymphocytes, and plasma cells are present. Macrophages associated with chronic inflammation of the lower respiratory tract are often large and multinucleated (Figures 15.44–15.46). Heterophilic inflammation in birds is associated with a suppurative inflammatory process that is often associated with infectious agents, especially when these leukocytes are degenerate. Close examination of the heterophils for infectious agents should be made when this type of inflammation is present. Heterophilic inflammation can also be associated with noninfectious agents, such as inhalation of foreign material (e.g., smoke

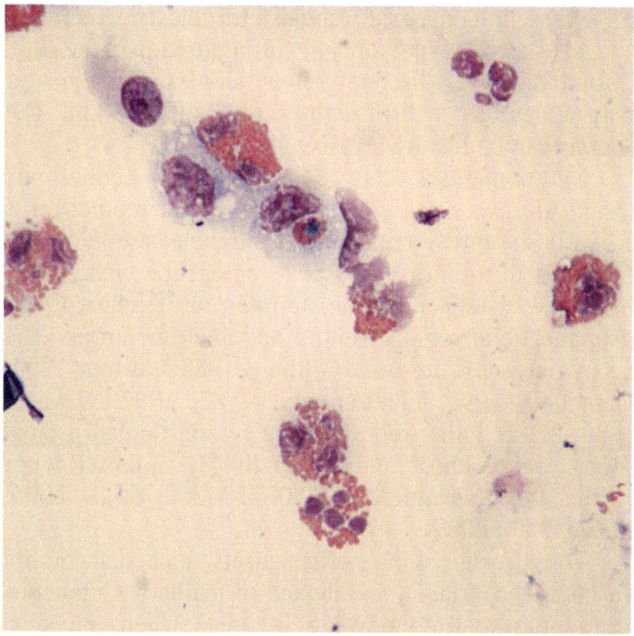

Fig. 15.44. Heterophils and macrophages (one exhibiting leukophagocytosis) in a tracheal wash from a domestic duck (*Anas platyrhynchos domestica*), Wright–Giemsa stain (100× oil). Source: Image from Campbell and Grant (2010, p. 77).

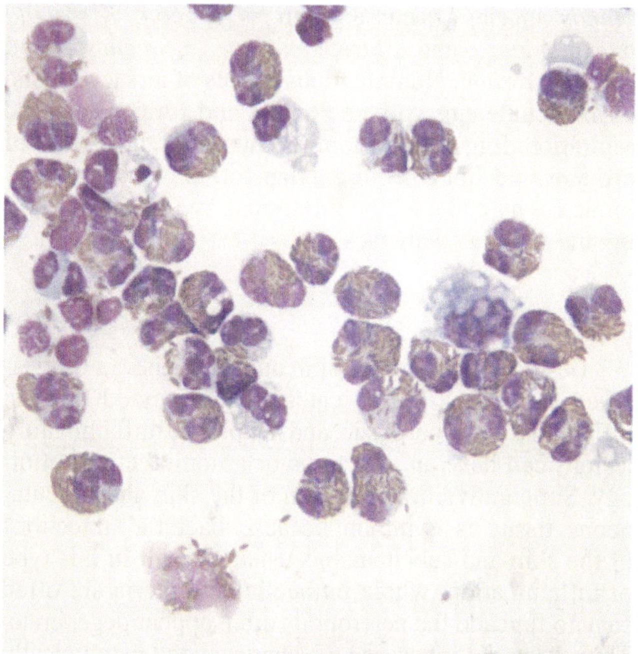

Fig. 15.45. Mixed cell inflammation (nondegenerate heterophils and macrophages) in a tracheal wash from an eclectus parrot (*Eclectus roratus*), Wright–Giemsa stain (1000×). Source: Image from Campbell and Grant (2010, p. 231).

inhalation), in some cases. Tracheal trauma, such as placement of an endotracheal tube, or rarely, tracheitis can result in tracheal stricture in birds (Doneley and Raidal, 2010). Degenerate ciliated respiratory epithelial cells (i.e., loss of cilia, cytoplasmic vacuolation, cell lysis, and karyolysis) may be seen with severe infections. Fragmented ciliated respiratory epithelial cells associated with a mononuclear leukocytic inflammatory response are suggestive of a viral etiology. Septic lesions are confirmed by the presence of leukocyte phagocytosis of bacteria.

A foreign body reaction or aspiration tracheobronchitis associated with the lower respiratory tract may reveal large reactive macrophages that form giant cells containing phagocytized foreign material (Figure 15.46). Macrophagic inflammation is common in certain avian diseases, such as mycobacterial and *Chlamydia* infections. Multinucleated giant cells are found in granulomatous lesions in inflammatory diseases such as tuberculosis (Montali et al., 1976; Pond and Rush, 1981; Sandford et al., 1994). Areas of macrophagic inflammation and heterophilic inflammation can occur together as macrophages respond to necrotic materials. Therefore, depending upon where the sample is obtained from the inflammatory lesion, a macrophagic inflammatory response may predominate the cytology.

Macrophagic inflammation associated with the tracheobronchial tract and lungs is often associated with fungal, foreign body, or mycobacterial lesions (Tully et al., 1995). The macrophages present may appear as reactive multinucleated giant cells, or as epithelioid cells.

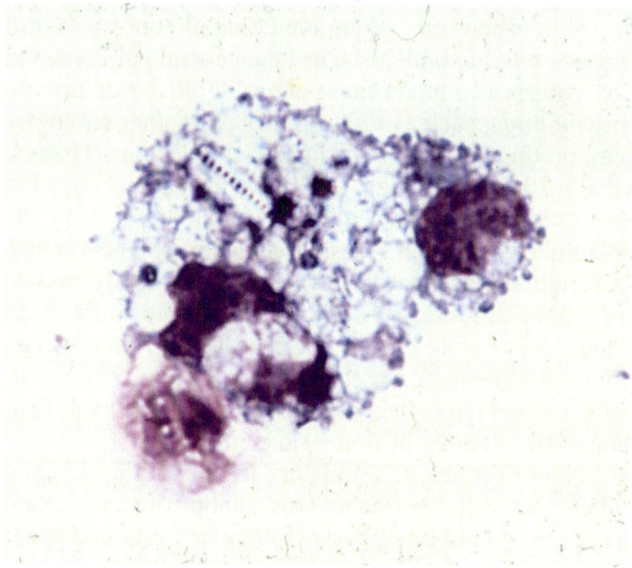

Fig. 15.46. A macrophage exhibiting phagocytosis of foreign material (likely plant material) in a tracheal wash sample from a barred owl (*Strix varia*), Diff–Quik stain (100× oil).

Inflammation of the air sacs, airsacculitis, can have an infectious or noninfectious etiology. Microorganisms that commonly cause airsacculitis in birds include *Chlamydia* species; fungi, such as *Aspergillus* and

Mucor species; bacteria, such as E. *coli*, *Klebsiella pneumoniae*, and *Streptococcus pyogenes*; and *Mycobacterium*. Noninfectious causes of airsacculitis in birds include egg yolk coelomitis and foreign material aspiration. Egg yolk coelomitis caused by the release of proteins and lipids from ovarian follicles into the coelomic cavity can elicit an inflammatory reaction involving the associated air sacs.

Inflammation of the Skin

Lesions involving the skin and subcutis can be classified using the basic categories of cytodiagnosis: inflammatory, hyperplasic, and neoplastic. Inflammatory lesions can have an infectious or a noninfectious etiology. Suppurative inflammation of the skin and subcutaneous tissue is common because bacterial infections of the skin and subcutaneous usually result in this type of inflammation, where intracellular bacteria are often easy to find and the heterophils often appear degenerate. Thus, bacterial infections are characterized cytologically by numerous degenerate heterophils, cellular debris, and bacteria. Septic inflammation is indicated by the presence of intracellular bacteria. The appearance of the bacteria may suggest the etiology; however, bacterial culture is necessary for a definitive diagnosis (Brandão et al., 2013).

Skin lesions are a common cause of concern to bird owners, wildlife biologists, and the general public. Avian pox virus is a common cause of proliferative skin disease in wild birds, such as turkeys; however, other etiologies may produce grossly indistinguishable lesions (Hydock et al., 2018). Although the gross appearance of skin lesions is often insufficient to determine the etiology, the anatomic distribution of lesions and temporal occurrence of certain diseases may offer insights into likely causes; for example, lesions involving or restricted to the head and neck are more likely to be caused by avian pox than other etiologies (Elsmo et al., 2016). Cytology is a cost-effective and rapid diagnostic tool to aid in the identification of the etiology of skin lesions in birds.

Noninfectious inflammatory lesions of the skin and subcutaneous tissues include foreign body reaction, xanthomatosis, epidermal cysts (follicular cysts or feather follicle cysts), and hematoma. Foreign bodies in the skin or subcutis cause mixed cell inflammation or macrophagic inflammation with multinucleated giant cells. The macrophages present in the cytology sample may contain phagocytized material. A secondary septic inflammation may also be present.

Differential diagnosis for large, soft to semisoft masses of the skin and subcutis of birds includes lipoma, xanthoma, fibrosarcoma, and myelolipoma (Nevarez et al., 2002). Cutaneous xanthomatosis is a granulomatous inflammation of the skin of birds (Campbell, 1995). Cutaneous xanthomatosis results from the accumulation of excess lipid material (cholesterol and triglycerides) and an associated macrophagic inflammation in the skin. Lesions occur as discrete yellow nodules or plaques or may appear as a diffuse thickening of the skin. The lesions can be locally invasive.

Xanthomatosis is common in budgerigars (*Melopsittacus undulates*), but may occur in other birds as well. In birds, cutaneous xanthomas are typically observed in the dorsal cervical region, the wattles, the back, the distal wings, the sternum, the feathered skin over the tibial region, ventral abdomen, or around the uropygial area (Petrak and Gilmore, 1982; Latimer, 1994; Campbell, 1995; Quesenberry et al., 1997; Nevarez et al., 2002). Other reports include periarticular, periosseous, oral, tracheal, and conjunctival locations (Raynor et al., 1999; Nevarez et al., 2002; Monks et al., 2006; Souza et al., 2009).

The affected skin is often raised, thickened, highly vascularized, friable, and devoid of feathers. Cutaneous xanthomas tend to develop in areas where physical trauma, local pressure, bleeding, or inflammation has occurred or is occurring (Latimer, 1994; Campbell, 1995).

Xanthomas are often classified as neoplastic processes; however, they are not true neoplasms (Nevarez et al., 2002). The etiology of xanthomatosis in birds is unknown. Possible causes of this condition include trauma and metabolic or nutritional disorders. A high-fat diet, disorder of lipid metabolism, metabolic conditions causing hypercholesterolemia, necrosis of the epithelium, and prior hemorrhage in the area of the lesion may be underlying factors in the development of this disorder (Bennett and Harrison, 1994). When abnormal lipid metabolism is suspected as a cause of xanthomas, hypercholesterolemia and hypertriglyceridemia are present in affected individuals (Jaensch et al., 2002; Souza et al., 2009).

Exposure to toxic fat-soluble substances (such as chlorinated hydrocarbons) that accumulate in the tissues inducing the inflammatory characteristics of xanthomatosis has also been proposed as a possible etiology (Peckham, 1955; Turrel et al., 1987; Latimer, 1994; Raynor et al., 1999). Xanthomas have also been associated with the skin overlying cysts and tumors, such as lipomas, osteosarcomas, and lymphoid leukosis lesions (Petrak and Gilmore, 1982; Campbell, 1995). Cutaneous xanthomatosis may also develop as a sequela following feather cyst removal in psittacine birds, where a significant amount of cutaneous hemorrhage may occur.

Cytological features of xanthomatosis include numerous highly vacuolated (foamy) macrophages, multinucleated giant cells, and cholesterol crystals (Figures 15.47–15.49). The background of the cytologic sample is often heavy with round, clear areas that resemble fat droplets. Cholesterol crystals appear as angular, variable shaped, negative-staining (clear), notched plates, which often appear stacked in the noncellular

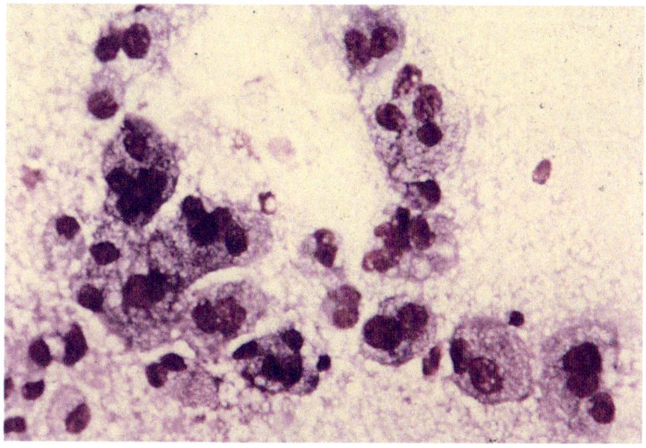

Fig. 15.47. Macrophagic inflammation associated with cutaneous xanthomatosis in a budgerigar (*Melopsittacus undulatus*), Diff–Quik stain (100× oil).

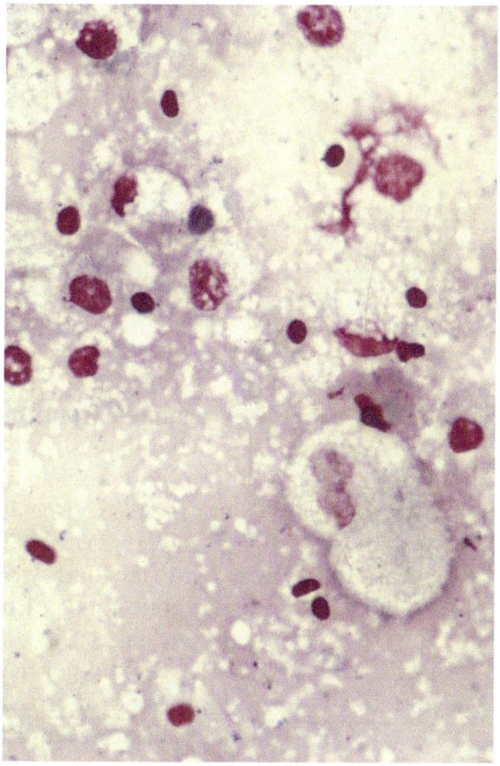

Fig. 15.48. Macrophagic inflammation with foamy macrophages associated with cutaneous xanthomatosis in a budgerigar (*Melopsittacus undulatus*), Diff–Quik stain (100× oil).

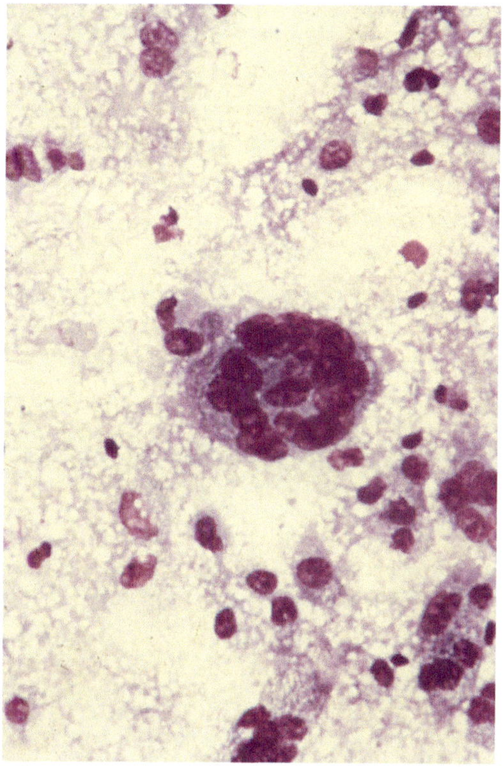

Fig. 15.49. Macrophagic inflammation with a multinucleated giant cell associated with cutaneous xanthomatosis in a budgerigar (*Melopsittacus undulatus*), Diff–Quik stain (100× oil).

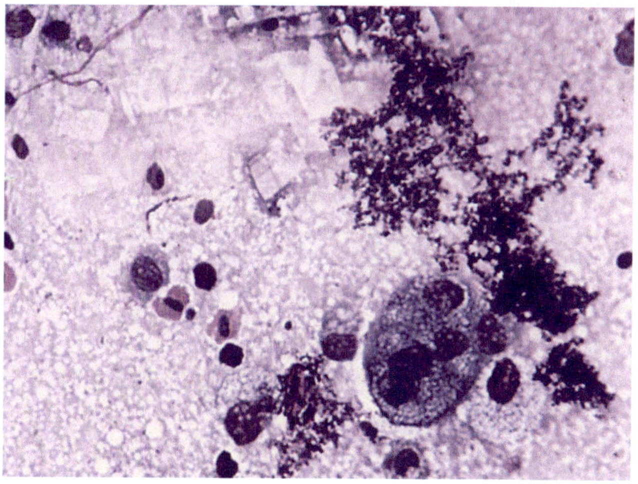

Fig. 15.50. Macrophagic inflammation with a multinucleated giant cell, cholesterol crystals (the angular clear crystals), and stain precipitate (the dark purple material) associated with cutaneous xanthomatosis in a budgerigar (*Melopsittacus undulatus*), Diff–Quik stain (400×).

background (Figures 15.50–15.52). These crystals will often dissolve in the alcohol fixatives of some stains and subsequently appear as a negative image in the cytology sample. The foamy macrophages (highly vacuolated) will stain positive with lipid stains.

The cytologic findings of xanthomatosis reflect what is observed on histology. Histological characteristic of cutaneous xanthogranulomas have features of both xanthomas and granulomas with numerous highly vacuolated, lipid-laden macrophages (called foam or xanthoma cells), cholesterol clefts, fibroblasts, and multinucleated giant cells (Raynor et al., 1999; Di Girolamo et al., 2014) (Figure 15.53).

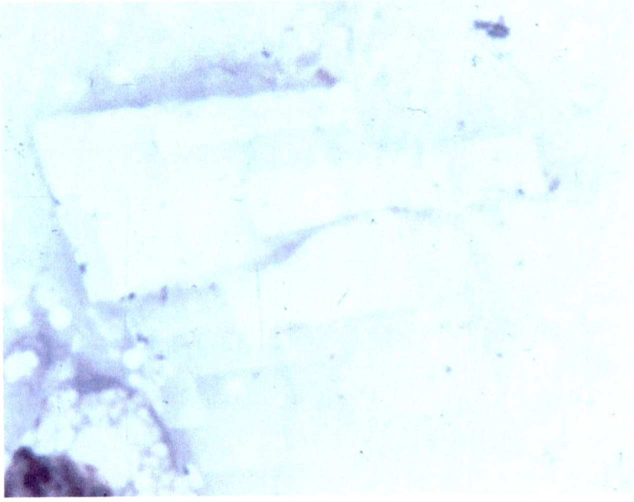

Fig. 15.51. Clear, angular cholesterol crystals associated with cutaneous xanthomatosis in a budgerigar (*Melopsittacus undulatus*), Diff–Quik stain (100× oil).

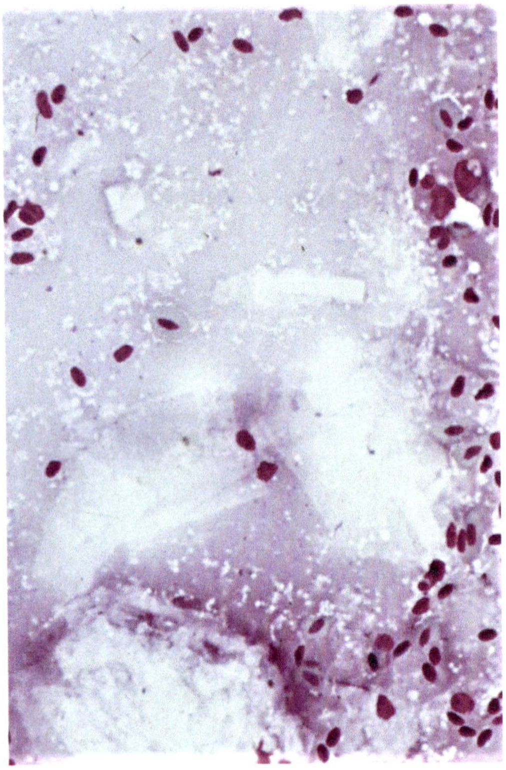

Fig. 15.52. Clear, angular cholesterol crystals associated with cutaneous xanthomatosis in a budgerigar (*Melopsittacus undulatus*), Diff– Quik stain (400×).

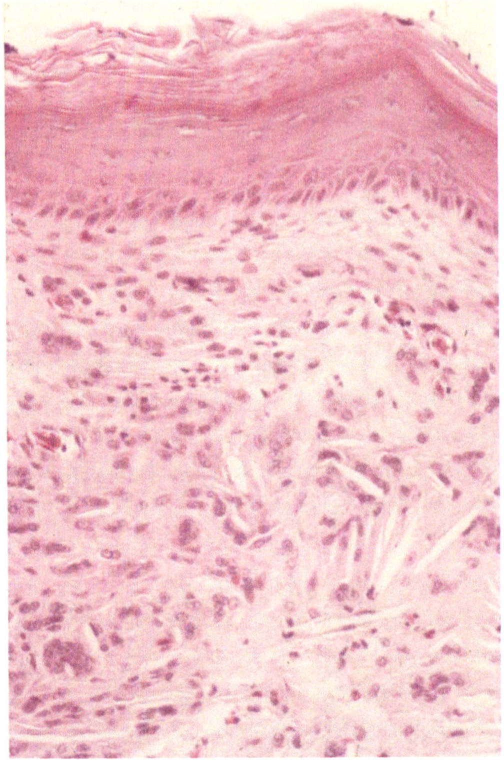

Fig. 15.53. Histopathology of cutaneous xanthomatosis revealing numerous highly vacuolated, lipid-laden macrophages (foam or xanthoma cells), cholesterol clefts, fibroblasts, and multinucleated giant cells in a skin biopsy of a budgerigar (*Melopsittacus undulatus*), H&E stain (10×).

Inflammation of Synovial Joints

Inflammatory joint disease can be caused by infectious agents such as bacteria, fungi, parasites, mycoplasmas, and viruses, or by noninfectious etiologies such as gout and immune-mediated disease. Microfilaria are occasionally found in the joint fluid of arthritic birds living in the wild or recently captured from the wild (Madani and Dorrestein, 2012). Cytology of inflammatory joint disease reveals an increase in heterophils, abnormal color and clarity, and reduced viscosity and mucin quality (Figures 15.54 and 15.55). The background of smears made from synovial fluid with poor mucin quality lacks the granular appearance of normal joint fluid. The presence of multinucleated osteoclasts or spindle-shaped fibroblasts indicates erosion of the articular cartilage, exposing underlying bone, or erosion into the fibrous layer of the articular capsule (Figures 15.56 and 15.57).

Septic arthritis is indicated by a high cell count and the presence of high numbers of heterophils. Extracellular bacteria are suggestive of bacterial involvement, and bacterial phagocytosis is considered diagnostic for septic joint disease (Malka et al., 2020) (Figures 15.55 and 15.58). Bacteria often are not inherently obvious on the slide; however, the presence of degenerative heterophils is suggestive of a septic lesion.

Mycoplasma spp.–induced arthritis and tenosynovitis is well documented in birds, especially in the Galliformes, where infection with *Mycoplasma synoviae* or M. *gallisepticum* causes articular and tendon lesions in populations of chickens and turkeys (Whitehear

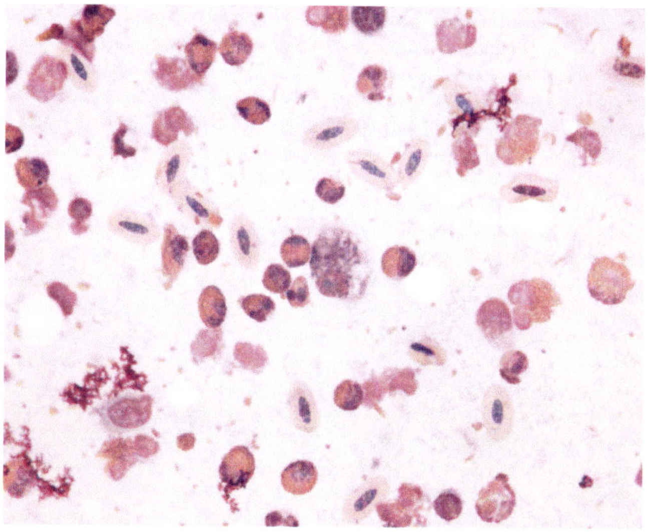

Fig. 15.54. Inflammatory cells (predominately nondegenerate heterophils, a macrophage, and a lymphocyte) and reduced granular background (mucin quality) in a joint fluid aspirate from a gyrfalcon (*Falco rusticolus*) with degenerative joint disease, Wright- Giemsa stain (100× oil).

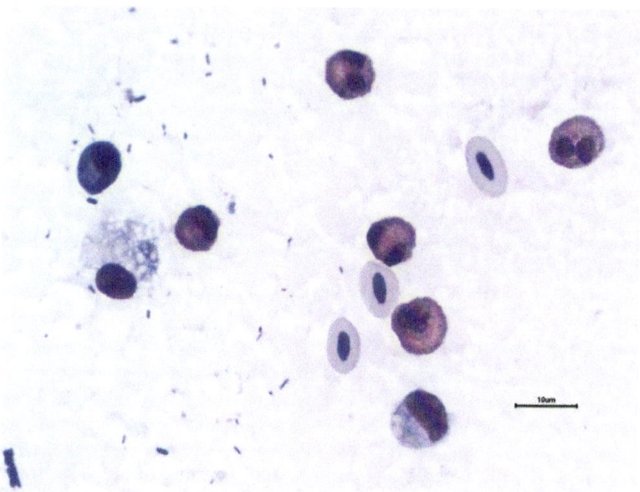

Fig. 15.55. An aspirate from a swelling on the dorsal aspect of the metatarsal joint of a Pekin duck (*Anas platyrhynchos domestica*) reveals mixed cell inflammation, extracellular bacteria, and reduce mucin quality indicative of septic arthritis, Wright–Giemsa stain.

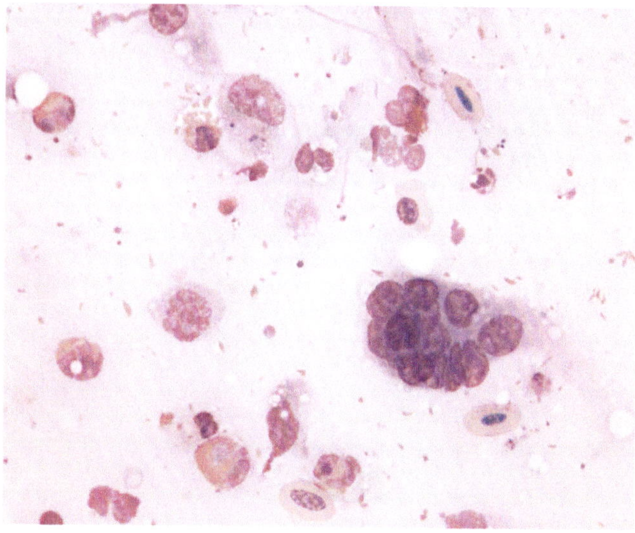

Fig. 15.56. A multinucleated osteoclast among the inflammatory cells (nondegenerate heterophils and macrophages) and reduced granular background (mucin quality) in a joint fluid aspirate from a gyrfalcon (*Falco rusticolus*) with degenerative joint disease, Wright–Giemsa stain (100× oil).

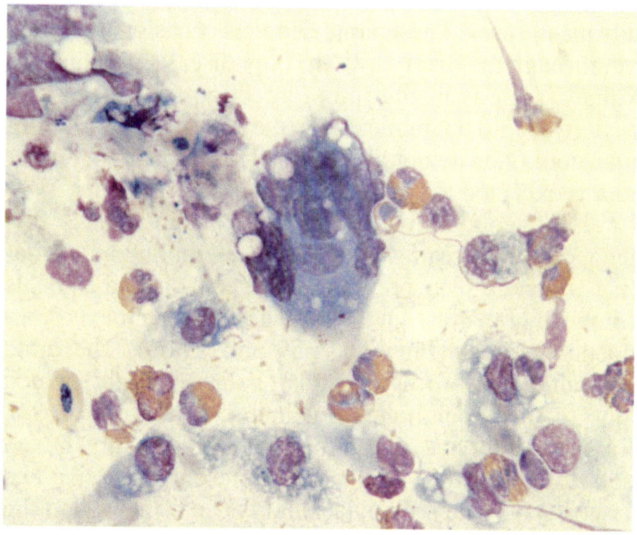

Fig. 15.57. A multinucleated osteoclast along with mixed cell inflammation and reduced granular background (mucin quality) in a joint fluid aspirate from a gyrfalcon (*Falco rusticolus*) with degenerative joint disease, Wright- Giemsa stain (100× oil).

et al., 2004; Van Wettere et al., 2012). Cytological examination of the synovial fluid of affected joints typically reveals a heterophilic (heterophilic arthritis) or mixed cell inflammation with no apparent etiologic agent. The cell count of the fluid can be (i.e., 42 000 to 55 000 leukocytes/µL) (Van Wettere et al., 2012).

Traumatic injury to the joint (traumatic arthritis) may reveal an increase in the number of inflammatory leukocytes, primarily heterophils in cases of acute trauma. Depending upon the degree of joint injury, synoviocytes and mesenchymal cells representing exfoliation of cells from the underlying cartilage may be present. Cartilage fragments may also be found. These are represented by the presence of amorphous material with variable staining characteristics on the Romanowsky-stained smear. The mucin clot test and viscosity of synovial fluid associated with acute traumatic arthritis is typically normal if hemarthrosis is not involved.

Articular gout, a common disorder of companion birds, is often diagnosed by the gross appearance of the

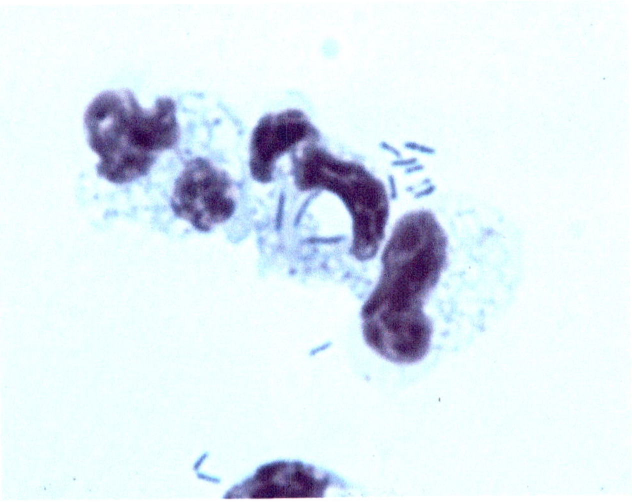

Fig. 15.58. Degenerate heterophils and extracellular and intracellular bacteria and reduced granular background (mucin quality) in a joint fluid aspirate from a great horned owl (*Bubo virginianus*) with septic arthritis, Wright–Giemsa stain (100× oil).

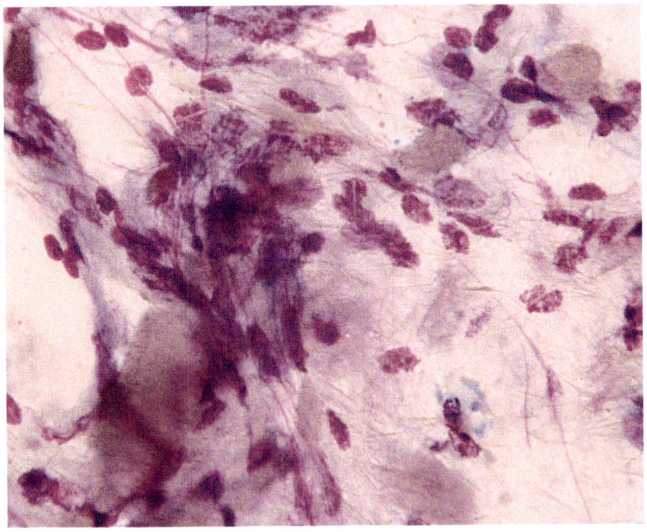

Fig. 15.59. Long, golden-colored, needle-shaped uric acid crystals in the joint fluid indicating articular gout in a Caribbean flamingo (*Phoenicopterus ruber*), Wright–Giemsa stain (100× oil).

affected joint. Cream-colored to yellow deposits (tophi) in the joint can be seen through the skin of birds in advanced cases. These urate deposits occasionally bulge out through the overlying skin. Any disease affecting the kidney, such as malnutrition, infectious processes, and toxicity, could be implicated in the development of articular gout (Nevarez et al., 2002). Therefore, hyperuricemia is expected to be associated with this disorder.

Early gout lesions may reveal a joint that is distended with a creamy, gritty fluid resembling an exudative effusion. The presence of needle-shaped crystals (monosodium urate) in the synovial fluid sample is diagnostic for gout (Figures 15.59 and 15.60). The urate crystals are birefringent under polarized light, which aids in their identification (Figures 15.61 and 15.62). Large numbers of inflammatory cells (usually mixed cell inflammation) are usually present as well. The viscosity of gouty synovial fluid is usually low, and the mucin clot test often provides poor results.

Joints affected by immune-mediated disease exhibit increased numbers of nondegenerate heterophils. Increased numbers of lymphocytes and plasma cells may also be seen. However, an easily recognized immune-mediated cause of joint disease in birds is rare.

Degenerative joint disease is represented by synovial fluid with mild increases in cell numbers compared to the marked increases observed with inflammatory joint disease. The cells in synovial fluid from a degenerative joint are represented primarily by mononuclear cells (greater than 90% of the cells), such as macrophages, lymphocytes, and synovial cells (Figure 15.63). Degenerative joint disease is more common, especially in captive waterfowl (Degernes et al., 2011). Joint aspirates associated with degenerative joint disease often

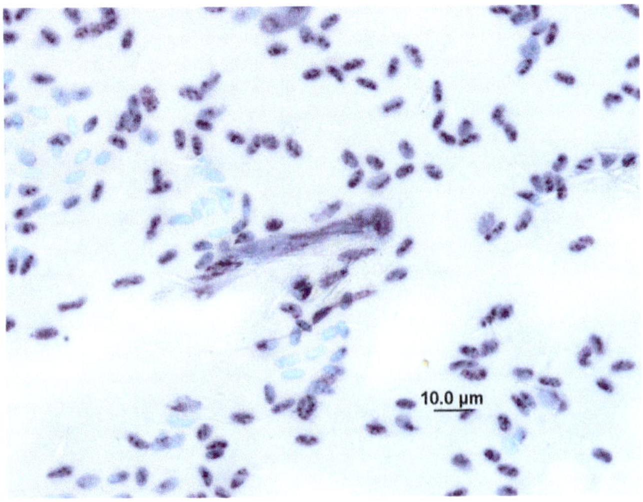

Fig. 15.60. Needle-shaped uric acid crystals in the joint fluid indicating articular gout in a cockatiel (*Nymphicus hollandicus*), Wright–Giemsa stain.

reveal synoviocytes, and mesenchymal cells representing exfoliation of cells from the underlying cartilage may be present. Cartilage fragments may also be found. These are represented by the presence of amorphous material with variable staining characteristics on the Romanowsky-stained smear. The viscosity and mucin clot tests may be normal or reduced with degenerative joint disease.

Inflammation of the Spleen

Splenitis is indicated by the presence of increased numbers of inflammatory cells in the splenic sample. When evaluating a splenic sample for splenitis, it is

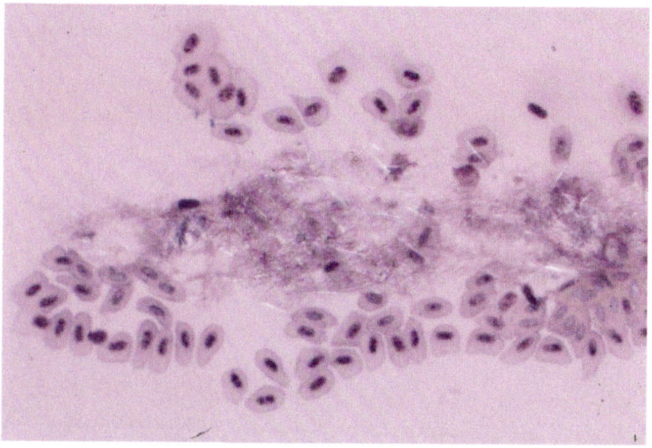

Fig. 15.61. Needle-shaped uric acid crystals from joint fluid indicating articular gout in a budgerigar (*Melopsittacus undulatus*), Diff–Quik stain (100× oil).

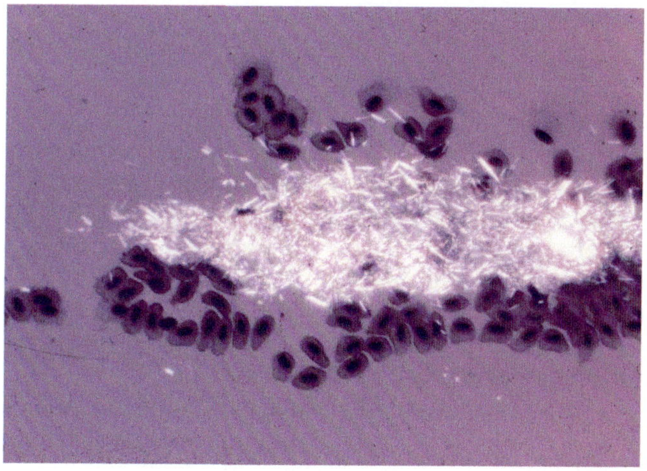

Fig. 15.62. The same needle-shaped uric acid crystals as in Figure 15.61 under polarized light from joint fluid indicating articular gout in a budgerigar (*Melopsittacus undulatus*), Diff–Quik stain (100× oil).

important to differentiate between true inflammatory changes in the spleen and contamination of the sample with peripheral blood that contains a peripheral leukocytosis. Cytologic specimens, splenic or otherwise, that are contaminated with peripheral blood having a marked leukocytosis appear to have an inflammatory response; however, the majority of heterophils present have originated from the blood and not from the tissue being examined.

Septicemia may reveal high numbers of small lymphocytes, large lymphoblasts, reactive lymphocytes, and macrophages on splenic preparations. Bacteremia and infectious splenitis may reveal numerous macrophages containing cytoplasmic bacteria with fewer organisms present in the background (Gartrell et al., 2005).

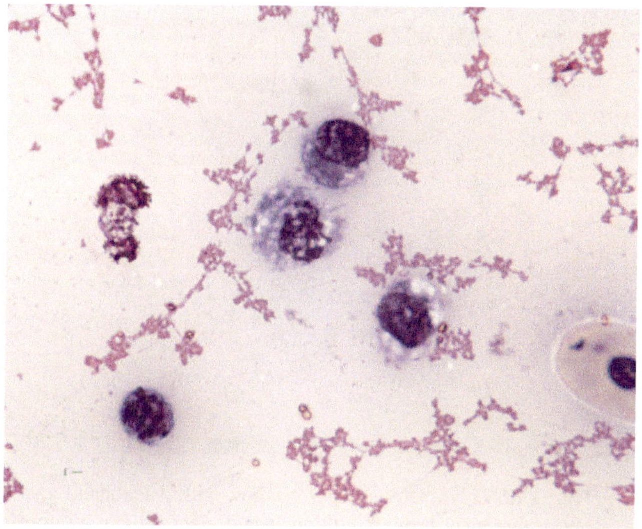

Fig. 15.63. Inflammatory cells (macrophages and lymphocyte) and reduced granular background (mucin quality) in a joint fluid aspirate from a bald eagle (*Haliaeetus leucocephalus*) with degenerative joint disease, Wright–Giemsa stain (100× oil).

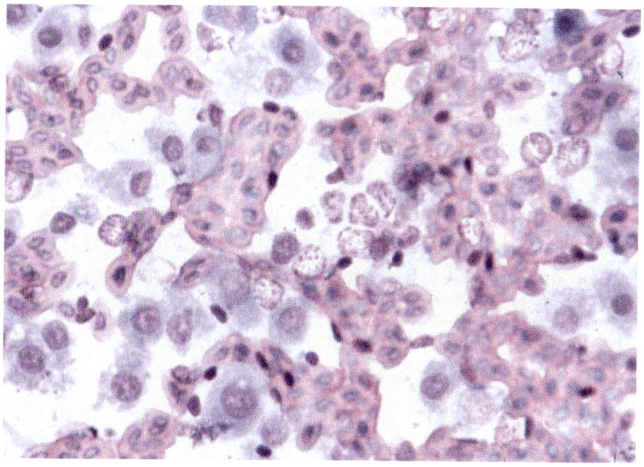

Fig. 15.64. An imprint of a liver biopsy shows numerous erythrocytes, hepatocytes, and mature heterophils in a budgerigar (*Melopsittacus undulatus*) with hepatitis. The number of heterophils present exceeds that expected from peripheral blood contamination of the sample alone, Diff–Quik stain (400×).

Inflammation of the Liver

Hepatitis (inflammatory responses involving the liver) is indicated by the presence of numerous leukocytes in the cytology specimen. Suppurative inflammation – that is, heterophilic inflammation – is suggested when high numbers of mature heterophils are observed relative to the red blood cell numbers (Figure 15.64). The presence of heterophils associated with aggregates of hepatocytes provides further cytologic support of suppurative inflammation. Heterophilic inflammation in birds may be differentiated from hepatic heterophil granulocytopoiesis by the presence of a predominance

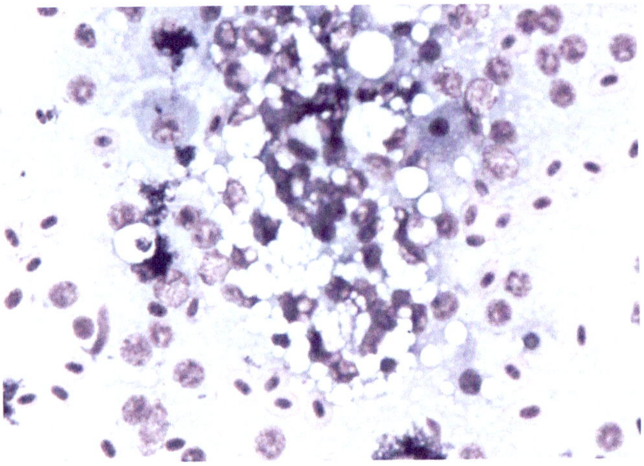

Fig. 15.65. Numerous macrophages with vacuolated cytoplasm that have formed multinucleated giant cells in a imprint of a liver biopsy from a red-tailed hawk (*Buteo jamaicensis*). The macrophagic inflammation is indicative of a granulomatous lesion. In this case the histopathology revealed a mycobacterial granuloma. Diff–Quik stain (100× oil).

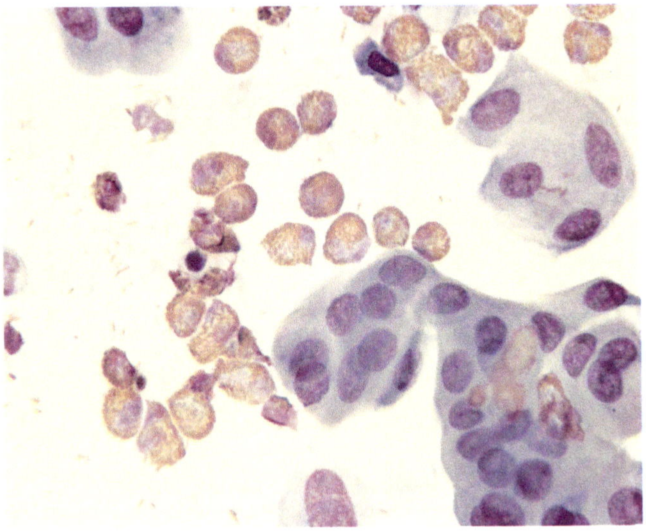

Fig. 15.66. Heterophilic inflammation with epithelial cells in a conjunctival swab from an emu (*Dromaius novaehollandiae*) with conjunctivitis, Wright–Giemsa stain (100× oil).

of mature heterophils and an absence of immature, developing heterophils. Septic inflammation is indicated by the presence of bacteria within leukocytes. Extracellular bacteria must be differentiated from "cadaver" bacteria or bacterial contamination of the sample when the sample is obtained during necropsy.

Mixed cell or macrophagic inflammation of the liver can be associated with mycotic, parasitic, or mycobacterial infections. Granulomatous lesions reveal macrophages that are often vacuolated and multinucleated giant cells (Figure 15.65).

Ophthalmic Inflammation

Corneal cytology is indicated whenever there are superficial erosions and progressive ulceration associated with infiltrations of inflammatory cells. Bacterial and fungal keratitis may occur in birds and corneal scraping may reveal bacteria or fungal hyphae or yeast with confirmation of the etiologic agent provided by microbial culture (Sadar et al., 2014; Schunk et al., 2017).

Obtaining an ophthalmic sample (cornea or conjunctiva) for cytology requires use of a topical anesthetic (1 or 2 drops), and after 60 seconds the sample can be obtained by gentle scraping; then the smear is stained with Giemsa or Diff–Quick. However, one should be aware that a topical anesthetic can cause systemic toxicity in birds; therefore, general anesthesia should be considered (Bayón et al., 2007).

Conjunctivitis is a common cause for sampling the conjunctiva for cytologic examination and is recognized by the presence of many inflammatory cells (Figure 15.66). Heterophilic inflammation of the conjunctiva can be caused by bacteria, viruses, or noninfectious agents, such as trauma, foreign bodies, and environmental irritants.

Degenerate heterophils are often associated with bacterial infections. Septic conjunctivitis is confirmed cytologically by the presence of phagocytosis of the bacterial pathogens. The epithelial cells in septic lesions may show degenerative changes such as cytoplasmic vacuolation, karyolysis, or karyorrhexis.

Bacterial conjunctivitis is the most commonly diagnosed cause of conjunctivitis in birds and is frequently associated with upper respiratory tract infections (Abrams et al., 2005). Numerous bacteria may be associated with this condition. Common isolates include *Pseudomonas* spp., *Staphylococcus* spp., *Pasteurella* spp., *Citrobacter* spp., *Escherichia coli*, *Klebsiella* spp., and *Haemophilus* spp. *Haemophilus* conjunctivitis is often associated with systemic disease in birds (Devriesc et al., 1988; Yamamoto, 1991). *Mycobacterium avium* has been associated with conjunctival granulomas of the nictitating membrane of birds (Hood, 1978; Pocknell et al., 1996). Bacterial conjunctivitis in birds has also been caused infectious by *Streptococcus* spp., *Erysipelothrix rhusiopathiae*, *Clostridium botulinum*, and *Bordetella avium* (Bayón et al., 2007).

Viruses associated with conjunctivitis in birds include Newcastle virus, paramyxovirus, poxvirus, cytomegalovirus, herpesvirus, adenovirus, and pneumovirus (Bayón et al., 2007). Parasites may also be associated with conjunctivitis in birds; for example, *Cryptosporidium*-like structures associated with *Cryptosporidium baileyi* in the conjunctival cells were reported in owls (Molina-López et al., 2010).

The mucopurulent discharge associated with a bacterial conjunctivitis in mammals is not typically seen in birds owing to the differences in the activities of mammalian neutrophils and heterophils of birds. Instead, bacterial infections in birds tend to be more caseous. Septic conjunctivitis is confirmed cytologically by the presence of phagocytosis of the bacterial pathogens. The epithelial cells in septic lesions may show degenerative changes such as cytoplasmic vacuolation, karyolysis, or karyorrhexis.

Chlamydia organisms may be seen on cytologic specimens from conjunctival scrapings. They appear as intracytoplasmic inclusion bodies in epithelial cells.

Mycoplasma is frequently overlooked as a cause for conjunctivitis because it can be difficult to diagnose. Mycoplasmal inclusions appear as small basophilic granules on the surface of epithelial cells (Figure 15.67).

Eyelid disorders can result from traumatic injury (i.e., lacerations, hemorrhages, and abrasions) or infectious disease. The most frequently described causes of infectious eyelid diseases are blepharoconjunctivitis caused by *Staphylococcus* in Amazon parrots; fibrinopurulent blepharoconjunctivitis secondary to *Escherichia coli*, *Streptococcus* spp., and *Pasteurella multocida*; *Actinobacillus* spp. in waterfowl; bilateral supraorbital abscesses due to *Pseudomonas* spp. in Amazon parrot; poxvirus in dove, parrots, canaries, mynas, and birds of prey; blepharitis due to parvovirus in geese; and protuberant lesions for *Knemidocoptes pilae* mites in parakeets (Bayón et al., 2007). Hypovitaminosis A can result in conjunctival hyperkeratosis and swelling of the eyelids, resembling lesions caused by poxvirus.

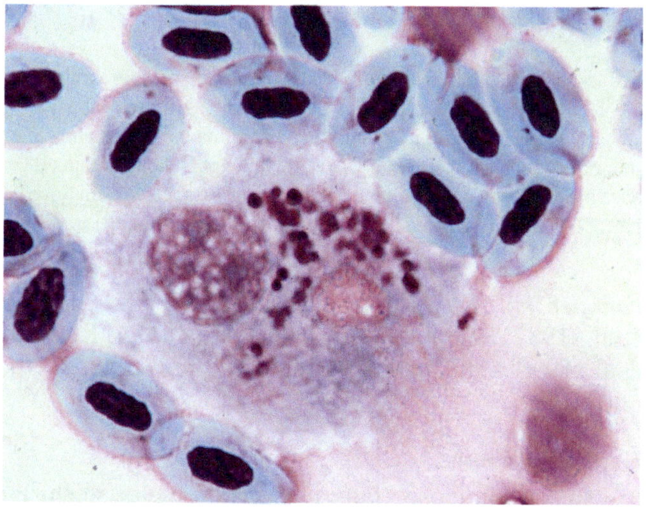

Fig. 15.67. An epithelial cell (one of several such cells) containing intracytoplasmic inclusions resembling those of *Mycoplasma* in the serous ocular and nasal discharge of a peach-faced lovebird (*Agapornis roseicollis*). *Mycoplasma gallisepticum* was isolated from the sample, Wright–Giemsa stain (100× oil).

Hyperplasia/Benign neoplasia

Examples of tissue hyperplasia or benign neoplasia that are frequently identified by cytodiagnosis in birds include squamous cell hyperplasia or metaplasia associated with hypovitaminosis A, lipomas, and lymphoid hyperplasia. Plasma cell hyperplasia is commonly found in lymphoid tissues in association with certain infectious diseases, such as avian chlamydiosis. Cells suggestive of hyperplasia of epithelial and connective tissue often occur in cytologic specimens of long-standing chronic inflammation.

Adipose

As in mammals, avian lipomas are benign, encapsulated accumulations of adipose tissue occurring in the subcutis that are composed of normal, mature adipocytes (fat cells), and can be difficult to differentiate histologically and cytologically from normal adipose tissue if the capsule is not observed (DeVoe et al., 2004; Blakey et al., 2018). Grossly, lipomas typically appear as pale yellow, soft, often freely movable subcutaneous masses that occur singly or as multiple masses. Lipomas are slow growing and can become quite large, causing epithelial ulceration from lack of blood supply, and if traumatized can become inflamed and necrotic. They may even become infiltrative (Mehler et al., 2007). Because it is often cytologically difficult to differentiate a lipoma from normal adipose tissue, accidental aspiration of normal adipose tissue should be considered a rule-out whenever lipocytes are identified in a cytology sample. The gross appearance of the tissue sample may aid in the diagnosis in some cases. Grossly, unstained aspirated material from a lipoma has a "greasy" appearance and does not dry completely on the slide due to the lipid content.

Avian adipocytes vary in size and can appear as large, round cells with an abundant foamy cytoplasm containing large vacuoles and are often blended with extracellular fat (Figures 15.68a–15.68d). The nucleus is typically located adjacent to the cell margin, as seen in mammalian adipocytes. Avian adipocytes differ from mammalian adipocytes in that they do not appear to have just one large cytoplasmic vacuole, but instead have numerous cytoplasmic vacuoles of variable sizes. These cells would be considered highly abnormal and perhaps an indicator of liposarcoma in a mammalian specimen.

Although relatively uncommon, lipomas and liposarcomas have been reported in the integument of birds (Tully et al., 1994; Romagnano and Heard, 2000; Gill, 2005). Lipomas are especially common neoplasms of the integument in budgerigars (*Melopsittacus undulatus*), rose-breasted cockatoos (*Eolophus roseicapilla*), cockatiels (*Nymphicus hollandicus*), and Amazon parrots (*Amazona* spp.) (Campbell, 1995; Schmidt, 1997; Romagnano and Heard, 2000; Gill, 2005; Zoller

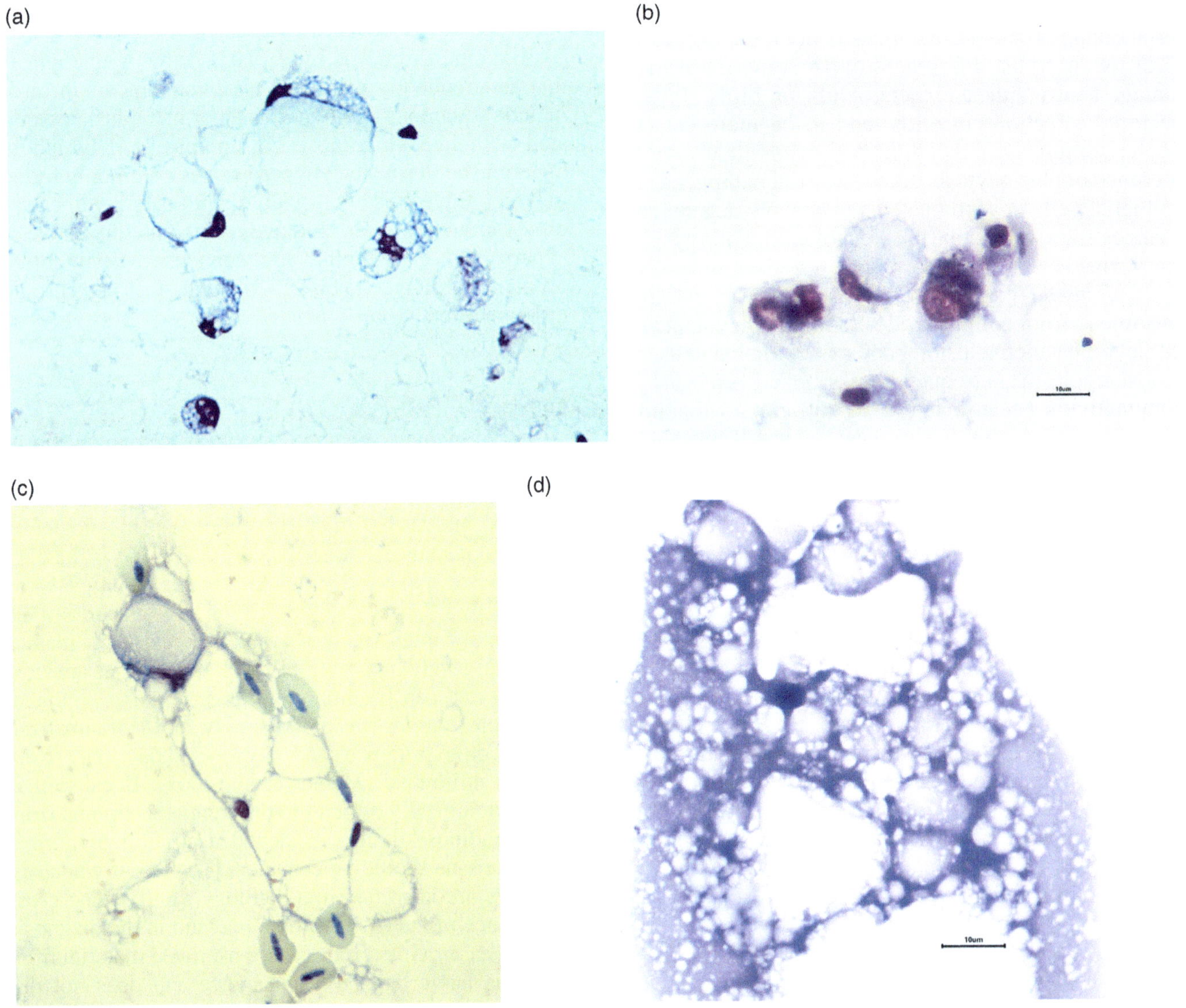

Fig. 15.68. (a) Adipocytes and a background containing fat droplets in a fine-needle aspiration biopsy of a soft tissue subcutaneous mass over the keel of a budgerigar (*Melopsittacus undulatus*), Diff–Quik stain (100× oil); (b) An adipocyte from a fine-needle aspiration biopsy of a lipoma in an umbrella cockatoo (*Cacatua alba*), Diff–Quik stain (100× oil). (c) Adipocytes and a background containing fat droplets in a fine-needle aspiration biopsy of a soft tissue mass in the coelomic cavity of an umbrella cockatoo bird (*Cacatua alba*), Wright–Giemsa stain (100× oil). Source: Image from Campbell and Grant (2010, p. 267). (d) Adipocytes blended with a background containing fat droplets in a fine-needle aspiration biopsy of a subcutaneous lipoma from a spectacled Amazon parrot (*Amazona albifrons*), Wright–Giemsa stain (100× oil).

et al., 2019). In companion birds, lipomas can occur anywhere on the body, but frequently are found in the sternal and ventral abdominal areas, between muscles, or within the coelomic cavity extending to the subcutaneous space. Lipomas, which occur frequently in psittacines, are rarely diagnosed in gallinaceous birds (Blakey et al., 2018).

Liposarcomas are rare neoplasms of birds, but have been reported in the budgerigar (*Melopsittacus undulatus*), cockatiel (*Nymphicus hollandicus*), Quaker parakeet (*Myiopsitta monachus*), green-cheek conure (*Pyrrhura molinae*), African gray parrot (*Psittacus erithacus*), pigeon (*Columba livia*), chukar partridge (*Alectoris chukar*), and Canada goose (*Branta canadensis*) (Petrak and Gilmore, 1982; Doster et al., 1987; Schmidt, 1992; Tully et al., 1994; Ritzman et al., 1996; Graham et al., 2003; Beaufrère et al., 2019).

Hepatic Lipidosis

Hepatic lipidosis (fatty liver syndrome or steatosis) is represented by the appearance of hepatocytes with many small or large clear cytoplasmic vacuoles, which represent lipid that has dissolved during the staining process (Figure 15.69). Unstained smears made from livers with fatty change may appear "greasy" on gross inspection of the slide.

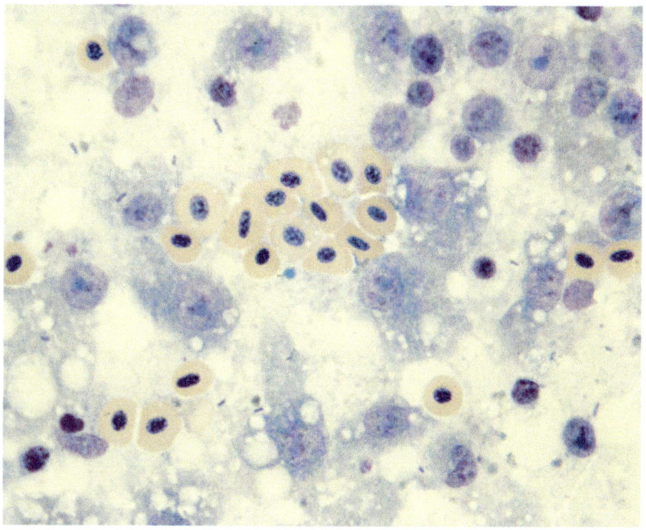

Fig. 15.69. Hepatocytes severely distended by small, clear vacuoles (presumed to be lipid) and a background containing numerous round structures presumed to be free lipid droplets in a contact smear of a liver from a bird (*Nymphicus hollandicus*), Wright–Giemsa stain (100× oil).

The liver of post-hatched birds may exhibit hepatocytes with cytoplasmic fat vacuoles because they are processing fat from the retained yolk as part of the normal post-hatching physiology.

Feather Cysts

Feather cysts and dermal cysts are often diagnosed in companion birds (Chaudary, 1987). Feather cysts present as subcutaneous swellings that may resemble a cutaneous neoplasm and result from the failure of a growing feather to erupt through the skin. As the feather continues to grow in its follicle, the cutaneous mass enlarges. Early feather cysts may exhibit numerous erythrocytes and erythrophagocytosis in the cytologic specimen. Chronic feather cysts contain keratinocytes, keratinaceous debris, feather fragments, and caseous exudation. The feather cysts commonly found in Norwich canaries are often considered to be benign basal cell tumors or feather folliculomas (Gill, 2005).

Papillomatosis

Cloacal and internal papillomatosis of psittacine birds is a disease of New World psittacines, such as macaws, Amazon parrots, conures, Pionus parrots, and hawk-headed parrots; however, it can also be found in Old World psittacines, such as cockatoos, as well (McDonald, 1988; Graham, 1991; Phalen et al., 1998, Gartrell et al., 2009). Papillomas are difficult to diagnose by cytology alone because they reveal predominantly cornified squamous epithelial cells on the cellular sample if they originate from cutaneous epithelium. However, if they originate from mucosal epithelium, nonsquamous epithelial cells will predominate.

Papillomas are commonly found on the mucosal surfaces of the cloaca, but may be found in the oral cavity, esophagus, crop, proventriculus, and ventriculus as well. Papillomatous lesions on mucosal surfaces are characterized by proliferation of the lining epithelium on a fibrovascular stalk. The resulting multiple fronds of epithelium varying from simple to pseudostratified columnar epithelium and proliferation of goblet cells with underlying well-vascularized connective tissue stroma infiltrated with mixed inflammatory cells (heterophils, macrophages, lymphocytes, plasma cells) (Gartrell et al., 2009). Therefore, cloacal (mucosal) papillomas are difficult to diagnose by cytology alone, because they reveal a variety of cell types (Figures 15.70a–15.70f).

Squamous Hyperplasia/Metaplasia

Hypovitaminosis A causes hyperkeratosis and hyperplasia of squamous epithelium and squamous metaplasia of nonsquamous epithelium in all species. Metaplasia is the transformation of nonsquamous epithelium into squamous epithelium.

This disorder is especially common in the oral cavity of companion psittacine birds. Cytology samples obtained by gently scraping the oral cavity of a normal animal reveal few squamous cells that have exfoliated singly or in small groups (Figure 15.71). When squamous cell hyperplasia or squamous metaplasia is present, scrapings from the oral cavity yield numerous squamous epithelial cells and small tissue fragments composed of tightly packed squamous epithelial cells that stain basophilic (indicating keratinization).

As with this condition in mammalian cytology, the cytology of early lesions in birds with hypovitaminosis A reveals many highly cornified squamous epithelial cells, little background debris, and no evidence of inflammation, yeast, or protozoa. Chronic lesions are often characterized by the presence of secondary infection and an associated neutrophilic, heterophilic, or mixed cell inflammatory response in addition to the squamous hyperplasia or metaplasia.

Squamous metaplasia of the epithelial cells of the upper respiratory tract may occur as a response to chronic inflammation, irritation, or hypovitaminosis A (commonly found in birds fed inadequate diets). Hypovitaminosis A causes squamous metaplasia of mucin-secreting epithelium as the simple or pseudostratified columnar epithelium changes to stratified squamous cells (Rosenthal et al., 1994; Kim et al., 2002). Squamous metaplasia in the cytologic sample is suggested by the presence of numerous squamous epithelial cells, small tissue fragments composed of tightly packed

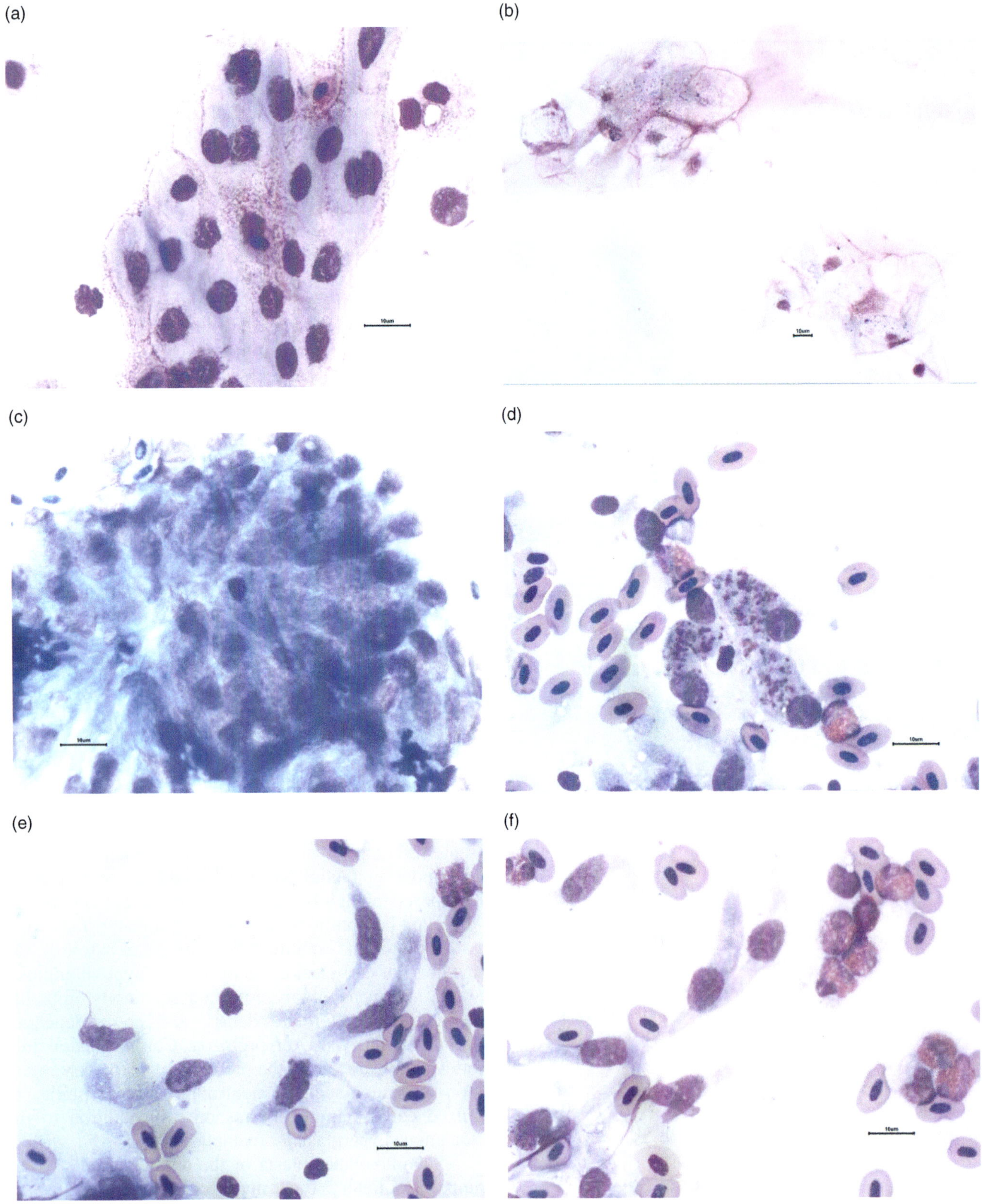

Fig. 15.70. (a) Simple epithelial cells from an imprint of the biopsy of a cloacal papilloma from an orange-wing Amazon parrot (*Amazona amazonica*), Wright–Giemsa stain (100× oil). (b) Simple epithelial cells from an imprint of the biopsy of a cloacal papilloma from an African gray parrot (*Psittacus erithacus*), Wright–Giemsa stain. (c) Columnar epithelial cells from an imprint of the biopsy of a cloacal papilloma from an African gray parrot (*Psittacus erithacus*), Wright–Giemsa stain (100× oil). (d) Goblet cells likely representing goblet cell proliferation in an imprint of the biopsy of a cloacal papilloma from an African gray parrot (*Psittacus erithacus*), Wright–Giemsa stain (100× oil). (e) Mesenchymal cells (fibroblasts) from the connective tissue stroma in an imprint of the biopsy of a cloacal papilloma from an African gray parrot (*Psittacus erithacus*), Wright–Giemsa stain (100× oil). (f) Mesenchymal cells (fibroblasts) from the connective tissue stroma and heterophils from the inflammatory response in an imprint of the biopsy of a cloacal papilloma from an African gray parrot (*Psittacus erithacus*), Wright–Giemsa stain (100× oil).

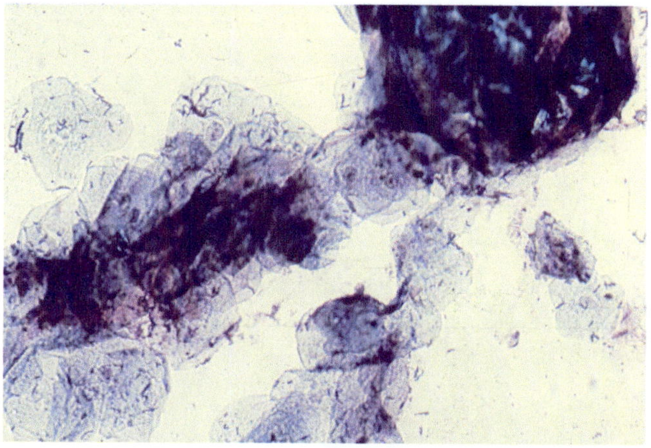

Fig. 15.71. Clusters of keratinized epithelial cells with no evidence of inflammation, yeast, or protozoa in a swab of cream-colored, raised lesion surrounding the choanal slit in a bird (*Amazona aestiva*), Diff–Quik stain (100× oil).

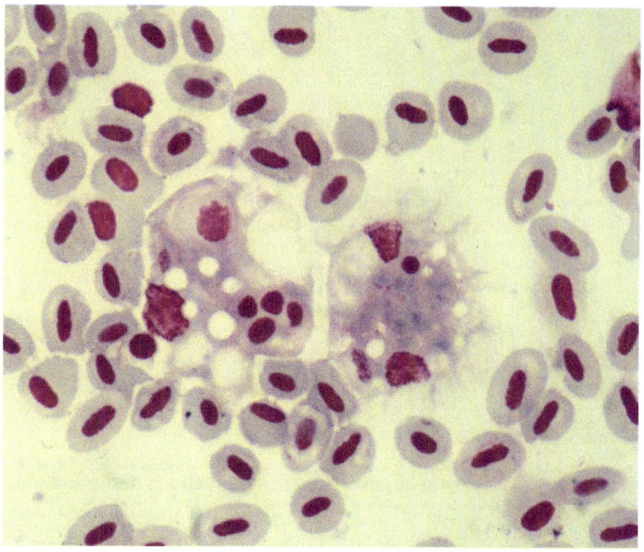

Fig. 15.72. Macrophages exhibiting erythrophagocytosis in the coelomic fluid from a cockatiel (*Nymphicus hollandicus*) diagnosed with an ovarian cystadenocarcinoma, Diff–Quik stain (100× oil).

squamous epithelial cells that stain basophilic (indicating keratinization), no evidence of inflammation, and little background debris.

Malignant Neoplasia

The same cytologic features of malignant neoplasia of mammals also apply to the avian cytology sample. For example, the cytological evidence of hemorrhage in an area without a history of trauma may suggest an erosive neoplasm. Erythrophagocytosis in such lesions would be indicative of chronic hemorrhage (Figure 15.72). A common location for this to occur is the coelomic cavity of birds. A chronic hemoperitoneum with radiographic evidence of a coelomic mass leads to the presumptive diagnosis of a neoplasm, although there may be no direct cellular evidence of malignant cells in the fluid.

Lymphoma/Lymphocytic Leukemia

Lymphoma is a common round cell tumor of birds, but other types, such as mast cell tumors and histiocytic tumors, have been rarely reported (Swayne et al, 1990; Sacre et al, 1992; Campbell and Grant, 2010). Lymphoma is the primary neoplasia of lymphocytes, and the cytology indicative of lymphoma reveals a predominance of medium or large lymphocytes representing 60% to 90% of the cell population (Figures 15.73a–15.73c). The neoplastic lymphocytes are often immature and are represented by lymphoblasts and prolymphocytes. Numerous classification schemes have been applied to lymphoid tumors in dogs, but none have been developed for lower vertebrates even as they are common neoplasms of birds, reptiles, amphibians, and fish (Heidenreich, 1997; Baker and Lumsden, 2000; Forbes et al., 2000; Kelly et al., 2004; Souza et al., 2008; Malka et al., 2008; Rivera et al., 2009; Nevarez et al., 2011; Schmidt et al., 2012). A viral etiology has been found as the cause of lymphoid neoplasia in poultry, but few have been described in other avian species (Halliwell, 1971; Drén et al., 1988; Haesendonck et al., 2015). Hypercalcemia and hyperglobulinemia associated with paraneoplastic syndrome commonly reported in domestic mammals with malignant lymphoma rarely occur in birds (de Wit et al., 2003; Lennox et al., 2014).

Multicentric T-cell lymphomas and lymphocytic leukemia are often reported in aged birds (Sinclair et al., 2015). Cytochemical and immunohistochemical staining allow for evaluation and differentiation of the neoplastic cell populations and a definitive diagnosis, such as either a T-cell or B-cell lymphoid leukemia.

Cytological findings associated with lymphoid neoplasia of birds are typically characterized by the same criteria described for this neoplasm in mammals: a monotypic, homogenous, or heterogeneous population of lymphocytes devoid of inflammatory cells. Cells from malignant lymphoid tissue exhibit a marked increase in the number of large lymphocytes, such as lymphoblasts; nuclear and cytoplasmic pleomorphism; cytoplasmic basophilia; and mitotic figures. Abnormal or multiple nucleoli are also frequently seen. In mammals, the cell size is estimated by comparing the average nuclear diameter of the abnormal lymphocytes to the size of a non-distorted red cell (i.e., the average diameter of a dog erythrocyte is 7 μm): however, because of the relatively large size of the oval erythrocytes of birds, cell size comparison with erythrocytes may be more difficult than with the spherical erythrocytes of mammals.

Lymphocytic leukemia, lymphoid neoplasia involving blood or bone marrow, is characterized by a marked

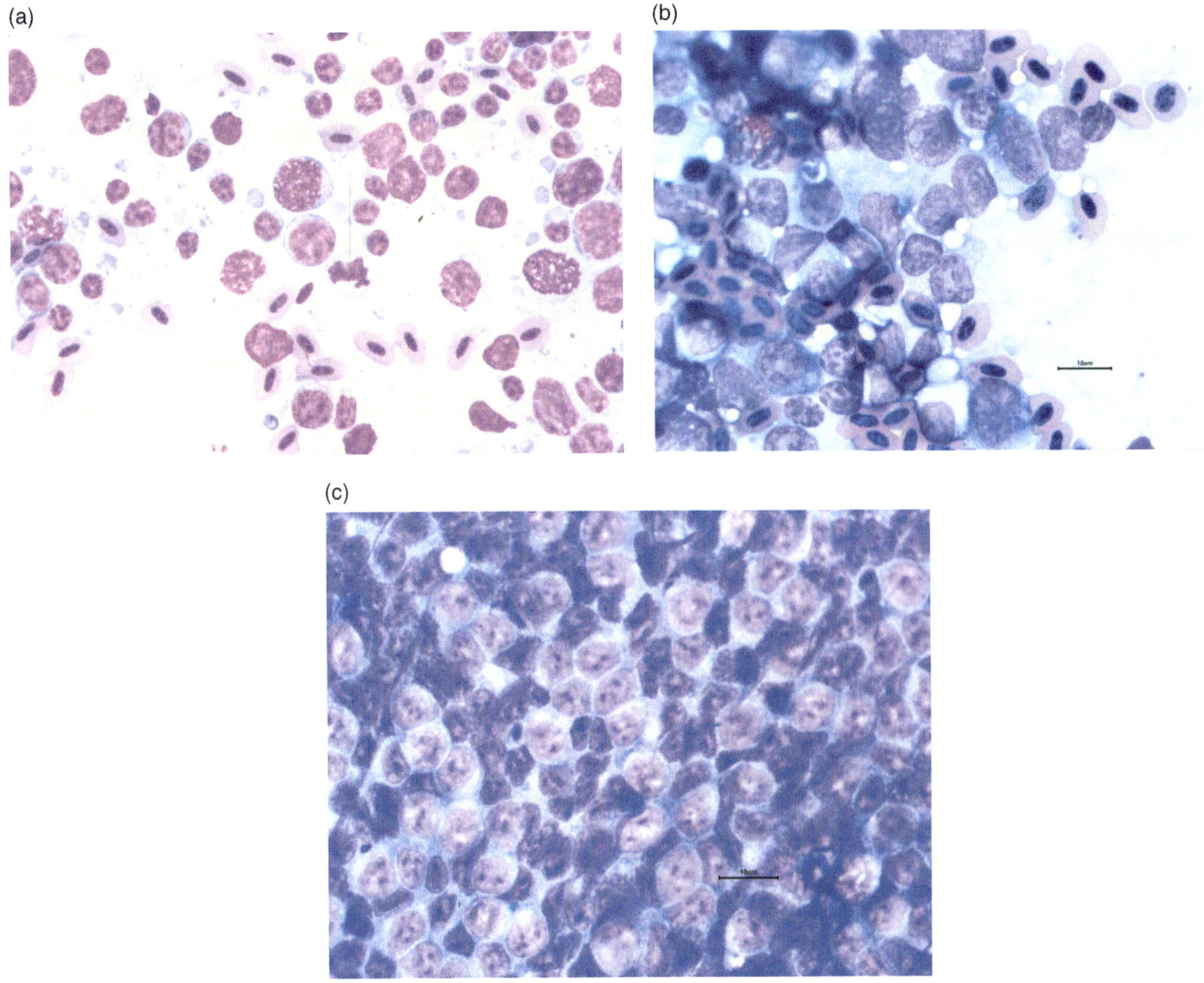

Fig. 15.73. (a) Numerous pleomorphic lymphocytes that exhibit marked anisocytosis with variable nuclear chromatin patterns and multiple prominent nucleoli in a fine-needle aspiration biopsy of a subcutaneous mass diagnosed as lymphoma from a spectacled Amazon parrot (*Amazona albifrons*), Diff–Quik stain (100× oil). (b) A predominance of large, immature lymphocytes in a fine-needle aspiration biopsy of an intracoelomic mass diagnosed as lymphoma from a blue and gold macaw (*Ara ararauna*), Wright–Giemsa stain. (c) A 50:50 mixture of mature and large immature lymphocytes in a fine-needle aspiration biopsy of an intracoelomic mass diagnosed as lymphoma from a cockatiel (*Nymphicus hollandicus*), Wright–Giemsa stain.

increase in lymphocytes in the peripheral blood, especially with the presence of abnormal lymphocyte morphology (Kelly et al., 2004; Campbell and Grant, 2010; Hammond et al., 2010; Osofsky et al., 2011; Gaharan et al., 2012). Important morphology includes large lymphocytes (larger than heterophils) with fine nuclear chromatin and a pale-staining nucleus. A prominent nucleolus and increased cytoplasmic volume are additional supportive features of malignant lymphocytes. Occasionally, neoplastic lymphocytes exhibit cytoplasmic vacuolation. Affected birds may exhibit anemia, leukocytosis, and thrombocytopenia as well as the presence of neoplastic lymphocytes in the peripheral blood (Coleman, 1995; Rivera et al., 2009). In some cases, most lymphocytes appear as small, mature lymphocytes with scalloped cytoplasmic margins (Purchase and Burmester, 1978; Campbell, 1984; Campbell and Ellis, 2007). Lymphocytosis, heterophilia, monocytosis, mild regenerative anemia, and a predominance of mature lymphocytes with scalloped cell margins have been associated with the sarcoma/leukosis complex of chickens (Ritchie, 1995a, 1995b).

Chronic myelogenous leukemia (CML) is a rare disease in birds. One case has been reported in an owl that presented with a severe leukocytosis that consisted primarily of mature heterophils (Wiley et al., 2009). A presumptive diagnosis of CML was made based on the persistence of the leukocytosis lasting longer than 3 months; lack of identifiable foci of inflammation; and lack of response to conventional therapy.

Carcinoma

Squamous cell carcinomas are common neoplasms in mammals, but are less common in birds: however, they have been reported in aged psittacines (especially cockatiels, Amazon parrots, conures, budgerigars, eclectus parrots, and macaws), storks, poultry, hornbills, flamingos, raptors, and penguins (Miller et al., 1985; Murtaugh et al., 1986; Leach, 1992; Lopez-Beceiro et al., 1998; Manucy et al., 1998; Pye et al., 1999; Ramis et al., 1999; Gill, 2005; Abu et al., 2009; Campbell and Grant, 2010; Zehnder et al., 2014; Halley et al., 2020). The most likely sites for development are the skin (patagial and axillary regions) and upper gastrointestinal tract, including the beak, oral cavity, esophagus, crop, and proventriculus (Ramis et al., 1999; Malka et al., 2005; Klaphake et al., 2006; Heatley et al., 2007; Suedmeyer et al., 2007; Le et al., 2011; Rettenmund et al., 2015; Schmidt et al., 2015; Zehnder et al., 2018; Staudenmaier et al., 2019) (Figures 15.74a–15.74e). Squamous cell carcinomas in birds usually arise from single or multiple sites in the skin, mucocutaneous junctions, uropygial gland, and upper gastrointestinal tract. They rarely originate at the beak; however, when this occurs, it leads to chronic non-healing wounds, beak deformities (cracking, peeling, irregular growth, overgrowth), and potential difficulty in prehending food and water (Halley et al., 2020). These neoplasms also cause osteolysis of the underlying bone as a result of local invasion. Squamous cell carcinomas frequently develop necrotic areas with secondary bacteria or fungal infections. Squamous cell carcinoma can also arise in the respiratory tract (Diaz-Figueroa et al., 2006). Avian poxvirus associated with squamous cell carcinoma has been reported in some cases (Fallavena et al., 2002; Pesaro et al., 2009). In some avian species, the cells of squamous cell carcinoma are strongly immunopositive for cytokeratin AE1/AE3 (Halley et al., 2020).

Adenocarcinomas have been reported in a variety of avian species and affect multiple tissues, including the gastrointestinal tract, reproductive tract, pancreas, liver, kidney, integument, and respiratory tract (Robertson et al., 2020). The cytologic examination of fine-needle aspirates of a pancreatic adenocarcinoma have revealed round to slightly polygonal cells loosely to tightly aggregated with small to moderate amounts of medium blue cytoplasm and oval nuclei with fine to coarsely stippled chromatin and multiple prominent nucleoli; and therefore, indicative of malignant neoplasia based upon the mild to moderate anisocytosis and anisokaryosis with occasional karyomegaly and multinucleation (Le Roux et al., 2020).

See Chapter 7 for cytologic descriptions of squamous cell carcinomas in mammals.

Basal cell tumors are dermal tumors that are also seen commonly in mammals, but rarely in birds (Tell et al., 1997; Bradford et al., 2009). Cytologic descriptions of basal cell tumors are presented in the mammalian section.

Sarcoma

Sarcomas commonly occur in birds (Figures 15.75 and 15.76a–15.76d). Fibromas and fibrosarcomas are frequently reported in birds (Reavill and Schmidt, 2000; Lamberski and Theon, 2002; Gill, 2005; Ochi et al., 2012) (Figures 15.77a–15.77c, 15.78, 15.79a–15.79c, 15.80a–15.80d, 15.81a and 15.81b).

See Chapter 7 for cytologic descriptions of fibromas and fibrosarcomas in mammals.

Rhabdomyosarcoma (a malignant tumor originating from rhabdomyoblasts) is rarely reported in birds (Maluenda et al., 2010). The cytology of rhabdomyosarcomas reveals spindle-shaped cells with features of malignancy and cytoplasmic cross-striations indicative of muscle cells.

Peripheral nerve sheath tumors (neurofibromas, schwannomas, neurilemmomas, and perineuromas) are rare in birds (Carvalho et al., 2016). Cytologic preparations reveal neoplastic spindle cells.

Hemangiomas and hemangiosarcomas have been reported in a variety of locations in a variety of avian species (Suedmeyer et al., 2001b; Hanley et al., 2005; Headley, 2005; Sledge et al., 2006; Campbell and Ellis, 2007; Mickley et al., 2009; Campbell and Grant, 2010; Nakano and Une, 2012; Kline et al., 2016; Piccione et al., 2017). These neoplasms may have a viral etiology (subgroup J avian leukosis virus) in domestic chickens (Sun et al., 2010; Lai et al., 2011). Cytologic samples from these tumors contain heavy amounts of peripheral blood contamination with erythrophagocytosis and/or macrophages that contain hemosiderin pigment indicative of chronic hemorrhage. Thrombocytes are usually not present in the cytology sample owing to the long-standing nature of the hemorrhagic lesion. Additional cytologic features of hemangiomas may include an occasional small basophilic endothelial cell. The cytology of hemangiosarcomas tends to be more cellular, although the overall cellularity is poor. Aggregates of pleomorphic mesenchymal cells with high N:C ratios, basophilic cytoplasm, indistinct cell margins, and oval nuclei containing coarse chromatin and prominent multiple nucleoli among a background of peripheral blood cells is suggestive of a hemangiosarcoma (Figures 15.82a, 15.82b, 15.83a, and 15.83b).

Mesenchymal neoplasms, such as epithelioid hemangiosarcomas that have an epithelial-like appearance, may be misidentified as epithelial tumors based on cytology alone (Piccione et al., 2017). Neoplastic cells of epithelioid hemangiosarcomas can be small, round to polygonal with indistinct borders, and arranged in variably sized clusters, even with pseudo-acinar arrangements (Figure 15.84). The cells have scant amount of

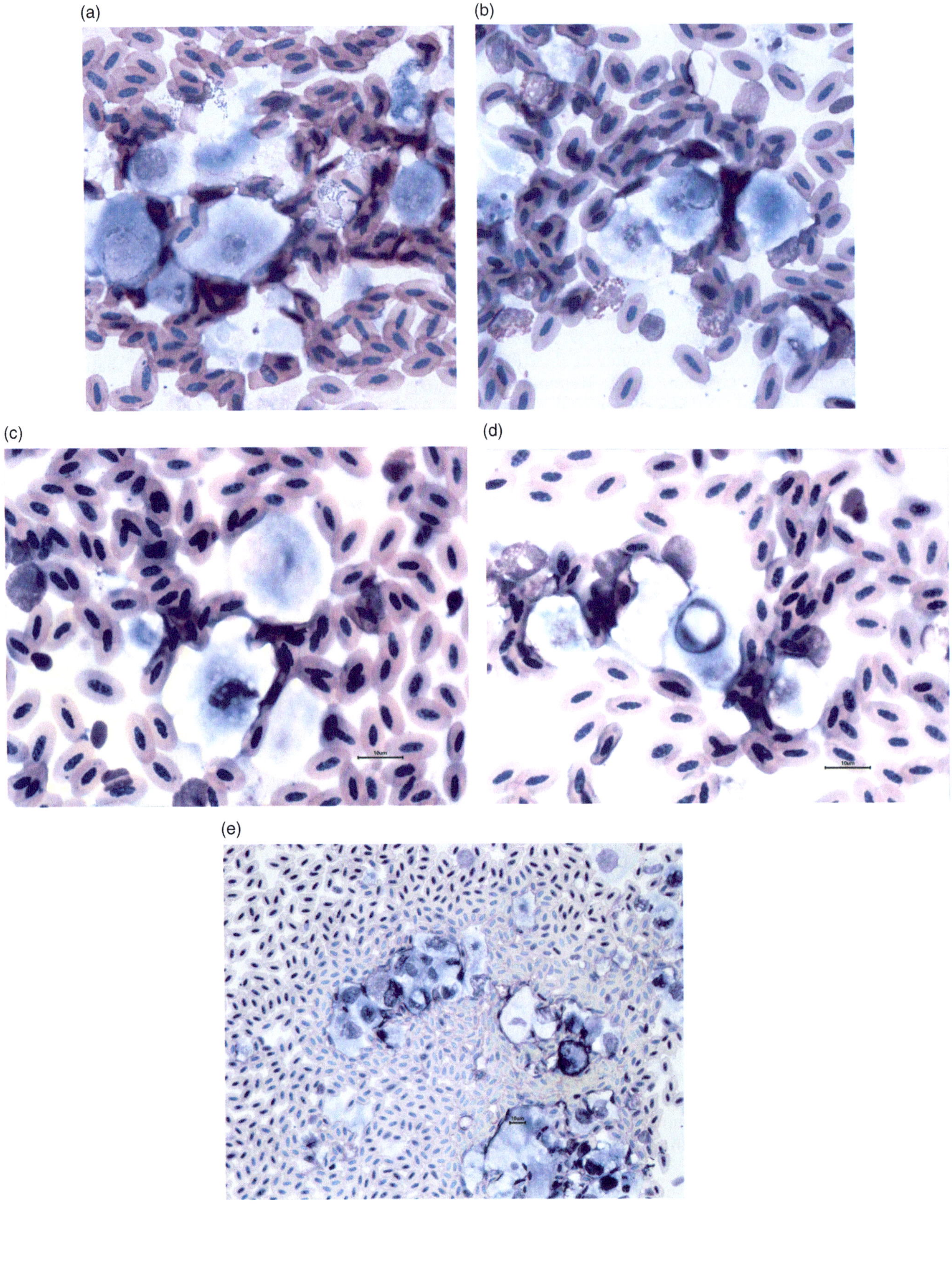
(a)
(b)
(c)
(d)
(e)

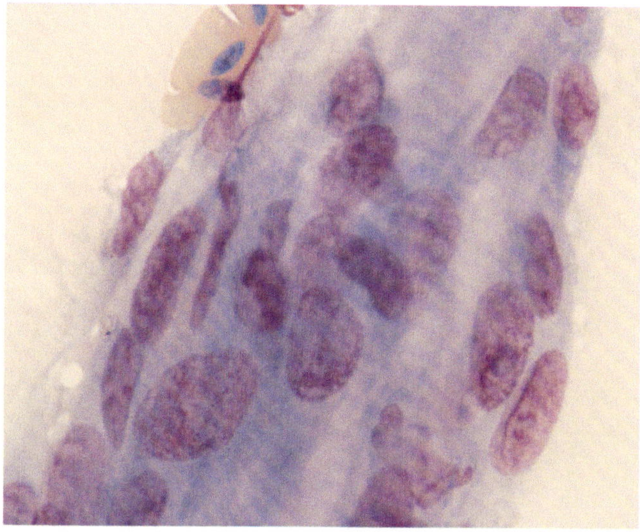

Fig. 15.75. Spindle-shaped mesenchymal cells showing anisokaryosis with oval to spindle-shaped nuclei from a leiomyosarcoma from a peregrine falcon (*Falco peregrinus*), Diff–Quik stain (100× oil).

pale blue cytoplasm and a centrally located round to irregularly round nucleus with finely stippled chromatin and indistinct nucleoli.

Chondromas and chondrosarcomas are neoplasia of cartilage (chondrocytes and cartilaginous cells). The cytology often reveals mesenchymal cells embedded in a bright, pink, smooth to slightly granular background material (chondroid). The cells resemble those found in osteosarcomas (primary neoplasia of bone) and can vary from round to fusiform with large nuclei and deeply basophilic cytoplasm. Like cells from osteosarcomas, chondrosarcomas can contain small intracytoplasmic vacuoles and fine eosinophilic granules.

Osteosarcoma and chondrosarcoma are uncommon tumors of chickens and other avian species (Bossa et al., 2015). The avian leukosis/sarcoma virus (ALSV) group is associated with sarcomas of all types in chickens, including chondromas, osteomas, and osteosarcomas (Fadly and Nair, 2008; Dittmer et al., 2012).

Neoplasia of the Gastrointestinal Tract

A variety of neoplastic diseases involving the gastrointestinal tract have been reported in birds: most are associated with the liver (Cork and Stockdale, 1995). Gastrointestinal neoplasms commonly reported in birds include lymphoid neoplasia, squamous cell carcinomas, adenocarcinomas, and sarcomas (Dillehay et al., 1985; Anderson and Steinberg, 1989; Leach et al., 1989; Leach, 1992; Reece, 1992; Cork and Stockdale, 1995; Cho et al., 1998; Hatkin et al., 2002; Vazquez et al., 2003; Yonemaru et al., 2004; Hafner et al., 2007; Kummrow et al., 2007; Palmieri et al., 2011; Weyna et al., 2021). Esophageal lymphomas have been reported in birds (Schmidt et al., 2012) Reviews have revealed that gastric carcinomas are more common than sarcomas in birds (Langlois, 2005). Although the etiology for gastric neoplasms is generally unknown, macrorhabdiosis (*Macrorhabdus ornithogaster*) may be an associated factor for proventricular adenocarcinoma in psittacines (Powers et al., 2019).

Papillomas arising from mucosal surfaces of the oral cavity, pharynx, choanal slit, and cloaca (a condition commonly referred to as “internal papillomatosis of parrots”) are common in psittacine birds, especially in macaws, Amazon parrots, conures, Pionus parrots, and hawk-headed parrots (McDonald, 1988; Graham, 1991; Phalen et al., 1998; Jones et al., 2020). Although papillomas are found most commonly on the mucosal surfaces of the cloaca, they may also be found in the oral cavity, esophagus, crop, proventriculus, and ventriculus. Cloacal papillomas are difficult to diagnose by cytology alone because they reveal predominantly cornified squamous epithelial cells on the cellular sample (Figures 15.70a–15.70f).

Neoplasia of the Respiratory Tract

Neoplasia of the avian upper respiratory tract has been reported, most commonly in budgerigars (*Melopsittacus undulatus*). Neoplasms involving the oral cavity include basal cell carcinoma, fibroma,

Fig. 15.74. (a) The large epithelial cells in both Figures 15.74a and 15.74b from a scraping of an oral lesion in an orange-winged amazon parrot (*Amazona amazonica*) exhibit squamous differentiation based upon their polygonal shapes and baby blue cytoplasm indicating keratinization. These epithelial cells demonstrate anisokaryosis, pleomorphic nuclei, nuclear chromatin clumping, high nucleus to cytoplasm ratio, and multinucleation. Some cells have a dark blue cytoplasm suggestive of inappropriate keratinization (dyskeratosis). The histopathologic diagnosis was squamous cell carcinoma, Wright–Giemsa stain (100× oil). Source: Image from Campbell and Grant (2010, p. 255). (b) See description in Figure 15.74a, Wright–Giemsa stain (100× oil). Source: Image from Campbell and Grant (2010, p. 255). (c) Imprint of a uropygial mass diagnosed as a squamous cell carcinoma in a budgerigar (*Melopsittacus undulatus*) revealing squamous epithelial cells with features of malignancy, Wright–Giemsa stain (100× oil). (d) Imprint of a uropygial mass diagnosed as a squamous cell carcinoma in a budgerigar (*Melopsittacus undulatus*) revealing squamous epithelial cells with features of malignancy from the same sample as Figure 15.74c, Wright–Giemsa stain (100× oil). (e) Imprint of a mass in the nares of a cockatiel (*Nymphicus hollandicus*) revealing squamous epithelial cells with features of malignancy with a histologic diagnosis of squamous cell carcinoma, Wright–Giemsa stain.

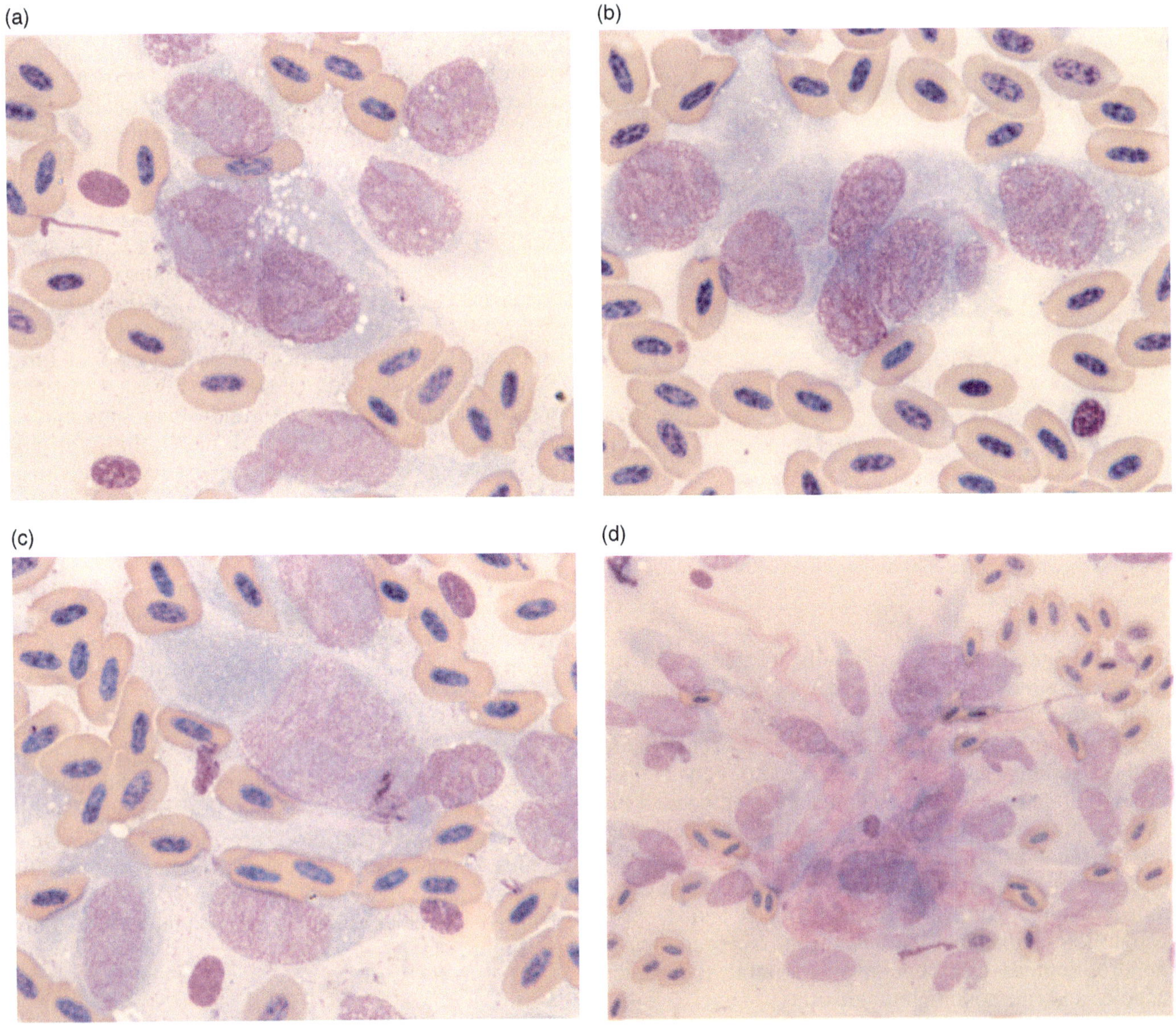

Fig. 15.76. (a) Neoplastic cells with large nuclei from a poorly differentiated sarcoma from a gray-cheeked parakeet (*Brotogeris pyrrhoptera*), Diff–Quik stain (100× oil). (b) Malignant mesenchymal cells exhibiting high N:C ratios from the same sample as Figure 15.76a. The cell in the center has either three nuclei (two large and one small) or two nuclei (a large nucleus with a deep cleft and a small nucleus) from a poorly differentiated sarcoma from a gray-cheeked parakeet (*Brotogeris pyrrhoptera*), Diff–Quik stain (100× oil). (c) Abnormal nucleoli (multiple pale-staining, large nucleoli) in the nucleus (smooth chromatin pattern) of cells from a poorly differentiated sarcoma from a gray-cheeked parakeet (*Brotogeris pyrrhoptera*) from the same sample as Figure 15.76a, Diff–Quik stain (100× oil). (d) Pleomorphic mesenchymal cells within an eosinophilic background substance in an imprint from a poorly differentiated sarcoma from a gray-cheeked parakeet (*Brotogeris pyrrhoptera*) from the same sample as Figure 15.76a, Diff–Quik stain (500×).

fibrosarcoma, papilloma, and squamous cell carcinoma; may occur in the oropharynx; and may involve the beak (Miller et al., 1985; Leach, 1992; Manucy et al., 1998; Suedmeyer et al., 2001a). Melanoma has been reported in the nasal sinus and syrinx of psittacine birds, and a poorly differentiated sarcoma in the periorbital sinus of a budgerigar with clinical signs of chronic rhinorrhea, exophthalmia, and swollen head was diagnosed based on cytology of a fine-needle aspirate that demonstrated variably sized mesenchymal cells with moderate numbers of mitotic figures (Leach, 1992; Andre et al., 1993; Colby, 1998; Shrader et al., 2016). Carcinomas of the infraorbital sinus can be associated with the formation of cystic fluid (Stiles and Greenacre, 2001; Baine et al., 2014). Fibrosarcomas have been reported in the syrinx of birds (Latimer, 1994; Spira, 1996; Dorrestein, 1997).

The lungs and air sacs of birds have been associated with a variety of neoplasms. These include adenocarcinoma, fibrosarcoma, hemangiosarcoma, malignant

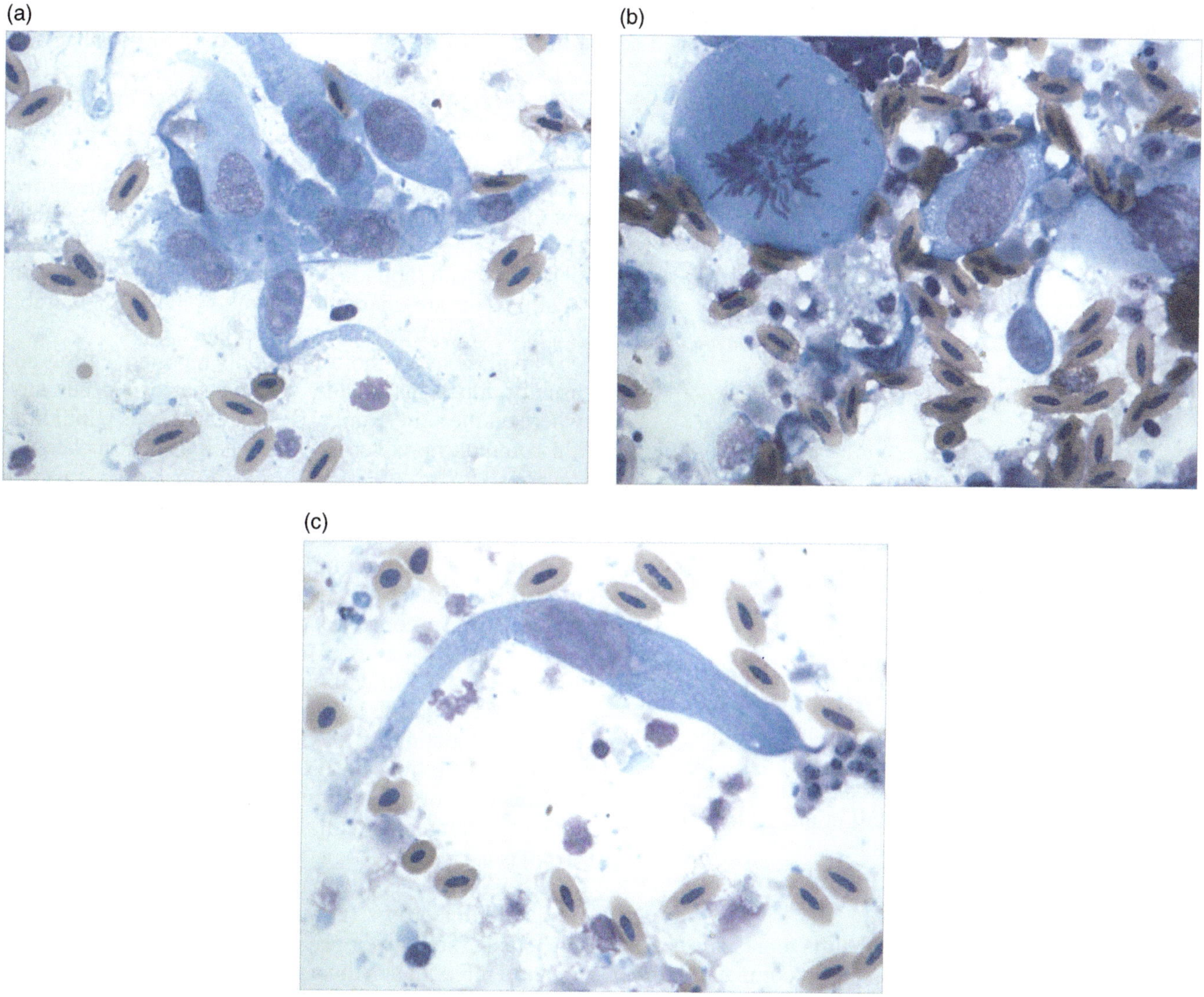

Fig. 15.77. (a) Nuclear and cellular pleomorphism in mesenchymal cells obtained from a contact smear of a fibrosarcoma in a military macaw (*Ara militaris*), Wright–Giemsa stain (100× oil). (b) An abnormal mitotic figure among malignant mesenchymal cell obtained from a contact smear of a fibrosarcoma in a military macaw (*Ara militaris*) from the same sample as Figure 15.77a, Wright–Giemsa stain (100× oil). (c) A mesenchymal cell exhibiting dark cytoplasmic basophilia along with other features of malignant neoplasia (large size, large nucleus, and multiple nucleoli) in a fine-needle aspiration biopsy of a fibrosarcoma in a military macaw (*Ara militaris*) from the same sample as Figure 15.77a, Wright–Giemsa stain (100× oil).

melanoma, mesothelioma, and osteosarcoma (Swartout and Wymann, 1987; Latimer, 1994; Loukopoulos et al., 2014). Pulmonary adenocarcinomas are neoplasms arising from the bronchial epithelium involving the lungs and usually have a unilateral presentation. Although they are rarely reported in poultry and other birds, they occur more frequent in ducks, which are believed to have a natural predisposition (Zafra et al., 2011). Pulmonary adenocarcinomas has been reported in a bird also suffering from silicosis, suggesting a possible cause for the neoplasia (Zafra et al., 2011). Other neoplasms associated with the lower respiratory tract include hemangiosarcoma, leiomyosarcoma, lymphosarcoma, bronchiolar adenoma, adenocarcinoma, papillomas, myxoma, myxosarcomas, and poorly differentiated mesenchymal neoplasm (Griner, 1983; Graham, 1991; Leach, 1992; Burgmann, 1994; Latimer, 1994; Powers et al., 1998; Ellis, 2001; Newman and West, 2001; Schmidt et al., 2003; Marshall et al., 2004). Primary neoplasms of the lungs of birds include bronchial and bronchiolar adenomas and adenocarcinomas (Effron et al., 1977; Reece, 1992; Andre and Delverdier, 1999; Jones et al., 2001). Osseous metastasis has been associated with primary bronchial carcinoma in psittacine birds (Andre and Delverdier, 1999; Jones et al., 2001). Metastatic tumors to the respiratory tract, especially the lungs, are reported more commonly than primary tumors of the respiratory tract

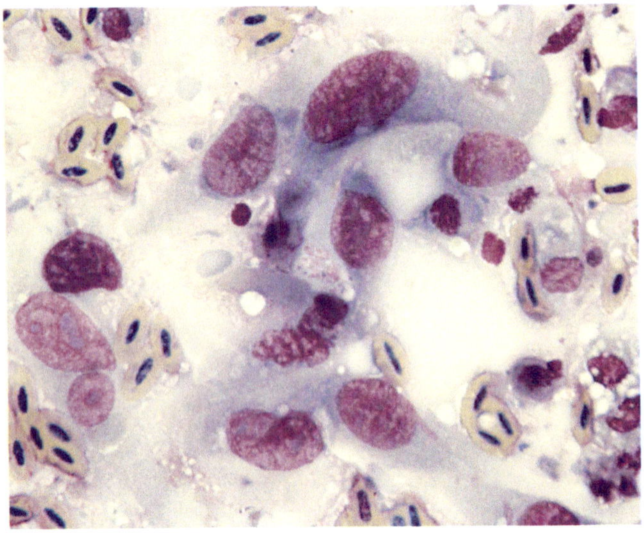

Fig. 15.78. Nuclear and cellular pleomorphism in mesenchymal cells obtained from a contact smear of a fibrosarcoma in a rose-ringed parakeet (*Psittacula krameri*), Wright–Giemsa stain (100× oil).

(Effron et al., 1977; Campbell, 1995; Reece, 1992; Burgmann, 1994; Latimer, 1994). A primary mucinous adenocarcinoma of the humeral air sac has been reported in a cockatoo; however, the cytology of a fine-needle aspirate revealed mixed cell inflammation, but no neoplastic cells (Marshall et al., 2004).

Cutaneous Neoplasms

Neoplasia of the skin and subcutis represents nearly one-third of the neoplasms reported in companion birds (Campbell and Coles, 1986; Bauck, 1992). Some, such as basal cell tumors and melanomas, are rarely reported, while others are more common (Bradford et al., 2009; Schmidt et al., 2012). Granular cell tumors are rare benign skin tumors of birds. They likely are myogenic in origin in psittacine birds, as a muscular origin of this type of neoplasia has also been suggested for mammals (dog, cat, and rat) (Hernández et al., 2012). The neoplastic cells are round to polygonal in shape with abundant slightly eosinophilic cytoplasm with numerous granules and well-defined borders. The nuclei tend to be round to oval with fine granular chromatin and exhibit marked anisokaryosis.

Fibromas and fibrosarcomas are common neoplasms of the integument of birds (Romagnano and Heard, 2000). Cutaneous sarcomas, such as rhabdomyosarcomas and fibrosarcomas, can be locally invasive and have the potential to metastasize to internal organs (Ijzer et al., 2002; Fernandez-Bellon et al., 2003; Gill, 2005).

Benign and malignant neoplasms of melanin-producing cells are reported in a variety of avian species and in a variety of tissues (Smith et al., 2002; Rambaud et al., 2003; Barlow and Girling, 2004; Campbell and Ellis, 2007; Crosset, 2007; Irizarry-Rovira et al., 2007; Guthrie et al., 2010; Kajigaya et al., 2010; Costagliola et al., 2011; Williams et al., 2012; Duncan et al., 2014). Melanoma has rarely been reported in the subcutaneous tissue of birds (Stern and Lamm, 2009). The cells tend to be round to oval with brown or pale blue to blue-brown cytoplasmic pigment (Campbell and Grant, 2010) (Figure 15.85). Fewer cells tend to be more stellate to dendritic with abundant amounts of brown pigment granules or are markedly pleomorphic with variable amounts of pigment, even amelanistic.

Papillomas are more commonly reported in birds and usually appear as solitary lesions that can occur anywhere on the skin (Rupley, 1997). Cutaneous papillomas are common in passerine birds, such as chaffinches and canaries (Jones et al., 2020). Papillomas of companion birds have been reported on the skin around the eyes, eyelids, beak, oral cavity, feet, legs, and cloaca (Rupley, 1997). Papillomas of all species of animals are often identified by the gross appearance of a wart-like lesion; however, other conditions may at times resemble papillomas. Examples of these include chronic inflammatory lesions with fibrous proliferation, pox lesions, and other neoplastic lesions. Cytology may be helpful in the differentiation of these conditions. The cytology of the wart-like lesions of squamous papillomas reveals predominately normal, mature squamous epithelial cells; a lack of inflammatory cells; cells with obvious features of neoplasia; or an etiologic agent, such as pox inclusions. The cauliflower-shaped papillomas, or warts are caused by papillomaviruses (Family: Papillomaviridae), which are small, non-enveloped viruses that cause skin and mucosa infections in diverse vertebrates. Seven complete genomes, corresponding to five papillomavirus genera, have been detected from various sample types, including skin, internal epithelium, and fecal material, from seven highly diverse wild and captive avian species (Truchado, 2018). Papillomavirus has also been detected in avian tissue with no apparent lesions, similar to findings in mammals.

Cutaneous lymphoma and lymphosarcoma have been reported in many species of companion birds. Lymphoid skin neoplasia in birds is typically of B lymphocyte origin, and is often associated with lymphosarcoma (Gamble, 1999; Rivera et al., 2009). The lymphocytes present in avian cytology specimens have features of malignant neoplasia, as mentioned earlier, and lack a uniform appearance (Reavill and Schmidt, 2000; Campbell and Ellis, 2007) (Figures 15.86a–15.86c).

Mast cell tumors are rarely reported in birds (Swayne et al, 1990; Schmidt, 1992; Dallwig et al., 2012). The cells exfoliate easily, but are fragile and often rupture during preparation of cytology slides, where the released granules are found scattered throughout the background. Intact mast cells are recognized on Romanowsky-stained

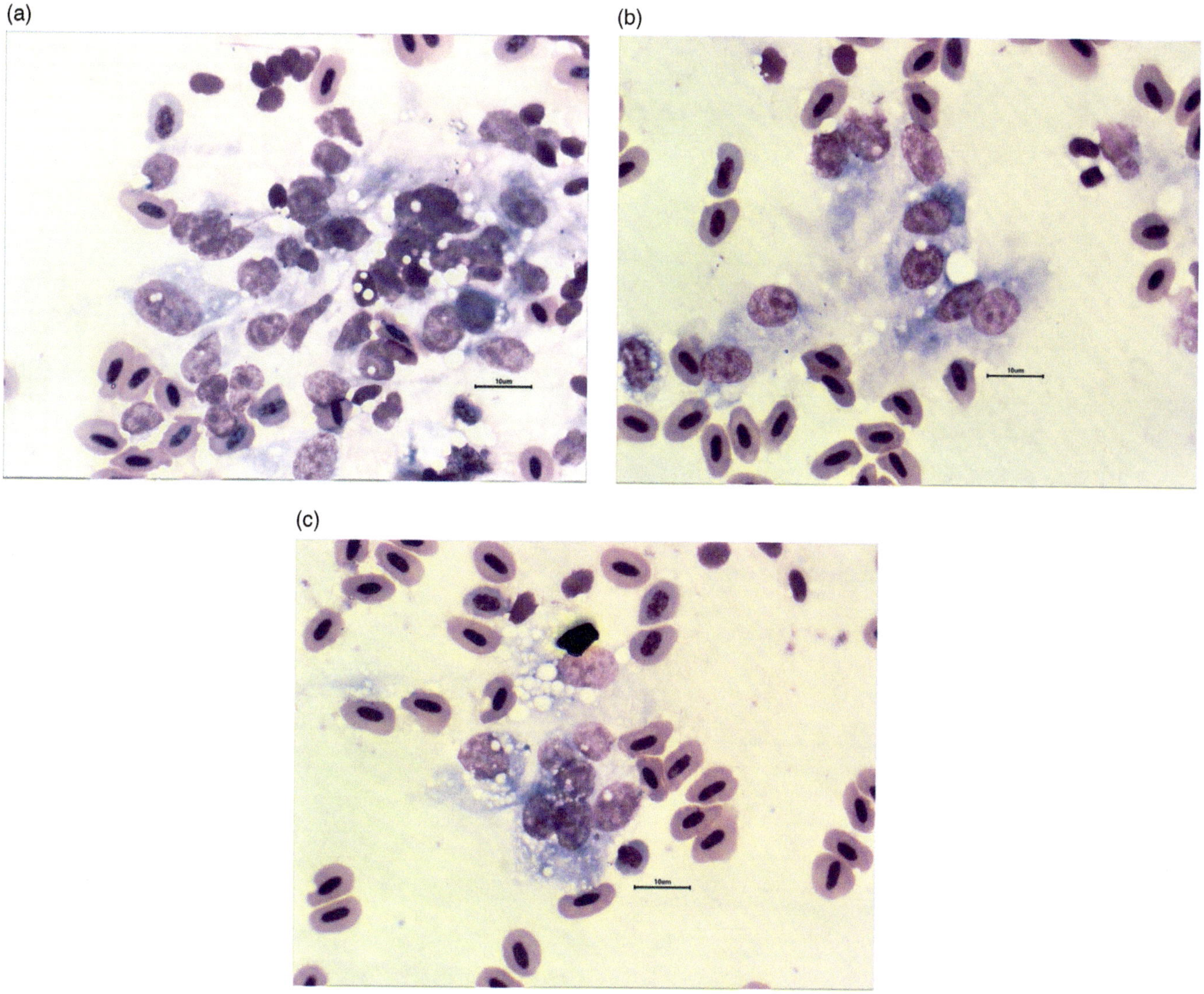

Fig. 15.79. (a) Nuclear and cellular pleomorphism in mesenchymal cells obtained from a contact smear of a poorly differentiated sarcoma in a cockatiel (*Nymphicus hollandicus*), Wright–Giemsa stain. (b) Nuclear and cellular pleomorphism in mesenchymal cells obtained from a contact smear of a poorly differentiated sarcoma in a cockatiel (*Nymphicus hollandicus*) from the same sample as Figure 15.79a, Wright–Giemsa stain. (c) Nuclear and cellular pleomorphism in mesenchymal cells obtained from a contact smear of a poorly differentiated sarcoma in a cockatiel (*Nymphicus hollandicus*) from the same sample as Figure 15.79a, Wright–Giemsa stain.

cytologic specimens as discrete, round cells with pale, eccentric nuclei and inconspicuous nucleoli. The cytoplasm contains numerous distinct purple or metachromatic cytoplasmic granules ranging in size from 0.2 to 5.0 μm in diameter. The cells in cutaneous mast cell tumors may disseminate to other tissues (Dallwig et al., 2012).

Dermal squamous cell carcinoma has been reported in young chicken. The high incidence of cutaneous squamous cell carcinoma in these chickens may have been related to their breed, use of reused litter, and possibly the season (Nakamura et al., 2010).

Adenocarcinomas have been reported in the ears of birds and are likely associated with the external ear glands (Moreno et al., 2015; Houck et al., 2016). Cytology preparations reveal epithelial cells with features of adenocarcinomas, and reactive osteoblasts may also be found (Houck et al., 2016).

Neoplasms that affect the uropygial gland include carcinomas (most commonly squamous cell carcinoma), adenocarcinomas, and adenomas (Robertson et al., 2020).

Ocular Neoplasms

Ocular and retrobulbar neoplasia is rarely reported in birds. Reports from a few species include adenoma, cystadenoma, adenocarcinoma, carcinoma, adenofibroma, lipoma, teratoma, osteosarcoma, and rhabdomyosarcoma (Simova-Curd et al., 2009; Fordham et al., 2010). Retrobulbar adenomas in birds may arise

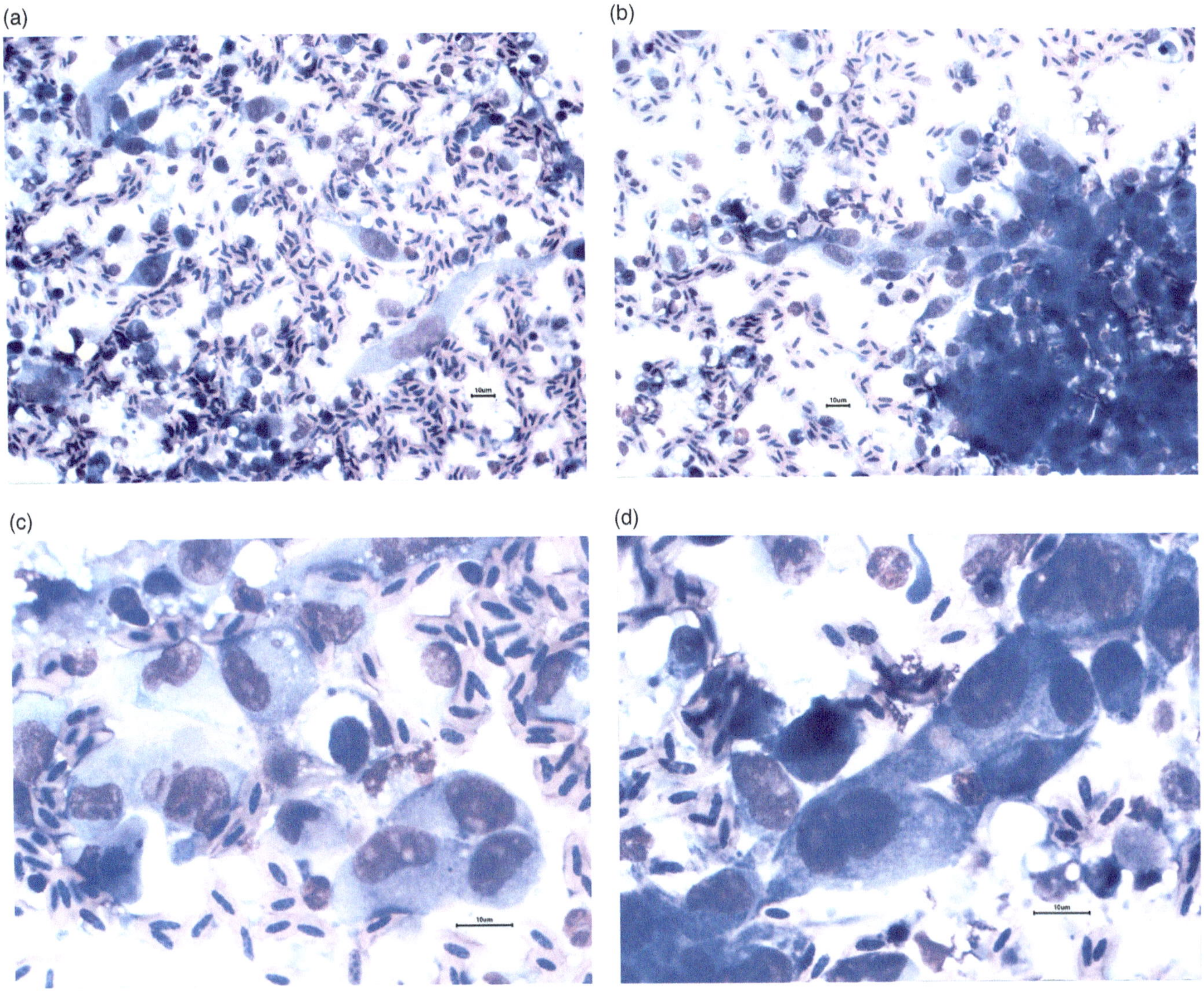

Fig. 15.80. (a) Nuclear and cellular pleomorphism in mesenchymal cells obtained from a contact smear of a poorly differentiated sarcoma in a blue and gold macaw (*Ara ararauna*), Wright–Giemsa stain. (b) Mesenchymal cells obtained from a contact smear of a poorly differentiated sarcoma in a blue and gold macaw (*Ara ararauna*) from the same sample as Figure 15.80a, Wright–Giemsa stain. (c) Mesenchymal cells with features of malignant neoplasia obtained from a contact smear of a poorly differentiated sarcoma in a blue and gold macaw (*Ara ararauna*) from the same sample as Figure 15.80a, Wright–Giemsa stain. (d) Nuclear and cellular pleomorphism with binucleation in mesenchymal cells obtained from a contact smear of a poorly differentiated sarcoma in a blue and gold macaw (*Ara ararauna*) from the same sample as Figure 15.80a, Wright–Giemsa stain.

from one of the orbital glands (glandula lacrimalis, glandula membranae nictitantis or Harderian gland, and glandula nasalis). Cytologic evaluation of an aspirate of a retrobulbar adenocarcinoma in a parrot revealed cuboidal to columnar cells with high nuclear-to-cytoplasmic ratio; scant, basophilic cytoplasm; a central, round to oval nucleus, with finely stippled chromatin; and exfoliating individually or in variably sized clusters with occasional acinar structures (Watson et al., 2013). Squamous cell carcinomas have been rarely reported on the third eyelid of birds (Le et al., 2011).

Conjunctival neoplasia is rarely reported in birds and other lower vertebrates; however, those that have been reported include lymphoma, various sarcomas, epidermoid carcinoma, hibernoma, and basal cell carcinoma (Murphy et al., 1986; Sacre et al., 1992; Kern et al., 1996; Ramos-Vara et al., 1997). Benign palpebral and conjunctival neoplasms of basophil cells have been reported in a parakeet; histiocytic sarcoma in an owl; mastocytoma and cystadenoma in juncos; and subconjunctival hibernoma in a goose (Bayón et al., 2007). Neoplasia involving the conjunctival epithelium may be difficult to differentiate from the atypical and often hyperplastic epithelial cells associated with severe inflammation (Raskin, 2001). Cells with cytologic features of malignant neoplasia should always be viewed with suspicion.

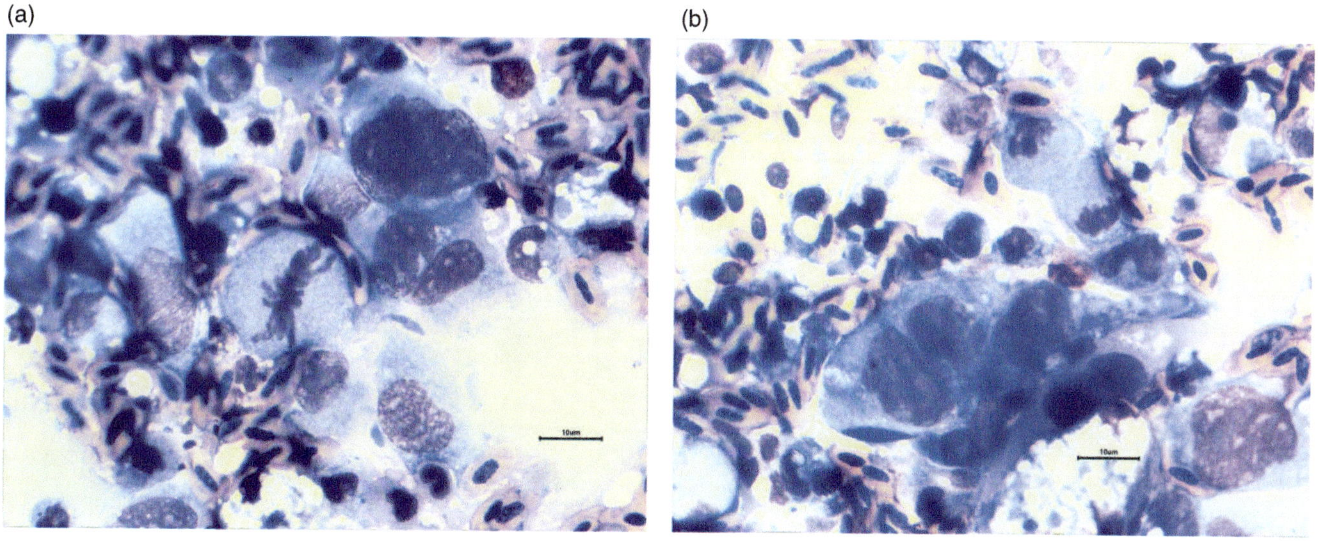

Fig. 15.81. (a) Nuclear and cellular pleomorphism with a mitotic figure in mesenchymal cells obtained from a contact smear of a poorly differentiated sarcoma in a blue and gold macaw (*Ara ararauna*) from the same sample as Figure 15.80a, Wright–Giemsa stain. (b) Nuclear and cellular pleomorphism with binucleation and a mitotic figure in mesenchymal cells obtained from a contact smear of a poorly differentiated sarcoma in a blue and gold macaw (*Ara ararauna*) from the same sample as Figure 15.80a, Wright–Giemsa stain.

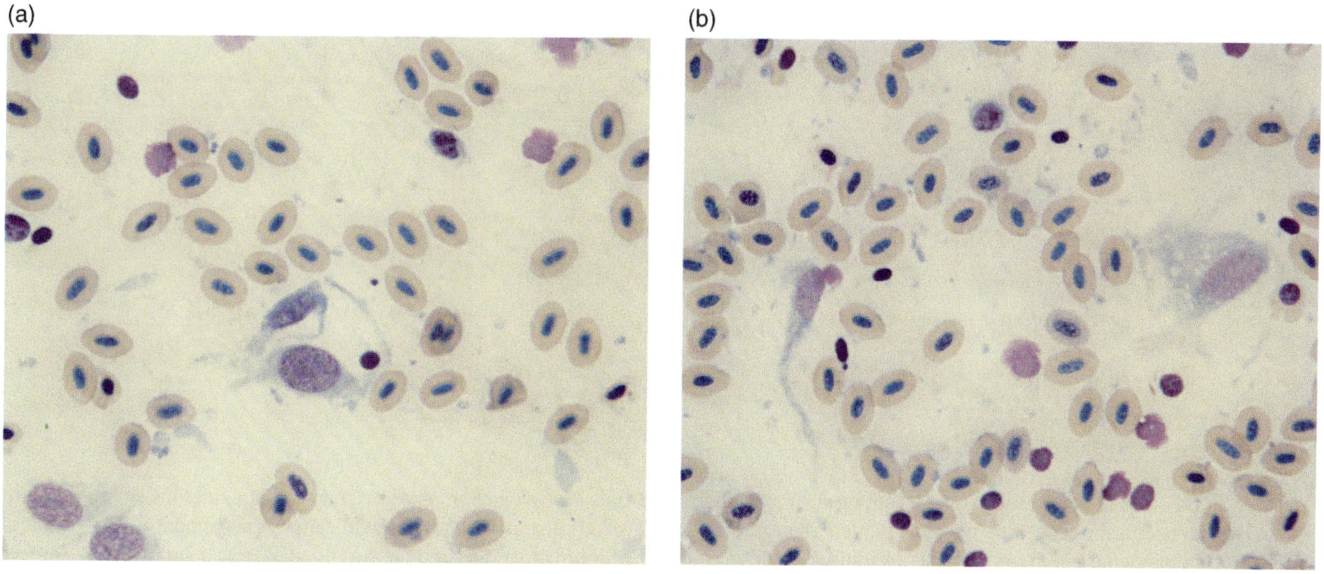

Fig. 15.82. (a) Pleomorphic mesenchymal cells in an imprint from a mass with a histologic diagnosis of a hemangiosarcoma removed from the ear of a cockatiel (*Nymphicus hollandicus*), Wright–Giemsa stain. (b) Mesenchymal cells from the same imprint of the mass in Figure 15.82a, Wright–Giemsa stain.

Neoplasms of Joints and Bone

Neoplasia involving joints are rarely reported in birds (Howard et al., 1996; Daigle et al., 1999). Synovial cell sarcoma is an uncommon tumor that arises from primitive mesenchymal precursor cells outside the synovial membrane (Liu and Moroff, 1993). A case reported in an African gray parrot (*Psittacus erithacus*) revealed a soft tissue mass around the femur (Daigle et al., 1999). Cytologic examination of the mass was supportive of a mesenchymal neoplasm. Many round to spindle-shaped cells with pale-staining cytoplasm, indistinct cytoplasmic margins, increased N:C ratios, and prominent and multiple nucleoli were present as individual cells or in clusters. A pink extracellular matrix was incorporated into many of the cell clusters, and many erythrocytes, few heterophils, and rare macrophages were present. Following amputation of the leg, histology revealed a synovial cell sarcoma.

Primary bone tumors are rarely reported in avian species, and their behavior appears to be less aggressive

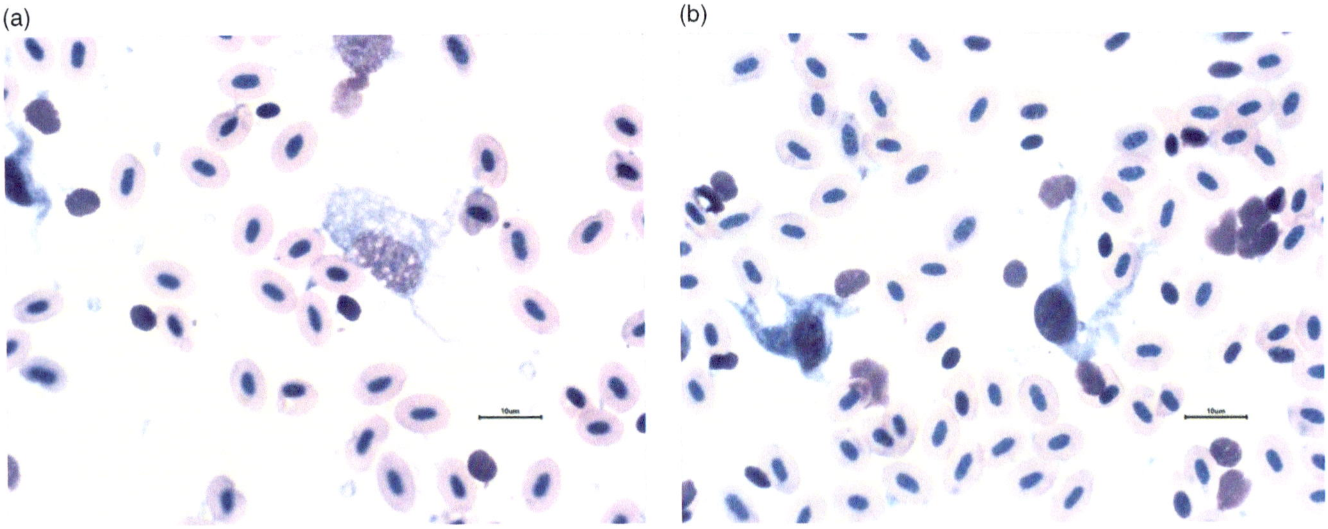

Fig. 15.83. (a) Mesenchymal cell with characteristics of a cell from a hemangioma in an aspirate from a mass with a histologic diagnosis of a hemangiosarcoma in a green-cheeked conure (*Pyrrhura molinae*), Wright–Giemsa stain. (b) Pleomorphic mesenchymal cells from the same aspirate as in Figure 15.83a, Wright–Giemsa stain.

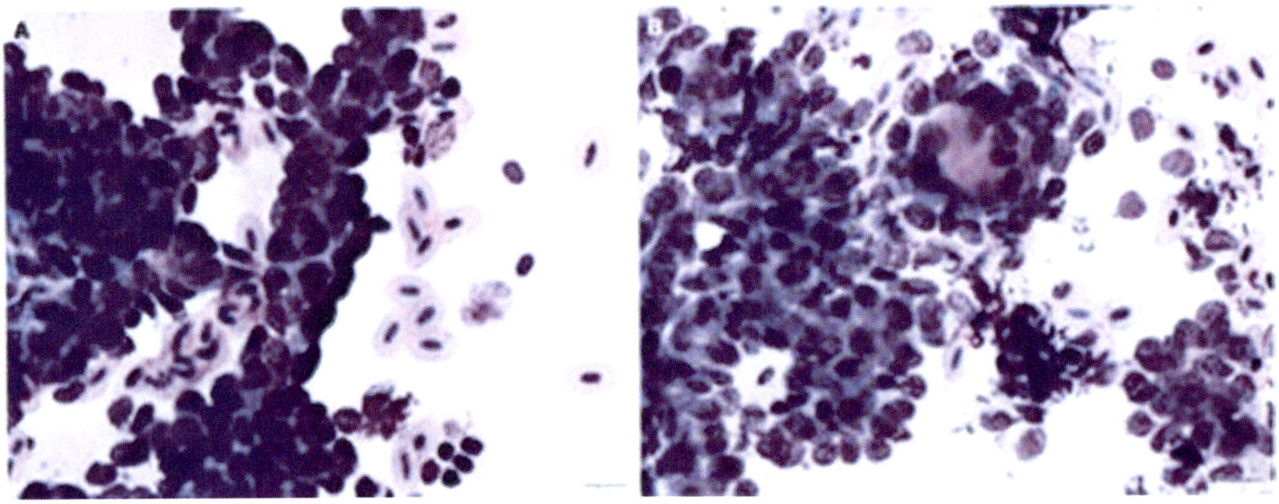

Fig. 15.84. A fine-needle aspirate of a foot mass in a Peking duck (*Anas platyrhynchos domestica*) revealing numerous small, round to polygonal neoplastic cells with indistinct borders arranged in variable-sized clusters with rare pseudo-acinar arrangements that are indicative of an epithelial neoplasm. The histopathology indicated an epithelioid hemangiosarcoma, Modified Wright's stain (60×). Source: Image from Piccione et al. (2017, figure 1).

than those in mammals (Reece, 2008; Dittmer et al., 2012). The presence of spindle-shaped mesenchymal cells and many multinucleated giant cells (resembling osteoclasts) is suggestive of giant cell tumor of bone (Amann et al., 2007).

Reproductive Tract Neoplasia

Ovarian cystadenocarcinomas and adenocarcinomas have been reported in birds. The cytology is characterized by neoplastic epithelial cells associated with cystic structures.

Testicular tumors reported in birds include Sertoli cell tumor, interstitial cell tumor, and seminoma, as well as lymphosarcoma, undifferentiated sarcoma, and teratoma (Schmidt et al., 2003; Reavill, 2004; Bédard et al., 2007; Pardini et al., 2012; Barger et al., 2020). Although these tumors are uncommon in birds, they have a higher incidence in budgerigars (*Melopsittacus undulates*).

Feminization secondary to hyperestrogenism from functional Sertoli cells and other germ cell testicular tumors has been reported in both mammalian and avian species (Uetsuka et al., 2012). In such cases, birds may

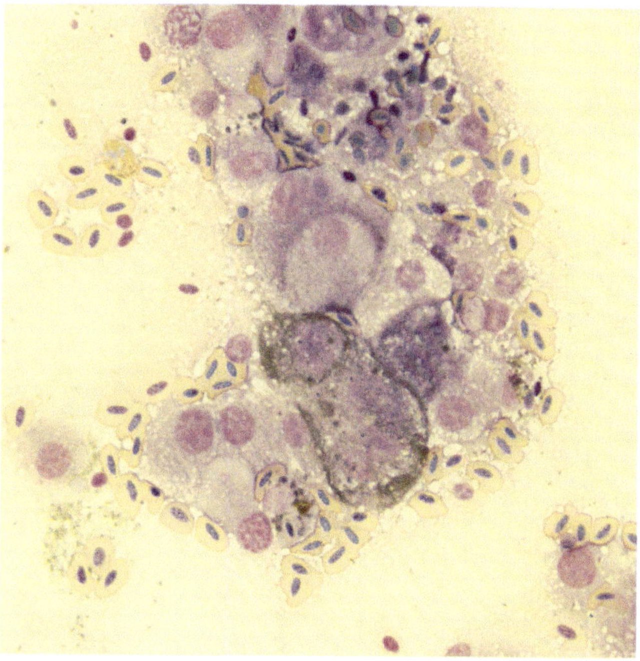

Fig. 15.85. Melanocytes containing variable amounts of brown-black melanin cytoplasmic granules with nuclei exhibiting features of malignant neoplasia in a fine-needle aspiration biopsy of a black mass with a histologic diagnosis of malignant melanoma from a white-winged wood duck (*Cairina scutulata*), Wright–Giemsa stain (100× oil). Source: Image from Campbell and Grant (2010, p. 274).

demonstrate changes in the cere color (blue to brown in budgerigars), polyostotic hyperostosis, pancytopenia, and female plumage characteristics. Fine-needle aspiration biopsy of a Sertoli cell tumor reveals aggregates of round cells with moderate amounts of basophilic cytoplasm that contains many punctate vacuoles; round to oval nuclei with finely stippled chromatin; and a heavy eosinophilic fibrillar background (Barger et al., 2020).

Seminomas originate from immature germ cells that form the spermatogenic epithelium within the seminiferous tubules of the testis. They have been reported in captive and wild birds (guinea fowl, black swan, pigeons, cockerels, and budgerigars) and are normally unilateral with occasional atrophy of the contralateral testis. Seminomas in dogs and birds have a characteristic cytological appearance revealing numerous pleomorphic round to slightly polygonal cells arranged in dense clusters of varying size with large nuclei and prominent nucleoli; moderate to marked anisocytosis and anisokaryosis; atypical mitoses; occasional binucleation; and multinucleation (Bédard et al., 2007). Intact cells generally have poorly to moderately distinct cell borders and a variable amount of slightly basophilic amorphous to finely granular cytoplasm with occasional small clear vacuoles. Lymphocytic infiltrates are frequently observed in seminomas in dogs, but are not a prominent feature in avian specimens.

Neoplasia of the Liver

Hepatic neoplasia occurs as a primary neoplasm of the hepatocytes or bile duct epithelium, or as a secondary neoplasia, such as metastatic disease or hepatic lymphoma (Figures 15.87 and 15.88).

Avian species (i.e., chickens and penguins) that have melanin pigment within their viscera can develop melanocytic neoplasms in the liver, with these melanocytes serving as the points of origin (Rambaud et al., 2003; Duncan et al., 2014; Culligan and Craig, 2020). In avian species, melanomas appear to be highly malignant. Microscopically, the neoplastic melanocytes tend to be large, oval to slightly polygonal or spindle-shaped mononuclear cells with moderate to abundant pale blue cytoplasm containing innumerable small, rod-shaped, green-black granules (Browning et al., 2020). The nucleus is typically round with finely stippled chromatin and a single, small, round distinct nucleolus. Moderate anisocytosis and anisokaryosis are expected as well as macrophages containing variably sized, globular, green-black cytoplasmic pigment.

Further evidence for a diagnosis of melanoma may be aided by special stains. The cytoplasm of these cells may show strong immunopositivity for Melan-A and S-100 in some species (i.e., seagull and budgerigar), but be negative in others (i.e., zebra finches and penguins) (Browning et al., 2020). In penguins, immunohistochemical analysis for PNL-2, a common melanocytic marker, has been shown to be highly useful in the identification of poorly pigmented (amelanotic) melanomas (Rambaud et al., 2003; Duncan et al., 2014). Examination of fine-needle aspirates of the liver with a melanoma may also reveal other types of intracellular pigment. Hemosiderin, or bile pigment, for example, is more amorphous and has different tinctorial properties from melanin pigment.

Neoplasia of the Kidney

Renal adenomas and adenocarcinomas arise from epithelial cells of the kidney. Embryonal nephromas or nephroblastomas arise from pluripotential embryonal renal tissue. Embryonal nephromas of budgerigars often contain neoplastic cuboidal epithelial cells with a fibrous stroma. The fibrous stroma contains spindle-shaped cells dispersed among large amounts of mucinous material. It may undergo metaplasia to form bone or cartilage. The noncellular background may contain a heavy eosinophilic substance suggestive of a cellular attempt to produce a matrix, such as chondroid or osteoid (Figures 15.89a–15.89c, and 15.90a–15.90c).

Neoplasia of the Thyroid

Thymoma has been rarely described in birds. It appears as a soft tissue mass in the cervical region. Cytologic preparations may reveal clustered polygonal

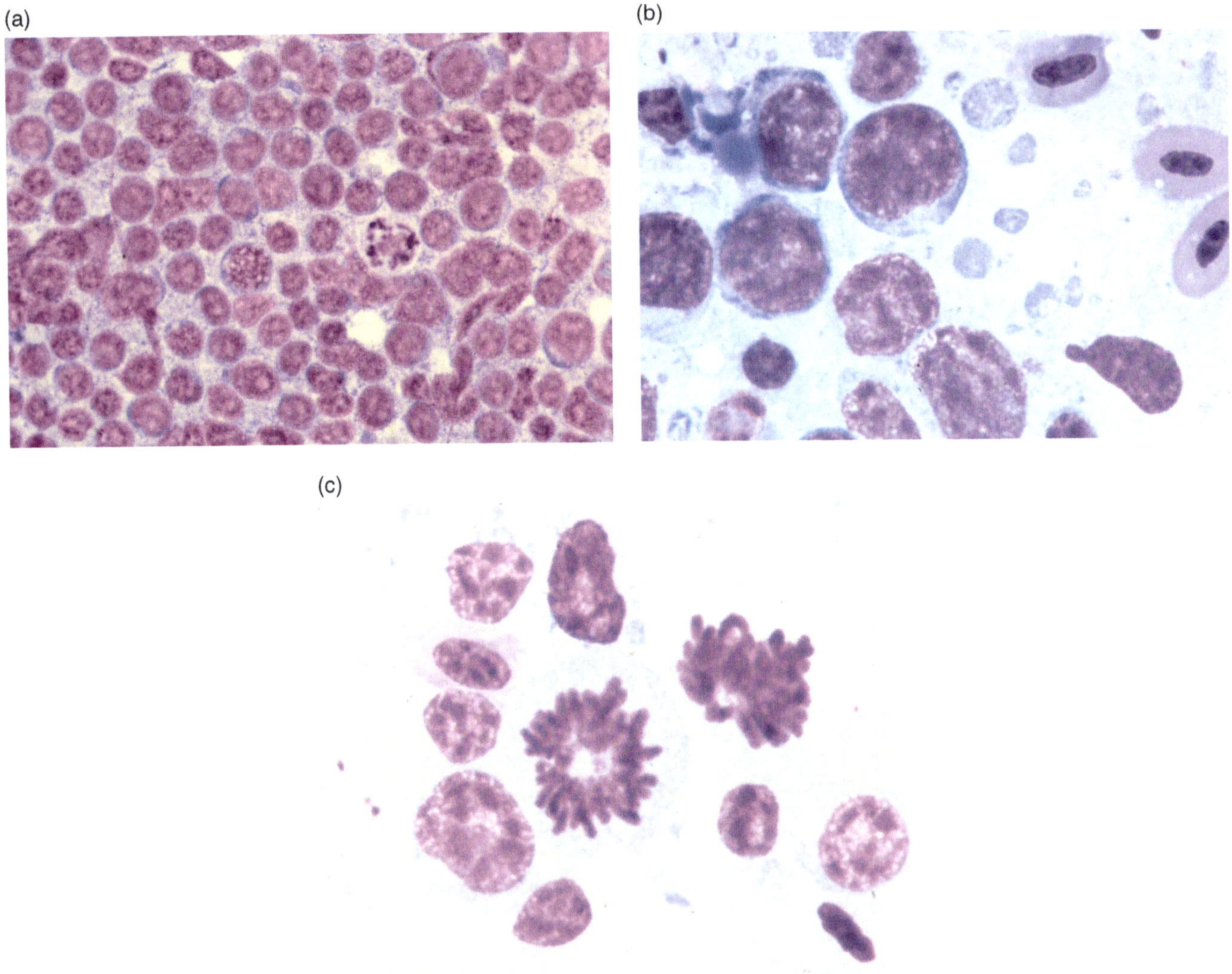

Fig. 15.86. (a) Numerous discrete round cells with round nuclei, high N:C ratios, prominent nucleoli, and mitotic figures in a fine-needle aspiration biopsy of a subcutaneous lymphoma in a spectacled Amazon parrot (*Amazona albifrons*), Diff–Quik stain (400×). (b) A predominance of large lymphocytes with variable chromatin patterns and nucleoli in the same fine-needle aspiration biopsy of a subcutaneous lymphoma as in Figure 15.86a in a spectacled Amazon parrot (*Amazona albifrons*), Diff–Quik stain (100× oil). (c) Mitotic activity in large lymphocytes in the same fine-needle aspiration biopsy of a subcutaneous lymphoma as in Figure 15.86a in a spectacled Amazon parrot (*Amazona albifrons*), Diff–Quik stain (100× oil).

epithelial cells (occasionally arranged in acinar formations) and small lymphocytes, and the definitive classification of the lesion as a thymoma is provided by positive immunohistochemistry for pancytokeratin and CD3 (Blakey et al., 2021).

Effusions

The coelomic cavity of birds is divided into five distinct peritoneal cavities: the intestinal, right and left ventral hepatic, and right and left dorsal hepatic. These "cavities" are potential spaces created by the air sacs that invaginate into and occupy most of the space within the coelom (King and McLelland, 1984; Bezuidenhout, 1988). The intestinal peritoneal cavity occurs as a single midline space that extends from the liver to the vent. The left and right ventral hepatic spaces are large, blind pouches that extend lateroventrally from the liver to the caudal body wall. The two dorsal hepatic cavities are small spaces located craniodorsally in the coelom. The right dorsal cavity is blind, but the left dorsal hepatic peritoneal cavity communicates with the intestinal peritoneal cavity. In normal birds, these spaces are small and contain little fluid for sampling.

Causes of coelomic effusions in birds include right heart failure (Julian, 1987, 1993; Sedacca et al., 2009), liver failure (Campbell, 1986, 1995; Degernes, 1991; O'Connor and Garner, 2018), mycobacteriosis (Dolphin et al., 1979), polyomavirus (Ritchie, 1995b), viral serositis (Gaskin et al., 1991), reproductive tract disorders

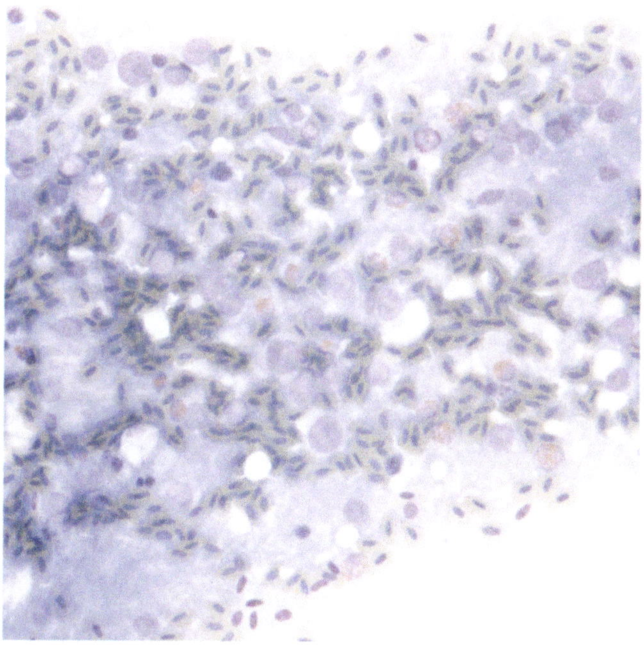

Fig. 15.87. Normal hepatocytes, erythrocytes, and heterophils in a fine-needle aspiration biopsy of a normal liver in a peach-faced lovebird (*Agapornis roseicollis*), Wright–Giemsa stain (40×). Source: Image from Campbell and Grant (2010, p. 226).

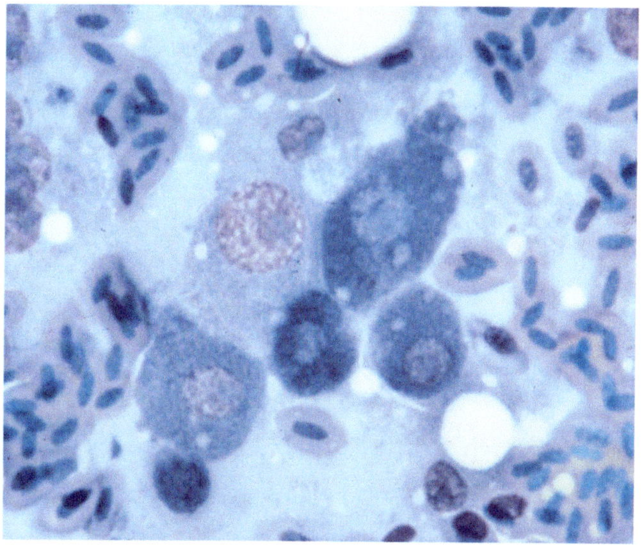

Fig. 15.88. Pleomorphic hepatocytes showing marked anisocytosis, moderate anisokaryosis, nuclear pleomorphism, large nucleoli, variable nuclear chromatin patterns, and deeply basophilic cytoplasm in an imprint of a liver biopsy with a histologic diagnosis of a hepatoma from a Java rice bird (*Lonchura oryzivora*), Diff–Quik stain (100× oil).

such as egg-related peritonitis and cystic ovary (Joyner, 1994; Campbell, 1995), and neoplastic diseases of other coelomic organs (Campbell, 1986, 1995; McCleery et al., 2015.).

Iron storage disease is caused by high dietary iron levels or increased absorption of dietary iron (Klasing et al., 2012). The increased iron in the blood is stored in the liver as hemosiderin and eventually results in hepatocellular damage once the iron load exceeds the liver's storage capacity and the development of ascites (Cork, 2000; O'Connor and Garner, 2018). This disorder is most commonly encountered in frugivorous or nectivorous species such as starlings, mynas, toucans, birds of paradise, and lorikeets and is rarely reported in other species of psittacine birds (O'Connor and Garner, 2018).

Ascites fluid in the avian patient may accumulate within one or more of the five peritoneal cavities, compressing the caudal thoracic and abdominal air sacs laterally and increasing the peritoneal cavity space, resulting in abdominal enlargement (Lumeij, 1994; Redrobe, 2000). Portal hypertension secondary to chronic liver disease is a common cause of ascites with a transudative effusion in birds, and results from increased capillary and lymphatic hydrostatic pressure, which increases fluid flow into the hepatic sinusoids (Grauer and Nichols, 1985; Degernes, 1991; Julian, 1993; Wheeler and Webber, 2002). The lymphatic system is unable to return this fluid to the plasma, so it escapes into the adjacent peritoneal space.

Long-standing transudates in birds, as with mammals, become modified with the increase in the number of cells or protein content. Modified transudates are often associated with cardiac insufficiency, cardiomyopathy, compression of vascular structures from neoplasia, inflammation or torsion of an organ, and the presence of sterile irritants (Shelly, 2001; Sedacca et al., 2009; Campbell and Grant, 2010). Modified transudates grossly resemble transudative effusions but contain either an increase in cellularity (1000–5000 cells/mL) or protein content (2.5–3.0 g/dL). The specific gravity is low (1.017–1.025) (Baker and Lunsden, 2000). The cells found in modified transudates are primarily macrophages and reactive mesothelial cells (Figures 15.91–15.96). Mitotic figures are frequently found (Figures 15.97a and 15.97b). Longer-standing modified transudates may appear as a mixed cell exudate (Knafo et al., 2011).

Hemorrhagic, exudative, and malignant effusions in birds occur in one or more of the five peritoneal cavities depending upon the location of the primary lesion (Figures 15.98–15.102). For example, egg-related coelomitis is generally confined to the intestinal peritoneal cavity.

Egg-related coelomitis of birds is indicated by the presence of a slightly yellow fluid in the coelomic cavity. The fluid usually has features of an exudative effusion, but may also appear noninflammatory or septic. The inflammatory component of the fluid consists of a mixture of heterophils, macrophages, lymphocytes, and plasma cells. Numerous round, dark blue, amorphous globules (protein globules) of variable size and staining

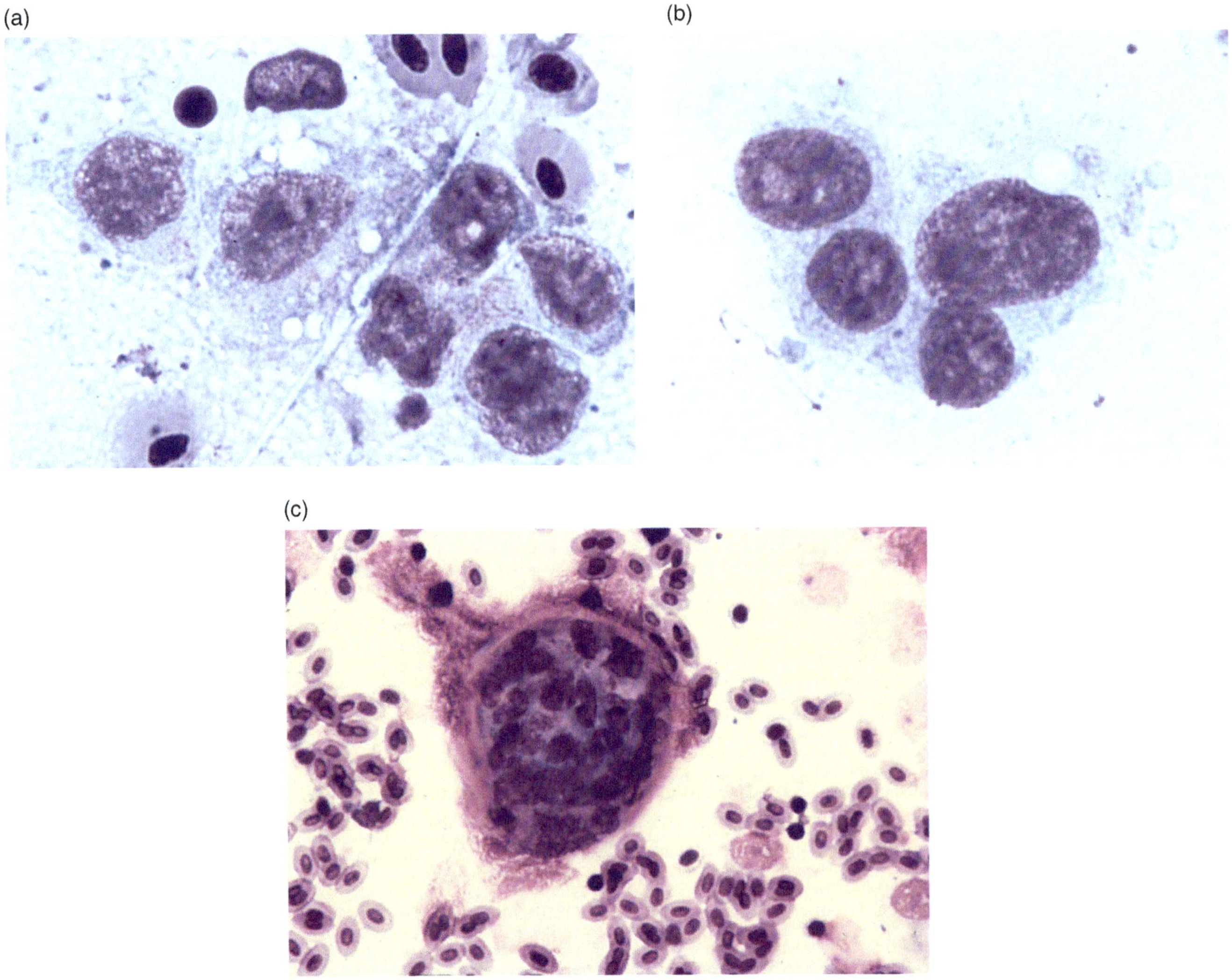

Fig. 15.89. (a) Pleomorphic mesenchymal cells in an imprint of a nephroblastoma (embryonal nephroma) from a budgerigar (*Melopsittacus undulatus*), Diff–Quik stain (100× oil). (b) Multinucleated giant cell with anisokaryosis and prominent irregular nucleoli in the same imprint of a nephroblastoma (embryonal nephroma) as Figure 15.89a from a budgerigar (*Melopsittacus undulatus*), Diff–Quik stain (100× oil) (c) A ball of cells surrounded by a heavy eosinophilic substance (possibly an attempt to produce either chondroid or osteoid) in the same imprint of a nephroblastoma (embryonal nephroma) as Figure 15.89a from a budgerigar (*Melopsittacus undulatus*), Diff–Quik stain (100× oil).

intensity are also present and are key findings in the identification of egg-related coelomitis (Figures 15.103–15.105). Fat globules are typically present in the background due to the high lipid content of egg yolk and appear as clear circular spaces. The high lipid and protein content of the fluid is likely associated with the presence of egg yolk (egg yolk is composed of 33% lipids, 17% protein, 48% water, 0.2% free carbohydrates, and 1% inorganic elements) in the coelomic cavity (Johnson, 1995).

The cytologic appearance of an early hematoma of the skin and subcutis initially resembles that of peripheral blood; early hematomas typically contain fluid that resembles blood without thrombocytes. Hemarthrosis or true hemorrhage into a joint is indicated by the presence of erythrocytes, erythrophagia, hematoidin crystals, hemosiderin, and lack of thrombocytes.

Hemorrhagic effusions present as red, turbid fluid, and often result from trauma or injury. Peracute hemorrhagic effusions may resemble peripheral blood (based on cell counts, leukocyte differentials, and the packed cell volume). Established hemorrhagic effusions contain a variable number of erythrocytes and leukocytes.

It is important to differentiate hemorrhagic effusions from peripheral blood contamination of the sample during collection. Observation of the sudden appearance of a red fluid in a clear fluid during sample collection indicates peripheral blood contamination of the sample. The

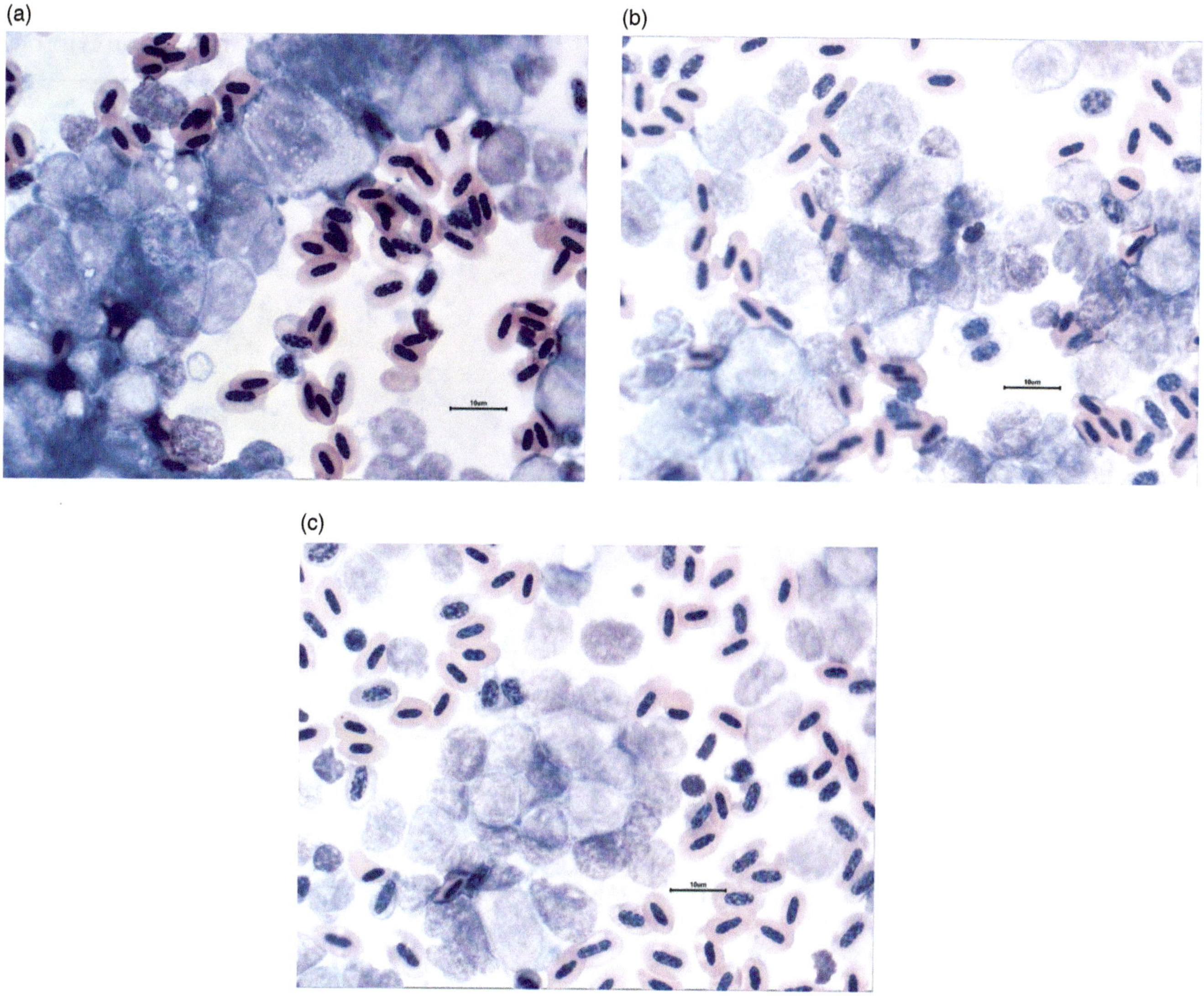

Fig. 15.90. (a) Pleomorphic epithelial cells in an imprint of a renal adenocarcinoma from a budgerigar (*Melopsittacus undulatus*), Wright–Giemsa stain. (b) Pleomorphic epithelial cells in the same imprint of a renal adenocarcinoma as in Figure 15.90a from a budgerigar (*Melopsittacus undulatus*), Wright–Giemsa stain. (c) Pleomorphic epithelial cells resembling lymphocytes or possibly epithelial cells in an acinar arrangement in the same imprint of a renal adenocarcinoma as in Figure 15.90a from a budgerigar (*Melopsittacus undulatus*), Wright–Giemsa stain.

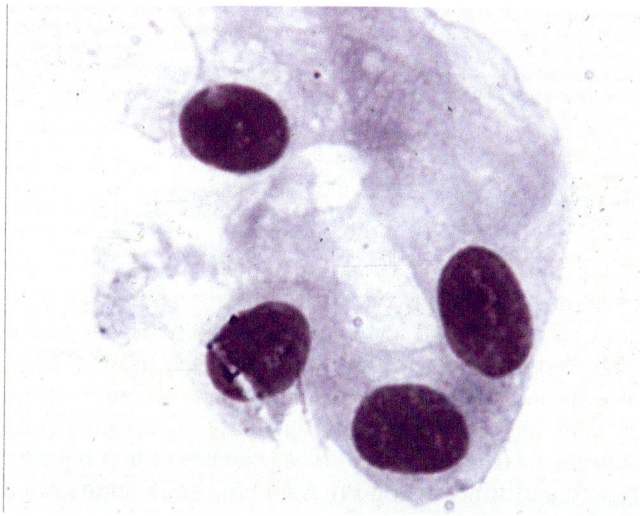

Fig. 15.91. Normal flat mesothelial cells in the coelomic fluid from a great horned owl (*Bubo virginianus*), Diff–Quik stain (100× oil).

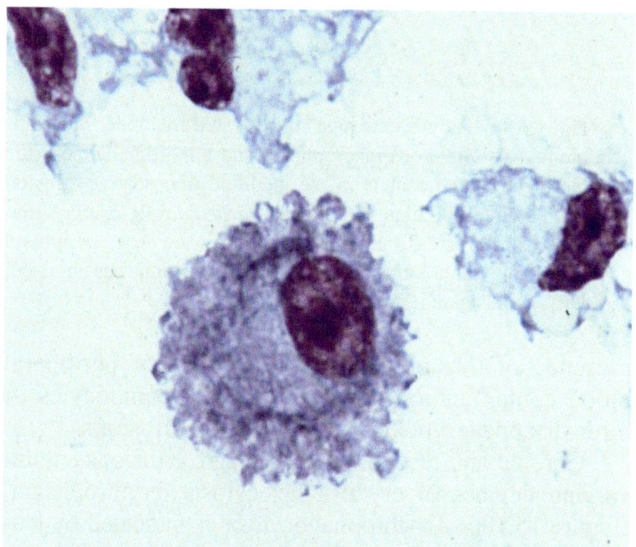

Fig. 15.92. A reactive mesothelial cell in the coelomic fluid (long-standing coelomic transudative effusion) from a blue-fronted Amazon parrot (*Amazona aestiva*), Diff–Quik stain (100× oil).

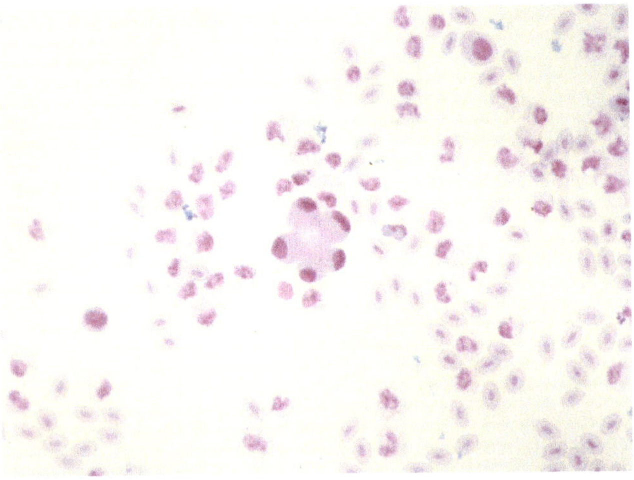

Fig. 15.93. An aggregate of mesothelial cells in the coelomic fluid (modified transudative effusion) from a bird (*Gracula religiosa intermedia*), Diff–Quik stain (100× oil).

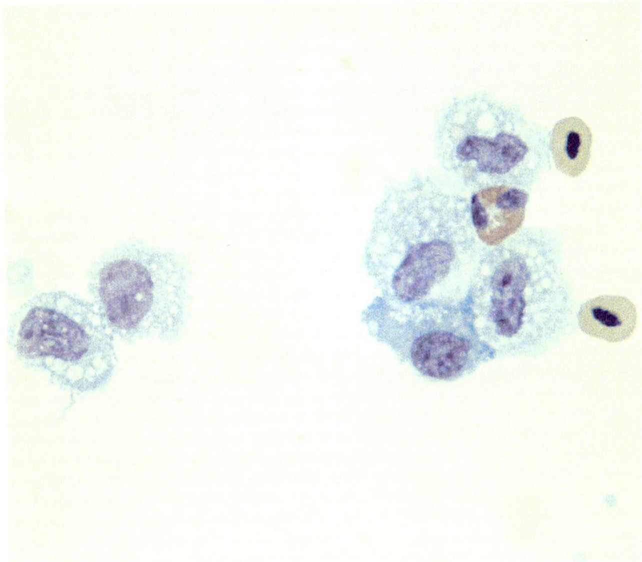

Fig. 15.95. A cytocentrifuge concentrated coelomic fluid sample reveals numerous macrophages and a nondegenerate heterophil in the modified transudative effusion from an African gray parrot (*Psittacus erithacus*) with heart failure, Wright–Giemsa stain (100× oil). Source: Image from Campbell and Grant (2010, p. 211).

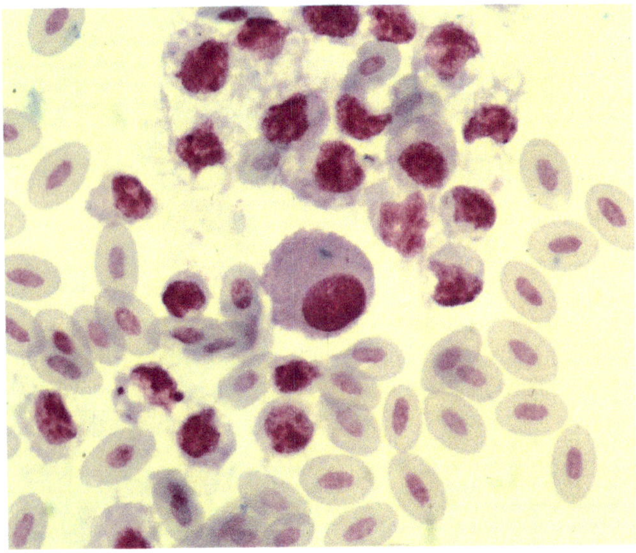

Fig. 15.94. A cytocentrifuge concentrated coelomic fluid sample reveals numerous macrophages and a mesothelial cell (the large cell in the center) in the modified transudative effusion from a Greater Indian Hill Mynah (*Gracula religiosa intermedia*) with liver failure. The erythrocytes are from peripheral blood contamination of the fluid when the sample was obtained, Diff–Quik stain (100× oil).

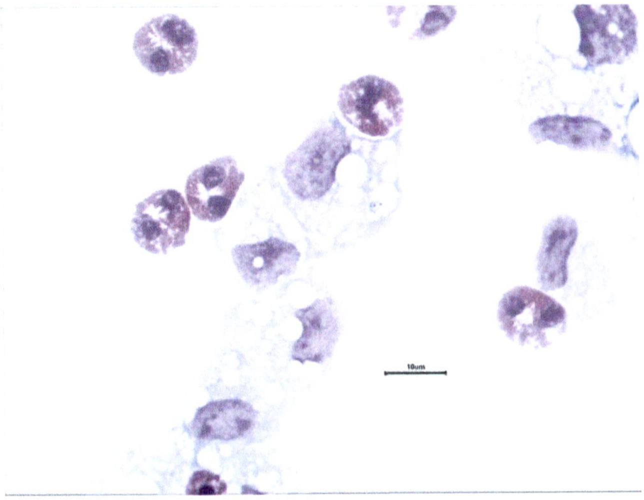

Fig. 15.96. A cytocentrifuge concentrated coelomic fluid sample reveals numerous macrophages and nondegenerate heterophils in the modified transudative effusion from a green-cheeked conure (*Pyrrhura molinae*), Wright–Giemsa stain.

presence of thrombocytes is suggestive of peripheral blood contamination as well because thrombocytes of birds disappear quickly in hemorrhagic effusions.

Chronic and resolving hemorrhagic effusions exhibit varying degrees of erythrophagocytosis (erythrophagia) (Figure 15.106). Erythrophagocytosis is indicated by leukocytic (usually macrophagic) phagocytosis of intact erythrocytes, or macrophages containing remnants of erythrocytes such as red cell fragments and iron pigment (Figures 15.107–15.110). Iron pigment results from the breakdown of erythrocytes and appears as blue-black to gray pigment in the cytoplasm of macrophages stained with Wright's stain. Hemosiderin crystals also indicate iron from erythrocyte degradation. Hemosiderin appears as diamond-shaped crystals that have a refractile gold appearance (Figure 15.110). The presence of iron pigment can be confirmed using Prussian blue stain applied to a Wright's stained smear. A spontaneous hemorrhagic effusion in a bird without a history of trauma provides

(a) (b)

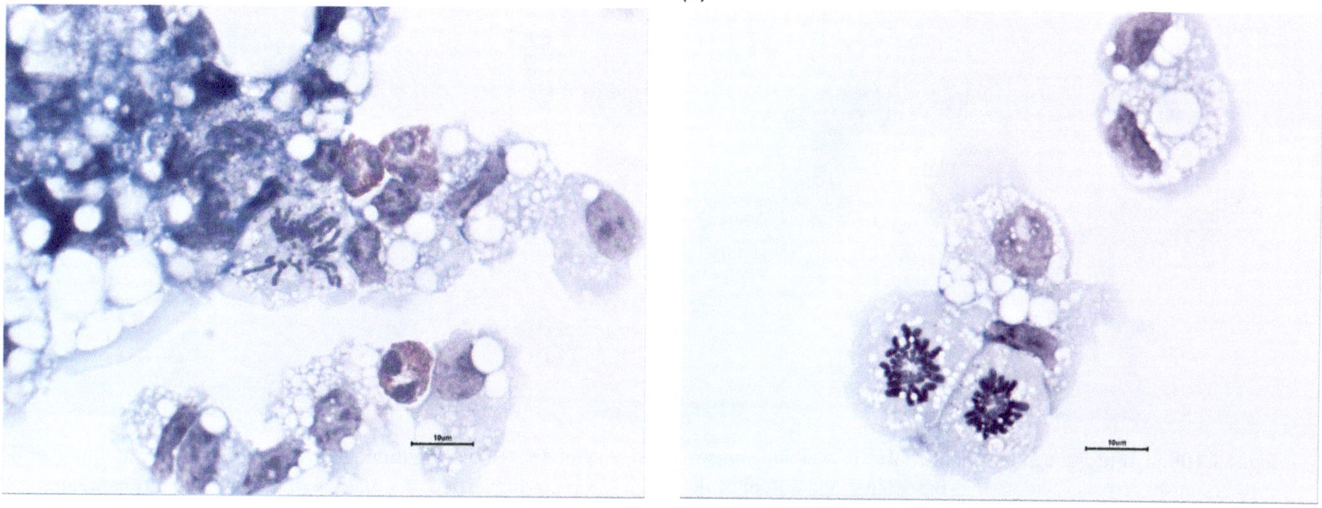

Fig. 15.97. (a) A cytocentrifuge concentrated coelomic fluid sample reveals numerous macrophages, nondegenerate heterophils, and a mitotic figure in the modified transudative effusion from a green-cheeked conure (*Pyrrhura molinae*), Wright–Giemsa stain (100× oil). (b) A cytocentrifuge concentrated coelomic fluid sample reveals macrophages and a mitotic figure in the modified transudative effusion from a green-cheeked conure (*Pyrrhura molinae*), Wright–Giemsa stain (100× oil).

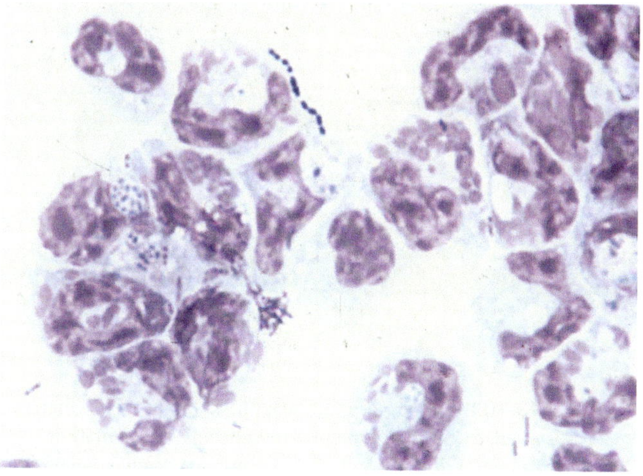

Fig. 15.98. Numerous degranulated and partially degranulated heterophils indicating heterophilic inflammation in the coelomic fluid (exudative effusion) from a lesser sulfur crested cockatoo (*Cacatua sulphurea*). The wide variety of both extracellular and intracellular bacteria present indicates a septic coelomitis and suggests leakage of gastrointestinal fluid contents into the coelomic cavity. Necropsy revealed an acute duodenal rupture. Diff–Quik stain (100× oil).

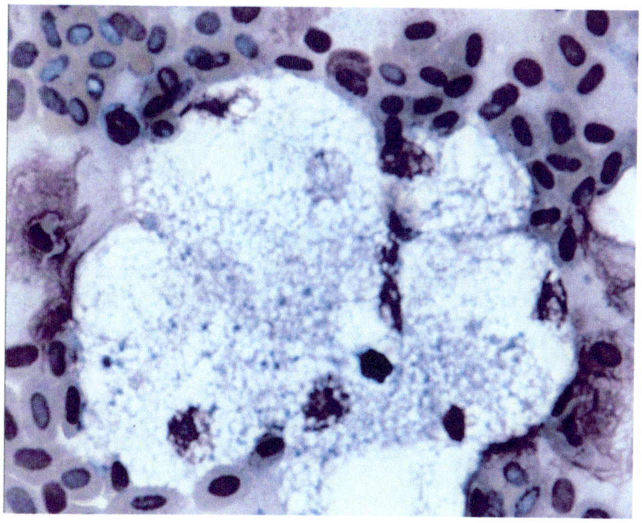

Fig. 15.99. Large foamy giant cells, presumed to be secretory epithelial cells from a neoplasm, in the coelomic fluid from a cockatiel (*Nymphicus hollandicus*) diagnosed with an ovarian cystadenocarcinoma, Diff–Quik stain (100× oil).

circumstantial evidence for an intracoelomic lesion that is hemorrhaging (Mickley et al., 2009) (Figure 15.108).

Accidental Aspiration of the Liver

During a coelomic aspiration for intracoelomic fluid evaluation, the liver may be accidentally aspirated, especially if it is enlarged. The cytologic sample in this situation will reveal hepatocytes. Hepatocytes appear as individual or clusters of large cells with abundant, lightly basophilic cytoplasm and round nuclei among numerous erythrocytes (Figures 15.87 and 15.111). The nuclei of normal hepatocytes appear uniform in size and shape with coarsely granular chromatin and prominent large nucleoli (Campbell and Grant, 2010).

Synovial Cyst

Synovial cysts are uncommon, but have been reported in birds (Pirie and Heatley, 2001; Campbell and Grant, 2010). Cytology of the fluid aspirated from a synovial cyst resembles normal synovial fluid unless

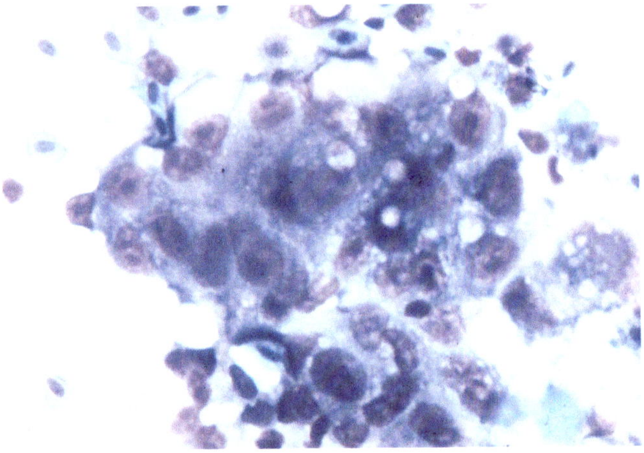

Fig. 15.100. Large aggregates of epithelial cells exhibiting anisocytosis, anisokaryosis, cytoplasmic basophilia, and cytoplasmic vacuolation in the coelomic fluid of a cockatiel (*Nymphicus hollandicus*) with an ovarian cystadenocarcinoma. These cells are not normally found in coelomic fluid and are indicative of a malignant effusion, Wright–Giemsa stain (100× oil).

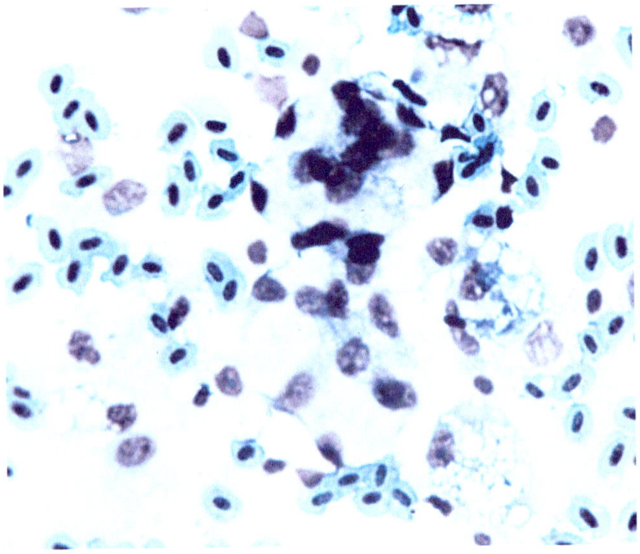

Fig. 15.101. Rosettes or balls of cells in the malignant effusion are suggestive of a coelomic adenocarcinoma (such as an ovarian cystadenocarcinoma) in a budgerigar (*Melopsittacus undulatus*), Wright–Giemsa stain (100× oil).

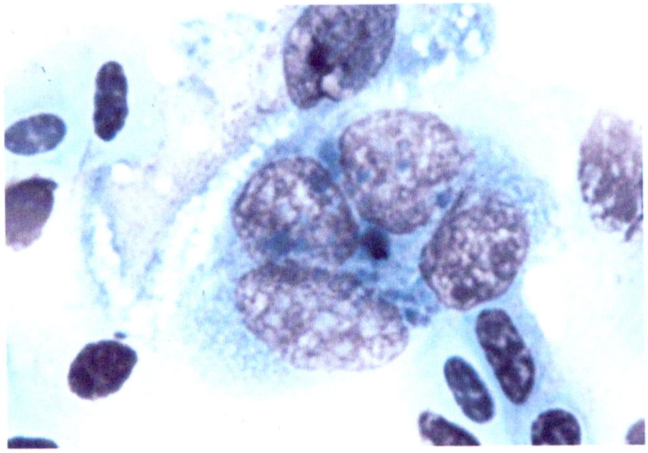

Fig. 15.102. A multinucleated giant cell in the coelomic effusion is suggestive of a malignant effusion (in this case, an ovarian cystadenocarcinoma) in a cockatiel (*Nymphicus hollandicus*), Wright–Giemsa stain (100× oil).

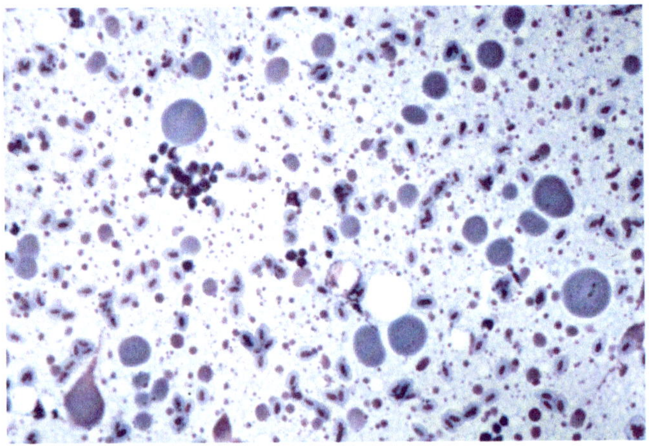

Fig. 15.103. Large, round, basophilic amorphous material (presumed to be egg protein), mixed cell inflammation, and clear round fat droplets in the background are indicative of egg-related coelomitis in a female cockatiel (*Nymphicus hollandicus*), Diff–Quik stain (200×).

secondary inflammation is present; therefore, synoviocytes with an eosinophilic granular background would be expected (Figure 15.112).

Mucocele

Mucoceles are rarely reported in birds. When aspirated, cytologic preparation of the clear, pale yellow fluid reveals erythrocytes, moderate numbers of heterophils, and numerous foamy mononuclear cells against a mucoid background (Huynh et al., 2014).

Infectious Agents

Avian Pox

Avian pox is a slow-spreading viral disease of many species of birds (reported in 278 of the approximately 9800 bird species) caused by viruses of the family Poxviridae and the genus *Avipoxvirus* (Hernández et al., 2001; Van Riper and Forrester, 2007; Shivaprasad and Fanca, 2011; Slocombe et al., 2013; Williams et al., 2014). Avian poxvirus is an enveloped double-stranded DNA virus that may be transmitted to birds by arthropod vectors or mucosal membrane contact with infectious particles (Godoy et al., 2013). There are 10 species of Avipoxviruses: Fowlpox virus, Canarypox virus, Juncopox virus, Mynahpox virus, Psittacinepox virus, Sparrowpox virus, Starlingpox virus, Pigeonpox

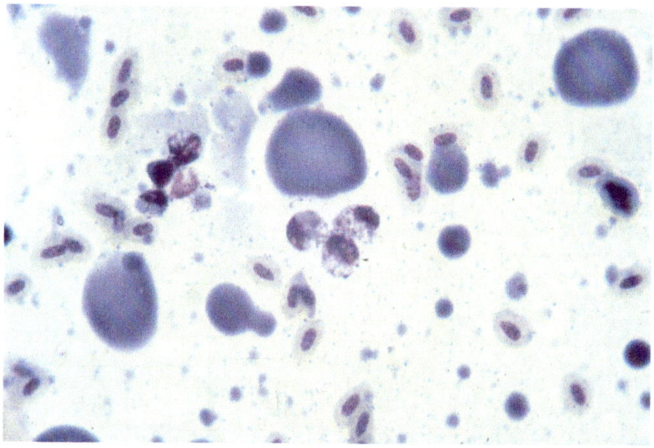

Fig. 15.104. Large, basophilic globular material (presumed to be egg protein aggregates) and mixed cell inflammation in the coelomic fluid are indicative of egg-related coelomitis in a female cockatiel (*Nymphicus hollandicus*), Diff–Quik stain (400×).

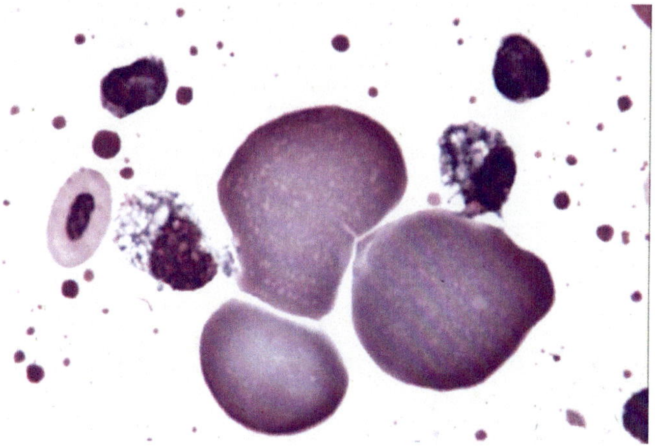

Fig. 15.105. Large, basophilic globular material (presumed to be egg protein aggregates) and clear, round fat droplets in the background are indicative of egg-related coelomitis in a female cockatiel (*Nymphicus hollandicus*), Diff–Quik stain (100× oil).

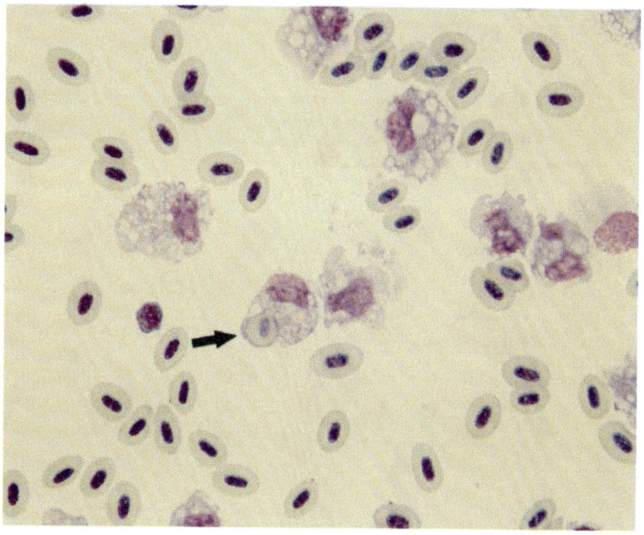

Fig. 15.106. A macrophage exhibiting erythrophagocytosis (arrow) in the coelomic fluid of a budgerigar (*Melopsittacus undulatus*), Diff–Quik stain (100× oil).

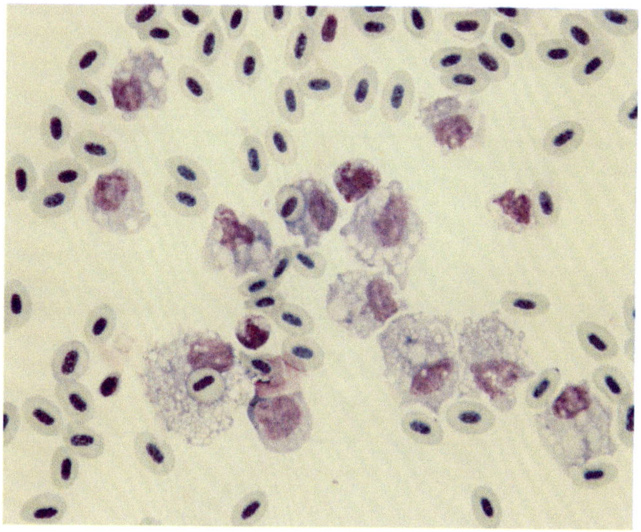

Fig. 15.107. A macrophage exhibiting erythrophagocytosis in the coelomic fluid of a budgerigar (*Melopsittacus undulatus*), Diff–Quik stain (100× oil).

virus, Turkeypox virus, and Quailpox virus (Van Riper and Forrester, 2007; Suepaul et al., 2019). Phylogenetic analysis indicates that species fall into three main clades: clad A "Fowlpox-like viruses" being mainly isolated from Galliformes that appear to be fairly host-specific; clad B "Canarypox-like viruses" from passerines that seem to infect a wide range of species; and clad C Psittacinepox viruses (Williams et al., 2014; Giotis and Skinner, 2019; Suepaul et al., 2019). However, new isolates that may represent new species, strains, or variants of Avipoxviruses continue to be identified in other avian species (Gyuranecz et al., 2013).

Cutaneous pox, the more common form, can occur separately or concurrently with the diphtheritic manifestation (Bolte et al, 1999; Sentíes-Cué et al., 2010). Grossly, avian poxvirus, in general, causes cutaneous papules or raised crusty lesions on unfeathered areas of the integument (Figures 15.113a and 15.113b). Lesions often appear on the head around the eyes, beak, and nares, and on legs on the tarsometatarsus and feet (Beaufrère et al., 2009; Chen et al., 2011; Slocombe et al., 2013). However, pox lesions can also be found in feathered areas as well as the uropygial gland in some cases (Hsieh et al., 2005).

Canary pox in canaries is often septicemic in nature and capable of producing nearly 100% mortality in affected aviaries (Shivaprasad and Fanca, 2011). Canary pox manifests itself in three different forms: (i) cutaneous (dry), characterized by nodular proliferative lesions on the unfeathered skin; (ii) diphtheritic (wet), when

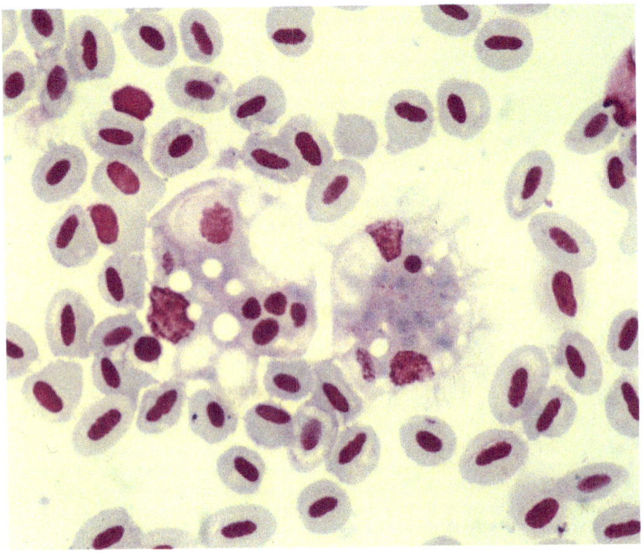

Fig. 15.108. A macrophage exhibiting erythrophagocytosis in the coelomic fluid of a cockatiel (*Nymphicus hollandicus*) with an ovarian cystadenocarcinoma, Diff–Quik stain (100× oil).

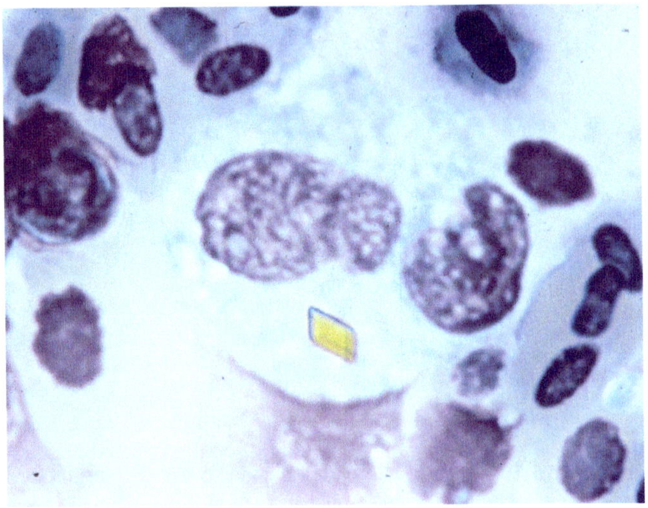

Fig. 15.110. A macrophage containing a golden hemosiderin crystal in the cytoplasm from erythrocyte degradation indicating previous erythrophagocytosis in the coelomic fluid of a bird (*Agapornis roseicollis*), Diff–Quik stain (100× oil).

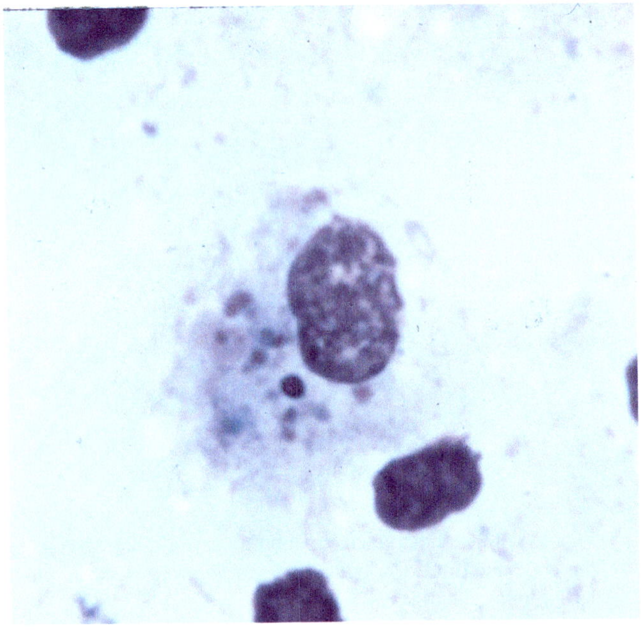

Fig. 15.109. A macrophage exhibiting iron pigment in the cytoplasm indicating previous erythrophagocytosis in the coelomic fluid of a peach-faced lovebird (*Agapornis roseicollis*), Diff–Quik stain (100× oil).

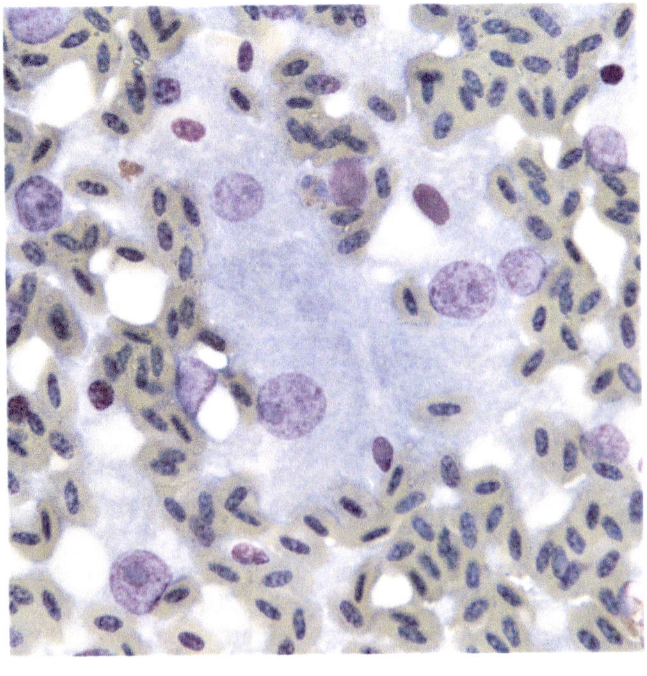

Fig. 15.111. Hepatocytes indicating accidental aspiration of the liver in fluid obtained by celiocentesis from a peach-faced lovebird (*Agapornis roseicollis*) with hepatomegaly, Wright–Giemsa stain (100× oil). Source: Image from Campbell and Grant (2010, p. 226).

fibrinonecrotic and proliferative lesions develop on the mucous membrane of the upper respiratory and digestive tracts; and (iii) the respiratory or peracute form, which causes a severe, peracute, fatal pneumonia and high mortality (Catania et al., 2017).

Cytology has been shown to be a sensitive and specific diagnostic method for the diagnosis of avian pox that is as reliable as histopathology (Hydock et al., 2018). Cytological examination of these lesions reveals ballooning degeneration of the epithelial cells, which is typified by swollen squamous epithelial cells containing one or more large cytoplasmic vacuoles that push the cell nucleus to the margin of the cell, peripheralized nuclei (Figures 15.114–5.116). This ballooning degeneration can be easily seen with low magnification

(Campbell and Grant, 2010). The large cytoplasmic vacuoles (A-type cytoplasmic inclusion bodies or Bollinger bodies) contain tiny, round, pale eosinophilic inclusions (Borrel bodies) on slides stained with Wright's stain (Deem et al., 1997; Campbell and Ellis, 2007; Campbell and Grant, 2010; Hydock et al., 2018).

An inflammatory response does not usually accompany avian pox virus. When numerous inflammatory cells are present in the cytology sample, they are often the result of a superimposed bacterial (or fungal) infection.

Cellular inclusions of other viral diseases involving the skin are rare. Viral agents associated with conjunctivitis have been reported in birds; however, conjunctivitis is rarely the only clinical sign (Abrams et al., 2005). Avian poxviruses are the most important viral agents that cause conjunctivitis in birds.

Mycoplasmosis

Mycoplasma spp. conjunctivitis is often associated with sinusitis or other respiratory disorders and is commonly reported in several species of free-ranging birds (Cookson and Shivaprasod, 1994; Fisher et al., 1997; Hartnup et al., 1998; Sydenstricker et al., 2006). *Mycoplasma* is frequently overlooked as a cause of

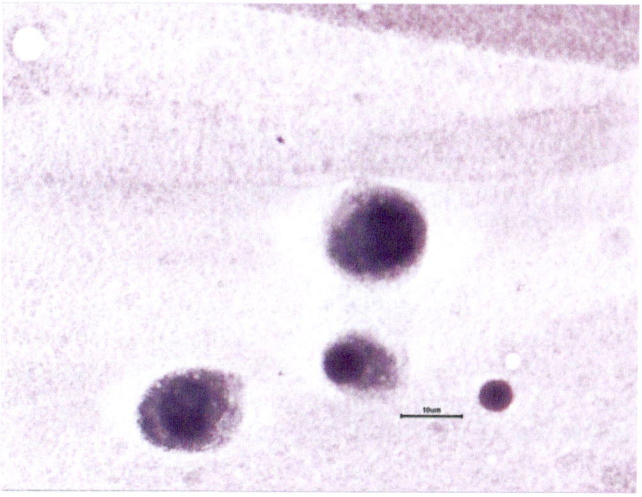

Fig. 15.112. Synoviocytes in a heavy eosinophilic granular background from fluid aspirated from a synovial cyst from a barn owl (*Tyto alba*), Wright–Giemsa stain (100× oil).

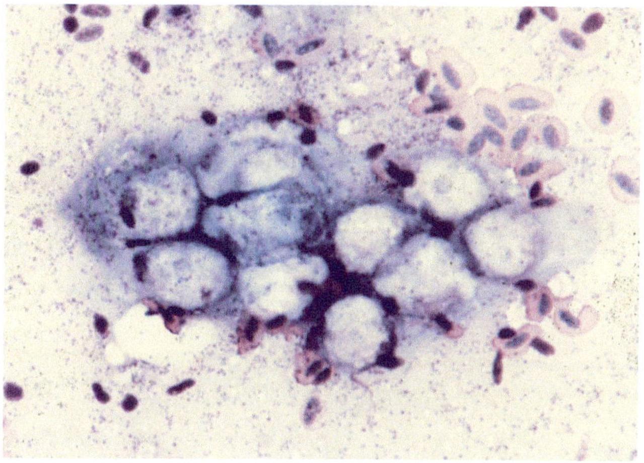

Fig. 15.114. Ballooning degeneration of the squamous epithelial cells, indicative of avian pox from a scraping of a cutaneous lesion, Diff–Quik stain (400×).

(a) (b)

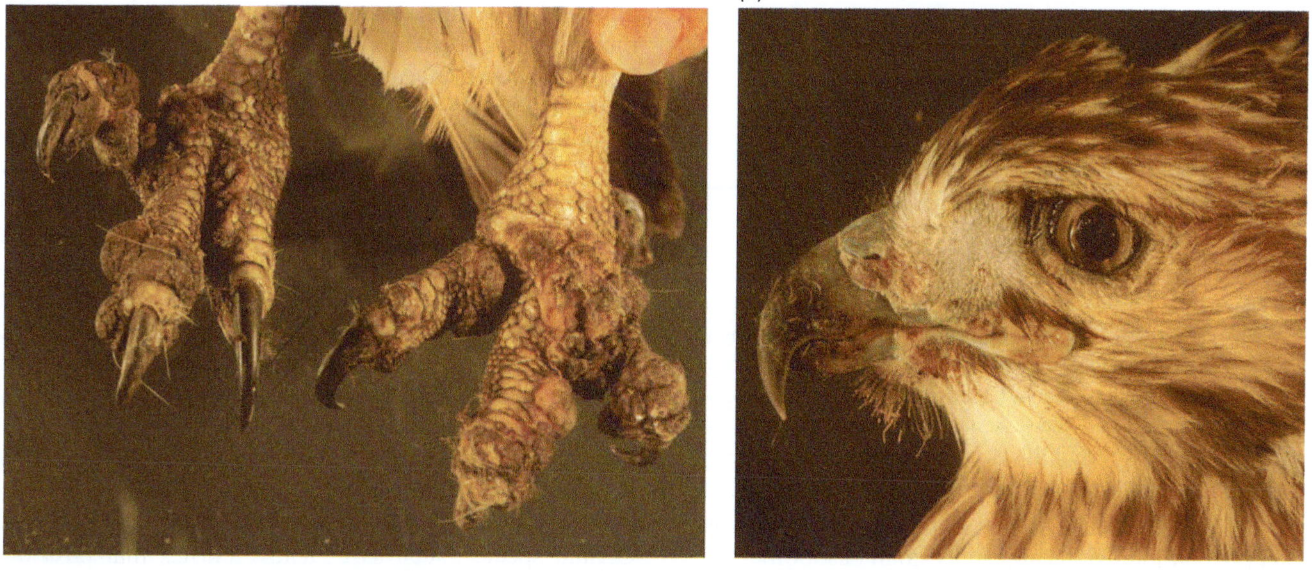

Fig. 15.113. (a) Gross appearance of avian pox lesions (hawk pox) on the feet of a red-tailed hawk (*Buteo jamaicensis*). (b) Gross appearance of avian pox lesions (hawk pox) on the mucocutaneous margins of the mouth, eyelid, and cere of a red-tailed hawk (*Buteo jamaicensis*).

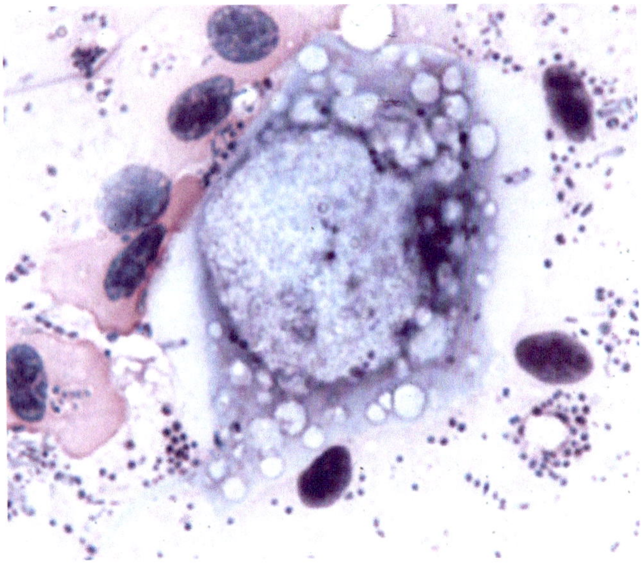

Fig. 15.115. A squamous epithelial cell with a large cytoplasmic vacuole (Bollinger body) forcing the nucleus to the periphery of the cell. The small, round, pale eosinophilic inclusions (Borrel bodies) can be seen inside the large vacuole, indicative of avian pox from a scraping of a cutaneous lesion, Diff–Quik stain (100× oil)

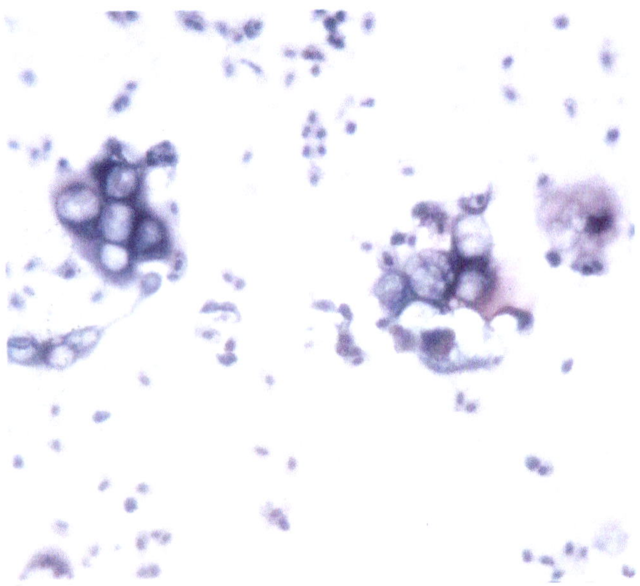

Fig. 15.116. Lower magnification of squamous epithelial cell with a large cytoplasmic inclusion (Bollinger body), forcing the nucleus to the periphery of the cell from a fine-needle aspiration biopsy of a pox lesion in a Chilean flamingo (*Phoenicopterus chilensis*), Wright–Giemsa stain (50×). Source: Image from Campbell and Grant (2010, p. 277).

conjunctivitis because it can be difficult to diagnose. *Mycoplasma* inclusions appear as small basophilic granules on the surface of epithelial cells (Figure 15.67).

Lymphoplasmacytic inflammation and epithelial hyperplasia in conjunctivae, nasal sinuses, and trachea is

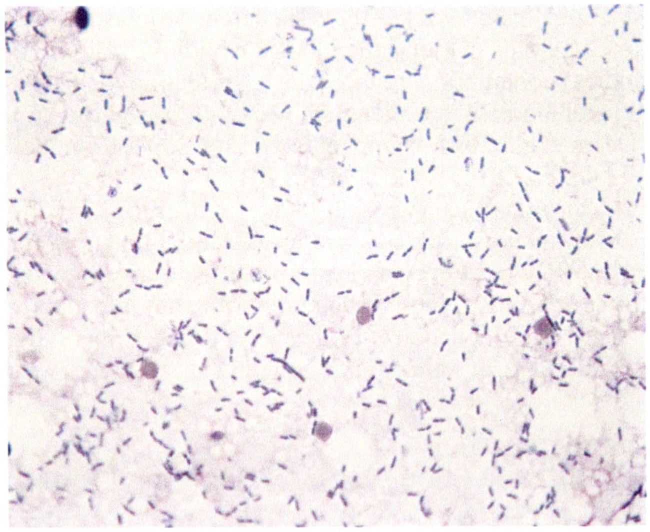

Fig. 15.117. A uniform population of bacteria in a fecal swab cytology from an umbrella cockatoo (*Cacatua alba*) with diarrhea. A heavy growth of *Klebsiella pneumoniae* was isolated from the sample, Diff–Quik stain (100× oil).

typical of M. *gallisepticum* infection in wild passerine species (Hawley et al., 2011; Ley et al., 2012). However, in another species, *M. sturni*, a heterophilic inflammation with ulceration of conjunctival epithelium was reported in a European starling (Frasca et al., 1997).

Clostridium

Bacteria are commonly found in cloacal or fecal samples of birds and are typically represented by a wide variety of morphological types. Heterophils and other inflammatory cells are not normally found in these samples and, when present, suggest an active infection. A monomorphic population of bacteria, *Clostridium*-like bacteria, *Candida*-like yeast, protozoa, parasite ova, and fungal elements are also abnormal cytologic findings in the cloacal or fecal samples of birds (Figures 15.117 and 15.118).

Clostridia bacteria appear as large, rod-shaped bacteria with a clear center and an increased density on one end (the endospore) on cytologic preparations. This bacterium is a gram-positive anaerobic bacillus that forms cylindrical, subterminal spores. This is often referred to as a "safety pin" or "tennis racquet" appearance (Figure 15.119). Clostridia are not considered to be normal enteric flora in birds that lack ceca, such as psittacine birds. Certain species of *Clostridium* are known to be highly pathogenic. For example, C. *colinum* in game birds causes severe, fatal ulcerative enteritis, known as quail disease.

Clostridia can produce disease in one of two ways. Certain species, such as *C. tetani* and *C. botulinum* (an important avian pathogen, especially affecting waterfowl), produce extremely potent toxins outside the host or in localized areas within the host. Other clostridial species,

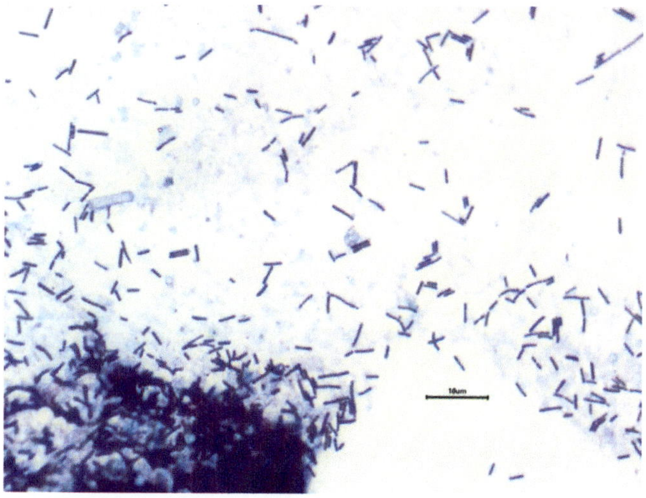

Fig. 15.118. A uniform population of bacteria in a fecal swab cytology from a yellow-naped Amazon parrot (*Amazona auropalliata*) with diarrhea. A heavy growth of *E. coli* was isolated from the sample, Wright–Giemsa stain (100× oil).

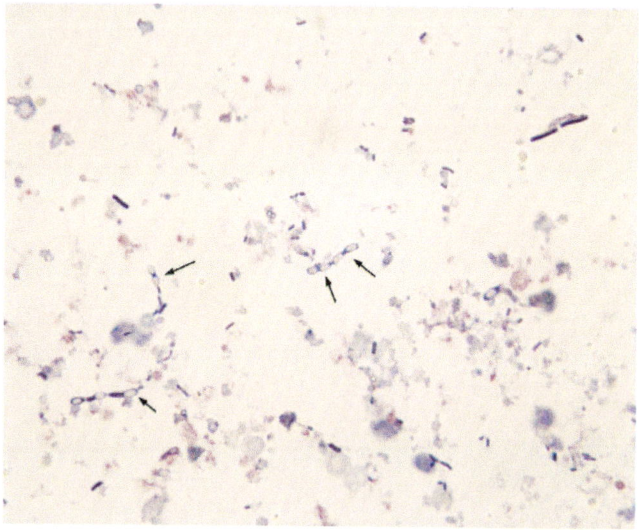

Fig. 15.119. Numerous clostridium-like bacteria (a few indicated by arrows) in a fecal swab cytology from a ferruginous hawk (*Buteo regalis*) with diarrhea. Wright–Giemsa stain (100× oil).

such as *C. perfringens*, *C. colinum*, *C. septicum*, *C. tertium*, and *C. novyi*, are invasive and produce less potent toxins. Invasion of the intestinal tract can damage the gastrointestinal mucosa by direct colonization, resulting in a fatal enteritis and enterotoxemia (Kolmstetter et al., 1995; Ferrell and Tell, 2001). Necrotic enteritis caused by *Clostridium perfringens* is one of the most prevalent and severe enteric diseases of poultry (Cooper et al., 2013). *Clostridium perfringens* is responsible for diseases that include necrotic or ulcerative enteritis, gaseous gangrene, necrotic dermatitis, and enterotoxemia. There are more than 17 potentially toxic exoproteins associated with *C. perfringens*, and the strains are classified into five toxinotypes (A, B, C, D, and E) according to the production of four major toxins: alpha, beta, epsilon, and iota (Guimarães et al., 2014). *C. perfringens* type A produces alpha toxin and is associated with necrotic or ulcerative enteritis in poultry. Ulcerative enteritis, produced by *C. colinum*, also known as quail disease, has been described in many avian species, but is most common in quail, where large gram-positive rods with subterminal spores can be found in the liver, spleen, and/or intestinal smears (Cooper et al., 2013; Uzal et al., 2016). *C. sordellii* causes gangrenous dermatitis in chickens and turkeys as well as enteritis and hepatitis in ostriches (Clark et al., 2010). *C. difficile* has been associated with necrotizing enteritis in newly hatched ostriches (Shivaprasad, 2003). *C. tertium* has caused enteritis in a rainbow lorikeet (*Trichoglossus moluccanus*) (Ferrell and Tell, 2001).

Campylobacter

Several avian species are considered the main reservoirs of thermotolerant *Campylobacter* spp., primarily *Campylobacter jejuni* and *Campylobacter coli*, which are among the most common bacteria causing acute human gastroenteritis throughout the world (Dipineto et al., 2008; Dipineto et al., 2009: Dipineto et al., 2014). The detection rate based on microbial culture of fecal samples is low (15.3% in one study), and screening using fecal cytology is likely to be low as well; whereas a higher detection rate might be obtained using polymerase chain reaction (PCR) (Kwon et al., 2017).

See Chapter 7 for further description of the organism.

Spirochetes (Spirochaetes)

The spirochete species considered to be pathogenic for avian species are classified into the genus *Brachyspira*, family Brachyspiraceae, order Spirochaetales (Nemes et al., 2006). *Brachyspira* spp. are anaerobic, flagellated, and helically shaped (spirochete) bacteria involved in enteric infections in chickens, pheasants, turkeys, partridges, ducks, geese, and rheas (Shivaprasad and Duhamel, 2005; Nemes et al., 2006; Uzal et al., 2016). *Borrelia anserina* is the causative agent of avian spirochetosis, an acute septicemia that can affect several species of birds, especially Galliformes and waterfowl (see Chapter 11). A non-classified spirochete has been reported in the choanal and tracheal mucus of cockatiels (*Nymphicus hollandicus*) with mild upper respiratory tract disease (Figures 15.120a and 15.120b) (Gerlach, 1994).

Chlamydiosis

Avian chlamydiosis (frequently called psittacosis in birds) primarily involves the respiratory, pharyngeal, and cloacal epithelia of a wide range of avian species worldwide and is generally caused by *Chlamydia psittaci*, an obligate intracellular gram-negative bacterium that

(a) (b)

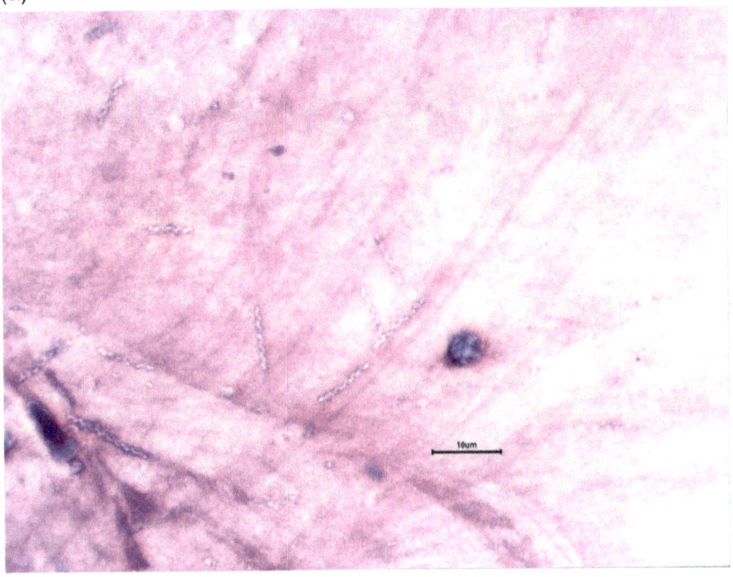

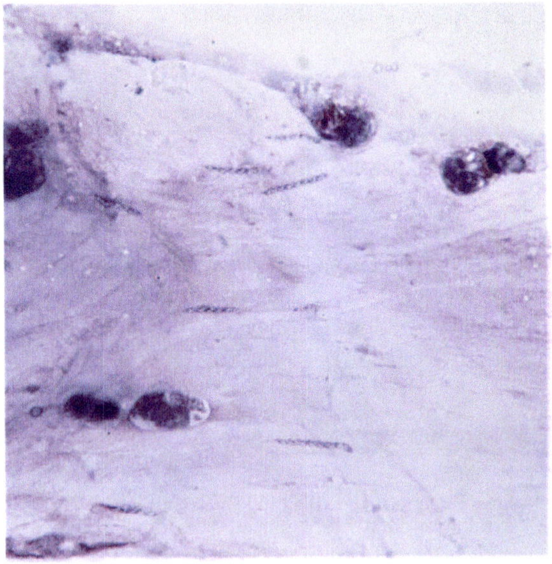

Fig. 15.120. (a) Spiral-shaped bacteria that have failed to stain in a sinus wash sample from a cockatiel (*Nymphicus hollandicus*) with a thick nasal discharge, Diff–Quik stain (100× oil). (b) Spiral-shaped bacteria in a sinus wash sample from a cockatiel (*Nymphicus hollandicus*) with a thick nasal discharge, Wright–Giemsa stain (100× oil).

belongs to the Chlamydiaceae family; however, other avian *Chlamydia* species, such as *C. avium* and *C. gallinacean*, can infect birds (Blomqvist et al., 2012; Luján-Vega et al., 2018). Three distinct morphologic stages occur in its life cycle: elementary bodies, the extracellular infective and metabolically inactive form; reticular bodies, larger structures that divide by binary fission and result from elementary body differentiation when they enter a cell via endocytosis; and intermediate bodies, a transitional stage between reticular bodies and elementary bodies (Longbottom and Coulter, 2003). Captive and wild birds are important reservoirs of *C. psittaci* and may be subclinically infected asymptomatic shedders.

Chlamydia psittaci infections are often associated with an inflammatory sinusitis and airsacculitis. The inflammatory response is represented as a mixed cell inflammation with heterophils, macrophages, lymphocytes, and plasma cells. Cytology samples stained with Wright's stain may reveal macrophages and occasionally epithelial cells that contain one of two types of inclusions that may be found depending upon the stage of development of the *Chlamydia* organism (Figures 15.121 and 15.122). Special staining using Giménez or Macchiavello's stains aid in the detection of the *Chlamydia* inclusions within the cells (Çelebi and Seyyal, 2006). The small (0.2–0.3 μm) basophilic elementary bodies are the infectious stage and will develop into the larger (0.9–1.0 μm) initial bodies, which proliferate to become large, membrane-bound reticulate bodies. The elementary and initial bodies stain red, and the host cells stain blue-green with Giménez stain (Figures 15.123 and 15.124). With Macchiavello's stain, the elementary bodies stain red and the initial bodies and host cells stain blue (Figure 15.125). Certain host cell structures, such as heterophil granules, may stain red with Macchiavello's stain and should not be confused with *Chlamydia* inclusions.

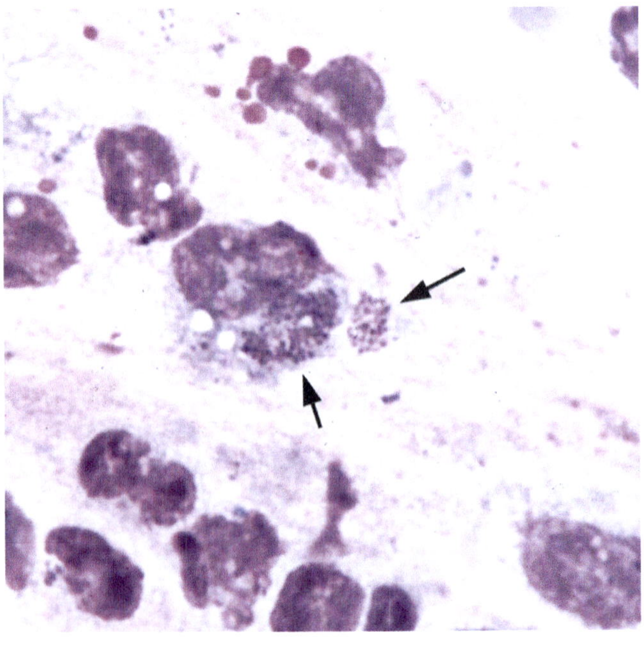

Fig. 15.121. Small, round, purple *Chlamydophila* intracytoplasmic inclusions (arrows) in a macrophage in a sinus aspirate with mixed cell inflammation from a blue-fronted Amazon parrot (*Amazona aestiva*). *Chlamydophila psittaci* was isolated from the sample, Diff–Quik stain (100× oil).

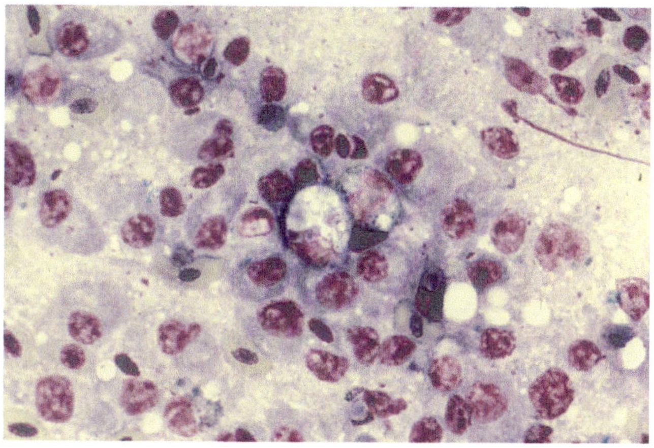

Fig. 15.122. Small, round, purple *Chlamydophila* intracytoplasmic inclusions in macrophages in a liver imprint that also exhibited a marked number of plasma cells from a yellow-naped Amazon parrot (*Amazona auropalliata*) that tested positive for *Chlamydophila psittaci*, Wright–Giemsa stain (100× oil).

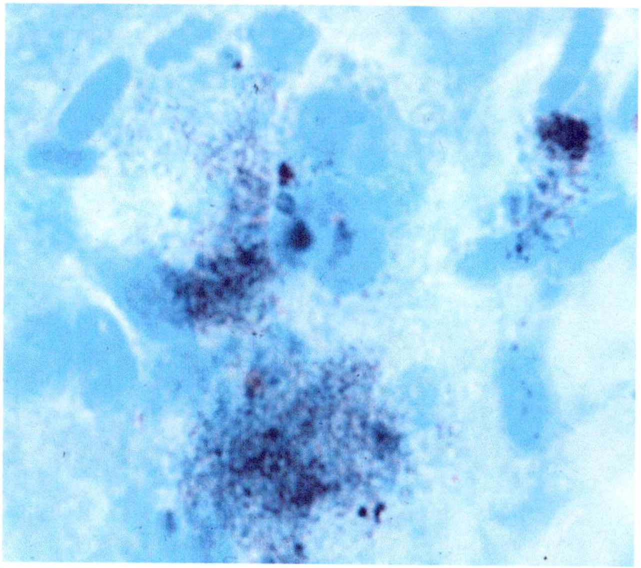

Fig. 15.123. Small, red *Chlamydophila* elementary bodies in a sinus aspirate from a blue-fronted Amazon parrot (*Amazona aestiva*) that was positive for *Chlamydophila psittaci*, Giménez stain (100× oil).

The spleen often provides an excellent cytological specimen for the detection of *Chlamydia* infections in birds. A marked number of plasma cells and macrophages containing *Chlamydia* inclusions are often present in the cytology sample.

Chlamydiosis frequently involves the liver, resulting in hepatomegaly. Hepatic cytology reveals an inflammatory response consisting primarily of macrophages, lymphocytes, and plasma cells. The *Chlamydia* organism appears as small, blue to purple, spherical, intracytoplasmic inclusions within the macrophages (Figures 15.121 and 15.122). Giménez or Macchiavello's stains can be used to confirm the *Chlamydia* inclusions (Figures 15.123–15.125).

With high sensitivity and specificity, microbial culture is the gold standard for the identification of *C. psittaci* infections even though it is time consuming and requires professional laboratory techniques and equipment (Wang et al., 2019). Use of PCR-based assays that amplify and detect small pieces of DNA and nonspecific serologic assays have been used to screen birds for *C. psittaci* as well as other Chlamydiaceae (Kaleta and Taday, 2003; Luján-Vega et al., 2018). Monoclonal antibodies against the major outer membrane protein have been used to identify eight serotypes (A to F, WC and M56) of C. *psittaci*, with serotypes WC and M56 being isolated solely from mammals and serotypes A, B, C, D, E, and F being roughly associated with different types of birds, such as psittacines, pigeons, waterfowl, turkeys, ratites and pigeons, and a parakeet, respectively (Madani and Peighambari, 2013; Wang et al., 2019).

Mixed cell inflammation with nondegenerate heterophils of the conjunctiva may be associated with *Chlamydia* infections. In birds, conjunctivitis has been reported as the sole clinical sign of *Chlamydia* infection, although often this condition is associated with other clinical signs (Surman et al., 1974; Farmer et al., 1982). Cytological findings include mixed cell inflammation and the presence of small (0.1–0.3 µm) basophilic intracytoplasmic inclusions in the epithelial cells or macrophages. Granulomatous inflammation with giant cells also may be seen in birds with a conjunctivitis associated with other bacterial pathogens, such as *Moraxella phenylpyruvica* (Grurel et al., 2004).

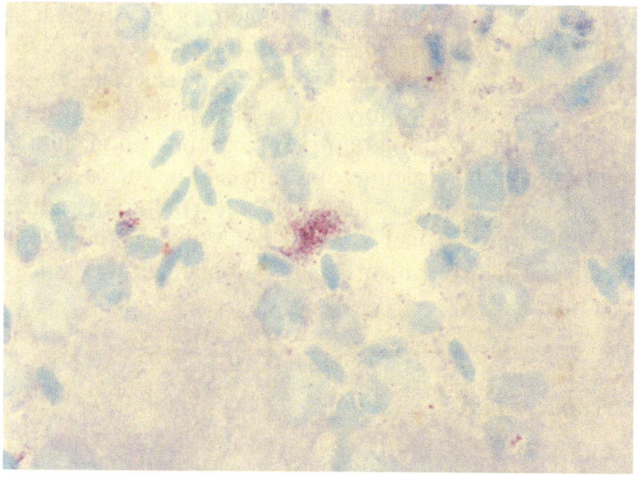

Fig. 15.124. Small, red *Chlamydophila* inclusions in a liver imprint from a yellow-naped Amazon parrot (*Amazona auropalliata*) that tested positive for *Chlamydophila psittaci*. Giménez stain (100× oil).

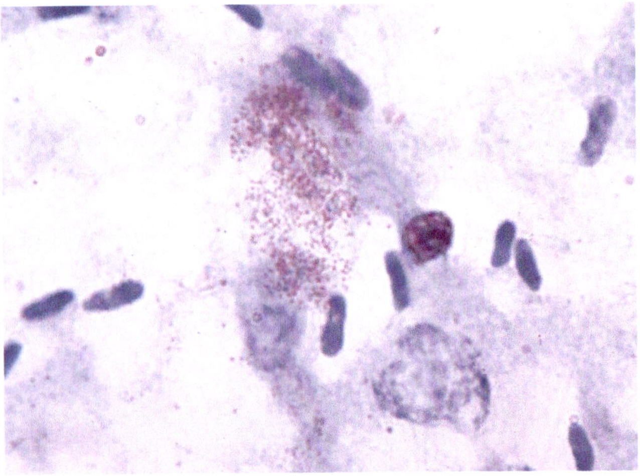

Fig. 15.125. Small, red, and blue *Chlamydophila* inclusion bodies in a sinus aspirate from a blue-fronted Amazon parrot (*Amazona aestiva*) that was positive for *Chlamydophila psittaci*, Macchiavello stain (100× oil).

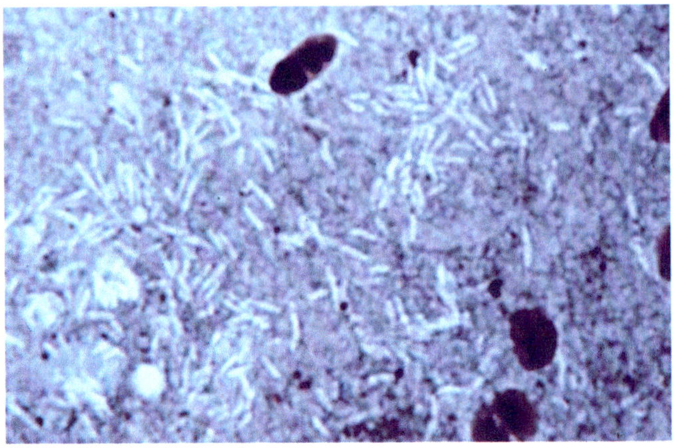

Fig. 15.126. Numerous bacterial rods that fail to stain (negative staining) in a liver imprint stained with routine cytology stains from a pine siskin (*Carduelis pinus*) with mycobacteriosis, Wright–Giemsa stain (100× oil).

Microsporidia

Microsporidial conjunctivitis caused by *Encephalitozoon hellem* has been identified in conjunctival scrapings in companion birds (primarily in lovebirds) (Kemp and Kluge, 1975; Novilla and Kwapien, 1978; Lowenstein and Petrak, 1980; Randall et al., 1986; Powell et al., 1989; Norton and Prior, 1994; Steinhort, 1995; Black et al., 1997; Gray et al., 1998; Canny et al., 1999). Cytology may reveal small (1–2 µm) gram-positive, round, intracellular and extracellular structures, presumed to be microsporidian organisms. Microsporidia closely resemble chlamydial and mycoplasmal inclusions; a definitive diagnosis for microsporidian organisms must be obtained using electron microscopy.

Mycobacterium

Avian mycobacteriosis is a severe disease affecting various domestic and wild bird species (the disease has been diagnosed in almost every avian order) and is primarily caused by several species and subspecies of the genus *Mycobacterium*, mainly members of the *Mycobacterium avium* complex (MAC; *Mycobacterium avium* subsp. *avium*, *Mycobacterium avium* subsp. *hominissuis*, and *Mycobacterium intracellulare*) and *Mycobacterium genavense* (Witte et al., 2008; Quinn et al., 2011; Fulton and Sanchez, 2013; Kriz et al., 2013; Palmieri et al., 2013; Haridy et al., 2014; Rindi and Garzelli, 2014; McRee et al., 2017). *Mycobacterium avium* subsp. *avium* is considered ubiquitous in nature, and there have been no reports of its spread from birds to humans (Burgdorf-Moisuk et al., 2009). *Mycobacterium genavense* is the primary cause of mycobacteriosis in psittacine birds (Palmieri et al., 2013). Other *Mycobacterium* species associated with clinical disease have been identified in birds at a lower incidence including *Mycobacterium tuberculosis*, *Mycobacterium gordonae*, *Mycobacterium nonchromogenicum*, *Mycobacterium fortuitum*, and *Mycobacterium bovis* (Steinmetz et al., 2006; Lennox, 2007; Lanteri et al., 2011; Kelly et al., 2013; Sáncheza et al., 2016).

Avian mycobacteriosis is characterized primarily by enterohepatic lesions with dissemination to other organs, such as the spleen, lung, air sacs, bone marrow, and skin, suggesting the oral route as the most common route of entry. Avian mycobacteriosis is a chronic disease that is represented by granulomatous lesions primarily involving the liver, spleen, and intestine; however, unusual manifestations of this disease have involved the respiratory system, especially involving *M. tuberculosis* (Steinmetz et al., 2006; Saggese et al., 2007; Kriz et al., 2011; Lanteri et al., 2011; Sáncheza et al., 2016).

Romanowsky-stained cytologic specimens of affected livers or granulomatous lesions in other locations in the body reveal macrophages and multinucleated giant cells and a background that contains numerous negative images of rod-shaped bacteria (Figure 15.126). Acid-fast staining is required to demonstrate the tubercle bacilli because the waxy cell wall of the organism prevents penetration of the Romanowsky stains (Figures 15.127 and 15.128). Demonstration of acid-fast positive bacilli provides only a strong presumptive diagnosis of mycobacteriosis. However, because other bacteria may also stain positive with acid-fast staining, definitive diagnosis requires a positive identification of the *Mycobacterium* spp. using special culture techniques or PCR testing.

Thus, a cytologic specimen that contains mixed cell or macrophagic inflammation and negative-staining slender rods in the cytoplasm of macrophages is suggestive of *Mycobacterium* spp. infection. The presence of numerous acid-fast positive bacilli is typically caused by

Mycobacterium, especially *M. avium*; however, human–avian transmission of *M. tuberculosis* is possible (Steinmetz et al., 2006; Lanteri et al., 2011). Antemortem diagnosis of mycobacteriosis and screening of birds for the disease can be challenging, as many exposed birds are likely to remain uninfected (Witte et al., 2010).

Candidiasis

Candidiasis is an infection caused by the fungus of the genus *Candida* that can affect many types of birds, especially those with a gastrointestinal dysbiosis or are immunocompromised, which allow the growth of opportunistic yeast that are a part of the normal gastrointestinal tract microbiota. C. *albicans* is the common organism involved with candidiasis of companion birds. This opportunistic fungal pathogen is involved in infections ranging from superficial mucosal infections to systemic candidiasis (Proenca et al., 2014; Sokół et al., 2018). Other species such as *Candida parapsilosis*, *Candida rugosa*, *Candida famata*, *Candida tropicalis*, and *Candida krusei* have also been isolated from poultry with candidiasis (Sokół et al., 2018). Typical lesions associated with candidiasis include caseous material and small pseudo-caseous nodules in the mucosa of the crop or glandular stomach. Although rare, pulmonary candidiasis can occur in birds (Proenca et al., 2014).

Candidiasis is detected by the presence of many oval, thin-walled, narrowly based budding yeast that measure 2–6 µm in diameter (Campbell and Grant, 2010) (Figures 15.129a and 15.129b). Candida typically stain deeply basophilic in color with Wright's stain and

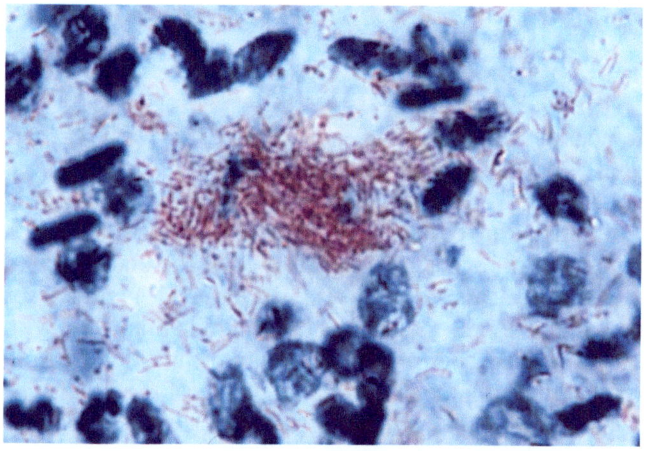

Fig. 15.127. Numerous red-staining, acid-fast positive bacterial bacilli in a liver contact smear from a pet bird (*Amazona aestiva*) with *Mycobacterium*, acid-fast stain (100× oil).

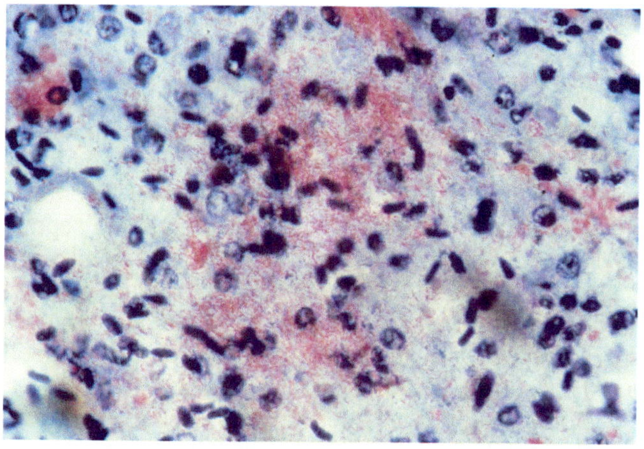

Fig. 15.128. Numerous red-staining, acid-fast positive bacterial bacilli in a liver contact smear from a wild bird (*Bubo virginianus*) with *Mycobacterium*, acid-fast stain (100× oil).

(a) (b)

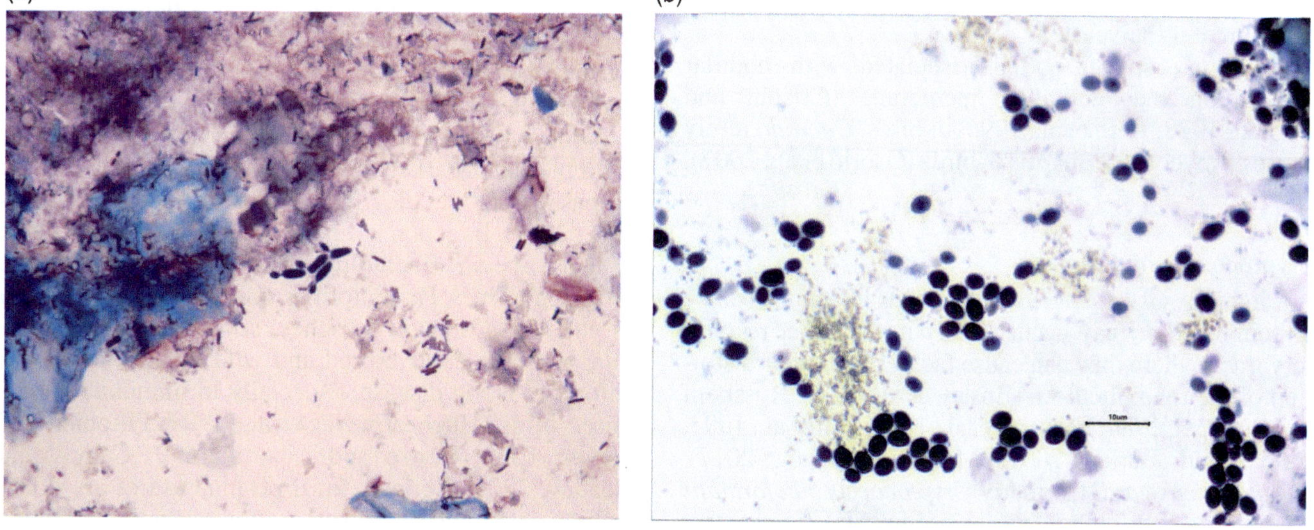

Fig. 15.129. (a) Several budding *Candida*-like yeast in a fecal cytology from a hyacinth macaw (*Anodorhynchus hyacinthinus*) with diarrhea, Wright–Giemsa stain (100× oil). (b) Numerous *Candida*-like yeast in a fecal cytology from a military macaw (*Ara militaris*) with weight loss, Wright–Giemsa stain.

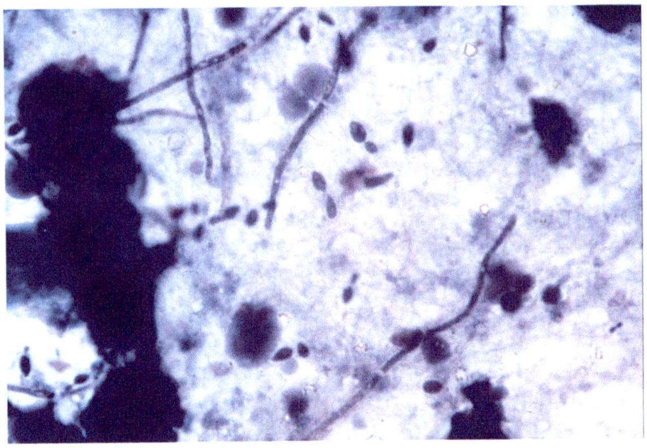

Fig. 15.130. Several budding *Candida*-like yeast and hyphae in a crop aspirate from a young cockatiel (*Nymphicus hollandicus*) with delayed emptying of the ingluvies (crop). This finding is indicative of candidiasis, Wright–Giemsa stain (100× oil).

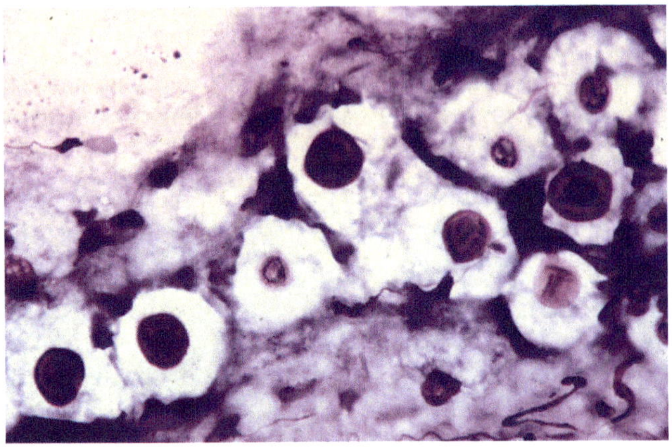

Fig. 15.131. Numerous round to oval yeast characterized by a colorless capsule of varying thicknesses and deep-purple to blue content in a sinus aspirate of an orange-winged Amazon parrot (*Amazona amazonica*) with *Cryptococcus neoformans* sinusitis, Diff–Quik stain (100× oil).

gram-positive with Gram's stain, although occasionally the yeast and hyphae stain poorly. A marked amount of background debris is often present, but few inflammatory cells are typically noted unless mucosal ulceration has occurred. The presence of short tubular septate hyphae and blastospores indicate tissue invasion by the *Candida* organism (Figure 15.130). The appearance of *Candida* hyphae provides a poor prognosis and indicates the need for systemic therapy for the yeast (Campbell and Ellis, 2007; Caliendo and Bull, 2011).

Some food products fed to birds contain yeast as a supplemental source of B vitamins. Cytologic samples obtained from the alimentary tracts of animals fed such foods may reveal large numbers of nonbudding yeast. These yeasts are not associated with lesions or other clinical signs of illness and are considered incidental findings. A sample of the food can be stained to confirm the source of the yeast.

Candida spp. is often associated with nodular lesions on the nictitating membrane (Crispin and Barnett, 1978; Kern et al., 1996) of birds. *Candida* rarely causes a mycotic dermatitis in birds (Osorio et al., 2007).

Cryptococcus neoformans

In birds, *Cryptococcus neoformans* infections can be disseminated or may occur focally in the upper respiratory tract, where they can cause facial swelling or distortion of the rhamphotheca (Ensley et al., 1979; Rosskopf and Woerpel, 1984; Fenwick et al., 1985; Hill et al., 1995; Raidal and Butler, 2001; Maccolini et al., 2017). *Cryptococcus gattii* (formerly *Cryptococcus neoformans* var. *gattii*) is a pathogenic environmental fungus that infects immunocompetent (in contrast to C. *neoformans*, which typically infects immunocompromised hosts) tropical and semitropical animals; however, animals in temperate climates can be infected as well (Lester et al., 2011; Molter et al., 2014).

Choanal smears or smears made from fine-needle aspirates of the paraorbital sinuses stained with Wright's stain contain occasional aggregates of the encapsulated yeast organisms (Raidal and Butler, 2001). Sheets of round to irregular yeast cells (5–15 μm in diameter) with narrow-based budding encased in a clear, thick capsule (5–10 μm in diameter) is characteristic of *Cryptococcus* spp. (Molter et al., 2014) (Figure 15.131). Macrophages may also be present.

See Chapter 7 for further description of the organism.

Macrorhabdus ornithogaster in Birds

Macrorhabdus ornithogaster is often present in greatest numbers in the superficial mucosal glands of the proventricular isthmus, the narrow transition zone between the oxynticopeptic glands of the proventriculus and the straight, koilin-producing ventricular glands (Filippich and Parker, 1994; Phalen and Moore, 2003; Tomaszewski et al., 2003; Phalen, 2005; Powers et al., 2019). Infection has been described in a wide range of avian species (including Anseriformes, Galliformes, Struthioniformes, Passeriformes, and Psittaciformes), such as chickens, turkeys, ostriches, several species of parrots, and both captive-bred and wild finches, causing a chronic wasting disease, especially in immunocompromised birds (Huchzermeyer et al., 1993; Filippich and Parker, 1994; Conzo and Liberti, 1999; Camus and Heatley, 2001; Gerlach, 2001; Hannafusa et al., 2007; Robinoa et al., 2019). Disease often occurs in passerine and psittacine birds from chick to 1–5 years of age. In ostriches, the disease appears to be limited to chicks less than 20 weeks old (Gerlach, 2001).

The organism is shed intermittently, which may hinder the diagnosis, but is typically diagnosed based on observation of symptoms and microscopic detection of the organism in feces, crop swabs or proventricular washings or scrapings collected from brush cytology, biopsy, or a postmortem examination (Camus and Heatley, 2001; Phalen, 2014; Püstow and Krautwald-Junghanns, 2017). Feces made into a slurry with water or saline can be scanned for *M. ornithogaster* using 40× as a wet mount preparation, or fecal smears can be stained with a Quick stain or Gram stain (Phalen, 2014). Confirmation of the disease is made with molecular methods, where cloacal swab PCR has been found to diagnose the presence of the organism better than fecal Gram's stain (Sullivan et al., 2017).

Macrorhabdus ornithogaster was previously referred to as Megabacteria and was once considered to be a bacterium; however, research has confirmed that it is a fungal organism (yeast) containing a eukaryotic nucleus, and the ribosomal RNA gene sequence of yeast (Moore et al., 2001; Tomaszewski et al., 2003; Marlier et al., 2006). The organism is rod shaped, microaerophilic, gram-positive, argyrophilic, and periodic acid–Schiff (PAS) positive and is the only species of this genus in the phylum Ascomycota (Schmidt et al., 2015). The organism is a large (20–80 μm long × 2–3 μm wide), stiff, straight rod with rounded ends that stains positive with Gram's and periodic acid–Schiff stains (Hargreaves, 1981; Lublin et al., 1998; Hannafusa et al., 2007). It is commonly found using routine fecal cytology methods with Romanowsky stains, where the organism appears as a very large blue-staining rod; hence, the early misidentification as a bacterium (Campbell and Grant, 2010) (Figures 15.132 and 15.133). Because the organism frequently stains poorly with quick stains and Gram stain, where the contents of the cell stain but the cell wall does not, heat fixing the slide preparation may improve stain uniformly (Phalen, 2014).

M. ornithogaster is also readily demonstrated in hematoxylin- and eosin-stained sections of the isthmus where the eosinophilic organisms appear as a "log-jam" or "haystack" pattern on the surface of and between the mucosal glands. Calcofluor White-M2R (a stain specific for chitin and cellulose, substances present in fungi) is an inexpensive stain that provides a rapid method of visualization of a *M. ornithogaster* in air-dried smears of feces and other samples. The caveat to the use of this stain is that it does require a microscope with ultraviolet fluorescent and barrier filter capabilities (Moore et al., 2001; see reference for preparation). The organism also stains positive with silver stains and the periodic acid shift stain.

Aspergillosis

Aspergillus spp. is a common fungal agent that affects the respiratory tract of wild and domestic birds worldwide. Most infections occur through inhalation when birds are exposed to high levels of spores and damp conditions and/or if the birds are immunosuppressed, resulting in three main diseases: infiltrative bronchopneumonia, granulomatous pneumonia and airsacculitis, and open fungal plaques in the air sacs (Beernaert et al., 2010; Glare et al., 2014; Fischer et al., 2018). The infection depends on spore size and where it settles in the respiratory tract, and the fungus frequently invades blood vessels, resulting in dissemination throughout the body (Beernaert et al., 2010). Leukocytosis is a parameter with a high sensitivity (88.9%) and specificity (75%) in birds with aspergillosis (Fischer and Lierz, 2015).

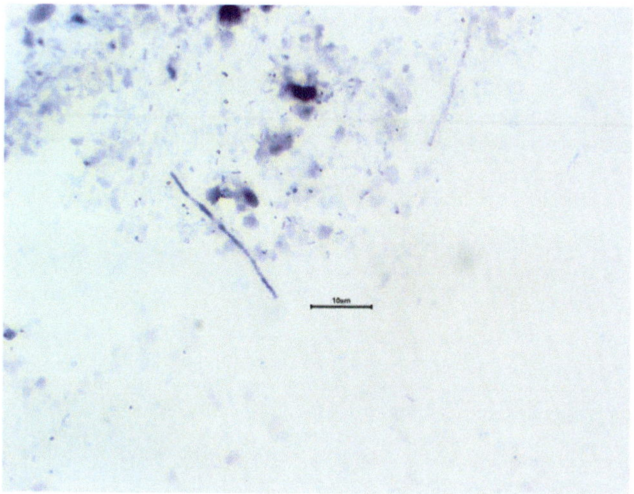

Fig. 15.132. *Macrorhabdus ornithogaster* organisms in a fecal sample from a budgerigar (*Melopsittacus undulatus*) exhibiting chronic weight loss, Wright–Giemsa stain (100× oil).

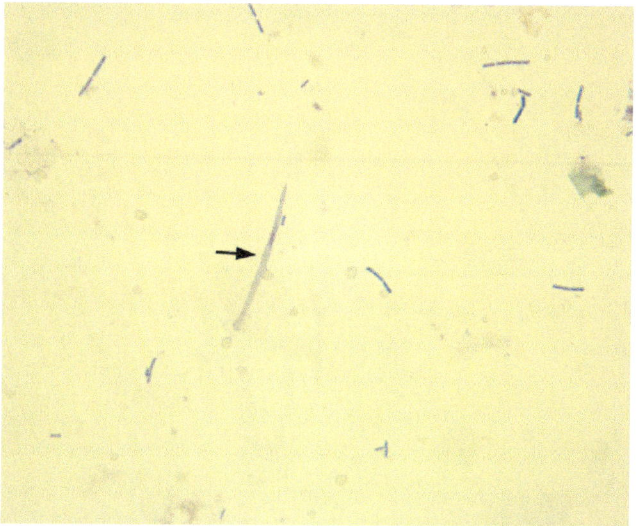

Fig. 15.133. *Macrorhabdus ornithogaster* organism (arrow) in a fecal sample from a cockatiel (*Nymphicus hollandicus*) exhibiting chronic weight loss. Diff–Quik stain (100× oil).

Aspergillosis should be suspected when cytologic specimens reveal septate hyphae (5–10 µm in width) that have straight parallel sides with a ball-shaped terminal end, and branch at 45° angles (Figures 15.134– 15.138). The hyphae may fail to stain, or may stain deeply basophilic with a thin, clear outer cell wall. Round to oval blue-green fungal spores may also be present with or without the appearance of the hyphae (Figure 15.139). The associated inflammatory response often contains moderately degenerate heterophils intermixed with macrophages and lymphocytes. Definitive diagnosis of *Aspergillus* is based on a positive culture. Although *Aspergillus fumigatus* is commonly isolated from aspergillosis cases in avian species, *A. flavus*, *A. niger*, and other species may be isolated, but less frequently (Haucka et al., 2020).

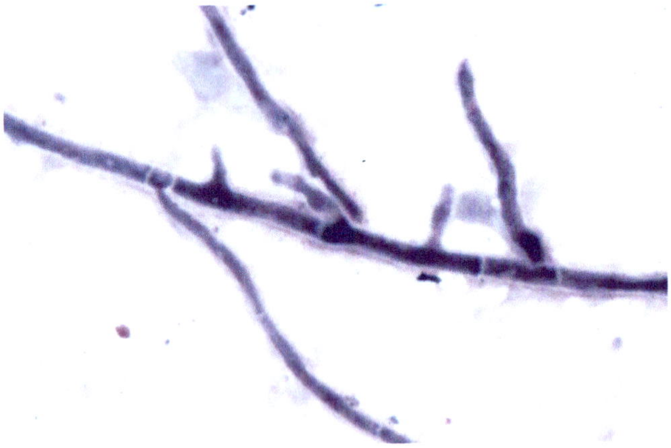

Fig. 15.134. Septate branching hyphae in a sinus aspirate that had a positive culture for *Aspergillus fumigates* in an Atlantic puffin (*Fratercula arctica*), Diff–Quik stain (100× oil).

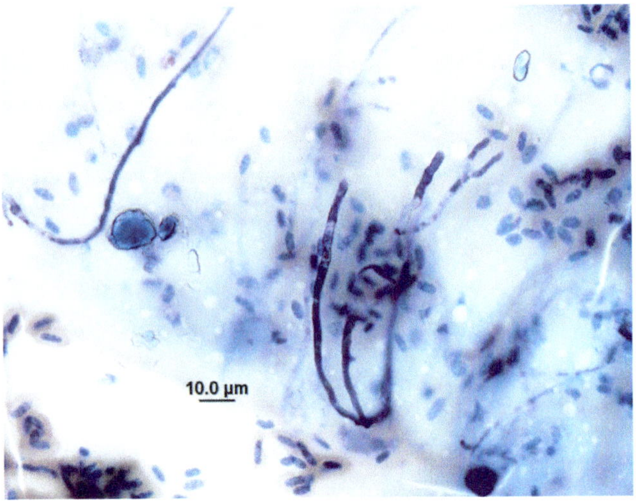

Fig. 15.135. Septate branching hyphae in a tracheal wash that had a positive culture for *Aspergillus fumigates* in a green-winged macaw (*Ara chloropterus*), Wright–Giemsa stain (100× oil).

Mycotic tracheobronchial or syrinx lesions of birds may reveal fungal elements along with mixed cell or macrophagic inflammation in the wash fluid (Campbell and Grant, 2010). *Aspergillus* spp. and phycomycetes fungi (e.g., *Mucor* spp.) are opportunistic fungi that may infect immunocompromised birds (e.g., captive birds of prey, waterfowl, and immunosuppressed companion birds with systemic illnesses). *Aspergillus* is the most common fungal agent involving the avian respiratory tract.

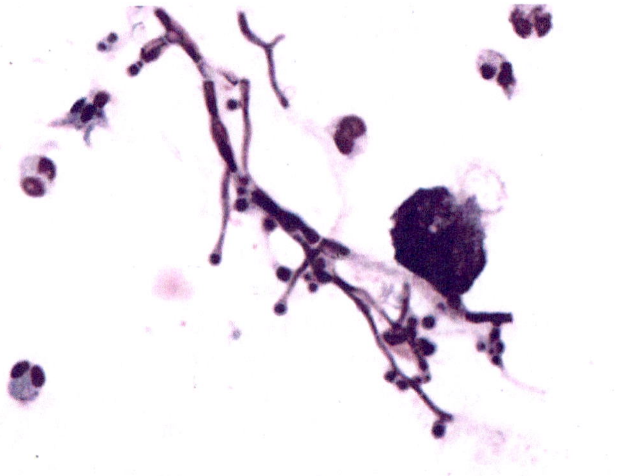

Fig. 15.136. Septate branching hyphae in a tracheal wash that had a positive culture for *Aspergillus fumigates* in Timneh African gray parrot (*Psittacus erithacus timneh*), Wright–Giemsa stain (100× oil).

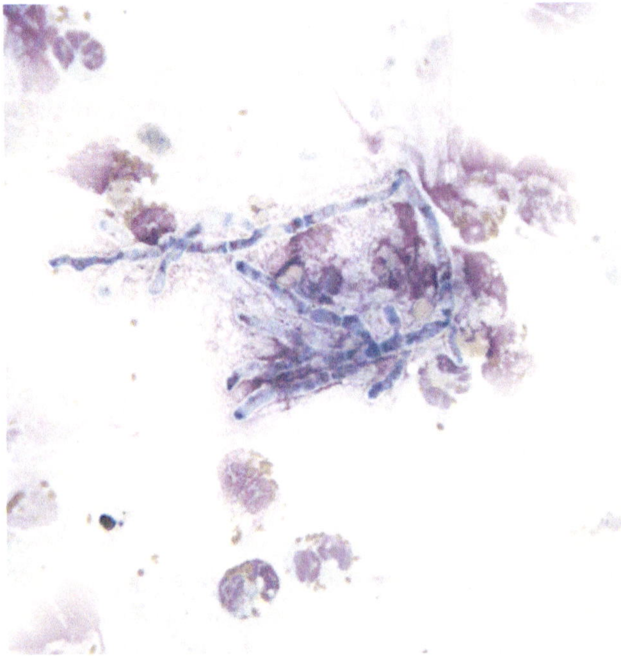

Fig. 15.137. Septate branching hyphae in a tracheal wash that had a positive culture for *Aspergillus fumigates* in an eclectus parrot (*Eclectus roratus*), Wright–Giemsa stain (100× oil). Source: Image from Campbell and Grant (2010, p. 232).

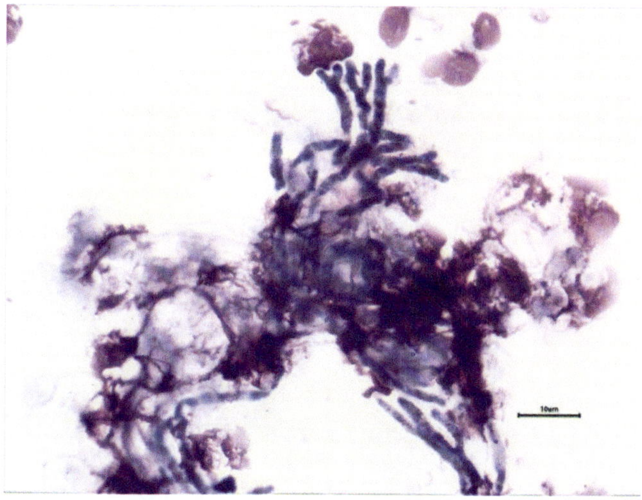

Fig. 15.138. Septate branching hyphae in a tracheal wash that had a positive culture for *Aspergillus fumigates* in an eclectus parrot (*Eclectus roratus*), Wright–Giemsa stain (100× oil).

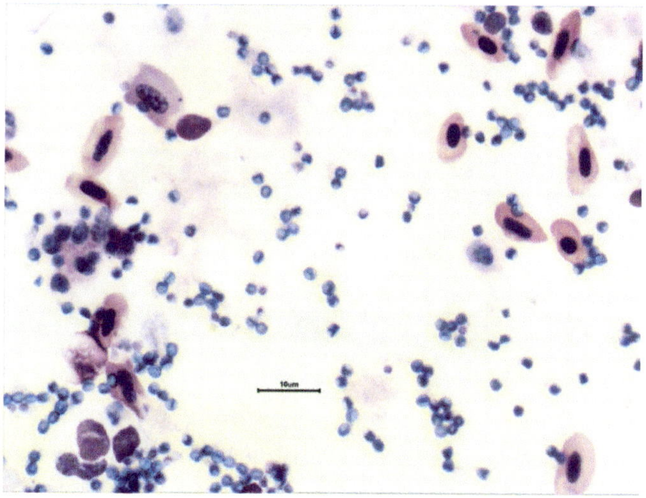

Fig. 15.139. Round to oval blue-green fungal spores in a tracheal wash that had a positive culture for *Aspergillus fumigates* in ferruginous hawk (*Buteo regalis*), Wright–Giemsa stain.

Gross lesions in the lungs and air sacs can occur as granulomas with blue-green fungal colonies. *Aspergillus* is characterized on cytological samples by thick, septate branching hyphae compared to the nonseptate, branching hyphae of phycomycosis (mucormycosis).

Although mycotic conjunctivitis rarely occurs in birds, *Aspergillus* spp. has been reported to cause mycotic conjunctivitis in birds (Pal and Mehrotra, 1986; Beckman et al., 1994).

Trichomoniasis

Trichomoniasis is a common disease of birds (especially pigeons, doves, raptors, and soft-billed birds) that affects the upper alimentary tract. A strong seasonal pattern is often associated with epizootics in wild birds (Neimanis et al., 2010). Birds infected with *Trichomonas* spp. typically have lesions that include chronic pyogranulomatous inflammation and ulcerations in the oral cavity and esophagus (Carpenter et al., 1998). When the organism enters the digestive tract, depending upon the virulence, it can migrate to the liver, lungs, heart, and pancreas via the circulatory system, resulting in death of the bird (Brobey et al., 2017).

Trichomonas gallinae is a well-documented and important pathogen of columbids (order Columbiformes), raptors (orders Falconiformes and Accipitriformes), and passerines (order Passeriformes). This parasite is transmitted to birds through various routes, including crop feeding of nestlings, billing or feeding courtship rituals, congregation at birdfeeders or birdbaths, and consumption of infected birds (Grunenwald et al., 2018). Birds of prey acquire the disease when they ingest infected prey as the parasite is in the upper alimentary and respiratory tracts of pigeons and doves (Harden, 1996; Stimmelmayr et al., 2012; Zadravec et al., 2017). Prey species such as pigeons and doves are typically asymptomatic carriers of the organism. One study revealed that the prevalence of trichomoniasis in mourning dove populations approaches 25% without affecting the population (Ostrand et al., 1995). Pigeons and doves can be the major dietary component of urban nesting raptors. Therefore, nestlings of urban birds of prey have higher infection rates compared to exurban locations, and trichomoniasis can be one of the most important single nestling mortality factors of these birds (Boal et al., 1998; Real et al., 2000). Latent *Trichomonas* infection has been reported in turkeys, chickens, and certain species of wild fowl (Nemes et al., 2006; Grunenwald et al., 2018).

Cytologic preparations of trichomonad lesions of the upper alimentary tract of birds stained with Romanowsky stains often reveal numerous basophilic pyriform to leaf-shaped organisms with a round nucleus (Figures 15.140 and 15.141). Eosinophilic flagella, undulating membrane, and axostyle may also be seen. Wet mount preparations reveal the highly mobile organisms with movement of the undulating membrane and flagella.

The pathogenicity of *Tetratrichomonas gallinarum* in birds is controversial as it is a nonpathogenic, commensal organism of the lower intestinal tract in anseriform and gallinaceous birds (Grunenwald et al., 2018).

An immunochromatographic capillary flow enzyme immunoassay dipstick test developed for rapid diagnosis of human *T. vaginalis*, the OSOM Trichomonas Rapid Test (OSOM Trich; Genzyme Diagnostics, Cambridge, MA) is not able to distinguish between *Trichomonas* species; however, it has proved to be a suitable test for the rapid detection of *Trichomonas* spp. infection in pigeons (Campbell et al., 2008; Brobey et al., 2017).

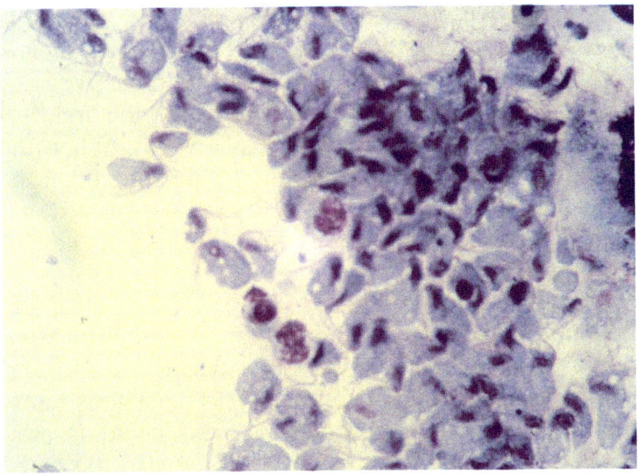

Fig. 15.140. Numerous piriform-shaped organisms with anterior flagella, undulating membrane, and axostyle supportive of a diagnosis of trichomoniasis in a crops aspirate from a budgerigar (*Melopsittacus undulatus*), Diff–Quik stain (100× oil).

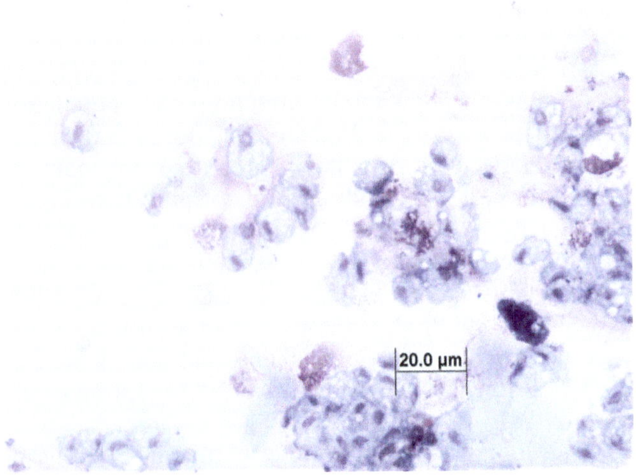

Fig. 15.141. Numerous piriform-shaped organisms with eosinophilic anterior flagella and axostyle indicative of trichomoniasis in a swab of an ulcerative lesion in the mouth of a barn owl (*Tyto alba*), Wright–Giemsa stain.

See Chapter 7 for further description of the organism.

Giardia

Trophozoites of Giardia may be found in the feces or in samples obtained from cloacal swabs or washes (Reuschel et al., 2020). On stained smears, the trophozoites appear as binucleated piriform flagellate protozoa, with a deeply notched adhesive disk that is present at the rounded end, a single caudal flagellum, and a single, round median body (Figures 15.142 and 15.143).

See Chapter 7 for further description of the organism.

Fig. 15.142. A *Giardia* trophozoite (arrow) in a fecal smear from a budgerigar (*Melopsittacus undulatus*), Lugol's iodine solution (100× oil).

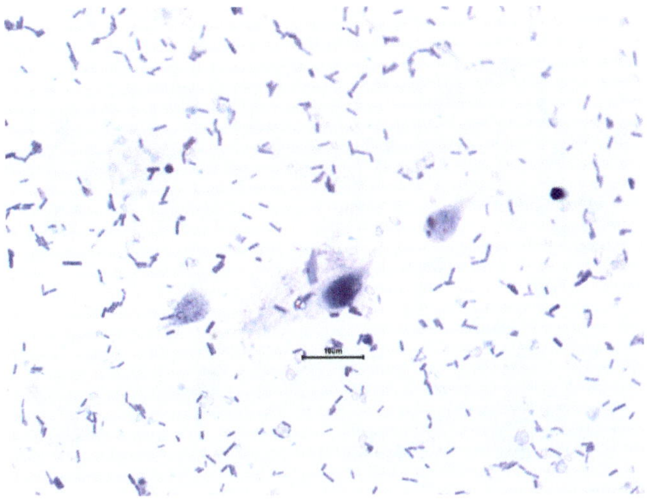

Fig. 15.143. Poorly staining *Giardia* trophozoites in a fecal smear from a budgerigar (*Melopsittacus undulatus*), Diff–Quik stain.

Cryptosporidiosis

Protozoal parasites, such as *Giardia*, *Cryptosporidium*, and *Microsporidium*, are present in the gastrointestinal tracts of many animal species and are often found in fecal samples of birds (Greiner, 1997; Page and Haddad, 1995; Franssen et al., 2000). Cryptosporidiosis has been reported in more than 30 avian species worldwide (Molina-López et al., 2010; Nakamura and Meireles, 2015). *Cryptosporidium* is a coccidian protozoal parasite that affects the gastrointestinal and respiratory tracts of birds (Goodwin and Krabill, 1989; Page and Haddad, 1995; Greiner, 1997). The species of *Cryptosporidium* that are reported in birds include *C. meleagridis*, *C. baileyi*, *C. parvum*, and *C. galli* (Molina-López et al., 2010; Bougiouklis et al., 2013; Krindges et al., 2013; Oliveira et al., 2017; Azmanis et al., 2018). *Cryptosporidium* avian genotype V has been reported in several avian species, and although it is considered nonpathogenic, it can be associated with clinical disease in birds (Curtiss et al., 2015). Fecal smears stained with negative malachite green have been used to reveal the coccidian oocysts (Oliveira et al., 2017). Acid-fast stain can also be used to reveal the organism in cytologic preparations (Azmanis et al., 2018).

The genus *Cryptosporidium* (Apicomplexa: Conoidasida) comprises protozoal parasites that develop in the epithelial cells in the digestive, respiratory, and urinary tracts of vertebrates. More than 25 species and genotypes of *Cryptosporidium* have been documented infecting birds (Hurtado et al., 2020). Birds are infected through the ingestion or inhalation of oocysts present in the environment (feces, water, dust, nesting materials, etc.), and the infection causes enteritis, respiratory disease, and renal disease.

Cryptosporidium spp. infections in the respiratory tract of chickens, turkeys, and quail result in varying degrees of epithelial hyperplasia and mixed cell inflammation (lymphocytes, macrophages, and heterophils) in the lamina propria, like that observed in mycoplasmal infections (Ley et al., 2012). Cryptosporidial infections of the urinary tract have also been identified in chickens (*Gallus gallus domesticus*), a black-throated finch (*Poephila cincta*), and a junglefowl (*Gallus sonneratii*), and a cockatoo (*Lophochroa leadbeateri*) (Curtiss et al., 2015).

See Chapter 23 for further description of the organism.

Blastocystis

Blastocystis is a single-celled protist found in the intestinal tract of birds and other animals, including humans (Yoshikawa, 2012; Alfellani et al., 2013). *Blastocystis* belongs to the branch of Eukarya known as Stramenopiles or Heterokonta, which also includes brown algae, water molds, and diatoms and is an obligate anaerobe with several morphologic forms: cyst, vacuolar, granular, and amoeboid, which may correspond to different phases of the life cycle (Tan, 2008; Ilchyshyn and Monti, 2019). Cytologic examination of direct smears and a cytocentrifugation preparation from an aspirate from the facial swelling in a duck revealed large numbers of round protist cysts, 10–15 μm in diameter, that contain a large single (or occasionally 2–4 smaller) central, clear to faintly basophilic vacuole(s) and a peripheral rim of mildly basophilic, grainy cytoplasm that contains a small oval aggregate of nuclear material (Ilchyshyn and Monti, 2019) (Figure 15.144). Large numbers of bacteria (a mixture of cocci and bacilli) were present, but no inflammatory cells were observed.

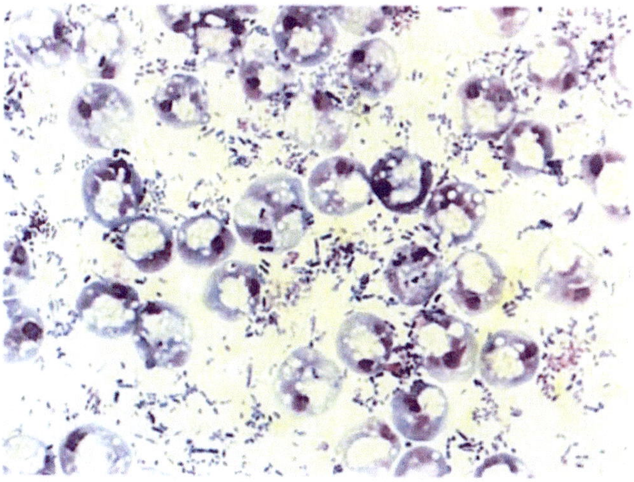

Fig. 15.144. Numerous vacuolar forms of *Blastocystis* and large numbers of bacteria (predominantly bacilli) in an aspirate from the facial swelling in domestic duck (*Anas platyrhynchos domestica*), Wright–Giemsa stain (50×). Source: Image from Ilchyshyn and Monti (2019).

Atoxoplasmosis

Atoxoplasmosis is a form of coccidian infection, also known as systemic isosporosis (Cushing et al., 2011). *Isospora* spp. with extra-intestinal proliferative stages cause atoxoplasmosis, primarily in passerine birds (Jamriška et al., 2013). The host becomes infected after the ingestion of sporulated oocysts in feces. The organism has an asexual lifecycle that occurs in leukocytes (primarily lymphocytes and monocytes) and a sexual stage, gametogony, occurring in the enterocytes of the duodenum (Sánchez-Cordo´ et al., 2007). Therefore, atoxoplasmosis is generally detected by the presence of sporozoites in mononuclear blood cells or oocysts in feces. It is not possible to distinguish *Atoxoplasma* spp. oocysts from those of enteric species of *Isospora* by microscopic examination of feces, because oocysts from both organisms contain two sporocysts, each with four sporozoites (Schrenzel et al., 2005; Mohr et al., 2017). Atoxoplasmosis can be diagnosed using histopathologic examination of tissue samples, buffy coat smears, impression smears, transmission electron microscopy, and PCR analysis (Adkesson et al., 2005).

See Chapter 11 for further description of the organism.

Microfilaria

Microfilaria are commonly found on blood films or cytologic preparations of the skin of clinically healthy wild birds from many families, and at least 16 genera of filariae occur in avian species (Bartlett, 2009; Huang et al., 2017; Sekiguchi et al., 2018). Reports of host reactions to microfilariae are uncommon and limited to cases in which the larval nematodes are located outside the blood vessel lumen (Bartlett, 2009). Adult filariid nematodes, which can be found in various tissues, are generally considered nonpathogenic in birds; however, reports of clinical disease have been made when the parasites invade major organs (Larrat et al., 2012).

Microfilaria on cytologic preparations stained with Romanowsky-type stains appear irregularly curved with relatively uniform widths over the length of their bodies, except for one end (the anterior end), which is gradually tapered. The nuclei stain pinkish-violet, and the cuticle fails to stain and appears as a colorless covering (Huang et al., 2017).

See Chapter 11 for further description of the organism.

References

Abrams GA, Paul-Murphy J, Murphy CJ. 2005. Conjunctivitis in birds. In: Rupley A (ed), *The Clinics Collection Veterinary Clinics of North America, Exotic Animal Practice, Avian Pet Medicine*. Philadelphia, PA: WB Saunders.

Abu J, Wünschmann A, Redig PT, Feeney D. 2009. Management of a cutaneous squamous cell carcinoma in an American flamingo (*Phoenicopterus ruber*). *J Avian Med Surg* 23(1):44–48.

Adkesson MJ, Zdziarski JM, Little SE. 2005. Atoxoplasmosis in tanagers. *J Zoo Wildl Med* 36:265– 272.

Alfellani MA, Taner-Mulla D, Jacob AS, et al. 2013. Genetic diversity of *Blastocystis* in livestock and zoo animals. *Protist* 164:497–509.

Amann O, Meij BP, Westerhof I, et al. 2007. Giant cell tumor in the bone in a scarlet macaw (Ara macao). Avian Dis 51(1):146–149.

Anderson NL. 1993. Candida/megabacteria proventriculitis in a lesser sulfur-crested cockatoo (*Cacatua sulphurea sulphurea*). *J Assoc Avian Vet* 7:197–201.

Anderson WI, Steinberg H. 1989. Primary glossal squamous-cell carcinoma in a Spanish Cochin hen. *Avian Dis* 33:827–828.

Andre JP, Delverdier M, Cabanie P, et al. 1993. Malignant melanoma in an African grey parrot (*Psittacus erithacus erithacus*). *J Assoc Avian Vet* 7:83–85.

Andre JP, Delverdier M. 1999. Primary bronchial carcinoma with osseous metastasis in an African grey parrot (*Psittacus erithacus*). *J Avian Med Surg* 13:180–186.

Awadhiya R P, Vegad JL, Kolte GN. 1980. Studies on acute inflammation in the chicken using mesentery as a test system. *Res Vet Sci* 29:172–180.

Awadhiya R P, Vegad JL, Kolte GN. 1981. A microscopic study of increased vascular permeability and leucocyte emigration in the chicken wing web. *Res Vet Sci* 31:231–235.

Azmanis P, di Somma A, Pappalardo L, Sivanose CD, Bangoura B. 2018. First detection of *Cryptosporidium parvum* in falcons (Falconiformes): diagnosis, molecular sequencing, therapeutic trial, and epidemiological assessment of a possible emerging disease in captive falcons. *Vet Parasitol* 252:167–172.

Baine K, Nobrega-Lee M, Jones MP, et al. 2014. Branchial cyst with carcinoma in an Umbrella cockatoo (Cacatua alba). *J Avian Med Surg* 28(3):232–239.

Baker R, Lumsden JH. 2000. Cytopathology techniques and interpretation. In: Baker R, Lumsden J (eds), *Color Atlas of the Dog and Cat*. St. Louis: Mosby.

Banks WJ. 1974. Histology and comparative organology. In: Banks WJ (ed*), Histology and Comparative Organology: A Text Atlas*. Baltimore: Williams and Wilkins.

Barger AM, Welle K, Athey JM, Hamel P, Bailey K. 2020. What is your diagnosis? A coelomic mass in a duck. *Vet Clin Pathol* 49:684–685.

Barlow AM, Girling TR. 2004. Malignant melanoma in a merlin (*Falco columbarius*). *Vet Rec* 154(22):696–697.

Bartlett CM. 2009. Filarioid nematodes. In: Atkinson CT, Thomas NJ, Hunter DB (eds), *Parasitic Diseases of Wild Birds*. Ames, IA: Wiley-Blackwell, pp. 439–462.

Bauck LD. 1992. A clinical approach to neoplastic disease in the pet bird. *Semin Avian Exotic Pet Med* 1:65–72.

Bayón A, Almela RM, Talavera J. 2007. Avian ophthalmology. *EJCAP* 17(3):1–13.

Beaufrère H, Bhaskaran M, Jankowski G, Tully TN. 2009. What is your diagnosis? *J Avian Med Surg* 23(4):325–328.

Beaufrère H, Reavill D, Heatley J, Susta L. 2019. Lipid-related lesions in Quaker parrots (*Myiopsitta monachus*). *Vet Pathol* 56(2):282–288.

Beckman BJ, Howe CW, Trampel DW, et al. 1994. *Aspergillus fumigatus* keratitis with intra-ocular invasion in 15-day-old chicks. *Avian Dis* 38:660–665.

Bédard C, Lair S, Langlois I. 2007. What is your diagnosis? coelomic mass in a rock dove (*Columba livia*).*Vet Clin Pathol* 36:303–305.

Beernaert LA, Pasmans F, Van Waeyenberghe L, Haesebrouk F, Martel A. 2010. Aspergillus infections in birds: a review. *Avian Pathol* 39:325–331.

Bennett RA, Harrison GJ. 1994. Soft tissue surgeries. In: Ritchie B, Harrison G, Harrison L (eds), *Avian medicine: principles and application*. Lake Worth, FL: Wingers.

Bezuidenhout AJ. 1988. Ascites and the anatomy of the peritoneal sacs of broilers: Ondersterpoort. *J Vet Res* 55:23–25.

Black SS, Steinhort LA, Bertucci DC, et al. 1997. *Encephalitozoon helium* in budgerigars (*Melopsittacus undulatus*). *Vet Pathol* 34:189–198.

Blakey J, Crispo M, Bickford A, Stoute S. 2018. Liposarcoma in a backyard silkie and retrospective summary of neoplasms diagnosed in backyard chickens submitted to the California animal health and food safety laboratory system, 2008–2017. *Avian Dis* 62:124–129.

Blakey J, Jerry C, da Silva A, Stoute S. 2021. Thymoma in an aged backyard leghorn chicken, with reviews of a database and literature. *J Vet Diagn Invest* 33(2):336–339.

Blomqvist M, Christerson L, Waldenström J, Herrmann B, Olsen B. 2012. *Chlamydia psittaci* in Swedish wetland birds: a risk to zoonotic infection? *Avian Dis* 56:737–740.

Boal CW, Mannan RW, Hudelson KS. 1998. Trichomoniasis in Cooper's hawks from Arizona. *J Wildl Dis* 34(3):590–593.

Bolte AL, Meurer J, Kaleta EF. 1999. Avian host spectrum of avipoxviruses. *Avian Pathol* 28:415–432.

Bossa LMDL, Mennonna G, Meomartino L, et al. 2015. Polyostotic chondroblastic osteosarcoma in a Kestrel (*Falco tinnunculus*). *J Avian Med Surg* 29(4):336–339.

Bougiouklis PA, Weissenbock H, Wells A, et al. 2013. Otitis media associated with *Cryptosporidium baileyi* in a Saker falcon (*Falco cherrug*). *J Comp Pathol* 148:419–423.

Boydell IP, Forbes NA. 1996. Diseases of the head (including the eye). In: Beynon P, Forbes N, Harcourt-Brown N (eds), *Manual of Raptors, Pigeons, and Waterfowl*. Cheltenham, England: British Small Animal Veterinary Association Ltd.

Bradford C, Wack A, Trembley S, et al. 2009. Two cases of neoplasia of basal cell origin affecting the axillary region in anseriform species. *J Avian Med Surg* 23(3):214–221.

Brandão J, Wong C, Kurotaki T, et al. 2013. Chronic dermatitis caused by *Lactobacillus jensenii* infection in a blue and gold macaw (*Ara ararauna*). *J Am Vet Med Assoc* 243(7):1030–1034.

Brobey B, Kucknoor A, Armacost J. 2017. Prevalence of Trichomonas, Salmonella, and Listeria in wild birds from southeast Texas. *Avian Dis* 61:347–352.

Browning GR, Eshar D, Springer NL, Bouschor J, Ganta C. 2020. Pathology in practice. *J Am Vet Med Assoc* 256(10): 1115–1118.

Burgdorf-Moisuk A, Whittington JK, Gilor S, Coleman D. 2009. What is your diagnosis? *J Avian Med Surg* 23(3):227–232.

Burgmann PM. 1994. Pulmonary fibrosarcoma with hepatic metastases in a cockatiel (*Nymphicus hollandicus*). *J Assoc Avian Vet* 8:81–84.

Burkhard MJ, Valenciano A, Barger A. 2001. Respiratory tract. In: Raskin R, Meyer D (eds), *Atlas of Canine and Feline Cytology*. Philadelphia, PA: WB Saunders.

Caliendo V, Bull A. 2011. Case report: ventricular candidiasis in stone curlews (*Burhinus oedicnemus*). *Avian Dis* 55:509–512.

Campbell L, Woods V, Lloyd T, Elsayed S, Church DL. 2008. Evaluation of the OSOM trichomonas rapid test versus wet preparation examination for detection of *Trichomonas vaginalis* vaginitis in specimens from women with a low prevalence of infection. *J Clin Microbiol* 46:3467–3469.

Campbell TW.1983. Disorders of the avian crop. *Compend Cont Ed Pract* 5(10):813–824.

Campbell TW. 1984. Lymphoid leukosis in an Amazon parrot—a case report. In: Proceedings of the Annual Conference of the Association of Avian Veterinarians.

Campbell TW, Coles EH. 1986. Avian clinical pathology. In: Coles EH (ed), *Veterinary Clinical Pathology*, 4th edn. Philadelphia, PA: WB Saunders Co.

Campbell TW. 1995. Avian hematology and cytology. In: Ritchie B, Harrison G, Harrison L (eds), *Avian medicine: principles and application*, 2nd edn. Ames: Iowa State University Press.

Campbell TW, Ellis CS. 2007. *Avian and Exotic Animal Hematology and Cytology*, 3rd edn. Ames, IA: Blackwell Publishing.

Campbell TW, Grant KR. 2010. *Clinical Cases in Avian and Exotic Animal Hematology and Cytology*. Ames: Wiley-Blackwell.

Camus AC, Heatley JJ. 2001. What is your diagnosis? *J Avian Med Surg* 15(1):54–57.

Canny CJ, Ward DA, Patton A, Orosz SE. 1999. Microsporidian keratoconjunctivitis in a double yellow-headed Amazon parrot (*Amazona ochrocephala oratrix*). *J Avian Med Surg* 13(4):279–286.

Catania S, Carnaccini S, Mainenti M, et al. 2017. Isolation of avipoxvirus from tongue of canaries (*Serinus canaria*) show severe localized proliferative glossitis. *Avian Dis* 61:531–535.

Carlson HC, Allen JR. 1969. The acute inflammatory reaction in chicken skin: blood cellular response. *Avian Dis* 14:817–833.

Carpenter JW, Pye GW, Cornwell D, DeBey BM. 1998. What is your diagnosis? *J Avian Med Surg* 12(3):211–213.

Carvalho MPN, Fernandes NCCA, Nemer VC, et al. 2016. Benign peripheral nerve sheath tumor of wild toco toucan (*Ramphastos toco*). *J Avian Med Surg* 30(3):280–285.

Cazzini P, Watson VE, Brown HM. 2013. Laboratory medicine: yesterday – today- tomorrow: the many faces of Mott cells. *Vet Clin Pathol* 42/2:125–126.

Çelebi BS, Seyyal Ak. 2006. A comparative study of detecting *Chlamydophila psittaci* in pet birds using isolation in embryonated egg and polymerase chain reaction. *Avian Dis* 50(4):489–493.

Chad N, Eyre P. 1978. Immunological release of histamine and SRS in domestic fowl. *Can J Comp Med* 42:519–524.

Chaudary C. 1987. Neoplasms, cysts, and obstructive diseases. In: Burr E (ed), *Companion Bird Medicine*. Ames: Iowa State University Press.

Chen CC, Pei KJC, Lee FR, Tzeng MP, Chang TC. 2011. Avian pox infection in a free-living crested serpent eagle (*Spilornis cheela*) in southern Taiwan. *Avian Dis* 55:143–146.

Cho K-O, Kimura T, Ochiai K, Itakura C. 1998. Gizzard adenocarcinoma in an aged Humboldt penguin (*Spheniscus humboldti*). *Avian Pathol* 27:100–102.

Clark S, Porter R, Mc Comb B, et al. 2010. Clostridial dermatitis and cellulitis: an emerging disease of turkeys. *Avian Dis* 54:788–794.

Colby SFM. 1998. What is your diagnosis? *J Avian Med Surg* 12(1):43–44.

Coleman CW. 1995. Lymphoid neoplasia in pet birds: a review. *J Avian Med Surg* 9:3–7.

Conzo G, Liberti L. 1999. Megabacterium infections of the proventriculus in recently imported pet birds to Italy. In: Proceedings of the European Conference of the Association of Avian Veterinarian.

Cookson KC, Shivaprasod HL. 1994. *Mycoplasma gallisepticum* in chukar partidges, pheasants, and peafowl. *Avian Dis* 38:914–921.

Cooper J. E. 1978. Veterinary aspects of captive birds of prey. In: Cooper J E (ed), *Veterinary Aspects of Captive Birds of Prey*. Saul, England: Standfast Press.

Cooper JE, Harrison GJ. 1997. Dermatology. In: Ritchie B, Harrison G, Harrison L (eds), *Avian Medicine Principles and Applications*. Lake Worth, FL: Wingers.

Cooper KK, Songer JG, Uzal FA. 2013. Diagnosing clostridial enteric disease in poultry. *J Vet Diagn Invest* 25:314–327.

Cork SC, Stockdale PHG. 1995. Case report: carcinoma with concurrent haemosiderosis in an Australian bittern (*Botaurus poidloptilus*). *Avian Pathol* 24:207–213.

Cork SC. 2000. Iron storage diseases in birds. *Avian Pathol* 29:7–12.

Costagliola A, Britti D, Russo V, et al. 2011. Malignant melanoma in a Seagull (*Larus fuscus*): morphological and immunohistochemical approach. *Avian Dis* 55:147–150.

Cotter PF, Bakst MR. 2017. A comparison of Mott cell morphology of three avian species. II. Bad behavior by plasmacytes? *Poultry Sci* 96:325–331.

Crespo R, Stirtzinger T, Hunter DB. 1998. Evaluation of different procedures for processing avian air sac lavage fluid. *Avian Dis* 42:20–27.

Crispin SM, Barnett KC. 1978. Ocular candidiasis in ornamental ducks. *Avian Pathol* 7:49–59.

Crispo M, Shivaprasad HL, Cooper GL, Bickford AA, Stoute ST. 2018. Streptococcosis in commercial and noncommercial avian species in California: 95 Cases (2000–2017). *Avian Dis* 62:152–162.

Crosset VR. 2007. Malignant melanoma in a rock hopper penguin (*Eudyptes chrysocome*). *Annu Proc Am Zoo Vet Tech*, p. 112.

Culligan CM, Craig LE. 2020. Pathology in practice. *J Am Vet Med Assoc* 257(4):383–385.

Curtiss JB, Leone AM, Wellehan JFX, et al. 2015. Renal and cloacal cryptosporidiosis (*Cryptosporidium* avian genotype V) in a major Mitchell's cockatoo (*Lophochroa leadbeateri*). *J Zoo Wildl Med* 46(4):934–937.

Cushing TL, Schat KA, States SL, et al. 2011. Characterization of the host response in systemic isosporosis (atoxoplasmosis) in a colony of captive American goldfinches (*Spinus tristis*) and house sparrows (*Passer domesticus*). *Vet Pathol* 48:985–992.

Daigle JC, LeBlanc CJ, Tully Tn, Mitchell MA. 1999. What is your diagnosis? *J Avian Med Surg* 13(1):50–54

Dallwig RK, Whittington JK, Terio K, Barger A. 2012. Cutaneous mast cell tumor and mastocytosis in a black-masked lovebird (*Agapornis personata*). *J Avian Med Surg* 26(1):29–35.

Deem SL, Heard DJ, Fox JH. 1997. Avian pox in eastern screech owls and barred owls from Florida. *J Wildl Dis* 33(2):323–327.

Degernes LA. 1991. A clinical approach to ascites in pet birds. In: Proceedings of the Annual Conference of the Association of Avian Veterinarian. Chicago, pp. 131–136.

Degernes LA, Lynch PS, Shivaprasad HL. 2011. Degenerative joint disease in captive waterfowl. *Avian Pathol* 40(1):103–110.

DeVoe RS, Trogdon M, Flammer K. 2004. Preliminary assessment of the effect of diet and L-carnitine supplementation on lipoma size and body weight in budgerigars (*Melopsittacus undulatus*). *J Avian Med Surg* 18(1):12–18.

Devriesc LA, Viaene N, Uyttebrock E, et al. 1988. Three cases of infection by *Haemophilus*-like bacteria in psittacines. *Avian Pathol* 17:741–744.

de Wit M, Schoemaker NJ, Kik MJL,Westerhof I. 2003. Hypercalcemia in two Amazon parrots with malignant lymphoma. *Avian Dis* 47(1):223–228.

Diaz-Figueroa O, Tully TN, Williams J, Evans D. 2006. Squamous cell carcinoma of the infraorbital sinus with fungal tracheitis and ingluvitis in an adult Solomon Eclectus parrot (*Eclectus roratus solomonensis*). *J Avian Med Surg* 20(2):113–119.

Di Girolamo N, Lane EP, Reyers F, Gardner BR. 2014. Subcutaneous xanthomatosis in a great white pelican (*Pelecanus onocrotalus*). *J Zoo Wildl Med* 45(1):153–156.

Dillehay DL, Schoeb TR, Ranglack GS. 1985. Mucinous adenocarcinoma of the tongue in a great horned owl. *Vet Pathol* 22:520–521.

Dipineto L, Gargiulo A, De Luca Bossa LM, et al. 2008. Prevalence of thermotolerant *Campylobacter* in pheasants (*Phasianus colchicus*). *Avian Pathol* 37:507–508.

Dipineto L, Gargiulo A, De Luca Bossa LM, et al. 2009. Prevalence of thermotolerant campylobacter in partridges (*Perdix perdix*). *Lett Appl Microbiol* 49:351–353.

Dipineto L, De Luca Bossa LM, Russo TP, et al. 2014. *Campylobacter* spp. and birds of prey. *Avian Dis* 58:303–305.

Dittmer KE, French AF, Thompson DJ, Buckle KN, Thompson KG. 2012. Case report: primary bone tumors in birds: a review and description of two new cases. *Avian Dis* 56:422–426.

Dolphin RE, Olsen DE, Gallina AM. 1979. Tubercular infection in a sulfur-crested cockatoo. *Vet Med Small Anim Clin* 74:833–835.

Doneley RJT, Raidal SR. 2010. Tracheal resection and anastomosis in a red-tailed black cockatoo (*Calyptorhynchus banksia banksia*). *Aust Vet J* 88(1):451–454.

Dorrestein GM. 1997. Physiology of avian respiration. In: Altman R, Clubb S, Dorrestein G, Quesenberry k (eds), *Avian Medicine and Surgery*. Philadelphia, PA: WB Saunders

Doster A, Johnson J, Duhamel G, et al. 1987. Liposarcoma in a Canada goose (*Branta canadensis*). *Avian Dis* 31:918–920.

Drén CsN, Németh I, Sári I, et al. 1988. Isolation of a reticuloendotheliosis-like virus from naturally occurring lyphoreticular tumours of domestic goose. *Avian Pathol* 17:259–277.

Duncan AE, Smedley R, Anthony S, Garner MM. 2014. Malignant melanoma in the penguin: characterization of the clinical, histologic, and immunohistochemical features of malignant melanoma in 10 individuals from three species of penguin. *J Zoo Wildl Med* 45(3):534–549.

Effron M, Gringer L, Benirschke K. 1977. Nature and rate of neoplasia found in captive wild mammals, birds, and reptiles at necropsy. *J Natl Cancer Inst* 59:185–198.

Ellis C. 2001. What is your diagnosis? *J Avian Med Surg* 15(1):60–63.

Elsmo EJ, Allison AB, Brown JD. 2016. Retrospective study of causes of skin lesions in wild turkeys (*Meleagris gallopavo*) in the eastern USA, 1975–2013. *J Wildl Dis* 52(3):582–591.

Ensley PK, Davis CE, Anderson MP, Fletcher KC. 1979. Cryptococcosis in a male Beccari's crowned pigeon. *JAVMA* 175:992–994.

Evans EE, Mitchell MA, Whittington JK, Roy A, Tully TN. 2014. Measuring the level of agreement between cloacal Gram's stains and bacterial cultures in Hispaniolan Amazon parrots (*Amazona ventralis*). *J Avian Med Surg* 28(4):290–296.

Fadly AM, Nair V. 2008. Leukosis/sarcoma group. In: Saif YM, Fadly AM, Glisson JR, McDougald LR, Nolan LK, Swayne DE, Editorial Board for the American Association of Avian Pathologists (eds), *Diseases of Poultry*, 12th edn. Ames, IA: Blackwell Publishing, pp. 514–568.

Fallavena LC, Canal CW, Salle CTP, et al. 2002. Presence of avipoxvirus DNA in avian dermal squamous cell carcinoma. *Avian Pathol* 31(3):241–246.

Farmer H, Chalmers WSK, Coolcock PR. 1982. Chlamydia psittaci isolated from the eyes of domestic ducks (*Anas platyrynchos*) with conjunctivitis and rhinitis. *Vet Rec* 110:346–347.

Fenwick B, Takeshita K, Wong A. 1985. A moluccan cockatoo with disseminated cryptococcosis. *JAVMA* 187:1210–1212.

Fernandez-Bellon H, Martorell J, Rabanal R, Ramis A. 2003. Rhabdomyosarcoma in a racing pigeon (*Columba livia*). *Avian Pathol* 32:613–616.

Ferrell ST, Tell LA. 2001. *Clostridium terium* infection in a rainbow lorikeet (*Trichoglossus haematodus haematodus*) with enteritis. *J Avian Med Surg* 14(3):204–208.

Filippich LJ, Parker MG. 1994. Megabacteriosis and proventricular/ventricular disease in psittacines and passerines. In: *Proceedings of the annual conference of Avian veterinarians*.

Fisher DJ. 2001. Musculoskeletal system. In: Raskin R, Meyer D (eds), *Atlas of Canine and Feline Cytology*, Philadelphia, PA: WB Saunders.

Fischer D, Lierz M. 2015. Diagnostic procedures and available techniques for the diagnosis of aspergillosis in birds. *J Exotic Pet Med* 24:283–295.

Fischer D, Van Waeyenberghe L, Failing K, Martel A, Lierz M. 2018. Single tracheal inoculation of *Aspergillus fumigatus* conidia induced aspergillosis in juvenile falcons (*Falco* spp.). *Avian Pathol* 47(1):33–46.

Fisher JR, Stallknecht DE, Luttrell MP, et al. 1997. Mycoplasmal conjunctivitis in wild songbirds: the spread of a new contagious disease in a mobile host population. *Emerg Infect Dis* 3:69–72.

Forbes NA, Cooper JE, Higgins RJ. 2000. Neoplasms of birds of prey. In: Lumeij JT (ed), *Raptor Biomedicine III*. Lake Worth, FL: Zoological Education Network, Inc. pp.127–145.

Fordham M, Rosenthal K, Durham A, et al. 2010. Intraocular osteosarcoma in an umbrella cockatoo (*Cacatua alba*). *Vet Ophthalmol* 13(suppl):103–108.

Franssen FFJ, Hooimeijer J, Blankenstein B, Houwers DJ. 2000. Giardiasis in a white stork in the Netherlands. *J Wildl Dis* 36:764–766.

Frasca S, Hinckley L, Forsyth MH, et al. 1997. Mycoplasmal conjunctivitis in a European starling. *J Wildl Dis* 33:336–339.

Fulton RM, Sanchez S. 2013. Tuberculosis. In: Swayne DE, Glisson JR, McDougald LR, et al. (eds), *Diseases of Poultry*, 13th edn. Hoboken, New Jersey: John Wiley & Sons, Inc. pp. 1008–1017.

Gaharan S, Gupta A, Boudreaux B, Beaufrère H. 2012. What is your diagnosis? *J Avian Med Surg* 26(1):45–48.

Gamble KC. 1999. What is your diagnosis? *J Avian Med Surg* 13(3):214–217.

Gartrell BD, Alley MR, Mack H, et al. 2005. Erysipelas in the critically endangered kakapo (*Strigops habroptilus*). *Avian Pathol* 34(5):383–7.

Gartrell BD, Morgan KJ, Howe L, Munday JS, McFadden AMJ. 2009. Cloacal papillomatosis in the absence of herpesvirus and papillomavirus in a sulphur-crested cockatoo (*Cacatua galerita*). *N Z Vet J* 57(4):241–243.

Gaskin JM, Homer BL, Eskelund KH. 1991. Preliminary findings in avian viral serositis: a newly recognized syndrome of psittacine birds. *J Assoc Avian Vet* 5(1):27–34.

Gerlach H. Bacterial. 1994. In: Ritchie BW, Harrison GJ, Harrison LR (eds), Avian Medicine: Principles and Application. Lake Worth, FL: Wingers Publication, pp. 349–383.

Gerlach H. 2001. Megabacteriosis. *Semin Avian Exotic Pet Med* 10:12–19.

Gill JH. 2005. Avian skin diseases. In: Rupley A (ed), *The Clinics Collection Veterinary Clinics of North America, Exotic Animal Practice, Avian Pet Medicine*. Philadelphia, PA: WB Saunders.

Giotis ES, Skinner MA. 2019. Spotlight on avian pathology: fowlpox virus. *Avian Pathol* 48(2):87–90.

Gill KS, Helmer PJ. 2020. Cloacal diseases in companion parrots: a retrospective study of 43 cases (2012–2018). *J Avian Med Surg* 34(4):364–370.

Glare TR, Gartrell BD, Brookes JJ, Perrott JK. 2014. Isolation and identification of *Aspergillus* spp. from brown kiwi (*Apteryx mantelli*) nocturnal houses in New Zealand. *Avian Dis* 58:16–24.

Godoy LA, Dalbeck LS, Tell LA, et al. 2013. Characterization of avian poxvirus in Anna's hummingbird (*Calypte anna*) in California, USA. *J Wildl Dis* 49(4):978–985.

Goodwin MA, Krabill VA. 1989. Diarrhea associated with small-intestinal cryptosporidiosis in a budgerigar and a cockatiel. *Avian Dis* 33(4):829–833.

Graham A. 1994. Nasal flushes for diagnosis and treatment. In: Proceedings of the Association of Avian Veterinarians. Reno.

Graham DL. 1991. Internal papillomatosis disease: a pathologist's view of cloacal papillomas and then some! In: Proceedings of the Annual Conference of Association of Avian Veterinarians.

Graham JE, Werner JA, Lowenstine LJ, et al. 2003. Periorbital liposarcoma in an African grey parrot (*Psittacus erithacus*). *J Avian Med Surg* 17:147–153.

Grauer GF, Nichols CE. 1985. Ascites, renal abnormalities, and electrolyte and acid-base disorders associated with liver disease. *Vet Clin North Am, Sm Anim Pract* 15(1):197–214.

Gray ML, Puette M, Latimer KS. 1998. Microsporidiosis in a young ostrich (*Struthio camelus*). *Avian Dis* 42:832–836.

Green L. 1992. Gastrointestinal cytology. In: Atkinson B (ed), Atlas of Diagnostic Cytopathology. Philadelphia, PA: WB Saunders.

Griner LA. 1983. Pathology of zoo animals. In: Griner LA (ed), *Pathology of Zoo Animals*. San Diego: Zoological Society of San Diego.

Greiner EC. 1997. Parasitology. In: Altman R, Clubb S, Dorrestein G, Quesenberry K (eds), *Avian Medicine and Surgery*. Philadelphia, PA: WB Saunders.

Grunenwald C, Sidor I, Mickley R, Dwyer C, Gerhold R. 2018. *Tetratrichomonas* and *Trichomonas* spp.-associated disease in free-ranging Common eiders (*Somateria mollissima*) from Wellfleet Bay, MA and description of ITS1 region genotypes. *Avian Dis* 62:117–123.

Grurel A, Gulcubuk A, Turan N. 2004. A granulomatous conjunctivitis associated with *Morexella phenylpyruvica* in an ostrich (*Struthio camelus*). *Avian Pathol* 33:196–199.

Guimarães MB, Torres LN, Mesquita RG, et al. 2014. *Clostridium perfringens* type A enteritis in blue and yellow macaw (*Ara ararauna*). Avian Dis 58:650–653.

Guthrie AL, Gonzalez-Angulo C, Wigle WL, deMaar TW. 2010. Clinical reports: radiation therapy of a malignant melanoma in a thick-billed parrot (*Rhynchopsitta pachyrhyncha*). *J Avian Med Surg* 24(4):299–307.

Gyuranecz M, Foster JT, Dán A, et al. 2013. Worldwide phylogenetic relationship of avian poxviruses. *J Virol* 87(9):4938– 4951.

Haesendonck R, Garmyn A, Dorrestein GM, et al. 2015. Marek's disease virus associated ocular lymphoma in roulroul partridges (*Rollulus rouloul*). *Avian Pathol* 44(5):347–351.

Hanley CS, Wilson HG, Latimer KS, et al. 2005. Interclavicular hemangiosarcoma in a double yellow-headed Amazon parrot (Amazona ochrocephala oratrix). *J Avian Med Surg* 19(2):130–137.

Hannafusa Y, Bradley A, Tomaszewski EE, Libal MC, Phalen DN. 2007. Growth and metabolic characterization of Macrorhabdus ornithogaster. *J Vet Diagn Invest* 19:256–265.

Hänse M, Krautwald-Junghanns M-E, Reitemeier S, Einspanier A, Schmidt V. 2013. Testicular biopsy in psittacine birds (Psittaciformes): comparative evaluation of testicular reproductive status by endoscopic, histologic, and cytologic examination. *J Avian Med Surg* 27(4):247–257.

Haridy M, Fukuta M, Mori Y, et al. 2014. An outbreak of *Mycobacterium genavense* infection in a flock of captive diamond doves (*Geopelia cuneate*). *Avian Dis* 58:383–390.

Headley SA. 2005. Intrathoracic haemangiosarcoma in an ostrich (*Struthio camelus*). *Vet Rec* 156(11):353–354.

Heatley JJ, Bellah J, Brawner W, Reavill D. 2007. Radiation therapy of squamous cell carcinoma in a golden eagle. In: *Proceedings of the Annual Conference of Association of Avian Veterinarian*, pp. 327–328.

Hafner S, Williams SM, Sutton MT. 2007. Retroviral inclusions in the enteric smooth muscle of a tumor-bearing young chicken. *Avian Dis* 51(1):133–136.

Halley MA, Stilwell JM, Comolli JR, et al. 2020. Mandibular squamous cell carcinoma in 2 psittacines. *J Vet Diagn Invest* 32(2):344–347.

Halliwell WH. 1971. Lesions of Marek's disease in a great horned owl. *Avian Dis* 15:49–55.

Hammond EE, Guzman DS-M, Garner MM, et al. 2010. Long-term treatment of chronic lymphocytic leukemia in a green-winged macaw (*Ara chloroptera*). *J Avian Med Surg* 24(4):330–338.

Harden J. 1996. Trichomoniasis in raptors, pigeons, and doves. *J Wildl Rehabil* 19:8–17.

Hargreaves RC. 1981. A fungus commonly found in the proventriculus of small pet birds. In: Proceedings of the 30th Western Poultry Conference and 15th Poultry Healthy Symposium.

Hatkin J, Styler E, Miller D. 2002. Ingluvial squamous cell carcinoma in a game chicken. *Avian Dis* 46:1070–1075.

Hartnup BK, Mohammed HO, Kollias GV, et al. 1998. Risk factors associated with mycoplasmal conjunctivitis in house finches. *J Wildl Dis* 34:281–288.

Haucka R, Cray C, França M. 2020. Spotlight on avian pathology: aspergillosis. *Avian Pathol* 49(2):115–118.

Hawley DM, Grodio J, Frasca S, Kirkpatrick L, DH. 2011. Experimental infection of domestic canaries (*Serinus canaria domestica*) with *Mycoplastna gallisepticum*: a new model system for a wildlife disease. *Avian Pathol* 40:321–327.

Heidenreich M. 1997. Infectious diseases. In: Heidenreich M (ed), *Birds of prey: medicine and management*. Osney Mead, Oxford: Blackwell Science, pp.103–129.

Hernández M, Sánchez C, Galka ME, et al. 2001. Avian pox infection in Spanish imperial eagles (*Aquila adalberti*). *Avian Pathol* 30(1):91–97.

Hernández V, Carrera E, Méndez A, et al. 2012. Histopathologic, immunohistochemical and ultrastructural features of a granular cell tumour in an Australian parakeet (*Melopsittacus undulatus*). *Avian Pathol* 41(5):437–440.

Hill F, Woodgyer A, Lintott M. 1995. Cryptococcosis in a North Island brown kiwi (*Apteryx australis mantelli*). *N Z J Med Vet Mycology* 33(5):305–309.

Hood HB. 1978. Eye pathology in an adult male ostrich (*Struthio camelus*). In: *Proceedings American Association of Zool Veterinarians*.

Houck EL, Keller KA, Hawkins MG, et al. 2016. Bilateral aural adenocarcinoma in a Congo African grey parrot (Psittacus erithacus erithacus). *J Avian Med Surg* 30(3):257–262.

Howard MO, Nieves MA, Miles KG. 1996. Synovial chondromatosis in a great horned owl (*Bubo virginianus*). *J Wildl Dis* 32:370–372.

Hsieh C, Chen SH, Wang CW, et al. 2005. Unusual pox lesions found in Chinese jungle mynahs (*Acridotheres cristatellus*). *Avian Pathol* 34(5):415–417.

Huang Y-L, Tsai S-S, Thongchan D, Khatri-Chhetri R, Wu H-Y. 2017. Filarial nematode infection in Eclectus parrots (*Eclectus roratus*) in Taiwan. *Avian Pathol* 46(2):188–194.

Huchzermeyer FW, Henton MM, Keffen RH. 1993. High mortality associated with megabacteriosis of proventriculus and gizzard in ostrich chicks. *Vet Rec* 7:143–144.

Hurtado R, Parsons NJ, Gous TA, et al. 2020. Outbreak of cryptosporidiosis in African penguins *Spheniscus demersus*. *Dis Aquat Org* 140:143–149.

Huynh M, Brandão J, Sabater M, Stidworthy MF, Forbes NA. 2014. Mucocele in a Spectacled owl (*Pusilatrix perspicillata*). *J Avian Med Surg* 28(1):45–49.

Hydock K, Brown H, Nemeth N, et al. 2018. Evaluation of cytology for diagnosing avian pox in wild turkeys (*Meleagris gallopavo*). *Avian Dis* 62(1):45–49.

Ijzer J, Dorrestein GM, van der Hage MH. 2002. Metastatic subcutaneous sarcoma and abdominal carcinoma in a peach-faced lovebird (*Agapornis roseicollis*). *Avian Pathol* 31:101–104.

Ilchyshyn NP, Monti P. 2019. Extra-enteric blastocystis infection in a duck. *J Vet Diagn Invest* 31(3):382–384.

Irizarry-Rovira AR, Lennox AM, Ramos-Vara JA. 2007. Malignant melanoma in a zebra finch (*Taeniopygia guttata*): cytologic, histologic, and ultrastructural characteristics. *Vet Clin Pathol* 36(3):297–302.

Jaensch SM, Butler R, O'Hara A, Raidal SR, Wyatt K. 2002. Atypical multiple, papilliform, xanthomatous, cutaneous neoplasia in a goose (*Anser anser*). *Aust Vet J* 80:277–280.

Jamriška J, Lavilla LA, Thomasson A, et al. 2013. Treatment of atoxoplasmosis in the Blue-crowned laughing thrush (*Dryonastes courtoisi*). *Avian Pathol* 42(6):569–571.

Johnson AL. 1995. Reproduction in the female. In: Whittow G (ed), *Sturkie's Avian Physiology*, 5th edn. San Diego: Academic Press.

Jones AL, Suárez-Bonnet A, Mitchell JA, et al. 2020. Avian papilloma and squamous cell carcinoma: a histopathological, immunohistochemical and virological study. *J Comp Pathol* 175:13–23.

Jones MP, Orosz SE, Richman K, Daniel GB, et al. 2001. Pulmonary carcinoma with metastases in a Moluccan cockatoo (*Cacatua moluccensis*). *J Avian Med Surg* 15(2):107–113.

Joyner KL. 1994. Theriogenology. In: Ritchie B, Harrison G, Harrison L (eds), *Avian medicine: principles and application*. Lake Worth, FL: Wingers.

Julian RJ. 1987. The effect of sodium in the drinking water on right ventricular hypertrophy, right ventricular failure, and ascites in broiler chickens. *Avian Pathol* 16:61–71.

Julian RJ. 1993. Ascites in poultry. *Avian Pathol* 22:419–454.

Kajigaya H, Konagaya K, Ejima H, et al. 2010. Case report: metastatic melanoma appearing to originate from the beak of a racing pigeon (*Columba livia*). *Avian Dis* 54:958–960.

Kaleta EF, Taday EM. 2003. Avian host range of *Chlamydophila* spp. based on isolation, antigen detection and serology. *Avian Pathol* 32:435–461.

Kelly P, Jahns H, Power E, et al. 2013. Mycobacteriosis in ostriches (*Struthio camelus*) due to infection with *Mycobacterium bovis* and *Mycobacterium avium* complex. Avian Dis 57:808–811.

Kelly TR, Vennen KM, Duncan R, Sleeman JM. 2004. Lymphoproliferative disorder in a great horned owl (*Bubo virginianus*). *J Avian Med Surg* 18:263–268.

Kern TJ, Paul-Murphy J, Murphy CJ, et al. 1996. Disorders of the third eyelid in birds. *J Avian Med Surg* 10:8–12.

Kemp RL, Kluge JP. 1975. *Encephalitozoon* sp. in the blue-masked lovebird (Agapornis *personata*): first confirmed report of microsporidian infection in birds. *J Protozool* 22:489–491.

Kim YS, Hwang SM, Lee SJ, Jung JS. 2002. Differential expression of a WD protein during squamous differentiation of tracheal epithelial cells. *J Cell Biochem* 86:194–201.

King AS, McLelland J. 1984. Integument. In: King AD, McLelland J (eds), *Birds: their structure and function*, 2nd edn. London: Bailliere Tindall.

Klaphake E, Beazley-Keane SL, Jones M, Shoieb A. 2006. Multi-site integumentary squamous cell carcinoma in an African grey parrot (Psittacus erithacus erithacus). *Vet Rec* 158(17):593–596.

Klasing K. 1991. Avian inflammatory response: mediation by macrophages. *Poult Sci* 70:1176–1186.

Klasing KC, Dierenfeld ES, Koutsos EA. 2012. Avian iron storage disease: variations on a common theme? *J Zoo Wildl Med* 43(3S):S27–S34.

Kline ZF, Whittington JK, Coleman DA. 2016. Cutaneous hemangiosarcoma in a Pacific parrotlet (*Forpus coelestis*). *J Avian Med Surg* 30(2):152–158.

Knafo SE, Rapoport G, Williams J, et al. 2011. Clinical reports: cardiomyopathy and right-sided congestive heart failure in a red-tailed hawk (*Buteo jamaicensis*). *J Avian Med Surg* 25(1):32–39.

Kolmstetter C, Carpenter JW, Ernst S. 1995. What is your diagnosis? *J Avian Med Surg* 9(3):195–197.

Krindges MM, Almeida AB, Araujo DN, Stefani LM, da Silva AS. 2013. Parasitological and molecular detection of *Cryptosporidium parvum* in Rheas (*Rhea Americana*). *ACTA Scientiae Veterinariae* 41(1):10.

Kriz P, Slana I, Kralik P, et al. 2011. Case report - outbreak of *Mycobacterium avium* subsp. *avium* infection in one flock of domestic pigeons. *Avian Dis* 55:503–508.

Kriz P, Kaevska M, Bartejsova I, Pavlik I. 2013. *Mycobacterium avium* subsp. *avium* found in raptors exposed to infected domestic fowl. *Avian Dis* 57:688–692.

Kummrow M, Murray M, Garner M. 2007. What is your diagnosis? *J Avian Med Surg* 21:162–166.

Kwon Y-K, Oh J-Y, Jeong O-M, et al. 2017. Prevalence of *campylobacter* species in wild birds of south Korea. *Avian Pathol* 46(5):474–480.

Lai H, Zhang H, Ning Z, et al. 2011. Isolation and characterization of emerging subgroup J avian leukosis virus associated with hemangioma in egg-type chickens. *Vet Microbiol* 151(3–4):275–283.

Lamberski N, Theon Ap. 2002. Concurrent irradiation and intratumoral chemotherapy with cisplatin for treatment of a fibrosarcoma in a blue and gold macaw (Ara ararauna). J Avian Med Surg 16(3):234–238

Langlois I. 2005. The anatomy, physiology, and diseases of the avian proventriculus and ventriculus. In: Rupley A (ed), *The Clinics Collection Veterinary Clinics of North America, Exotic Animal Practice, Avian Pet Medicine*. Philadelphia, PA: WB Saunders.

Lanteri G, Marino F, Reale S, et al. 2011. *Mycobacterium tuberculosis* in a red-crowned parakeet (*Cyanoramphus novaezelandiae*). *J Avian Med Surg* 25(1):40–43.

Larrat S, Dallaire AD, Lair S. 2012. Emaciation and larval filarioid nematode infection in boreal owls (*Aegolius funereus*). *Avian Pathol* 41(4):345–349.

Latimer KS. 1994. Oncology. In: Ritchie B, Harrison G, Harrison L (eds), *Avian medicine: principles and application*. Lake Worth, FL: Wingers.

Le K, Nevarez J. 2011. What is your diagnosis? *J Avian Med Surg* 25(4):301–303.

Leach MW. 1992. A survey of neoplasia in pet birds. *Semin Avian Exotic Pet Med* 1:52–64.

Leach MW, Paul-Murphy J, Lowenstine LJ. 1989. Three cases of gastric neoplasia in psittacines. *Avian Dis* 33(1):204–210.

Lennox AM. 2007. Mycobacteriosis in companion psittacine birds: a review. *J Avian Med Surg* 21(3):181–187.

Lennox A, Clubb D, Romagnano S, Altman NH, Cray C. 2014. Monoclonal hyperglobulinemia in lymphosarcoma in a cockatiel (*Nymphicus hollandicus*) and a blue and gold macaw (*Ara ararauna*). *Avian Dis* 58:326–329.

Le Roux AB, Quesenberry K, Donnelly KA, Donovan TA. 2020. Disseminated pancreatic adenocarcinoma in an eclectus parrot (*Eclectus roratus*). *J Am Vet Med Assoc* 257(6):635–641.

Lester SJ, Malik R, Bartlett KH, Duncan CG. 2011. Cryptococcosis: update and emergence of *Cryptocccus gattii*. *Vet Clin Pathol* 40:4–17.

Ley DH, Moresco A, Frasca D. 2012. Conjunctivitis, rhinitis, and sinusitis in cliff swallows (*Petrochelidon pyrrhonota*) found in association with *Mycoplasma sturni* infection and cryptosporidiosis. *Avian Pathol* 41(4):395–401.

Liu SK, Moroff S. 1993. Case report 805: synovial sarcoma, epithelial hyperplasia in the humeral air sac, and formation of medullary bone. *Skeletal Radiol* 22:473–475.

Longbottom D, Coulter LJ. 2003. Animal chlamydioses and zoonotic implications. *J Comp Pathol* 128:217–244.

Lopez-Beceiro Am, Pereira JL, Barreiro A, Nieto JM, Lopez-Pena M. 1998. Squamous cell carcinoma in an immature common stork (*Ciconia Ciconia*). *J Zoo Wildl Med* 29:84–86.

Loukopoulos P, Okuni JB, Micco T, et al. 2014. Air sac adenocarcinoma of the sternum in a quaker parrot (*Myiopsitta monachus*). *J Zoo Wildl Med* 45(4):961–965.

Lowenstein LJ, Petrak ML. 1980. Microsporidiosis in two peach-faced lovebirds. In: Montali R, Migaki G (eds), *The Comparative Pathology of Zoo Animals*. Washington, DC: Smithsonian Institution Press.

Lublin A, Mechani S, Malkinson M, et al. 1998. A five-year survey of megabacteriosis in birds of Israel and a biological control trial. In: Proceedings of the Annual Conference of Association of Avian Veterinarians.

Lucas AM, Stettenheim PR. 1972. Avian anatomy, integument. In: Lucas AM, Stettenheim PR (eds), *Agriculture Handbook, 362*. Washington, DC: Department of Agriculture.

Luján-Vega C, Hawkins MG, Johnson CK, et al. 2018. A typical chlamydiaceae in wild populations of hawks (*Buteo* spp.) in California. *J Zoo Wildl Med* 49(1):108–115.

Lumeij JT. 1994. Gastroenterology. In: Ritchie B, Harrison G, Harrison L (eds), *Avian medicine: principles and application*. Lake Worth, FL: Wingers.

Maccolini EO, Dufresne PJ, Aschenbroich SA, et al. 2017. A disseminated *Cyptococcus gattii* VGIIa infection in a citron-crested cockatoo (*Cacatua sulphurea citrinocristata*) in Québec, Canada. *J Avian Med Surg* 31(2):142–151.

Madani SA, Dorrestein GM. 2012. Filarial tenosynovitis caused by Pelecitus species (Spirurida, Filarioidea, Onchocercidae) in the legs of a Channel-billed toucan (*Ramphastos vitellinus*). *J Avian Med Surg* 26(1):36–39.

Madani SA, Peighambari SM. 2013. PCR-based diagnosis, molecular characterization and detection of atypical strains of avian *Chlamydia psittaci* in companion and wild birds. *Avian Pathol* 42(1):38–44.

Malka S, Keirstead ND, Gancz AY, et al. 2005. Ingluvial squamous cell carcinoma in a geriatric cockatiel (*Nymphicus hollandicus*). *J Avian Med Surg* 19(3):234–239.

Malka S, Crabbs T, Mitchell EB, et al. 2008. Disseminated lymphoma of presumptive T-cell origin in a great horned owl (*Bubo virginianus*). *J Avian Med Surg* 22(3):226–233.

Malka S, Goller M, Dennison-Gibby S. 2020. Septic arthritis and osteomyelitis caused by *Chryseobacterium indologenes* in a mute swan (*Cygnus olor*) and a ring-billed gull (*Larus delawarensis*). *J Avian Med Surg* 34(3):289–294.

Maluenda ACH, Casagrande RA, Kanamura CT, et al. 2010. Rhabdomyosarcoma in a yellow-headed caracara (*Milvago chimachima*). *Avian Dis* 54(2):951–954.

Manucy TK, Bennett RA, Greenacre C, et al. 1998. Squamous cell carcinoma of the mandibular beak in a Buffon's macaw (*Ara ambigua*). *J Avian Med Surg* 12:158–166.

Marlier D, Leroy C, Sturbois M, et al. 2006. Increasing incidence of megabacteriosis in canaries (*Serinus canarius domesticus*). *Vet J* 172(3):549–552.

Marshall K, Daniel G, Patton C, Greenacre C. 2004. Humeral air sac mucinous adenocarcinoma in a salmon-crested cockatoo (*Cacatua moluccensis*). *J Avian Med Surg* 18(3):167–174.

Maxwell MH. 1987. The avian eosinophil—a review. *World's Poultry Sci* 43:190–207.

Maxwell MH, Robertson GW. 1998. The avian heterophil leucocyte: a review. *World's Poultry Sci* 54:155–178

Maxwell MH, Robertson GW. 1995. The avian basophilic leukocyte: a review. *World's Poultry Sci* 51:307–325.

McCleery B, Jones MP, Manasse J, et al. 2015. Pericardial mesothelioma in a yellow-naped Amazon parrot (*Amazona auropalliata*). *J Avian Med Surg* 29(1):55–62.

McDonald SE. 1988. Clinical experiences with cloacal papillomas. In: Proceedings of the Association of Avian Veterinarians. Houston (TX).

McLelland J. 1991. External features and integument. In: McLelland J (ed), *A Color Atlas of Avian Anatomy*. Philadelphia, PA: WB Saunders.

McRee AE, Higbie CT, Nevarez JG, Rademacher NT, Tully TN. 2017. Mycobacteriosis in captive psittacines: a brief review and case series in common companion species (*Eclectus roratus*, *Amazona oratrix*, and *Pionites melanocephala*). *J Zoo Wildl Med* 48(3):851–858.

Mehler SJ, Briscoe JA, Hendrick MJ, Rosenthal KL. 2007. Infiltrative lipoma in a blue-crowned conure (*Aratinga acuticaudata*). *J Avian Med Surg* 21(2):146–149.

Menon, GK, Menon, J. 2000. Avian epidermal lipids: functional considerations and relationship to feathering. *Am Zool* 40:540–552.

Mickley K, Buote M, Kiupel M, Graham J, Orcutt C. 2009. Ovarian hemangiosarcoma in an orange-winged Amazon parrot (*Amazona amazonica*). *J Avian Med Surg* 23(1):29–35.

Miller RE, Trampel DW, Boever WJ, Kling MA. 1985. Squamous cell carcinoma in a great Indian hornbill (*Buceros bicornis*). *J Zoo Wildl Med* 16:131–136.

Mohr F, Betson M, Quintard B. 2017. Investigation of the presence of *Atoxoplasma* spp. in blue-crowned laughingthrush (*Dryonastes courtoisi*) adults and neonates. *J Zoo Wildl Med* 48(1):1–6.

Molina-López R, Ramis A, Martín-Vázquez S, et al. 2010. *Cryptosporidium baileyi* infection associated with an outbreak of ocular and respiratory disease in Otus owls (*Otus scops*) in a rehabilitation centre. *Avian Pathol* 39(3):171–176.

Molter CM, Zuba JR, Papendick R. 2014. Cryptococcus gattii osteomyelitis and compounded itraconazole treatment failure in Pesquet's parrot (*Psittrichas fulgidus*). *J Zoo Wildl Med* 45(1):127–133.

Monks DJ, Zsivanovits HP, Cooper JE, Forbes NA. 2006. Successful treatment of tracheal xanthogranulomatosis in a red-tailed hawk (*Buteo jamaicensis*) by tracheal resection and anastomosis. *J Avian Med Surg* 20:247–252.

Montali RJ. 1988. Comparative pathology of inflammation in the higher vertebrates (reptiles, birds, and mammals). *J Comp Pathol* 99:1–26.

Montali RJ, Bush M, Thoen CO, Smith E. 1976. Tuberculosis in captive exotic birds. *JAVMA* 169:169–920.

Moore RP, Snowden KF, Phalen DN. 2001. A method of preventing transmission of so-called "megabacteria" in budgerigars (*Melopsittacus undulatus*). *J Avian Med Surg* 15(4):283–287.

Moreno AC, Modesto F, Huynh M, Shivaprasad L. 2015. External ears glands adenocarcinoma in a common goose (*Anser anser domesticus*). *Proc Int Conf Avian Herpetolog Exot Mamm Med*, p. 405.

Murphy CJ, Bellhorn RW, Buyukmihei NC. 1986. Subconjuctival hibernoma in a goose. *JAVMA* 189:1109–1112.

Murtaugh RJ, Ringler DJ, Petrak ML. 1986. Squamous cell carcinoma of the esophagus in an Amazon parrot. *J Am Vet Med Assoc* 188:872–873.

Nair MK. 1973. The early inflammatory reaction in the fowl-light microscopical, ultrastructural and autoradiographic study. *Acta B Veterinaria Scandinavica (Supplement)* 42:1–103.

Nakamura K, Ito M, Fujino K, et al. 2010. Case report: pathology and microbiology of dermal squamous cell carcinoma in young brown chickens reared on reused litter. *Avian Dis* 54:1120–1124.

Nakamura AA, Meireles MV. 2015. Cryptosporidium infections in birds: a review. *Revista Brasileira De Parasitologia Veterinaria* 24(3):253–267.

Nakano Y, Une Y. 2012. Hemangiosarcoma with widespread metastasis that originated on the metatarsal pad of a Java sparrow (*Padda oruzivora*). *J Vet Med Sci* 74(5):6221–623.

Neimanis AS, Handeland k, Isomursu M, et al. 2010. Case report: first report of epizootic trichomoniasis in wild finches (Family Fringillidae) in southern Fennoscandi. *Avian Dis* 54:136–141.

Nemes CS, Glavits R, Dubos-Kovacs M, et al. 2006. Typhlocolitis associated with spirochaetes in goose flocks. *Avian Pathol* 35:4–11.

Nevarez J, Tully TN, Hananeh W, Paulsen DB. 2002. What is your diagnosis? *J Avian Med Surg* 16(2):154–158.

Nevarez JG, Cho D-Y, Tully TN. 2011. What is your diagnosis? Lymphosarcoma. *J Avian Med Surg* 25(3):231–233.

Newman SJ, West K. 2001. Pulmonary leiomyosarcoma in a white carneau pigeon (*Columba livia*). *J Avian Med Surg* 15(4):293–296.

Norton JH, Prior HC. 1994. Microsporidiosis in a peach-faced lovebird (*Agapornis roseicollis*). *Aust Vet J* 71:23–24.

Novilla MN, Kwapien RP. 1978. Microsporidian infection in the pied peach-faced lovebird (*Agapornis roseicollis*). *Avian Dis* 22:198–204.

Nunoya T, Kanai K, Yagihashi T, et al. 1997. Natural case of salpingitis apparently caused by *Mycoplasma gallisepticum* in chickens. *Avian Pathol* 26:391–398.

Ochi A, Ochiai K, Nakamura S, et al. 2012.Molecular characteristics and pathogenicity of an avian leukosis virus isolated from avian neurofibrosarcoma. *Avian Dis* 56(1):35–43.

O'Connor MR, Garner MM. 2018. Iron storage disease in African grey parrots (*Psittacus erithacus*) exposed to a carnivorous diet. *J Zoo Wildl Med* 49(1):172–177.

Oliveira BCM, Ferrari ED, da Cruz Panegossi MF, et al. 2017. First description of *Cryptosporidium parvum* in carrier pigeons (*Columba livia*). *Vet Parasitol* 243:148–150.

Osofsky A, Hawkins MG, Foreman O, et al. 2011. Chronic lymphocytic leukemia in a double yellow-headed Amazon parrot (*Amazona ochrocephala oratrix*). *J Avian Med Surg* 25(4):286–294.

Osorio C, Fletcher O, Dykstra MJ, Post K, Barnes HJ. 2007. Comb candidiasis affecting roosters in a broiler breeder flock. *Avian Dis* 51(2):618–622.

Ostrand WD, Bissonette JA, Conover MR. 1995. Trichomoniasis as a factor in mourning dove population decline in Fillmore, Utah. *J Wildl Dis* 31(1):87–89.

Padrid PA, Feldman BF, Funk K, et al. 1991. Cytologic, microbiologic and biochemical analysis of bronchoalveolar lavage fluid obtained from 24 healthy cats. *Am J Vet Res* 52:1300–1307.

Page CD, Haddad BA. 1995. Coccidial infections in birds. *Semin Avian Exotic Pet Med* 3:138–144.

Pal M, Mehrotra BS. 1986. Studies on the association of *Aspergillus fumigatus* with ocular infections in animals. *Vet Rec* 118:42–44.

Palmieri C, Cusinato I, Avallone G, et al. 2011.Cloacal fibrosarcoma in a canary (*Serinus canaria*). *J Avian Med Surg* 25(4):277–280.

Palmieri C, Roy P, Dhillon AS, Shivaprasad HL. 2013. Avian mycobacteriosis in psittacines: a retrospective study of 123 cases. *J Comp Pathol* 148:126–138.

Pardini V, Schlanser J, Hanley CS. 2012. What is your diagnosis? *J Avian Med Surg* 26(4):267–269.

Peckham MC. 1955. Xanthomatosis in chickens. *Am J Vet Res* 16:580–583.

Pesaro S, Biancani B, Fabbrizi G, Rossi G. 2009. Squamous cell carcinoma with presence of poxvirus-like inclusions in the foot of a pink-backed pelican (*Pelecanus rufescens*). *Avian Pathol* 38(3):229–231.

Petrak ML, Gilmore C. 1982. Neoplasms. In: Petrak M (ed), Diseases *of Cage and Aviary Birds*. Philadelphia, PA: Lea & Febiger.

Phalen DN, Tomaszewski EK, Wilson VG. 1998. Internal papillomatosis: a herpesvirus connection? In: Proceedings of the Association of Avian Veterinarians. St. Paul (MN).

Phalen DN, Moore RP. 2003. Experimental infection of white-leghorn cockerels with *Macrorhabdos ornithogaster* (Megabacterium). *Avian Dis* 47:254–260.

Phalen DN. 2005. Diagnosis and management of *Macrorhabdus ornithogaster* (formerly megabacteria). *Vet Clin Exot Anim* 8:299–306.

Phalen DN. 2014. Update on the diagnosis and management of Macrorhabdus ornithogaster (formerly Megabacteria) in avian patients. *Vet Clin Exot Anim* 17:203–210.

Piccione J, Bryan LK, Hoppes S, Levine GJ. 2017. What is your diagnosis? Mass on the foot of a duck. *Vet Clin Pathol* 46(1):191–192.

Pirie G, Heatley JJ. 2001. What is your diagnosis? *J Avian Med Surg* 15(4):323–324.

Pocknell AM, Miller DJ, Neufeld JL, et al. 1996. Conjunctival mycobacteriosis in two emus (*Dromaius novaehollandiae*). *Vet Pathol* 33:346–348.

Pond CL, Rush HG. 1981. Infection of white carneaux pigeons (*Columbia livia*) with *Mycobacterium avium. Lab Anim Sci* 31:196–199.

Powell S, Tang KN, Chandler F, et al. 1989. Microsporidiosis in a lovebird. *J Vet Diagn Invest* 1:69–71.

Powers LV, Merrill CL, Degeneres LA, et al. 1998. Axillary cystoadenocarcinoma in a Molluccan cockatoo (*Cacatua moluccensis*). *Avian Dis* 42:408–412.

Powers LV, Mitchell MA, Garner MM. 2019. Macrorhabdus ornithogaster infection and spontaneous proventricular adenocarcinoma in Budgerigars (*Melopsittacus undulatus*). *Vet Pathol* 56(3):486–493.

Preziosi DE, Morris DO, Johnston MS, et al. 2006. Distribution of *Malassezia* organisms on the skin of unaffected psittacine birds and psittacine birds with feather-destructive behavior. *J Am Vet Med Assoc* 228(2):216– 221.

Proenca LM, Mayer J, Schnellbacher R, et al. 2014. Antemortem diagnosis and successful treatment of pulmonary candidiasis in a Sun conure (*Aratinga solstitialis*). *J Avian Med Surg* 28(4):316–321.

Purchase GH, Burmester BD. 1978. Leukosis/sarcoma group. In: Hofstad M (ed), *Diseases of Poultry*. Ames: Iowa State University Press.

Püstow R, Krautwald-Junghanns M-E. 2017. The incidence and treatment outcomes of *Macrorhabdus ornithogaster* infection in Budgerigars (*Melopsittacus undulatus*) in a veterinary clinic. *J Avian Med Surg* 31(4):344–350.

Pye GW, Carpenter JW, Goggin JM, Bacmeister C. 1999. Metastatic squamous cell carcinoma in a salmon-crested cockatoo (*Cacatua moluccensis*). *J Avian Med Surg* 13(3); 192–200.

Quereshi MA. 1998. Role of macrophages in avian health and disease. *Poult Sci* 77:978–982.

Quesenberry KE, Orosz SE, Dorrenstein GM. 1997. Musculoskeletal system. In: Altman R, Clubb S, Dorrestein G, Quesenberry K (eds), *Avian medicine and surgery*. Philadelphia, PA: WB Saunders.

Quinn PJ, Markey BK, Leonard FC, et al. 2011. *Veterinary Microbiology and Microbial Disease*, 2nd edn. New York: Wiley-Blackwell.

Raidal SR, Butler R. 2001. Chronic rhinosinusitis and rhamphothecal destruction in a major mitchell's cockatoo (*Cacatua leadbeateri*) due to *Cryptococcus neoformans* var *gattii*. *J Avian Med Surg* 15(2):121–125.

Rambaud YF, Flach EJ, Freeman KP. 2003. Malignant melanoma in a Humboldt penguin (Spheniscus humboldti). *Vet Rec* 153(7):217–218.

Ramis A, Gibert X, Majo N, Grifols J. 1999. Metastatic oral squamous cell carcinoma in a Montagu's harrier (*Cirus pigarus*). *J Vet Diagn Invest* 11(2):191–194.

Ramos-Vara JA, Smith EJ, Watson GL. 1997. Lymphosarcoma with plasmacytoid differentiation in a scarlet macaw (*Ara macao*). *Avian Dis* 41:499–504.

Randall CJ, Less S, Higgins RJ, Harcourt-Brown NH. 1986. Microsporidian infection in lovebirds (*Agapornis* spp.). *Avian Pathol* 15:223–231.

Raskin RE. 2001. Eyes and adnexa. In: Raskin R, Meyer D (eds), *Atlas of Canine and Feline Cytology*. Philadelphia, PA: WB Saunders.

Raynor PL, Kollias GV, Krook L. 1999. Periosseous xanthogranulomatosis in a fledgling great horned owl (*Bubo virginianus*). *J Avian Med Surg* 13(4):269–274.

Real J, Manosa S, Munoz E. 2000. Trichomoniasis in a Bonelli's eagle population in Spain. *J Wildl Dis* 36:64–70.

Reavill DR. Tumors of pet birds. 2004. *Vet Clin North Am Exot Anim Pract* 7:537–560.

Reavill DR, Schmidt RE. 2000. Avian surgical pathology. In: Fudge A (ed), *Laboratory Medicine: Avian and Exotic Pets*. Philadelphia, PA: WB Saunders.

Rebar AH, DeNicola DB, Muggenburg BA. 1980. Bronchopulmonary lavage cytology in the dog: normal findings. *Vet Clin North Am (Sm Anim)* 22:1065–1085.

Redrobe S. 2000. Treatment of avian liver disease. *Semin Avian Exotic Pet Med* 9:136–145.

Reece RL. 1992. Observation on naturally occurring neoplasms in birds in the state of Victoria, Australia. *Avian Pathol* 21:3–32.

Reece RL. 2008. Other tumours of unknown etiology. In: Saif YM, Fadly AM, Glisson JR, McDougald LR, Nolan LK, Swayne DE, Editorial Board for the American Association of Avian Pathologists (eds), *Diseases poultry*, 12th edn. Ames, IA: Blackwell Publishing, pp. 593–616.

Rettenmund CL, Newton AL, Calle PP. 2015. Uropygial gland squamous cell carcinoma in Chinstrap (Pygoscelis antarcticus) and Gentoo (Pygoscelis papua) penguins at the Wildlife Conservation Society's Central Park Zoo. *J Zoo Wildl Med* 46(1):113–119.

Reuschel M, Pantchey N, Vrhovec G, et al. 2020. Occurrence and colecular typing of *Giardia psittaci* in parakeets in Germany—a case study. *Avian Dis* 64(2):228–233.

Rindi L, Garzelli C. 2014. Genetic diversity and phylogeny of *Mycobacterium avium*. *Infect Genet Evol* 21:375–383.

Ritchie BW. 1995a. Avian viruses, function and control. In: Ritchie BW (ed), *Avian viruses, function and control*. Lake Worth, FL: Wingers.

Ritchie BW. 1995b. Papovaviridae. In: Ritchie BW (ed), *Avian viruses, function and control*. Lake Worth, FL: Wingers.

Ritzman TK, Hawley SB, Schulman FY. 1996. Liposarcoma in a green-cheeked conure. In: Proceedings of the Annual Conference of Association of Avian Veterinarians.

Rivera S, McClearen JR, Reavill DR. 2009. Treatment of nonepitheliotropic cutaneous B-cell lymphoma in an umbrella cockatoo (*Cacatua alba*). *J Avian Med Surg* 23(4):294–302.

Robertson J, Guzman DS-M, Sinnott D, et al. 2020. Clinical report: modified tail amputation technique in a blue and gold macaw (*Ara ararauna*) with uropygial gland adenocarcinoma. *J Avian Med Surg* 34(1):57–64.

Robinoa P, Ferrocinob I, Rossic G, et al. 2019. Changes in gut bacterial communities in canaries infected by *Macrorhabdus ornithogaster*. *Avian Pathol* 48(2):111–120.

Romagnano A, Heard DJ. 2000. Avian dermatology. In: Olsen G, Orosz S (eds), *Manual of Avian Medicine*. St. Louis: Mosby.

Rosenthal D, Lancilloti F, Darwiche N, Sinha R, et al. 1994. Regulation of epithelial differentiation by retinoids. In: Blomhoff R (ed), *Vitamin A in Health and Disease*. New York: Marcel Dekker, Inc.

Rosenthal KL, Morris DO, Mauldin EA, Ivey ES, Piekes H. 2004. Cytologic, histologic, and microbiologic characterization of the feather pulp and follicles of feather-picking psittacine birds: a preliminary study. *J Avian Med Surg* 18(3):137-143.

Rosskopf WJ, Woerpel RW. 1984. Cryptococcosis in a thick-billed parrot. In: Proceedings of the Association of Avian Veterinarians.

Royal AB, Jochems B. 2018.What is your diagnosis? Tongue lesion in a great horned owl. *Vet Clin Pathol* 47(3):505–506.

Rupley AE. 1997. *Manual of Avian Practice*. Philadelphia, PA: WB Saunders.

Sacre BJ, Oppenheing YC, Steinburg H, et al. 1992. Presumptive histiocytic sarcoma in a great horned owl (*Bubo virginianus*). *J Zoo Wildl Med* 23:113–121.

Sadar MJ, Guzman DS-M, Burton AG, et al. 2014. Mycotic keratitis in a khaki campbell duck (Anas platyrhynchos domesticus). *J Avian Med Surg* 28(4):322–329.

Saggese MD, Riggs G, Tizard I, et al. 2007. Gross and microscopic findings and investigation of the aetiopathogenesis of mycobacteriosis in a captive population of white-winged ducks (*Cairina scutulata*). *Avian Pathol* 36(5):415–422.

Sáncheza FD, Yelab IJ, Alfonsecab E, et al. 2016. Respiratory tract infection caused by *Mycobacterium bovis* in a black swan (*Cygnus atratus*). *Avian Pathol* 45(1):126–131.

Sánchez-Cordo´ n PJ, Gómez-Villamandos JC, Gutiérrez J, et al. 2007. Atoxoplasma spp. infection in captive canaries (*Serinus canaria*). *J Vet Med A Physiol Pathol Clin Med* 54:23–26.

Sandford SE, Rehmtulla AJ, Josephson GK. 1994. Tuberculosis in farmed rheas (*Rhea americana*). *Avian Dis* 38:193–196.

Schlein LJ, Wycislo KL, Barger AM. 2019. What is your diagnosis? Impression smear from the uropygial gland of an African gray parrot. *Vet Clin Pathol* 48:140–142.

Schmidt RE. 1992. Mast cell tumors in two owls. *J Assoc Avian Vet* 6:23–24.

Schmidt RE. 1997. Neoplastic diseases. In: Altman R, Clubb S, Dorrestein G, Quesenberry K (eds), *Avian Medicine and Surgery*. Philadelphia, PA: WB Saunders.

Schmidt RE, Reavill DR, Phalen DN. 2003. Pathology of pet and aviary birds. In: Schmidt R, Reavill D, Phalen D (eds), *Pathology of Pet and Aviary Birds*. Ames: Iowa State University Press.

Schmidt V, Philipp H-C, Thielebein J, et al. 2012. Malignant lymphoma of T-cell origin in a humboldt penguin (*Spheniscus humboldti*) and a pink-backed pelican (*Pelecanus rufescens*). *J Avian Med Surg* 26(2):101–106.

Schmidt RE, Reavill DR, Phalen DN. 2015. Respiratory system. In: Schmidt RE, Reavill DR, Phalen DN, (eds), *Pathology of pet and aviary birds*, 2nd edn. Ames, IA: Wiley-Blackwell, pp. 21–94.

Schrenzel MD, Maalouf GA, Gaffney PM, et al. 2005 Molecular characterization of isosporoid coccidia (*Isospora* and *Atoxoplasma* spp.) in passerine birds. *J Parasitol* 91:635–647.

Schunk RS, Sitinas NE, Quesenberry KE, Grodio JL. 2017. Multicentric cryptococcosis in a Congo African grey parrot (*Psittacus erithacus erithacus*). *J Avian Med Surg* 31(4):373–381.

Sedacca CD, Campbell TW, Bright JM, et al. 2009 Chronic cor pulmonale secondary to pulmonary atherosclerosis in an African grey parrot. *JAVMA* 234(8):1055–9.

Sekiguchi M, Nonaka N, Adachi M, Sekiya T, Yamamoto Y. 2018. Avian filariasis in backyard chickens in Japan. *Avian Dis* 62:326–329.

Senties-Cué CG, Charlton BR, Woolcock P, et al. 2010. Atypical distribution of fowl pox lesions in broilers. *Avian Dis Digest* 5(4):e58–e60.

Shelly SM. 2001. Body cavity fluids. In: Raskin R, Meyer D (eds), *Atlas of Canine and Feline Cytology*. Philadelphia, PA: WB Saunders.

Shivaprasad HL. 2003. Hepatitis associated with *Clostridium difficile* in an ostrich chick. *Avian Pathol* 32:57–62.

Shivaprasad HL, Duhamel GE. 2005. Cecal spirochetosis caused by *Brachyspira pilosicoli* in commercial turkeys. *Avian Dis* 49:609–613.

Shivaprasad HL, Fanca M. 2011. Unusual disseminated lesions of poxvirus in psittacines resembling canary pox. *Proc Annu Conf Assoc Avian Vet*, pp. 275–276.

Shrader TC, Carpenter JW, Cino-Ozuna AD, Andrews GA. 2016. Malignant melanoma of the syrinx and liver in an African grey parrot (*Psittacus erithacus erithacus*). *J Avian Med Surg* 30(2):165–171.

Simova-Curd S, Richter M, Hauser B, Hatt J-M. 2009. Clinical reports: surgical removal of a retrobulbar adenoma in an African grey parrot (*Psittacus erithacus*). *J Avian Med Surg* 23(1):24–28.

Sinclair KM, Hawkins MG, Wright L, et al. 2015. Chronic T-cell lymphocytic leukemia in a black swan (*Cygnus atratus*): diagnosis, treatment, and pathology. *J Avian Med Surg* 29(4):326–335.

Sledge DG, Radi ZA, Miller DL, Lynn BS. 2006. Subcutaneous haemangiosarcoma in a cockatiel (*Nymphicus hollandicus*). *J Vet Med A Physiol Pathol Clin Med* 53(6):293–295.

Slocombe RF, McCowan C, Wang J, Holz P. 2013. Avian pox in crimson rosellas (*Platycercus elegans*) in southern Australia. *Avian Pathol* 42(2):147–150.

Smith SH, Goldschmidt MH, McManus PM. 2002. A comparative review of melanocytic neoplasms. *Vet Pathol* 39:651–678.

Sokół I, Gaweł A, Bobrek K. 2018. The prevalence of yeast and characteristics of the isolates from the digestive tract of clinically healthy turkeys. *Avian Dis* 62:286–290.

Souza MJ, Newman SJ, Greenacre CB, et al. 2008. Diffuse intestinal T-cell lymphosarcoma in a yellow-naped Amazon parrot (*Amazona ochrocephala auropalliata*). *J Vet Diagn Invest* 20(5):656–660.

Souza MJ, Johnstone-McLean NS, Ward D, Newkirk K. 2009. Conjunctival xanthoma in a blue and gold macaw (*Ara ararauna*). *Vet Ophthalmol* 12:53–55.

Spira A. 1996. Disorders of the respiratory system. In: Rosskopf W, Woerpel R (eds), *Diseases of Cage and Aviary Birds*. Baltimore, MD: Lea and Febiger.

Staudenmaier AM, Simone-Freilicher EA, Noonan BP, Ewing PJ. 2019. Antemortem diagnosis of esophageal squamous cell carcinoma in a blue-fronted Amazon parrot *(Amazona aestiva)* and a mealy Amazon parrot *(Amazona farinosa)*. *J Am Vet Med Assoc* 254(11):1324–1328

Steinhort LA. 1995. Microsporidiosis in budgerigars. In: Proceedings of the Annual Conference of the Association of Avian Veterinarians.

Steinmetz HW, Rutz C, Hoop RK, et al. 2006. Case report: possible human-avian transmission of *Mycobacterium tuberculosis* in a green-winged macaw (*Ara chloroptera*). *Avian Dis* 50:641–645.

Stern AW, Lamm CG. 2009. Malignant melanoma of the subcutaneous tissues in an umbrella cockatoo (*Cacatua alba*). *J Avian Med Surg* 23(4):303–306.

Stiles J, Greenacre C. 2001. Infraorbital cyst in a white cockatoo (*Cacatua alba*). *J Avian Med Surg* 15:40–43.

Stimmelmayr R, Stefani LM, Thrall MA, et al. 2012. Case report: Trichomonosis in free-ranging eurasian collared doves (*Streptopelia decaocto*) and African collared dove hybrids (*Streptopelia risoria*) in the Caribbean and description of ITS-1 region genotypes. *Avian Dis* 56:441–445.

Suedmeyer WMK, McCaw D, Turnquist S. 2001a. Attempted photodynamic therapy of squamous cell carcinoma in the casque of a great hornbill (*Buceros bicornis*). *J Avian Med Surg* 15:44–49.

Suedmeyer WK, Witter RL, Bermudez A. 2001b. Hemangiosarcoma in a golden pheasant (*Chrysolophus pictus*). *J Avian Med Surg* 15(2):126–130.

Suedmeyer WK, Henry C, McCaw D, Boucher M. 2007. Attempted photodynamic therapy against patagial squamous cell carcinoma in an African rose-ringed parakeet (*Psittacula krameri*). *J Zoo Wildl Med* 38(4):597–600.

Suepaul RB, Seetahal JFR, Oura C, et al. 2019. Novel poxviral infection in three finch species illegally imported into Trinidad, West Indies, with implications for native birds. *J Zoo Wildl Med* 50(1):231–237.

Sullivan PJ, Ramsay EC, Greenacre CB, et al. 2017. Comparison of two methods for determining prevalence of *Macrorhabdus ornithogaster* in a flock of captive budgerigars (*Melopsittacus undulates*). *J Avian Med Surg* 31(2):128–131.

Summa NM, Guzman DS-M. 2017. Evidence-based advances in avian medicine. *Vet Clin Exot Anim* 20:817–837.

Sun H, Qin M, Xiao Y, et al. 2010. Haemangiomas, leiomyosarcoma and myeloma caused by subgroup J avian leukosis virus in a commercial layer flock. *Acta Vet Hung* 58(4):441–451.

Surman PG, Schultz DJ, Tham VL. 1974. Keratoconjunctivitis and chlamydiosis in caged birds. *Aust Vet J* 50:346–362.

Swartout MS, Wymann M. 1987. Pancreatic carcinoma in a cockatiel. *JAVMA* 4:451–452.

Swayne DF, Weisbrode SF. 1990. Cutaneous mast cell tumor in a great horned owl (*Bubo virginianus*). *Vet Pathol* 27:124–126.

Sydenstricker KV, Dhondt AA, Hawley DM, et al. 2006. Characterization of experimental *Mycoplasma gallisepticum* infection in captive house finch flocks. *Avian Dis* 50(1):39–44.

Tan KS. 2008. New insights on classification, identification, and clinical relevance of *Blastocystis* spp. *Clin Microbiol Rev* 21:639–665.

Tell LA, Woods L, Mathews KG. 1997. Basal cell carcinoma in a blue-fronted Amazon parrot (*Amazona aestiva*). *Avian Dis* 41:755–759.

Tomaszewski EK, Logan KS, Snowden KF, et al. 2003. Phylogenic analysis identifies the "megabacterium" of birds as a novel anamorphic ascomycetous yeast, *Macrorhbdus ornithogaster* gen. nov., sp. nov. *Int J Syst Evol Microbiol* 53:1201–1205.

Truchado DA, Williams RAJ, Benítez L. 2018. Natural history of avian papillomaviruses. *Virus Res* 252:58–67.

Tully TN, Morris JM, Veazey RS, et al. 1994. Liposarcoma in a monk parakeet (*Myiopsitta monachus*). *J Assoc Avian Vet* 8:120–124.

Tully TN, Morris JM, Pechman RD, Taylor HW. 1995. What is your diagnosis? *J Avian Med Surg* 9:57–58.

Turrel JM, McMillan MC, Paul-Murphy J. 1987. Diagnosis and treatment of tumors of companion birds. *AAV Today* 1:109–116.

Uetsuka K, Suzuki T, Doi K, Nunoya T. 2012. Case report: Malignant sertoli cell tumor in a goose (*Anser cygnoides domesticus*). *Avian Dis* 56:781–785.

Uzal FA, Sentíes-Cué CG, Rimoldi G, Shivaprasad HL. 2016. Non-clostridium perfringens infectious agents producing necrotic enteritis-like lesions in poultry. *Avian Pathol* 45(3):326–333.

Vail DM, Mahler PA, Soergel SA. 1995. Differential cell analysis and phenotypic subtyping of lymphocytes in bronchoalveolar lavage fluid from clinically normal dogs. *Am J Vet Res* 56:282–285.

Van Riper C, Forrester DJ. 2007. Avian Pox. In: Thomas N, Hunter B, Atkinson CA (eds), *Infectious and Parasitic Diseases of Wild Birds*. Ames, Iowa: Blackwell Publishing Professional, pp. 131–176.

Van Wettere AJ, Ley DH, Scott DE, Buckanoff HD, Degernes LA. 2012. *Mycoplasma corogypsi*–associated polyarthritis and tenosynovitis in Black vultures (*Coragyps atratus*). *Vet Pathol* 50(2):291–298.

Vazquez S, Quiroga MI, Aleman N, et al. 2003. Squamous cell carcinoma of the oropharynx and esophagus in a Japanese bantam rooster. *Avian Dis* 47:215–217.

Villaverde-Morcillo S, García-Sánchez R, Castaño C, et al. 2015. Characterization of natural ejaculates and sperm cryopreservation in a golden eagle (*Aquila chrysaetus*). *J Zoo Wildl Med* 46(2):335–338.

Walberg J, Loar AS. 2004. Cytology and hematology of small mammals. In: Carpenter J, Quesenberry K (eds), *Ferrets, Rabbits, and Rodents Clinical Medicine and Surgery*. St. Louis: Saunders Elsevier.

Wang C, Li L, Xie Y, et al. 2019. Isolation and characterization of avian *Chlamydia psittaci* from symptomatic pet birds in Southern Hunan, China. *Avian Dis* 63:31–37.

Watson VE, Murdock JH, Cazzini P, et al. 2013. Retrobulbar adenocarcinoma in an Amazon parrot (*Amazona autumnalis*). *J Vet Diagn Invest* 25(2):273–276.

Weyna A, Watrud M, Elsmo E. 2021. Pathology in practice. *J Am Vet Med Assoc* 258(1):51–54.

Wheeler CL, Webber RA. 2002. Localized ascites in a cockatiel (*Nymphicus hollandicus*) with hepatic cirrhosis. *J Avian Med Surg* 16:300–305.

Whitehear KL, Browning GF. 2004. Mycoplasma. In: Gyles CL, Prescott JF, Songer G, et al. (eds), *Pathogenesis of Bacterial Infections in Animals*, 3rd edn. Ames, IA: Blackwell Publishing, pp. 397–414.

Williams RAJ, Duch CE, Pérez-Tris J, Benítez L. 2014. Polymerase chain reaction detection of avipox and avian papillomavirus in naturally infected wild birds: comparisons of blood, swab and tissue samples. *Avian Pathol* 43(2):130–134.

Wiley JL, Whittington JK, Wilmes CM, Messick JB. 2009. Chronic myelogenous leukemia in a great horned owl (*Bubo virginianus*). *J Avian Med Surg* 23(1):36–43.

Williams SM, Zavala G, Hafner S, Collett SR, Cheng S. 2012. Metastatic melanomas in young broiler chickens (*Gallus gallus domesticus*). *Vet Pathol* 49(2):288–291.

de Wit M, Schoemaker NJ, Kik MJL, Westerhoff I. 2003. Hypercalcemia in two Amazon parrots with malignant lymphoma. *Avian Dis* 47(1):223–228.

Witte CL, Hungerford LL, Papendick R, Stalis IH, Rideout BA. 2010. Investigation of factors predicting disease among zoo birds exposed to avian mycobacteriosis. *J Am Vet Med Assoc* 236 (2):211–218.

Witte CL, Hungerford LL, Papendick R, Stalis IH, Rideout BA. 2008. Investigation of characteristics and factors associated with avian mycobacteriosis in zoo birds. *J Vet Diagn Invest* 20:186–196.

Yamamoto R. 1991. Infectious coryza. In: Calnek B (ed), *Diseases of Poultry*, 9th edn. Ames: Iowa State University Press.

Yonemaru K, Sakai H, Asaoka Y, et al. 2004. Proventricular adenocarcinoma in a Humboldt penguin (*Spheniscus humboldti*) and a great horned owl (*Bubo virginianus*): identification of origin by mucin histochemistry. *Avian Pathol* 33:75–79.

Yoshikawa H. 2012. Epidemiology, transmission, and zoonotic potential of *Blastocystis* in human and animals. In: Melhorn H, Tan KSW, Yoshikawa H (eds), *Blastocystis: pathogen or passenger?* Heidelberg: Springer. pp. 37–49.

Zadravec M, Slavec B, Krapež U, et al. 2017. Trichomonosis outbreak in a flock of canaries (*Serinus canaria* f. *domestica*) caused by a finch epidemic strain of *Trichomonas gallinae*. *Vet Parasitol* 239:90–93.

Zafra R, Pe´rez J, Mozos E, Galk M, Bautista MJ. 2011. Case report: concurrent pulmonary adenocarcinoma and silicate pneumoconiosis in a red-legged partridge (*Alectoris rufa*). *Avian Dis* 55:128–132.

Zehnder A, Swift L, Sundaram A, et al. 2014. Multi-institutional survey of squamous cell carcinoma in birds. In: Proceedings of the Annual Conference of the Association of Avian Veterinarian, p. 3.

Zehnder AM, Swift LA, Sundaram A, et al. 2018. Clinical features, treatment, and outcomes of cutaneous and oral squamous cell carcinoma in avian species. *J Am Vet Med Assoc* 252(3):309–315.

Zoller G, Cavoizy J, Devaux L, et al. 2019. Multiple infiltrative intraosseous lipomas in the appendicular skeleton of a rose-breasted cockatoo (*Eolophus roseicapilla*) with a humeral fracture. *J Avian Med Surg* 33(1):65–71.

16 Avian Cytology and Clinical Chemistry: Clinical Case Presentations

Case 1: Lethargic Parrot

Signalment

5-year-old wild-caught intact female Cape parrot (*Poicephalus robustus*)

History

The parrot presented with a few days' duration of a distended crop and suspected crop infection. The parrot was lethargic and not perching, vocalizing, or eating. She had been owned for 2.5 years and was one of the various breeding parrots housed in an aviary. She was fed a mixture of Zupreem pellets/cockatoo seeds and vegetables/fruits, and had a watering system. She was housed in an 8 × 8 ft hanging cage with perches. In the breeding facility, the hanging cages were separated by dividers and special lighting and heating were provided.

Physical Examination

The parrot was bright, alert, and responsive, but appeared mildly lethargic. On physical exam, she regurgitated food particles after palpation of the distended fluid-filled, flaccid ingluvies (crop). The bird weighed 282 g three months earlier and now weighed 326 g, which likely represented a weight gain due to retention of fluid in the gastrointestinal tract since she appeared to have a moderate reduction of the pectoral muscle mass. A reddened area was noted on the ventral left tibial tarsal joint, most likely resulting from being on the bottom of her cage and not perching. She was not lame. The oral cavity was normal, and no other abnormalities were noted.

Diagnostic involving a complete blood profile, crop aspirate, and fecal swab for cytodiagnosis, and whole-body radiographs were offered (Tables 16.1 and 16.2; Figures 16.1a, 16.1b, 16.2a, and 16.2b). The radiographic examination was declined at that time.

Interpretive Discussion

The hemogram appeared to be within normal expected limits; however, the plasma biochemistry profile revealed hyperuricemia, likely associated with renal

Table 16.1. Cape parrot hematology results (Case 1).

		Decision level[a]
PCV (%)	46	35–55
Leukocytes		
WBC (×10³/μL)	8.8	5.0–20.0
Heterophils (×10³/μL)	4.1	2.1–10.0
(%)	51	—
Lymphocytes (×10³/μL)	2.9	1.7–10.0
(%)	37	—
Monocytes (×10³/μL)	0.6	0–0.7
(%)	8	—
Eosinophils (×10³/μL)	0.2	0–0.4
(%)	2	—
Basophils (×10³/μL)	0.2	0–0.4
(%)	2	—
Thrombocytes		
Estimated number	Adequate	1–5/1000× field
Morphology	Normal	
Plasma protein (refractometry) (g/dL)	5.5	3–5

[a] Decision levels used by authors when reference values are unavailable.

Exotic Animal Hematology and Cytology, Fifth Edition. Terry W. Campbell and Krystan R. Grant.

Companion website: www.wiley.com/go/campbell/exotic

disease, and hypophosphatemia likely associated with decreased dietary intake, gastrointestinal loss of phosphorus, or both.

The crop aspirate sample stained with Wright–Giemsa–Romanowsky stain revealed numerous narrowly based budding-yeast-compatible *Candida albicans* and bacteria. The fecal sample revealed an identical cytological finding (Figures 16.2a and 16.2b). The cytological findings indicated an overgrowth of yeast indicative of candidiasis. A secondary bacterial overgrowth was also likely and associated with the crop stasis.

Table 16.2. Cape parrot plasma biochemical results (Case 1).

		Reference[a]
Glucose (mg/dL)	236	200–500
BUN (mg/dL)	4	<10
Uric acid (mg/dL)	16.5	<15
Total protein (biuret) (g/dL)	4.5	2.5–4.0
Albumin (g/dL)	1.7	—
Globulin (g/dL)	2.8	—
Aspartate aminotransferase (IU/L)	133	<275
Creatine kinase (IU/L)	518	<500
Calcium (mg/dL)	8.8	8–11
Phosphorus (mg/dL)	2.3	5–7
Sodium (mEq/L)	152	130–160
Potassium (mEq/L)	3.4	2–4
Chloride (mEq/L)	111	111–120
Bicarbonate (mEq/L)	20.5	—
Anion gap (calculated)	23	—
Cholesterol (mg/dL)	185	<200
Calculated osmolality	303	---

[a] Decision levels used by the authors when reference values are unavailable.

Summary

The bird was treated with an oral broad-spectrum antibiotic (trimethoprim-sulfa) and antifungal (itraconazole) for the suspected candidiasis and bacterial ingluvitis. Candidiasis is generally considered to be secondary to immunosuppression in an adult bird, and the underlying cause of that is unknown but could be related to kidney disease based upon the plasma biochemistry findings. The prognosis for this bird is guarded to poor due to the loss of body condition and possible renal disease.

During the following two weeks, the bird's overall health had improved, and it was no longer lethargic. The bird stopped regurgitating and was behaving normally when evaluated on a follow-up examination. The client declined a recheck of the blood profile, but it was assumed that the plasma chemistry profile had also improved based upon the bird's physical appearance.

Case 2: Macaw with Periorbital Swelling

Signalment

22-year-old male blue and gold macaw (*Ara ararauna*)

History

The macaw was presented for evaluation of a periorbital mass of a few days' duration. During that time, the bird had been mildly lethargic and quiet with a decreased appetite. The owner had noticed mild swelling in the same area a month prior; however, it resolved after a couple of days.

(a) (b)

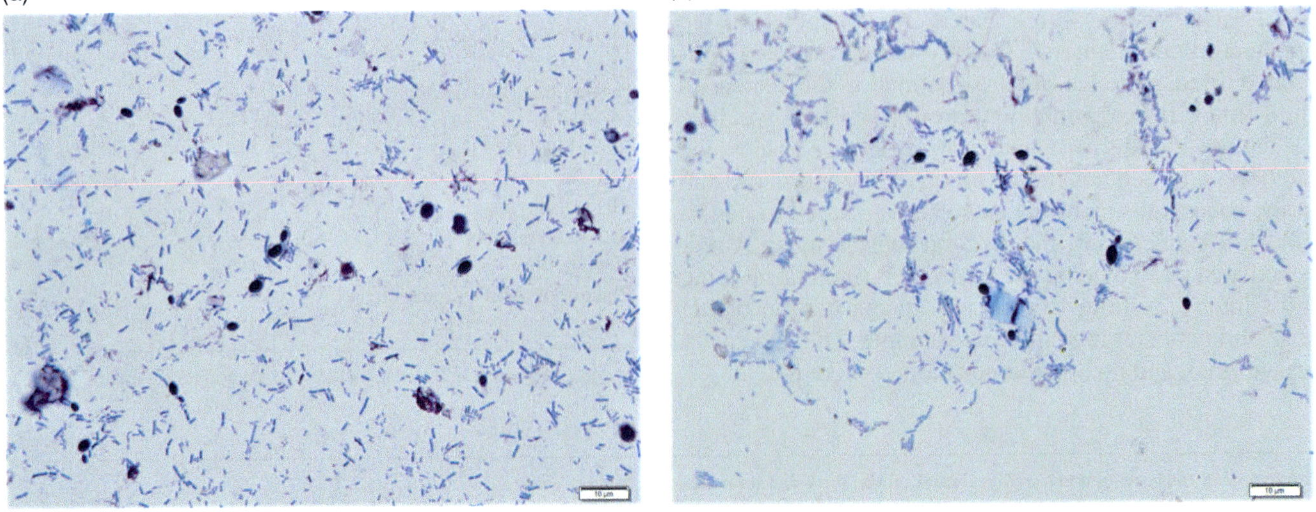

Fig. 16.1. (a), (b) Crop aspirate (Wright–Giemsa stain, 100× oil).

(a)

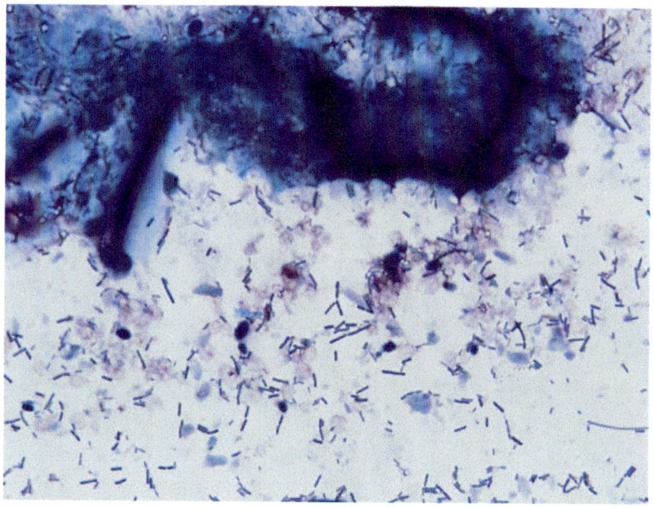

(b)

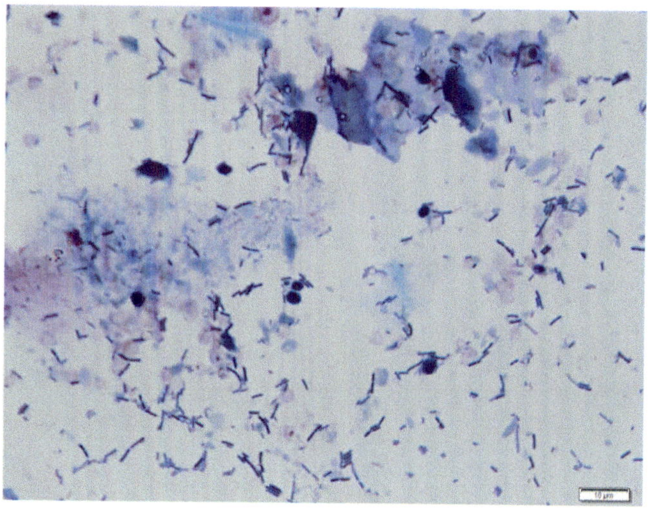

Fig. 16.2. (a), (b) Fecal sample (Wright–Giemsa stain, 100× oil).

Table 16.3. Macaw hematology results (Case 2).

	1/17	Reference[a]
PCV (%)[*]	38	47–55
Leukocytes		
WBC (×10³/μL)	87.4	7.0–22.0
Heterophils (×10³/μL)[**]	83.0	—
(%)	95	40–60
Lymphocytes (×10³/μL)	1.7	—
(%)	2	35–60
Monocytes (×10³/μL)	2.6	—
(%)	3	0–3
Eosinophils (×10³/μL)	0	—
(%)	0	0–1
Basophils (×10³/μL)	0	—
(%)	0	0–1
Thrombocytes		
Estimated number	Adequate	1–5/1000× field
Morphology	Normal	
Plasma protein (refractometry)		
(g/dL)	6.1	3–5

[*] 2% polychromasia
[**] Moderate heterophil toxicity
[a] Campbell and Ellis (2007).

Table 16.4. Macaw plasma biochemical results (Case 2).

		Reference[a]
Glucose (mg/dL)	294	290–750
BUN (mg/dL)	1	—
Uric acid (mg/dL)	3.1	1–6
Total protein (biuret) (g/dL)	4.1	3.4–4.2
Albumin (g/dL)	2.0	1.3–1.7
Globulin (g/dL)	2.1	1.3–1.9
Aspartate aminotransferase (IU/L)	552	90–180
Creatine kinase (IU/L)	4,539	180–500
Calcium (mg/dL)	9.6	9.5–10.5
Phosphorus (mg/dL)	4.5	4.6–6.4
Sodium (mEq/L)	148	148–156
Potassium (mEq/L)	2.46	2.2–3.9
Chloride (mEq/L)	109	105–113
Bicarbonate (mEq/L)	15.5	—
Cholesterol (mg/dL)	317	100–300

[a] Pollack et al. (2005).

Physical Examination

The macaw was bright, alert, and responsive. He was mildly underweight owing to a slight reduction of the pectoral muscle mass. His feathers were tattered. A 2-cm-diameter periorbital swelling caused ventrolateral displacement of the globe.

During an ophthalmic examination, a small portion of the iris could be examined after retraction of palpebrae. The iris and conjunctiva appeared healthy. An ultrasound examination revealed a soft tissue mass with multiple fluid pockets.

Whole-body radiographs, a complete blood profile, and fine-needle aspiration of the mass for cytology were performed (Tables 16.3 and 16.4; Figures 16.3a–16.3c).

Radiographic images revealed a moderately enlarged spleen (suggestive of either metastatic disease, a reactive spleen, or perhaps an insignificant finding) and increased opacity of the great vessels of the heart (consistent with atherosclerosis).

Interpretive Discussion

The hemogram revealed a severe heterophilic leukocytosis with moderately toxic heterophils, which is indicative of a severe inflammatory response, likely associated with an infectious agent. The hematology

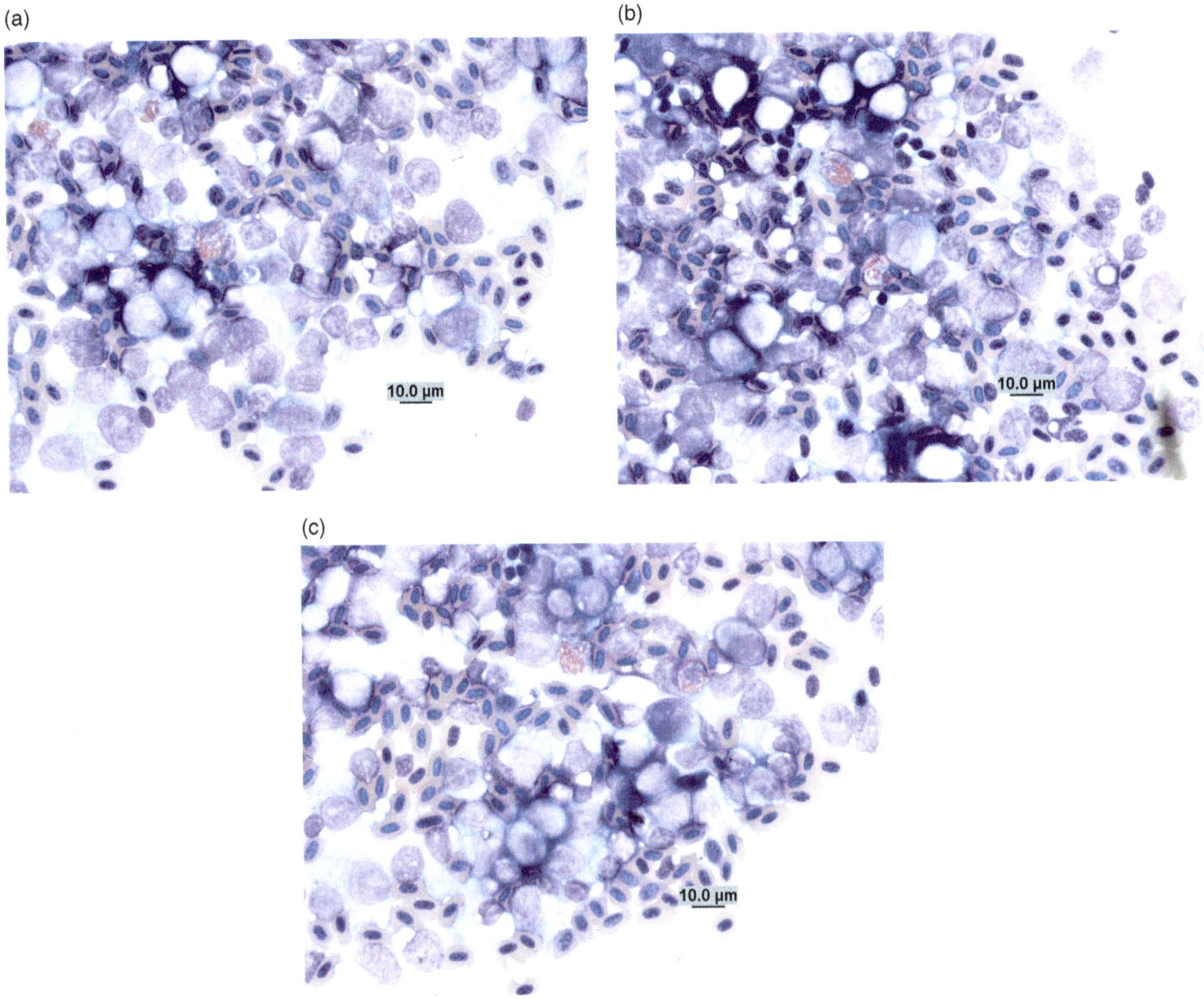

Fig. 16.3. (a)–(c) Cytology of a fine-needle aspiration of the mass (Wright–Giemsa stain, 100× oil).

also revealed anemia with 2% polychromasia observed on the blood film. The anemia was nonregenerative as the degree of polychromasia would be expected to be 10% or greater with a regenerative response. The hyperproteinemia based on an elevated plasma protein value (refractometer) was not supported by the plasma chemistry profile.

The plasma biochemistry profile was normal except for a markedly elevated creatine kinase and moderately elevated aspartate aminotransferase activities. These degrees of activity were suggestive of skeletal muscle injury.

The aspirate of the mass sample stained with Wright–Giemsa–Romanowsky stain revealed a predominantly homogenous lymphocyte population. The cells were approximately 1.5–2 times the size of a heterophil. Nuclei were round, contain finely stippled chromatin, and occasionally displayed a single indistinct nucleolus. Cytoplasm was scant, round, and mildly basophilic. Lymphoglandular bodies were abundant. There was a moderate amount of blood in the background. A few small lymphocytes and thrombocytes were present. No microorganisms were seen. The cytology was indicative of lymphoma.

Summary

The cytology and hematology were indicative of lymphoma with a possible suppurative inflammation.

Treatment recommendations included palliative radiation therapy and chemotherapy for the periorbital mass (lymphoma). Further diagnostic directed at the enlarged spleen included an exploratory celiotomy with splenic biopsy, to evaluate for metastatic disease. However, the client declined that option and was not willing to risk surgery. The client also did not agree to the chemotherapy.

The macaw was hospitalized and given six fractions of radiation therapy divided into biweekly treatments along with a broad-spectrum antibiotic (orbifloxacin) and pain management (meloxicam for the first week and flurbiprofen for the following two weeks).

The bird responded well to radiation therapy, and at the end of treatment, there was no evidence of the mass. The skin around the eye remained mildly erythematous and inflamed due to the bird scratching at the area. There was no evidence of radiation damage to the eye, and the globe returned to normal position. Serial ophthalmic examinations indicated the macaw had vision in that eye. A small central cataract and signs of previous uveitis that likely occurred years prior were also noted.

The hemogram at 4 weeks post treatment indicated significant improvement with a moderate leukocytosis ($31.5\times10^3/\mu L$), heterophilia ($29.9\times10^3/\mu L$), relative lymphopenia ($1.3\times10^3/\mu L$), and normal monocyte numbers ($0.3\times10^3/\mu L$). No toxic changes to the heterophils were noted. The plasma total protein value had decreased to a normal 4.6 g/dL. The PCV improved to 40% with increased polychromasia (10%).

Three months following treatment, the bird's health began to deteriorate. The client indicated that the bird had been "slowing down" during the past four days, which included not talking, decreased climbing with occasional loss of balance, and increased sleeping. The bird had been seeking more attention from his owner and scratching at both eyes. An increase in the respiratory effort was also noted as indicated by "bobbing" of the tail while breathing. Although the bird's appetite remained normal, he appeared to be losing weight. No abnormalities around the right eye (previous periocular lymphoma) were reported.

On physical exam, the macaw was quiet, lethargic, but responsive and had lost 16% of his body weight from the initial presentation. The feathers were slightly fluffed, and he had a moderate increase in respiratory effort. Whole-body radiographs, a blood profile, and ophthalmic examination were performed under general anesthesia. The previously noted periocular swelling had resolved, and the tissue surrounding the eye appeared healthy. Whole-body radiographs showed a large coelomic mass in the areas of the liver, spleen, and gonad restricting the air sacs. Fine-needle aspirates were obtained and were consistent with lymphoma. The blood profile revealed an improved leukocyte count (15 000/μL) and mild to moderate elevation of aspartate aminotransferase (AST) activity.

The bird died a few days later, and the necropsy revealed disseminated lymphoma involving the right eye, liver, spleen, and kidneys.

Case 3: Eagle with Swollen Right Foot

Signalment

Adult female golden eagle (*Aquila chrysaetos*)

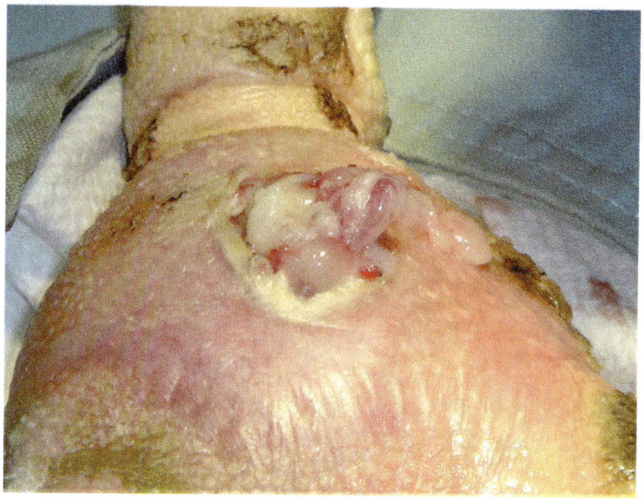

Fig. 16.4. Gross lesion of the right foot.

History

The eagle was a long-term resident of a raptor rehabilitation facility, and was presented for evaluation of a recurrent swollen right foot.

Physical Examination

The eagle was alert but lethargic. The right metatarsus was swollen with a cutaneous scab in the center of the metatarsal pad. Proliferative tissue protruded through the opening in the metatarsal pad after the scab was removed (Figure 16.4).

A biopsy of the proliferative tissue was obtained for histopathology. Fluid from this area was aspirated and submitted for bacterial culture, and a smear was prepared for cytodiagnosis (Figures 16.5a–16.5c). The colorless fluid appeared slightly cloudy and was not viscous.

Interpretive Discussion

The fluid aspirate sample stained with Wright–Giemsa–Romanowsky stain revealed a marked number of inflammatory cells, many multinucleated giant cells, and occasional spindle-shaped cells suggestive of fibroblasts. The multinucleated giant cells were indicative of osteoclasts. The inflammatory cells were predominately degenerate and nondegenerate heterophils with occasional macrophages. The noncellular background lacked the granular appearance of healthy joint fluid. The cytology findings were indicative of degenerative joint disease and supportive of chronic pododermatitis.

Summary

The histopathologic finding from the tissue obtained from the metatarsal pad indicated a severe, acute, diffuse, suppurative pododermatitis with intralesional bacteria.

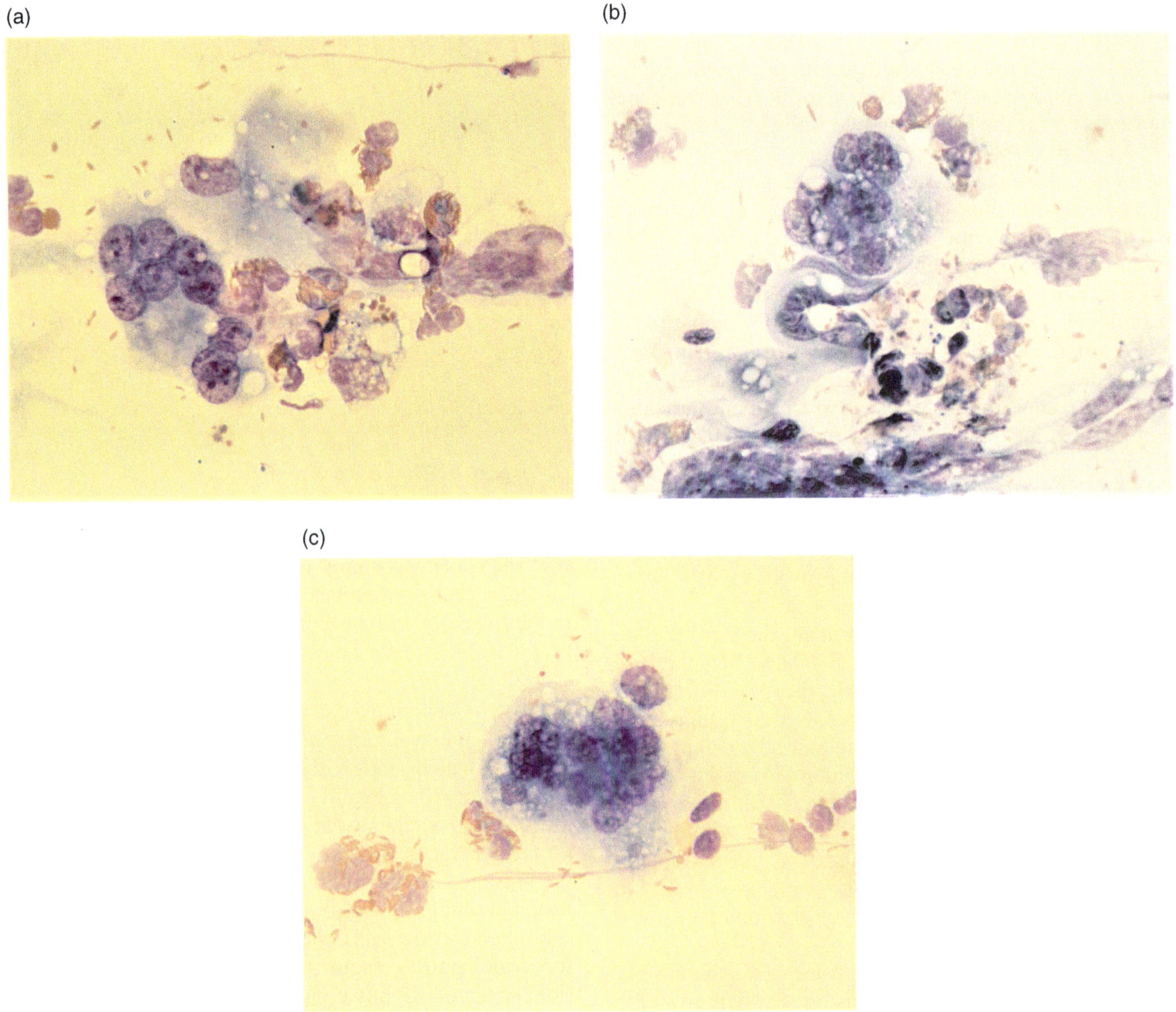

Fig. 16.5. (a)–(c) Cytology of the joint fluid (Wright–Giemsa stain, 100× oil).

The bacterial culture of the fluid revealed multiple isolates that included light growths of *Staphylococcus* and *Enterococcus* species.

Case 4: Owl with Oral Lesions

Signalment

Adult great horned owl (*Bubo virginianus*)

History

Recent acquisition to a raptor rehabilitation facility and presented for evaluation of large masses in the oral cavity.

Physical Examination

The owl was alert but mildly lethargic. Two large masses were seen in the choanal slit in the oral cavity (Figure 16.6). Manipulation of the lesions revealed caseous material, a sample of which was obtained for cytodiagnosis (Figures 16.7a and 16.7b).

Interpretive Discussion

An impression smear of the sample stained with Wright–Giemsa–Romanowsky stain revealed numerous heterophils (often degenerate) and piriform-shaped organisms with pale blue, somewhat foamy, cytoplasm. The organisms contained an eosinophilic nucleus, axostyle, and flagella that occur at the nuclear end of the cell. An eosinophilic undulating membrane could be occasionally seen. The cytology indicates trichomoniasis with pyogranulomatous inflammation.

Summary

In raptors, trichomoniasis is typically associated with *Trichomonas gallinae*. The owl was placed on supportive care along with a 5-day metronidazole treatment for the trichomonads and a 10-day treatment with a broad-spectrum antibiotic to protect the bird against opportunistic bacterial pathogens. The lesions disappeared within 10 days, and the owl fully recovered. It was released back into the wild a month later.

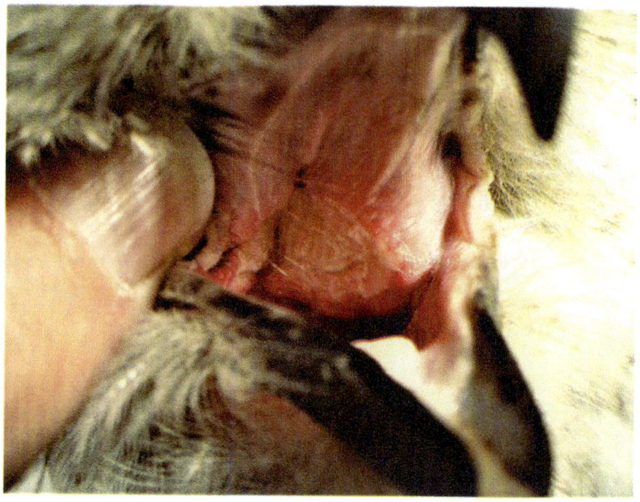

Fig. 16.6. Gross lesion in oral cavity.

Case 5: Hawk with Skin Lesions

Signalment

Adult male red-tailed hawk (*Buteo jamaicensis*)

History

The hawk was a recent acquisition to a raptor rehabilitation facility and presented for evaluation of numerous raised skin lesions on the feet and face.

Physical Examination

The hawk was alert but lethargic. He was mildly underweight owing to a slight reduction of the pectoral muscle mass. Multiple raised and sometimes crusty and ulcerated cutaneous lesions involved the feet, the lateral commissures of the mouth, and eyelids (Figures 16.8a and 16.8b).

A complete blood profile, a serum protein electrophoresis, and a fine-needle aspiration of one of the foot lesions for cytology were performed (Tables 16.5–16.7; Figures 16.9a–16.9c, 16.10a, and 16.10b).

Interpretive Discussion

The hemogram revealed a marked leukocytosis with heterophilia, monocytosis, and marked eosinophilia. There was moderate heterophil toxicity (Figures 16.9a and 16.9b). The marked eosinophilia was unusual and likely represented misinterpretation of toxic heterophils as eosinophils. The leukogram indicated a severe inflammatory response, and the presence of toxic heterophils provided a poor prognosis.

(a) (b)

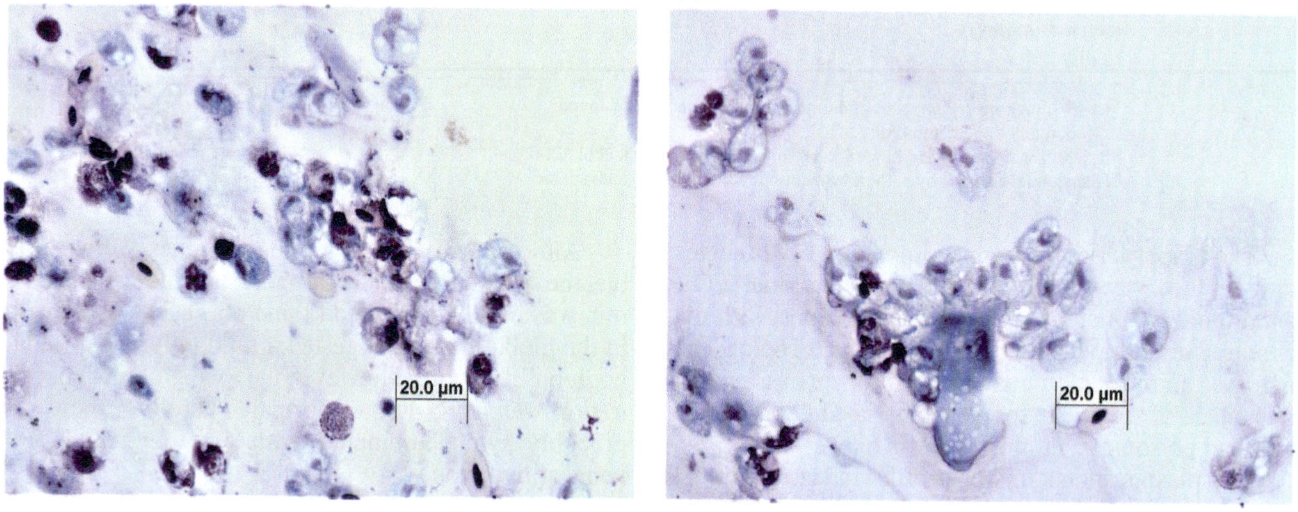

Fig. 16.7. (a), (b) Impression smear of the sample (Wright–Giemsa stain, 100× oil).

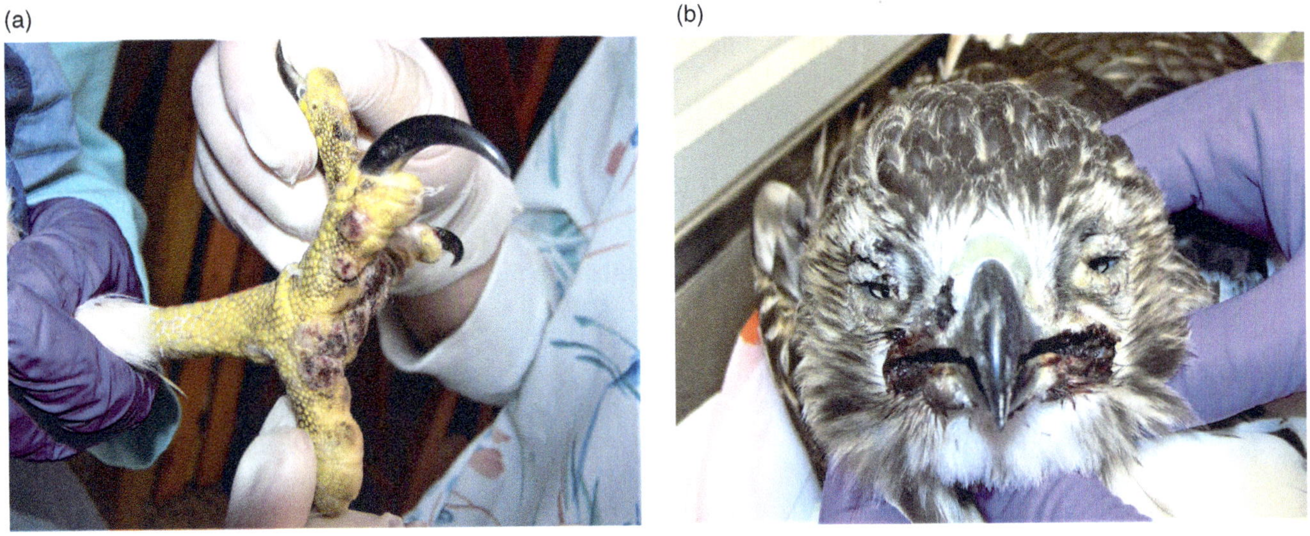

Fig. 16.8. (a) Gross lesions on feet. (b) Gross lesions on face.

Table 16.5. Hawk hematology results (Case 5).

		Reference[a]	Decision level[b]
PCV (%)*	36	31–43	35–55
Leukocytes			
WBC (×10³/μL)	116.6	19.1–33.4	5.0–20.0
Heterophils (×10³/μL)**	35.0	—	2.1–10.0
(%)	30	—	—
Lymphocytes (×10³/μL)	8.2	—	1.7–10.0
(%)	7	—	—
Monocytes (×10³/μL)	2.3	—	0–0.7
(%)	2	—	—
Eosinophils (×10³/μL)	71.1	—	0–0.4
(%)	61	—	—
Basophils (×10³/μL)	0	—	0–0.4
(%)	0	—	—
Thrombocytes			
Estimated number	Adequate	1–5/1000× field	
Morphology	Normal, clumped		
Plasma protein (refractometry)			
(g/dL)	4.6		3–5

* Many immature erythrocytes and mitotic erythrocytes can be found.
** Moderately toxic heterophils.
[a] Ranges for the red-tailed hawk (*Buteo jamaicensis*). Pollack et al. (2005).
[b] Decision levels used by authors when reference values are unavailable.

The inappropriate release of immature erythrocytes with erythrocyte mitotic figures with a normal PCV could represent increased erythropoiesis along with the increased granulopoiesis (Figures 16.9b and 16.9c). The increased number of immature erythrocytes associated with a lack of significant polychromasia could also indicate lead poisoning, but this was less likely.

The plasma biochemistry profile appeared normal except for a hypokalemia that was likely associated with decreased dietary intake.

Although no normal reference values were available, the serum protein electrophoresis indicated the albumin was mildly decreased (Table 16.7). The asymmetry in the globulin area suggested a mild polyclonal immunoglobulin response; however, the total globulin concentration was likely low or normal. Therefore, there was probably hypoalbuminemia with some degree of antigenic stimulation.

The aspirate of the mass sample stained with Wright–Giemsa–Romanowsky stain revealed swollen

Table 16.6. Hawk plasma biochemical results (Case 5).

		Reference[a]
Glucose (mg/dL)	365	292–390
BUN (mg/dL)	4	—
Uric acid (mg/dL)	7.1	8.1–16.8
Total protein (biuret) (g/dL)	3.8	3.9–6.7
Albumin (g/dL)	0.7	—
Globulin (g/dL)	2.3	—
Aspartate aminotransferase IU/L)	259	76–492
Creatine kinase (IU/L)	644	—
Calcium (mg/dL)	9.2	10.0–12.8
Phosphorus (mg/dL)	5.7	1.9–4.0
Sodium (mEq/L)	158	143–162
Potassium (mEq/L)	1.8	2.6–4.3
Chloride (mEq/L)	116	118–129
Bicarbonate (mEq/L)	19.1	—
Anion gap (calculated)	25	—
Calculated osmolality	319	—

[a]Pollack et al. (2005).

squamous epithelial cells containing one or more large cytoplasmic vacuoles that push the cell nucleus to the margin of the cell. This ballooning degeneration of squamous epithelial cells was indicative of avian pox.

Summary

The hawk was placed on supportive care along with treatment with a broad-spectrum antibiotic. Avian pox is frequently a self-limiting disease, and an inflammatory

Table 16.7. Hawk protein electrophoresis results (Case 5).

Total protein (g/dL)	4.0
A/G	1.32
Albumin, 33% (g/dL)	0.7
Alpha 1, 1.6% (g/dL)	0.06
Alpha 2, 9.9% (g/dL)	0.40
Beta, 12.1 (g/dL)	0.48
Gamma, 43.3 (g/dL)	1.74

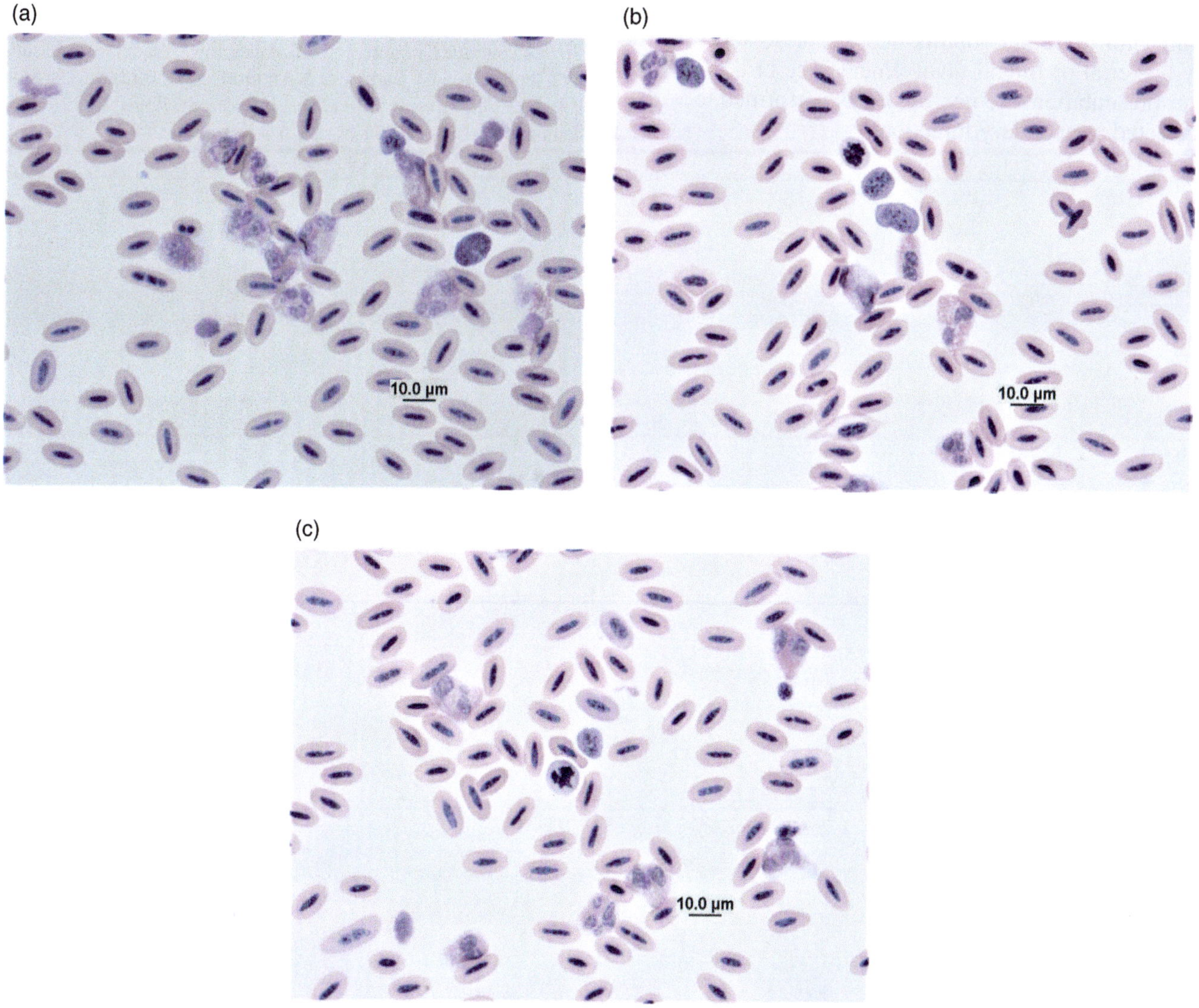

Fig. 16.9. (a)–(c) Blood film (Wright–Giemsa stain, 100× oil).

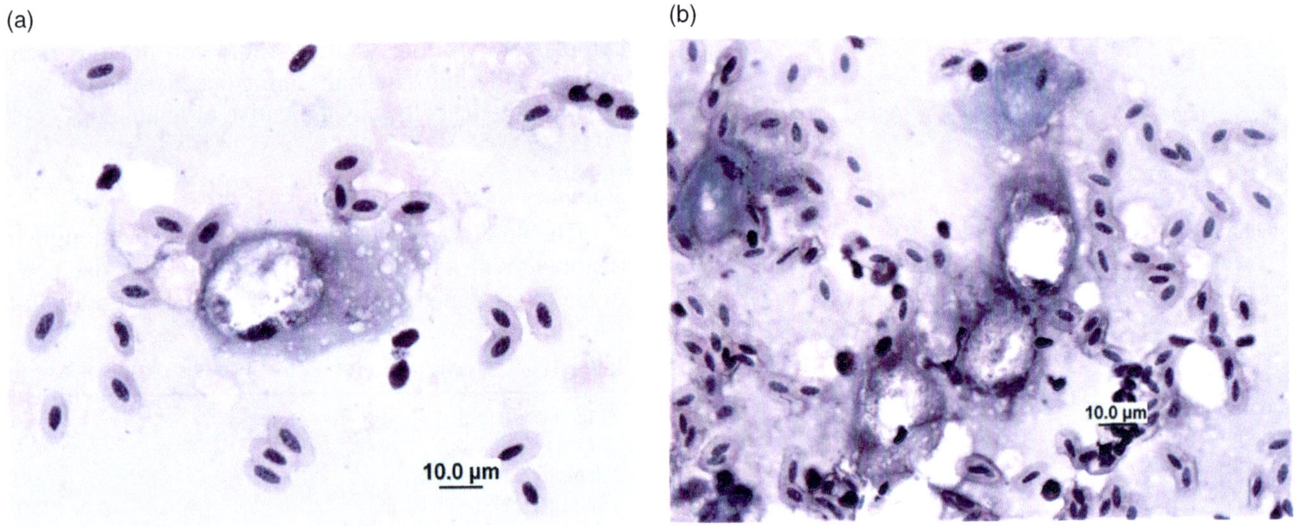

Fig. 16.10. (a), (b) Fine-needle aspiration cytology of a foot lesion (Wrights-Giemsa stain, 100× oil).

response does not typically accompany the disease; however, in this case, the severe inflammatory leukogram with toxic heterophils likely represented secondary bacterial or fungal involvement. The bird died 48 h after presentation. No necropsy was performed to verify suspected a secondary infection.

References

Campbell TW, Ellis CK. 2007. *Avian and Exotic Animal Hematology and Cytology*, 3 rd edn. Ames, Iowa: Blackwell Publishing.

Pollack, C, JW Carpenter, N Antinoff. 2005. Birds. In: Carpenter J (ed), *Exotic Animal Formulary*, 3rd edn. St. Louis, MO: Elsevier Saunders, p. 268 and 277.

SECTION III

Herptile

17 Blood and Bone Marrow Sample Collection and Preparation in Reptiles and Amphibians

For the chapters in this section (Section III, "Herptiles"), it is noteworthy that the animals discussed here include reptiles (of orders Testudines or Chelonia, Squamata, and Crocodilia) and amphibians (of orders Anura and Caudata).

Blood Sample Collection

General Considerations

Diagnostic testing, such as hematology, biochemistry profiles, or cytology, is useful for evaluating the reptile or amphibian patient. These diagnostic tests may be used as baseline information for apparently healthy individuals or to evaluate health status, disease progression, or prognosis against reliable sources or established reference intervals. When using reference intervals, it is important to note that many intrinsic and extrinsic factors can influence parameters in reptiles and amphibians; therefore, care should be exercised during comparison.

Blood samples for hematologic and blood biochemical studies can be collected from reptiles by a variety of methods depending upon the peculiarities of the species, volume of blood needed, size of the reptile, physical condition of the patient, and preference of the collector. The site of blood sample collection will influence the hematologic values because lymphatic vessels often accompany blood vessels in reptiles; frequently a mixture of blood and lymph occurs with venipuncture of peripheral vessels (Gottdenker and Jacobson, 1995; Crawshaw, 1996). Lymph often appears as transparent fluid entering the syringe immediately prior to the appearance of blood. If this occurs, discard the syringe and attempt sample collection again. The quantity of lymphatic fluid that mixes with the blood sample is variable and will dilute the cellular components of the blood, resulting in lower packed cell volume (PCV), hemoglobin concentration (Hb), erythrocyte count (TRBC), and leukocyte count (TWBC) (Gottdenker and Jacobson, 1995).

The use of a general anesthetic may be required as a method of restraint for blood collection in some reptiles, such as chelonians that can hide within their carapace and plastron. Ketamine hydrochloride used alone or in combination with xylazine or midazolam are commonly used anesthetics for this purpose. It has been shown that this anesthetic does not affect the hemogram in red-eared sliders (*Trachemys scripta elegans*) (Holz and Holz, 1994). Anesthetic agents, such as alfaxalone, midazolam, and dexmedetomidine, have also been used in snakes for minor procedures like venipuncture (Yaw et al., 2020).

Some amphibians may be manually restrained for blood collection, and others may require sedation or anesthesia. Submersion of the amphibian in a 0.05% solution of tricaine methanesulfonate (Tricaine, MS222, Sigma Chemical Co., St. Louis, MO) is one method of restraint that may be considered for use in blood sample collection of amphibian patients. Moistened powder-free nitrile gloves should be worn when handling amphibians for examination, restraint, or blood collection in order to protect their skin. Small-gauge needles and small syringes are typically used to collect blood samples from amphibians. Consequently, blood flow into the syringe is usually slow. Many amphibian patients are small, making it necessary to use microhematocrit

Exotic Animal Hematology and Cytology, Fifth Edition. Terry W. Campbell and Krystan R. Grant.

Companion website: www.wiley.com/go/campbell/exotic

tubes with inner diameters that are smaller than regular hematocrit tubes in order to obtain a PCV. Use of these small microhematocrit tubes will also help maximize the amount of hematologic testing that can be performed on small blood samples.

Blood Volume Collection

Reptiles

The total blood volume of reptiles is estimated to range between 5% and 8% of the body weight. For example, the total blood volume of desert tortoises (*Gopherus polyphemus*), a freshwater turtle (*Chelydra serpentina*), and marine turtles is 4.9–7.2%, 3.8–5.6%, and 5.2–7.9% of the body weight, respectively (Thorson, 1968a, 1968b). Most reptile species can tolerate withdrawal of up to 10% of the total blood volume (1% of the body weight) without detrimental effects (Jacobson, 1993a; Sykes and Klaphake, 2015). The maximum blood sample volume recommended for collection from chelonians is 3 mL/kg body weight (Wilkinson, 2004). Typically, only 0.2–0.3 mL of blood is required for routine hematologic studies; most reptiles will tolerate this loss. A summary of collection sites is listed in Table 17.1.

Amphibians

The approximate blood volume of many species of aquatic amphibians ranges between 13% and 25%, and ranges between 7% and 10% for most terrestrial amphibians (Thorson, 1964; Boutilier et al., 1992; Wright, 2001). In general, it is considered "safe" to draw a blood sample equaling 1% of the total body weight of an individual amphibian at one time. Sites for blood collection include the ventral abdominal vein, ventral caudal vein, heart, femoral, and lingual vein (Table 17.1).

Table 17.1. Blood collection sites for select herptiles.

Herptile	Collection sites
Chelonians	Jugular vein Dorsal or ventral coccygeal (tail) vein Subcarapacial sinus Supravertebral sinus (sea turtles)
Lizards	Jugular vein Ventral coccygeal (tail) vein Ventral abdominal vein
Snakes	Dorsal vertebral vein Ventral coccygeal (tail) vein Cardiac
Crocodilians	Supravertebral sinus Ventral coccygeal (tail) vein
Amphibians	Ventral coccygeal (tail) vein Ventral abdominal vein Femoral vein Lingual vein Facial vein

Sources: Campbell (2015); Heatley and Russell (2020).

Restraint and Collection Sites

Chelonians

The challenge with chelonians is their ability to retract into their shell. Before handling, the approach for isolating the anatomy for venipuncture and blood sample collection should be determined considering the safety of the handlers and the animal. For example, many turtles have a strong bite (e.g., snapping turtles, *Chelydra* spp., and *Macrochelys* spp.), and caution should be taken by distracting them or restraining their head (Figure 17.1).

Jugular venipuncture can be used to collect blood from reptiles, especially chelonians (turtles and tortoises), and is the preferred site of blood collection by some authors (Gottdenker and Jacobson, 1995; Jenkins, 1996; Lloyd and Morris, 1999).

The jugular vein of certain species of tortoises (e.g., desert tortoise (*Gopherus agassizii*)) may be visible; however, this vein is rarely visible in most species. Some species of chelonians have dorsal and ventral jugular veins that lie on either side of a large cervical lymphatic vessel (superficial jugular trunk), and the right jugular vein may be larger than the left in some species of reptile (Jenkins, 1996; Barrows et al., 2004). Chelonians may be restrained by an assistant with the head and neck extended to expose the lateral aspect of the neck (Figure 17.2). Chemical restraint may be required to aid

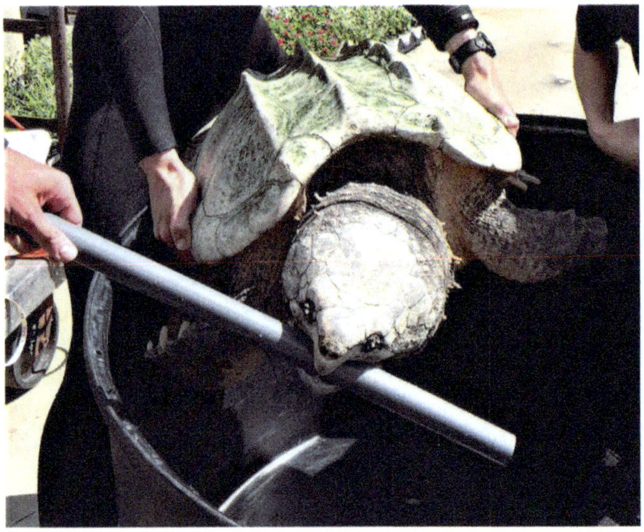

Fig. 17.1. Restraining an alligator snapping turtle (*Macrochelys temminckii*) and distracting the bite with a heavy-duty pipe.

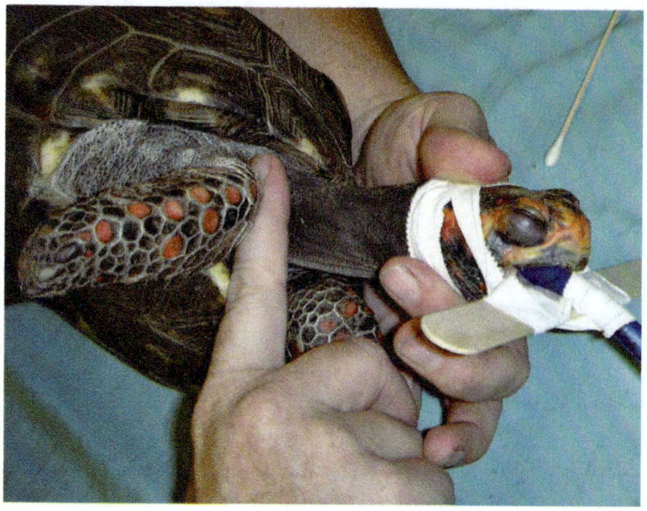

Fig. 17.2. An anesthetized red-footed tortoise (*Chelonoidis carbonaria*) in preparation for a jugular catheter. The head is extended, and pressure is applied to the thoracic inlet to encourage the vessel to fill for visualization.

in sample collection in some chelonians. The jugular vein (or veins) courses caudally in a line extending from the angle of the mandible to the cranial carapacial inlet. The dorsal jugular vein extends from the dorsal edge of the tympanic membrane to the carapacial inlet when present. The jugular veins are relatively superficial; deep insertion of a needle may result in sample collection from the carotid artery (Jacobson et al., 1992).

Placement of a polyurethane central catheter provides long-term venous access that allows for serial blood sampling and administration of medications, anesthetic agents, and fluids in chelonians. This can be accomplished by suturing in place a 4 Fr. 13-cm polyurethane double-lumen central venous catheter that has been inserted using a modified Seldinger technique, which allows placement of a 0.018-in.-diameter wire, over which the polyurethane catheter is guided in place (Pardo and Divers, 2016). The appropriate length of the catheter is determined by measuring from the point of entry into the jugular vein to the cranial border of the pectoral scutes (this allows the catheter to be cranial to the heart).

A dorsal coccygeal venous sinus (dorsal coccygeal vein) is present in many species of chelonians and is located on the dorsal midline of the tail. Blood collected from this site is often diluted with lymph (Marks and Citino, 1990; Jacobson et al., 1992). Venipuncture requires an assistant to restrain the chelonian. Insert a 22–25-gauge needle attached to a 1–3 mL syringe on the dorsal midline at the base of the tail at a 30–60° angle (Knotkova et al., 2002) (Figures 17.3a–17.3d).

The subcarapacial (subvertebral) venous sinus may be used for blood collection in chelonians (Hernandez-Divers et al., 2001, 2002). The subcarapacial venous sinus is located caudal to the nuchal scute at the level of the eighth cervical vertebra, and is made up of a collection of blood vessels (internal jugular vein, anterior pulmonic vein and artery, vertebral veins and arteries, and subclavian veins and arteries) and lymphatic vessels (Hernandez-Divers et al., 2002; Barrows et al., 2004). Blood collected from this site may not be adequate for hematologic evaluation because marked dilution with lymphatic fluid may occur (Barrows et al., 2004). For sample collection, insert a needle dorsal to the neck at the carapacial inlet and angle it up toward the ventral aspect of the carapace (Figures 17.4a and 17.4b). This can be performed with the head and neck extended or retracted. If the needle touches bone (either a vertebra or the carapace) before blood enters the syringe, withdraw the needle slightly and redirect it caudally. The major lymphatic vessels are located cranial to the venous sinus; therefore, subsequent attempts at sample collection should be made caudal to the site of the first attempt (Barrows et al., 2004).

The supravertebral sinus (dorsal cervical venous, post-occipital, or occipital sinus) is a common location for obtaining blood samples in sea turtles (Campbell, 1996, 2012; Whitaker and Krum, 1999; Wyneken et al., 2006). With the neck extended and the head held downward slightly, the sinus can be located just lateral to the cervical vertebrae. The sinus is approached by inserting the needle into the neck at a location one-third the distance from the base of the head to the carapace and one-third the distance from the dorsal midline to the lateral edge of the neck (Campbell, 1996) (Figure 17.5). This site can also be located sonographically, after which an ultrasound-guided technique is used to insert the needle (Figure 17.6). This site can also be used for blood collection in freshwater turtles. A 20–22-gauge, 1–1.5-inch needle is inserted at a 30° angle, and the blood sample is collected with a syringe or evacuated tube. While the head is restrained, the needle is inserted just lateral to the dorsal midline on the right side of the neck (Martinez Silvestre et al., 2002).

Lizards

The approach to restraining a lizard for venipuncture considers safety for the handler(s) and the animals and is consistent with the approach during physical examinations (Divers, 2019a). The primary weapons of the lizards, in general, are their bite, claws, and tails. Items often used to assist with restraint include towels, tape, or other bandaging materials.

Jugular venipuncture is a useful method for obtaining blood samples from large lizards, such as green iguanas (*Iguana iguana*) and monitor lizards (*Varanus* spp.). One advantage of jugular venipuncture is that the chances of sample hemodilution with lymphatic fluid are minimized owing to the size of the vessels.

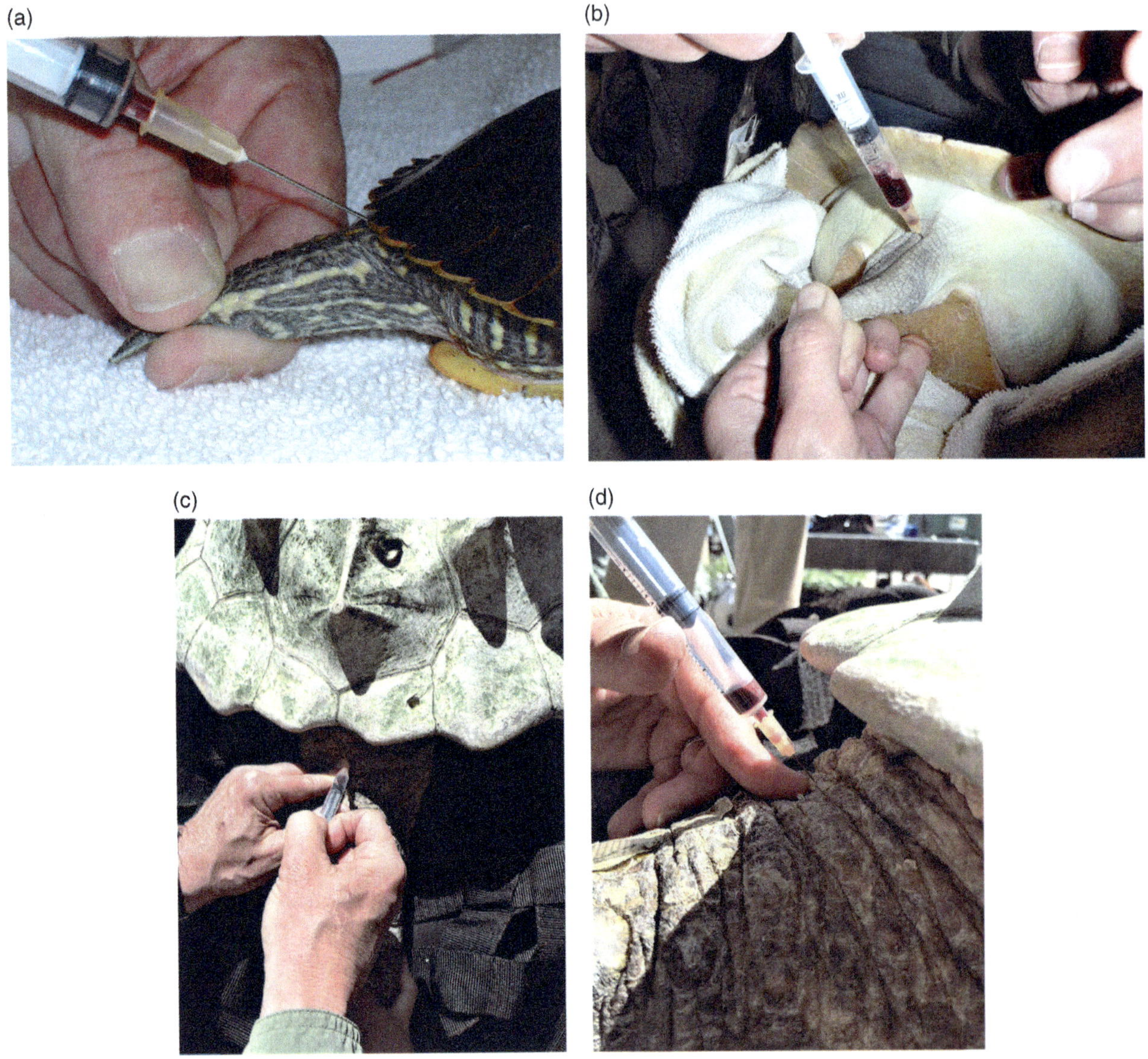

Fig. 17.3. Obtaining blood from the dorsal coccygeal venous sinus of a(n) (a) red-eared slider (*Trachemys scripta elegans*), (b) New Guinea snapping turtle (*Elseya novaeguineae*), (c) alligator snapping turtle (*Macrochelys temminckii*) dorsal view, and (d) alligator snapping turtle (*Macrochelys temminckii*) lateral view.

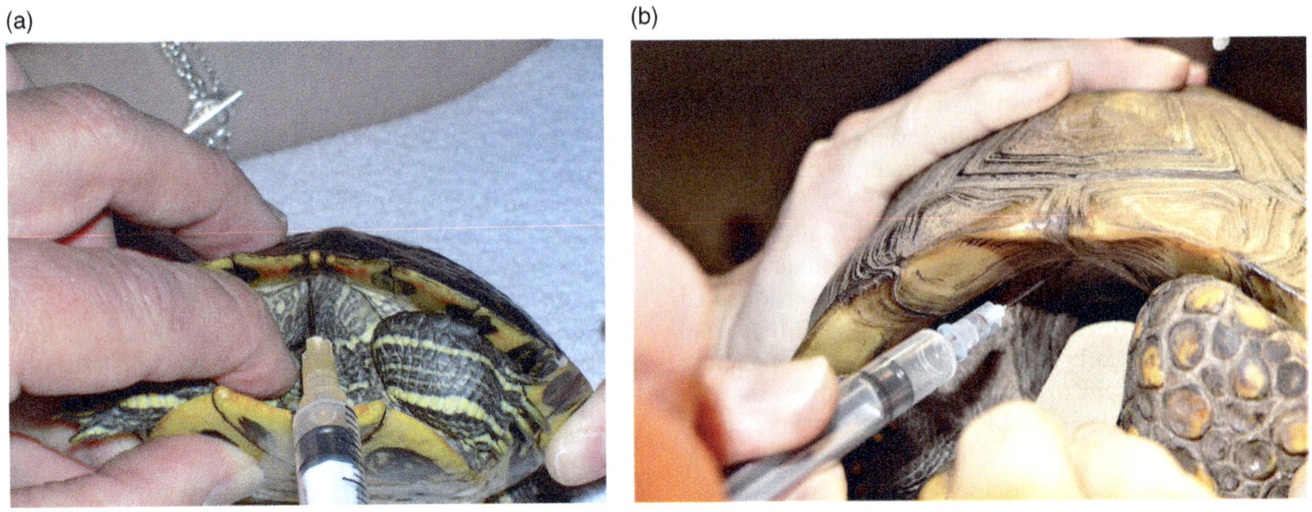

Fig. 17.4. Obtaining blood from the subcarapacial (subvertebral) venous sinus of a (a) red-eared slider (*Trachemys scripta elegans*) and a (b) yellow-footed tortoise (*Chelonoidis denticulata*) while using a tongue depressor to hold the head inside the shell.

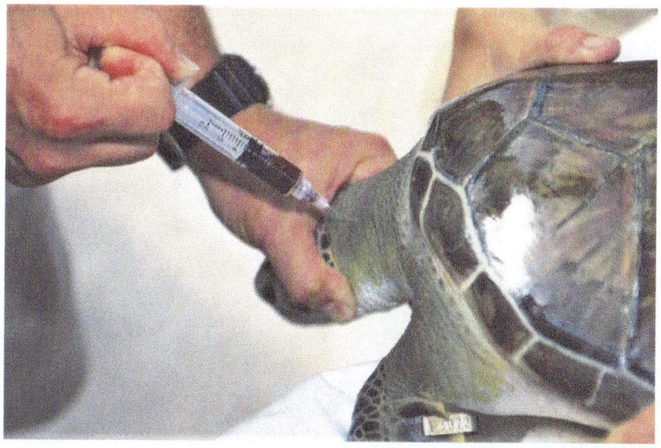

Fig. 17.5. Obtaining blood from the supravertebral sinus of a juvenile sea turtle (*Chelonia mydas*) by inserting the needle into the neck at a location one-third the distance from the base of the head to the carapace and one-third the distance from the dorsal midline to the lateral edge of the neck.

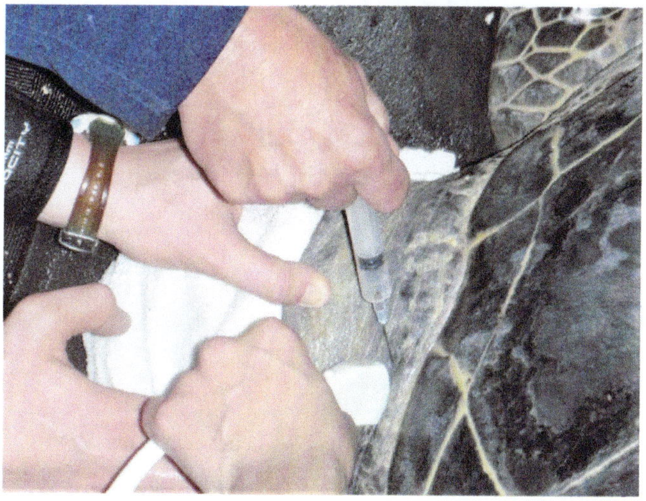

Fig. 17.6. Obtaining blood from the supravertebral sinus of a green sea turtle (*Chelonia mydas*) using an ultrasound-guided technique.

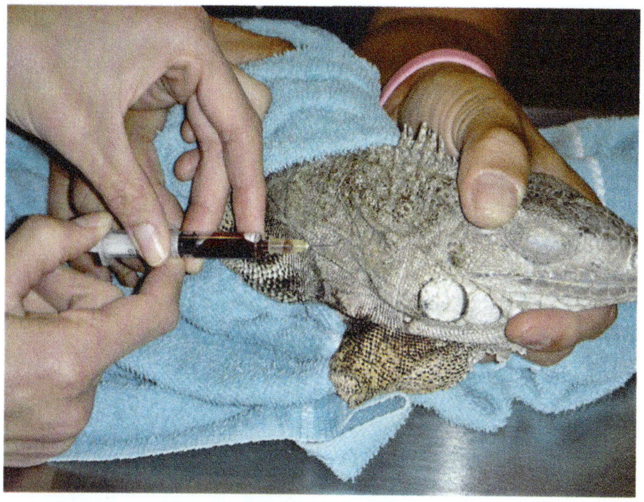

Fig. 17.7. Jugular venipuncture is approached blindly by directing the needle along a line that runs behind the tympanum along the stretched neck of a green iguana (*Iguana iguana*).

The jugular vein of lizards lies deep along the lateral aspect of the neck. The vein is rarely visible and is approached blindly by directing the needle along a line that runs behind the tympanum along the stretched neck of the lizard held in lateral recumbency (Figure 17.7). The right jugular vein is generally larger than the left, which is an aid to blood collection.

The caudal vein (ventral tail vein) lies just ventral to the caudal vertebrae and is a common site for blood collection in lizards (Jacobson, 1993a, 1993b). Lizards can be restrained for this procedure by holding them vertically, by allowing them to cling to a cage door, or by allowing the lizard to sit on a table with the tail extending over the edge. Blood samples may be collected using a 22–23-gauge, 1-inch needle inserted under a ventral scale on the ventral midline and directed toward the vertebrae (Figures 17.8a–17.8c). These methods of restraint are better tolerated by the reptile compared to restraining them in dorsal recumbency. A lateral approach can also be used by inserting the needle along the middle of the lateral aspect of the tail in an area where a natural groove or line created by muscles in the tail occurs (Figure 17.9). The needle tip should be placed just beneath the caudal vertebra and into the vein. It should be noted that some lizards have tail autotomy (the ability to quickly shed the tail, usually as a defensive mechanism); therefore, part of the tail could be lost during the mishandling of these lizards for blood collection.

Lizards also have a large ventral abdominal vein present on the ventral midline of the abdomen. This vein is easily located and even seen in some species (Figure 17.10a), but can be easily lacerated, and hemostasis following venipuncture can be problematic. The needle is inserted through the ventral midline usually just cranial to the umbilicus in a cranial–dorsal direction to reach the vein just below the body wall (Figure 17.10b). The vein can be cannulated with a needle and blood collected from the needle hub into a microcollection tube or aspirated into a syringe.

Snakes

The primary weapon of snakes is their bite; therefore, controlling the head is necessary to ensure the safety of the animal and those involved with the procedure. Aggressive or venomous snakes should be restrained using a tube, contained, or sedated prior to the procedure (Figure 17.11). Handling techniques for snakes and other

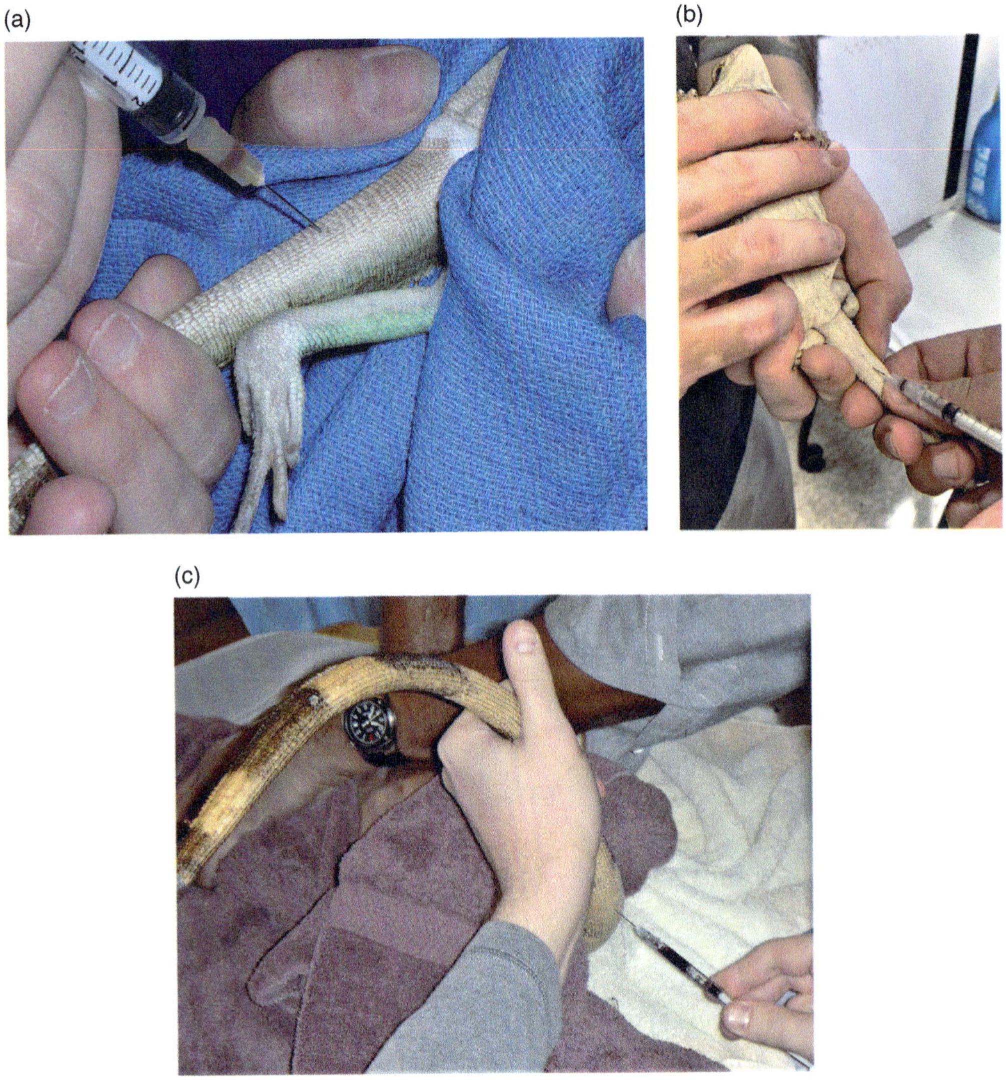

Fig. 17.8. (a) Venipuncture of the caudal vein using the ventral approach in a green iguana (*Iguana iguana*) being held in dorsal recumbency. (b) Venipuncture of the caudal vein using the ventral approach in a juvenile bearded dragon (*Pogona vitticeps*) being held to expose the ventral surface of the tail. (c) Venipuncture of the caudal vein using the ventral approach in a large green iguana (*Iguana iguana*) being restrained in ventral recumbency and lifting the tail to access the ventral aspect.

reptiles can be reviewed in more detail in other texts (Divers, 2019a).

The caudal vein (ventral tail vein) lies just ventral to the caudal vertebrae and is a common site for blood collection in large snakes (Jacobson, 1993a, 1993b). Blood samples may be collected using a 22–23-gauge, 1-inch needle inserted under a ventral scale on the ventral midline and directed toward the vertebrae (Figure 17.12). The location of the needle insertion should be some distance caudal to the vent (e.g., 25–50% of the distance from the vent to the tip of the tail in snakes) to avoid the hemipenes of males or musk glands of snakes (Divers, 2019b). Slight negative pressure should be applied to the syringe as the needle is advanced. If the needle contacts bone (a vertebra) before blood enters the needle, withdraw the needle slowly and change the direction of the needle (either cranially, caudally, left, or right) until blood flows into the syringe.

Cardiocentesis is commonly performed for blood collection from snakes. The exact location of the heart varies depending on the species, but in general lies in the cranial one-third of the body. With the snake held in dorsal recumbency, the heart is located by palpation, by observing the movement of the ventral scutes for heartbeats, or by use of a Doppler (Figures 17.13a and 17.13b). The heart can move cranially and caudally and should be stabilized at the apex and base during sample collection (Figure 17.13c) (Jacobson, 1993b). A 22–23-gauge needle attached to a 3–6-cc syringe needle is inserted under (not through) the scute and advanced into the heart (Figure 17.13d). The syringe typically fills slowly as the heart pulsates. Sedation of the snake prior to cardiocentesis is recommended to avoid excessive movement and possible cardiac trauma (Divers, 2019b).

A dorsal vertebral blood vessel can be used to obtain a blood sample from large boid snakes. With the back of the snake held in a tight flexed position, a needle is inserted between the vertebrae while negative pressure is applied to the syringe as the needle advances (Figure 17.14). Once blood enters the syringe, advancement of the needle is stopped, and blood is collected into the syringe.

Crocodilians

The caudal vein (ventral tail vein) lies just ventral to the caudal vertebrae and is a common site for blood collection in crocodilians (Jacobson, 1993a, 1993b). Crocodilians may be restrained on a tabletop, and either the ventral or lateral approach may be used. A lateral approach can also be used, especially in lizards and crocodilians, by inserting the needle along the middle of the lateral aspect of the tail in an area where a natural

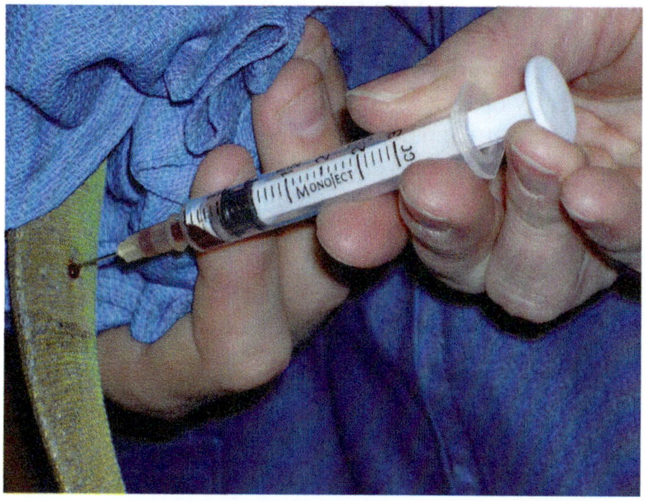

Fig. 17.9. Venipuncture of the caudal vein using the lateral approach in a green iguana (*Iguana iguana*).

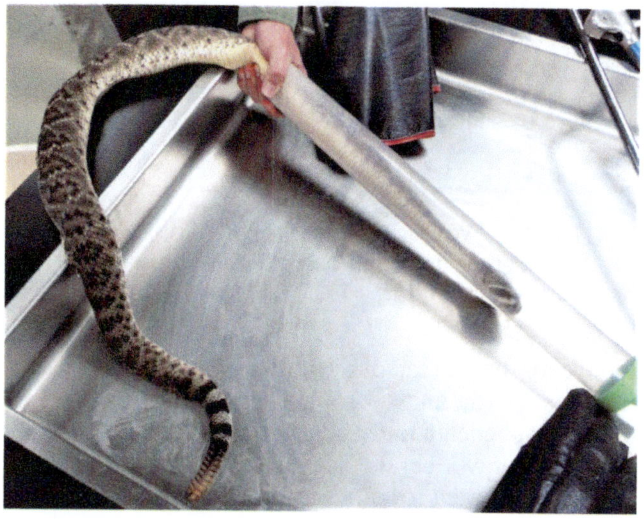

Fig. 17.11. Restraint of a venomous Western diamondback rattlesnake (*Crotalus atrox*) using a tube.

(a) (b)

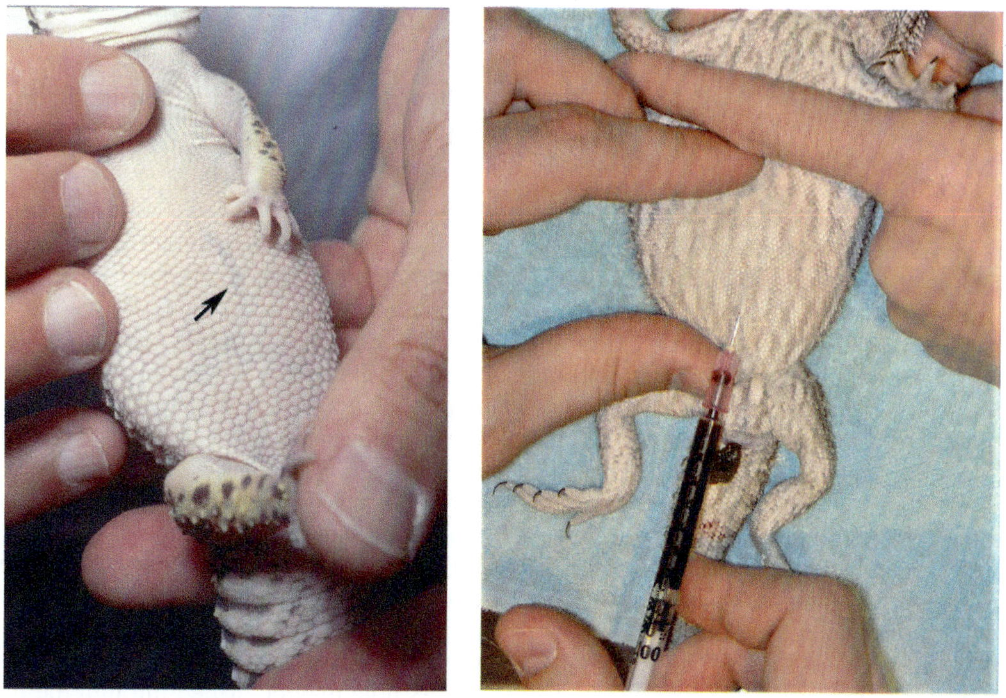

Fig. 17.10. (a) The ventral abdominal vein (arrow) seen through the skin of a leopard gecko (*Eublepharis macularius*). (b) Venipuncture of the ventral abdominal vein of a bearded dragon (*Pogona vitticeps*).

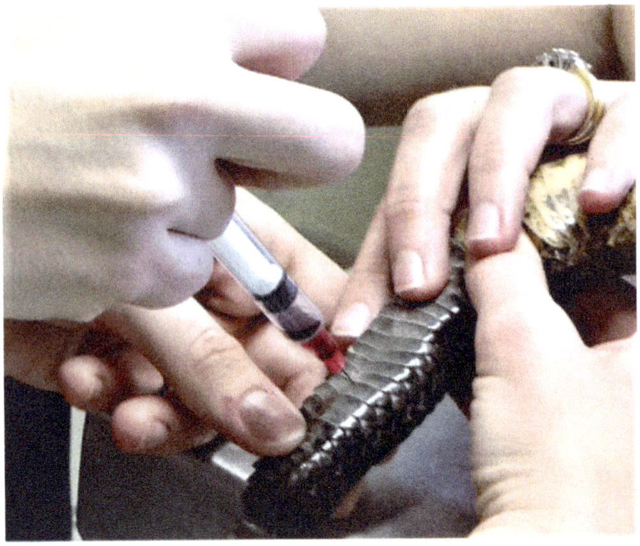

Fig. 17.12. Venipuncture of the caudal vein using the ventral approach in a timber rattlesnake (*Crotalus horridus*). Source: Photo courtesy of Joseph Tsang.

groove or line created by muscles in the tail occurs (Figures 17.15a and 17.15b). The needle tip should be placed just beneath the caudal vertebra and into the vein.

The supravertebral vein/sinus or post-occipital sinus is commonly used for blood collection in large crocodilians. The needle used for blood collection is inserted just behind the nuchal crest or occiput on the dorsal midline (Figure 17.16) (Olson et al., 1975; Myburgh et al., 2014). Slight negative pressure is applied to the syringe as the needle is advanced until the sinus is entered. Spinal trauma is possible if the needle is inserted too deeply (Divers, 2019b).

Amphibians

The ventral abdominal vein lies under the linea alba along the ventral midline of the coelomic cavity. Venipuncture is performed by inserting a 25–30-gauge needle in a craniodorsal direction midway along a line of sight extending from the sternum and pelvis (Figures 17.17a and 17.17b). A Doppler probe may be needed to locate this vein in species where the vein is not clearly visible. Blood may then be collected by the drip method or by aspiration of blood into a small syringe. Lymph contamination of the blood sample is not uncommon when blood is collected from the ventral abdominal vein, as the lymphatic vessels runs parallel, and may occur when venipuncture is performed from other blood vessels as well. Mixing of lymphatic fluid with the blood sample is variable and will dilute the cellular components of the blood, resulting in a lower PCV, hemoglobin concentration, and erythrocyte and leukocyte concentrations.

Venipuncture of the ventral caudal vein (ventral coccygeal vein, tail vein) may be used for blood collection from some species of salamanders and newts, and is performed in the same manner described for venipuncture of the ventral caudal vein in reptiles. This technique should not be performed in salamanders and newts that have tail autotomy (a natural ability to lose their tails) because their tails may break off during the procedure. The salamander or newt is held in dorsal recumbency to perform a venipuncture of the ventral coccygeal vein. A 25-gauge needle is inserted into the ventral midline of the tail and directed to a point just below the coccygeal vertebrae. The needle is then advanced while applying negative pressure to the syringe until blood can be aspirated into the syringe barrel.

Venipuncture of the lingual vein may be performed after gently opening the patient's mouth and moving the tongue forward and upward using a cotton tip applicator to expose the lingual venous plexus that lies on the ventral aspect of the tongue on the floor of the mouth (Baranowski-Smith and Smith, 1983) (Figure 17.18). Excess saliva must be swabbed from below the tongue prior to puncturing the largest vessel in the plexus with a 25- or 27-gauge needle to avoid contamination of the blood sample with fluid from the oral cavity (Wright, 2006; Forzan et al., 2017). Blood should be collected by the drip method into a microcollection tube or microhematocrit tube instead of by aspiration into a syringe in order to minimize the potential for hematoma formation. Amphibians must be handled delicately when performing this method of blood collection, and care must be taken to avoid fracture of the mandibular bones while holding the mouth open to collect blood from the lingual vein.

Other Collection Sites and Considerations

Reptiles

Blood may be collected from the ulnar (radiohumeral) venous sinus of reptiles (Rosskopf, 1982; Barrows et al., 2004). Blood is collected by extending the front leg of the reptile and inserting a needle at a perpendicular angle to the body behind the tendon that lies on the caudal aspect of the radiohumeral joint. Advance the needle toward the radiohumeral joint while applying gentle pressure to the attached syringe.

Cardiocentesis may be performed in other reptile species as well. Cardiocentesis of chelonians is performed by passing a needle through the plastron on the ventral midline at the junction of the humeral and pectoral scutes. A needle can be passed through the soft plastron of soft-shelled turtles (*Trionyx* spp.), neonates, or those affected by secondary nutritional hyperparathyroidism (Figure 17.19a) (Divers, 2019b). Otherwise, an access hole may be drilled through the plastron with an 18–20-gauge needle in small chelonians; a sterile drill bit may be required for larger chelonians (Mautino and

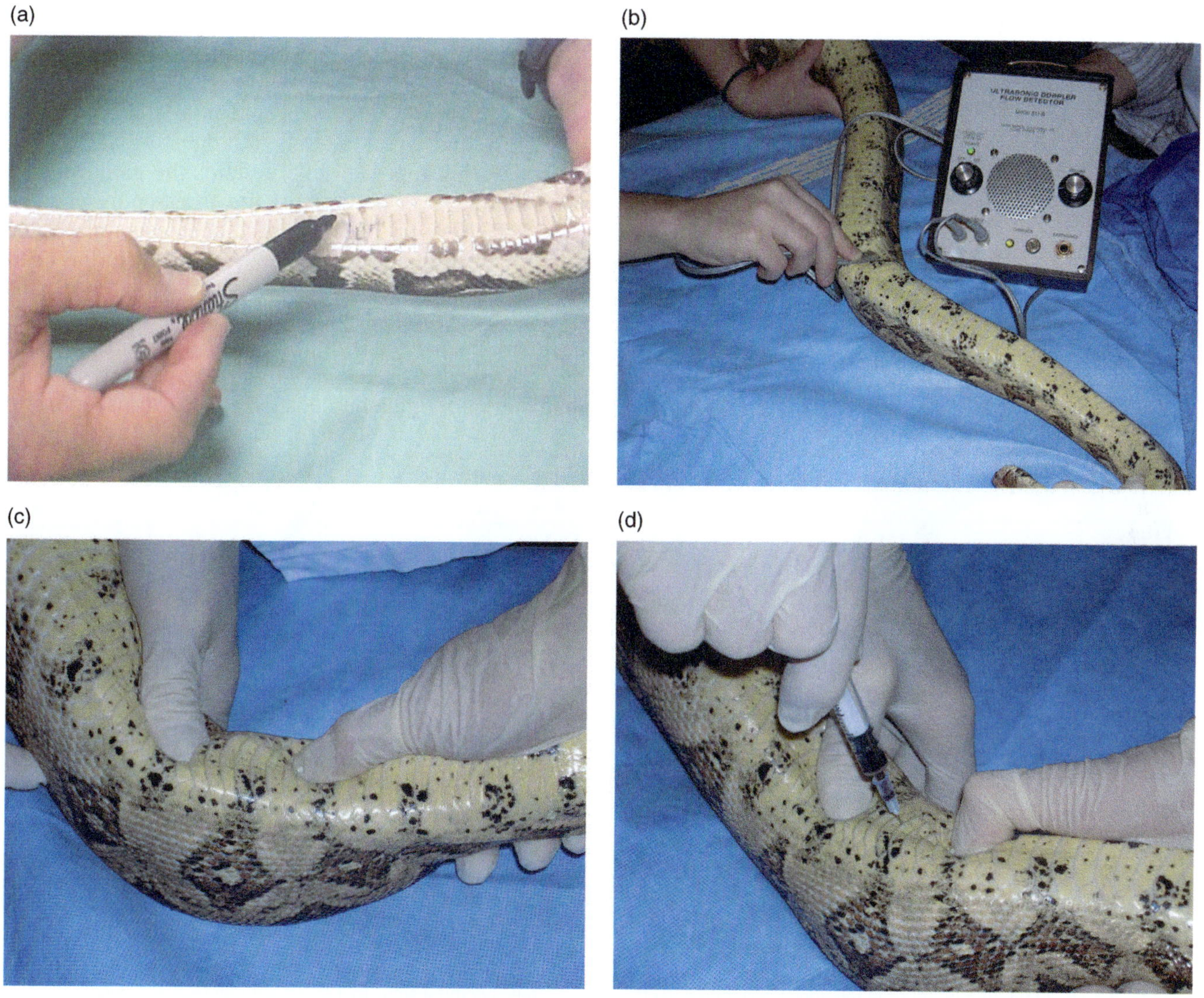

Fig. 17.13. (a) Obtaining blood via cardiocentesis from a common boa (*Boa constrictor*) begins with locating the heart, which can be visualized by the movement of the overlying scutes. Once the heart has been located, its position can be tagged by making a mark over the ventral scutes that overlie the heart. (b) A Doppler can be used to locate the heart of a common boa (*Boa constrictor*) if the heartbeat cannot be visualized. (c) Once the heart of the common boa (*Boa constrictor*) has been located, it should be held in position before performing a cardiocentesis to prevent the heart from moving away from the advancing needle. (d) Blood is collected from the heart of the common boa (*Boa constrictor*) by inserting the needle between the ventral scutes and advancing it into the heart.

Page, 1993). Following sample collection, the hole should be sealed with an epoxy. If multiple samples are required, a larger hole can be drilled through the plastron and plugged with a rubber stopper from a blood collection tube (Johnson et al., 1998) (Figure 17.19b). The rubber stopper must then be sealed in position with epoxy, and serves as an access port to the heart for blood collection (Campbell, 2012, 2022). Cardiocentesis is not recommended for routine blood collection from lizard species.

Other less commonly used blood collection sites include the brachial vein or artery, the palatine-pterygoid vein, and toenails. Blood collection from the brachial vein or artery is a blind approach and may be attempted in chelonians or lizards. Samples obtained by this method are often diluted with lymph, although blood collected from this site in tortoises may be more reliable for hematologic study than blood collected from the dorsal coccygeal vein (Marks and Citino, 1990; Jackson, 1991; Jacobson et al., 1992; Gottdenker and Jacobson, 1995; Lopez-Olvera et al., 2003). Blood can be collected from the palatine-pterygoid veins in the oral cavity of medium- to large-sized snakes, but will require general anesthesia or an extremely cooperative patient. These veins are fragile and easily lacerated. Blood can be collected by syringe or by allowing the blood to flow from the needle hub into a microcollection tube. Blood collected from capillary beds (toenails) do not provide optimal samples for hematologic studies, but may be the only procedure available for blood collection in very small reptiles (<30 g). The humane and ethical aspects of toenail clipping should be considered as this method causes pain and trauma to the patient and other locations are available (Mader, 1998; Divers, 2019b).

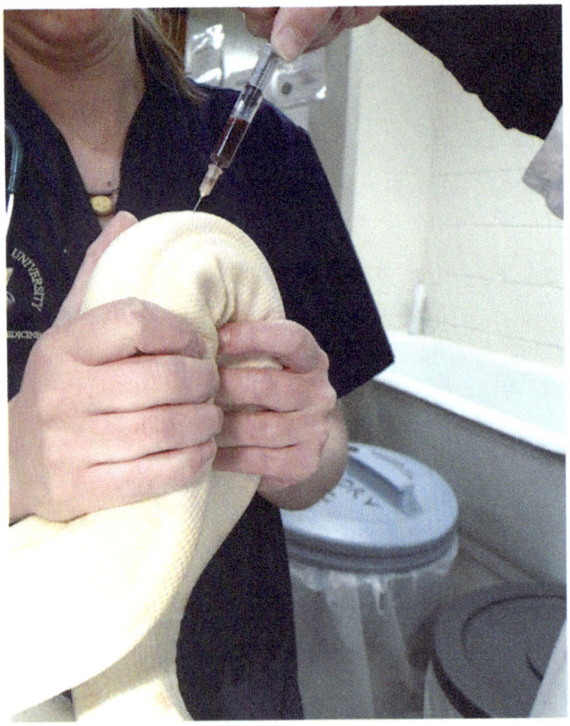

Fig. 17.14. Obtaining blood from the dorsal vertebral vessels from a common boa (*Boa constrictor*).

Amphibians

Cardiocentesis in amphibians often requires sedation or general anesthesia using tricaine methanesulfonate to prevent movement and potential damage to the heart and great vessels (Cathers et al., 1997). Although this approach likely yields the greatest sample volume, it is potentially life-threatening (Forzan et al., 2017). To perform cardiocentesis, place the amphibian in dorsal recumbency, and locate the heart by visualization of the pulsing heart as it raises and lowers the skin, use of a Doppler probe, or by transillumination. Internal illumination of the heart may also be performed in some amphibians by passing a small-diameter cool light source, such as an arthroscope, into

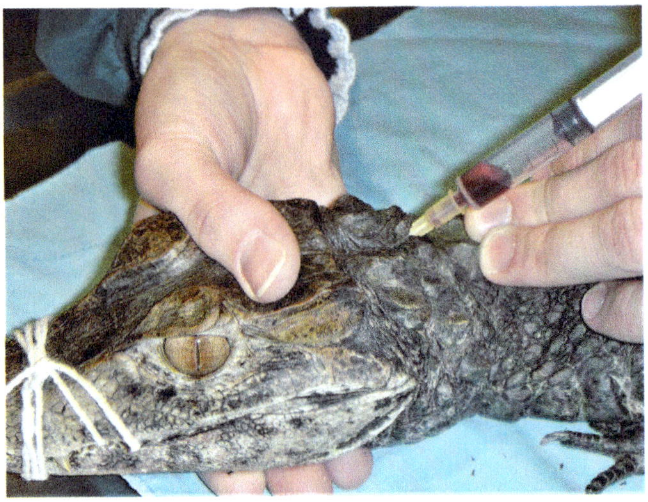

Fig. 17.16. Venipuncture of the supravertebral vein or post-occipital sinus in a dwarf caiman (*Paleosuchus palpebrosus*).

(a) (b)

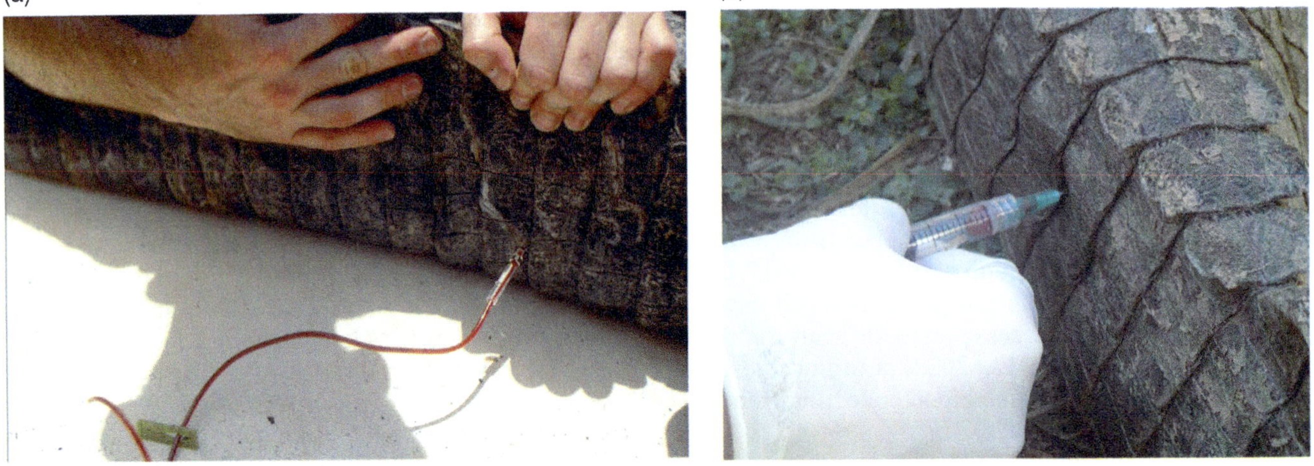

Fig. 17.15. (a) Venipuncture of the caudal vein using the lateral approach in an American alligator (*Alligator mississippiensis*). (b) Venipuncture of the caudal vein using the lateral approach in a caiman (*Caiman crocodiles*).

(a) (b)

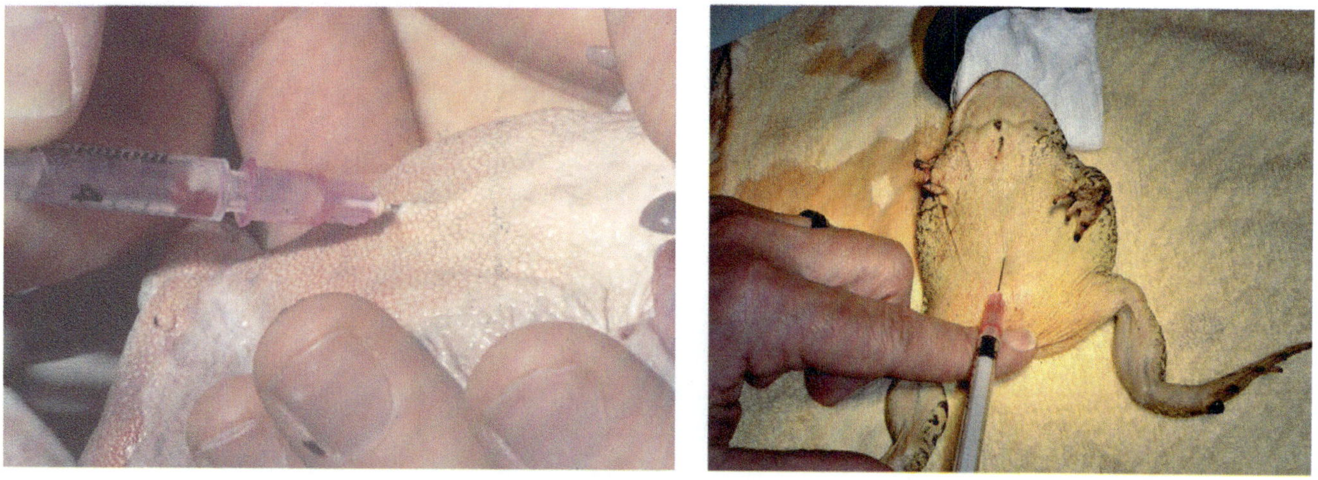

Fig. 17.17. (a) Obtaining blood from the ventral abdominal vein of a green tree frog (*Litoria caerulea*). (b) Obtaining blood from the ventral abdominal vein of an anesthetized Woodhouse's toad (*Bufo woodhousii*).

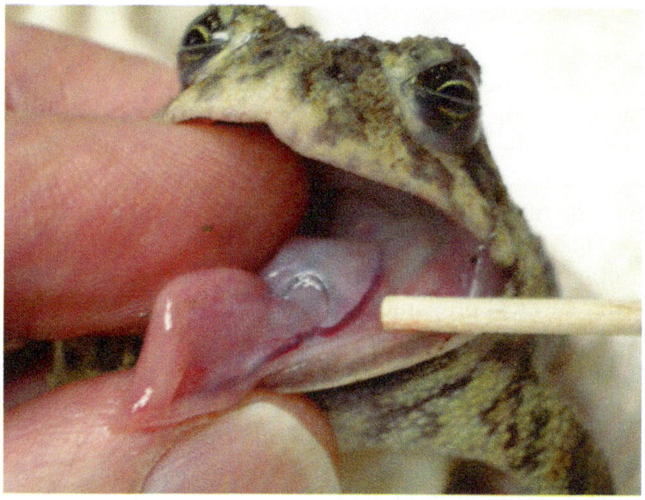

Fig. 17.18. Lingual vein of a Woodhouse's toad (*Bufo woodhousii*).

the stomach (Wright, 2001). Once you locate the heart, insert a 25-gauge needle into the ventricle and aspirate blood into the syringe.

Other methods of amphibian blood collection that are commonly used in field research studies include tail amputation and digit amputation. Collection of blood using these methods is not recommended for clinical practice, and should not be employed as a means of blood collection. They are painful procedures and yield small sample volumes (Forzan et al., 2017).

Blood Sample Handling and Preparation

Anticoagulant

The sample volume collected will help in determining testing prioritization and therefore sample processing. For example, if a very small sample volume is collected, a drop should be used to make a blood film. Larger or adequate sample volumes can be used for multiple diagnostics, and blood should be collected into an anticoagulant for hematologic evaluation. Lithium heparin is the anticoagulant of choice for many reptilian and amphibian blood samples intended for hematologic evaluation because ethylenediaminetetraacetic acid (EDTA) can cause hemolysis, especially in blood samples collected from chelonian and several amphibian species (McArthur, 1996; Muro et al., 1998; Knotkova et al., 2002; Campbell, 2012; Klein et al., 2020). A 3% EDTA solution with distilled water may be used as an anticoagulant in some amphibian species without causing hemolysis (Zwemer, 1991). Syringes may be pretreated with lithium heparin prior to collection, or blood can be allowed to drip from the needle hub into microcollection tubes that contain lithium heparin. In reptiles, lithium heparin will cause clumping of leukocytes and thrombocytes, which can make it difficult to obtain accurate cell counts. Evaluation of cell morphology may be difficult as well due to the clumping and because lithium heparin imparts a blue tinge to blood films. Blood samples collected in lithium heparin do not stain well if several hours pass prior to processing. In some species of reptiles, such as the green iguana (*Iguana iguana*), Chinese water dragon (*Physignathus cocincinus*), and perhaps most species of lizards, EDTA can be used and is considered to be the anticoagulant of choice, allowing for better staining of the cells and, therefore, making cell identification easier than cells exposed to heparin (Mayer et al., 2005).

To minimize these effects, the blood sample should be processed as soon as possible after collection. Blood film slides should be quickly prepared from a drop of blood containing no anticoagulant taken from the needle immediately following collection to avoid interference during staining (Walberg, 2001).

(a)

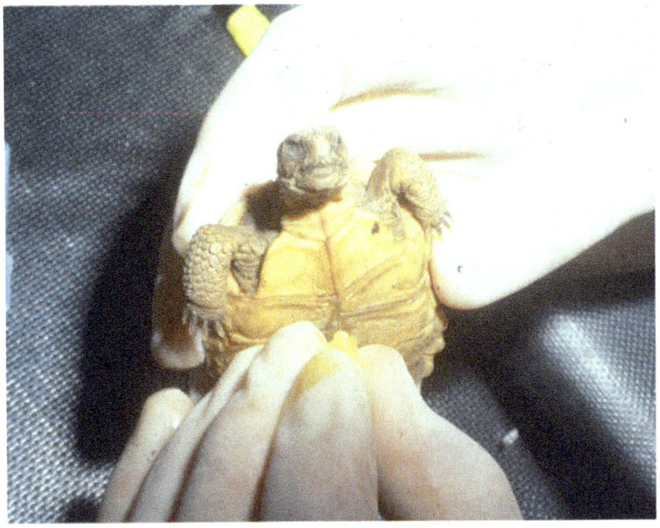

(b)

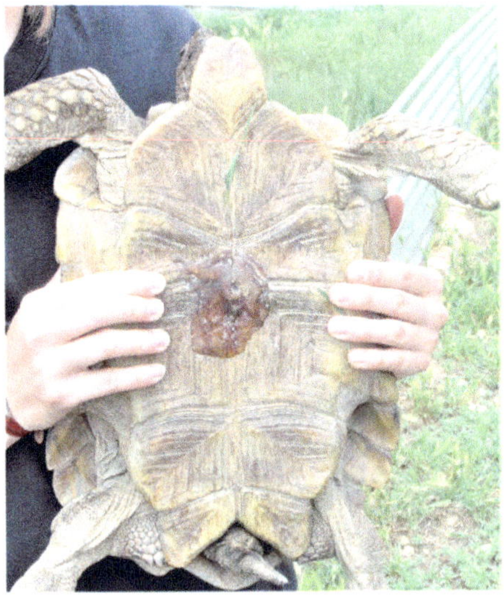

Fig. 17.19. (a) A needle being inserted through the plastron overlying the heart for blood collection via cardiocentesis in a juvenile chelonian. (b) A sealed hole from a tortoise used in a study that required repeated blood samples collected via cardiocentesis.

Blood Film Techniques

There are several methods for preparing blood films, such as the push-slide technique (or wedge smear or slide-to-slide technique) (Figures 9.9a and 9.9b in Chapter 9), the alternative push-slide technique (Figures 9.10a–9.10c in Chapter 9), the coverslip-to-slide technique, or the coverslip-to-coverslip technique (Russell and Heatley, 2020). Some authors feel that preparation of blood films using the two-microscope slide wedge method is more likely to cause cell lysis than use of a coverslip method (Raskin, 2000). Experienced medical technologists working with blood collected from lower vertebrates, such as reptiles, routinely prepare blood films using the conventional methods employing two microscope slides without creating cell lysis. It has been the experience of the authors of this book that coverslip smears can also result in excessive cell lysis; therefore, the method chosen appears to be a matter of technical skill.

Stains

Stains used to evaluate avian blood films, such as Wright, Wright–Giemsa, Wright–Leishman, and May Grünwald–Giemsa are commonly used for reptile and amphibian blood films.

Bone Marrow Collection

Bone marrow samples can be collected from the femur or tibia of lizards, crocodilians, and perhaps, some chelonians. When performing a bone marrow aspiration biopsy, a general anesthetic or infiltration of the subcutis and periosteum with a local anesthetic is used to control pain. Commercially available pediatric bone marrow biopsy needles or spinal needles are required for small patients. These needles contain a stylet to facilitate passage of the aspiration needle through the cortical bone into the marrow space.

The intertrochanteric fossa of the proximal femur is a common site for bone marrow collection in lizards. After surgical preparation of the skin, the skin is incised to facilitate passage of the needle through the skin. Once the needle has reached the cortical bone, it is rotated in a clockwise-counterclockwise manner until firmly seated and then advanced into the marrow space. The stylet is removed, a syringe (3–6 mL) is attached, and slight negative pressure is applied to draw the small marrow sample into the needle's lumen. Excessive aspiration should be avoided to prevent peripheral blood contamination. The sample should not appear just beyond the hub of the needle, as is the technique for bone marrow collection in mammals.

The cranial aspect of the proximal tibia just below the knee joint is a suitable location for bone marrow aspiration in lizards (Figures 17.20a and 17.20b). The site is prepared for bone marrow sampling as described above. The needle with a stylet is placed against the bone adjacent to the tibial crest and advanced through the cortex and into the marrow cavity using gentle pressure and rotary movements. The hand not used for manipulating the needle is used to stabilize the tibia. Once the needle is positioned into the marrow cavity, the stylet is removed and the sample is gently aspirated inside the lumen of the needle using a 3–6 mL syringe attached to the hub of the needle.

Bone marrow samples may be obtained by drilling the biopsy needle into the plastocarapacial bridge of

(a) (b)

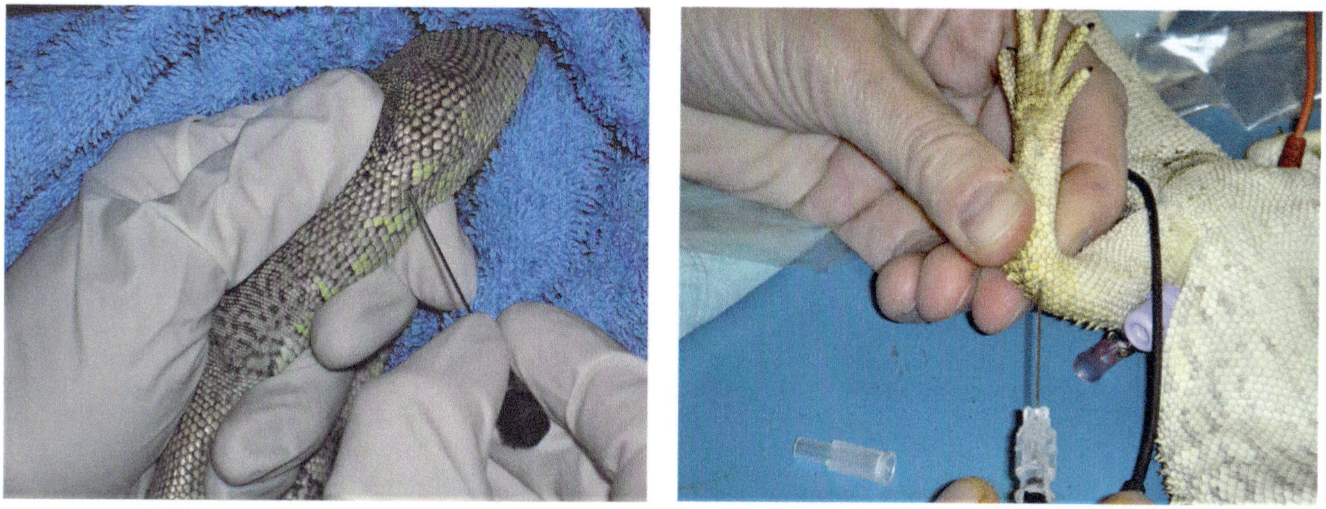

Fig. 17.20. (a) The location at the proximal tibia for obtaining a bone marrow aspiration biopsy from a green iguana (*Iguana iguana*). (b) The location at the proximal tibia for obtaining a bone marrow aspiration biopsy from a bearded dragon (*Pogona vitticeps*).

some chelonians (Frye, 1991; Divers, 2019b). The sampling procedure follows the same method described for obtaining a bone marrow sample for long bones.

The bone marrow of some reptiles, especially chelonians (i.e., sea turtles), is not gelatinous, and hematopoietic cells may be difficult to sample for study. A saline soak technique can be used to harvest hematopoietic cells from reptiles that lack a gelatinous bone marrow. A 2 mm thickness of bone is allowed to soak for 18–24 h at 4°C, followed by agitation for 30 min, and the solution is centrifuged to obtain the hematopoietic cells (Garner et al., 1996).

Slides of the marrow sample are made quickly before clotting occurs. Pull films are prepared by placing a drop of marrow on a glass slide, gently placing a spreader slide directly on top with a little or no manual pressure, and then pulling the two glass slides apart after the drop has been allowed to spread. Air-dried slides are stained with a Romanowsky stain.

Bone marrow samples diluted with peripheral blood are difficult to interpret. Romanowsky-stained bone marrow films are evaluated for cellularity and the maturation of the myeloid and erythroid cells. A myeloid:erythroid (M:E) ratio is obtained as part of the routine bone marrow evaluation. Examination of other cells, such as macrophages, plasma cells, lymphocytes, and osteoclasts, is also part of bone marrow evaluations.

References

Baranowski-Smith LL, Smith CJV. 1983. A simple method for obtaining blood samples from mature frogs. *Lab Anim Sci* 33(4):338–339.

Barrows M, McArthur S, Wilkinson R. 2004. Diagnosis. In: McArthur S, Wilkinson R, Meyer J (eds), *Medicine and Surgery of Tortoises and Turtles*. Oxford: Blackwell Publishing Ltd.

Boutilier RG, Stiffler DF, Toews DP. 1992. Exchange of respiratory gases, ions, and water in amphibious and aquatic amphibians. In: Feder M, Burggren W (eds), *Environmental Physiology of Amphibians*. Chicago, IL: University of Chicago Press.

Campbell TW. 1996. Sea turtle rehabilitation. In: Mader D (ed), *Reptile Medicine and Surgery*. Philadelphia, PA: WB Saunders.

Campbell TW. 2012. Hematology of reptiles. In: Thrall MA, Weiser G, Allison RW, Campbell TW (eds), *Veterinary Hematology and Clinical Chemistry*, 2nd edn. Ames, IA: Wiley-Blackwell, pp. 277–297.

Campbell TW. 2015. Hematology. *Veterinary Clinics of North America: Exotic Animal Practice*. Philadelphia, PA: Elsevier.

Campbell TW. 2022. Hematology of reptiles. In: Thrall MA, Weiser G, Allison RW, Campbell TW (eds), *Veterinary Hematology and Clinical Chemistry*, 3rd edn. Ames, IA: Wiley-Blackwell.

Cathers T, Lewbart GA, Correa M, Stevens JB. 1997. Serum chemistry and hematology values for anesthetized American bull frogs (*Rana catesbeiana*). *J Zoo Wildl Med* 28(2):171–174.

Crawshaw GJ. 1996. Comparison of plasma biochemical values in blood and blood-lymph mixtures from red-eared sliders, *Trachemys scripta elegans*. *Bull Assoc Rept Amphib Vet* 6:7–9.

Divers SJ. 2019a. Medical history and physical examination. In: Divers SJ, Stahl SJ (eds), *Mader's Reptile and Amphibian Medicine and Surgery*, 3rd edn. St. Louis, MO: Elsevier, pp. 385–404.

Divers SJ. 2019b. Diagnostic techniques and sample collection. In: Divers SJ, Stahl SJ (eds), *Mader's Reptile and Amphibian Medicine and Surgery*, 3rd edn. St. Louis, MO: Elsevier, pp. 405–421.

Forzan MJ, Heatley J, Russell KE, Horney B. 2017. Clinical pathology of amphibians: a review. *Vet Clin Pathol* 46(1):11–33.

Frye FL. 1991. Hematology as applied to clinical reptile medicine. In: Frye FL (ed), *Biomedical and Surgical Aspects of Captive Reptile Husbandry*, Vol. 1, 2nd edn. Malabar, FL: Krieger Publishing Co.

Garner MM, Homer BL, Jacobson ER, et al. 1996. Staining and morphologic features of bone marrow hematopoietic cells in desert tortoises (*Gopherus agassizii*). *Am J Vet Res* 57:1608–1615.

Gottdenker NL, Jacobson ER. 1995. Effect of venipuncture sites on hematologic and clinical biochemical values in desert tortoises (*Gopherus agassizii*). *Am J Res* 56:19–2.

Heatley JJ, Russell KE. 2020. *Exotic Animal Laboratory Diagnosis*. Hoboken, NJ: John Wiley & Sons, Inc.

Hernandez-Divers SJ, Hernandez-Divers SM, Wyneken J. 2001. Clinical applications of a supravertebral (subcarapacial) vein in chelonia. In: Proceedings of the Association of Zoo Veterinarians. Orlando, FL.

Hernandez-Divers SJ, Hernandez-Divers SM, Wyneken J. 2002. Angiographic, anatomic, and clinical techniques descriptions of a subcarapacial venipuncture site for chelonians. *J Herpatol Med Surg* 12:32–37.

Holz P, Holz RM. 1994. Evaluation of ketamine, ketamine/xylazine, and ketamine/midazolam anesthesia in red-eared sliders (*Trachemys scripta elegans*). *J Zoo Wildl Med* 25(4):531–537.

Jackson OF. 1991. Reptiles, part one. chelonians. In: Beynon P, Cooper J (eds), *Manual of Exotic Pets*. Cheltenham, UK: British Small Animal Veterinary Association.

Jacobson ER. 1993a. Blood collection techniques in reptiles: laboratory investigations. In: Fowler M (ed), *Zoo and Wild Animal Medicine, Current Therapy 3*. Philadelphia, PA: WB Saunders.

Jacobson ER. 1993b. Snakes. *Vet Clin North Am (Small Anim Pract)* 23(6):1179–1212.

Jacobson ER, Schumacher J, Green M. 1992. Field techniques and clinical techniques for sampling and handling blood for haematologic and selected biochemical determinations in the desert tortoise. *Copiea* 1:237–241.

Jenkins JR. 1996. Diagnostic and clinical techniques. In: Mader D (ed), *Reptile Medicine and Surgery*. Philadelphia, PA: WB Saunders.

Johnson JD, Mangone B, Wimsatt J. 1998. Placement of cardiac access ports for repeated blood sampling in chelonians. In: Proceedings of 5th Association of Reptilian and Amphibian Veterinarians Conference. Kansas City, MO.

Klein K, Gartlan B, Doden G, et al. 2020. Comparing the effects of lithium heparin and dipotassium ethylenediaminetetraacetic acid on hematologic values in Eastern box turtles (*Terrapene carolina carolina*). *J Zoo Wildl Med* 51(4):999–1006.

Knotkova Z, Doubek J, Knotek Z, Hajkova P. 2002. Blood cell morphology and plasma biochemistry in Russian tortoises (*Agrionemys horsfieldi*). *Acta Vet Brno* 71:191–198.

Lloyd M, Morris P. 1999. Chelonian venipuncture techniques. *Bull Assoc Reptil Amphib Vet* 9:26–29.

Lopez-Olvera JR, Montane J, Marco I, et al. 2003. Effect of venipuncture site on hematologic and serum biochemical parameters in marginated tortoise (*Testudo marginata*). *J Wildl Dis* 39(4):830–836.

Mader DR. 1998. Laboratory sampling in reptile patients: do's and don'ts. In: Proceedings of 5th Association of Reptilian and Amphibian Veterinarians Conference. Kansas City, MO

Marks SK, Citino SB. 1990. Hematology and serum chemistry of the Radiated tortoise (*Testudo radiata*). *J Zoo Wildl Med* 21:342–344.

Martinez Silvestre A, Perpinan D, Marco I, Lavin S. 2002. Venipuncture technique of the occipital venous sinus in freshwater aquatic turtles. *J Herp Med Surg* 12:31–32.

Mautino M, Page CD. 1993. Biology and medicine of turtles and tortoises. *Vet Clin North Am (Small Anim Pract)* 23(6):1251–1270.

Mayer J, Knoll J, Innis C, Mitchell MA. 2005. Characterizing the hematologic and plasma chemistry profiles of captive Chinese water dragons, *Physignathus cocinicinus*. *J Herp Med Surg* 15(3):45–52.

McArthur S. 1996. Veterinary management of tortoises and turtles. In: McArthur S, Wilkinson R, Meyer J (eds), *Medicine and Surgery of Tortoises and Turtles*. Oxford: Blackwell Publishing Ltd.

Muro J, Cuenca R, Pastor J, et al. 1998. Effects of lithium heparin and tripotassium EDTA on hematologic values of Hermann's tortoises *Testudo hermanni*. *J Zoo Wildl Med* 29:40–44.

Myburgh JG, Kirberger RM, Steyl JCA, et al. 2014. The post-occipital spinal venous sinus of the Nile crocodile (*Crocodylus niloticus*): its anatomy and use for blood sample collection and intravenous infusions. *Journal of the South African Veterinary Association* 85(1), Art. #965, 10 pages. http://dx.doi.org/10.4102/jsava.v85i1.965.

Olson GA, Hessler JR, Faith RE. 1975. Techniques for blood collection and intravascular infusion of reptiles. *Lab Anim Sci* 25:783–786.

Pardo MA, Divers S. 2016. Jugular central venous catheter placement through a modified Seldinger technique for long-term venous access in chelonians. *J Zoo Wildl Med* 47(1):286–290.

Raskin RE. 2000. Reptilian complete blood count. In: Fudge A (ed), *Laboratory Medicine: Avian and Exotics*. Philadelphia, PA: WB Saunders.

Rosskopf WJ. 1982. Normal hemogram and blood biochemistry values for California desert tortoises. *Vet Med/Small Anim Clin* 77:85–87.

Russell KE, Heatley JJ. 2020. Introduction. In: Russell KE, Heatley JJ (eds), *Exotic Animal Laboratory Diagnosis*. Hoboken, NJ: John Wiley & Sons, Inc.

Sykes JM, Klaphake E. 2015. Reptile hematology. In: Campbell TW (ed), *Vet Clin North Am: Exotic Animal Practice*. 18(1):63–82.

Thorson TB. 1964. The partitioning of body water in Amphibia. *Physiol Zool* 37:395–399.

Thorson TB. 1968a. Body fluid partitioning in freshwater, marine, and terrestrial chelonia. *Am Zool* 3:529.

Thorson TB. 1968b. Body fluid partitioning in reptilians. *Copiea* 2:592–601.

Walberg J. 2001. White blood cell counting techniques in birds. *Semin Avian Exotic Pet Med* 10:72–76.

Whitaker BR, Krum H. 1999. Medical management of sea turtles in aquaria. In: Fowler M, Miller R (eds), *Zoo and Wild Animal Medicine, Current Therapy 4*. Philadelphia, PA: WB Saunders.

Wilkinson R. 2004. Clinical pathology. In: McArthur S, Wilkinson R, Meyer J (eds), *Medicine and Surgery of Tortoises and Turtles*. Oxford: Blackwell Publishing Ltd.

Wright KM. 2001. Amphibian hematology. In: Wright K, Whitaker B (eds), *Amphibian Medicine and Captive Husbandry*. Malabar, FL: Krieger Publishing Co.

Wright KM. 2006. Overview of amphibian medicine. In: Mader D (ed), *Reptile Medicine and Surgery*, 2nd edn. St. Louis, MO: Saunders Elsevier.

Wyneken J, Mader DR, Weber III ES, Merigo C. 2006. Medical care of sea turtles. In: Mader DR (ed), *Reptile Medicine and Surgery*, 2nd edn. St. Louis, MO: Saunders Elsevier.

Yaw TJ, Mans C, Bunke L, Doss GA, Sladky KK. 2020. Evaluation of subcutaneous administration of alfaxalone-midazolam and dexmedetomidine-midazolam for sedation of ball pythons (*Python regius*). *JAVMA* 256(5):573–579.

Zwemer CF. 1991. An effective acquisition and stable containment technique for *Ambystoma mexicanum* whole blood. *Axolotl Newsletter* 20:39–40.

18

Hematologic Techniques for Quantitative Assessment in Reptiles and Amphibians

The in-house veterinary laboratory evaluation of the blood sample of reptiles and amphibians, collectively referred to as herptiles, involves the same routine procedures used in mammalian hematology, with a few modifications. Similar to mammalian and avian hematology, hematologic evaluation of herptile blood samples begins after the sample is prepared with preferred stains and solutions and centrifuges, microhematocrit tubes, refractometers, hemacytometers, and slides. The systematic approach to evaluating the herptile hemogram involves an assessment of cell and plasma parameters, morphologic features of the cells, and intra- and extracellular parasites. This chapter focuses on obtaining the sample parameter counts or concentrations and interpreting the herptile hemogram. Chapters 19 and 20 will continue with procedures on the herptile hemograms with a focus on evaluating the blood film by identifying the morphologic features of the cells and parasites, and interpreting the findings.

Erythrocyte and Plasma Parameters

The same basic, primary hematologic procedures used for mammals and birds can be applied to reptiles and amphibians. They include a packed cell volume (PCV) by centrifugation (or hematocrit by calculation), a plasma total protein estimation by refractometry, determination of hemoglobin concentration by spectrophotometry or hemoglobinometer, erythrocyte concentration by Natt and Herrick's solution dilution and use of a hemacytometer, and a stained blood film evaluation. Erythrocytes of reptiles and amphibians are larger compared to mammals and birds, and therefore the parameters and indices reflect this difference (Heatley and Russell, 2019). Tables B.7 and Table B.10, Appendix B, provide guidelines for evaluating reptile and amphibian erythrocytes, respectively.

PCV

The PCV provides the percentage of whole blood that is composed of erythrocytes. Determination of the PCV via the microhematocrit method is the most commonly used method for evaluating the red cell mass of reptiles and amphibians. The total erythrocyte count (TRBC) or erythrocyte concentration value, described later in the chapter, is commonly reported as well, but it is not as useful for clinical interpretation and generally parallels the PCV and the hemoglobin concentration (Weiser, 2012). The TRBC may be useful in calculating red cell indices or for calculating the hematocrit (HCT) when instrument determinations are used.

Preparation of the microhematocrit tube with the blood sample can be done as described for mammals (Weiser, 2012). It is determined using the standard manual technique that employs microhematocrit tubes, tube sealant, a microhematocrit centrifuge (12 000 *g* for 5 min), and a tube-reading card or device. The three distinct layers observed in the spun microhematocrit tube of mammals are also present in blood samples from herptiles. The plasma column is located at the top of the tube, and the packed erythrocytes are located at the bottom. The buffy coat appears as a small, white band located just above the erythrocyte column, and consists of leukocytes and thrombocytes. The buffy coat typically increases in size when the leukocyte concentration increases.

Exotic Animal Hematology and Cytology, Fifth Edition. Terry W. Campbell and Krystan R. Grant.

Companion website: www.wiley.com/go/campbell/exotic

Much as in mammals and birds, the PCV of herptiles is affected by the number and size of the erythrocytes, as well as changes in the plasma volume that do not affect the total cell mass. These changes include increased plasma volume (hemodilution), decreased plasma volume (hemoconcentration), improper blood sampling (hemodilution), and epinephrine administration and hypothermia, which may result in hemoconcentration. The normal PCV of many species of reptiles and amphibians ranges between 20% and 40% (see Appendix B for PCV ranges of selected species), but intrinsic and extrinsic factors may impact several values. Generally, a PCV less than 15% is suggestive of anemia, and a PCV greater than 40% suggests dehydration or erythrocytosis (polycythemia). Anemia and erythrocytosis are described in more detail in Chapters 19 and 20.

Erythrocyte Sedimentation Rate (ESR)

The ESR is the time in which erythrocytes settle from the plasma, and is usually measured as millimeters per hour. The ESR is commonly used in human medicine, as well as in marine mammal medicine in a limited way, as an indirect marker to identify or monitor inflammatory conditions (Bossart et al., 2001; Tishkowski and Gupta, 2020). Inflammatory processes increase the amount of protein in the blood, thereby promoting erythrocyte aggregation and faster settling times (Tishkowski and Gupta, 2020). In addition to an increase of proteins (fibrinogen, haptoglobin, immunoglobulins, etc.) in the blood, other factors that may affect the ESR include erythrocyte number, size, or shape; leukocyte count; or viscosity, which may be affected by anticoagulant.

Commercial kits are available for the determination of the ESR; however, due to the volume required (Westergren (2 mL) or Wintrobe (1 mL) tubes), these methods are not suitable for many smaller species. For larger reptile species in which the volume of blood for the ESR can be obtained, it has been used to assess health in Chinese alligators (*Alligator sinensis*) and gopher tortoises (*Gopherus polyphemus*) (Peng et al., 2018; Rosenberg et al., 2018). Some researchers have modified the assessment for use in smaller reptile species by using microhematocrit tubes, which are readily available, require a smaller volume, and are cost-effective for field study (Adamovicz et al., 2020).

Hemoglobin

The two methods used for determining the total hemoglobin concentration for birds can be used for reptiles and amphibians: the cyanmethemoglobin method (using alkaline Drabkin's solution), which estimates hemoglobin from methemoglobin with a spectrophotometer, and the hemoglobinometer method, which estimates hemoglobin from azide-methemoglobin (Clark et al., 2008; Velguth et al., 2010; Young et al., 2012; Andrewartha et al., 2016; Hopkins et al., 2016). Total hemoglobin concentration for reptiles and amphibians using the standard cyanmethemoglobin method is similar to that used for mammals, with one modification: the cyanmethemoglobin reagent–blood mixture should be centrifuged prior to analysis. The free nuclei from lysed erythrocytes are removed before obtaining the optical density value, in order to avoid overestimating the hemoglobin concentration. Using a hemoglobinometer, such as the HemoCue® (HemoCue America, Brea, CA), allows the blood to be mixed with a dry reagent within a cuvette prior to inserting into the device that reads the sample with a built-in photometer. The use of the HemoCue system has been validated for the blue-tongued skink, but overestimates the hemoglobin concentration compared to the Drabkin's method and therefore requires correction (Andrewartha et al., 2016).

Published hemoglobin concentration values for reptiles and amphibians are usually low; often less than 10 g/dL (Diethelm and Stein, 2006; Klaphake et al., 2018; Whitaker and McDermott, 2018).

Total Erythrocyte Concentration

The total erythrocyte concentration in reptiles can be determined using the same automated or manual methods used for the determination of total erythrocyte counts in mammalian blood. Electronic impedance cell counters provide a rapid, reliable method of obtaining total red blood cell concentrations. Erythrocyte counts with electronic cell counters are slightly inflated owing to the inclusion of leukocytes and thrombocytes in the count; however, these additional cells are not significant in most samples as they make up approximately 0.1% of the peripheral blood cell population. An option for a more accurate count when sampling frog blood is to adjust the automated erythrocyte count by subtracting the manual white blood cell and thrombocyte counts and dividing the result by 1000 (Maxham et al., 2016). Progress toward automated counting includes identification of distinct groups of cells using flow cytometry and erythrocyte identification using image processing in reptiles (Carvalho et al., 2016; Govind et al., 2018). Image processing is used to detect the number of cells from the image.

Previously, two manual methods for obtaining total red blood cell counts in reptiles were the erythrocyte Unopette (Unopette, Becton-Dickinson, Rutherford, NJ) method used in mammalian hematology and Natt and Herrick's method, which involves the preparation of Natt and Herrick's solution to be used as a stain and diluent (Natt and Herrick, 1952) (Appendix A). In 2009, the erythrocyte Unopette system was discontinued, but a similar kit is available for manual red cell counts in mammals (Erythro-pette™, Exotic Animal Solutions,

Inc. Hueytown, AL, USA), which has been used for counting avian red blood cells (Ferreyra et al., 2015). Natt and Herrick's solution is commercially available as a stain (Vetlab Supply, Palmetto Bay, FL) or within a kit (Natt-pette™, Exotic Animal Solutions LLC, Rockledge, FL USA). Another staining option for manual cell counting that is used with red-eared sliders (*Trachemys scripta*) is the crystal violet stain and 0.45% sodium chloride. This proposed option was used to better identify cell types such as lymphocytes and thrombocytes, which are challenging to differentiate (Tsai et al., 2014).

Manual red cell counts using Natt and Herrick's method involves making a 1:200 dilution of the blood using Natt and Herrick's solution and red-blood-cell diluting pipettes. Alternatively, commercially prepared Natt and Herrick's solution kits can be used to easily obtain accurate dilutions for the total erythrocyte determination, because dilutions are made using a provided capillary tube and not a diluting pipette. After mixing, the diluted blood is discharged into a hemacytometer counting chamber (Figure 18.1), and the cells are allowed to settle for 5 min to the ruled surface before counting (Figure 10.2). Erythrocytes located in the four corner squares and the central square within the large center square of the Neubauer-ruled hemacytometer chamber are counted when one of the manual methods is used (Figures 10.3a and 10.3b). Using the 40× objective, the cells can be identified for counting (Figure 18.2). Cells on the borders of the squares should be counted on the top and left, but such cells should not be counted on the bottom and right borders, to avoid redundancy. Both sides of the hemacytometer should be counted separately. If the count totals from each side are within 10% of each other, then the total red blood cell count can be calculated. The number obtained from either side, or an average of the two sides, is multiplied by 10 000 to calculate the total red blood cell count per cubic millimeter (mm^3) or microliter (μL) of blood:

$$\text{RBC/mm}^3 = (\text{Average count from both sides of chamber}) \times 10\,000$$

This method, as with all manual counting methods, may have an inherent error of 10%; however, it is commonly used in clinical practice. The other method mentioned above, using crystal violet stain, is similar to Natt and Herrick's method for finding the total erythrocyte concentration; however, the blood sample is diluted at a ratio of 1:75, and therefore the average count from both sides would be multiplied by 3750 (Tsai et al., 2014). The TRBC count in reptiles is usually lower than in mammals, averaging 0.3 to 2.5 x 10^6/μL (Table B.7, Appendix B) (Cital and Goodnight, 2016).

Erythrocyte Indices

After the primary hematologic parameters (PCV, erythrocyte count, and hemoglobin concentration) have been determined, the erythrocyte indices can be calculated. These include the mean cell volume (MCV) or mean erythrocyte volume (MEV), mean cell hemoglobin (MCH) or mean erythrocyte hemoglobin (MEH), and mean cell hemoglobin concentration (MCHC) or mean erythrocyte hemoglobin concentration (MEHC). The MCV is an index of the red cell volume and is calculated similarly to mammalian MCV (Stacy and Harr, 2021):

$$\text{MCV}(\text{fL}) = (\text{PCV}(\%) \times 10)/\text{TRBC}$$

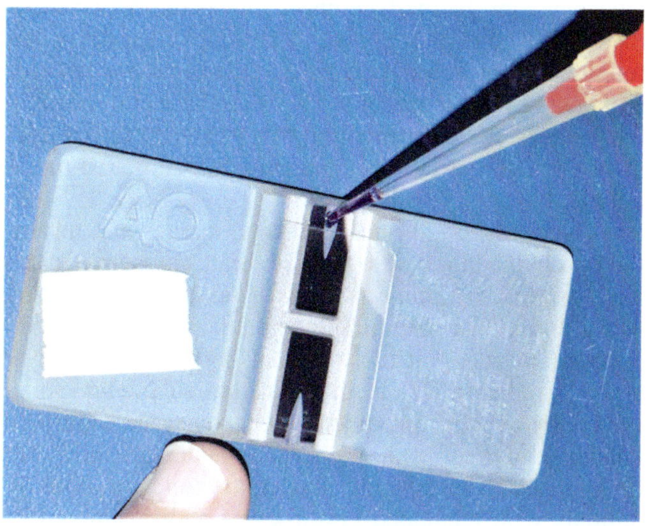

Fig. 18.1. This image shows the diluted blood with Natt and Herrick's solution being discharged into a Neubauer hemacytometer.

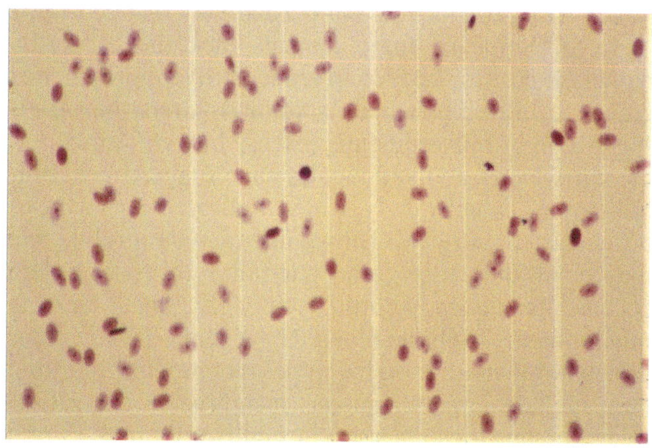

Fig. 18.2. Erythrocytes, including immature erythrocytes, and leukocytes in the blood from a chelonian (*Chelonia mydas*) diluted and stained with Natt and Herrick's solution in the Neubauer-ruled hemacytometer counting chamber (Natt and Herrick's solution, 40×).

The MCH is an index of hemoglobin content in an average red blood cell and is calculated similarly to mammalian MCH, although it is not commonly used (Stacy and Harr, 2021):

$$\text{MCH}(\text{pg}) = (\text{Hb}(\text{g/dL}) \times 10)/\text{TRBC}$$

The MCHC is an index denoting the proportion of hemoglobin present in an average erythrocyte and is calculated as follows (Stacy and Harr, 2021):

$$\text{MCHC}(\text{g/dL}) = (\text{Hgb}(\text{g/dL}) \times 100)/\text{PCV}(\%)$$

Erythrocyte parameters for selected reptile and amphibian species can be found in Appendix B (Tables B.7 and B.10).

Published MCV values for reptiles and amphibians generally range between 160 and 950 fL (femtoliters, μm^3) and 370 and 920 fL, respectively. Published MCHC values typically range between 20 and 40 g/dL and between 20 and 30 g/dL for reptiles and amphibians, respectively (Diethelm and Stein, 2006; Klaphake et al., 2018; Whitaker and McDermott, 2018). Although published references are available for the erythrocyte indices of reptiles and amphibians, the assessment of abnormal values has not been properly evaluated in these species.

Plasma Appearance and Protein

The color and clarity of the plasma column above the packed erythrocytes should be noted. Normal plasma is typically colorless; however, in some amphibians and reptiles, it may be light blue, green, yellow, or orange depending upon the species (Wright, 2001; Allender and Fry, 2008; Young et al., 2012). In some cases, colored plasma may be an indication of disease, such as hepatobiliary disease. The color of plasma may be due to bile pigment. Some of these animals lack the biliverdin reductase enzyme needed to reduce biliverdin (which is green) to bilirubin (which is yellow). Green plasma is suggestive of biliverdinemia (excess biliverdin bile pigment in blood), and yellow plasma is suggestive of bilirubinemia, which is typically indicative of a poor prognosis for survival. Biliverdinemia or bilirubinemia may be an indication of hepatic failure or renal failure because the kidney is normally very efficient at clearing bile pigments from the blood. Other clinical indications of hepatobiliary disease in reptiles that produce bilirubin may include icterus (mucous membranes) or yellow-tinged urates; those that produce biliverdin may exhibit green-tinged urates (Divers, 2019). Further evaluation using biochemical testing may be done on reptiles that produce bilirubin. Currently, biochemical tests exist to confirm the presence of biliverdin, but are not commercially available (Divers, 2019). Lipemia may be noted in some samples and is most commonly associated with postprandial conditions. In some cases, lipemic samples may reflect disorders involving lipid metabolism. Hemolysis may occur and usually results from lysis of erythrocytes during blood collection or sample handling. Intravascular hemolysis may also cause hemolysis of the sample in some instances. If the PCV is normal, then the presence of the hemolysis is probably associated with artifactual lysis of erythrocytes.

Plasma protein concentration is typically determined using handheld refractometers, which have been the standard instruments for determining protein concentration in plasma and body cavity fluid samples since the 1960s (George and O'Neill, 2001). Some authors report good correlation between protein estimation by refractometry and biuret protein in turtle samples (Santos Schmidt et al., 2011; Pessoa et al., 2017). Major discrepancies found between biuret and refractometric results may be due to differences in the brand of refractometers used in the study, changes in the alteration of the chemical composition of the biuret reagent, use of different standards, or changes in reaction conditions (George and O'Neill, 2001). Sample-related causes of error in protein determination by refractometric methods include increased nonprotein solids, such as cholesterol, urea, lipoproteins, and glucose (George and O'Neill, 2001). These compounds can increase the refractometric protein measurements by 0.5–1.0 g/dL (5–10 g/L) (George and O'Neill, 2001).

Leukocyte Parameters

As with erythrocyte parameters, methods used for leukocyte counts in avian blood samples are applied to other lower vertebrates. Leukocyte counts may be obtained using manual and automated methods. However, significant differences may occur between the manual absolute and relative microscopic leukocyte differential count and the automated absolute and relative leukocyte count techniques (Post et al., 2003). Manual methods for the determination of a leukocyte differential have a greater variability compared to automated methods (Russo et al., 1986).

The presence of nucleated erythrocytes and thrombocytes in the blood of lower vertebrates presents a challenge when attempting to apply the automated counting methods used for obtaining mammalian white blood cell counts. The fact that these animals have an erythrocyte that is similar in size to many of the leukocytes, small lymphocytes, and thrombocytes presents an additional challenge. Direct and semidirect manual methods for obtaining absolute (total) leukocyte concentrations in animals with nucleated erythrocytes and thrombocytes have been developed, although a gold standard for leukocyte counts in reptiles and amphibians is not established. One study investigated agreement between a direct method and semidirect method, as described below, for obtaining total leukocyte counts in Galapagos tortoises (*Chelonoidis* spp.) (Sheldon et al., 2016). The direct method consistently showed agreement with the estimated leukocyte count from the direct smear compared to semidirect method. Another study investigated agreement between two methods of obtaining leukocyte counts in eastern box turtles (*Terrapene carolina carolina*). The quantification from the direct method, as described later, was significantly higher than the estimation directly from the blood film (Winter et al., 2019). Both studies used the method of quantifying leukocyte counts from the blood film as described in Chapter 10 for birds.

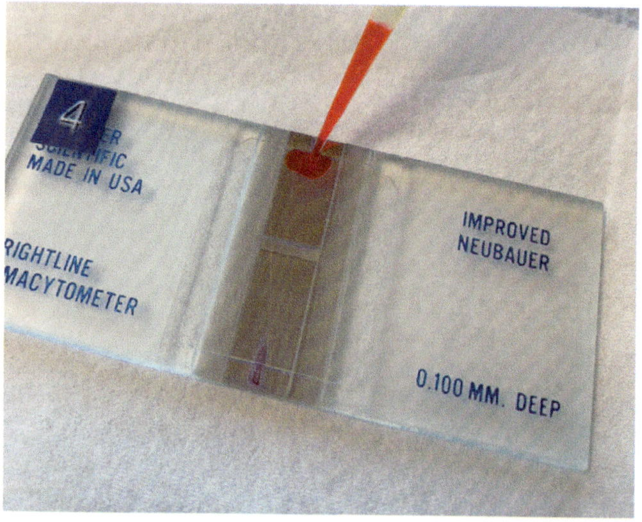

Fig. 18.3. This image shows the diluted blood with eosin (phloxine) solution being discharged into a Neubauer hemacytometer.

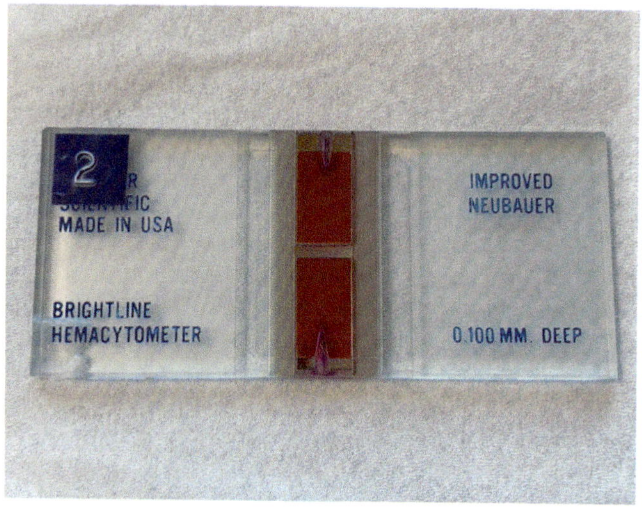

Fig. 18.4. This image shows the diluted blood with eosin (phloxine) solution loaded into a Neubauer hemacytometer in preparation for cell counting.

Semidirect Method for Manual Leukocyte Concentration

A commonly used semidirect method involves the staining of heterophils and eosinophils using eosin or phloxine B (a specific stain for mammalian eosinophils) as the diluent. The procedure was simplified utilizing the Eosinophil Unopette 5877 System (Becton-Dickinson, Rutherford, NJ), which was developed for determining total eosinophil concentrations in mammalian blood but was discontinued in 2007. When it was available, the blood sample was diluted 1:32 with the phloxine B solution in the Unopette vial using the 25 µL pipette provided. The Eopette™ Test Kit (Exotic Animal Solutions LLC, Rockledge, FL) is now available as a substitute for the Eosinophil Unopette 5877 System and eliminates the need for a manual pipette to make the dilutions.

After a Neubauer-ruled hemacytometer chamber has been properly loaded with the blood–eosin or phloxine mixture (Figures 18.3 and 18.4) and allowed to stand in a humid chamber for a minimum of 5 min, the eosin-stained heterophils and eosinophils are counted in both sides of the chamber (18 large squares) (Figures 10.5, 10.6 and 18.5). It is important to load the hemacytometer immediately following proper mixing of the blood and phloxine diluent, because red blood cells may also stain following prolonged exposure. Next, the total leukocyte concentration (TWBC/mm^3) is calculated after completing a leukocyte differential to obtain the percent heterophils and eosinophils on the stained blood film using the following equation:

$$\text{WBC/mm}^3 = \frac{\begin{array}{c}(\text{Total count in both sides of}\\ \text{hemacytometer}) \times 1.1 \times 16 \times 100\end{array}}{\begin{array}{c}\%\text{Heterophils} + \%\text{Eosinophils}\\ \text{from differential}\end{array}}$$

For example, if the total number of eosin-stained cells counted in the nine large squares on both sides of a Neubauer-ruled hemacytometer chamber (total of 18 squares) was 73 and the differential leukocyte count revealed 16% heterophils and 2% eosinophils, then using the above formula, the TWBC/mm^3 is calculated to be 7138/mm^3 when rounded to the nearest whole number.

The phloxine B semidirect method is relatively easy to perform and has been shown to be more precise for hemacytometer counting than Natt and Herrick's method (see next section) (Dein et al., 1994). A disadvantage of this method is that the determination of total leukocyte count depends on an accurate leukocyte differential (in particular, the number of heterophils and eosinophils present), and the count often becomes less accurate when the mononuclear leukocytes exceed the granulocytes.

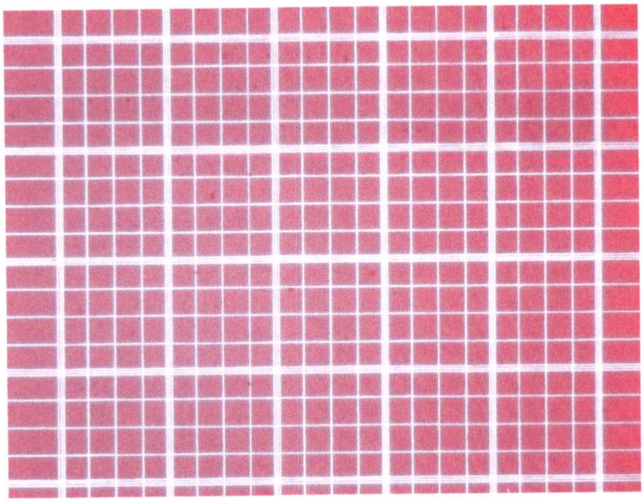

Fig. 18.5. The blood from a bearded dragon (*Pogona vitticeps*) diluted and stained with eosin (Phloxine) solution in the Neubauer-ruled hemacytometer counting chamber focused on the large middle square (eosin stain, 10×).

Direct Methods for Manual Leukocyte Concentration

Natt and Herrick's Solution

A direct method for obtaining total leukocyte concentrations in reptile and amphibian blood is to make a 1:200 dilution with Natt and Herrick's solution (Appendix A) using a standard red-blood-cell diluting pipette. An alternative method would be to add 20 µL of blood to 4 mL of Natt and Herrick's solution. It is easy to obtain accurate dilutions for the total leukocyte determination using commercially prepared Natt and Herrick's solution kits because dilutions are made using a provided capillary tube and not a diluting pipette. The leukocytes in the sample will stain dark blue (Figures 10.4 and 18.2). The total leukocyte concentration is obtained by counting all the leukocytes (dark blue cells) in the nine large squares in the ruled area of the Neubauer-ruled hemacytometer chamber (Figure 10.5) using the following equation:

$$\text{TWBC/mm}^3 = \left(\text{total cells in nine large squares} + 10\%\right) \times 200$$

The advantage of using this method is that a total erythrocyte and thrombocyte count can also be obtained using the same charged hemacytometer. A disadvantage is that it is often difficult to differentiate thrombocytes from small lymphocytes, which produces errors in the counts. It has been recommended that staining the blood sample for 60 min in Natt and Herrick's solution improves the differentiation between small lymphocytes and thrombocytes (Robertson and Maxwell, 1990). An alternative approach to the problem of differentiating lymphocytes and thrombocytes using this method is to include thrombocytes in the leukocyte differential and subtract the absolute thrombocyte count from the total count to obtain the total leukocyte count.

Crystal Violet

Crystal violet stain in conjunction with diluting the sample with 0.45% sodium chloride has been used with red-eared slider (*Trachemys scripta*) blood samples with promising results compared to the Liu staining method and the Unopette method (no longer available) (Tsai et al., 2014). The procedure is similar to Natt and Herrick's method described above with the exception that the four large corner squares were counted in the study. This is a standard approach to obtaining the leukocyte count using a hemocytometer, and therefore the calculation is similar: the product of the counted cells (or the average of the two chambers) and the dilution rate (75) divided by the product of 4 mm^2 (area of four large squares) and the depth of the chamber (0.1 mm) (Tsai et al., 2014).

Leukocyte Differential

The differential leukocyte count and leukocyte morphology are obtained by microscopic evaluation of stained blood films. A variety of hematologic stains are available (see Appendix A). Rapid stains (i.e., Diff–Quik, Dade Diagnostics, Aguada, Puerto Rico) or Hemacolor (Miles Laboratories, Inc., Elkhart, IN) have a shorter staining time, but do not always provide adequate differentiation between the various leukocytes. Additionally, heterophil granules tend to coalesce more with rapid stains, especially those of reptiles, making evaluation of these cells difficult (Muro et al., 1998). Stains such as Wright's and May–Grünwald–Giemsa stains are more time consuming, but provide better differentiation of the leukocytes, thrombocytes, and immature erythrocytes (Alleman et al., 1992; Muro et al., 1998).

The leukocyte differential is performed during the microscopic evaluation of Romanowsky-stained blood films. Blood samples collected into heparin make it necessary to prepare the blood films immediately following sample collection in order to decrease the incidence of cell clumping. Whenever possible, preparing blood films using blood containing no anticoagulant is preferred. The differential leukocyte count is performed by counting a minimum of 100 leukocytes in a monocellular area in the blood film. The cells counted are those consecutively encountered as one moves from one counting field to the next. The cells are classified as heterophils in reptiles (Figure 19.10), neutrophils in amphibians (Figure 20.3), eosinophils (Figures 19.11 and 20.4), basophils (Figures 19.12 and 20.5), lymphocytes (Figures 19.13 and 20.6), and monocytes (Figures 19.15 and 20.7). The number of each cell type becomes a fraction of the total or a percentage of the leukocyte population. Absolute numbers of each cell type are obtained by multiplying the total leukocyte concentration by the percentage of that type of leukocyte from the differential count.

Thrombocyte Parameters

The concentrations of thrombocytes in the blood of lower vertebrates vary. Thrombocytes typically occur in numbers that range between 25 and 350 thrombocytes per 100 leukocytes in the blood film of normal reptiles (Sypek and Borysenko, 1988). The actual thrombocyte concentration is difficult to determine because thrombocytes tend to clump; therefore, thrombocyte concentration is often reported as normal, increased, or decreased, based upon estimates from peripheral blood films.

Blood films may be used to assess thrombocyte numbers. Approximately 1–5 thrombocytes can be seen in a monolayer 1000× (oil-immersion) field in a blood film from a normal herptile, unless the thrombocytes clump excessively during preparation.

The absolute thrombocyte concentration can be obtained using the same hemacytometer used for obtaining total leukocyte and erythrocyte counts with Natt and Herrick's method. The number of thrombocytes counted in the central large square on both sides of the Neubauer-ruled hemacytometer is multiplied by 1000 to obtain the number of thrombocytes per microliter of blood (Figure 10.8).

Thrombocytopenia is suggested by thrombocyte numbers less than one per monolayer 1000× field. Thrombocytosis is suggested by numbers greater than five in an average monolayer 1000× field.

References

Adamovicz L, Baker SJ, Kessler E, et al. 2020. Erythrocyte sedimentation rate and hemoglobin-binding protein in free-living box turtles (*Terrapene* spp.). *PLOS ONE* https://doi.org/10.1371/journal.pone.0234805

Alleman AR, Jacobson ER, Raskin RE. 1992. Morphologic and cytochemical characteristics of blood cells from the desert tortoise (*Gopherus agassizii*). *Am J Vet Res* 53:1645–1651.

Allender MC, Fry MM. 2008. Amphibian hematology. *Vet Clin Exot Anim* 11(3):463–480.

Andrewartha SJ, Munns SL, Edwards A. 2016. Calibration of the HemoCue point-of-care analyser for determining haemoglobin concentration in a lizard and a fish. *Conserv Physiol* 4:10.1093/conphys/cow006.

Bossart GD, Reidarson TH, Dierauf LA, Duffield DA. 2001. Clinical pathology. In: Dierauf LA, Gulland FMD (eds), *CRC Handbook of Marine Mammal Medicine*, 2nd edn. CRC Press LLC.

Carvalho MPN, Queiroz-Hazarbassanov NGT, Massoco CO, et al. 2016. Flow cytometric characterization of peripheral blood leukocyte populations on2 neotropical snake species: *boa constrictor, bothrops jararaca,* and *Crotalus durissus*. *Vet Clin Pathol* 45(2):271–280.

Cital S, Goodnight A. 2016. Reptile and amphibian transfusion medicine. In: Yagi K, Holowaychuk MK (eds), *Manual of Veterinary Transfusion Medicine and Blood Banking*. Ames, IA: John Wiley & Sons.

Clark TD, Eliason EJ, Sandblom E, Hinch SG, Farrell AP. 2008. Calibration of a hand-held haemoglobin analyser for use on fish blood. *J Fish Biol* 73(10):2587–2595.

Dein FJ, Wilson BA, Fischer MT. 1994. Avian leucocyte counting using the hemocytometer. *J Zoo Wildl Med* 25:432–437.

Diethelm G, Stein G. 2006. Hematologic and blood chemistry values in reptiles. In: Mader D (ed), *Reptile Medicine and Surgery*, 2nd edn. St. Louis, MO: Saunders Elsevier.

Divers SJ. 2019. Hepatology. In: Divers SJ, Stahl SJ (eds), *Mader's Reptile and Amphibian Medicine and Surgery*, 3rd edn. St. Louis, MO: Elsevier.

Ferreyra H, Beldomenico PM, Marchese K, et al. 2015. Lead exposure affects health indices in free-ranging ducks in Argentina. *Exotoxicology* DOI: 10.1007/s10646-015-1419-7.

George JW, O'Neill SL. 2001. Comparison of refractometer and biuret methods for total protein measurement in body cavity fluids. *Vet Clin Pathol* 30:16–18.

Govind D, Lutnick B, Tomaszewski JE, Sarder P. 2018. Automated erythrocyte detection and classification from whole slide images. *J Med Imaging* 5(2):027501.

Heatley JJ, Russell KE. 2019. Hematology. In: Divers SJ, Stahl SJ (eds), *Mader's Reptile and Amphibian Medicine and Surgery*, 3rd edn. St. Louis, MO: Elsevier, pp. 301–318.

Hopkins WA, Fallon JA, Beck ML, Coe BH, Jachowski CMB. 2016. Haematological and immunological characteristics of easter hellbenders (*Cryptobranchus alleganiensis alleganiensis*) infected and co-infected with endo- and ectoparasites. *Conserv Physiol* 4:10.1093/conphys/cow006.

Klaphake E, Gibbons PM, Sladky KK, Carpenter JW. 2018. Reptiles. In: Carpenter JW (ed), *Exotic Animal Formulary*, 5th edn. St. Louis, MO: Elsevier.

Maxham LA, Forzan MJ, Hogan NS, Vanderstichel RV, Gilroy CV. 2016. Hematologic reference intervals for *Xenopus tropicalis* with partial use of automatic counting methods and reliability of long-term stored-samples. *Vet Clin Pathol* 45(2):291–299.

Muro J, Cuenca R, Pastor J, Vinas L, Lavin S. 1998. Effects of lithium heparin and tripotassium EDTA on hematologic values of Hermann's tortoises (*Testudo hermanni*). *J Zoo Wildl Med* 29:40–44.

Natt MP, Herrick CA. 1952. A new blood diluent for counting erythrocytes and leucocytes of the chicken. *Poult Sci* 31:735–738.

Peng F, Chen X, Meng T, at al. 2018. Hematology and serum biochemistry parameters of captive Chinese alligators (*Alligator sinensis*) during the active and hibernating periods. *Tissue Cell* 51:8–13.

Pessoa LMB, Lima MGdM, Carneiro FT, et al. Refractometry as an alternative to the biuret method for measuring total serum proteins in *Podocnemis expansa* (Podocnemididae) and *Phrynops geoffroanus* (Chelidae). *Acta Amazonica* 47(1):83–86.

Post J, Rebel JMJ, Ter Huurne AAHM. 2003. Automated blood cell count: a sensitive and reliable method to study corticosterone-related stress in broilers. *Poult Sci* 82:591–595.

Robertson GW, Maxwell MH. 1990. Modified staining techniques for avian blood cells. *Br Poult Sci* 31:881–886.

Rosenberg JF, Hernandez JA, Wellehan JFX, et al. 2018. Diagnostic performance of inflammatory markers in gopher tortoises (*Gopherus polyphemus*). *J Zoo Wildfl Med* 49(2):765–769.

Russo EA, McEntee L, Applegate I, Baker JS. 1986. Comparison of two methods for determination of white blood cell counts in macaws. *J Am Vet Med Assoc* 189:1013–1016.

Santos Schmidt EM, Lange RR, Paulillo AC. 2011. Determination of snake-necked turtle *Hydromedusa tectifera* (Cope, 1870) (Testudines: Chelidae) plasma protein concentrations by refractometry and the biuret method. *Comp Clin Pathol* 20:487–489.

Sheldon JD, Stacy NI, Blake S, Cabrera F, Deem SL. 2016. Comparison of total leukocyte quantification methods in free-living Galapagos tortoises (*Chelonoides* spp.). *J Zoo Wildl Med* 47(1):196–205.

Stacy NI, Harr KE. 2021. Hematology of reptiles with a focus on circulating inflammatory cells. In: Jacobson ER, Garner MM (eds), *Infectious Diseases and Pathology of Reptiles Color Atlas and Text*, 2nd edn. Boca Rotan, FL: Taylor and Francis Group, LLC.

Sypek J, Borysenko M. 1988. Reptiles. In: Rowley A, Ratcliffe N (eds), *Vertebrate Blood Cells*. Cambridge: Cambridge University Press.

Tishkowski K, Gupta V. 2020. Erythrocyte sedimentation rate. In: StatPearls [Internet], Treasure Island (FL): StatPearls Publishing; Available from: https://www.ncbi.nlm.nih.gov/books/NBK557485/.

Tsai CY, Yu JF, Wang YW, et al. 2014. An alternative staining method for counting red-eared slider turtle (*Trachemys scripta*) blood cells using crystal violet in cells diluted with 0.45% sodium chloride. *J Vet Diagn Investig* 26(5):610–615.

Velguth KE, Payton ME, Hoover JP. 2010. Relationship of hemoglobin concentration to packed cell volume in avian blood samples. *J Avian Med Surg* 24(2):115–121.

Weiser G. 2012. Laboratory technology for veterinary medicine. In: Thrall M, Weiser G, Allison RW, Campbell T (eds), *Veterinary Hematology and Clinical Chemistry*, 2nd edn. Ames, IA: Wiley-Blackwell, pp. 3–33.

Whitaker BR, McDermott CT. 2018. Amphibians. In: Carpenter JW (ed), *Exotic Animal Formulary*, 5th edn. St. Louis, MO: Elsevier.

Winter JM, Stacy NI, Adamovicz LA, Allender MC. 2019. Investigating the analytical variability and agreement of manual leukocyte quantification methods in eastern box turtles (*Terrapene carolina carolina*). *Front Vet Sci* 6:398 DOI: 10.3389/fvets.2019.00398.

Wright KM. 2001. Amphibian hematology. In: Wright K, Whitaker B (eds), *Amphibian Medicine and Captive Husbandry*. Malabar, FL: Krieger Publishing Co.

Young S, Warner J, Speare R, et al. 2012. Hematologic and plasma biochemical reference intervals for health monitoring of wild Australian tree frogs. *Vet Clin Pathol* 41(4):478–492.

19

Evaluation and Interpretation of the Peripheral Blood and Bone Marrow of Reptiles

Evaluation of the hemograms and blood film is a valuable diagnostic tool that can be used to assess the response of a reptilian patient to disease or therapy. Hematologic evaluation involves examination of the erythrocytes, leukocytes, and thrombocytes in the peripheral blood. This chapter continues the hemogram assessment by reviewing the blood film components and interpreting the results. In addition to evaluating the peripheral blood, hematopoiesis and examination of the bone marrow sample are also covered. Representative hemic cells found in reptile blood films can be found in Appendix C.

The Interpretation of the Reptile Hemogram

Hematology is used to detect conditions such as anemia, inflammatory disease, parasitemia, hematopoietic disorders, and hemostatic alterations. An example of a favorable response in the leukogram would be a shift from leukocytosis or leukopenia to a normal leukocyte concentration. A normal heterophil, eosinophil, or monocyte count following heterophilia, eosinophilia, or monocytosis, respectively, would usually indicate improvement as well. The disappearance of toxic heterophils, reactive lymphocytes, and plasma cells from a blood film during or after therapy indicates improvement and a favorable response to therapy. Anemic reptiles that exhibit an erythrocytic regenerative response have a better prognosis compared to those with little or no response. Similarly, a normal thrombocyte concentration following thrombocytopenia indicates a favorable response.

Reptiles have adapted to a wide variety of environments (i.e., aquatic, terrestrial, fossorial, and alpine), and their normal hematologic parameters vary accordingly. When evaluating the hematologic responses of reptiles, the effects that intrinsic and extrinsic factors may have on the animal's response to disease cannot be overlooked. Hematologic evaluation may be used to monitor the health status of a reptile if the reported reference intervals and interpretations account for the intrinsic and extrinsic factors that affect the hemic response. The cellular responses in reptilian blood are less predictable than those of endothermic mammals and birds, whose cellular microenvironments are more stable.

Reptilian hemogram values may be affected by several sample-handling factors as well. The blood collection site, type of anticoagulant used, method of cell counting, type of stain used, and the experience of the technician add to the variability of reptilian hemogram values. All of these factors can complicate the establishment and validation of normal reference intervals in reptiles. Because of this variability, total and differential leukocyte counts must demonstrate twofold or greater increase or decrease from normal reference values to be considered significant.

Reptile Erythrocytes

Morphology and Color

Mature erythrocytes of reptiles are typically larger than the erythrocytes of birds, bony fish, and mammals, but are smaller than the erythrocytes of most amphibians. Erythrocytes of reptiles are blunt-ended ellipsoidal cells with permanent, centrally positioned, oval to round nuclei containing dense, purple chromatin (Figures 19.1a–c). Unlike the smooth nuclear margins of avian erythrocytes,

Exotic Animal Hematology and Cytology, Fifth Edition. Terry W. Campbell and Krystan R. Grant.

Companion website: www.wiley.com/go/campbell/exotic

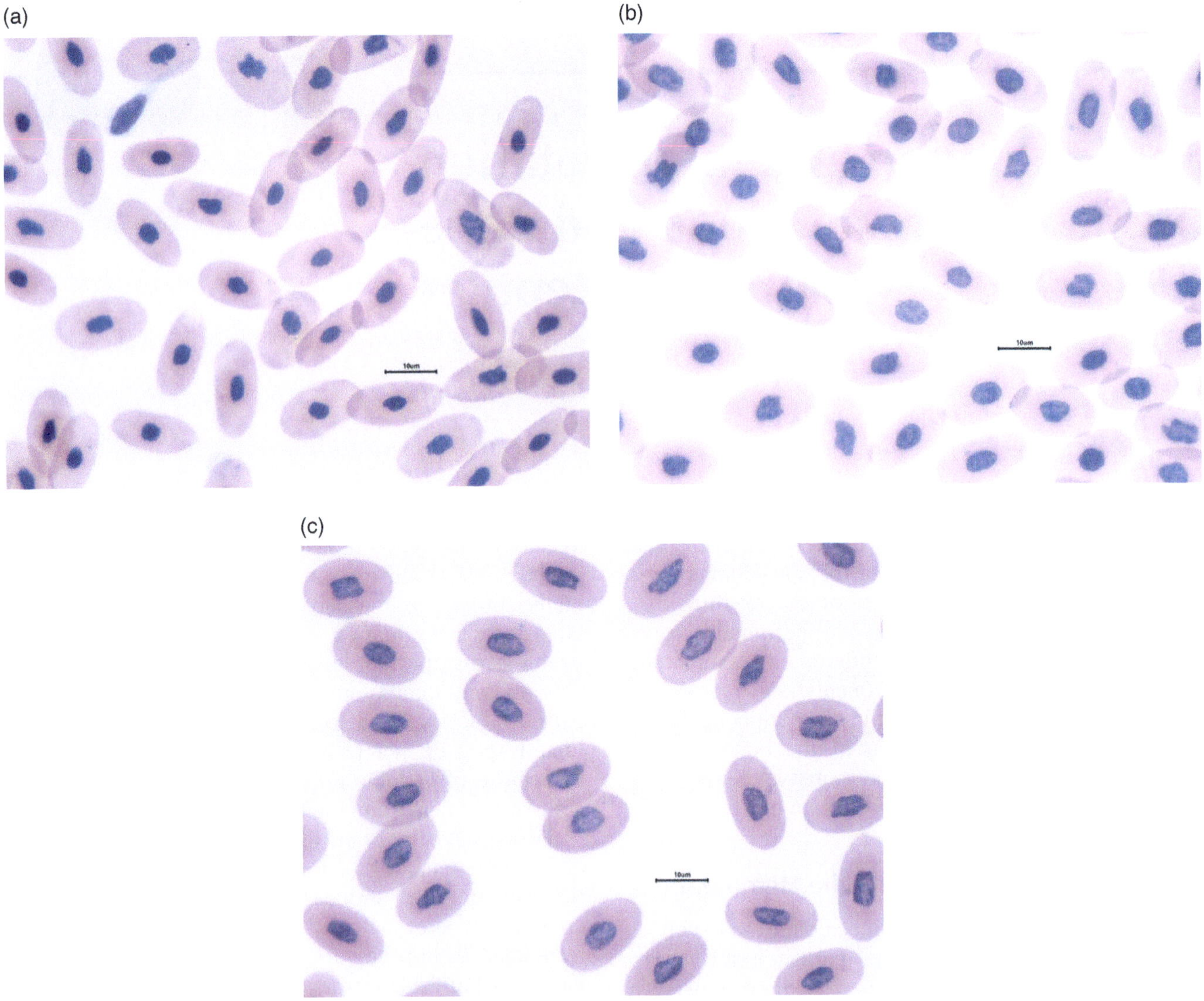

Fig. 19.1. (a) Normal erythrocytes in the blood film of a crocodilian (*Caiman* spp.), Wright–Giemsa stain. (b) Normal erythrocytes in the blood film of a Gila monster (*Heloderma suspectum*), Wright–Giemsa stain. (c) Normal erythrocytes in the blood film of a California kingsnake (*Lampropeltis getula californiae*), Wright–Giemsa stain. Bar = 10 μm.

those of reptiles tend to be irregular. The cytoplasm stains uniformly orange pink with Romanowsky stains such as Wright's stain. Polychromatophilic erythrocytes have nuclear chromatin that is less dense and cytoplasm that is more basophilic than those of mature erythrocytes (Figures 19.2a–c). Immature erythrocytes are occasionally seen in the peripheral blood of reptiles, especially very young animals or those undergoing ecdysis. Immature erythrocytes are round to slightly irregular cells with large, round nuclei and basophilic cytoplasm (Campbell and Grant, 2010) (Figures 19.3a and 19.3b). The nucleus lacks the dense chromatin clumping of the mature cell. Immature erythrocytes often appear smaller than mature erythrocytes, probably because they are spherical in shape and have yet to become flattened ellipsoid cells. Mitotic activity associated with erythrocytes is common in the peripheral blood of reptiles (Figures 19.4a and 19.4b).

Reticulocytes

Reticulocytes are detected by staining cells with a vital stain, such as new methylene blue. Reptilian reticulocytes, like avian reticulocytes, have a distinct ring of aggregated reticulum that encircles the red cell nucleus. These cells best correspond to polychromatophilic erythrocytes found in Romanowsky-stained blood films and are probably cells recently released from erythropoietic tissues (Figure 19.5). Basophilic stippling commonly occurs in reticulocytes stained with Romanowsky stains.

Cytoplasm Inclusions

Round to irregular basophilic inclusions are frequently seen in the cytoplasm of erythrocytes in peripheral blood films from many species of reptiles (Figures 19.1c and 19.6). These inclusions most likely

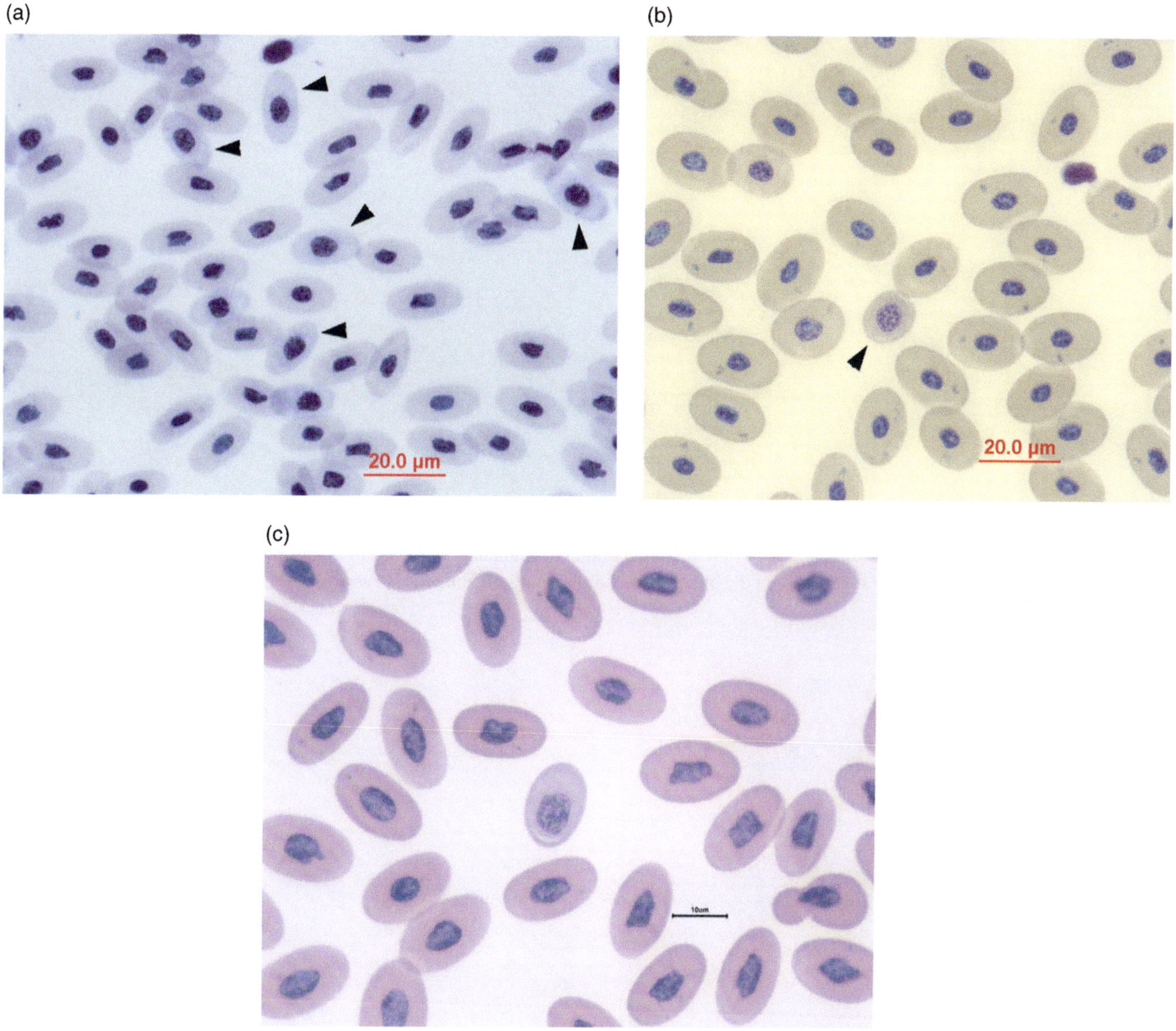

Fig. 19.2. (a) Polychromatic erythrocytes (arrowheads) in the blood film of a green iguana (*Iguana iguana*), Wright–Giemsa stain. (b) Polychromatic erythrocyte (arrowhead) in the blood film of a green sea turtle (*Chelonia mydas*), Wright–Giemsa stain. (c) Polychromatic erythrocyte in the blood film of a California kingsnake (*Lampropeltis getula californiae*), Wright–Giemsa stain.

represent an artifact of slide preparation since blood films made repeatedly from the same blood sample often reveal varying degrees of these inclusions and are not considered to be clinically significant. Electron microscopy suggests that these inclusions are degenerate organelles, such as clumping of the endoplasmic reticulum (Alleman et al., 1992; Clark et al., 2001). Other artifacts found in the erythrocyte cytoplasm include vacuoles and refractile clear areas (Figure 19.7). These can be minimized with careful blood film preparation. Erythrocyte inclusions may also be seen in reptiles with viral infections, such as those caused by arenaviruses and iridoviruses (see subsection "Inclusions" in section "Erythrocyte Response to Disease" later in chapter) (Sykes and Klaphake, 2015; Marschang, 2019).

Factors Affecting the Reptile Erythrogram

Reference intervals for the total red blood cell count (TRBC), hemoglobin (Hb), and packed cell volume (PCV) are difficult to establish for reptiles and other ectotherms, because profound physiologic adaptations may occur in response to several intrinsic and extrinsic factors (Appendix B, Table B.7). Intrinsic factors include species, sex, age, and the physiologic status of the reptile. Extrinsic factors include season, temperature, habitat, diet, disease, stress associated with captivity, and the venipuncture site (Mussachia and Sievers, 1956; Duguy, 1970; Saint Girons, 1970; Lawrence and Hawkey, 1986; Sypek and Borysenko, 1988; Frye, 1991; Gottdenker and Jacobson, 1995; Christopher et al., 1999;

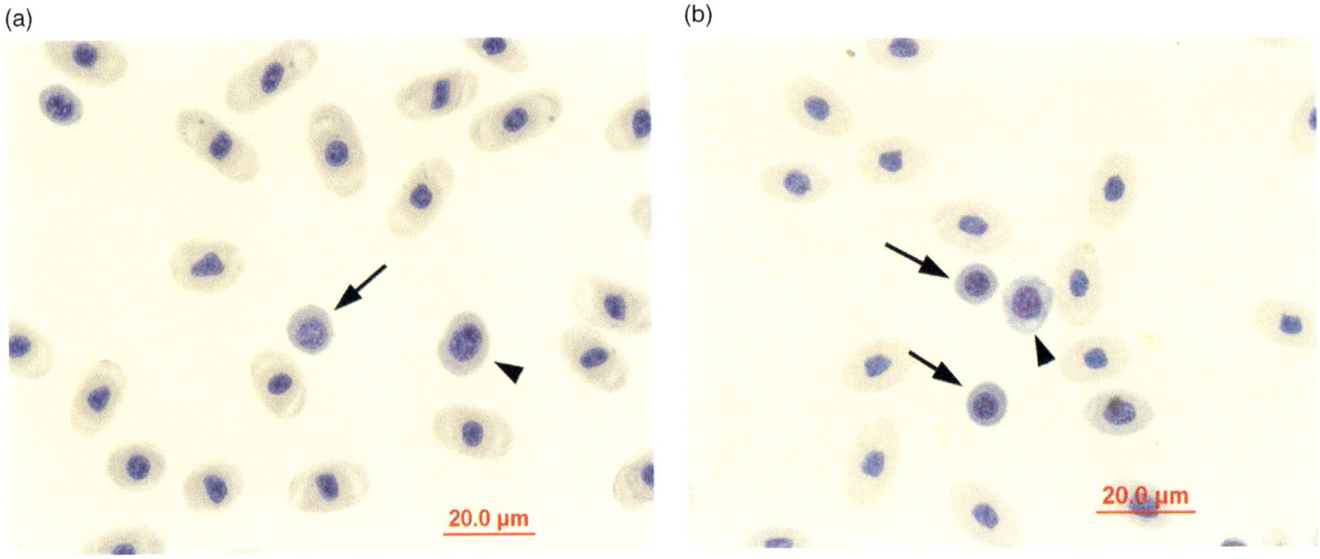

Fig. 19.3. (a) Immature erythrocyte – a late polychromatic rubricyte (arrow) and polychromatic erythrocyte (arrowhead) in the blood film of a painted terrapin (*Batagur borneoensis*), Wright–Giemsa stain. (b) Immature erythrocytes – mid-polychromatic rubricytes (arrows) and polychromatic erythrocyte (arrowhead) in the blood film of a pond turtle (*Chinemys reevesii*), Wright–Giemsa stain.

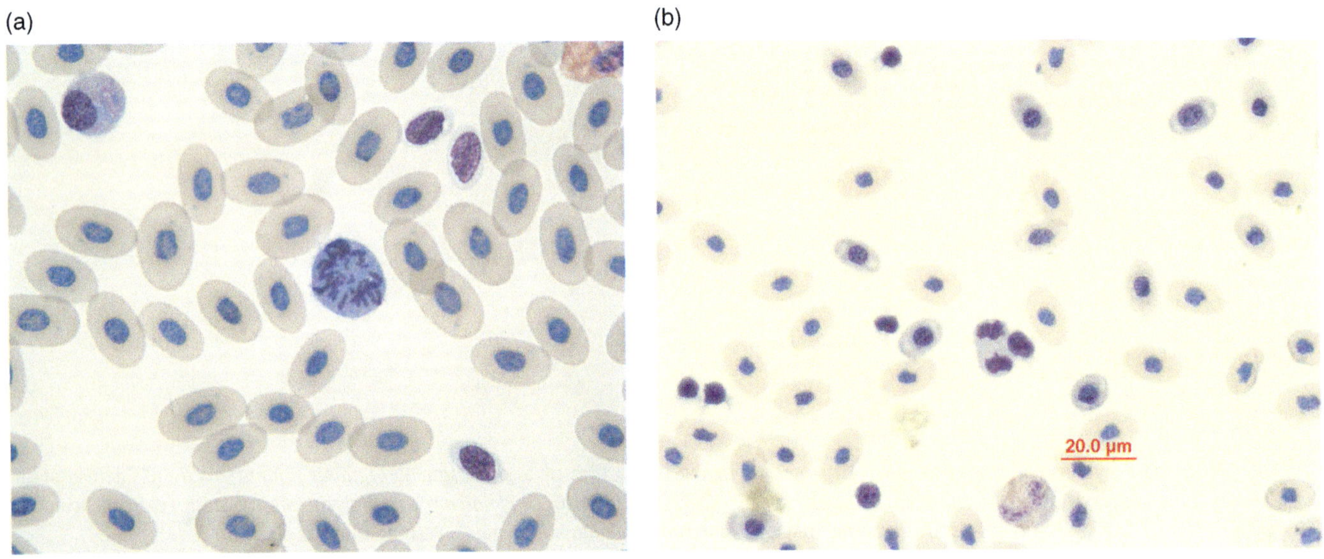

Fig. 19.4. (a) A mitotic figure in the blood film of a three-toed box turtle (*Terrapene carolina triunguis*), Wright–Giemsa stain (100× oil). (b) Erythrocyte mitotic activity in the blood film of a pond turtle (*Chinemys reevesii*), Wright–Giemsa stain.

Lopez-Olvera et al., 2003; Wilkinson, 2004; Sykes and Klaphake, 2015).

When establishing reference intervals, the intrinsic and extrinsic factors affecting the reference population must be documented to ensure that the physiologic data are collected under consistent circumstances (Lopez-Olvera et al., 2003). A minimum of 97 samples from a reference population is recommended to provide statistically meaningful intervals (Walton, 2001). Allowances for 20 or 40 samples to be used in the establishment of reference intervals have been recommended by the American Society of Veterinary Clinical Pathology (ASVCP); however, the preferred standard is use of 120 samples or more (Geffre et al., 2009; Friedrichs et al., 2012; Weiser and Allison, 2012).

Intrinsic Factors

Species

Hemoglobin of most vertebrates has four iron-containing heme subunits, two alpha-globin chains, and two beta-globin chains. The interaction between subunits, largely determined by amino acid sequence, alters

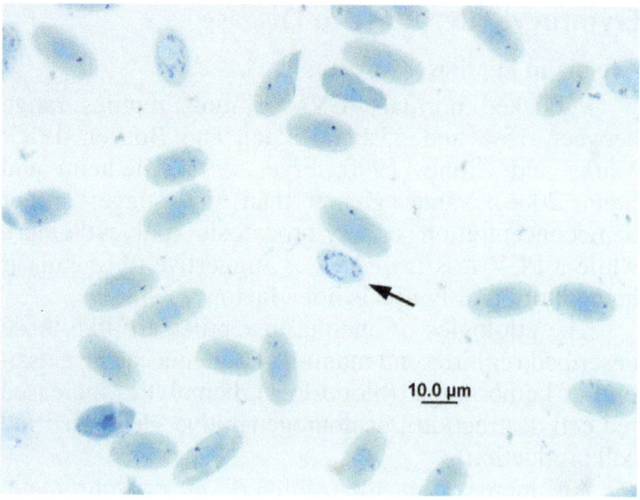

Fig. 19.5. A reticulocyte with a ring of aggregated reticulum encircling the nucleus (arrow) in the blood film of a common boa (*Boa constrictor*), new methylene blue stain.

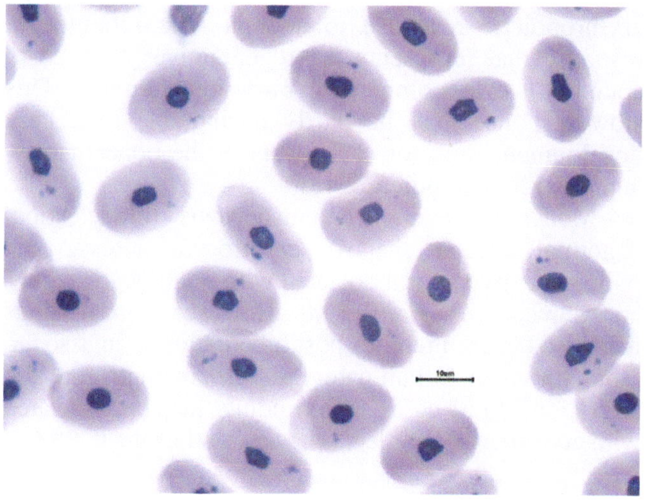

Fig. 19.6. Irregular basophilic inclusions in the cytoplasm of erythrocyte are artifacts in the blood film of a green sea turtle (*Chelonia mydas*), Wright–Giemsa stain. Bar = 10 µm.

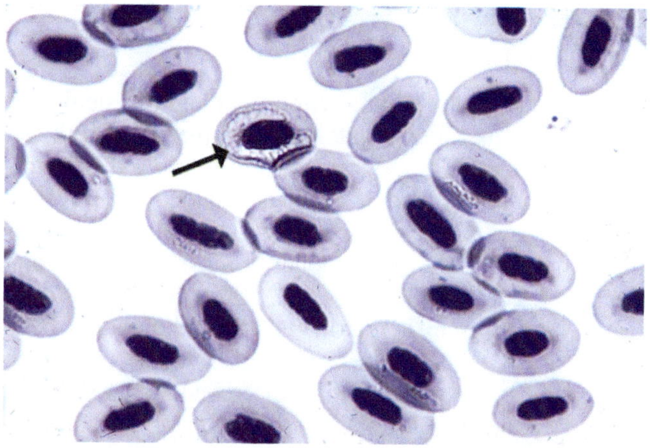

Fig. 19.7. Clear refractile spaces in the cytoplasm of erythrocytes (arrow) of lower vertebrates, such as reptiles and birds, are an artifact of slide preparation. Wright–Giemsa stain (100× oil).

the structure and the oxygen binding properties (Sanyal et al., 2013). The genes in the globin chains are expressed differently in the embryonic and postnatal life stages of mammals and birds as well as in the larval and adult stages of the *Xenopus* genus of amphibians, but not between life stages of the green anole lizard (Storz et al., 2011). In reptiles, the molecular changes in hemoglobin structure have allowed the variations required to adapt to environmental conditions related to altitude, hibernation, and temperature (Storz et al., 2011; Damsgaard et al., 2013; Lu et al., 2015). One study compared hematologic values of a toad-headed agama species living at high altitude (*Phrynocephalus erythrurus*) and a species (*Phrynocephalus przewalskii*) living at a lower altitude and found that the one at higher altitude had a higher oxygen-carrying capacity from the increased TRBC count, hemoglobin concentration, and hematocrit (Lu et al., 2015).

Sex

Disparity in erythrocytic values may be related to sex in some reptile species. Male reptiles typically have higher erythrocytic values than females; however, this is not always the case. For example, male forest hinge-back turtles (*Kinixys erosa*), New Guinea snapping turtles (*Elseya novaeguineae*), and Hermann's tortoise (*Testudo hermanni*) have higher PCV and Hb concentrations compared to females, and some red blood cell parameters are higher in male grass snakes (*Natrix natrix*) and Louisiana pine snakes (*Pituophis ruthveni*) than in the females (Wojtaszek, 1991; Anderson and Wack, 1996; Anderson et al., 1997; Wilkinson, 2004; Andreani et al., 2014; Giori et al., 2019). In another study, female green iguanas (*Iguana iguana*), either gravid or nongravid, had higher hemoglobin concentrations, PCVs, and MCHC values compared to males (Harr et al., 2001). Significant differences may not always be present in other species (Taylor and Jacobson, 1982; Bolten and Bjorndal, 1992; Raphael et al., 1994; Mayer et al., 2005).

Age

Age can affect the hematologic parameters of reptiles. For example, adult marsh crocodiles (*Crocodylus palustris*) have higher red blood cell counts compared to juveniles (Christopher et al., 1999; Stacy and Whitaker, 2000; Dickinson et al., 2002). Young reptiles or those undergoing ecdysis may also exhibit an increase in polychromasia and immature erythrocyte concentration.

Extrinsic Factors

Season and Environment

Seasonal changes in environment and physical condition can affect the hematologic parameters of reptiles. For example, the hemogram of free-ranging desert tortoises (*Gopherus agassizii*) is influenced by physical condition, availability of forage, and the rainfall patterns of the environment (Christopher et al., 1999; Stacy and Whitaker, 2000; Dickinson et al., 2002). Significant seasonal variations in hematologic values have also been reported in rattlesnakes (*Crotalus* spp.) (Troiano et al., 1997). The normal PCVs of green iguanas (*Iguana iguana*) housed outdoors with significant exposure to direct sunlight and a slightly higher environmental temperatures (80°F–100°F) exhibit a slightly wider range (28–46%) compared to the PCV (25–38%) of the same species housed indoors exposed to artificial lighting and lower environmental temperature (74°F–95°F) (Divers et al., 1996; Harr et al., 2001).

Hibernation will affect erythrocytic values in some reptile and amphibian species. In general, erythrocyte indices are highest prior to and lowest immediately after hibernation, although some reptile species do not appear to be affected by hibernation. For example, no differences were observed between pre- and post-hibernation erythrocytic values in several temperate species of snakes (Dutton and Taylor, 2003). In Chinese alligators, TRBC counts were greater during active periods, whereas MCV and MCH values were significantly greater in hibernating alligators, which may be due to lower blood flow with sufficient oxygen availability during hibernation (Peng et al., 2018).

Chronic Stressors

Chronic stressors such as captivity and inappropriate habitat or diet will affect the hemogram (Wilkinson, 2004). The effects of acute stressors, such as capture, handling, and restraint for venipuncture, are unknown but are likely to affect erythrocyte values as well. In one study, captive-bred king cobras (*Ophiophagus hannah*) had higher red blood cell parameters compared to wild-caught king cobras (Salakij et al., 2002).

Blood Collection Site

The site and method of blood collection can affect the hemogram. Lymphatic vessels often accompany blood vessels in reptiles, commonly resulting in a mixture of blood and lymph during venipuncture (Gottdenker and Jacobson, 1995; Crawshaw, 1996). The subsequent lymphodilution of the blood sample will affect the hemogram by decreasing the PCV, Hb concentration, TRBC, and TWBC (Gottdenker and Jacobson, 1995).

Erythrocyte Response to Disease

Anemia in Reptiles

Published normal PCVs of most reptiles range between 15% and 55% (Wallach and Boever, 1983; Marks and Citino, 1990; Frye, 1991; Diethelm and Stein, 2006). Values greater than 55% suggest either hemoconcentration or erythrocytosis (polycythemia), while a PCV less than 15% is suggestive of anemia if hemodilution of lymph is not a factor.

The etiologies of anemia in reptiles are like those described for birds and mammals. Anemia can be classified as hemorrhagic (blood loss), hemolytic (increased red cell destruction), or nonregenerative (decreased red cell production).

An increase in the numbers of polychromatic erythrocytes and increased numbers of reticulocytes are indications of increased erythropoietic activity and occur in reptiles responding to anemic conditions (Figures 19.2, 19.3, and 19.5). The presence of immature erythrocytes such as rubriblasts indicates a marked erythropoietic response to anemia. The reticulocyte response that represents the regenerative response to anemia is slower compared to birds and mammals. This slow response may be partly attributable to a long development time for rubriblasts in the bone marrow and other hematopoietic sites.

Moderate to marked anisocytosis (binucleation, abnormal nuclear shapes), erythrocyte mitosis, and poikilocytosis can be associated with erythrocytic regenerative responses (Figure 19.8). However, these findings may also occur in reptiles post hibernation or in association with severe inflammatory disease, malnutrition, and starvation. In rare cases, these findings may be associated with erythrocyte disorders (Hawkey and Dennett, 1989).

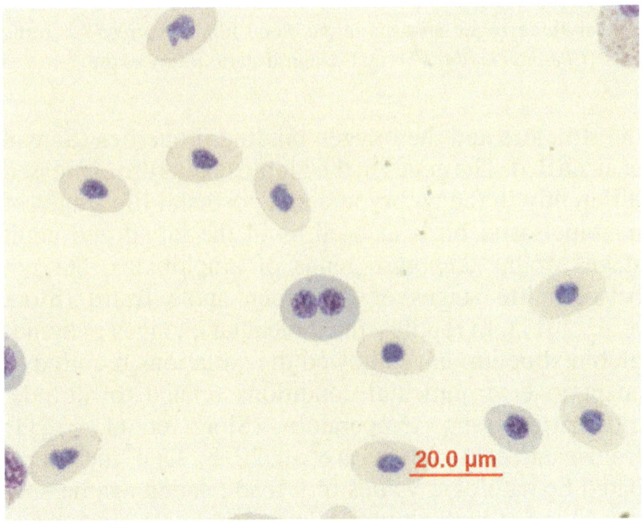

Fig. 19.8. Binucleated erythrocyte in the blood film of a pond turtle (*Chinemys reevesii*), Wright–Giemsa stain.

Hemorrhagic Anemia

Hemorrhagic anemias are typically caused by traumatic injuries or blood-sucking parasites; however, etiologies such as a coagulopathy or an ulcerative lesion should also be considered. In severe cases of hemorrhagic anemia, homologous blood transfusions have been used without adverse reactions in some species (Wack and Anderson, 2004; Louis et al., 2020).

Hemolytic Anemia

Hemolytic anemias may commonly result from sepsis or blood parasites; however other conditions such as autoimmune disease or toxemia should also be considered.

Nonregenerative (Depression) Anemia

Nonregenerative anemia is usually associated with chronic inflammatory diseases, especially those associated with infectious agents. Other etiologies that should be considered as a cause for nonregenerative anemia include chronic renal or hepatic disease, neoplasia, chemical or drug reactions, or potentially hypothyroidism.

Nonregenerative anemia may be associated with chronic infectious disease. Severe anemia has been associated with viral fibropapillomatosis in green sea turtles (*Chelonia mydas*) (Work and Balazs, 1999). Juvenile green sea turtles with fibropapillomatosis showed a significant decrease in hematocrit, hemoglobin, and erythrocyte count compared to turtles without fibropapillomatosis, although the hematocrit values may not be considered consistent with anemia (de Mello and Alvarez, 2020). Tortoises with herpesvirus infection and desert tortoises (*Gopherus agassizii*) with mycoplasma infection and resultant chronic upper respiratory disease develop a normocytic–normochromic, nonregenerative anemia (Jacobson et al., 1990; Muro et al., 1998). Erythrocytes from herpesvirus-infected tortoises stained with May-Grünwald/Giemsa stains demonstrated eccentric, pale blue, long intracytoplasmic inclusions as well. The significance of this finding is unknown (Muro et al., 1998).

Basophilic Stippling

Basophilic stippling usually suggests an erythrocyte regenerative response, but may occur in patients with iron deficiency or, less commonly, lead toxicosis. Hypochromatic erythrocytes are associated with iron deficiency or chronic inflammatory disease (presumably in association with iron sequestration).

Inclusions

In response to viral disease and hemoparasites, erythrocyte inclusion bodies may be present. Other differential diagnoses for observing intracellular inclusions may be bacteria, hemoglobin crystals, or staining artifact.

Erythrocytic Iridovirus

Reptiles with iridoviral infections may exhibit intracytoplasmic erythrocytic inclusion bodies in the hemogram. Reptile erythrocytic iridovirus has been reported in central bearded dragons (*Pogona vitticeps*), as well as in other squamates (Grosset et al., 2014). Reptiles with this disease may exhibit a wide variety of clinical signs such as dehydration, conjunctivitis, tongue lesions, pale mucous membranes, or no clinical signs at all. In addition to intracytoplasmic erythrocytic inclusion bodies, other observed changes on the hemogram may include polychromasia, hypochromasia, or anemia (Grosset et al., 2014).

Inclusion Body Disease

Inclusion body disease (IBD) is a common and highly contagious disease seen worldwide in snakes of the families Boidae and Pythonidae (Schumacher et al., 1994; Chang and Jacobson, 2010). The exact cause of the disease remained unknown for some time; however, it is now believed that IBD is caused by an arenavirus, specifically a reptarenavirus (Latney and Wellehan, 2013, Hetzel et al., 2015, Marschang, 2019). Blood films from boid snakes affected with IBD may reveal inclusions within the cytoplasm of erythrocytes, lymphocytes, or heterophils (Chang and Jacobson, 2010; Banajee et al., 2012). IBD inclusions stained with Wright–Giemsa appear as lightly basophilic homogenous intracytoplasmic inclusions of varying size and shape (Figure 19.9a). These inclusions tend to stain darkly basophilic with quick stains, such as Diff–Quik stain (Figure 19.9b). A lymphocytosis may also be present, presumably due to chronic antigenic stimulation from the infectious agent.

Reptile Leukocytes

Classification of reptilian leukocytes can be problematic in part due to the presence of morphologic variation among the different reptilian species. Classification can be further complicated by the presence of differing descriptive nomenclature in the literature. For example, some sources differentiate the reptilian granulocytes into three cell groups – eosinophils, azurophils, and neutrophils – whereas other sources only differentiate into two: eosinophils and heterophils, or eosinophils and neutrophils (Saint Girons, 1970; Mateo et al., 1984; Wood and Ebanks, 1984; Sypek and Borysenko, 1988; Knotkova et al., 2002).

In general, the leukocytes of reptiles can be divided into two groups: the granulocytes and the mononuclear

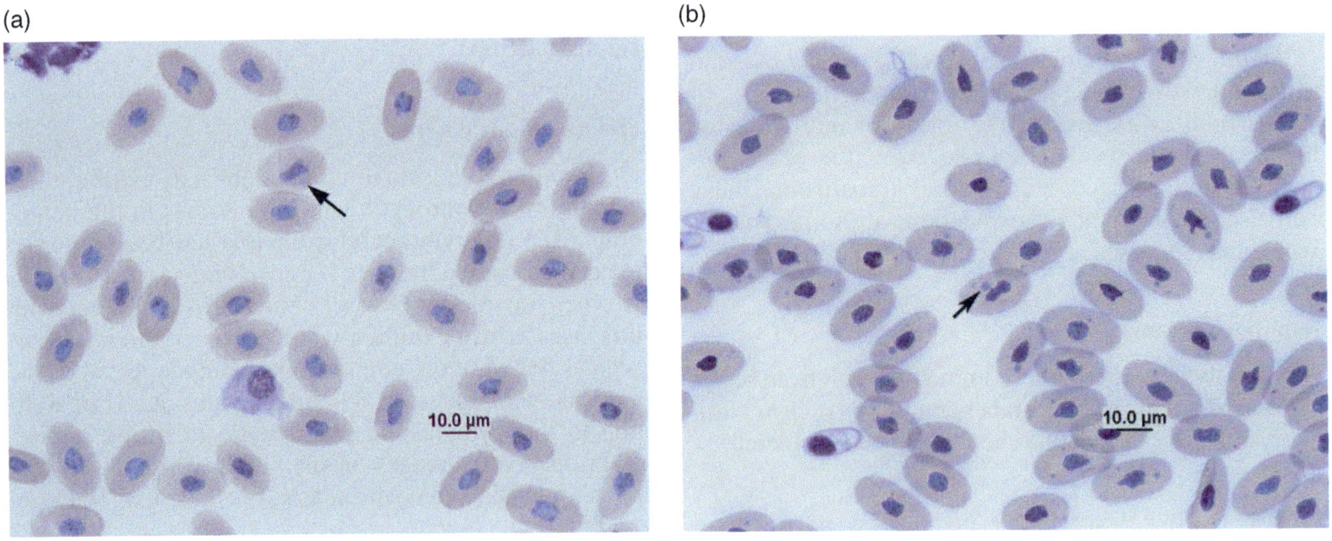

Fig. 19.9. (a) Intracytoplasmic inclusions (arrow) within erythrocytes in the blood film of a common boa (*Boa constrictor*) with IBD, Wright–Giemsa stain. (b) Diff–Quik stain.

leukocytes. The granulocytes of reptiles can be further classified into two groups –acidophils and basophils – based upon their appearance in blood films stained with Romanowsky stains. The acidophils are further divided into heterophils and eosinophils. Heterophils and eosinophils may then be distinguished from each other by the shape and color of their granules. The basophils, lymphocytes, and monocytes found in reptilian blood closely resemble those of mammals and birds and are classified accordingly. A sixth cell type, the azurophil, is often described in the literature and could be a monocyte with azurophilic granules. Attempts using cytochemical staining reactions for normal leukocytes and thrombocytes in various reptiles have been made to help in the classification of reptilian leukocytes (Appendix B, Table B.8).

Heterophils

Reptilian heterophils may be described as large (10–23 µm), round cells with a colorless cytoplasm containing eosinophilic (bright orange), refractile, rod- to spindle-shaped cytoplasmic granules (Saint Girons, 1970) (Figures 19.10a–d). Occasionally, degranulated heterophils can be found in the blood film of normal reptiles (Harr et al., 2001). The cell margins may appear irregular, and pseudopodia may be present under certain circumstances. The nucleus of the mature heterophil is typically eccentrically positioned in the cell and is round to oval with densely clumped nuclear chromatin. Some species of lizards (i.e., green iguanas, *Iguana iguana*) have heterophils with lobed nuclei (Saint Girons, 1970). When toxic changes are present, the cytoplasm appears blue in color and contains abnormal, purple-colored granules and vacuoles. Reptilian heterophils are functionally equivalent to mammalian neutrophils, but probably behave like avian heterophils in that they rely primarily on oxygen-independent mechanisms to destroy phagocytized microorganisms. Reptilian heterophils do not stain for alkaline phosphatase and are usually peroxidase negative, except for a few species of snakes and lizards (Caxton-Martins and Nganwuchu, 1978; Egami and Sasso, 1988; Montali, 1988; Sypek and Borysenko, 1988; Alleman et al., 1992; Work et al., 1998). The heterophils of the green iguana (*Iguana iguana*) and rainbow lizard (*Agama agama*) have cytochemical staining properties like mammalian neutrophils in that they stain positive with benzidine peroxidase (Caxton-Martins and Nganwuchu, 1978; Harr et al., 2001).

Eosinophils

Eosinophils in most reptilian blood films are large (11–17 µm), round cells with light blue cytoplasm, a round to oval (maybe lobed in some species of lizards), slightly eccentric nucleus, and large numbers of spherical eosinophilic cytoplasmic granules (Saint Girons, 1970) (Figures 19.11a–f). Some reptilian species, observed and reported primarily in aquatic or semiaquatic turtles, have a higher prevalence of eosinophils, and may have small (10–16 µm) and large (14–22 µm) eosinophils (Work et al., 1998; Stacy and Harr, 2021) (Figure 19.11f). The cytoplasmic granules of some reptilian species, such as iguanas, stain blue with Romanowsky stains, and will stain positive for peroxidase in some species of reptiles, allowing differentiation between eosinophils and heterophils (Alleman et al., 1992; Harr et al., 2001) (Figures 19.11d and 19.11e). The nucleus is typically centrally located, but may be eccentrically located in

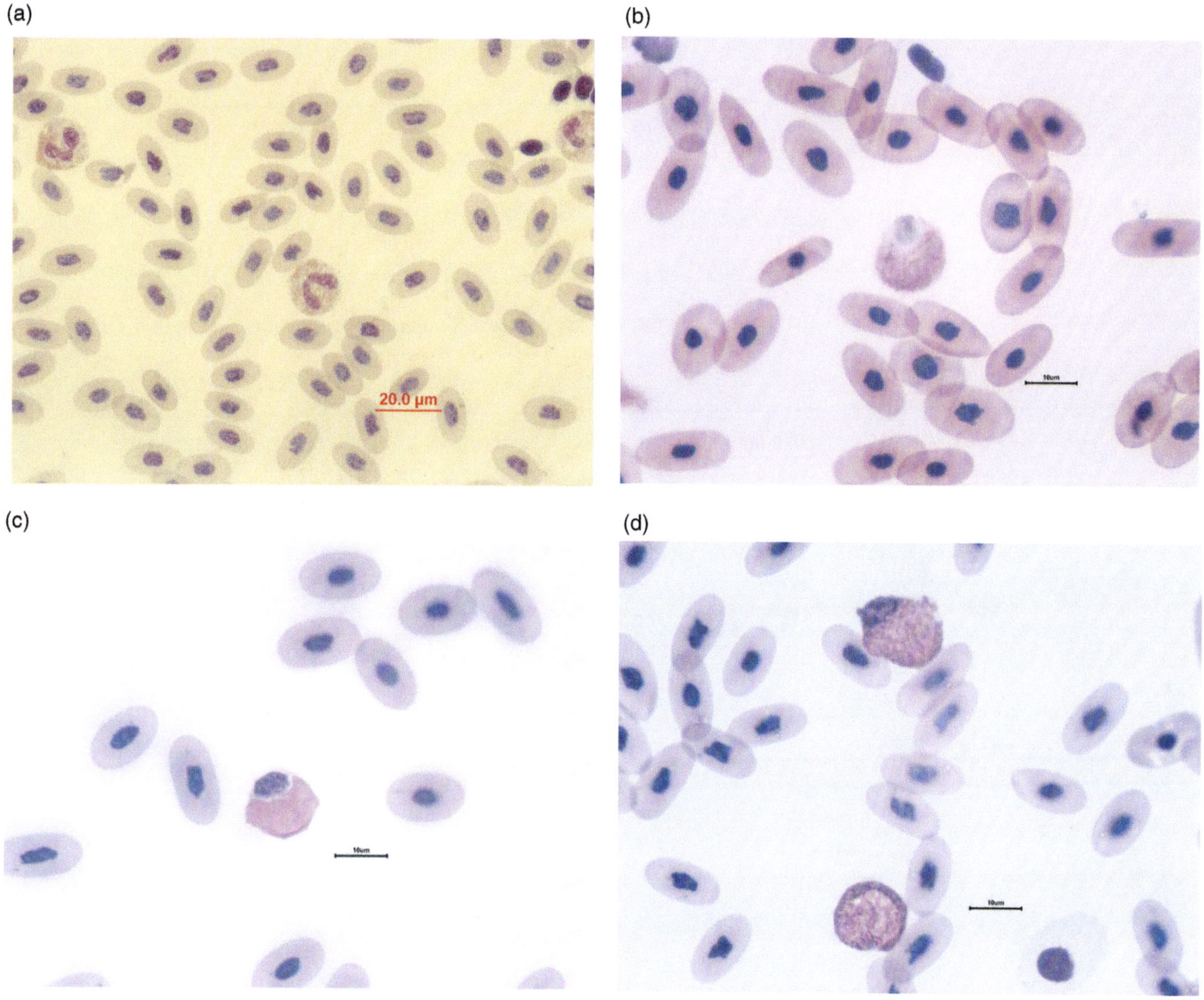

Fig. 19.10. (a) Heterophils in the blood film of a green iguana (*Iguana iguana*), Wright–Giemsa stain. (b) Heterophils in the blood film of a crocodilian (*Caiman* spp.), Wright–Giemsa stain. (c) Heterophils in the blood film of a sulcata tortoise (*Centrochelys sulcata*), Wright–Giemsa stain. (d) Heterophils in the blood film of a green tree python (*Morelia viridis*), Wright–Giemsa stain.

some cases. The size of the eosinophil is species variable. For example, snakes have the largest eosinophils and lizards have the smallest (Saint Girons, 1970).

Basophils

Basophils are small (8–15 µm), round cells (typically smaller than heterophils and eosinophils in the same blood film) that contain variable numbers of round, basophilic (i.e., dark blue to purple), metachromatic cytoplasmic granules (Saint Girons, 1970) (Figures 19.12a–c). The nucleus is often obscured by the granules, but when visible is nonlobed and slightly eccentric in position. Alcohol fixation and use of Romanowsky stains provide the best staining for reptilian basophils because basophil granules are frequently affected by water-based stains and will partially dissolve. Species differences in basophil sizes do occur; lizards tend to have smaller basophils than those observed in turtles and crocodiles (Saint Girons, 1970).

Lymphocytes

Reptilian lymphocytes resemble those of birds and mammals. Lymphocytes are round cells varying in size from small (5–10 µm) to large (15 µm or larger) and exhibit irregularity when they mold around adjacent cells in the blood film or fold at their cytoplasmic margin (Saint Girons, 1970; Sypek and Borysenko, 1988) (Figures 19.13a–d). The nucleus is round and is centrally or slightly eccentric in its position in the cell. Nuclear chromatin is heavily clumped in mature lymphocytes.

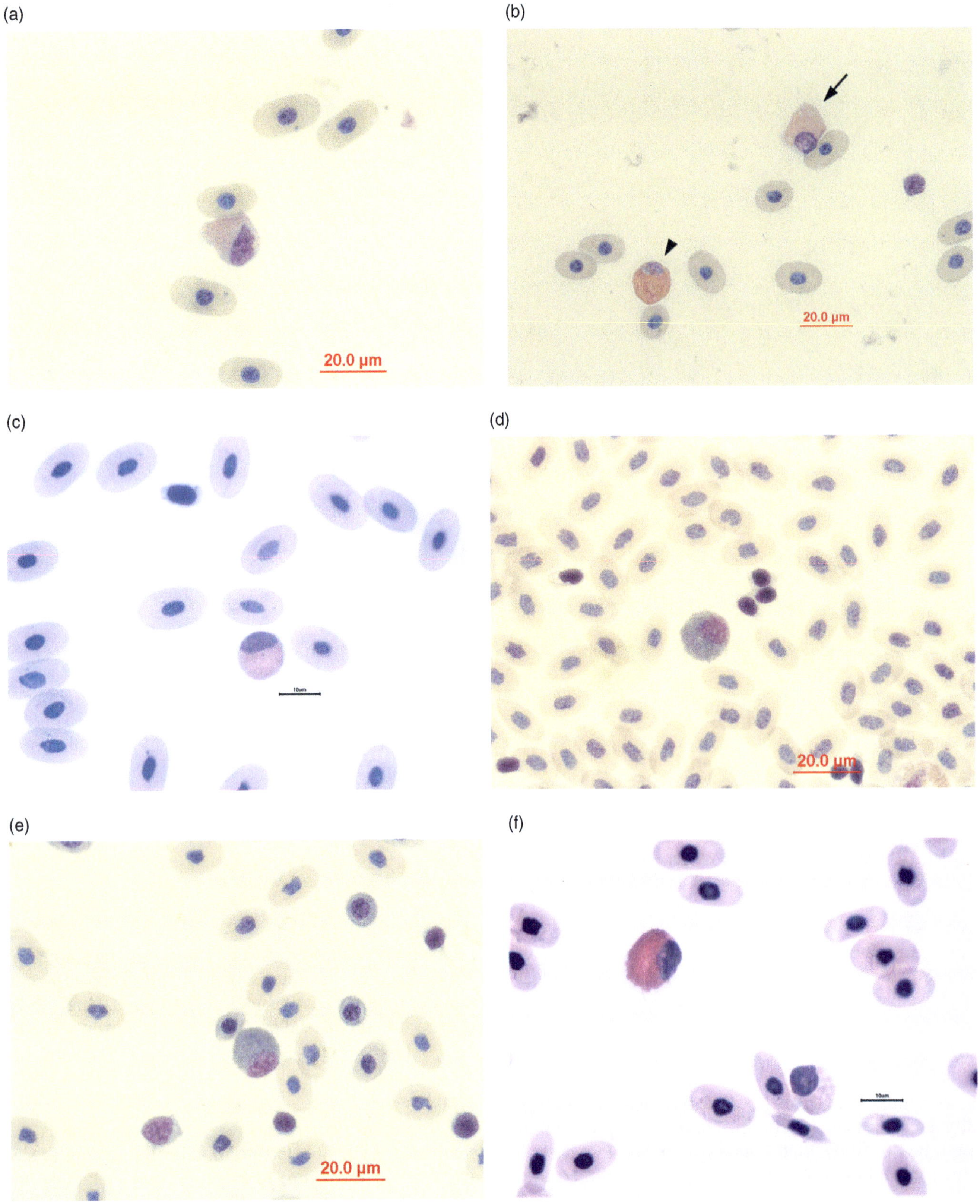

Fig. 19.11. (a) Eosinophil in the blood film of a wood turtle (*Glyptemys insculpta*), Wright–Giemsa stain. (b) A heterophil (arrowhead) and an eosinophil (arrow) in the blood film of a wood turtle (*Glyptemys insculpta*), Wright–Giemsa stain. (c) Eosinophil in the blood film of a sulcate tortoise (*Centrochelys sulcata*), Wright–Giemsa stain. (d) An eosinophil with blue cytoplasmic granules in the blood film of a green iguana (*Iguana iguana*), Wright–Giemsa stain. (e) An eosinophil with blue cytoplasmic granules in the blood film of a pond turtle (*Chinemys reevesii*), Wright–Giemsa stain. (f) A small and a large eosinophil in the blood film of a red-eared slider (*Trachemys scripta elegans*), Wright–Giemsa stain.

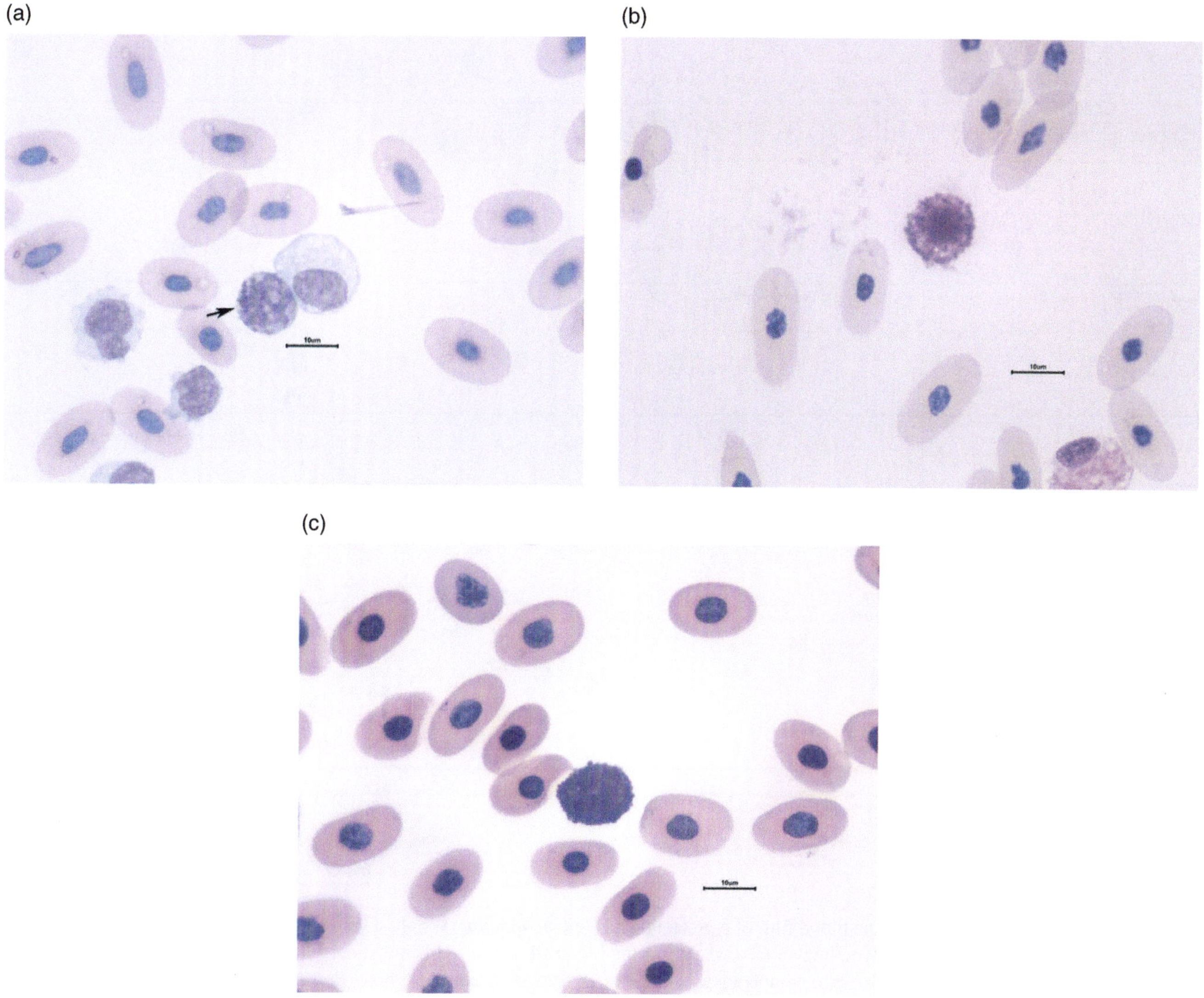

Fig. 19.12. (a) Basophil (arrow) in the blood film of a jungle carpet python (*Morelia spilota cheynei*), Wright–Giemsa stain. (b) Basophil in the blood film of an American alligator (*Alligator mississippiensis*), Wright–Giemsa stain (100× oil). (c) Basophils in the blood film of a Gila monster (*Heloderma suspectum*), Wright–Giemsa stain. Bar = 10 µm.

The cytoplasm of a normal lymphocyte appears homogenous, generally lacks vacuoles and granules, and is slightly basophilic (pale blue) in the typical small, mature lymphocyte. Small azurophilic cytoplasmic granules may be found in some lymphocytes. Large lymphocytes have more cytoplasmic volume compared to small lymphocytes, and the nucleus is often pale staining. Lymphocytes typically have a large nucleus to cytoplasm ratio (N:C).

Plasma cells may be observed in the blood film of reptiles and are slightly larger than normal lymphocytes. The nucleus is eccentrically placed, is round to oval, and contains clumped chromatin. The cytoplasm of plasma cells stains deep blue, and a perinuclear halo (Golgi) is present (Figures 19.14a and 19.14b).

Monocytes

Reptilian monocytes resemble those of birds and mammals and are generally the largest leukocytes in peripheral blood (often one-half to two times the size of erythrocytes in the same blood film) (Figures 19.15a–f). Monocytes vary in shape from round to amoeboid and contain a variably shaped nucleus that ranges from round to oval to lobed (bean shaped). The nuclear chromatin of the monocyte is less condensed and paler staining compared to the nuclear chromatin of lymphocytes. The cytoplasm is abundant, stains pale blue-gray, and may be slightly opaque or foamy in appearance. Phagocytized material, vacuoles, or fine eosinophilic or azurophilic granules may be present in the cytoplasm of some monocytes. Monocytic cells of reptiles have been referred to

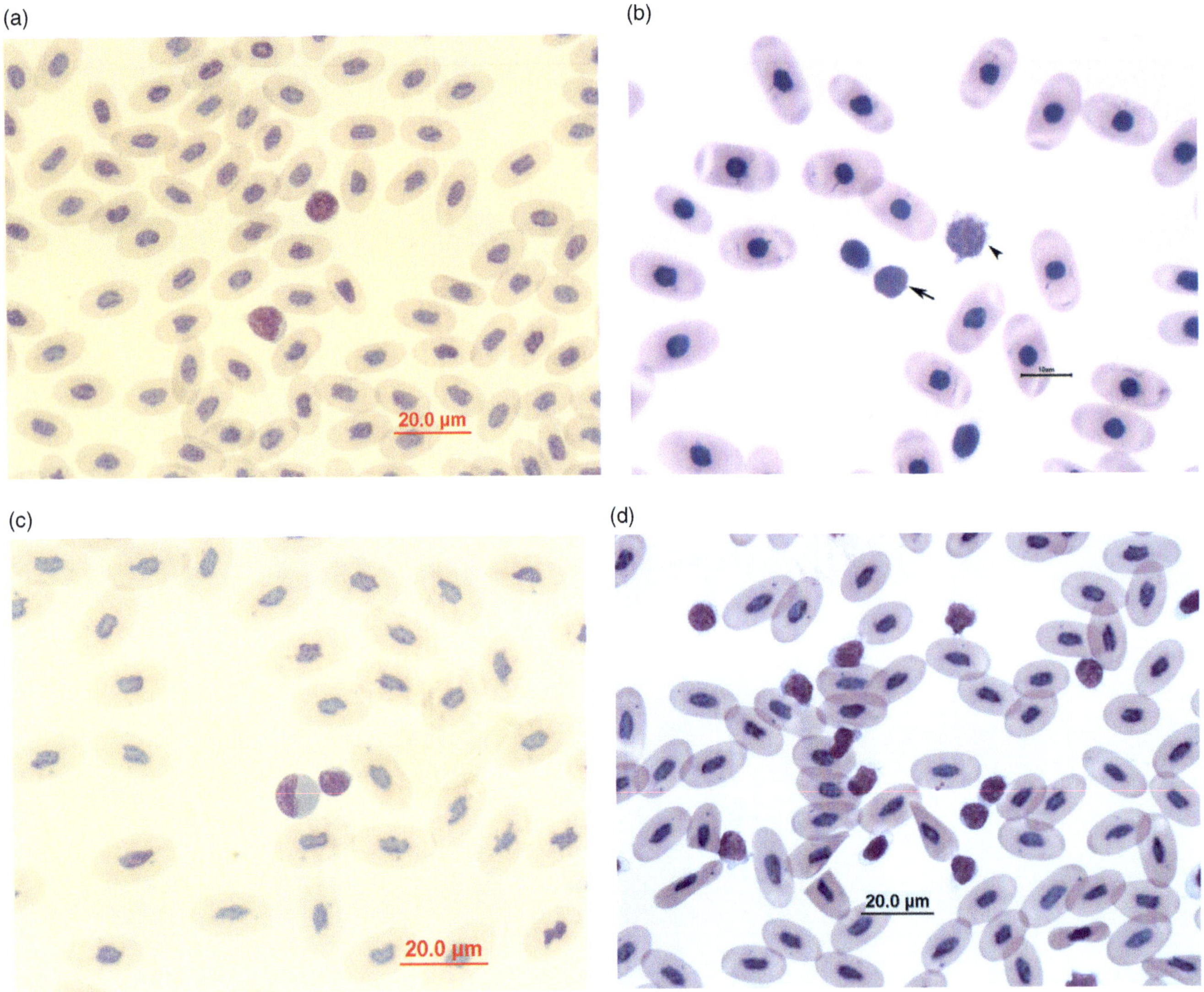

Fig. 19.13. (a) Lymphocytes in the blood film of a green iguana (*Iguana iguana*), Wright–Giemsa stain. (b) A thrombocyte, small lymphocyte (arrow), and a medium lymphocyte (arrowhead) in the blood film of a red-eared slider (*Trachemys scripta elegans*), Wright–Giemsa stain. (c) A small and a large lymphocyte in the blood film of a common boa (*Boa constrictor*), Wright–Giemsa stain. (d) Lymphocytosis in the blood film of a bearded dragon (*Pogona vitticeps*), Wright–Giemsa stain.

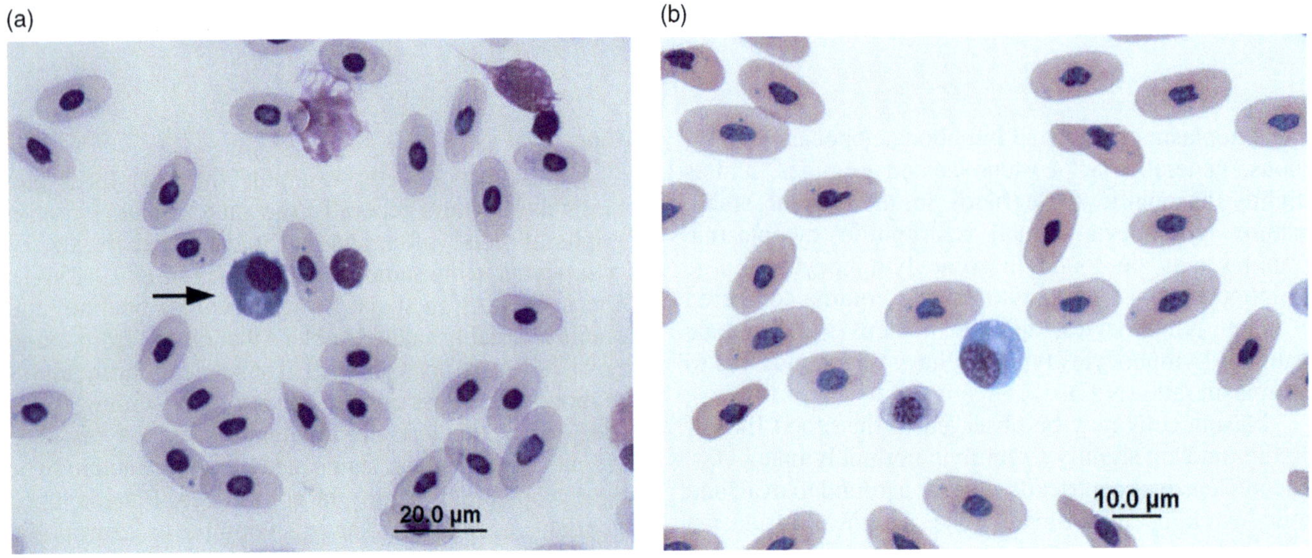

Fig. 19.14. (a) A plasma cell (arrow) in the blood film of a three-toed box turtle (*Terrapene carolina triunguis*), Wright–Giemsa stain. (b) A plasma cell in the blood film of a common boa (*Boa constrictor*), Wright–Giemsa stain.

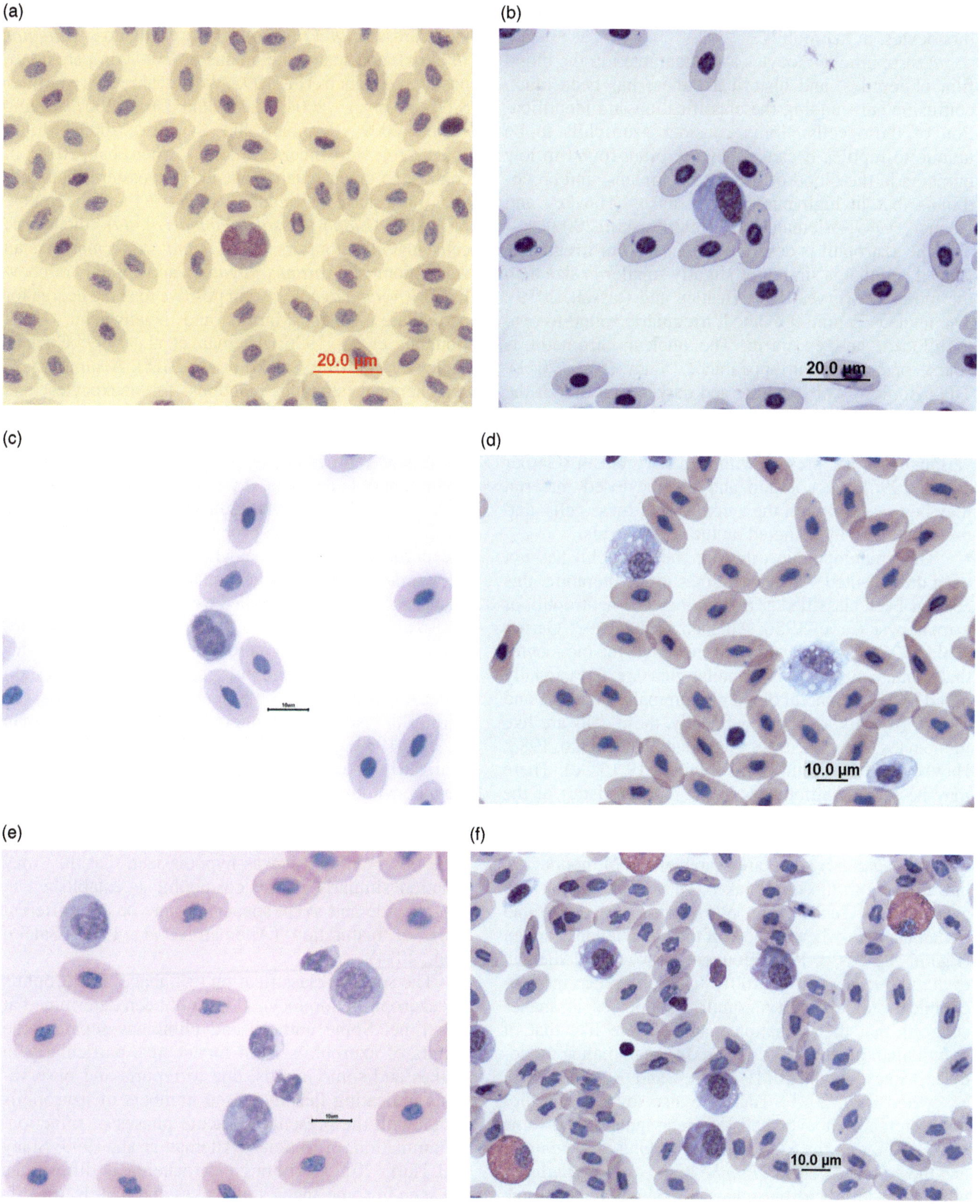

Fig. 19.15. (a) Monocyte in the blood film of a green iguana (*Iguana iguana*), Wright–Giemsa stain. (b) Monocyte in the blood film of a three-toed box turtle (*Terrapene carolina triunguis*), Wright–Giemsa stain. (c) Monocyte in the blood film of a sulcate tortoise (*Centrochelys sulcata*), Wright–Giemsa stain. (d) Monocytes in the blood film of a common boa (*Boa constrictor*), Wright–Giemsa stain. (e) Monocytes in the blood film of a California kingsnake (*Lampropeltis getula californiae*). (f) Monocytosis in the blood film of a green tree python (*Morelia viridis*), Wright–Giemsa stain.

as monocytes, monocytoid azurophils, azurophilic monocytes, or azurophils.

Azurophilic leukocytes are often noted in the blood film of reptiles, and historically there has been much confusion surrounding the classification and identification of these cells. Some consider azurophils to be unique to reptiles because they are often found in low numbers in the blood of lizards, chelonians, and crocodilians, but in high numbers in snakes (Hawkey and Dennett, 1989; Alleman et al., 1992; Raskin, 2000).

The azurophil is described as a round or irregularly shaped cell that is similar or slightly smaller in size than the monocyte (Frye, 1991; Heatley and Russell, 2019). The nucleus is nonsegmented, irregularly round to oval to bilobed, and eccentric. The nuclear chromatin is coarse or clumped in appearance (Stacy et al., 2011). The cytoplasm is basophilic and darker than that of the monocyte and may be described as blue to lavender in color. Small numbers of dull azurophilic granules of various sizes are present within the cytoplasm (Garner et al., 1996). Vacuolation and phagocytosed material may be present within the cytoplasm of these cells, and pseudopodia may be noted on the cell margins.

The granulopoietic origin of the azurophil has not been documented. At various times in the literature, this cell has been classified as a granulocyte, a neutrophil, or a monocyte (Frye, 1986; Alleman et al., 1992; Garner et al., 1996). Grossly, azurophils resemble the monocytes that contain azurophilic granules that are occasionally noted in the peripheral blood of mammals and birds, and ultrastructurally and cytochemically, these cells are like monocytes (Montali, 1988; Sypek and Borysenko, 1988; Hawkey and Dennett, 1989) (Figures 19.16a–c). There may be species differences in the characteristics of the cells. For example, the cytochemical properties of all monocytic cells (monocytes and azurophils) of green iguanas (*Iguana iguana*) are characteristic of monocytes, but differ from those of snakes (Harr et al., 2001). The azurophils of snakes stain positive for peroxidase and Sudan black B, whereas those of the green iguanas do not (Egami and Sasso, 1988; Bounous et al., 1996; Alleman et al., 1999; Harr et al., 2001). This difference in cytochemical staining of azurophilic monocytes in snakes suggests that their function may be more like that of mammalian neutrophils compared to mammalian monocytes (Stacy et al., 2011; Heatley and Russell, 2019; Stacy and Harr, 2021). There are also some similarities between the monocytic cells of green iguanas and some snakes, such as the king cobra (*Ophiophagus hannah*) and the yellow rat snake (*Elaphe obsoleta quadrivittata*), which all stain acid phosphatase positive and to some degree stain PAS positive (Bounous et al., 1996; Harr et al., 2001; Salakij et al., 2002). Monocytic cells of other reptiles also have cytochemical properties like those of green iguanas (*Iguana iguana*); however, there is some variability. For example, like green iguanas, the monocytic cells in giant lizards (*Gallotia simonyi*), bobtail lizards (*Tiliqua rugosa*), Chinese alligators (*Alligator sinensis*), and many chelonians do not stain peroxidase positive (Alleman et al., 1992; Work et al., 1998; Martinez Silvestre et al., 2004; Casal and Oros, 2007; Chung et al., 2009; Perpinan and Sanchez, 2009; Moller et al., 2016; Hernandez et al., 2017; Chen et al., 2018). In contrast to green iguanas but like the eastern diamondback rattlesnake (*Crotalus adamanteus*) and the yellow rat snake (*Elaphe obsolete quadrivitatta*), monocytic cells in Gila monsters (*Heloderma suspectum*), Asian water monitors (*Varanus salvator*), and possibly rainbow lizards (*Agama agama*), stain positive to some degree for peroxidase (Caxton-Martins and Nganwuchu, 1978; Bounous et al., 1996; Alleman et al., 1999; Cooper-Bailey et al., 2011; Salakij et al., 2014). A summary of cytochemical staining reactions for leukocytes and thrombocytes for the aforementioned species are in Appendix B, Table B.8.

In the reptile studies reviewed for cytochemical evaluation of leukocytes, it was observed that almost all species whose monocytes/azurophils were perioxidase positive were within the proposed clade Toxicofera (all except for the green iguana, which was peroxidase negative), order Squamata; other squamates as well as chelonians and crocodilians studied were peroxidase negative. It also appears that many of the aforementioned species within the group with peroxidase-positive monocytes (azurophils) lack eosinophils; or eosinophils as established in avian and reptile species were not observed during the studies (Bounous et al., 1996; Alleman et al., 1999; Cooper-Bailey et al., 2011; Salakij et al., 2014). Another observation of commonality is that they are within families identified with nonlobed heterophils (Blofield et al., 1992). In some studies, two types of heterophils, based on granulation and granule shape, were observed, and it was hypothesized that they may function similarly to the eosinophil as established in other reptile and avian species or may be at a different stage of maturation (Alleman et al., 1999; Salakij et al., 2014).

The specific classification or lineage of azurophils (or azurophilic monocytes) has not been determined at this time. Some authors and clinicians separate the counts of azurophils from monocytes, particularly in snakes and some lizards, due to reports and observations indicating that increased numbers of azurophils occur with the presence of acute phases of infection, inflammation, or toxicity (Alleman et al., 1999; Stacy and Harr, 2021). Although cytochemical differences are seen in some species of snakes and lizards, the difficulty in counting azurophils separately from azurophilic monocytes or monocytes is knowing which species it would be appropriate in, as general functional differences have not been distinctly identified (Origgi and Tecilla, 2021).

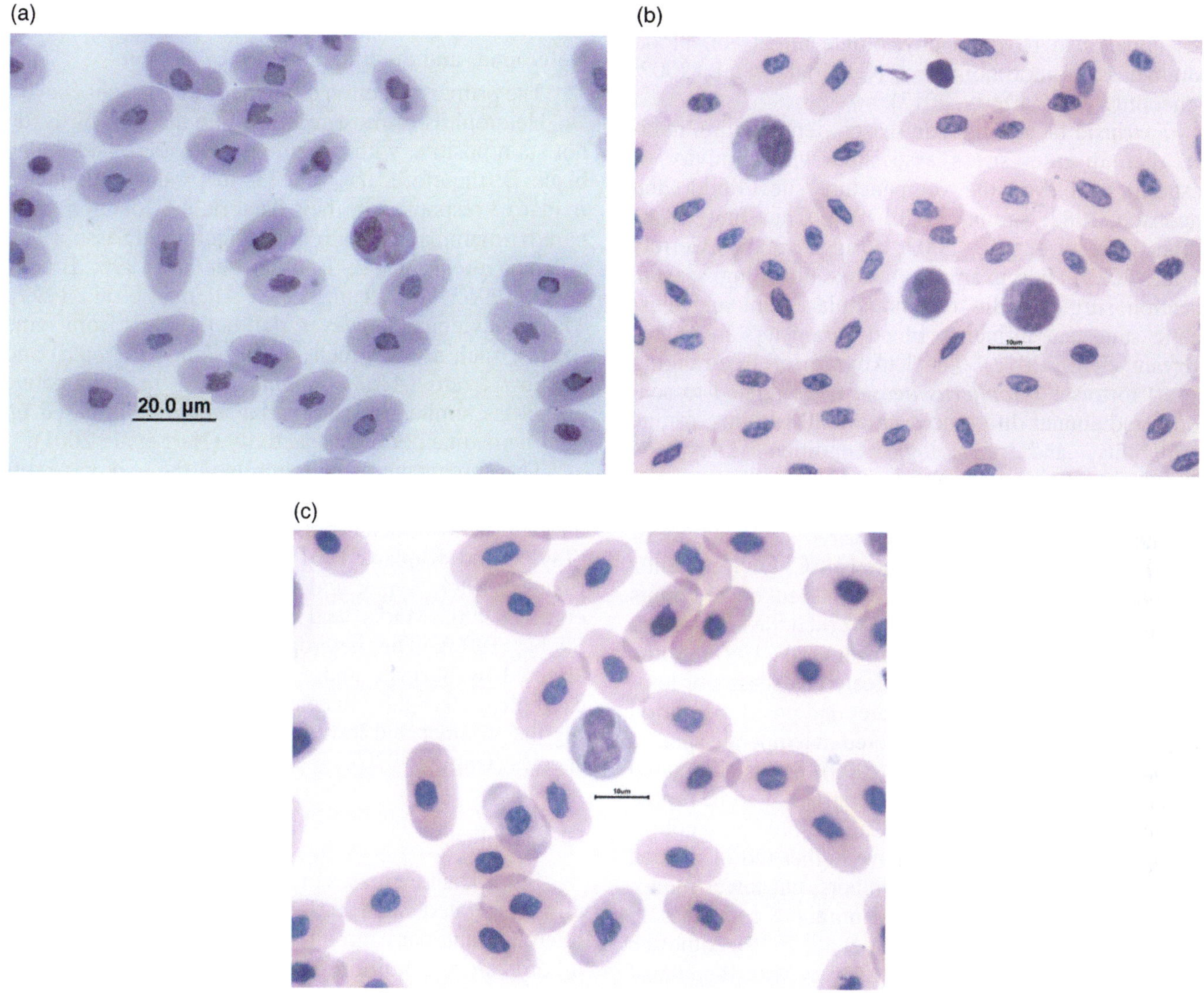

Fig. 19.16. (a) Monocyte with azurophilic granules (azurophil) in the blood film of a common boa (*Boa constrictor*), Wright–Giemsa stain. (b) Monocytes with azurophilic granules (azurophils) in the blood film of a California kingsnake (*Lampropeltis getula californiae*), Wright–Giemsa stain. (c) Monocyte with azurophilic granules (azurophil) in the blood film of a Gila monster (*Heloderma suspectum*), Wright–Giemsa stain.

Normal Variation to the Leukogram of Reptiles

Reference Intervals

Establishment of reference intervals for the total leukocyte count and leukocyte differential is difficult in reptiles and other ectotherms for the same reasons described in the erythrocyte section (Appendix B, Tables B.9a and B.9b) Physiologic adaptations to the intrinsic and extrinsic factors previously described may affect the leukogram of the individual reptile. The same guidelines used for establishing erythrocyte intervals should be considered when developing meaningful statistically accurate leukocyte intervals. Guidelines for establishing reference intervals have been described elsewhere (Weiser and Allison, 2012; Cray, 2015)

Intrinsic factors such as species, sex, age, and the physiologic status of the reptile will affect the leukogram. Differences in the leukogram may occur broadly across the reptile species, but can occur within the same genus as well. For example, significant differences in heterophil, monocyte, and lymphocyte counts have been documented among different species of *Gallotia* lizards (Martinez Silvestre et al., 2004). Sex and age differences may affect the leukocyte parameters. Male crocodiles (*Crocodylus palustris*) have higher total leukocyte and heterophil counts compared to females, and adult crocodiles have lower total leukocyte counts compared to juveniles (Stacy and Whitaker, 2000). The reproductive status of a reptile may influence the hemogram. For example, female chameleons may demonstrate heterophilia after egg laying; however, gravidity in turtles appears to have no physiologic effects on blood parameters or morphometrics (Cuadrado et al., 2002; Scheelings and Rafferty, 2012).

Extrinsic factors include season, temperature, habitat, diet, disease, stress associated with captivity or restraint, and even the venipuncture site (Taylor and Jacobson, 1982; Samour et al., 1986; Crawshaw, 1996; Lopez-Olvera et al., 2003; Origgi, 2007; Cerreta et al., 2020). For example, factors including season, location, surgical radio transmitter placement, and anesthetic state can influence blood parameters in snakes (Bryant et al., 2012). The leukogram of free-ranging desert tortoises (*Gopherus agassizii*) is related to seasonal and annual differences in rainfall patterns, forage availability, and physiologic condition (Dickinson et al., 2002). Young crocodiles housed in low-temperature (28°C) environments for 10 days had lower total leukocyte and lymphocyte counts compared to young crocodiles housed in high-temperature (38°C) environments, and both sets of these crocodiles had leukocyte counts that were abnormal compared to crocodiles housed at normal temperature (32°C) (Turton et al., 1997). Some species of reptile may not be affected by season or temperature; no differences in the pre- and post-hibernation hematologic parameters were noted in temperate species of snakes (Dutton and Taylor, 2003). Stress associated with captivity may affect the leukogram of some reptile species (Cerreta et al., 2020b). Captive-bred king cobras (*Ophiophagus hannah*) may have higher red blood cell parameters and lymphocyte numbers, but lower monocyte (azurophil) and heterophil numbers compared to wild-caught king cobras (Salakij et al., 2002). Although the results of the hemogram may vary with the site of venipuncture in some species, it may have no effect on others (Stewart et al., 2012).

Other considerations when establishing or referring to reference intervals are the methods and techniques used. For example, in a comparison of hematological values in the eastern indigo snake (*Drymarchon couperi*), the percentage of heterophils was shown to be significantly higher in heparin-preserved samples compared to samples collected without anticoagulant, the percentage of azurophils was significantly higher in heparin and EDTA samples compared to those without anticoagulant, and PCV and TS were significantly lower in samples prepared with trisodium citrate compared to other anticoagulants (heparin and EDTA) and no anticoagulant (Bogan et al., 2020). Another factor that may influence reference interval results is the method used to determine the total leukocyte count. Differences in total white cell count in eastern box turtles (*Terrapene carolina carolina*) have varied between manual counts using the avian Leukopet™ (Vetlab Supply, Palmetto Bay, FL) method compared to estimating the count from the blood film, with significantly higher counts reported using the Leukopet™ method (Winter et al., 2019).

Leukocyte Response to Disease

Heterophils and the Inflammatory Leukogram

The primary function of the heterophil is phagocytosis. Heterophils of most reptiles, like those of birds, do not stain positive with benzidine peroxidase and Sudan black B; therefore, they appear to produce attenuated oxidative responses in their bactericidal function compared to mammalian neutrophils (Egami and Sasso, 1988; Alleman et al., 1992; Bounous et al., 1996; Brooks et al., 1996; Work et al., 1998; Alleman et al., 1999). There is evidence, however, that heterophils from some lizards, such as the green iguana (*Iguana iguana*) and rainbow lizard (*Agama agama*), may have oxidative properties similar to mammalian neutrophils based on their benzidine peroxidase activity (Harr et al., 2001).

The percentage of heterophils in the leukocyte differential is species variable. Some normal reptiles may have up to 40% heterophils present in the differential (Taylor and Kaplan, 1961; Duguy, 1970; Wood and Ebanks, 1984; Sypek and Borysenko, 1988; Jacobson et al., 1990; Marks and Citino, 1990; Wright and Skeba, 1992). The heterophil concentration may be affected by intrinsic and extrinsic factors as well. For example, heterophil concentration is often highest during the summer and lowest during hibernation in some species (Duguy, 1970).

Heterophilia

Significant increases in the heterophil count are usually associated with inflammatory diseases such as microbial and parasitic infections or tissue injury. Noninflammatory conditions that may result in heterophilia include stress (glucocorticosteroid excess), neoplasia, and heterophilic leukemia. Noninfectious and infectious agents can result in an inflammatory response in reptiles. For example, extensive inflammatory response with heterophilia and monocytosis to implanted radiotransmitters with and without an associated anaerobic and gram-negative bacterial infection can occur in reptiles (Lentini et al., 2011). The high initial leukocyte counts that commonly occur in cold-stunned turtles are likely a reflection of inflammation, immune response, physiologic stress, or systemic pathologic conditions (Campbell, 2006; Innis et al., 2009).

Abnormal-Appearing Heterophils

Heterophils may appear abnormal in reptiles suffering from disease. Varying degrees of heterophil toxicity may be noted when inflammatory diseases are present, especially those involving infectious agents such as bacteria. Toxic heterophils exhibit increased cytoplasmic basophilia, increased cytoplasmic vacuolation, and abnormal granulation (i.e., dark blue to purple granules,

granules with abnormal shapes, abnormal staining) (Campbell and Grant, 2010) (Figures 19.17a–f). The presence of nuclear lobation in reptile species that normally do not have lobulated heterophil nuclei is another finding suggestive of severe inflammation (Figure 19.17e). Degranulated heterophils may be noted on some blood films and may represent toxic changes or are artifacts associated with preparation of the blood film slide.

Another possible distinct type of abnormal heterophil morphology resulting from disease is a heterophil projection resembling that of a heterophil extracellular trap (HET) (Stacy et al., 2017a; Flanders et al., 2021; Stacy and Harvey, 2021). The heterophilic projections were described in a case involving a gopher tortoise with anemia and acute inflammatory disease based on immature and toxic heterophils. The heterophilic projections were primarily observed in mature, non-toxic heterophils.

Immature Heterophils

The presence of immature heterophils (left shift) in the blood film of reptiles exhibiting a heterophilia is indicative of an inflammatory disease (Figure 19.18). A left shift in the presence of a heteropenia is indicative of an overwhelming inflammatory response that is likely associated with an infectious etiology. Reptiles often develop a marked leukocytosis and heterophilia with the presence of many immature heterophils, often as early as progranulocytes or myeloblasts, with severe inflammatory diseases, especially those with a bacterial etiology.

Disease and exposure to environmental or chemical toxins can affect the leukogram of reptiles. Tortoises affected with herpesvirus infection often demonstrate heteropenia and lymphocytosis in the leukogram; toxic heterophils; and lymphocytes with pale blue, eccentric intracytoplasmic inclusions (Muro et al., 1998). Abnormal heterophil:lymphocyte ratios appear to be related to the circulating blood concentration of organochlorines in loggerhead sea turtles (*Caretta caretta*) (Keller et al., 2004).

Eosinophilia in Reptiles

The number of circulating eosinophils in normal reptiles is variable. In general, lizards tend to have lower numbers of eosinophils compared to some species of turtles, which may have up to 20% eosinophils (Taylor and Kaplan, 1961; Duguy, 1970; Wood and Ebanks, 1984; Sypek and Borysenko, 1988; Jacobson et al., 1990; Marks and Citino, 1990; Wright and Skeba, 1992). Like most other hematologic parameters, the eosinophil count is influenced by intrinsic and extrinsic factors such as environmental and seasonal changes. In general, the number of eosinophils is lower during the summer and highest during hibernation in some species (Duguy, 1970). Eosinophilia may be associated with parasitic infections and stimulation of the immune system (Mead and Borysenko, 1984).

Basophilia in Reptiles

The percentage of basophils in the differential leukocyte count of normal reptiles can range between 0% and 40% (Taylor and Kaplan, 1961; Duguy, 1970; Wood and Ebanks, 1984; Sypek and Borysenko, 1988; Jacobson et al., 1990; Marks and Citino, 1990; Wright and Skeba, 1992). For example, some species of chelonians (i.e., desert tortoises, *Gopherus agassizii*) typically have high circulating basophil numbers (up to 40% of the leukocyte differential at times), although the reason for this is unknown (Mead et al., 1983; Sypek et al., 1984). Seasonal variation in basophil concentration is minimal compared to the heterophil and eosinophil concentrations (Saint Girons, 1970).

Cytochemical and ultrastructural studies show that reptilian basophils most likely function in a manner similar to that of mammalian basophils by processing surface immunoglobulins and releasing histamine upon degranulation (Mead and Borysenko, 1984; Sypek et al., 1984; Sypek and Borysenko, 1988). Basophilia has been associated with parasitic and viral infections (Sypek and Borysenko, 1988).

Lymphocytes

Lymphocyte concentration in the blood of reptiles is variable and can represent over 80% of the normal leukocyte differential in some species (Sypek and Borysenko, 1988). Many healthy reptiles have a higher lymphocyte count than heterophil count (Duguy, 1970; Harr et al., 2001; International Species Information System, 2002).

Lymphocyte numbers are influenced by several intrinsic and extrinsic factors. Environmental and physiologic factors such as seasonal change and hibernation may affect the lymphocyte count. In general, lymphocyte counts tend to be lowest during the winter and highest during the summer (Duguy, 1970; Sypek and Borysenko, 1988; Jacobson et al., 1990). Temperate reptiles often exhibit a decrease or absence of lymphocytes during hibernation. After hibernation, the lymphocyte concentration increases (Hussein et al., 1978, 1979a, 1979b; Wright and Cooper, 1981). Tropical reptiles that do not hibernate often demonstrate a decrease in circulating lymphocytes during the winter as well (Sypek and Borysenko, 1988). Lymphocyte numbers are also affected by sex. Females of some species may have significantly greater lymphocyte concentrations than males of the same species (Duguy, 1970; Sypek and Borysenko, 1988).

Reptilian lymphocytes function in a manner like those of birds and mammals. Reptiles have the same two

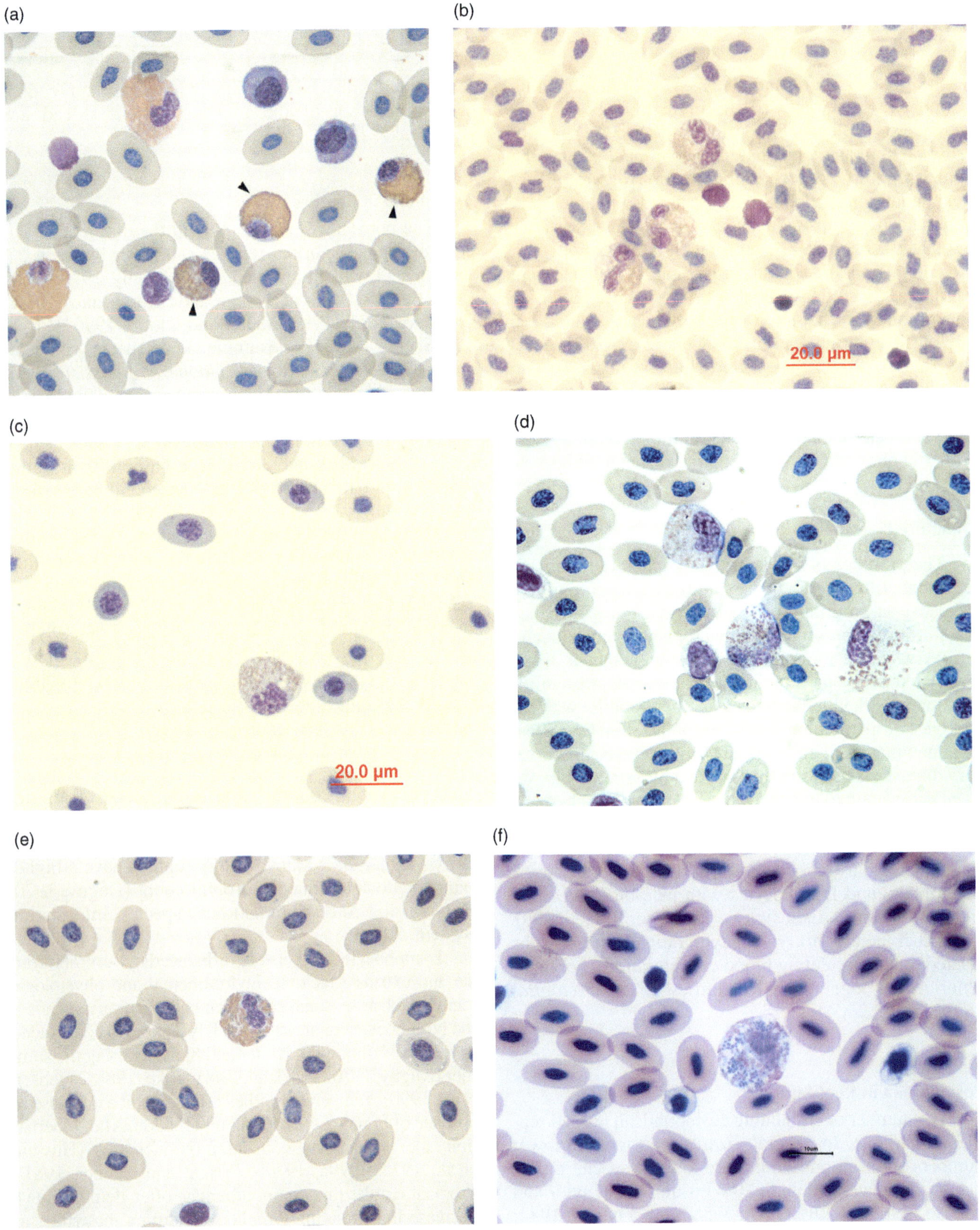

Fig. 19.17. (a) 1 + toxic heterophils (arrowheads) in the blood film of a three-toed box turtle (*Terrapene carolina triunguis*), Wright–Giemsa stain (100× oil). (b) Toxic heterophils (2+ toxicity) in the blood film of a green iguana (*Iguana iguana*), Wright–Giemsa stain. (c) Toxic heterophil (2+ toxicity) in the blood film of a pond turtle (*Chinemys reevesii*), Wright–Giemsa stain. (d) Toxic heterophils (3+ toxicity) in the blood film of a green iguana (*Iguana iguana*), Wright–Giemsa stain (100× oil). (e) Toxic heterophil (3+ toxicity) with partial nuclear lobation in a species that does not have lobate granulocyte nuclei in the blood film of a three-toed box turtle (*Terrapene carolina triunguis*), Wright–Giemsa stain (100× oil). (f) Toxic heterophil (4+ toxicity) with intracellular bacteria in the blood film of a bearded dragon (*Pogona vitticeps*), Wright–Giemsa stain.

major classes of lymphocytes (B- and T-lymphocytes) involved in immunologic function. However, unlike endothermic birds and mammals, the immunologic responses of ectothermic reptiles are greatly influenced by the environment. For example, low temperatures may suppress or inhibit the immune response in reptiles.

Lymphopenia

Lymphopenia often occurs secondary to a number of diseases associated with immunosuppression, chronic stress, and chronic malnutrition. Lymphocytosis often occurs during wound healing, inflammatory disease, parasitic infection (e.g., anisakiasis and spirorchidiasis), and viral infection. Lymphocytosis may also be present during ecdysis (Wallach and Boever, 1983).

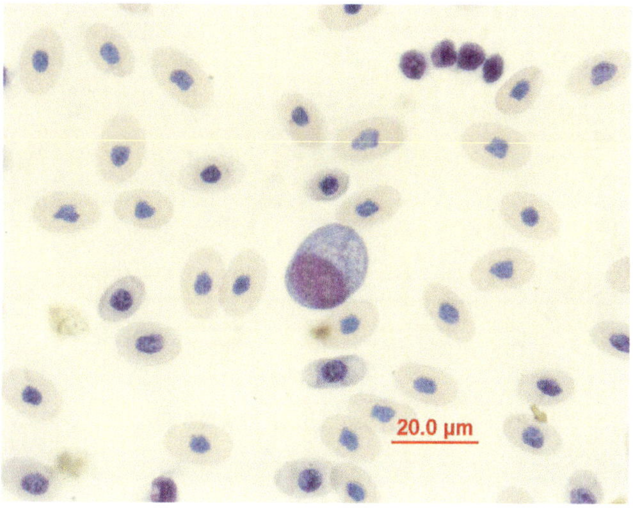

Fig. 19.18. Progranulocyte (promyelocyte) in the blood film of a pond turtle (*Chinemys reevesii*), Wright–Giemsa stain.

Reactive Lymphocytes

The presence of reactive lymphocytes and, less commonly, plasma cells, suggests stimulation of the immune system (Figures 19.19a and 19.19b). Reptilian reactive lymphocytes and plasma cells resemble those of birds and mammals. Reactive lymphocytes may be differentiated from normal lymphocytes by the presence of more abundant, deeply basophilic cytoplasm. The nuclear chromatin of the reactive lymphocyte is comparatively less condensed. Plasma cells have abundant, intensely basophilic cytoplasm that contains a distinct Golgi zone and an eccentrically positioned nucleus (Figures 19.14a and 19.14b).

Leukemia

Lymphoid leukemia and other hematopoietic neoplasia have been reported in reptiles (Frey and Carney, 1972; Frey and Carney, 1973; Langenberg et al., 1983; Goldberg and Holshuh, 1991; Oros et al., 2001; Tocidlowski et al., 2001; Garner et al., 2004; Silverstone et al., 2007; Campbell and Grant, 2010; Bezjian et al., 2013; Rousselet et al., 2017; Kubiak et al., 2019). Although the etiology of leukemias is generally unknown, lymphoblast lymphoma with a leukemic blood profile and concurrent IBD has been reported in a boa (Schilliger et al., 2011).

Myeloproliferative diseases of reptiles are classified in the same manner as in mammals (Figures 19.20a–d). Special cytochemical studies may be required to identify the abnormal cells. Affected animals frequently present with a marked to severe leukocytosis due to high numbers of atypical cells, usually blasts. Lymphoid leukemia is indicated by the presence of a large number of immature and abnormal lymphocytes. The lymphocytes can be medium-sized cells with round to pleomorphic nuclei, slightly clumped chromatin, indistinct nucleoli, and scant

(a) (b)

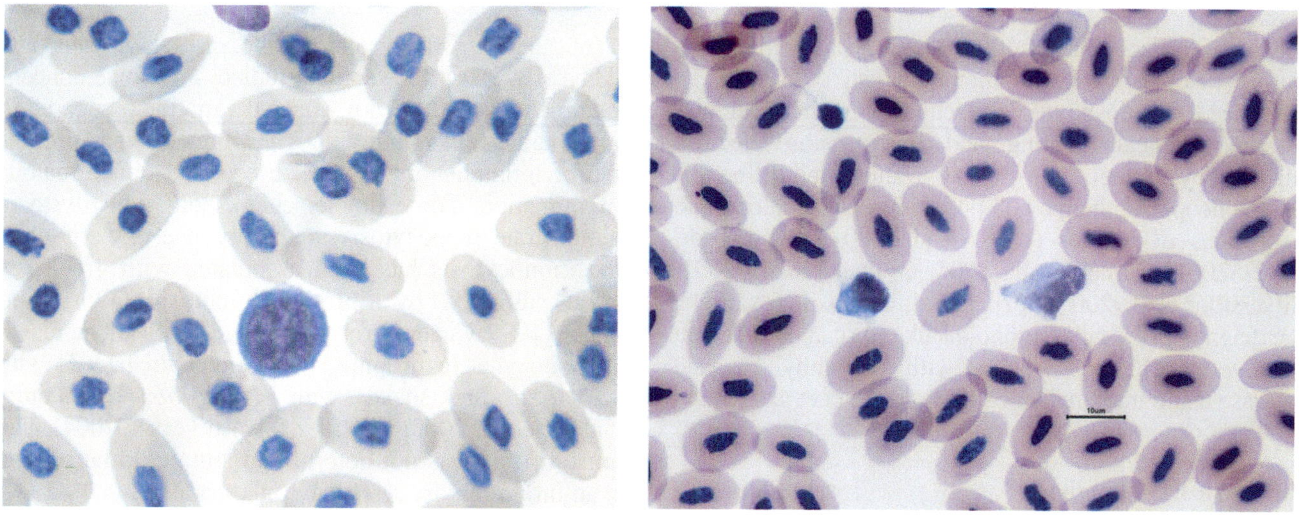

Fig. 19.19. (a) Reactive lymphocyte in the blood film of a green iguana (*Iguana iguana*), Wright–Giemsa stain (100× oil). (b) Reactive lymphocyte (left) in the blood film of a bearded dragon (*Pogona vitticeps*), Wright–Giemsa stain.

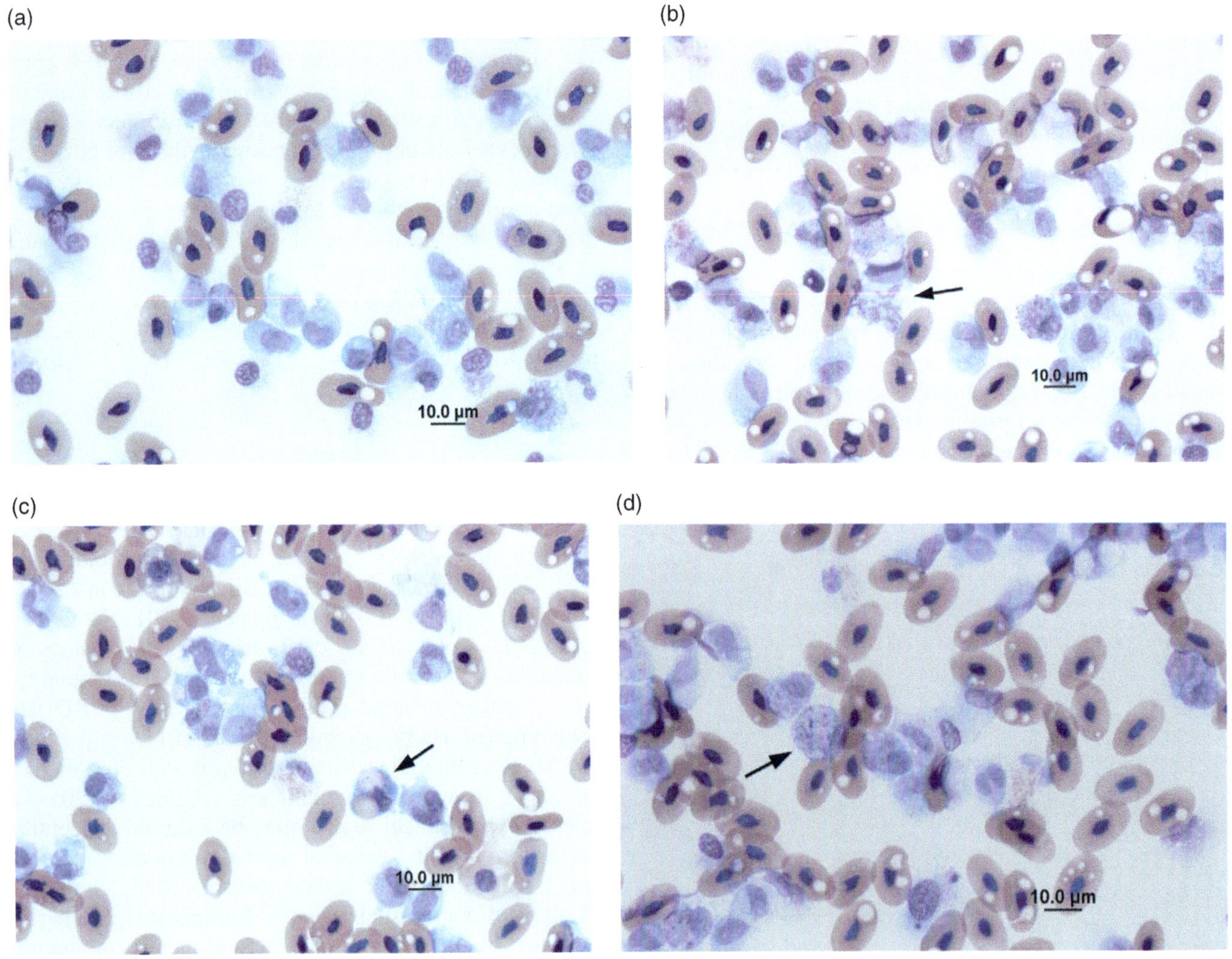

Fig. 19.20. (a) Numerous monocytes in the blood film of a lizard (*Pogona* sp.) with myelomonocytic leukemia, Wright–Giemsa stain. (b) Numerous monocytes and a mitotic figure (arrow) in the blood film of a lizard (*Pogona* sp.) with myelomonocytic leukemia, Wright–Giemsa stain. (c) Numerous monocytes and erythrophagocytosis (arrow) in the blood film of a lizard (*Pogona* sp.) with myelomonocytic leukemia, Wright–Giemsa stain. (d) Numerous monocytes and monocyte with melanin pigment (arrow) in the blood film of a lizard (*Pogona* spp.) with myelomonocytic leukemia, Wright–Giemsa stain.

moderate-to-dark blue cytoplasm with occasional red-to-purple cytoplasmic granulation (Bezjian et al., 2013). Advanced diagnostic tools, such as cytochemical and immunochemical staining and transmission electron microscopy, are needed to further evaluate and differentiate the neoplastic hemic cell population of hematopoietic neoplasms of reptiles (Oros et al., 2001; Tocidlowski et al., 2001; Garner et al., 2004; Gyimesi et al., 2005; Silverstone et al., 2007; Bezjian et al., 2013). For example, the diagnosis of T-cell lymphoid leukemia can be based on positive cytochemical staining with α-naphthyl butyrate esterase using mammalian controls (Bezjian et al., 2013).

Monocytosis in Reptiles

Monocytes typically occur in low numbers ranging from 0% to 10% in the leukocyte differential (Taylor and Kaplan, 1961; Taylor et al., 1963; Duguy, 1970; Wood and Ebanks, 1984; Sypek and Borysenko, 1988; Jacobson et al., 1990; Marks and Citino, 1990; Wright and Skeba, 1992). Of the reptiles studied, monocyte concentration changes little with seasonal variation compared to other hemic cells (Duguy, 1970). Monocytosis is suggestive of inflammatory disease, especially granulomatous inflammation. For example, chameleons with dystocia demonstrate monocytosis in the absence of peritonitis, and monocytosis has been associated with green sea turtles affected by fibropapillomatosis (Work and Balazs, 1999; Cuadrado et al., 2002). Significant increases in monocytes (azurophils) were noted in lizards with *Karyolysus* and snakes with *Hepatozoon* parasitemia (Salakij et al., 2002; Martinez Silvestre et al., 2004). The cause of this was not determined, but could be related to an inflammatory response to the parasites.

Monocytes in the peripheral blood of reptiles often reveal phagocytic activity. Erythrophagocytosis and leukophagocytosis by monocytes in the peripheral blood of reptiles can be associated with anemia and infectious

(a) (b)

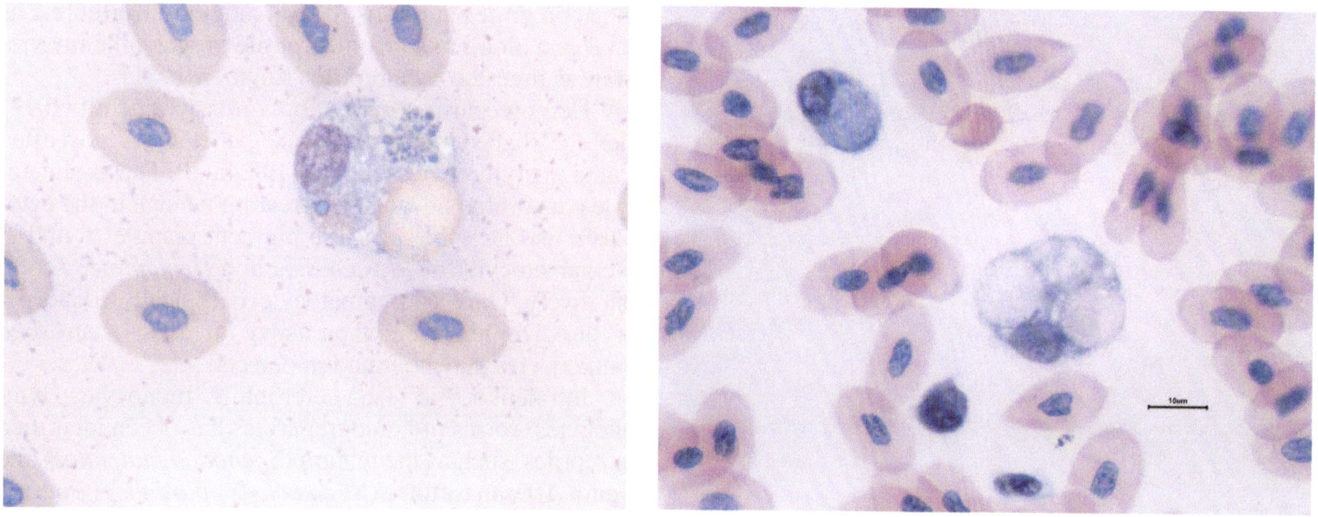

Fig. 19.21. (a) A monocyte showing erythrophagocytosis in the blood film of a green iguana (*Iguana iguana*), Wright–Giemsa stain (100× oil). (b) A monocyte showing erythrophagocytosis in the blood film of a California kingsnake (*Lampropeltis getula californiae*), Wright–Giemsa stain.

diseases (Figures 19.20c, 19.21a and 19.21b). Circulating siderophagocytes and erythrophagocytes can be transiently found to be part of the postsurgical removal of extravasated blood in reptiles recovering from intracoelomic surgery during which time the PCV remains relatively stable (George et al., 2008). Circulating siderophagocytes in the blood may reflect differences in the circulation of macrophages in snakes compared with mammals, where intraperitoneal macrophages are drained via lymphatics to lymph nodes, where they accumulate in the sinuses, revealing posthemorrhagic lymph nodes that contain large numbers of hemosiderin-laden macrophages (Fry and McGavin, 2007). Because reptiles have no lymph nodes to filter out these cells, it is likely the coelomic macrophages reenter circulating blood from the lymphatic system to be transported either directly to bone marrow or to the spleen (Origgi, 2007). Therefore, circulating siderophagocytes in postoperative blood films in reptiles can be interpreted as recirculating macrophages involved in the removal of blood from the coelomic cavity following mild postsurgical hemorrhage (George et al., 2008).

Macrophages that contain a variable number of intracytoplasmic oval or elongated, infrequently refractile, golden to black, brown pigment granules (consistent with melanin granules) are referred to as melanomacrophages (Figure 19.22). Black granules in macrophages in blood films stained with Fontana–Masson stain confirm the presence of melanin pigment. Melanomacrophages are found in the liver, spleen, kidney, and sites of chronic inflammation in reptiles (also, fish, and amphibians); however, they are rarely seen in the peripheral blood. Therefore, if observed more frequent than rare cells in blood film, melanomacrophages are considered increased and indicative of chronic inflammation (or other chronic diseases), infection, cachexia, or stress (Stacy et al., 2017b).

Reptile Thrombocytes

Thrombocytes of reptiles are small (generally smaller than erythrocytes), elliptical to fusiform cells with a centrally located oval nucleus containing dense nuclear chromatin that stains purple (Figures 19.23a–h). Some nuclei may contain a pale line that extends across the width of the nucleus. The cytoplasm is typically colorless to pale blue in color and may contain a few azurophilic granules. Activated thrombocytes are common and appear as aggregated clusters of cells with decreased cytoplasmic volume, irregular cytoplasmic margins, and vacuoles. Indistinct cytoplasmic margins may be noted on some individual thrombocytes and are probably a product of age, artifact, or function (Knotkova et al., 2002).

Reptilian thrombocytes function similarly to avian thrombocytes and mammalian platelets and play a significant role in thrombus formation. Activated reptilian thrombocytes exhibit ultrastructural features such as pseudopodia with fine granular material and many fibrinlike filaments that radiate between and around the cells (Wright and Cooper, 1981; Sypek and Borysenko, 1988) (Figure 19.23g). Abnormal thrombocytes with polymorphic nuclei may be noted occasionally and are thought to be associated with severe inflammatory disease (Hawkey and Dennett, 1989).

Thrombocytopenias do occur in reptiles and are most likely to occur due to excessive peripheral utilization of thrombocytes, or a decrease in thrombocyte production (Campbell and Grant, 2010). The presence of immature thrombocytes in the blood film is indicative of a regenerative response. Immature reptilian thrombocytes resemble the immature thrombocytes of birds.

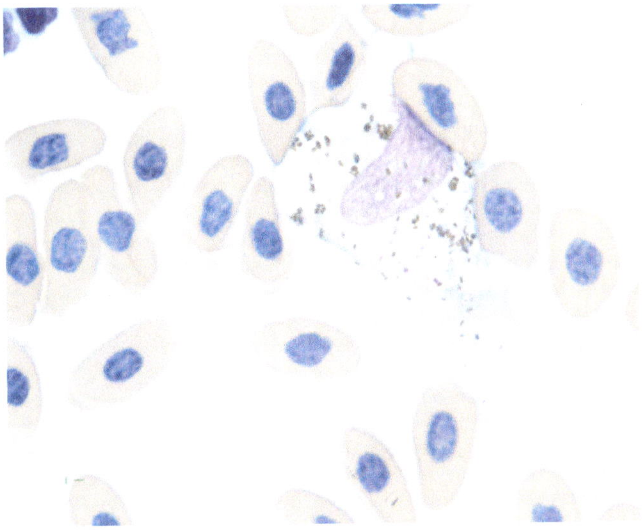

Fig. 19.22. A melanomacrophage in the blood film of a green iguana (*Iguana iguana*), Wright–Giemsa stain (100× oil).

Reptile Blood Parasites

Blood parasites are common in reptiles (Telford, 2009). Their presence is often considered an incidental finding; however, some blood parasites have the potential to cause diseases such as hemolytic anemia. Commonly encountered blood parasites include hemoprotozoa, piroplasmids, and microfilaria. Common hemoprotozoa include the hemogregarines, trypanosomes, and *Plasmodium* spp. Less commonly encountered hemoprotozoa include *Leishmania*, *Saurocytozoon*, *Hemoproteus*, *Schellackia*, and *Anaplasma*.

Hemogregarines

The hemogregarine parasites are the most common group of sporozoan hemoparasites affecting reptiles. The four genera of hemogregarines commonly found in reptiles are *Hemogregarina, Hepatozoon, Karyolysus*, and *Hemolivia* (Telford, 1984; Barnard and Upton, 1994; Cook et al., 2016; Stacy and Harr, 2021). The hemogregarines cannot be classified into the appropriate genus based upon the gross appearance of the gametocytes within the erythrocyte cytoplasm or by the examination of tissue schizonts (Keymer, 1981; Telford, 1984; Barnard and Upton, 1994). Therefore, the general term *hemogregarine* is used when reporting their presence in blood films during hematologic examinations.

Hemogregarines have a life cycle that involves sexual reproduction (sporogony) in an invertebrate host and asexual multiplication (merogony) in the reptilian host. A number of biting invertebrate hosts (i.e., mites, ticks, mosquitoes, flies) can transmit the parasite to terrestrial reptiles; leeches appear to be the primary intermediate host for hemogregarines of aquatic reptiles (Telford, 1984). The parasite infects a reptile host when the sporozoites are transmitted from the invertebrate as it takes a blood meal from a reptile or when the invertebrate is ingested by a reptile (Keymer, 1981).

Hemogregarines may be grossly identified as sausage-shaped intracytoplasmic gametocytes most often found in erythrocytes (Figures 19.24a–d). These gametocytes distort the host cell by creating a bulge in the cytoplasm and lack the refractile pigment granules found in the gametocytes of *Plasmodium* and *Hemoproteus* comparatively. Only one gametocyte is typically found per erythrocyte; however, when heavy infection occurs, two gametocytes may be found in one cell.

Intraleukocytic (i.e., heterophils, monocytes, lymphocytes) forms of hemogregarines have been identified in reptiles, such as the tuatara (*Spenodon punctatus*) and South African tortoise (*Stigmochelys pardalis*) (Godfrey et al., 2011; Cook et al., 2014). In the tuatara, they appear to be parasites phagocytized by leukocytes as part of an immune response in the vertebrate host. A high level of intraleukocytic hemogregarines may represent a stage in the infection cycle where the reptilian host is clearing the parasite infection from its blood cells (Godfrey et al., 2011). The increased number of intraleukocytic forms has a seasonal appearance that may represent a more efficient immune response during warmer months. Infection intensity varies with fluctuations in vector abundance, both seasonally and spatially, whereas patterns of infection within exposed populations can vary with host body size and perhaps reproductive status. For example, the hemogregarine parasitemia has been shown to decline with increasing host body size (Godfrey et al., 2011). In the tortoise, the suspected *Hepatozoon* species did not display evidence of intraerythrocytic or intraleukocytic division and was suspected to be transmitted by a tick vector (Cook et al., 2014).

In general, no significant differences in prevalence of hematozoan infections were found between sexes in surveys of wild reptiles (Madsen et al., 2005; Bonadiman et al., 2010), snakes (*Liasis fuscus*) (Madsen et al., 2005; Viana et al., 2010; Davis and Sterrett, 2011). However, sex differences can occur in certain localities. For example, the prevalence and severity of hemogregarine infections were higher in female alligators than in males living in a river in the southern United States (Davis et al., 2011).

Reptilian hemogregarines are well adapted to their natural hosts and typically do not cause clinical disease in these animals (Scheelings and Rafferty, 2012). This parasite is relatively non-host specific, however, and can cause significant clinical disease in unnatural or aberrant host species (Wozniak and Telford, 1991; Wozniak et al., 1994a). Clinical infection is associated with severe inflammatory lesions caused by schizonts in a variety of organs (Griner, 1983; Wozniak and Telford, 1991; Wozniak et al., 1994b).

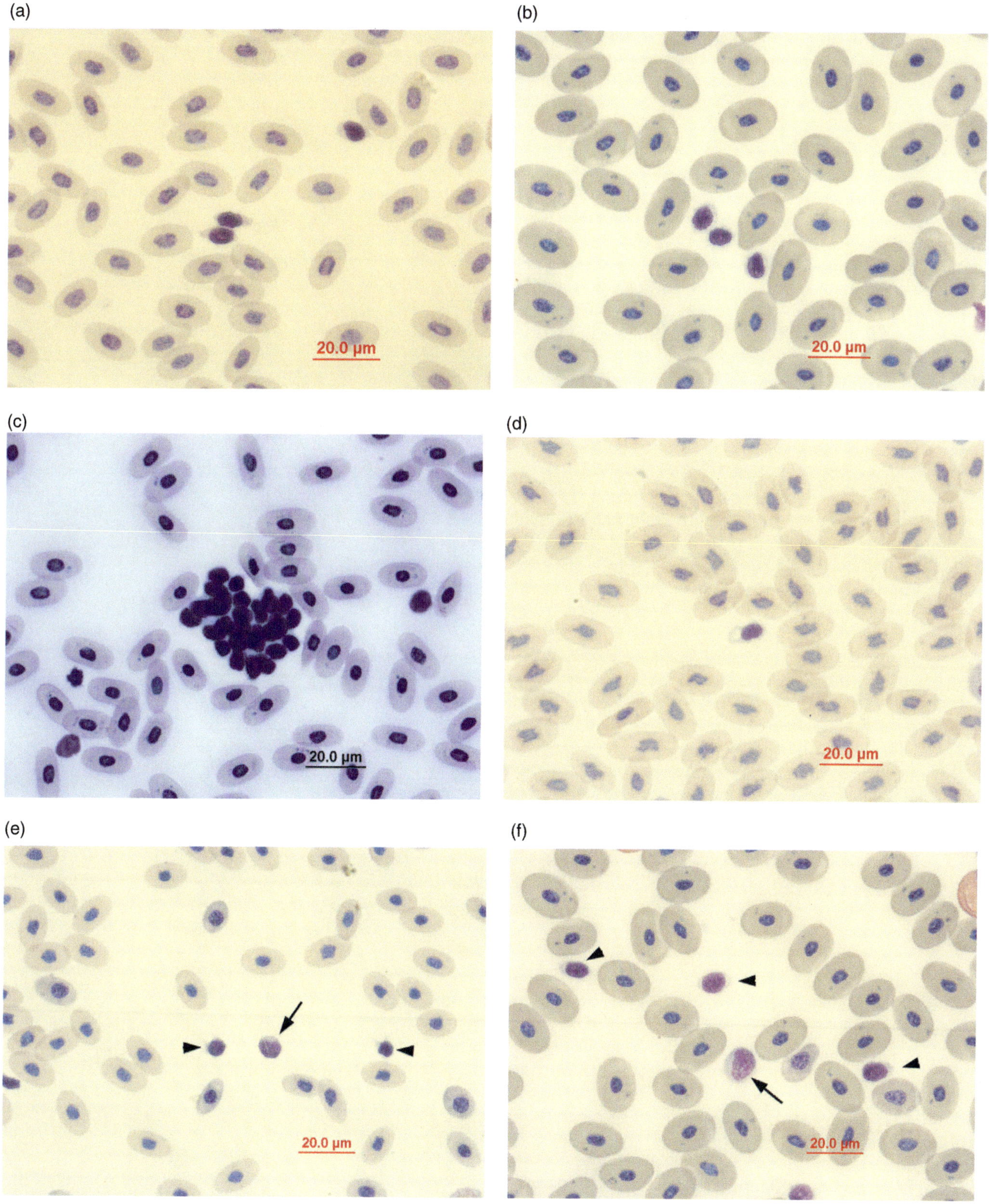

Fig. 19.23. (a) Thrombocytes in the blood film of a green iguana (*Iguana iguana*), Wright–Giemsa stain. (b) Thrombocytes in the blood film of a green sea turtle (*Chelonia mydas*), Wright–Giemsa stain. (c) Clumped thrombocytes in the blood film of a three-toed box turtle (*Terrapene carolina triunguis*), Wright–Giemsa stain. (d) Thrombocyte in the blood film of a common boa (*Boa constrictor*), Wright–Giemsa stain. (e) Thrombocytes (arrowheads) and small lymphocyte (arrow) in the blood film of a pond turtle (*Chinemys reevesii*), Wright–Giemsa stain. (f) Thrombocytes (arrowheads) and large lymphocyte (arrow) in the blood film of a green sea turtle (*Chelonia mydas*), Wright–Giemsa stain. (g) Thrombocyte (arrowhead), small lymphocyte (small arrow), and immature erythrocyte–mid-polychromatic rubricyte (large arrow) in the blood film of a pond turtle (*Chinemys reevesii*), Wright–Giemsa stain. (h) Thrombocyte (arrowhead) and small lymphocyte (arrow) in the blood film of a sulcate tortoise (*Centrochelys sulcata*), Wright–Giemsa stain.

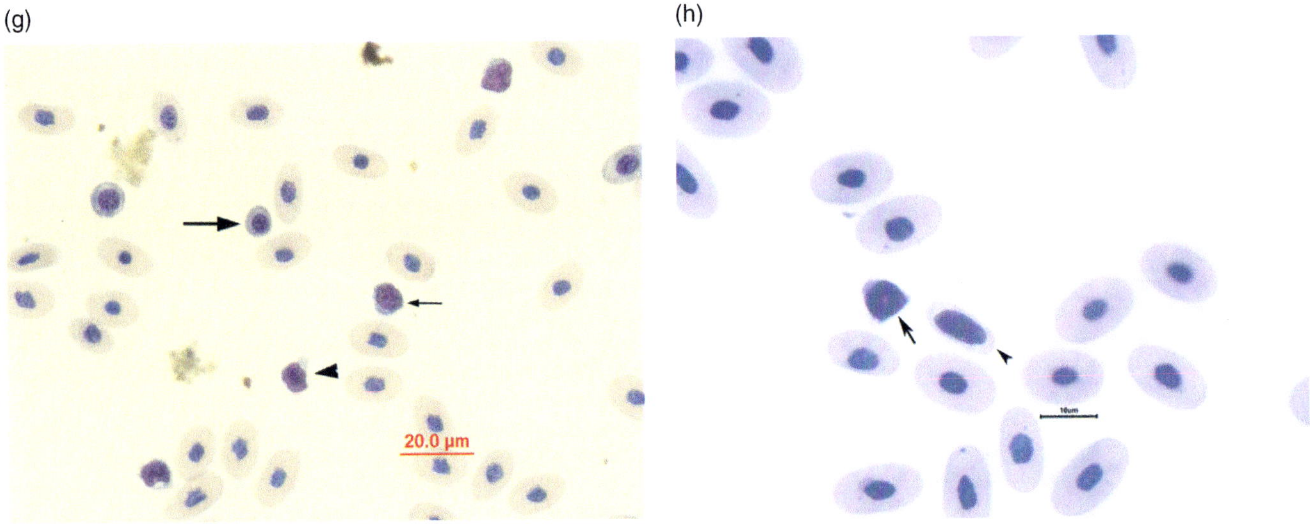

Fig. 19.23. (*Continued*)

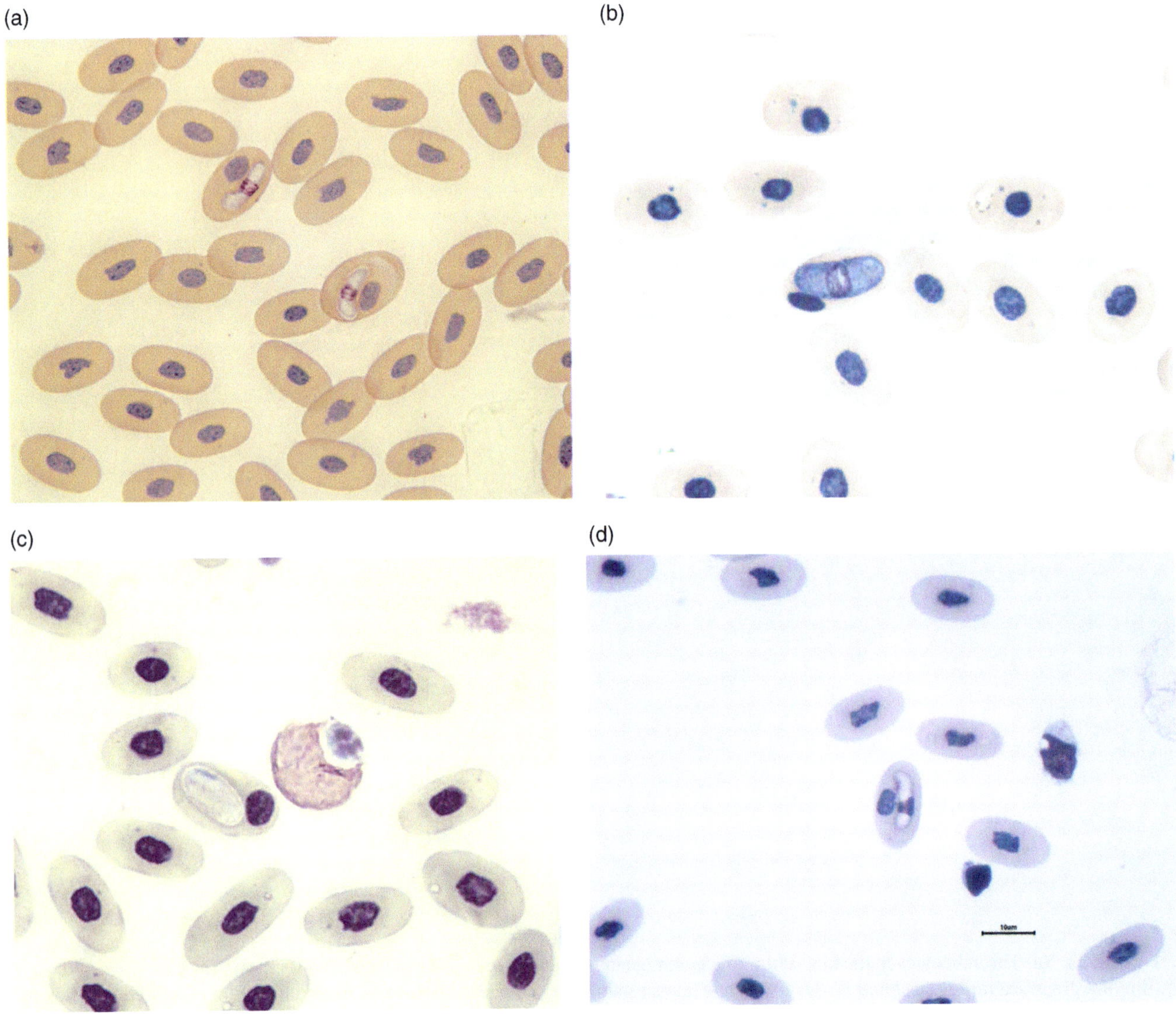

Fig. 19.24. (a) Hemogregarine gametocytes within two erythrocytes in the blood film of an emerald tree boa (*Corallus caninus*), Wright–Giemsa stain (100× oil). (b) Hemogregarine gametocyte within an erythrocyte in the blood film of a red-eared slider (*Trachemys scripta elegans*), Wright–Giemsa stain (100× oil). (c) Hemogregarine gametocytes within an erythrocyte in the blood film of a Asian forest tortoise (*Manouria emys*), Wright–Giemsa stain (100× oil). (d) Hemogregarine gametocytes within two erythrocytes in the blood film of a green tree python (*Morelia viridis*), Wright–Giemsa stain (100× oil).

Snakes are more commonly infected with hemogregarine parasites compared to other reptile species. The hemogregarines found in snakes are typically of the genus *Hepatozoon*. In one study, *Hepatozoon* infections were commonly noted in king cobras (*Ophiophagus hannah*) that were not exhibiting any clinical signs of severe hematologic abnormalities (Salakij et al., 2002). Hemogregarines may be found in semiaquatic freshwater turtles and are usually of the genus *Hemogregarina*. *Karyolysus* typically occurs in Old World lizards and possibly tree snakes (Keymer, 1981; Telford, 1984; Lowichik and Yeager, 1987; Frye, 1991). There are no reported cases of hemogregariniasis in sea turtles, and the parasites are rare in tortoises (Keymer, 1981). Hemogregarine parasites have been noted in the peripheral blood films of American alligators (*Alligator mississippiensis*) and are considered to be an incidental finding (Schoeb et al., 2002).

Hemoproteus

Hemoproteus (*Haemocystidium*) has been reported in lizards, turtles, and snakes and resembles the *Hemoproteus* species found in birds (Keymer, 1981; Jacobson, 1986; Barnard and Upton, 1994) (Figure 11.26). Only the gametocytes containing refractile pigment granules are found in the peripheral blood films of reptiles. This parasite can cause dehemoglobinization of the infected erythrocyte (Jacobson, 1986).

Plasmodium

Plasmodium infections can result in a severe hemolytic anemia and have the potential to cause significant illness in reptiles. Over 60 species of *Plasmodium* have been described in reptiles. Most *Plasmodium* species have been identified in lizards; a limited number have been identified in snakes (Telford, 1984; Jacobson, 1986; Barnard and Upton, 1994; Pereira et al., 2021). The life cycle of *Plasmodium* involves a sporogony stage in an invertebrate insect host (i.e., mosquito); the schizogony and gametogony stages occur in the reptile host.

Plasmodium trophozoites may be identified in the blood films as small, signet ring structures in the erythrocyte cytoplasm and resemble the *Plasmodium* spp. found in birds. The gametocytes have refractile pigment granules that can aid in the differentiation of *Plasmodium* from hemogregarine parasites (Figures 11.31–11.34). Packets of *Plasmodium* merozoites (schizogony stage) can sometimes be identified in red blood cells and may be used to differentiate this parasite from the hemogregarine parasites as well.

Saurocytozoon

Saurocytozoon is a parasite of lizards and is most likely transmitted by mosquitoes (Keymer, 1981). These parasites appear within the cytoplasm of leukocytes or immature erythrocytes as large, round gametocytes lacking pigment granules. Only the gametocyte stage is found in the peripheral blood; schizogony occurs in the tissues. The organism resembles avian *Leukocytozoon* because it grossly distorts the host cell that it parasitizes (Figures 11.35 and 11.36).

Microfilaria

Microfilaremia in reptiles is typically not associated with clinical signs of illness or changes in the hemogram or blood biochemical profile. Reptiles can survive for years with these parasites; microfilaria are often detected incidentally on examination of routine Romanowsky-stained blood films and resemble those found in birds and mammals (Figure 11.37). Microfilaria produced by adult female filariid nematodes can live in various locations in the body of a reptile and are ingested by a suitable blood-sucking arthropod or insect. The larval parasites reside within the insect host where they develop into the infective third-stage larval form. The life cycle is completed when the third-stage larva enters a new reptilian host during intermediate host feeding.

Piroplasmids

The piroplasmids of reptiles include *Babesia*, *Aegyptianella* (*Tunetella*), and *Sauroplasma* (*Serpentoplasma*) (Barnard and Upton, 1994). Transmission occurs by biting insects or arthropods, and reproduction occurs by either schizogony or binary fission. This group of parasites has been reported in chelonians, lizards, and snakes and appears as small (1–2 μm), round to piriform, nonpigmented signet-ring-like vacuoles in the cytoplasm of erythrocytes (Figure 19.25) (Keymer, 1981).

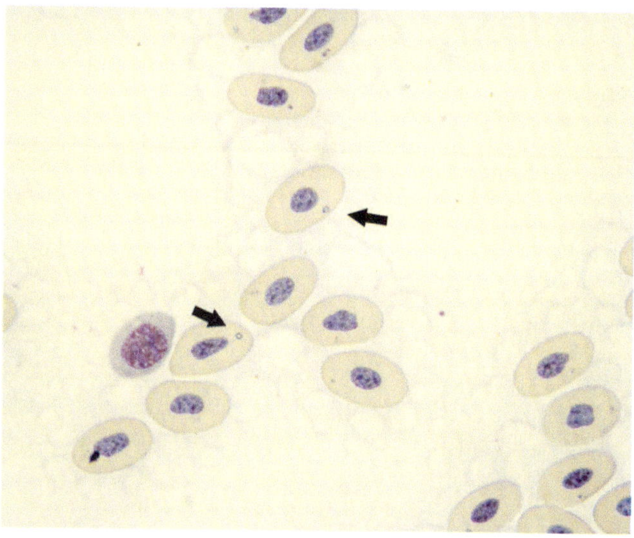

Fig. 19.25. Piroplasmid (*Serpentoplasma* spp.) inclusions within erythrocytes in a blood film from a emerald tree boa (*Corallus caninus*), Wright–Giemsa stain (100× oil).

The piroplasmids commonly found in the peripheral blood erythrocytes of lizards are referred to as *Sauroplasma*, whereas the same organisms in the blood of snakes are called *Serpentoplasma*.

Pirhemocyton

Pirhemocytonosis is characterized as the presence of red, punctate to oval, erythrocytic inclusions that increase in size (0.5–1.5 μm) as infection develops (Telford and Jacobson, 1993). Pirhemocytonosis is typically reported in lizards, although similar inclusions have been reported in snakes and turtles as well (Telford, 1984). Inclusions may be associated with vacuoles (albuminoid vacuoles) or irregular pale-staining areas in the cytoplasm of erythrocytes in Giemsa-stained blood films (Telford and Jacobson, 1993). A single inclusion per erythrocyte is typical; however, two inclusions per cell may occur on occasion.

These intraerythrocytic inclusions were previously considered to be piroplasmids and were referred to as *Pirhemocyton*, until ultrastructural studies revealed the presence of a virus consistent with the members of the Iridoviridae family (Telford and Jacobson, 1993). Natural infections with this erythrocytic virus appear to be nonfatal, even when high viremia is present (i.e., over 85% of the erythrocytes are infected) that result in the appearance of spindle-shaped or thin, elongated erythrocytes (Telford and Jacobson, 1993). One report of pirhemocytonosis in snakes was suggestive of an oncornavirus based upon ultrastructural studies (Daly et al., 1980).

Square to rectangular, pale, crystalline-like cytoplasmic inclusions are commonly found in the erythrocyte cytoplasm of green iguanas (*I. iguana*) (Figure 19.26). One report determined that 20% of the iguanas examined had these inclusions in 1–5% of their erythrocytes (Harr et al., 2001). Although some consider these to be viral or *Pirhemocyton* inclusions, the exact cause for these is unknown, and they do not appear to be associated with hematologic abnormalities or disease.

Lainsonia and Schellackia

Lainsonia and *Schellackia* are coccidian parasites of lizards and snakes that resemble avian *Atoxoplasma*. Transmission may occur via mites or possibly by ingestion of oocysts from feces. These parasites produce schizonts that can be found in the intestinal epithelium and sporozoites that are found in the peripheral blood (Keymer, 1981). The sporozoites appear as intracytoplasmic inclusions in erythrocytes and mononuclear leukocytes (primarily lymphocytes). The parasite can be identified as round to oval, pale-staining, nonpigmented inclusions that deform the host cell nucleus into a crescent shape (Figure 11.39). *Lainsonia iguanae* is frequently found in the blood of normal green iguanas (*Iguana iguana*) housed outdoors and is not associated with health problems (Harr et al., 2001).

Trypanosomes

The trypanosome parasites found in reptiles are large, extracellular, blade-shaped flagellate protozoa with a single flagellum and a prominent undulating membrane that closely resemble the trypanosome parasites of mammals and birds (Figure 19.27). Trypanosomes rarely cause clinical disease, have a worldwide distribution, and may be found in all orders of reptiles. Transmission requires a blood-feeding invertebrate host (i.e., biting flies) for transmission to terrestrial reptiles.

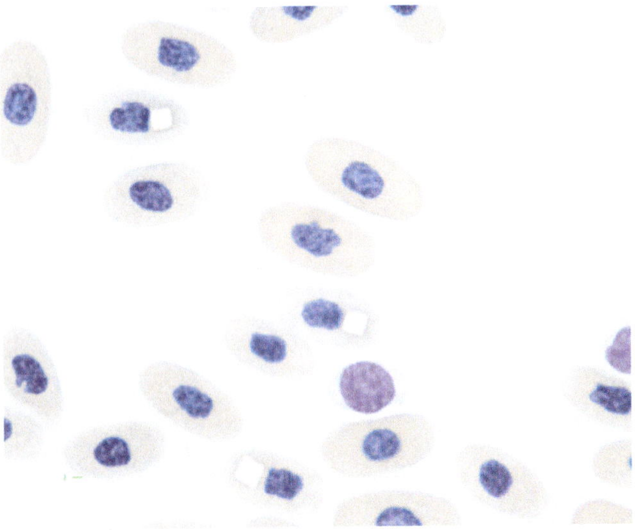

Fig. 19.26. Square vacuole-like inclusions within erythrocytes in a blood film from a green iguana (*Iguana iguana*), Wright–Giemsa stain (100× oil).

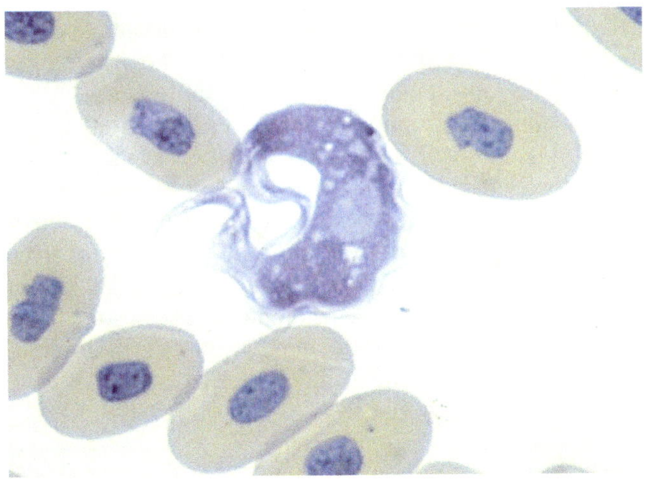

Fig. 19.27. A trypanosome (*Trypanosoma* spp.) in a blood film from an emerald tree boa (*Corallus caninus*), Wright–Giemsa stain (100× oil).

Leeches appear to be the invertebrate host involved in transmission to aquatic and semiaquatic reptiles (Keymer, 1981; Lowichik and Yeager, 1987).

Leishmania

Leishmania is related to the trypanosome parasites and is rarely seen in the blood films of reptiles. It is most often found in the blood films of lizards (Keymer, 1981). The organism appears in the amastigote (leishmanial) stage as a small (2.4 μm), round to oval inclusion with blue cytoplasm and an oval red nucleus within the cytoplasm of thrombocytes and mononuclear leukocytes. Leishmaniasis is primarily diagnosed using culture techniques (Campbell, 1996).

Anaplasmataceae

Erythrocytic inclusions associated with *Anaplasma* sp. are rarely observed in Wright–Giemsa-stained blood films from chelonians. The *Anaplasma* morulae are approximately 4 μm in diameter and tend to indent the nuclear membrane of erythrocytes (Raskin et al., 2020).

Reptile Hematopoiesis and Bone Marrow Evaluation

Bone marrow evaluation in reptiles as a diagnostic tool has received little attention in the literature; however, cytologic evaluation of a bone marrow aspiration biopsy is indicated whenever an unexplained hematologic abnormality is found. Common hematologic abnormalities evaluated by assessment of the bone marrow include nonregenerative anemia, heteropenia, thrombocytopenia, and suspicion of neoplasia.

Reptile Erythropoiesis

The bone marrow appears to be the primary site for erythropoiesis, granulopoiesis, and thrombopoiesis in adult reptiles. Erythropoiesis occurs within the vascular space of the reticular stroma, although foci of extramedullary erythropoiesis in the liver and spleen are common in some species (Meints et al., 1975; Alleman et al., 1992; Garner et al., 1996).

The stages of reptilian erythrocyte maturation appear to be like those of birds and mammals; however, during the final stages of maturation, the mature reptilian erythrocytes are often larger than the immature erythrocytes – a distinctive difference compared to mammals (Sheeler and Barber, 1965; Alleman et al., 1992; Campbell, 1996, 2012; Fry and McGavin, 2007). In general, there are seven recognizable stages of erythrocyte development: rubriblasts, prorubricytes, basophilic rubricytes, early polychromatic rubricytes, late polychromatic rubricytes, polychromatic erythrocytes, and mature erythrocytes. The morphologic features of the developing reptilian erythrocytes are basically similar to those described in birds.

The rubriblast (proerythroblast, pronormoblast) is the first progenitor cell that can be visually identified and appears as a round cell with a large, round nucleus; delicate uncondensed chromatin; and one or two nucleoli (Zapata et al., 1981; Pica et al., 1986; Hawkey and Dennett, 1989; Frye, 1991) (Figure 19.28). The cytoplasm is basophilic and agranular and typically appears as a narrow band surrounding the nucleus. Pinocytotic vesicles may be found along the cell margin and are a characteristic feature of early reptilian erythroid cells. These vesicles make up the process for ferritin incorporation used in hemoglobin synthesis.

The prorubricyte (basophilic erythroblast) is similar to the rubriblast. The cell is round, and the nucleus lacks nucleoli and contains a slightly more condensed chromatin network. The cytoplasm of the prorubricyte stains basophilic (Figure 19.28).

The rubricyte (polychromatic erythroblasts) is the third stage in erythrocyte maturation. During this stage of development, the cell is smaller in size and is still spherical or just beginning to develop an oval shape. The size of the nucleus is reduced, and the chromatin appears more condensed and clumped. The cytoplasm of the rubricyte is scant and lighter in color due to hemoglobin synthesis and may be classified as basophilic, early polychromatic, or late polychromatic (Figures 19.29 and 19.30). Reptilian erythrocytes are typically released into the peripheral circulation in the rubricyte stage (Efrati et al., 1970; MacMahon and Hamer, 1975; Pica et al., 1986; Canfield and Shea, 1988; Wojtaszek, 1992; Alibardi, 1994).

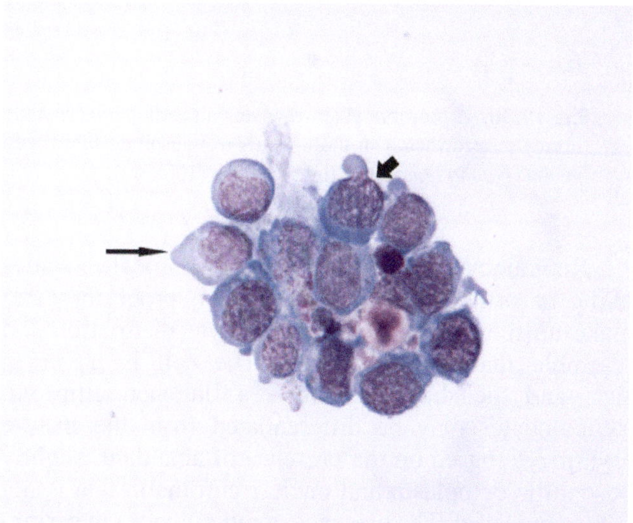

Fig. 19.28. Rubriblast (short arrow) and prorubricyte (long arrow) in the bone marrow aspirate of a green iguana (*Iguana iguana*), Wright–Giemsa (100× oil).

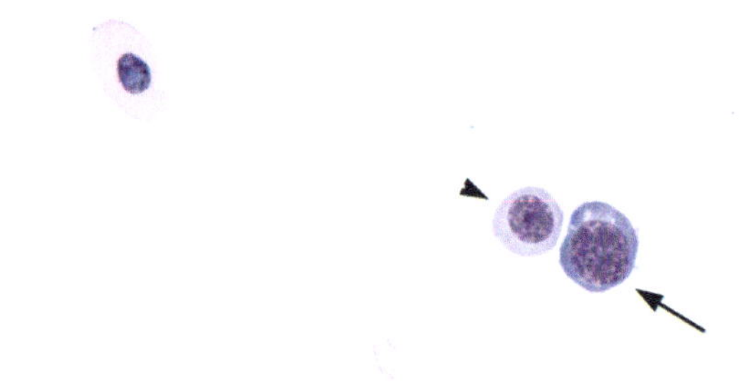

Fig. 19.29. A basophilic rubricyte (arrow) and late polychromatic rubricyte (arrowhead) in the bone marrow aspirate of a green iguana (*Iguana iguana*), Wright–Giemsa (100× oil).

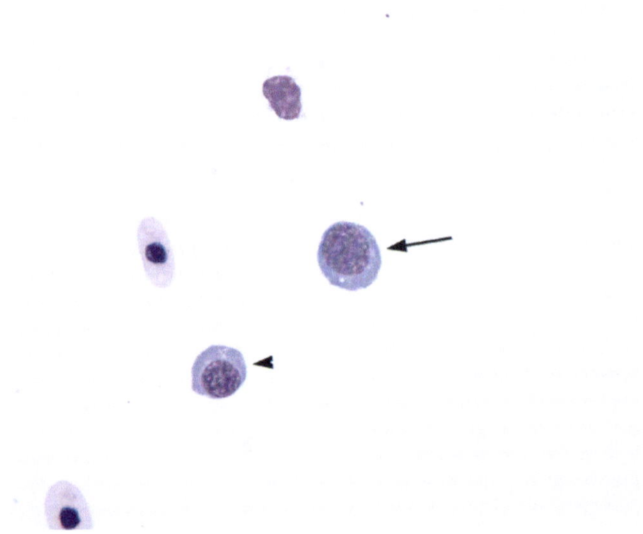

Fig. 19.30. A prorubricyte (arrow) and an early polychromatic rubricyte (arrowhead) in the bone marrow aspirate of a green iguana (*Iguana iguana*), Wright–Giemsa (100× oil).

Reticulocytes (polychromatic erythrocyte, acidophilic or orthochromatic erythroblast, proerythrocyte) make up the next stage of erythrocyte maturation and resemble mature erythrocytes. The cell is larger in size, and the shape resembles a flattened ellipsoid. Reticulocytes may be differentiated from the mature erythrocyte based on the presence of abundant, slightly basophilic cytoplasm and nuclear chromatin that is not fully condensed. The presence of reticulocytes in peripheral blood may vary with species. Some authors describe them as a common finding, and others describe them as rare (Sheeler and Barber, 1965; Efrati et al., 1970; Hawkey and Dennett, 1989; Campbell, 1996, 2012; Knotkova et al., 2002).

Mature erythrocytes (normocytes) are morphologically similar among most reptiles (Saint Girons, 1970). The mature erythrocyte is a flattened oval and has a centrally positioned nucleus with condensed nuclear chromatin. The nuclear margins may be irregular (Alleman et al., 1999). The nucleus is ellipsoid in many species of reptile; however, in some species (turtles, tortoises), the nucleus may appear round (Knotkova et al., 2002). The cytoplasm stains light red to yellowish in color. As erythrocytes age, the nucleus becomes more condensed and darker staining.

In summary, as reptilian erythrocytes mature, the cells tend to become larger; however, a clear size-related progression in erythrocyte development may not be evident in all species. The shape of the cell changes from spherical to a flattened ellipsoid, and the cytoplasm becomes increasingly eosinophilic due to increased hemoglobin synthesis. The erythrocyte nucleus decreases in size, the shape changes from round to ellipsoid in most species, and the nuclear chromatin becomes increasingly condensed as the cell matures. Sudan black B stains the cytoplasm of erythrocyte precursors and mature erythrocytes dark gray to black and may be used as an erythrocyte marker (Garner et al., 1996).

Reptile Granulopoiesis

Developing granulocytes are morphologically similar to mammalian granulocytes and are associated with the extravascular spaces of the bone marrow reticular stroma (Alleman et al., 1992). Maturing granulocytes of reptiles resemble those of birds and migrate through the endothelial cells of the sinusoids to enter the blood stream.

Granulopoiesis begins with the myeloblast. Myeloblasts have a moderate amount of agranular, slightly basophilic cytoplasm and a large, central to slightly eccentric ovoid, vesicular nucleus with a large nucleolus or prominent nucleoli (Figure 19.31). As maturation takes place, the cells decrease in size, the cytoplasm becomes less basophilic, the nuclear chromatin becomes increasingly condensed, and the nucleus changes shape from round to segmented in those reptile species with lobate nuclei. The acidophils (heterophils and eosinophils) are derived from separate cell lines, and their specific characteristic cytoplasmic granules appear in the myelocyte and metamyelocyte stages of development (Mateo et al., 1984) (Figures 19.31–33). These granules increase in number as maturation continues.

The cytoplasmic granules of the eosinophils of some reptiles are typically large, round, and stain pink with Romanowsky stains and golden brown with benzidine peroxidase, which helps differentiate eosinophil precursors from those of heterophils (Sypek and Borysenko, 1988; Cannon, 1992; Bounous et al., 1996; Garner et al., 1996). Mature and immature heterophils

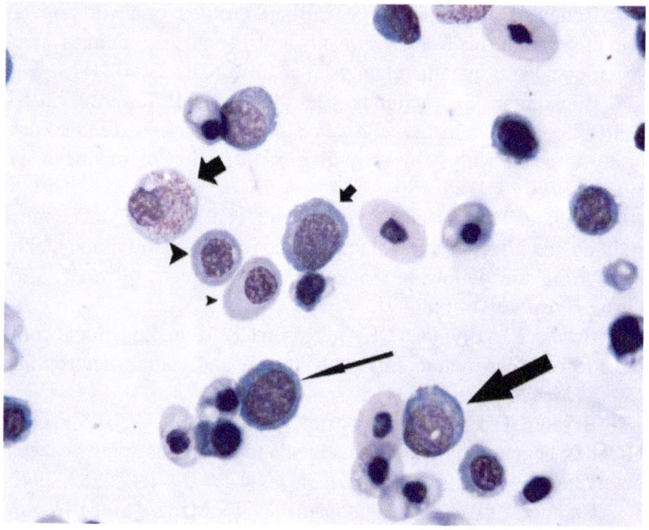

Fig. 19.31. A myeloblast (long thin arrow), a myeloblast transitioning into a progranulocyte (small arrow), a progranulocyte (large wide arrow), a heterophil myelocyte (short wide arrow), an early polychromatic rubricyte (large arrowhead), and a late polychromatic rubricyte (small arrowhead) in the bone marrow aspirate of a green iguana (*Iguana iguana*), Wright–Giemsa (100× oil).

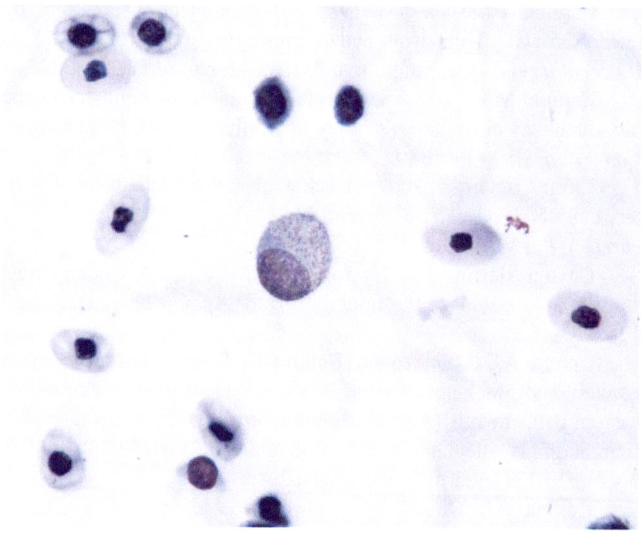

Fig. 19.32. A progranulocyte in the bone marrow aspirate of a green iguana (*Iguana iguana*), Wright–Giemsa (100× oil).

from some reptile species stain positive with chloroacetate esterase, α-naphthyl butyrate esterase, α-naphthyl acetate esterase, and leukocyte alkaline phosphatase chemical stains (Sypek and Borysenko, 1988; Cannon, 1992; Bounous et al., 1996; Garner et al., 1996).

Reptile Thrombopoiesis

Thrombopoiesis in reptiles is like that in birds. Reptilian thrombocytes are derived from a distinct line of mononuclear cells found in the bone marrow or other hematopoietic tissue. The thrombocyte series consists of thromboblasts, immature thrombocytes, and mature thrombocytes.

Thromboblasts appear as small, round to oval cells that resemble rubriblasts, and contain round nuclei with fine to punctate nuclear chromatin, and one or more nucleoli. Immature thrombocytes may be divided into three groups: early-, mid-, and late-immature thrombocytes, based upon their degree of maturity. As thrombocytes develop, they decrease in size, the cytoplasm becomes less basophilic, and the shape of the cell changes from round to elliptical. The nucleus changes from round to oval as well. In later stages of maturation, the nuclear chromatin becomes densely packed, and specific cytoplasmic granules may appear.

It is often difficult to differentiate thrombocytes from lymphocytes in hematopoietic specimens. Special chemical stains may be used to differentiate thrombocytes from lymphocytes in some reptile species. In general, thrombocytes will stain positive with periodic acid-Schiff, acid phosphatase, and α-naphthyl butyrate esterase stains, whereas lymphocytes will stain negatively (Sypek and Borysenko, 1988; Bounous et al., 1996; Garner et al., 1996).

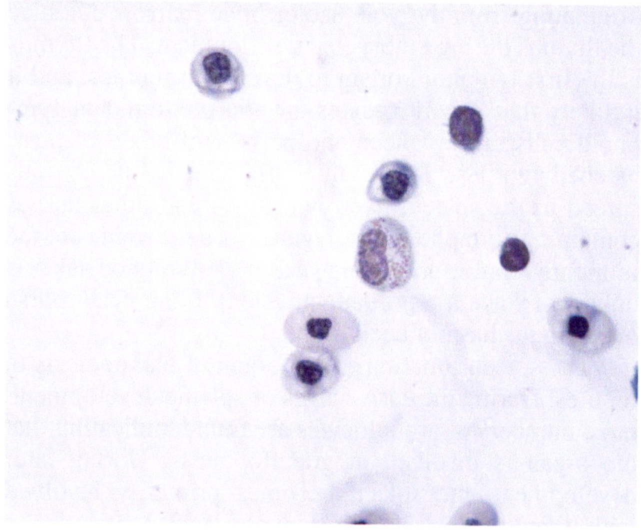

Fig. 19.33. A heterophil myelocyte in the bone marrow aspirate of a green iguana (*Iguana iguana*). Wright–Giemsa (100× oil).

Reptile Lymphopoiesis

Lymphopoiesis of reptiles resembles that of mammals and birds. Reptilian lymphoblasts, prolymphocytes, and mature lymphocytes appear identical to those found in birds and mammals and can be found in lymphopoietic tissues such as the spleen and liver.

The lymphocytes are derived from blood-borne stem cells, which most likely originated from the embryonic yolk sac (Alleman et al., 1992). Lymphoid precursors originating from the yolk sac or bone marrow colonize the thymus during embryonic development. The thymus is the first lymphoid organ to develop in reptiles, and it is likely that T-lymphocytes are the predominant lymphoid cells of the spleen and peripheral blood of post-hatched reptiles. T-cells that originate in the thymus spread to the spleen, liver, intestines, and other tissues containing lymphoid aggregates. The origin of the immunoglobulin-producing cells (B-lymphocytes) is unknown since a reptilian equivalent to the avian bursa of Fabricius has not been found.

The spleen functions as an organ of leukopoiesis in reptiles. During the early stages of splenic development, large numbers of granulocytes are found, indicating that the organ is involved in granulopoiesis. During later development, the spleen becomes primarily involved with lymphopoiesis (Alleman et al., 1992).

References

Alibardi L. 1994. Production of immature erythrocytes in lizard during tail regeneration. *Anim Biol* 3:139–147.

Alleman AR, Jacobson ER, Raskin RE. 1992. Morphologic and cytochemical characteristics of blood cells from the desert tortoise (*Gopherus agassizii*). *Am J Vet Res* 53:1645–1651.

Alleman AR, Jacobson ER, Raskin RE. 1999. Morphological, cytochemical staining, and ultrastructural characteristics of blood cells from eastern diamondback rattlesnakes (*Crotalus adamanteus*). *Am J Vet Res* 53:1645–1651.

Anderson NL, Wack R. 1996. The effects of temperature, sex, and sample type on hematology and serum/plasma chemistry values for captive New Guinea snapping turtles *Elseya novaeguineae*. In: Proceedings of the 3rd Annual Conference of the Association of Reptilian and Amphibian Veterinarians. Tampa, Florida.

Anderson NL, Wack R, Hatcher R. 1997. Hematology and clinical chemistry reference ranges for clinically normal captive New Guinea snapping turtles (*Elseya novaeguineae*) and the effects of temperature, sex, and sample type. *J Zoo Wildl Med* 28(4):394–403.

Andreani G, Carpene E, Cannavacciulolo A, et al. 2014. Reference values for hematology and plasma biochemistry variables, and protein electrophoresis of healthy Hermann's tortoises (*Testudo hermanni* ssp.). *Vet Clin Pathol* 43(4):573–583.

Banajee KH, Chang L-W, Jacobson ER, Rich GA, Royal AB. 2012. What is your diagnosis? Blood film from a boa constrictor. *Vet Clin Pathol* 41(1):158–159.

Barnard SM, Upton AJ. 1994. Protozoa. In: Barnard SM, Upton AK (eds), *Protozoa, A Veterinary Guide to the Parasites of Reptiles*. Malabar, FL: Krieger Publishing.

Bezjian M, Diep AN, De Matos R, Schaefer D. 2013. Chinese box turtle (*Cuora flavomarginata*) with lymphoid leukemia characterized by immunohistochemical and cytochemical phenotyping. *Vet Clin Pathol* 42(3):368–376.

Blofield BA, Short L, Samour HJ, Ball D, Hawkey CM. 1992. Phylogenetic and haematological implications of differences in the morphilocy of the heterophil nucleus in reptiles. *J Zool Lond* 226:539–549.

Bogan JE, Antonio F, Zachariah TT, Stacy NI. 2020. Comparison of the effects of three anticoagulants on heamtological analytes in the eastern indigo snake (*Drymarchon couperi*). *J Herpetolog Med Surg* 30(2):96–100.

Bolten AB, Bjorndal K. 1992. Blood profiles for a wild population of green turtles *Chelonia mydas* in the southern Bahamas: size-specific and sex-specific relationships. *J Wildl Dis* 28:407–413.

Bonadiman SF, Miranda FJB, Ribeiro MLS, et al. 2010. Hematological parameters of *Ameiva ameiva* (Reptilia: Teiidae) naturally infected with hemogregarine: confirmation of monocytosis. *Vet Parasitol* 171:146–150.

Bounous DI, Dotson TK, Brooks RJ, et al. 1996. Cytochemical staining and ultrastructural characteristics of peripheral blood leukocytes from the yellow rat snake (*Elaphe obsoleta quadrivitatta*). *Comp Haematol Int* 6:86–91.

Brooks RL, Bounous DI, Andreasen CB. 1996. Functional comparison of avian heterophils with human and canine neutrophils. *Comp Haemat Inter* 6:153–159.

Bryant GL, Fleming PA, Twomey L, Warren KA. 2012. Factors affecting hematology and plasma biochemistry in the southwest carpet python (*Morelia spilota imbricata*). *J Wildl Dis* 48(2):282–294.

Campbell TW. 1996. Hemoparasites. In: Mader D (ed), *Reptile Medicine and Surgery*. Philadelphia, PA: WB Saunders.

Campbell TW. 2006. Clinical pathology of reptiles. In: Mader D (ed), *Reptile Medicine and Surgery*, 2nd edn. St Louis, MO: Elsevier, pp. 453–470.

Campbell TW. 2012. Hematology of reptiles. In: Thrall M, Weiser G, Allison RW, Campbell TW (eds), *Veterinary Hematology and Clinical Chemistry*, 2nd edn. Ames, IA: Wiley-Blackwell, pp. 277–297.

Campbell TW, Grant KR. 2010. *Clinical Cases in Avian and Exotic Animal Hematology and Cytology*. Ames, IA: Wiley-Blackwell.

Canfield PJ, Shea GM. 1988. Morphological observations on the erythrocytes, leucocytes, and thrombocytes of blue tongue lizards (*Lacertilia scincidae*, Tiliqua). *Aant Histol Embryol* 17:328–342.

Cannon MS. 1992. The morphology and cytochemistry of the blood leukocytes of Kemp's ridley sea turtles (*Lepidochelys kempi*). *Can J Zool* 70:1336–1340.

Casal AB, Oros J. 2007. Morphologic and cytochemical characteristics of blood cells of juvenile loggerhead sea turtles (*Caretta caretta*). *Res Vet Sci* 82:158–165.

Caxton-Martins AE, Nganwuchu AM. 1978. A cytochemical study of the blood of the rainbow lizard (*Agama agama*). *J Anat* 125:477–480.

Cerreta AJ, Cannizzo SA, Smith DC, Minter LJ. 2020. Venous hematology, biochemistry, and blood gas analysis of free-ranging eastern copperheads (Agkistrodon contortrix) and eastern ratsnakes (Pantherophis alleghaniensis). PLoS one 15(2):e0229102. https://doi.org/10.1371/journal.pone.0229102

Cerreta AJ, Houck EL, Stowe DM, Lewbart GA. 2020b. Hematology of the keeled box turtle (*Cuora mouhotii*). *Vet Clin Pathol* 2020 49(2):227–231.

Chang L, Jacobson ER. 2010. Inclusion body disease, a worldwide infectious disease of boid snakes: a review. *J Exotic Pet Med* 19:216–225.

Chen Z, Wei Q, Wang J, et al. 2018. Cytochemical patterns of the peripheral blood cells in Chinese alligator (*Alligator sinensis*). *Tissue and Cell* 55:71–76.

Christopher MM, Berry KH, Wallis IR, et al. 1999. Reference intervals and physiologic alterations in hematologic and biochemical values of free-ranging desert tortoises in the Mojave desert. *J Wildl Dis* 35:212–238.

Chung CS, Cheng CH, Chin SC, Lee AH, Chi CH. 2009. Morphologic and cytochemical characteristics of Asian yellow pond turtle (*Ocadia sinensis*) blood cells and their hematologic and plasma biochemical reference values. *J Zoo Wild Med* 40(1):76–85.

Clark P, Hohnstone AC, Ellison R, Goold M. 2001. Inclusions in the erythrocytes of eastern water dragons (*Physignathus lesueurii*). *Aust Vet J* 79(1):61–62.

Cook CA, Smit NJ, Davies AJ. 2014. First record of an intraleucocytic haemogregarine (Adeleorina: Haemogregarinidae) from South African tortoises of the species Stigmochelys pardalis (Cryptodira: Testudinidae). *Afr Zool* 49(2):290–294.

Cook CA, Netherlands EC, Smit NJ. 2016. Redescription, molecular characterization, and taxonomic re-evaluation of a unique African monitor lizard haemogregarine *Karyolysus paradoxa* (Dias, 1954) n. comb. (*Karyolysidae*). *Parasites Vectors* 9:347–360.

Cooper-Bailey K, Smith SA, Zimmerman K, et al. 2011. Hematology, leukocyte cytochemical analysis, plasma biochemistry, and plasma electrophoresis of wild-caught and captive bred Gila monsters (*Heloderma suspectum*). *Vet Clin Pathol* 40(3): 316–323.

Crawshaw GJ. 1996. Comparison of plasma biochemical values in blood and blood-lymph mixtures from red-eared sliders, *Trachemys scripta elegans*. *Bull ARAV* 6:7–9.

Cray C. 2015. Reference intervals in avian and exotic hematology. *Veterinary Clinics of North America: Exotic Animal Practice* 18(1):105–116.

Cuadrado M, Diaz-Paniagua C, Quevedo MA, et al. 2002. Hematology and clinical chemistry in dystocic and healthy post-reproductive female chameleons. *J Wildl Dis* 38(2):395–401.

Daly JJ, Mayhue M, Menna JH, Calhon CH. 1980. Virus like particles associated with *Pirhemocyton* inclusion bodies in the erythrocytes of a water snake, *Nerodia erythrogster flavigaster*. *J Parasit* 66:82–87.

Damsgaard C, Storz JF, Hoffmann FG, Fago A. 2013. Hemoglobin isoform differentiation and allosteric regulation of oxygen in the turtle, *Trachemus scripta*. *Am J Physiol Regul Integr Comp Physiol* 305:R961–R967.

Davis AK, Sterrett SC. 2011. Prevalence of haemogregarine parasites in three freshwater turtle species in a population in northeast Georgia, USA. *Int J Zool Res* 7:156–163.

Davis AK, Horan RV, Grosse AM, et al. 2011. Gender differences in haemogregarine infections in American alligators (*Alligator mississippiensis*) at Savannah River, South Carolina, USA. *J Wildl Dis* 47(4):1047–1049.

de Mello DMD, Alvarez MCL. 2020. Health assessment of juvenile green turtles in southern Sao Paulo State, Brazil: a hematologic approach. *J Vet Diag Invest* 32(1):25–35.

Dickinson VM, Jarchow JL, Trueblood MH. 2002. Hematology and plasma biochemistry reference range values for free-ranging desert tortoises in Arizona. *J Wildl Dis* 38(1):43–53.

Diethelm G, Stein G. 2006. Hematologic and blood chemistry values in reptiles. In: Mader D (ed), *Reptile Medicine and Surgery*, 2nd edn. St. Louis, MO: Saunders Elsevier.

Divers SJ, Redmayne G, Aves EK. 1996. Haematological and biochemical values of 10 green iguanas (*Iguana iguana*). *Vet Rec* 138:203–205.

Duguy R. 1970. Numbers of blood cells and their variations. In: Gans C, Parsons T (eds), *Biology of the Reptilia*. New York: Academic Press.

Dutton CJ, Taylor P. 2003. A comparison between pre- and post-hibernation morphometry, hematology, and blood chemistry in viperid snakes. *J Zoo Wildl Med* 34(1):53–58.

Efrati P, Nir E, Yaari A. 1970. Morphological and cytochemical observations on cells of the hemopoietic system of *Agama stellio* (Linnaeus). *Israel J Med Sci* 6:23–91.

Egami MI, Sasso WS. 1988. Cytochemical observations of blood cells of *Bothrops jaracaca* (Reptilia, Squamata). *Rev Brasil Biol* 48:155–159.

Flanders AJ, Ossiboff RJ, Wellehan JFX, et al. 2021. Presumptive heterophil extracellular traps recognized cytologically in nine reptile patients with inflammatory conditions. *Veterinary Quarterly* 41(1):89–96.

Friedrichs KR, Harr KE, Freeman KP, et al. 2012. ASVCP reference interval guidelines: determination of de novo reference intervals in veterinary species and other related topics. *Vet Clin Pathol* 41(4):441–453.

Fry MM, McGavin MD. 2007. Bone marrow, blood cells, and lymphatic system. In: McGavin MD, Zachary JF (eds), *Pathologic Basis of Veterinary Disease*, 4th edn. St. Louis, MO: Mosby-Elsevier, pp. 743–832.

Frye FL. 1986. Hematology of captive reptiles. In: Fowler M (ed), *Zoo and Wild Animal Medicine*, 2nd edn. Philadelphia, PA: WB Saunders Co.

Frye FL. 1991. Hematology as applied to clinical reptile medicine. In: Frye FL (ed), *Vol. 1, Biomedical and Surgical Aspects of Captive Reptile Husbandry*, 2nd edn. Malabar, FL: Krieger Publishing Co.

Frye FL. 1991. Hemoparasites. In: Frye FL (ed), Vol. 1, *Biomedical and Surgical Aspects of Captive Reptile Husbandry*, 2nd edn. Melbourne, FL: Krieger Publishing Co.

Frey FL, Carney J. 1972. Myeloproliferative disease in a turtle. *J Am Vet Med Assoc* 161:595–599.

Frey FL, Carney J. 1973. Acute lymphocytic leukemia in a boa constrictor. *J Am Vet Med Assoc* 163:653–654.

Garner MM, Homer BL, Jacobson ER, et al. 1996. Staining and morphologic features of bone marrow hematopoietic cells in desert tortoises (*Gopherus agassizii*). *Am J Vet Res* 57:1608–1615.

Garner MM, Hernandez-Divers SM, Raymond JT. 2004. Reptile neoplasia: a retrospective study of case submissions to a specialty diagnostic service. *Vet Clin North Am Exotic Anim Pract* 7:653–671.

Geffre A, Friedrichs K, Harr K, et al. 2009. Reference values: a review. *Vet Clin Pathol* 38(3):288–298.

Giori L, Stacy NI, Ogle M, et al. 2019. Hematology, plasma biochemistry, and hormonal analysis of captive Louisiana pine snakes (*Pituophis ruthveni*): effects of intrinsic factors and analytical methodology. *Comp Clin Pathol* 29:145–154.

George JW, Holmberg TA, Riggs SM, Hawkins MG. 2008. Circulating siderophagocytes and erythrophagocytes in a corn snake (*Elaphe guttata*) after coelomic surgery. *Vet Clin Pathol* 37(3):308–311.

Godfrey SS, Nelson NJ, Bull CM. 2011. Ecology and dynamics of the blood parasite, *Hepatozoon tuatarae* (Apicomplexa), in Tuatara (*Sphenodon punctatus*) on Stephens Island, New Zealand. *J Wildl Dis* 47(1):126–139.

Goldberg SR, Holshuh HJ. 1991. A case of leukemia in the desert spiny lizard (*Sceloporus magister*). *J Wildl Dis* 27:521–525.

Gottdenker NL, Jacobson ER. 1995. Effect of venipuncture sites on hematologic and clinical biochemical values in desert tortoises (*Gopherus agassizii*). *Am J Res* 56:19–21.

Griner LA. 1983. Pathology of zoo animals. In: Griner LA (ed), *Pathology of Zoo Animals*. San Diego, CA: Zoological Society of San Diego.

Grosset C, Wellehan JFX, Owens SD, 2014. Intraerythrocytic iridovirus in central bearded dragons (*Pogona vitticeps*). *J Vet Diag Invest* 26(3):354–364.

Gyimesi ZS, Garner MM, Burns RB, et al. 2005. High incidence of lymphoid neoplasia in a colony of Egyptian spiny-tailed lizards (*Uromastyx aegyptius*). *J Zoo Wildl Med* 36:103–110.

Harr KE, Alleman AR, Dennis PM, Maxwell LK, et al. 2001. Morphologic and cytochemical characteristics of blood cells and hematologic and plasma biochemical reference ranges in green iguanas. *J Am Vet Med Assoc* 218(6):915–921.

Hawkey CM, Dennett TB. 1989. *A Colour Atlas of Comparative Veterinary Haematology*. London: Wolfe Medical Publications, Ltd.

Heatley JJ, Russell KE. 2019. Hematology. In: Divers SJ, Stahl SJ (eds), *Mader's Reptile and Amphibian Medicine and Surgery*, 3rd edn. St. Louis, MO: Elsevier, pp. 301–318.

Hernandez JD, Castro P, Saavedra P, Ramirez P, Oros J. 2017. Morphologic and cytochemical characteristics of the blood cells of the yellow-bellied slider (*Trachemus scripta scripta*). *Anat Histol Embryol* 46:446–455.

Hetzel U, Sironen T, Laurinmaki P, et al. 2015. Isolation, identification, and characterization of novel arnaviruses, the etiological agents of boid inclusion body disease. *J Virol* 87(20):10918–10935.

Hussein MF, et al. 1978. Differential effect of seasonal variation on lymphoid tissue of the lizard, *Chalecides ocellatus*. *Dev Comp Immunol* 2:297–310.

Hussein MF, et al. 1979a. Effect of seasonal variation on the immune system of the lizard, *Scinus scinus*. *J Exp Zool* 209:91–96.

Hussein MF, et al. 1979b. Lymphoid tissue of the snake, *Spalerosophis diadema* in the different seasons. *Dev Comp Immunol* 3:77–88.

Innis CJ, Ravich JB, Tlusty MF, et al. 2009. Hematologic and plasma biochemical findings in cold-stunned Kemp's ridley turtles: 176 cases (2001–2005). *J Am Vet Med Assoc* 235:426–432.

International Species Information System (ISIS) 2002. Currently Species360. Available at: https://www.species360.org/

Jacobson ER. 1986. Parasitic diseases of reptiles. In: Fowler M (ed), *Zoo and Wild Animal Medicine*, 2nd edn. Philadelphia, PA: WB Saunders Co.

Jacobson ER, Gaskin JM, Brown MB, et al. 1990. Chronic upper respiratory tract disease of free-ranging desert tortoises, *Xerobates agassizii*. *J Wildl Dis* 27(2):296–316.

Keller JM, Kucklick JR, Stamper MA, et al. 2004. Associations between organochlorine contamination concentration and clinical health parameters in loggerhead sea turtles from North Carolina, USA. *Environ Health Perspect* 112(10):1074–1079.

Keymer IF. 1981. Protozoa. I. In: Cooper J, Jackson O (eds), Vol. 1, *Diseases of Reptilia*. San Diego, CA: Academic Press.

Knotkova Z, Doubek J, Knotek Z, Hajkova P. 2002. Blood cell morphology and plasma biochemistry in Russian tortises (*Agrionemys horsfieldi*). *Acta Vet Brno* 71:191–198.

Kubiak M, Denk D, Stidworthy MF. 2019. Retrospective review of neoplasms of captive lizards in the United Kingdom. *Vet Rec* https://doi:10.1136/vetrec-2018–105308

Langenberg JA, Ramsay EC, Rotstein DS, et al. 1983. Hematopoietic and lymphoreticular tumors in zoo animals. *Lab Invest* 48:48A.

Latney LV, Wellehan J. 2013. Selective emerging infectious diseases of squamata. *Vet Clin N Am Exotic Anim Pract* 10(2): 319–338.

Lawrence K, Hawkey CM. 1986. Seasonal variations in haematological data from Mediterranean tortoises (*Testudo graeca* and *Testudo hermanni*) in captivity. *Res Vet Sci* 40:225–230.

Lentini AM, Crawshaw GJ, Licht LE, McLelland DJ. 2011. Pathologic and hematologic responses to surgically implanted transmitters in Eastern Massasauga rattlesnakes (*Sistrurus catenatus catenatus*). *J Wildl Dis* 47(1):107–125.

Lopez-Olvera JR, Montane J, Marco I, et al. 2003. Effect of venipuncture site on hematologic and serum biochemical parameters in marginated tortoise (*Testudo marginata*). *J Wildl Dis* 39(4): 830–836.

Louis MM, Cerreta AJ, Griffioen JA, et al. 2020. Homologous whole blood transfusion for treatment of severe anemia in five Eastern box turtles (*Terrapene carolina carolina*). *Journal of Exotic Pet Medicine* 35:27–33.

Lowichik A, Yeager RG. 1987. Ecological aspects of snake hemogregarine infections from two habitats in southern Louisiana. *J Parasitol* 73:1109–1115.

Lu S, Xin Y, Tang X, et al. 2015. Differences in hematological traits between high- and low-altitude lizards (Genus *Phrynocephalus*). PLOS one 10.1371/journal.pone.0125751.

MacMahon JA, Hamer AH. 1975. Hematology of the sidewinder (*Crotalus cerastes*). *Comp Biochem Physiol* 51A:53–58.

Madsen T, Ujvari B, Olsson M. 2005. Old pythons stay fit: effects of haematozoan infections on life history traits of a large tropical predator. *Oecologia* 142:407–412.

Marks SK, Citino SB. 1990. Hematology and serum chemistry of the radiated tortoise (*Testudo radiate*). *J Zoo Wildl Med* 21(3):342–344.

Marschang RE. 2019. Virology. In: Divers SJ, Stahl SJ (eds), *Mader's Reptile and Amphibian Medicine and Surgery*, 3rd edn. St. Louis, MO: Elsevier, pp. 247–269.

Martinez Silvestre A, Rodriguez DMA, Mateo JA, et al. 2004. Comparative haematology and blood chemistry of endangered lizards (*Gallotia* spp.) in the Canary Islands. *Vet Rec* 155:266–269.

Mateo MR, Roberts ED, Enright FM. 1984. Morphological, cytochemical, and functional studies of peripheral blood cells in young healthy American alligators (*Alligator mississippiensis*). *Am J Vet Res* 45:1046–1053.

Mayer J, Knoll J, Innis C, Mitchell MA. 2005. Characterizing the hematologic and plasma chemistry profiles of captive Chinese water dragons, *Physignathus cocincinus*. *J Herp Med Surg* 15(3):45–52.

Mead KF, Borysenko M. 1984. Surface immunoglobulins on granular and agranular leukocytes in the thymus and spleen of the snapping turtle, *Chelydra serpentina*. *Dev Comp Immunol* 8:109–120.

Mead KF, Borysenko M, Findlay SR. 1983. Naturally abundant basophils in the snapping turtle, *Chelydra serpentina*, possess cytophilic surface antibodies with reaginic function. *J Immunol* 130:384–340.

Meints RH, Carver FJ, Gerst JW, McLaughlin DW. 1975. Erythropoietic activity in the turtle: the influence of hemolytic anemia, hypoxia, and hemorrhage on hemopoietic function. *Comp Biochem Physiol* 50A:419–422.

Moller CA, Gaal T, Mills JN. 2016. The hematology of captive Bobtail lizards (*Tiliqua rugosa*): blood counts, light microscopy, cytochemistry, and ultrastructure. *Vet Clin Pathol* 45(4):634–647.

Montali RJ. 1988. Comparative pathology of inflammation in the higher vertebrates (reptiles, birds, and mammals). *J Comp Pathol* 99:1–26.

Muro J, Ramis J, Pastor R, et al. 1998. Chronic rhinitis associated with herpesviral infection in captive spur-thighed tortoises from Spain. *J Wildl Dis* 34(3):487–495.

Mussachia XJ, Sievers MI. 1956. Effects of induced cold torpor on blood of *Chrysemys picta*. *Am J Physiol* 187:99–102.

Origgi FG. 2007. Reptile immunology. In: Jacobson ER (ed), *Infectious Diseases and Pathology of Reptiles*. Boca Raton, FL: CRC Press, pp. 131–157.

Origgi FG, Tecilla M. 2021. Immunology of reptiles. In: Jacobson ER, Garner MM (eds), *Infectious Diseases and Pathology of Reptiles Color Atlas and Text*, 2nd edn. Boca Rotan, FL: Taylor and Francis Group, LLC.

Oros J, Torrent A, Espinosa de los Monteros A, et al. 2001. Multicentric lymphoblastic lymphoma in a loggerhead sea turtle (*Caretta caretta*). *Vet Pathol* 38:464–467.

Peng F, Chen X, Meng T, et al. 2018. Hematology and serum biochemistry parameters of captive Chinese alligators (*Alligator sinensis*) during the active and hibernating periods. *Tissue and Cell* 51:8–13.

Pereira FMAM, de Oliveira AR, Mattioli MP, Carneiro FT. 2021. Diagnosis and treatment of *Plasmodium* infection in captive black and white tegus. *J Comp Pathol* 183:9–12.

Pica A, Della Corte F, Grimaldi MC, D'Ippolito S. 1986. The blood cells of the common lizard (*Podarcis s. sicula* Raf.): morphocytochemistry, DNA amount of red cells and hemopoiesis. *Arch Ital Anat Embriol* 91:301–320.

Perpinan D, Sanchez C. 2009. Morphologic and cytochemical characteristics of blood cells from the european pond turtle (*Emys orbicularis*) and the Mediterranean pond turtle (*Mauremys leprosa*). *J Herp Med Surg* 19(4):119–127.

Raphael BL, Klemens MW, Moehlman P, et al. 1994. Blood values in free-ranging pancake tortoises *Malachochersus tornieri*. *J Zoo Wildl Med* 25:63–67.

Raskin RE. 2000. Reptilian complete blood count. In: Fudge A (ed), *Laboratory Medicine: Avian and Exotics*. Philadelphia, PA: WB Saunders.

Raskin RE, Crosby FL, Jacobson ER. 2020. Newly recognized *Anaplasma* sp. in erythrocytes from gopher tortoises (*Gopherus polyphemus*). *Vet Clin Pathol* 49(1):17–22.

Rousselet E, Norton TM, Wellman M, Kohart N, Stacy NI. 2017. Presumptive granulocytic leukemia in a hognose snake (*Heterodon platirhinos*). *Vet Q* 37(1):43–47.

Saint Girons MC. 1970. Morphology of the circulating blood cell. In: Gans C, Parsons T (eds), *Biology of the Reptilia, Vol. 3*. New York: Academic Press.

Salakij C, Salakij J, Apibal S, et al. 2002. Hematology, morphology, cytochemical staining, and ultrastructural characteristics of blood cells in king cobras (*Ophiophagus hannah*). *Vet Clin Pathol* 31(3):116–126.

Salakij C, Salakij J, Prihirunkit K, et al. 2014. Quantitative and qualitative morphologic, cytochemical, and ultrastructural characteristics of blood cells in captive Asian water monitors. *Vet Clin Pathol* 43(4):538–546.

Samour JH, Hawkey CM, Pugsley S, et al. 1986. Clinical and pathological findings related to malnutrition and husbandry in captive giant tortoises (*Geochelone* species). *Vet Rec* 15:299–302.

Sanyal M, Patil P, Jaiswal E, Deshmukh A. 2013. Structural and functional diversity of haemoglobin molecule properties amongst different classes and species of animals. *Acta Biologica Indica* 2(2):381–387.

Scheelings TF, Rafferty AR. 2012. Hematologic and serum biochemical values of gravid freshwater Australian chelonians. *J Wildl Dis* 48(2):314–321.

Schilliger L, Selleri P, Frye FL. 2011. Lymphoblastic lymphoma and leukemic blood profile in a red-tail boa (*Boa constrictor constrictor*) with concurrent inclusion body disease. *J Vet Diagn Invest* 23:159–162.

Schoeb TR, Heaton-Jones TG, Clemmons RM, Carbonneau DA, et al. 2002. Clinical and necropsy findings associated with increased mortality among American alligators of Lake Griffin, Florida. *J Wild Dis* 38(2):320–337.

Schumacher J, Jacobson ER, Homer BL, Gaskin JM. 1994. Inclusion body disease in boid snakes. *J Zoo Wildl Med* 25:511–524.

Sheeler P, Barber AA. 1965. Reticulocytosis and iron incorporation in the rabbit and turtle: a comparative study. *Comp Biochem Physiol* 16:63–76.

Silverstone AM, Garner MM, Wojcieszyn JW, Guillermo Couto C, Raskin RE. 2007. Acute lymphoblastic leukemia in a diamondback terrapin, *Malaclemys terrapin*. *J Herpetol Med Surg* 17:92–99.

Stacy BA, Whitaker N. 2000. Hematology and blood biochemistry of captive mugger crocodiles (*Crocodylus palustris*). *J Zoo Wildl Med* 31(3):339–347.

Stacy NI, Alleman AR, Sayler KA. 2011. Diagnostic hematology of reptiles. *Vet Lab Med* 21(1):87–108.

Stacy NI, Fredholm DV, Rodriquez C, Castro L, Harvey JW. 2017a. Whip-like heterophil projections in consecutive blood films from an injured gopher tortoise (*Gopherus polyphemus*) with systemic inflammation. *Vet Q* 37(1):162–165.

Stacy NI, Ranly M, Pelton C. 2017b. What is your diagnosis? Blood film from a Green turtle (*Chelonia mydas*). *Vet Clin Pathol* 46(1):193–194.

Stacy NI, Harr KE. 2021. Hematology of reptiles with a focus on circulating inflammatory cells. In: Jacobson ER, Garner MM (eds), *Infectious Diseases and Pathology of Reptiles Color Atlas and Text*, 2nd edn. Boca Rotan, FL: Taylor and Francis Group, LLC.

Stacy NI, Harvey JW. 2021. Whip-like heterophils projections: Best in show. *Vet Clin Path* 50(2):176–177.

Stewart K, Mitchell MA, Norton T, Krecek RC. 2012. Measuring the level of agreement in hematologic and biochemical values between blood sampling sites in Leatherback sea turtles (*Dermochelys coriacea*). *J Zoo Wildl Med* 43(4):719–725.

Storz JF, Hoffmann FG, Opazo JC, Sanger TJ, Moriyama H. 2011. Developmental regulation of hemoglobin synthesis in the green anole lizard *Anolis carolinensis*. *J Exp Biol* 214:575–581.

Sykes JM, Klaphake E. 2015. Reptile hematology. *Veterinary Clinics of North America: Exotic Animal Practice* 18(1):63–82.

Sypek JP, Borysenko M. 1988. Reptiles. In: Rowley A, Ratcliffe N (eds), *Vertebrate Blood Cells*. Cambridge: Cambridge University Press.

Sypek JP, Borysenko M, Findlay SR. 1984. Antiimmunoglobulin induced histamine release from naturally abundant basophils in the snapping turtle, *Chelydra serpentina*. *Dev Comp Immunol* 8:358–366.

Taylor K, Kaplan HM. 1961. Light microscopy of the blood cells of Pseudemyd turtles. *Herpetologica* 17:186–192.

Taylor KW, Kaplan HM, Hirano T. 1963. Electron microscope study of turtle blood cells. *Cytologia* 28:248–256.

Taylor R, Jacobson ER. 1982. Hematology and serum chemistry of the Gopher tortoise (*Gopherus polyphemus*). *Comp Biochem Physiol* 72A:425–428.

Telford SR. 1984. Haemoparasites of reptiles. In: Hoff G, Frye G, Jacobson E (eds), *Diseases of Amphibians and Reptiles*. New York: Plenum Book Co.

Telford SR. 2009. *Hemoparasites of the Reptilia: Color Atlas and Text*. New York: CRC Press.

Telford SR, Jacobson ER. 1993. Lizard erythrocytic virus in East African chameleons. *J Wild Dis* 29:57–63.

Tocidlowski ME, McNamara PL, Wojcieszyn JW. 2001. Myelogenous leukemia in a bearded dragon (*Acanthodraco vitticeps*). *J Zoo Wildl Med* 32:90–95.

Troiano JC, Vidal JC, Gould J, et al. 1997. Haematological reference intervals of the South American rattlesnake (*Crotalus durissus terrificus*, Laurenti, 1768) in captivity. *Comp Haemat Inter* 1:109–112.

Turton JA, Ladds PW, Manolis SC, Webb GJW. 1997. Relationship of blood corticosterone, immunoglobulin and haematological values in young crocodles (*Crocodylus porosus*) to water temperature, clutch of origin, and body weight. *Aust Vet J* 75(2):114–119.

Viana LA, Paiva F, Coutinho ME, Lourenco-De-Oliveira R. 2010. *Hepatozoon caimani* (Apicomplexa: Hepatozoidae) in wild caiman, *Caiman yacare*, from the Pantanal region, Brazil. *J Parasitol* 96:83–88.

Wack RF, Anderson NL. 2004. Resuscitation of a Hispaniolan slider, *Trachemys decorata*, using Oxyglobin® and a blood transfusion. *J Herpetological Med Surg* 14(1):4–5.

Wallach JD, Boever WJ. 1983. Diseases of exotic animals, medical and surgical management. In: Wallach JD, Boever WJ (eds), *Diseases of Exotic Animals, Medical and Surgical Management*. Philadelphia, PA: WB Saunders.

Walton RM. 2001. Establishing reference intervals: health as a relative concept. *Semin Avian Exot Pet Med* 10:66–71.

Weiser G, Allison RW. 2012. Perspectives in laboratory data interpretation and disease diagnosis. In: Thrall MA, Weiser G, Allison RW, Campbell TW (eds), *Veterinary Hematology And Clinical Chemistry*, 2nd edn. Ames, IA: Wiley-Blackwell.

Wilkinson R. 2004. Clinical pathology. In: McArthur S, Wilkinson R, Meyer J (eds), *Medicine and Surgery of Tortoises and Turtles*. Oxford: Blackwell Publishing.

Winter JM, Stacy NI, Adamovicz, Allender MC. 2019. Investigating the analytical variability and agreement of manual leukocyte quantification methods in eastern box turtles (*Terrapene carolina carolina*). *Front Vet Sci* 6:398. DOI: 10.3389/fvets. 00398.

Wojtaszek JS. 1991. Haematology of the grass snake *Natrix natrix natrix* L. *Comp Biochem Physiol* 100(4):805–812.

Wojtaszek JS. 1992. Seasonal changes of circulating blood parameters in the grass snake *Natrix natrix natrix* L. *Comp Biochem Physiol* 103A:461–471.

Wood FE, Ebanks GK. 1984. Blood cytology and hematology of the green sea turtle, *Chelonia mydas*. *Herpetologica* 40:331–336.

Work TM, Balazs GH. 1999. Relating tumor score to hematology in green turtles with fibropapillomatosis in Hawaii. *J Wildl Dis* 35(4):804–807.

Work TM, Raskin RE, Balazs GH, Whittaker SD. 1998. Morphological and cytochemical characteristics of blood cells from Hawaiian green turtles. *Am J Vet Res* 59:1252–1257.

Wozniak EJ, Telford SR. 1991. The fate of possibly two *Hepatozoon* species naturally infecting Florida black racers and watersnakes in potential mosquito and soft tick vectors: histological evidence of pathogenicity in unnatural host species. *Int J Parasitol* 21:511–516.

Wozniak EJ, McLaughlin GL, Telford SR. 1994a. Description of the vertebrate stages of a hemogregarine species naturally infecting Mojove Desert sidewinder rattlesnakes *(Crotalus cerastes cerastes)*. *J Zoo Wildl Med* 25:103–110.

Wozniak EJ, Telford SR, McLaughlin GL. 1994b. Employment of the polymerase chain reaction in the molecular differentiation of reptilian hemogregarines and its application to preventative zoological medicine. *J Zoo Wildl Med* 25:538–549.

Wright KM, Skeba S. 1992. Hematology and plasma chemistries of captive prehensile-tailed skinks (*Corucia zebrata*). *J Zoo Wildl Med* 23:429–432.

Wright RK, Cooper EL. 1981. Temperature effects on ectothermic immune responses. *Dev Comp Immunol* 5 (Suppl 1):117–122.

Zapata A, Leceta J, Villena A. 1981. Reptilian bone marrow: an ultrastructural study in the spanish lizard, *Lacerta hispanica*. *J Morph* 168:137–149.

20

Evaluation and Interpretation of the Peripheral Blood and Bone Marrow of Amphibians

Hematologic evaluation is not used routinely in veterinary medicine as a means of evaluating the health or diseased state of amphibian patients. Reasons why hematologic data are often not used include the difficulty in obtaining amphibian blood samples without affecting the hemogram results, the challenges involved in obtaining cell counts, and the lack of meaningful reference intervals. Many published reference ranges often fail to include information involving intrinsic (i.e., sex and age) and extrinsic (i.e., environmental temperature, photoperiod, water quality parameters, diet, population density, and season) factors, which may influence the hematology values (Harris, 1972; Singh, 1978; Mitruka and Rawnsley, 1981; Sinha, 1983; Wang and Herman, 1996). Some publications do include some of this information, and whenever possible these sources should be used when interpreting amphibian hematologic results.

Amphibians have adapted to a wide variety of environments (i.e., aquatic, terrestrial, fossorial, and alpine) and their normal hematologic parameters vary accordingly. Amphibians differ from other vertebrates in that their life cycle includes a metamorphosis from a larval form to an adult form; therefore, larval and adult stages should be considered separate entities when evaluating the hemograms, each with its own reference range.

Hematologic evaluation may be used to monitor the health status of an amphibian as long as the reported reference ranges and interpretations account for the intrinsic and extrinsic factors that affect the hemic response (Young et al., 2012). It should be remembered that absolute numbers of each cell type are expected to vary considerably with season, temperature, species, habitat, and a number of other extrinsic considerations (Allender and Fry, 2008).

Hematology can be useful in the detection of the diseases that affect the cellular components of blood, such as anemia, leukopenia, leukocytosis, thrombocytopenia, and other abnormal changes of blood cells, and may also be useful in following the progression of a disease or a response to therapy.

Interpretation of the amphibian hemogram may be challenging in some cases. Some amphibians, such as newts and salamanders, are more fishlike than other amphibians, making it necessary to interpret changes in their hemogram similar to the changes seen in the hemogram of fish. Changes in the hemogram of toads and frogs may be more similar to those of reptiles and can be interpreted as such. Representative hemic cells found in amphibian blood films can be found in Appendix C.

Amphibian Erythrocytes

The erythrocytes of amphibians are large compared to those of other vertebrates, with sizes vary from 10 to 70 μm in diameter and typically have MCV values ranging from 390 to 14 000 fL (Boutilier et al., 1992; Jerret and Mays, 1973; Cathers et al., 1997; Pfeiffer et al., 1990). The aquatic salamander (*Amphiuma* sp.) has the largest erythrocytes, with a length near 70 μm indicating the likelihood of a correspondingly long genome (Gregory, 2001; Forzán et al., 2017). Most amphibian erythrocytes are nucleated and elliptical in shape, have a distinct nuclear bulge, and often have irregular nuclear margins (Figures 20.1a and 20.1b). Some amphibians, such as the slender salamander (*Batrachoseps attenuatus*), do not have

Exotic Animal Hematology and Cytology, Fifth Edition. Terry W. Campbell and Krystan R. Grant.

Companion website: www.wiley.com/go/campbell/exotic

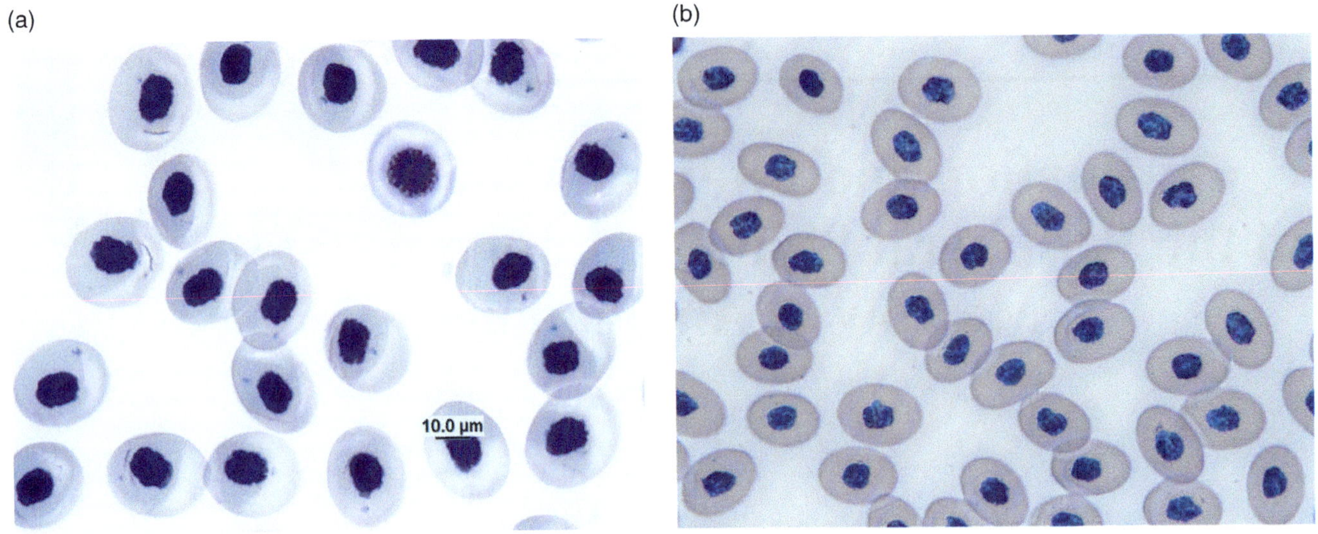

Fig. 20.1. (a) Normal erythrocytes in the blood film of a salamander (*Ambystoma tigrinum*), Wright–Giemsa stain. (b) Normal erythrocytes in the blood film of a toad (*Incilius alvarius*), Wright–Giemsa stain, 100× oil.

nucleated red blood cells (Cohen, 1982). The cytoplasm of frog and toad erythrocytes is homogenous and packed with hemoglobin. Ultrastructural studies of the cytoplasm of these cells reveal the presence of rare organelles. The erythrocytes of salamanders and newts complete their maturation in the peripheral circulation; therefore, the cytoplasm of immature erythrocytes is not homogenous, and ultrastructural examination demonstrates clusters of granular and vacuolar bodies (Turner, 1988). The cytoplasm of the immature cells also stains more basophilic compared to mature cells with Wright's stain (Figures 20.2a–20.2c). The blue staining of the amphibian erythrocyte cytoplasm may also be associated, in part, with the effects of heparin on Wright's-stained blood films, as heparin is a commonly used anticoagulant during blood collection in amphibians. The staining effects caused by heparin can be prevented if a blood film is made from a drop of blood remaining in the needle that does not contain heparin after blood collection.

The appearance of the nucleus of the amphibian erythrocyte also changes as the cell matures. The nuclear chromatin of immature erythrocytes lacks the dense chromatin clumping of the mature cell. Older senescent cells have pyknotic nuclei.

The packed cell volume (PCV) of amphibians is typically lower than that of mammals and birds (Appendix B, Table B.10) (Pfeiffer et al., 1990; Cathers et al., 1997). PCVs are affected by intrinsic and extrinsic factors and will vary depending on the species, age, sex, environmental temperature, photoperiod, season, and husbandry of the amphibian (Harris, 1972; Anvier and Pond, 1984; Allender and Fry, 2008). Captive amphibians may have more stable erythrocyte parameters than their wild counterparts due to the stability of the environment in which most captive amphibians reside.

The hemoglobin of most vertebrates has four iron-containing heme subunits, two alpha-globin chains, and two beta-globin chains. The interaction between subunits, largely determined by the amino acid sequence, alters the structure and the oxygen-binding properties (Sanyal et al., 2013). The genes in the globin chains are expressed differently in the embryonic and postnatal life stages of mammals and birds as well as in the larval and adult stages of the *Xenopus* genus of amphibians, but not between life stages of the green anole lizard (Storz et al., 2011). Environmental conditions also appear to affect the oxygen affinity for some amphibians, such as *Bufo* toads. For example, toads that live at high altitudes, like *Bufo spinulosus flavolineatus*, have a higher affinity to oxygen, which shifts the oxygen dissociation curve to the left, compared to other *Bufo* toads living at sea level or intermediate valleys (Ostojic et al., 2000).

Normal amphibian erythrocytes do exhibit slight anisocytosis; however, increased anisocytosis suggests an increased concentration of large red cells due to erythroid regeneration or erythroid dyscrasia. This may be seen in association with a regenerative response to a hemolytic or hemorrhagic anemia. The conditions that result in erythroid dyscrasia may indicate a nutritional deficiency or toxicity; however, these have not been documented in the literature. Increased numbers of immature erythrocytes may be indicative of a disease such as iridovirus infection or may indicate the presence of a regenerative response (Gruia-Gray and Desser, 1992; Graczyk et al., 1996). Iridovirus infections have been associated with disease outbreaks associated with high

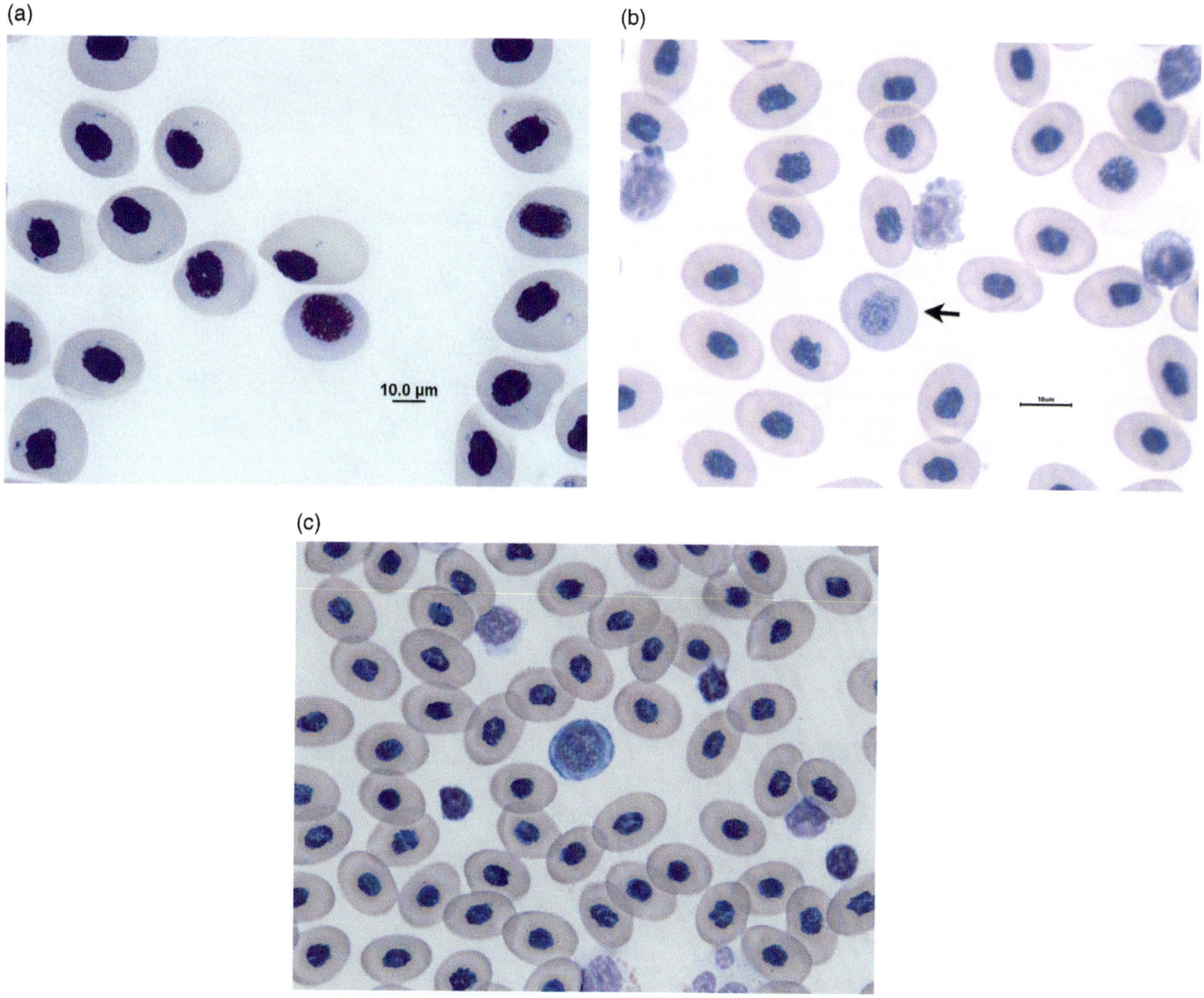

Fig. 20.2. (a) A polychromatic erythrocyte (cell in the center) that lacks the dense chromatin clumping of mature erythrocytes in the blood film of a salamander (*Ambystoma tigrinum*), Wright–Giemsa stain. (b) A polychromatic erythrocyte that lacks the dense chromatin clumping of mature erythrocytes in the blood film of a toad (*Incilius alvarius*), Wright–Giemsa stain, 100× oil. (c) An immature erythrocyte (cell in the center) in the blood film of a toad (*Incilius alvarius*), Wright–Giemsa stain, 100× oil.

mortalities in wild frogs and salamanders. Intranuclear inclusions of the iridovirus are found in the erythrocytes on histologic specimens (Green, 2001).

Irregular immature erythrocytes with characteristics reminiscent of cells in mammalian erythroid leukemia or exuberant responses can be found in blood films of clinically healthy frogs and may be indicative of rapid cell turnover or a result of environmental stressors (Barni et al., 2007; Bricker et al., 2012).

Amphibian Leukocytes

In general, amphibian leukocytes resemble those of mammals, but are comparatively larger (10 and 25 µm in diameter for most species) (Turner, 1988). Amphibian leukocytes are typically classified based upon their appearance in blood smears stained with Wright–Giemsa stain and their resemblance to mammalian leukocytes; therefore, they have been classified as neutrophils, eosinophils, basophils, lymphocytes, and monocytes (Forzán et al., 2017; Pessier, 2018). The literature sometimes classifies neutrophils as heterophils and identifies some cells as azurophils instead of or in addition to monocytes. Some references also include different combinations of heterophil, azurophil, and neutrophil to describe the granulocytic cells present (Jerret and Mays, 1973; Surbis, 1978; Cannon, 1979; Turner, 1988; Hawkey and Dennett, 1989; Pfeiffer et al., 1990).

Amphibian granulocytes (neutrophils or heterophils, eosinophils, and basophils) have multilobed nuclei with small cytoplasmic granules that are variable in size, shape, and ultrastructure depending on the species.

(a) (b) (c)

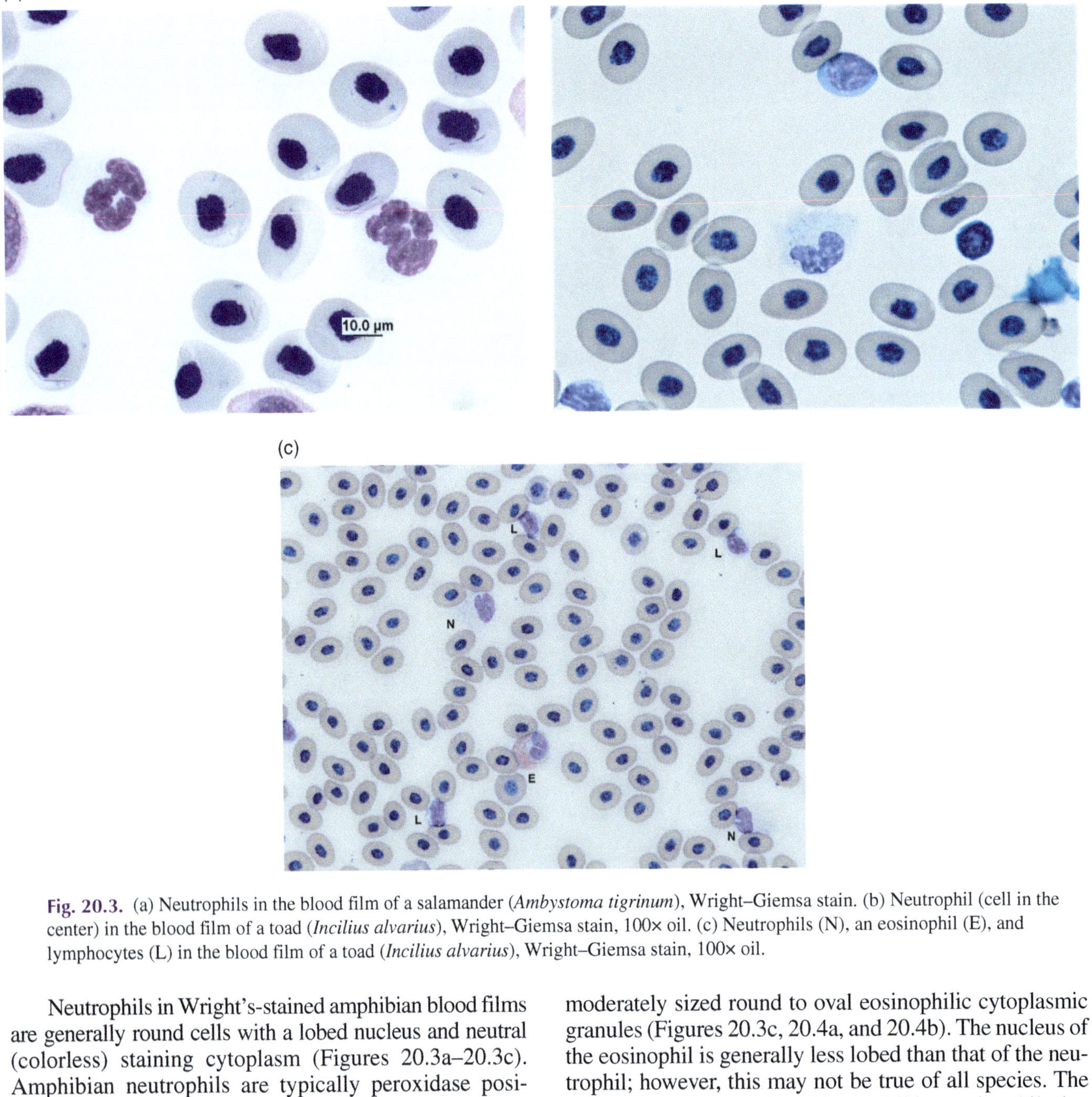

Fig. 20.3. (a) Neutrophils in the blood film of a salamander (*Ambystoma tigrinum*), Wright–Giemsa stain. (b) Neutrophil (cell in the center) in the blood film of a toad (*Incilius alvarius*), Wright–Giemsa stain, 100× oil. (c) Neutrophils (N), an eosinophil (E), and lymphocytes (L) in the blood film of a toad (*Incilius alvarius*), Wright–Giemsa stain, 100× oil.

Neutrophils in Wright's-stained amphibian blood films are generally round cells with a lobed nucleus and neutral (colorless) staining cytoplasm (Figures 20.3a–20.3c). Amphibian neutrophils are typically peroxidase positive, but phosphatase activity varies with the species (Turner, 1988). Some species may have cells that resemble neutrophils, but have distinct, small eosinophilic cytoplasmic granules. These cells are often referred to as heterophils. Some species of amphibians may exhibit neutrophils with large, irregular cytoplasmic granules that stain slightly eosinophilic (light pink). These cells resemble the neutrophils found in humans and other mammals with Chediak–Higashi syndrome.

Amphibian eosinophils are similar in size to or slightly larger than the neutrophils found in the same blood film. Eosinophils have a slightly basophilic cytoplasm compared to neutrophils and have small to moderately sized round to oval eosinophilic cytoplasmic granules (Figures 20.3c, 20.4a, and 20.4b). The nucleus of the eosinophil is generally less lobed than that of the neutrophil; however, this may not be true of all species. The eosinophilic granules found in amphibian eosinophils that have been studied exhibit a crystalloid ultrastructure that is typical of the ultrastructural morphology of eosinophils from higher vertebrates (Turner, 1988; Pfeiffer et al., 1990). Other amphibians such as the Japanese newt (*Cynops pyrrhogaster*) apparently lack these crystalloid structures. The eosinophils of amphibians are peroxidase negative, and the phosphatase activity varies with species (Turner, 1988). The eosinophils of some species, such as the Colorado River toad (*Bufo alvarius*), are negative for arylsulfatase and ß-glucuronidase activity.

Amphibian basophils typically have nonsegmented nuclei and large, metachromatic basophilic cytoplasmic

(a) (b)

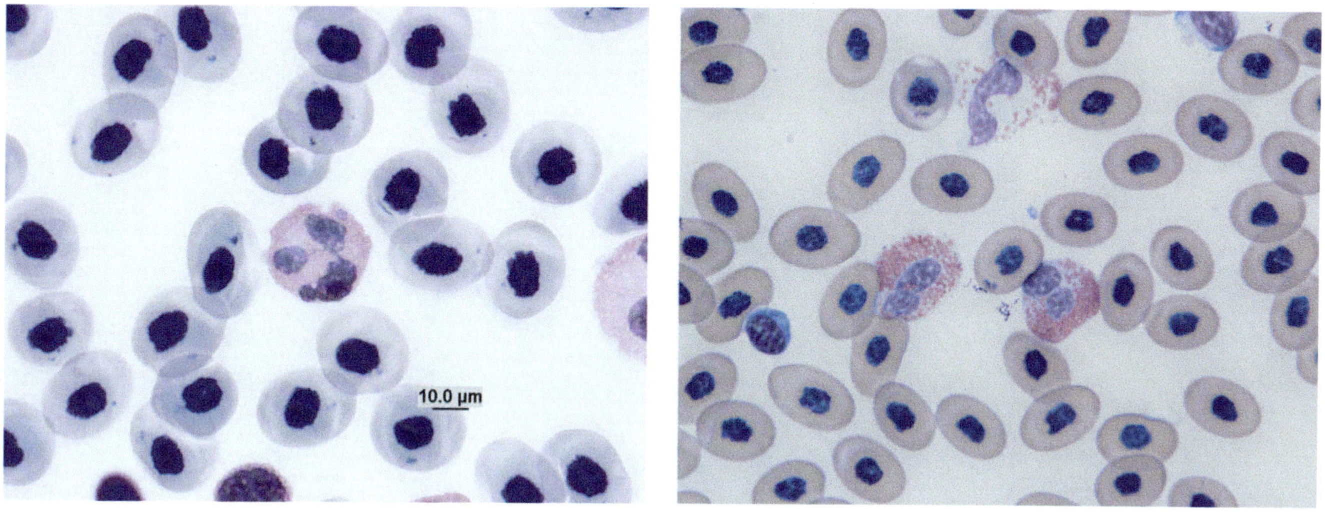

Fig. 20.4. (a) An eosinophil in the blood film of a salamander (*Ambystoma tigrinum*), Wright–Giemsa stain. (b) Eosinophils and a lymphocyte in the blood film of a toad (*Incilius alvarius*), Wright–Giemsa stain, 100× oil.

(a) (b)

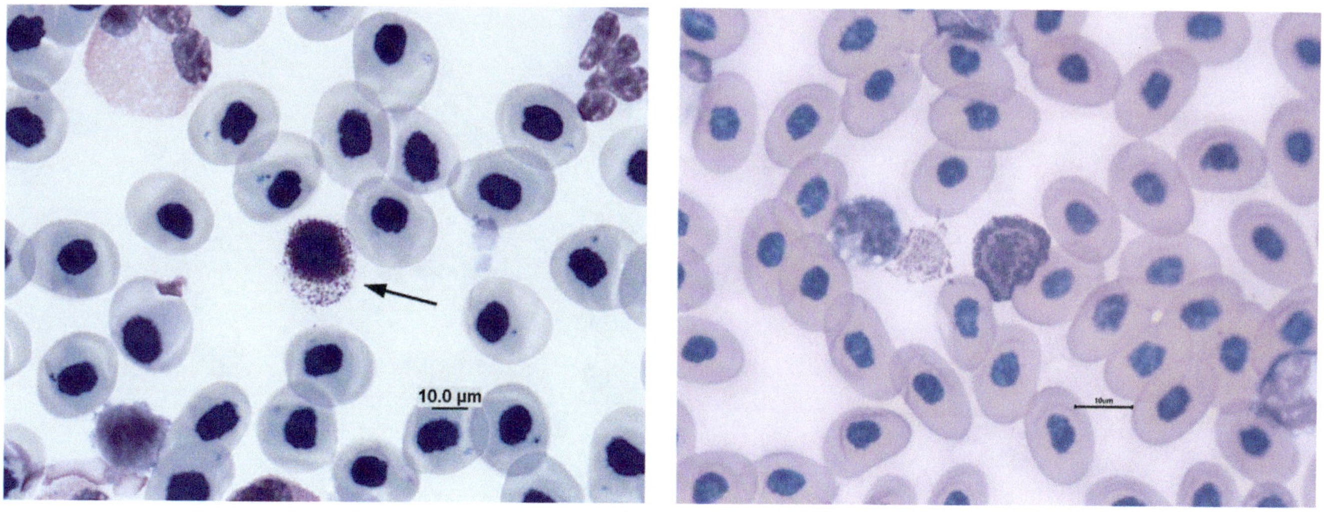

Fig. 20.5. (a) A basophil (arrow) in the blood film of a salamander (*Ambystoma tigrinum*), Wright–Giemsa stain. (b) A basophil (center) and a monocyte (left) in the blood film of a toad (*Incilius alvarius*), Wright–Giemsa stain, 100× oil.

granules (Figures 20.5a and 20.5b). The size of the cell varies with species. The nucleus is often obscured by the granules, but when visible is nonlobed and slightly eccentric in position. Alcohol fixation and use of Romanowsky stains provide the best staining for amphibian basophils because basophil granules are frequently affected by water-based stains and will partially dissolve. The basophilic granules contain acid mucopolysaccharides (glycosaminoglycans) that are less sulfated than the basophilic granules of mammals, and the histamine content is also lower than that of mammals (Turner, 1988). Ultrastructural studies demonstrate large numbers of membrane-bound cytoplasmic granules with small numbers of organelles.

The lymphocytes of amphibians morphologically resemble those of other vertebrates (Figures 20.3c, 20.4b, 20.6a, 20.6b, and 20.7b). Small lymphocytes are more abundant than the larger forms in the blood films of normal amphibians, and appear as round cells with scant amounts of pale blue cytoplasm and round nuclei. The nuclear chromatin is dense and clumped. Lymphocytes found in Ranidae frogs often contain distinct azurophilic granules. Amphibian lymphocytes are nonspecific esterase positive and peroxidase negative, much like the lymphocytes of mammals. Amphibian lymphocytes differ from mammalian cells, however, because they are negative for β-glucuronidase and aryl sulfatase (Turner, 1988).

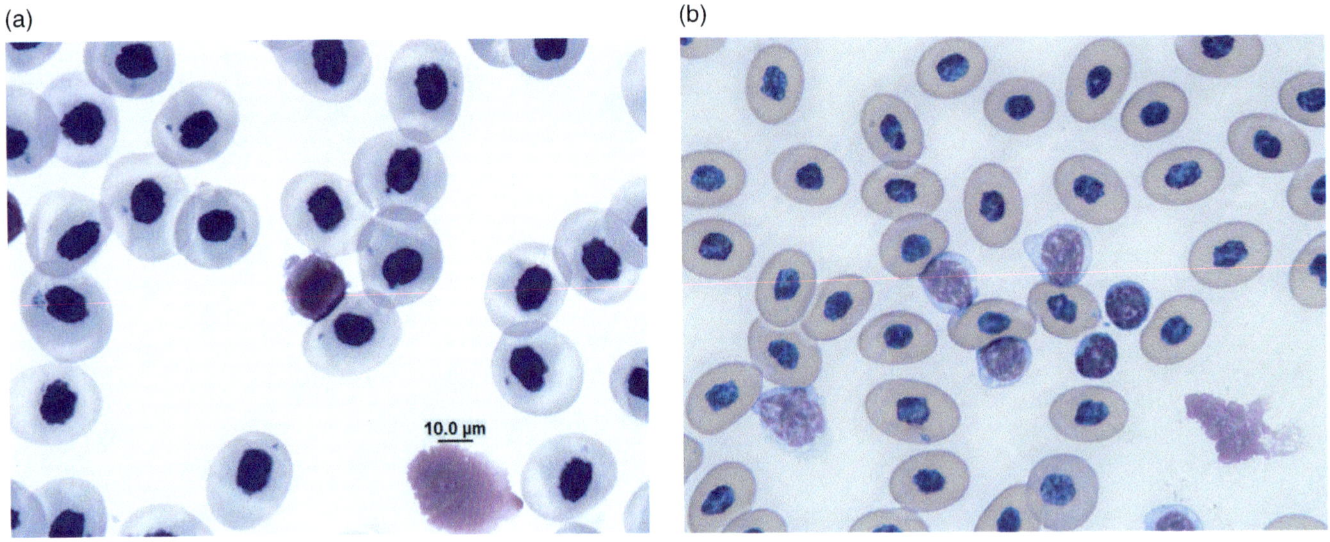

Fig. 20.6. (a) A lymphocyte in the blood film of a salamander (*Ambystoma tigrinum*), Wright–Giemsa stain. (b) Large and small lymphocytes in the blood film of a toad (*Incilius alvarius*), Wright–Giemsa stain, 100× oil.

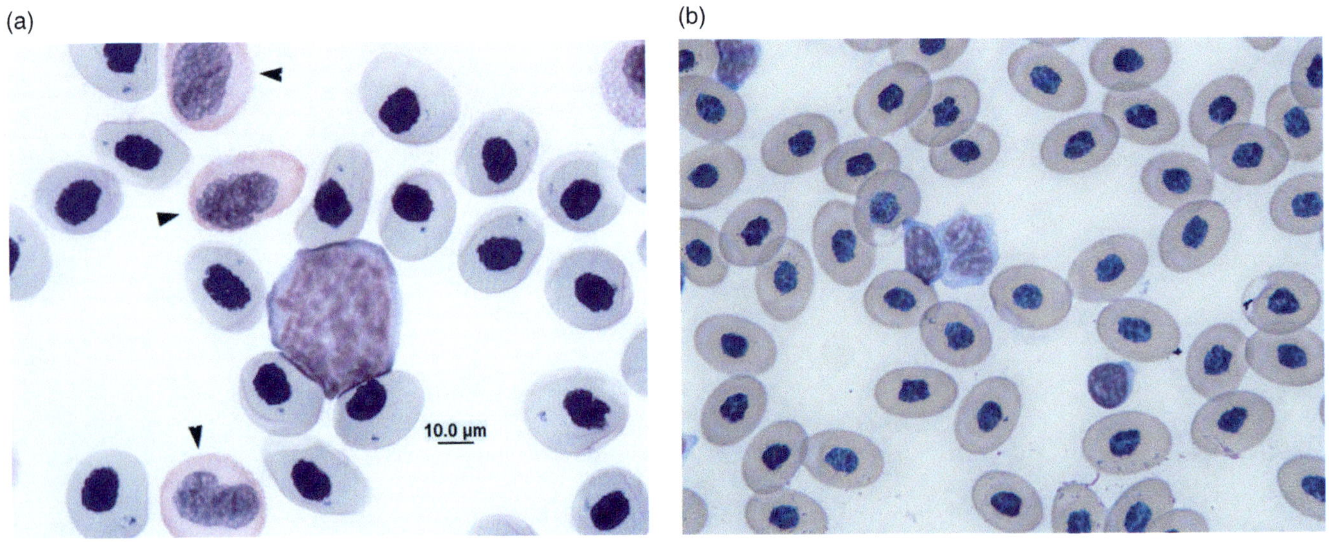

Fig. 20.7. (a) A monocyte with immature eosinophils (arrowheads) in the blood film of a salamander (*Ambystoma tigrinum*) with eosinophilic leukemia, Wright–Giemsa stain. (b) A monocyte (larger cell) adjacent to a lymphocyte in the center of the image from a blood film of a toad (*Incilius alvarius*), Wright–Giemsa stain, 100× oil.

Monocytes in amphibian blood films are similar in appearance to those of other vertebrates (Figures 20.7a and 20.7b). Monocytes are large in size and contain abundant blue-gray cytoplasm that may be foamy and vacuolated, or may contain fine azurophilic granules. The nucleus is variably shaped and demonstrates less chromatin clumping than is seen in the nuclei of lymphocytes (Cannon, 1979; Turner, 1988). Pseudopodia may be noted on some cells. Amphibian monocytes are peroxidase positive and do contain some of the same hydrolytic enzymes found in mammalian monocytes (Schermer, 1967; Turner, 1988).

Some amphibian leukocytes have been classified as azurophils. These cells have features commonly associated with monocytes and are considered to be monocytes by some authors (Montali, 1988). Other authors hypothesize that the amphibian azurophil is either an immature or senescent granulocyte or monocyte (Wright, 2001). There is little advantage in classifying these cells as separate cells from the monocyte population in the blood when interpreting the hemogram of amphibians. Therefore, they should be classified as monocytes until further evidence justifies classifying them as a different cell type.

Cytochemical characteristics have been applied to amphibian blood cells in an effort to characterize them as an aid for interpretation of cellular responses as performed in mammalian species, such as canines. Frog leukocytes have been described using a number of Romanowsky-type stains and cytochemical stains, including peroxidase, acid phosphatase, alkaline phosphatase, nonspecific esterase, basic protein, periodic acid-Schiff (PAS), Alcian blue, and toluidine blue, and by evaluating serotonin fluorescence (Turner, 1988; Wojtaszek and Adamowicz, 2003; Gutierre et al., 2008). For example, in the bullfrog (*Rana* (Aquarana) *catesbeiana*) and clawed frog (*Xenopus laevis*), neutrophils, eosinophils, and monocytes were positive for some or all of the following: α-naphthyl butyrate esterase (NBE), chloroacetate esterase (CAE), myeloperoxidase (PER), and Sudan black B (SBB) (Bricker et al., 2012). Lymphocytes were occasionally positive for CAE. Lymphocytes in these species were negative for all cytochemical stains, and leukocyte alkaline phosphatase (LAP) was not a useful marker for any leukocyte type. Peripheral blood lymphocytes in these frogs were strongly immunoreactive for CD3ε, CD79a, and BLA.36 (Bricker et al., 2012). Also, basophils from the African clawed frog had different enzymatic activity than basophils of the bullfrog, which may suggest different functions for the basophils of these two species (Bricker et al., 2012). Some cytochemical reactions, including PER and SBB in neutrophils, CAE in monocytes, and PER in eosinophils, were consistent across the species, suggesting they may be helpful in characterizing leukocytes from a variety of frog species. Some leukocytes were only noted occasionally in frogs, including azurophils, large granular lymphocytes, and, in the case of clawed frogs, eosinophils.

Little is known about the function of amphibian leukocytes; therefore, interpretation of the amphibian leukogram is typically based on the leukocytic responses to disease described for other vertebrates. For example, increases in neutrophil and monocyte counts are likely to suggest an inflammatory response because amphibian neutrophils and monocytes have migratory and phagocytic activity, participate in inflammation, and contain many of the same enzymes that occur in the neutrophils, heterophils, and monocytes of other vertebrates. More studies that evaluate the types of blood cells that increase or decrease during different disease states are needed to better determine the function of each cell type and its clinical importance.

The presence of a peripheral eosinophilia may be suggestive of parasitic infections. Amphibian eosinophils appear to have an inferior ability to phagocytize particles or microorganisms compared to neutrophils, but do respond to metazoan parasitic infections (Mitchell, 1982). Increased frequency of eosinophils has also been documented in frogs from polluted areas (Barni et al., 2007).

Amphibian basophils may function in a manner similar to those of mammals. They are rarely found in the peripheral blood of some amphibian species, such as the Colorado River toad (*Bufo alvarius*), but are abundant in others. For example, they occur in high numbers in the African clawed frog (*Xenopus laevis*), an aquatic species, compared to the bullfrog (*Rana* (Aquarana)), a semi-aquatic species, which may be reflective of their environment, as has been suggested for aquatic reptiles, such as aquatic turtles that are noted for their high numbers of circulating basophils (Wiechmann and Wirsiq-Wiechmann, 2003). Another example of this is in the Japanese newt (*C. pyrrhogaster*), which normally has a differential leukocyte count that includes up to 60% basophils (Pfeiffer et al., 1990). Basophils of this species are considered to play a significant role in immunosurveillance.

The lymphocytes of frogs and toads demonstrate immunologic sophistication similar to those of higher vertebrates (Turner, 1988). These lymphocytes can be classified as B-cells that produce immunoglobulins or T-cells with populations of functional diversity, such as helpers and different effectors. By contrast, the lymphocytes of newts and salamanders appear to lack such refinement (Turner, 1988). A lymphocytosis is suggestive of an excitement response, stimulation of the immune system, or possibly lymphoid leukemia. A transitory lymphocytosis following tail amputation for blood collection has been demonstrated in the Japanese newt (*C. pyrrhogaster*), suggesting either an excitement response or recruitment of lymphocytes (Pfeiffer et al., 1990).

Amphibian Thrombocytes

Amphibian thrombocytes are nucleated cells that resemble those described for birds, reptiles, and fish, although anucleated thrombocytes that resemble mammalian platelets have been described in certain species. Amphibian thrombocytes typically vary in shape from oval to spindle shaped (Figure 20.8). When the cells are in a nonreactive state, they tend to be oval in shape. Once activated, the cells become spindle shaped. The cytoplasm of the thrombocyte is abundant and colorless, and the nucleus is dense and round to oval; however, when they become reactive the cytoplasm may contain numerous eosinophilic granules (Figures 20.8 and 20.9). Amphibian thrombocytes are often confused with small, mature lymphocytes, but may be differentiated based on the appearance of the cytoplasm. The cytoplasmic volume of small lymphocytes tends to be small, and the cytoplasm stains blue. Ultrastructurally, the thrombocytes of some amphibian species, such as *Xenops* and *Rana*, are alkaline phosphatase positive, whereas the lymphocytes are negative (Turner, 1988).

Thrombocytes are functionally equivalent to mammalian platelets and participate in coagulation. Thrombocyte counts are typically interpreted in the

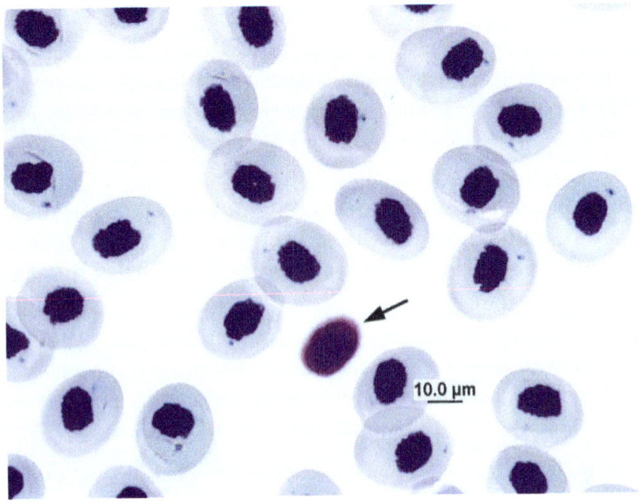

Fig. 20.8. A reactive thrombocyte with eosinophilic cytoplasmic granulation in the blood film of a salamander (*Ambystoma tigrinum*), Wright–Giemsa stain.

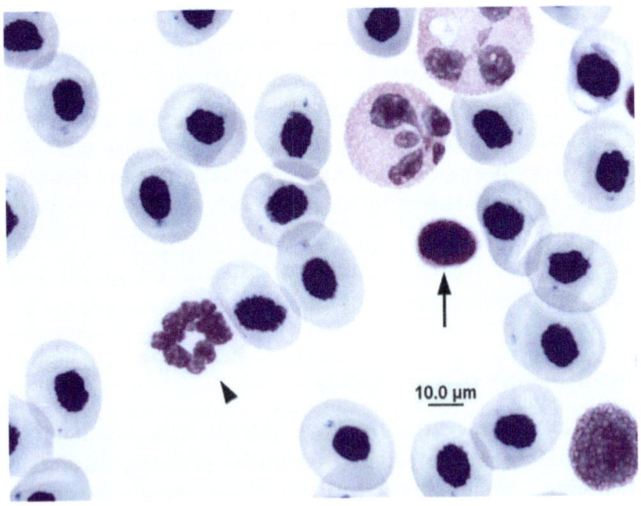

Fig. 20.9. A reactive thrombocyte (arrow) compared with erythrocytes, eosinophils, and a neutrophil (arrowhead) in the blood film of a salamander (*Ambystoma tigrinum*), Wright–Giemsa stain.

same manner as described for other nonmammalian vertebrates; an estimate of their number (reduced or adequate) is obtained, and the morphology is evaluated. Immature thrombocytes appear as round cells with round nuclei and are not normally found in the peripheral blood of amphibians. The presence of immature thrombocytes suggests either a regenerative response or dyscrasia.

Developing thrombocytes include thromboblasts, prothrombocytes, and immature thrombocytes. Thromboblasts are round to oval in shape, have weakly basophilic cytoplasm, and a round to oval nucleus that contains fine nuclear chromatin and a large irregular eccentric nucleolus. Prothrombocytes have elongated nuclei and vacuolated cytoplasm with pale blue granules (Turner, 1988). Immature thrombocytes resemble those described in avian hematology. They are intermediate in size between thromboblasts and the mature thrombocyte, and appear as round to oval cells containing more abundant cytoplasm than the thromboblasts. The color of the cytoplasm of immature thrombocytes varies with cell development and changes from a basophilic color in the early developing cells to a pale blue or colorless cytoplasm in the later stages. These cells may contain cytoplasmic vacuoles. The nuclear chromatin of the earlier immature thrombocytes is aggregated into irregular clumps that become more densely packed as the cell matures.

Amphibian Blood Parasites

Wet-mount evaluation of a whole blood sample may be utilized as a means to detect the movement of common extracellular blood parasites such as trypanosomes and microfilaria in amphibian blood (Woo, 1983; Wright, 2001). Common amphibian intraerythrocytic blood parasites include the hemogregarines (*Hepatozoon* spp.) and *Aegyptianella* spp. (Barta and Desser, 1984; Desser, 1987; Desser and Barta, 1989; Forzán et al., 2017). These organisms are considered to be an incidental finding. However, they may be pathogenic when they occur with anemia, suggesting a possible etiology for the anemia (Schmittner and McGhee, 1961; Graczyk et al., 1996).

Amphibian Hematopoiesis and Bone Marrow Evaluation

Amphibian Erythropoiesis

Development of the amphibian erythrocyte is essentially similar to that described for other vertebrates with nucleated erythrocytes. Erythropoiesis begins with rubriblasts, which go on to develop into mature erythrocytes, except in some amphibian species where the final stages of maturation may occur in the peripheral blood. Maturation of the rubriblast to the mature erythrocyte involves a progressive change of the cell from round to elongated in shape. The cytoplasm changes from basophilic to eosinophilic in color, and the nucleus decreases in size. The nuclear chromatin increases in density, and the size of the nucleolus decreases as well.

The primary site for erythropoiesis in most larval amphibians is the kidney, with some erythropoiesis occurring in the liver as well (Turner, 1988). Larval amphibians often have two populations of morphologically different erythrocytes that have arisen from these two different origins (Coates, 1975). Erythrocytes that originate in the kidney have a peripherally located nucleus. By comparison, the red blood cells that are derived from the liver contain a centrally positioned nucleus. These two different erythrocyte populations also contain different larval hemoglobins.

During metamorphosis, a third population of erythrocytes appears that will persist in the adult amphibian. Dark field illumination may be used to differentiate larval erythrocytes from adult erythrocytes. Larval erythrocytes have a white to gray granular luminescence compared to the adult erythrocytes, which lack luminescence.

Metamorphosis from larval to adult amphibians is also accompanied by the synthesis of hemoglobins with different oxygen affinities and various intracellular modulators of hemoglobin–oxygen affinity (Coates, 1975). For example, gilled larval amphibians have blood that has a higher affinity for oxygen than that of air-breathing adults. The tetramer hemoglobin of amphibians consists of two α-like and two β-like globin chains, creating four larval and four adult-type hemoglobins (Coates, 1975). No globin chains are shared between larval and adult amphibians.

The primary site of erythropoiesis in most adult amphibians is the spleen, with the kidney, liver, and bone marrow playing minor roles. Some species variability does exist; for example, the liver is the primary erythropoietic organ of certain frogs (Turner, 1988). In general, adult amphibians have higher hemoglobin concentrations and PCVs compared to larval forms. Metamorphosis also results in a decrease in adenosine triphosphate (ATP) and guanosine triphosphate (GTP) concentration in the erythrocytes, suggesting a change in the phosphate regulation of hemoglobin in adult amphibians compared to their larval counterparts.

Adult hemoglobin begins to appear in frogs and toads during tail regression as part of their metamorphism from the larval stage, and is the only hemoglobin found 3 weeks post metamorphosis. Metamorphosis in newts and salamanders, unlike in toads and frogs, is not always associated with a transition in hemoglobin. When the respiratory systems of newts and salamanders change from aquatic respiration to air breathing at metamorphosis, the larval and adult hemoglobins have the same affinity for oxygen; however, the reduced oxygen affinity of the blood in the adult is frequently achieved by an increase in the erythrocyte concentration of ATP (Coates, 1975). In some salamander and newt species, such as the tiger salamander (*Ambystoma tigrinum*), there is no decrease in the oxygen affinity of blood at metamorphosis, and the hemoglobin and total erythrocytic organic phosphate concentrations remain unchanged. Frogs and toads appear to differ in regard to their blood oxygen affinity. Frogs rely primarily on anaerobic respiration for energy production. Toads rely primarily on aerobic respiration and tend to have higher hemoglobin and erythrocyte phosphate concentrations and lower blood oxygen affinity compared to frogs.

Aquatic amphibians do not have the same association between high erythrocyte phosphate concentrations and dependence on aerobic production of energy for activity as terrestrial amphibians. This may be due in part to the fact that gaseous exchange occurs from the surrounding water to the blood through the skin of aquatic amphibians.

Amphibian Granulopoiesis

Granulopoiesis occurs in the liver, kidney, and bone marrow of most amphibians. Some species lack bone marrow; therefore, the liver and kidney are the major tissues for granulopoiesis (Curtis et al., 1979). Granulopoiesis in amphibians appears to be similar to that of other vertebrates, such as mammals, birds, and reptiles.

Myeloblasts and progranulocytes have not been positively described in amphibians; however, they are likely to occur as they do in other vertebrates. The immature neutrophil found in hematopoietic tissue and/or the peripheral blood has small granules of various shapes that increase in size and density with maturation until the larger definitive peroxidase-positive granules are formed.

Evidence is suggestive that the eosinophils of some amphibian species begin as round cells containing a round nucleus and scant cytoplasm with large, dense, round, primary granules (Turner, 1988). These cells resemble the eosinophil progranulocyte of other vertebrates. Further development of the eosinophil results in a mixture of the larger primary granules and smaller secondary granules. These cells would be comparable to the myelocytes of other vertebrate species.

The monocyte is the first leukocyte to appear in the peripheral blood of the bullfrog (*Rana catesbeiana*) larvae. Immature monocytes containing linear nuclear chromatin appear 15 days post hatch, and mature monocytes with round nuclei that go on to develop into kidney-shaped or lobed nuclei appear at 22 days post hatch. Definitive neutrophils, eosinophils, and basophils all appear at the same time in the peripheral blood during late development of larval bullfrogs (*R. catesbeiana*) (Surbis, 1978; Turner, 1988).

Lymphopoiesis in amphibians resembles that of other vertebrates. The spleen is the major lymphoid organ of amphibians, where small lymphocytes are the most common form seen on cytologic samples, but larger lymphocytes may also be seen.

References

Allender MC, Fry MM. 2008. Amphibian hematology. *Vet Clin North Am Exot Anim Pract* 11:463–480.

Anvier MR, Pond CL. 1984. Biology and diseases of amphibians. In: Fox J, Cohen B, Lowe F (eds), *Laboratory Animal Medicine*. Orlando, FL: Academic Press.

Barni SS, Boncompagni EE, Grosso AA, et al. 2007. Evaluation of *Rana* snk *esculenta* blood cell response to chemical stressors in the environment during the larval and adult phases. *Aquat Toxicol* 81:45–54.

Barta JR, Desser SS. 1984. Blood parasites of amphibians from Algonquin Park, Ontario. *J Wildl Dis* 180–189.

Boutilier RG, Stiffler DF, Toews DP. 1992. Exchange of respiratory gases, ions, and water in amphibious and aquatic amphibians. In: Feder M, Burggren W (eds), *Environmental Physiology of Amphibians*. Chicago, IL: University of Chicago Press.

Bricker NK, Raskin RE, Densmore CL. 2012. Cytochemical and immunocytochemical characterization of blood cells and immunohistochemical analysis of spleen cells from 2 species of frog, *Rana* (Aquarana) *catesbeiana* and *Xenopus laevis*. *Vet Clin Pathol* 41(3):353–361.

Cannon AM. 1979. The blood leukocytes of *Bufo alvarius*: a light, phase-contrast, and histochemical study. *Can J Zool* 57:314–322.

Cathers T, Lewbart GA, Correa M, Stevens JB. 1997. Serum chemistry and hematology values for anesthetized American bull frogs (*Rana catesbeiana*). *J Zoo Wildl Med* 28(2):171–174.

Cohen WD. 1982. The cytomorphic system of anucleate nonmammalian erythrocytes. *Protoplasma* 113:23–32.

Coates ML. 1975. Hemoglobin function in the vertebrates: an evolutionary model. *J Mol Evol* 6:285–307.

Curtis SK, Cowden RR, Nagel JW. 1979. Ultrastructure of the bone marrow of the salamander *Plethodon glutinosus* (Caudata: Plethodontidae). *J Morphol* 159:151–184.

Desser SS. 1987. *Aegyptianella ranarum* sp. n. (Rickettsiales, Anaplasmataceae): ultrastructure and prevalence in frogs from Ontario. *J Wildl Dis* 23:52–59.

Desser SS, Barta JR. 1989. The morphological features of *Aegyptianella bacterifera*: an intraerythrocytic rickettsia of frogs from Corsica. *J Wildl Dis* 25:313–318.

Forzán MJ, Heatley J, Russell KE, Horney B. 2017. Clinical pathology of amphibians: a review. *Vet Clin Pathol* 46(1):11–33.

Graczyk TK, Cranfield EJ, Bicknese EJ, Wisnieski AP. 1996. Progressive ulcerative dermatitis in a captive wild-caught South American giant treefrog (*Phyllomedusa bicolor*) with microsporidial septicemia. *J Zoo Wildl Med* 27:522–527.

Green DE. 2001. Pathology of amphibia. In: Wright K, Whitaker B (eds), *Amphibian Medicine and Captive Husbandry*. Malabar, FL: Krieger Publishing.

Gregory TR. 2001. The bigger the c-value, the larger the cell: genome size and red blood cell size in vertebrates. *Blood Cells Mol Dis* 27(5):830–843.

Gruia-Gray J, Desser SS. 1992. Cytopathological observations and epizootiology of frog erythrocytic virus in bullfrogs (*Rana catesbeiana*). *J Wildl Dis* 28:34–41.

Gutierre RC, Egami MI, Antoniazzi MM, et al. 2008. Cytochemistry and morphology of granulocytes of the caecilian *Siphonops annulatus* (Amphibia, Gymnophiona). *Comp Clin Pathol* 17:221–228.

Harris JA. 1972. Seasonal variation in some hematological characteristics of *Rana pipiens*. *Comp Biochem Physiol* 43A:975–989.

Hawkey CM, Dennett TB. 1989. *A Colour Atlas of Comparative Veterinary Haematology*. London: Wolfe Medical Publications, Ltd.

Jerret DP, Mays CE. 1973. Comparative hematology of the hellbender, *Cryptobranchus alleganiensis* in Missouri. *Copeia* 2:331–337.

Mitchell JB. 1982. The effect of host age on *Rana temporaria* and *Gorgoderina vitelliloba* interactions. *J Parasitol* 12:601–604.

Mitruka BM, Rawnsley HM. 1981. Clinical biochemical and hematological reference values in normal experimental animals. In: Mitruka BM, Rawnsley HM (eds), *Clinical Biochemical and Hematological Reference Values in Normal Experimental Animals*, 2nd edn. New York: Masson Publishing USA, Inc.

Montali RJ. 1988. Comparative pathology of inflammation in the higher vertebrates (reptiles, birds, and mammals). *J Comp Pathol* 99:1–26.

Ostojic H, Monge C, Cifuentes V. 2000. Hemoglobin affinity for oxygen in three subspecies of toads (*Bufo sp.*) living at different altitudes. *Biol Res* 33(1):1–9.

Pessier AP. 2018. Amphibia. In: Terio KA, McAloose D, St. Leger J (eds), *Pathology of Wildlife and Zoo Animals*. London, UK: Academic Press.

Pfeiffer CJ, Pyle H, Asashima M. 1990. Blood cell morphology and counts in the Japanese newt (*Cynops pyrrhogaster*). *J Zoo Wildl Med* 21(1):56–64.

Sanyal M, Patil P, Jaiswal E, et al. 2013. Structural and functional diversity of haemoglobin molecule properties amongst different classes and species of animals. *Acta Biologica Indica* 2(2):381–387.

Schermer S. 1967. The frog. In: Schermer S (ed), *Blood Morphology of Laboratory Animals*, 3rd edn. Philadelphia, PA: Davis Co.

Singh K. 1978. Hematology of the common Indian frog *Rana tigrina*. III. Hemoglobin and hematocrit. *Anat Anz* 143(2):161–166.

Sinha RC. 1983. Haematological studies on the prewintering and wintering frog, *Rana esclenta*. *Comp Biochem Physiol A*. 74(2):311–314.

Schmittner SM, McGhee RB. 1961. The intra-erythrocytic development of *Babesioma stableri* n. sp. in *Rana pipiens pipiens*. *J Protozool* 8:381–386.

Storz JF, Hoffmann FG, Opazo JC, et al. 2011. Developmental regulation of hemoglobin synthesis in the green anole lizard *Anolis carolinensis*. *J Exp Biol* 214:575–581.

Surbis AY. 1978. Ultrastructural study of granulocytes of *Bufo marinus*. *Fla Sci* 41:42–45.

Turner RJ. 1988. Amphibians. In: Rowley A, Ratcliffe N (eds), *Vertebrate Blood Cells*. Cambridge: Cambridge University Press, pp. 129–209.

Wang X, Herman C. 1996. Changes in blood cell numbers and formation of eicosanoids during clotting in warm- and cold-acclimated bullfrogs (*Rana catesbeiana*). *Gen Comp Endocrinol* 101(2):211–219.

Wiechmann AF, Wirsiq-Wiechmann CR. 2003. Lymphatic organs. In: Wiechmann AF, Wirsiq-Wiechmann CR (eds), *Color Atlas of Xenopus Laevis Histology*. Norwell, MA: Kluwer Academic Publishers, pp. 29–30.

Wojtaszek J, Adamowicz A. 2003. Haematology of the firebellied toad, *Bombina bombina* L. *Comp Clin Pathol* 12:129–134.

Woo PTK. 1983. Sensitivity of diagnostic techniques in determining the prevalence of anuran trypanosomes. *J Wildl Dis* 19:24–26.

Wright KM. 2001. Amphibian hematology. In: Wright K, Whitaker B (eds), *Amphibian Medicine and Captive Husbandry*. Malabar, FL: Krieger Publishing Co.

Young S, Warner J, Speare R, et al. 2012. Hematologic and plasma biochemical reference intervals for health monitoring of wild Australian tree frogs. *Vet Clin Pathol* 41(4):478–492.

21 Herptile Hematology and Clinical Chemistry: Clinical Case Presentations

Case 1: Snake with Nasal Discharge and Mites

Signalment

Adult female red-tailed boa (*Boa constrictor*)

History

The snake was acquired as an adult from another facility by a public aquarium approximately four months prior to presentation. Shortly after arrival, a physical examination revealed a serous nasal discharge (Figure 21.1) and mites. There were no other diagnostics performed, and the snake was treated with ceftazidime and ivermectin systemically, and pyrethroid solution was used to treat the environment. On follow-up visits to the aquarium, the snake exhibited no clinical signs or mites two months later. However, two months following the last examination, the snake presented with the complaint of regurgitating a partially digested rat.

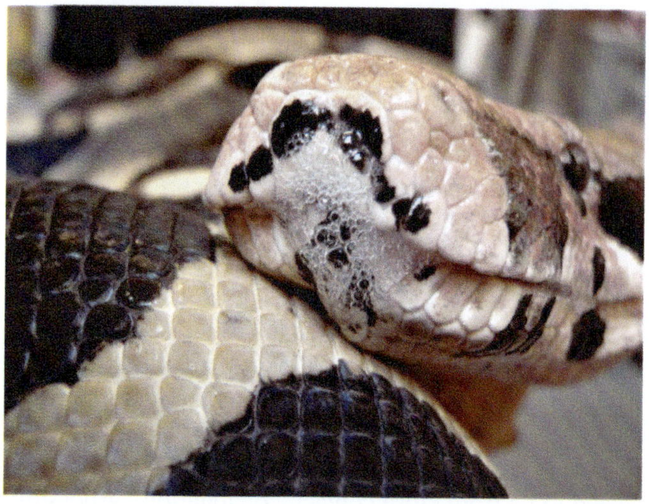

Fig. 21.1. Boa constrictor with serous nasal discharge.

Physical Examination

The physical examination revealed a 6.5-kg snake in good body condition, and there were no significant findings. A probe to determine its gender revealed that the snake was female. Regurgitation of one meal may be an isolated incident, but could also result from a snake feeling threatened, over-handling shortly after feeding, gastritis, or gastrointestinal parasites. Also, because this snake was in the family Boidae, the possibility of inclusion body disease (IBD) was considered. A blood sample was obtained by cardiocentesis to further evaluate health status. A fresh blood film (Figures 21.2a and 21.2b) was prepared, and samples were submitted for complete blood count (CBC) and plasma biochemistry profiles (Table 21.1).

Interpretive Discussion

The hemogram revealed a monocytosis and potential anemia (non-regenerative). Figure 21.2a revealed round pale blue inclusions within the cytoplasm of a few erythrocytes. It was noted on the hematology report that approximately 3% of the RBCs contained large, uniform, pale blue inclusions. Inclusions as seen here were suggestive of IBD of boid snakes. It is rare for inclusions to appear in the blood of affected snakes with this disease. Usually, the inclusions are found on histology from

Exotic Animal Hematology and Cytology, Fifth Edition. Terry W. Campbell and Krystan R. Grant.

Companion website: www.wiley.com/go/campbell/exotic

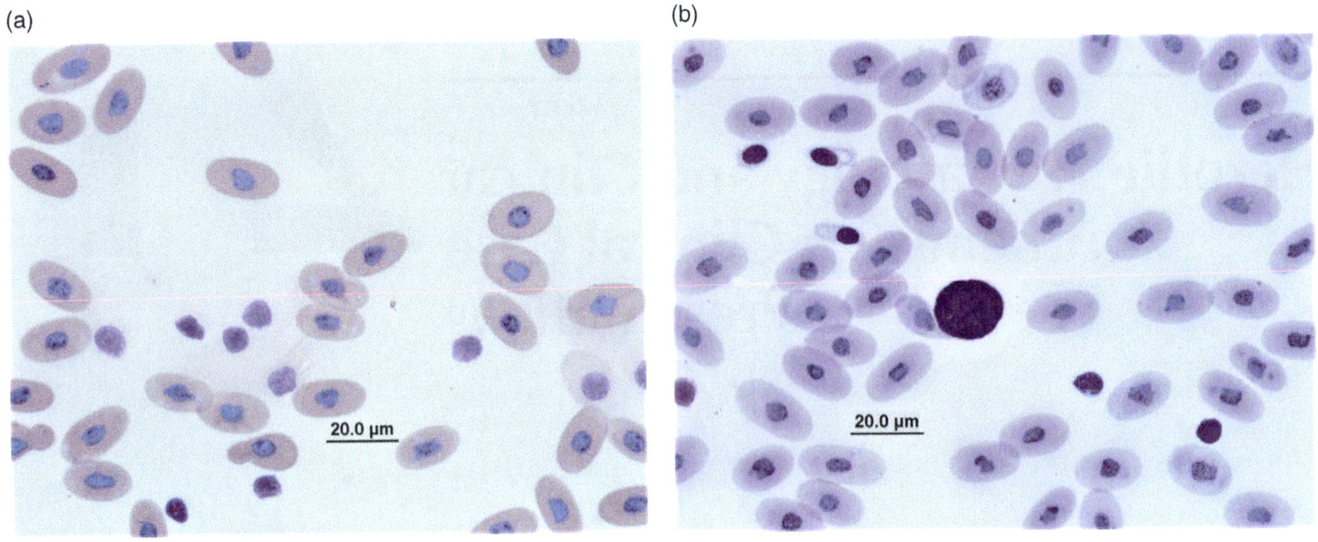

Fig. 21.2. (a), (b) Blood films (Wright–Giemsa stain, 100× oil).

Table 21.1. Boa hematology results (Case 1).

		Reference[a]
PCV(%)	15.0	29 (12–40)
Leukocytes		
WBC (×10³/µL)	14.5	7.37 (1.47–19.6)
Heterophils (×10³/µL)	1.3	1.93 (0.20–6.50)
S (%)	9	—
Lymphocytes (×10³/µL)	9.3	2.89 (0.34–11.9)
(%)	64	—
Monocytes (×10³/µL)	3.8	0.27 (0.03–2.38)
(%)	26	—
Eosinophils (×10³/µL)	0	0.13 (0–0.60)
(%)	0	—
Basophils (×10³/µL)	0.2	0.21 (0.03–1.01)
(%)	1	—
Thrombocytes		
Adequate thrombocytes	—	
Plasma protein (refractometry)		
(g/dL)	6.4	—
Notes		

[a]Carpenter (2018).

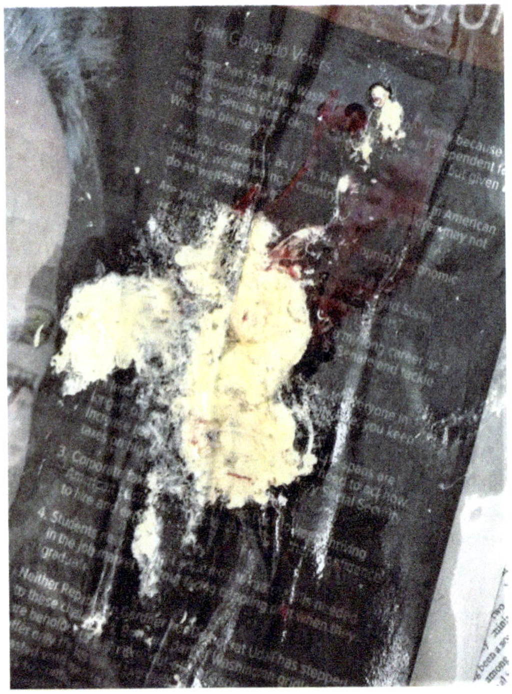

Fig. 21.3. Hematuria.

tissues obtained at necropsy or from biopsy samples. Also, on the blood film, it appeared that the thrombocytes also had inclusions, which was unusual (Figure 21.2b).

The plasma biochemistry profile (not shown) at the time revealed hypercalcemia (Ca 16 mg/dL) and possible hypoproteinemia (total protein 5.4 g/dL).

Summary

For confirmation of inclusion body disease, a blood sample was sent to an outside laboratory for immunohistochemical staining that confirmed IBD (Chang et al., 2013, Chang et al., 2016). IBD in boids and pythons is an immunosuppressive disease caused by an arenavirus (reptarenavirus). Transmission between snakes is suspected to be from close contact, cohabitation, or possibly from mites (Marschang, 2019). The snake was isolated from other snakes at the aquarium and was monitored over the next two years. Approximately 18 months later, the handler reported additional regurgitation episodes and, 23 months later, regurgitation and hematuria (Figure 21.3) were noted. Subsequent blood samples were collected, and blood films were evaluated for changes (Figures 21.4, 21.5a, 21.5b, 21.6a–21.6d). The snake was euthanized after two years, at which time she exhibited frequent regurgitation episodes and neurologic signs (ataxia, unable to right herself). The gross necropsy showed that she measured two meters in length and was in good body condition. Histopathology revealed disseminated cytoplasmic eosinophilic inclusion bodies and severe subacute necrotizing and ulcerative colitis with intralesional bacteria. The morphology and distribution throughout the body of eosinophilic cytoplasmic inclusion bodies was consistent with IBD of boids.

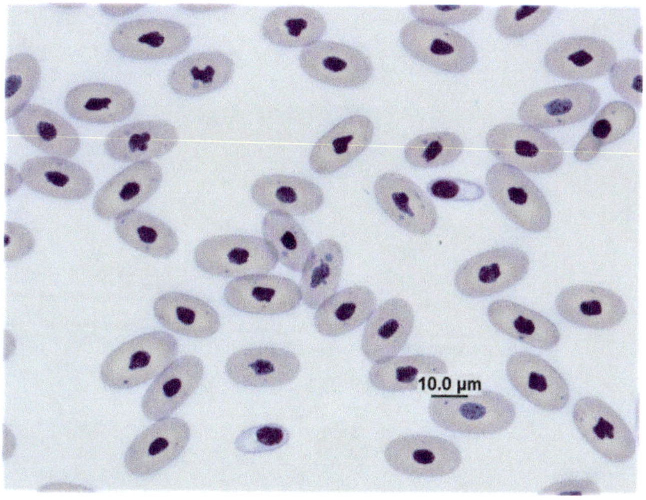

Fig. 21.4. Blood films after 18 months showing thrombocyte inclusions (Diff–Quik stain, 100× oil).

Case 2: Snake with Neurologic Behavior and Skin Nodules

Signalment

18-year-old intact male California kingsnake (*Lampropeltis getula californiae*)

History

The kingsnake was housed at a public aquarium and used as a program animal for educational purposes. Ten months prior to this presentation, the snake exhibited periodic episode of neurologic behavior that included being unable to right himself. On physical examination, the snake had two small, approximate 0.5 cm raised nodules on the left and right side of the caudal third of his body (Figure 21.7). A blood sample was collected during this examination. The sample was clotted, so only a plasma biochemical profile was performed, which revealed a hypercalcemia and hypercholesterolemia. Two months later (or 8 months prior to this case presentation), the snake was re-examined, and a blood profile at that time (shown in Tables 21.2 and 21.3, labeled "8 months prior") revealed similar findings of hypercholesterolemia, and leukocytosis and lymphocytosis. The snake was treated with an antibiotic (ceftazidime, 20 mg/kg IM q72h), and cryosurgery was performed to remove the nodules. The incision appeared to heal with a following shedding event. Five months later (or 3 months prior to case presentation), the snake was reevaluated due a recurrence of one of the masses and return of the neurologic behavior. A blood sample was collected, and the resulting CBC and plasma biochemistry profile are shown in Tables 21.2 and 21.3 (labeled "3 months prior").

(a) (b)

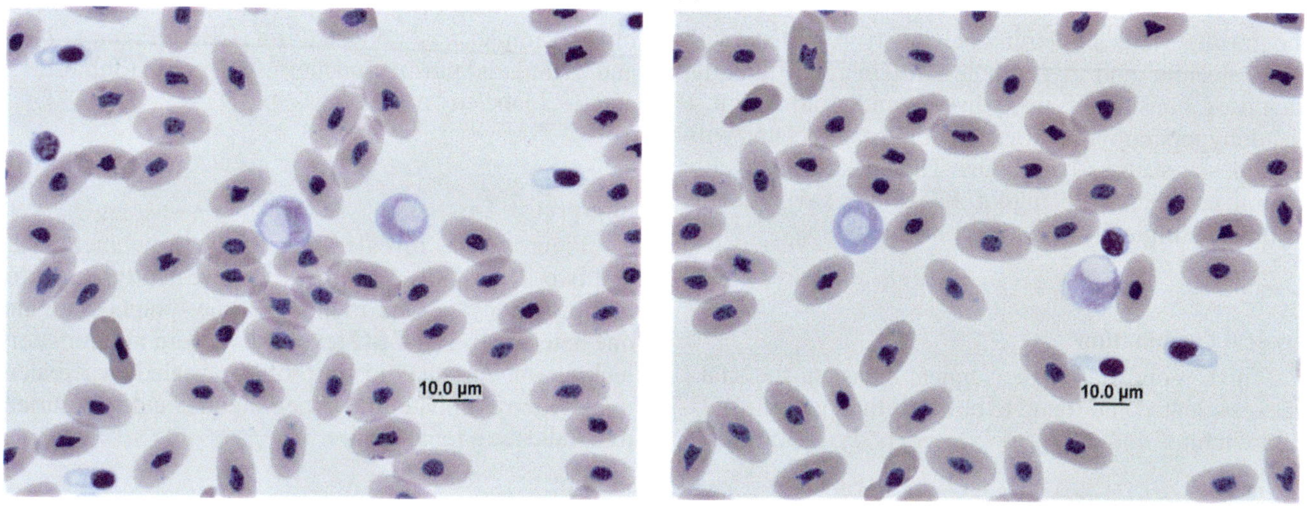

Fig. 21.5. (a), (b) Blood films after 18 months showing white blood cells with inclusions (Wright–Giemsa stain, 100× oil).

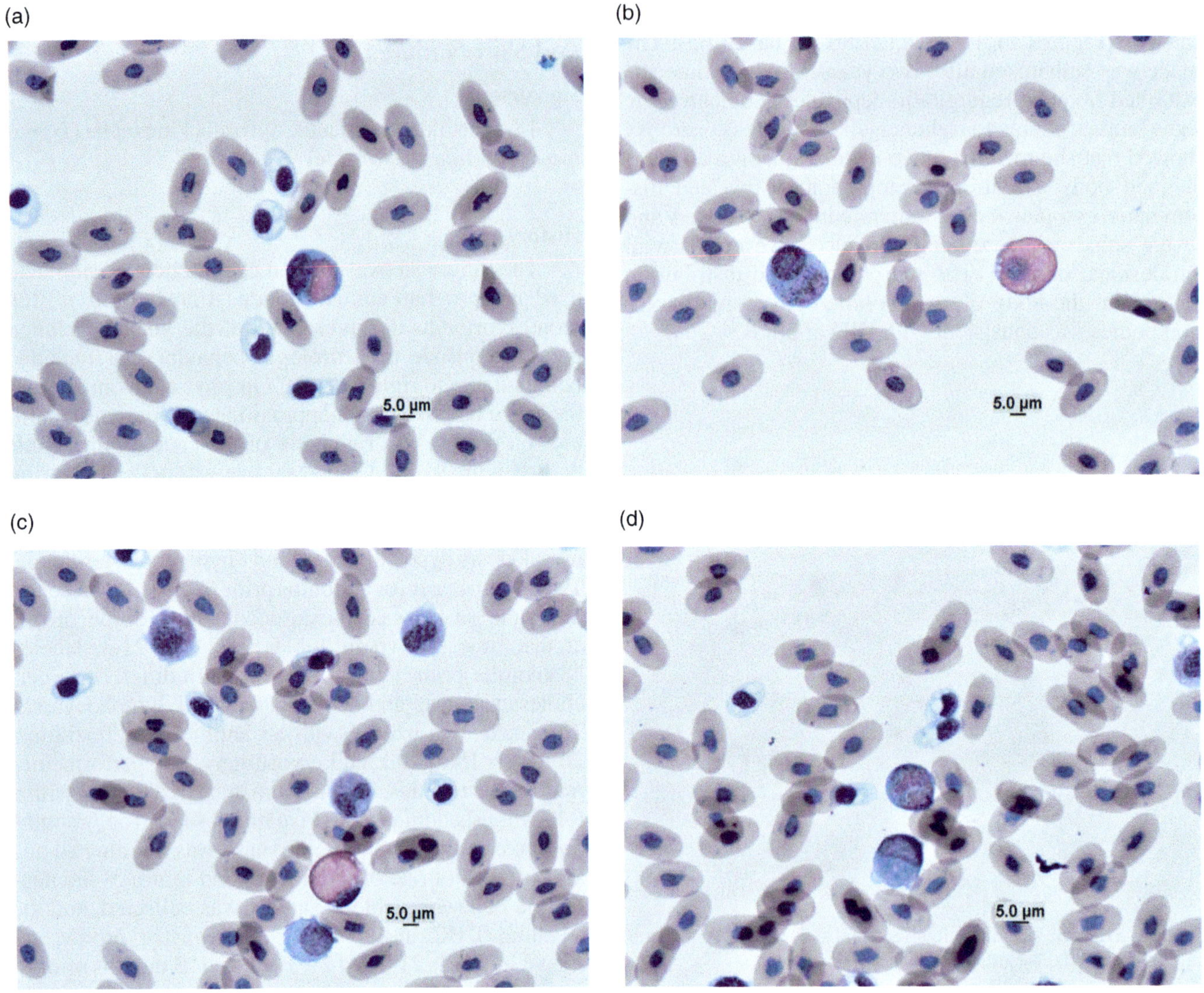

Fig. 21.6. a–d. Blood films after 23 months showing white blood cells with eosinophilic inclusions that likely represent leukophagocytosis of heterophils by monocytes (Wright–Giemsa stain, 100× oil).

The results were similar to previously reported, with hypercalcemia and hypercholesterolemia. Differential diagnoses considered were hyperparathyroidism or a pseudohypoparathyroidism that could be associated with a neoplasia, such as lymphoma. The snake was given a general anesthetic (25 mg/kg Alfaxalone IM), and the lesion was surgically excised for histopathology.

Physical Examination

Three months after the surgical excision, the snake was reevaluated and found to be exhibiting periodic muscle twitching and had a decreased body condition. A blood sample was collected for CBC (Figures 21.8a and 21.8b) and plasma biochemistry profile (Tables 21.2 and 21.3 labeled "present case").

Interpretive Discussion

Figure 21.8a revealed four azurophilic monocytes and two heterophils. Figure 21.8b revealed three azurophilic monocytes, one monocyte, one lymphocyte, and one heterophil. The CBC revealed a severe inflammatory leukogram. The diagnostic profile revealed hypercalcemia, hyperphosphatemia, hyperkalemia, and hyperuricemia indicating renal failure.

Summary

The histological diagnosis was an incompletely excised melanosarcoma. Due to a poor prognosis, the snake was euthanized and submitted for necropsy. Histopathology revealed a gastric neoplasm consistent with a gastric sarcoma with mesenteric and renal metastasis; pyogranulomatous and necrotizing hepatitis; and glomerular capillary fibrin thrombi and tubular necrosis (supporting the clinical diagnosis of renal failure). Liver sections with foci of granulomatous inflammation were stained with an acid-fast and Grocott-Gomori methenamine silver (GMS) stains, and no organisms were identified.

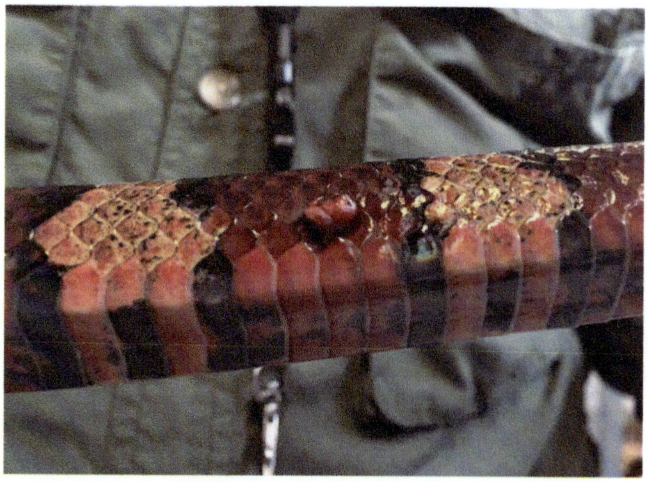

Fig. 21.7. California kingsnake with small, raised mass on body.

It is suspected that the recurrent dermal melanosarcoma metastasized to the viscera. The histological description of the mass was consistent with metastatic chromatophoromas described in the literature, which included infiltrative growth, spindle-shaped cells, anisokaryosis, 1–2 nucleoli, mitotic figures, and variable pigment (Heckers et al., 2012; Munoz-Gutierrez et al., 2016). Melanophoromas have also been shown to metastasize to the visceral organs with different morphological features (Heckers et al., 2012).

The rate of neoplasia in captive snakes at one zoo was 23% over a 10-year period (Ramsay et al., 1996). A study of chromatophoromas in snakes found that colubrid snakes were most represented at 55%, and of the cases of xanthophoromas, iridophoromas, melanocytic neoplasms, and mixed chromatophoromas submitted, melanocytic neoplasms were the most common (Munoz-Gutierrez et al., 2016). In this case, the indicators of a metastatic neoplasm included the negative righting reflex, monocytosis, hypercalcemia, and possibly the hyperuricemia (McNulty and Hoffman, 1995).

Table 21.2. Kingsnake hematology results (Case 2).

	8 months prior	3 months prior	Present case	Reference[a]
PCV (%)	30.0	34.0	19.0	31 (9–47)
Leukocytes				
WBC (×103/μL)	35.2	9.3	23.9	7.45 (1.55–27.7)
Heterophils (×103/μL)	1.1	1.6	1.4	1.01 (0.16–5.50)
(%)	3	17	6	—
Lymphocytes (×103/μL)	33.1	7.0	7.4	3.92 (0.35–20.9)
(%)	94	75	31	—
Monocytes (×103/μL)	1.1	0.7	14.6	1.98 (0.05–5.83)
(%)	3	7	61	—
Eosinophils (×103/μL)	0	0	0	0.08 (0.02–0.37)
(%)	0	0	0	—
Basophils (×103/μL)	0	0	0.5	0.27 (0.04–1.08)
(%)	0	1	2	—
Thrombocytes				
Adequate thrombocytes	Exist	—	Exist	
Plasma protein (refractometry)				
(g/dL)	7.0	9.0	7.2	
Notes				
			Present case: WBCC from smear higher. Many monocytes are erythrophagocytic, leukophagic, or contain phagocytized cellular debris	

[a]Gibbons et al. (2019, p. 336).

Table 21.3. Kingsnake plasma biochemical results (Case 2).

	8 months prior	3 months prior	Present	Reference[a]
Glucose (mg/dL)	26	42	10*	38 (8–92)
BUN (mg/dL)	1	2	6	2 (1–10)
Phosphorus (mg/dL)	2.0	7.5	9.9	3.8 (1.7–11.3)
Calcium (mg/dL)	15.6	35.6	17.7	14.9 (9.1–22.2)
Uric acid (mg/dL)	3.7	6.1	131.3	4.6 (1.4–16.0)
Total protein (biuret) (g/dL)	5.4	6.4	6.3	6.4 (3.8–10.3)
Albumin (g/dL)	1.6	1.5	1.3	1.8 (0.8–2.9)
Globulin (g/dL)	3.8	4.9	5.0	4.4 (2.1–7.2)
Cholesterol (mg/dL)	759	763	67	294 (75–513)
Creatine kinase (IU/L)	12	99	1072	406 (59–1909)
Aspartate aminotransferase (IU/L)	1	7	43	20 (4–107)
Sodium (mEq/L)	165	157	161	161 (140–180)
Potassium (mEq/L)	4.9	2.7	7.5	4.6 (2.3–9.2)
Chloride (mEq/L)	129	114	94.0	119 (97–141)

*Glucose falsely decreased due to one heparinized sample being shared between two departments.
[a]Gibbons et al. (2019, p. 336).

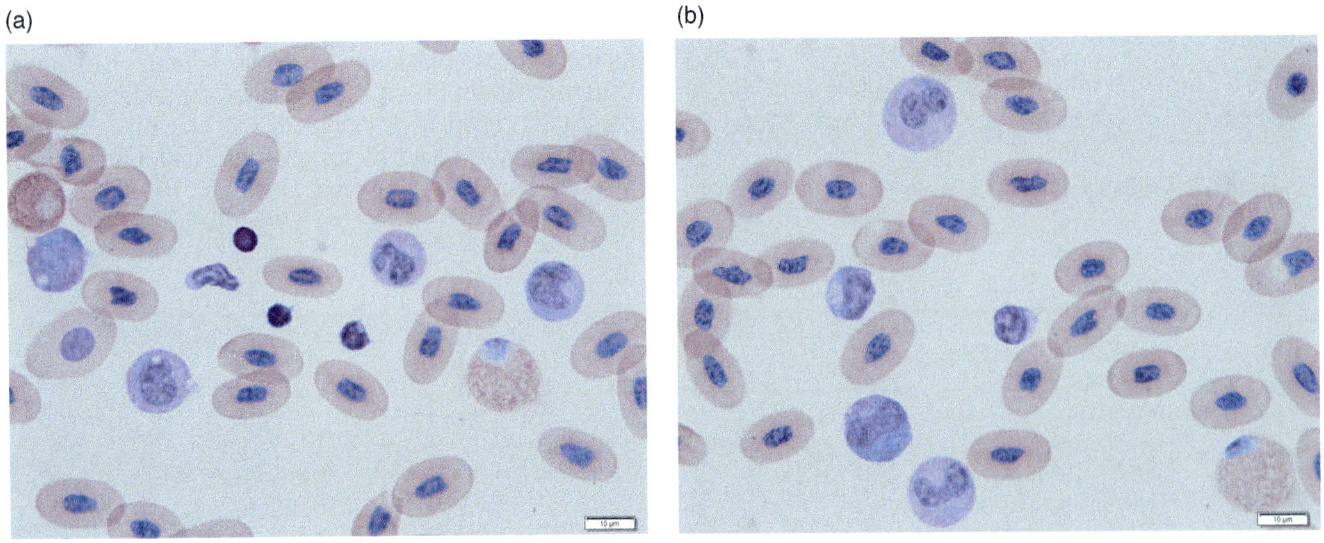

Fig. 21.8. (a), (b) Blood films (Wright–Giemsa stain, 100× oil).

Case 3: Comparison of two chelonian respiratory cases

	Tortoise	Turtle
Signalment	20-year-old intact male sulcata (African spurred) tortoise (*Centrochelys sulcata*)	5-year-old intact female red-eared slider (*Trachemys scripta elegans*)
History	The tortoise presented for urgent care with a two-day history of being "dumpy." The tortoise has access to both indoor and outdoor habitats and is fed a diet of fruit and vegetables. It was presented for lethargy and loud open mouth breathing.	A female red-eared slider from a cold freshwater exhibit in a public aquarium was placed in quarantine because she was less active and listing to the right side.
Physical Examination	Upon presentation, the 20.4 kg tortoise had marked pyramiding of the carapace (Figures 21.9 and 21.11). The tortoise was severely lethargic and offered no resistance when handled for blood collection. Diagnostics included a CBC (Table 21.4 and Figure 21.13), plasma biochemistry profile (Table 21.6), and whole-body radiographs (Figures 21.15–21.17)	Upon presentation, the approximate 2 kg turtle appeared normal. When observed in the aquatic exhibit, she listed to the right. There were no other abnormalities noted (Figures 21.10 and 21.12). Diagnostics included a CBC and plasma biochemistry profile (Tables 21.5 and 21.7) and whole-body radiographs (Figures 21.18 and 21.19).

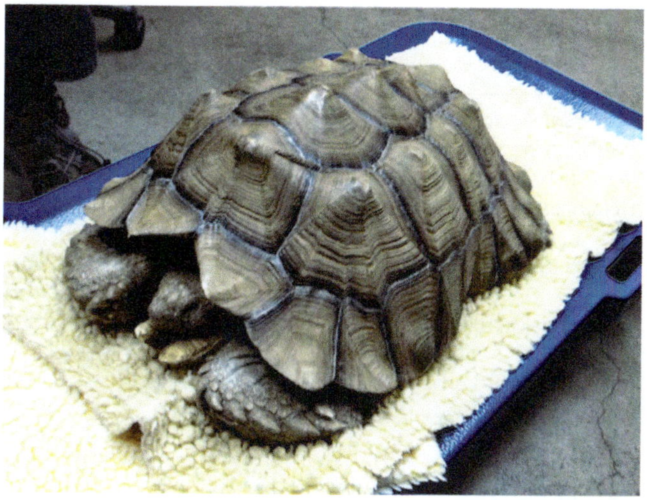

Fig. 21.9. Sulcata tortoise on presentation.

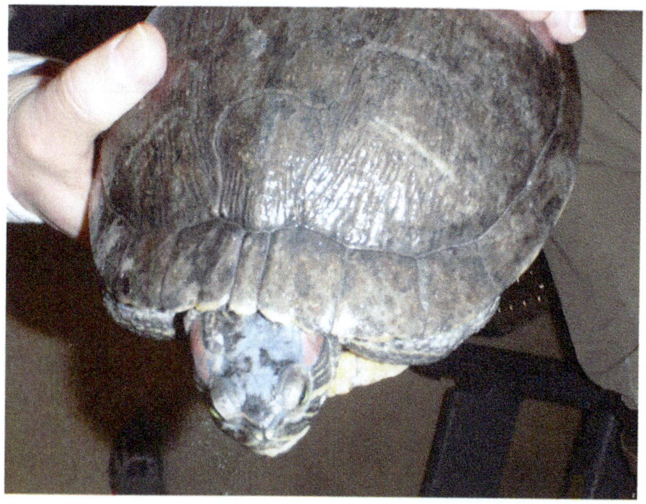

Fig. 21.10. Red-eared slider on presentation.

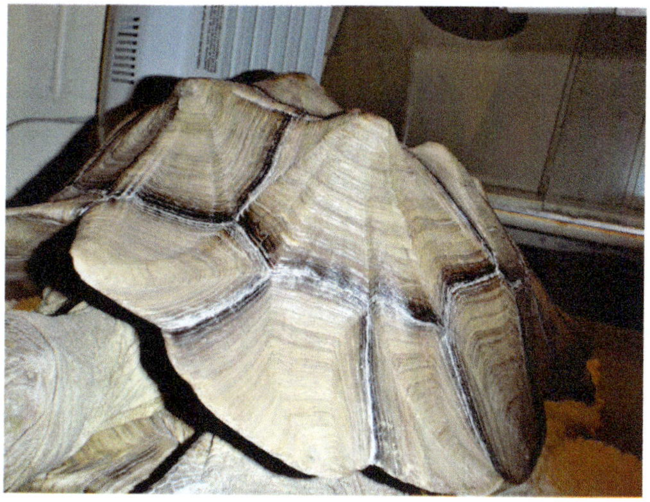

Fig. 21.11. Sulcata tortoise showing marked pyramiding on carapace.

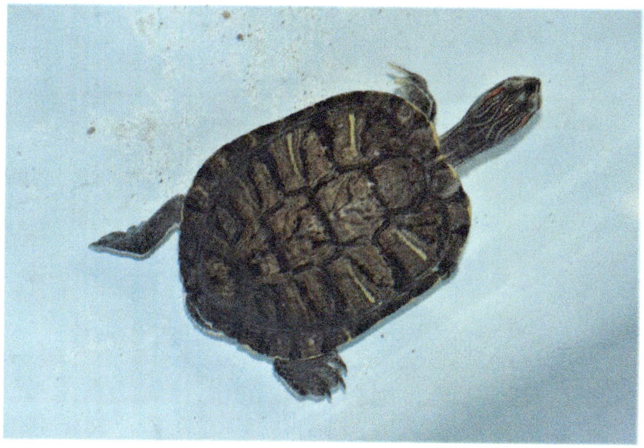

Fig. 21.12. Red-eared slider listing to the right while swimming in a pool.

	Tortoise	Turtle
Interpretive Discussion	A CBC was unable to be performed owing to marked toxicity of the heterophils and degeneration of other white blood cells (Table 21.4). Figures 21.13a–21.13d show toxic heterophils among erythrocytes. The toxicity of the heterophils is evident by the increased cytoplasmic basophilia, increased vacuolation, and abnormal granulation. Figure 21.13d also shows smudge cells, which are representative of the degenerate white blood cells that made completing a CBC difficult.	The CBC and biochemistry profile (Tables 21.5 and 21.7) were unremarkable. Figures 21.14a–21.14d are a representative set of normal blood film images. Figure 21.14a shows two heterophils, one eosinophil, and two thrombocytes. Figure 21.14b shows two heterophils, one eosinophil, one basophil, one immature erythrocyte, and one thrombocyte. Figure 21.14c shows two heterophils, one eosinophil, and two thrombocytes. Figure 21.14d shows two heterophils, one eosinophil, and four thrombocytes.

Table 21.4. Sulcata tortoise hematology results (Case 3).

		Reference[a]
PCV (%)	41.0	14–28
Plasma protein (refractometry)		
(g/dL)	5.0	—
Notes		

[a]Gibbons et al. (2019, p. 344).

Table 21.5. Red-eared slider hematology results (Case 3).

	Day 1	Day 55	Reference[a]
PCV (%)	26.0	22.0	26 (8–44)
Leukocytes			
WBC (×10³/μL)	14.2	13.0	6.73 (1.0–19.4)
Heterophils (×10³/μL)	5.4	4.9	2.33 (0.18–5.86)
(%)	38	38	—
Lymphocytes (×10³/μL)	3.7	3.5	2.28 (0.03–6.90)
(%)	26	27	—
Monocytes (×10³/μL)	0.4	0.4	0.18 (0.04–0.65)
(%)	3	3	—
Eosinophils (×10³/μL)	0	0.1	0.52 (0.01–3.06)
(%)	0	1	—
Basophils (×10³/μL)	4.7	4.0	1.07 (0.01–3.56)
(%)	33	31	—
Thrombocytes			
Adequate thrombocytes	Exist	—	
Plasma protein (refractometry)			
(g/dL)	7.4	4.2	
Notes			
	Normal morphology		

[a]Gibbons et al. (2019, p. 346).

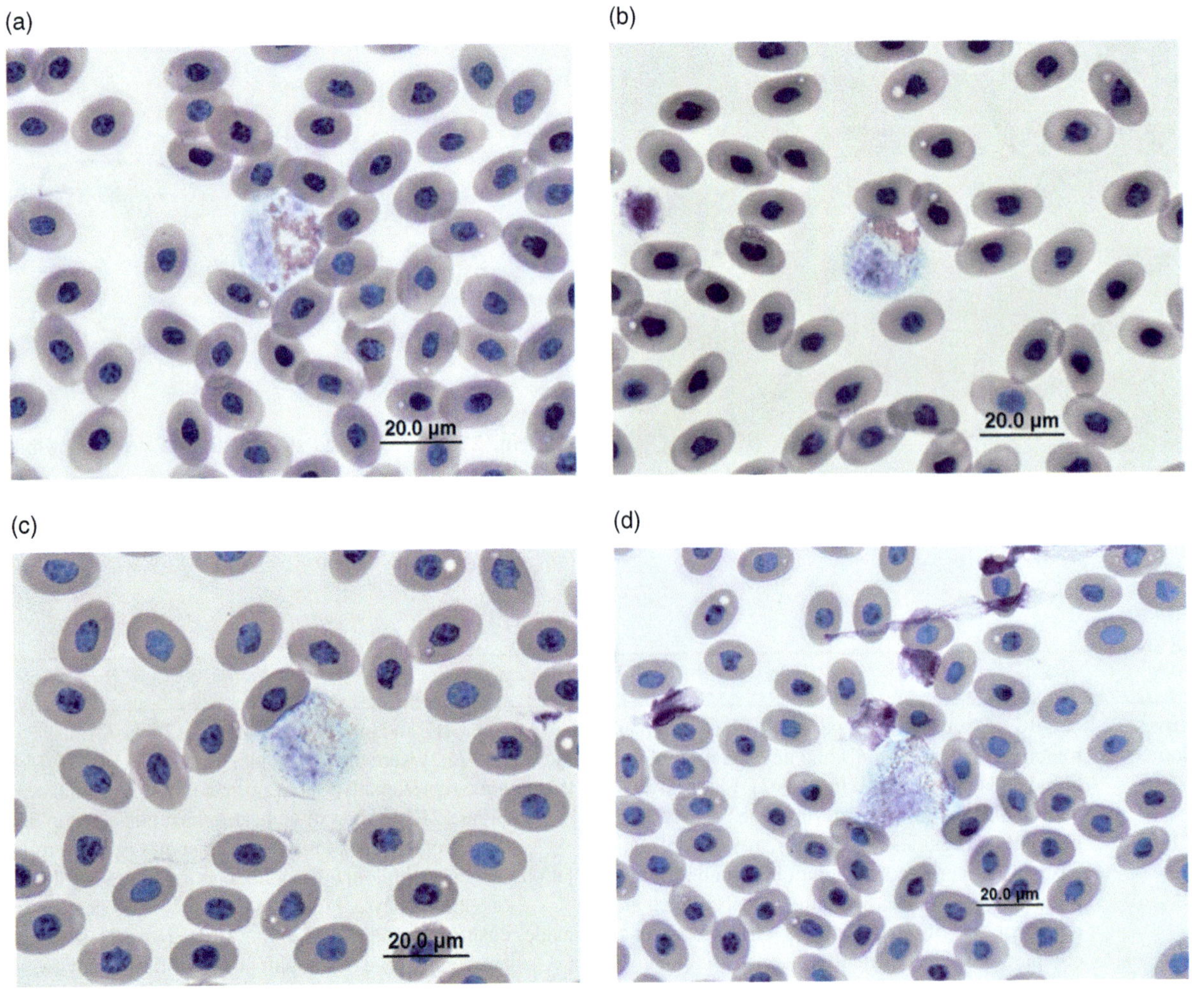

Fig. 21.13. (a)–(d) Blood films from the tortoise (Wright–Giemsa stain, 100× oil).

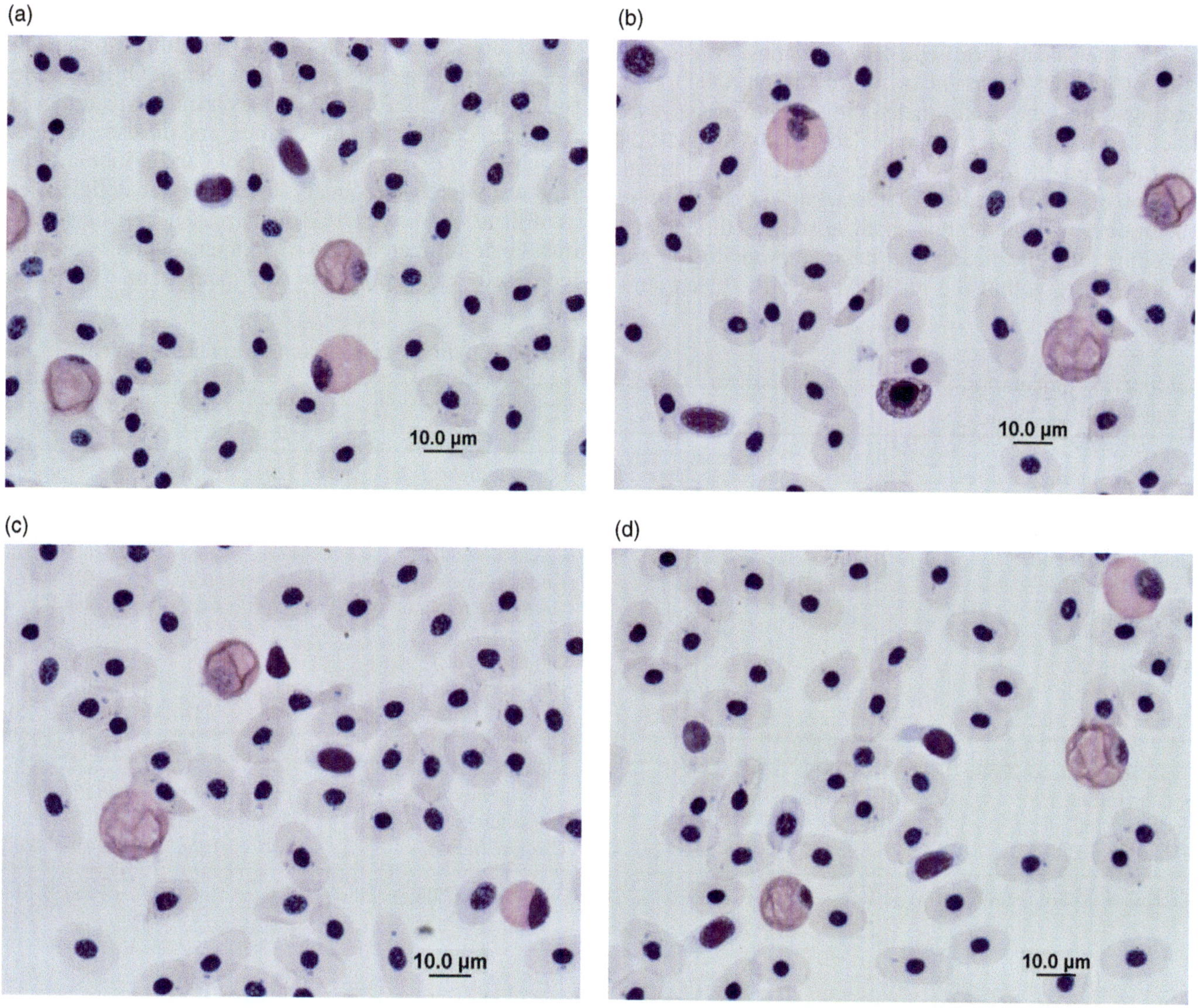

Fig. 21.14. (a)–(d) Blood films from a normal red-eared slider as a representative example (Wright–Giemsa stain, 100× oil).

	Tortoise	Turtle
	The most significant results on the plasma biochemistry profile were hypoglycemia and increased creatine kinase (CK) and aspartate aminotransferase (AST) (Table 21.6). The increased AST was likely associated with the increased CK values; however, in association with the hypoglycemia, hepatobiliary disease was also likely. The hyperuricemia can be the result of dehydration (as indicated by the elevated PCV) or renal disease. Radiographs, shown in Figures 21.15–21.17, revealed a diffuse bronchointerstitial pattern throughout the pulmonary parenchyma. There was gas throughout the intestines, and a moderate amount of heterogeneous material was visualized within the colon. The remaining osseous and soft tissue structures were normal. Radiographs indicated a diffuse bronchointerstitial pattern throughout the pulmonary parenchyma that could represent chronic, infectious, or allergic bronchitis.	Whole-body radiographs (Figures 21.18 and 21.19) revealed a diffuse interstitial pattern within the right lung lobes and a mild interstitial to bronchial pattern within the left lung lobes, best visualized on the craniocaudal view. Within the left caudal aspect of the celomic cavity, there was an ovoid opacity, surrounded by a rim of mineralized opacity. The marked interstitial pattern in the right lung lobe and mild interstitial to bronchial pattern in the left lung lobes represent interstitial pneumonia and/or fungal disease. There was also a mineralized egg within the left caudal celomic cavity.

Summary

For the sulcata tortoise, a grave prognosis was given with or without treatment owing to the physical exam findings and the toxic heterophils. Euthanasia was elected, and gross necropsy revealed copious amounts of mucoid fluid in the mouth and nasal cavity, minimal amount of visceral adipose stores, and severe diffuse pneumonia with numerous small abscesses throughout the lungs and the heart. The most relevant histologic findings were within the lung, liver, heart, spleen, and thymus revealing multiple, chronic, severe granulomas with a myriad of acid-fast bacilli (no fungal organisms were detected on GMS stain in the lung). Other diagnoses included chief cell hyperplasia of the parathyroid, lymphoid depletion of the thymus, and diffuse germ cell atrophy of the testes. The lymphoid and testicular atrophy were likely secondary to nutritional deficiencies, as well as the parathyroid hyperplasia. The nutritional imbalance ultimately caused immune suppression with increased susceptibility to pathogens such as

Table 21.6. Sulcata tortoise plasma biochemical results (Case 3).

		Reference[a]
Glucose (mg/dL)	25	63–155
BUN (mg/dL)	7	3 (1–6)
Phosphorus (mg/dL)	5.4	3.8 (1.5–6.5)
Calcium (mg/dL)	14.7	9.6–14.7
Uric acid (mg/dL)	13.7	1.5–5.1
Total protein (biuret) (g/dL)	4.5	3.8 (1.2–6.3)
Albumin (g/dL)	1.5	0.3–2.7
Globulin (g/dL)	3.0	2.3 (0.4–3.8)
Cholesterol (mg/dL)	27	129 (36–283)
Creatine kinase (IU/L)	19 301	191–3727
Aspartate aminotransferase (IU/L)	811	34–151
Sodium (mEq/L)	148	125–139
Potassium (mEq/L)	4.3	5.8–9.7
Chloride (mEq/L)	110	109 (93–124)

[a]Gibbons et al. (2019, p. 344).

Table 21.7. Red-eared slider plasma biochemical results (Case 3).

	Day 1	Day 55	Reference[a]
Glucose (mg/dL)	220	59	54 (21–143)
BUN (mg/dL)	15	20	23 (2–64)
Phosphorus (mg/dL)	7.4	5.1	4.0 (1.8–8.8)
Calcium (mg/dL)	18.4	13.8	12.6 (6.5–22.6)
Uric acid (mg/dL)	0.5	0.4	0.8 (0.1–1.9)
Total protein (biuret) (g/dL)	6.6	4.3	4.8 (1.1–8.8)
Albumin (g/dL)	2.1	1.5	1.8 (0.6–3.3)
Globulin (g/dL)	4.5	2.8	3.2 (1.1–5.9)
Cholesterol (mg/dL)	487	296	162 (106–227)
Creatine kinase (IU/L)	1929	237	516 (108–2125)
Aspartate aminotransferase (IU/L)	118	54	141 (44–358)
Sodium (mEq/L)	136	129	134 (123–147)
Potassium (mEq/L)	3.6	3.4	3.8 (2.4–7.5)
Chloride (mEq/L)	102	95	98 (88–112)

[a]Gibbons et al. (2019, pp. 346–347).

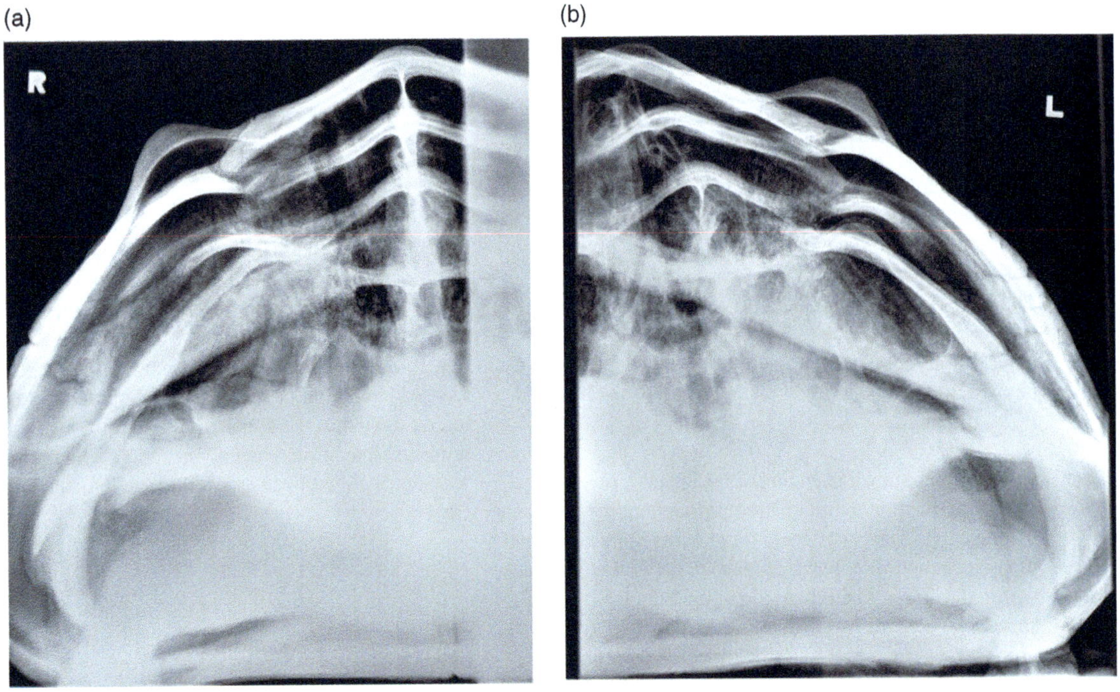

Fig. 21.15. (a), (b) Right and left craniocaudal radiograph.

(a) (b)

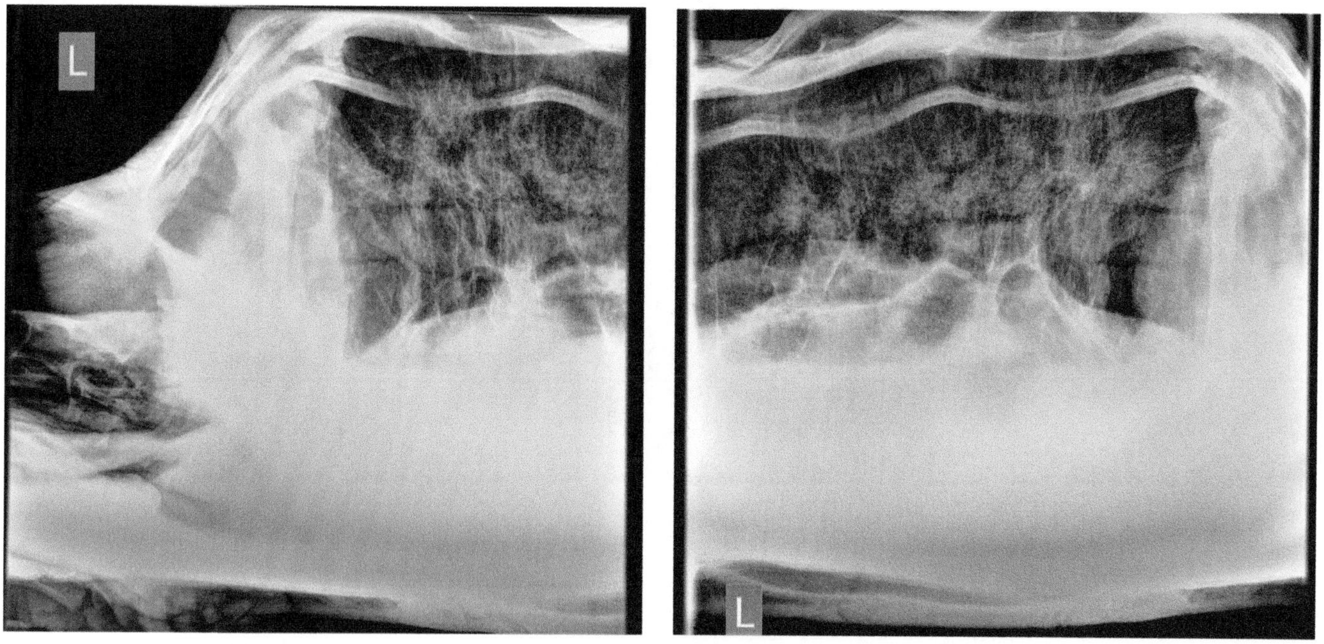

Fig. 21.16. (a), (b) Left lateral cranial aspect and caudal aspect radiograph.

(a) (b)

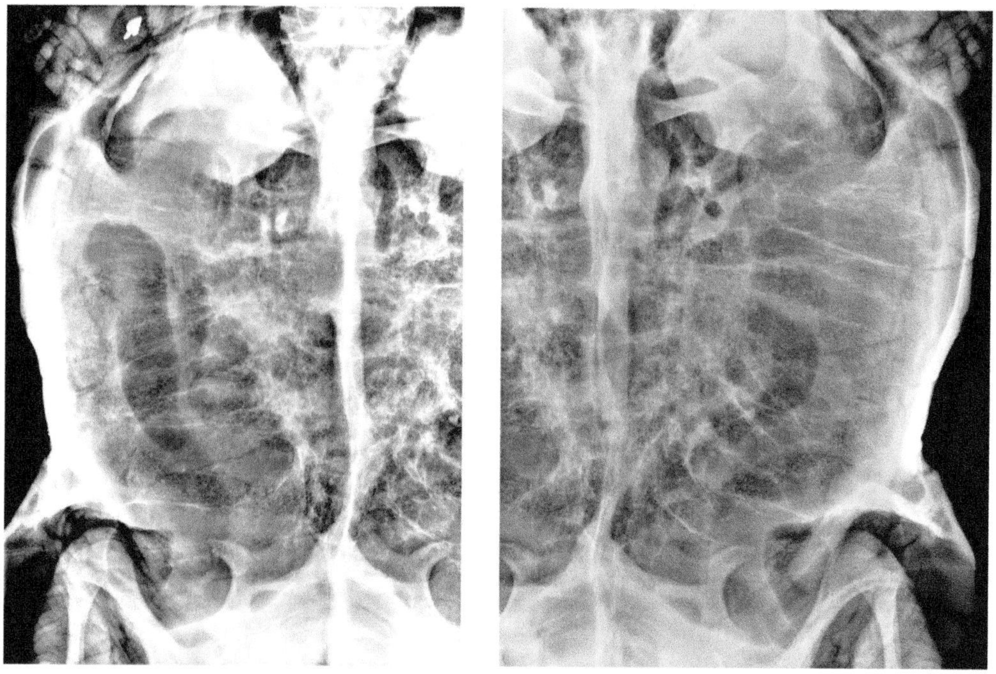

Fig. 21.17. (a), (b) Right and left dorsoventral radiograph.

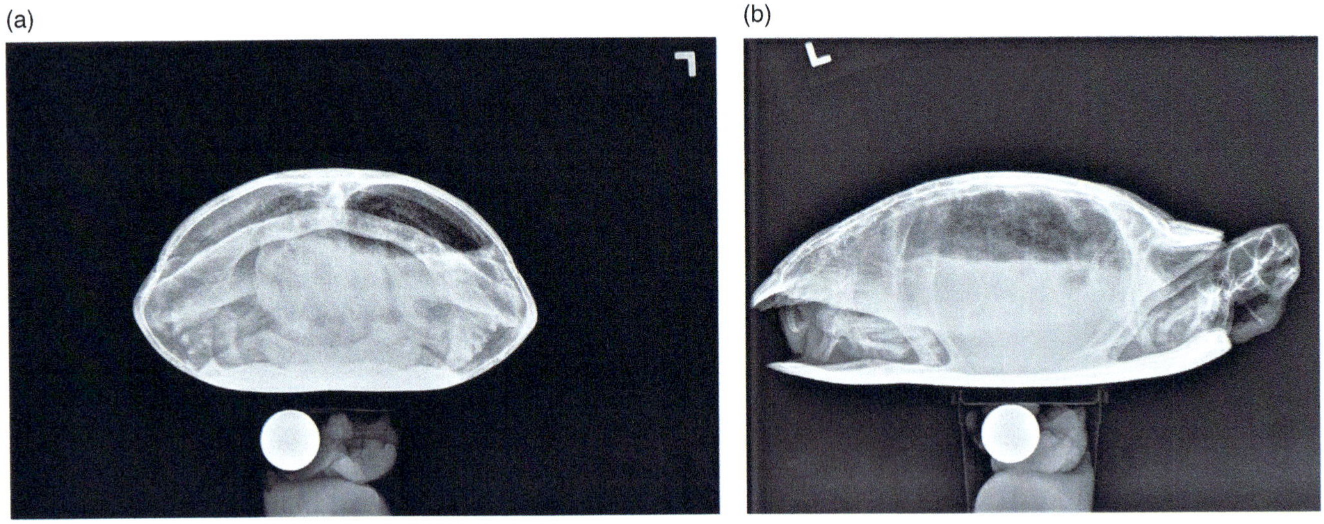

Fig. 21.18. (a) Craniocaudal radiograph. (b) Left lateral radiograph.

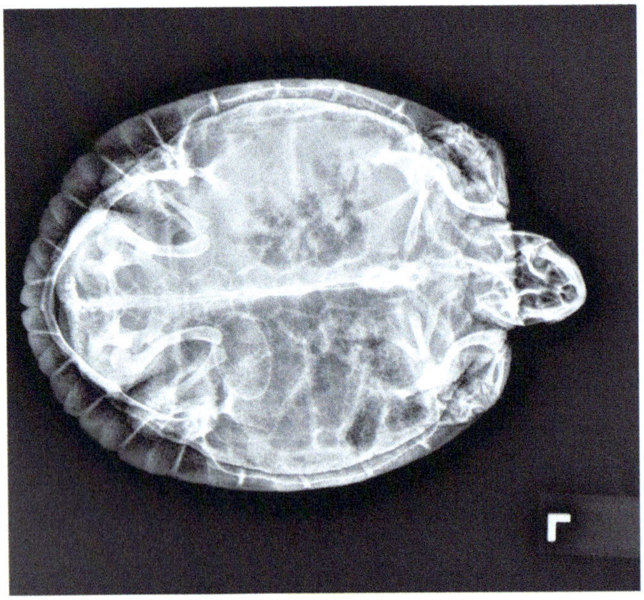

Fig. 21.19. Dorsoventral radiograph.

Mycobacterium species and subsequent bacteremia. Pneumonia cases associated with *Mycobacterium* (and *Chlamydia*) sp. are often chronic and have guarded to poor prognosis (Rodriguez et al., 2018; Knotek and Divers, 2019).

The prognosis for the red-eared slider was guarded to poor, given that pneumonia is a serious and, often, life-threatening disease of reptiles. In addition to the pneumonia, it was also unclear as to whether the egg was retained. The prescribed treatment included an antibiotic (Ceftazidime, 20 mg/kg IM q72h × 7 treatments) and to provide a heated haul-out area with substrate to encourage egg laying.

Follow-up examinations took place on days 14, 27, and 55. On day 14, the turtle continued isolation in a quarantine tank and appeared normal as she was observed walking normally on the bottom of the tank. She did, however, still list to the right side when rafting at the surface. She was still eating well, and there were no additional concerns. On day 27, she was reported to be doing well and no longer listed to one side when swimming. The only remaining concern at that time was the egg retention, so she remained in quarantine for one more month. On day 55, a blood sample was collected (Tables 21.5 and 21.7), and ultrasound was performed. There were no significant findings on the blood work results, and there was no egg seen on sonography. The turtle was returned to exhibit.

These two cases both presenting with pneumonia with similar findings on radiographs were managed differently in part with the assistance of the blood films.

Case 4: Case Series of Chelonian Dystocia and Follicular Stasis

Signalment

Turtle 1	Turtle 2	Turtle 3
10-year-old intact female Malayan box turtle (*Cuora amboinensis*)	At least 10-year-old intact female Malayan turtle (*Cuora amboinensis*)	30-year-old intact female yellow pond turtle (*Mauremys mutica*)

History

Turtle 1	Turtle 2	Turtle 3
The turtle was housed in a freshwater aquatic exhibit in a public aquarium with other turtles and fish. The patient presented with a history of chronic bilateral ocular discharge, "waxing and waning," lethargy, and anorexia. She sat hauled out of the water on a sandy area under the heat lamp for abnormally long periods of time.	This turtle was housed with Turtle 1 at the public aquarium. Two weeks after Turtle 1 died, there was concern that this turtle may be experiencing a similar problem due to an observed behavioral change. The turtle had been spending large amounts of time out of the water, which was unusual for her species.	This turtle was also housed with Turtle 1 and 2 in a turtle exhibit at a public aquarium. This turtle presented approximately nine months after Turtle 2 for anorexia and possible neurological issues (two-week duration). She had episodes of laying in her habitat showing no response to stimuli or food. She had lost weight in the past two months (811 g to 784 g).

Physical Examination

Turtle 1	Turtle 2	Turtle 3
Upon presentation, the 1.67 kg turtle appeared lethargic and was minimally interactive and responsive (Figure 21.20a). Skin ulcerations were noted along with loose and flaking skin around the neck and at the right commissure of the mouth (Figure 21.20b). White, multi-focal pinpoint to coalescing lesions or plaques were discovered throughout the inside of the mouth and on the tongue. The left nares was occluded, and the turtle was open mouth breathing intermittently. Blood was collected for a CBC (Table 21.8; Figures 21.22a–21.22d; Figures 21.23a–21.23c) and plasma biochemistry profile (Table 21.9) and whole-body radiographs (Figures 21.26a–1.26c) were obtained.	Upon presentation, the 1.97 kg turtle was bright, alert, and responsive. An attempt to collect a blood sample for a blood profile was challenging, and only enough was collected to prepare a blood film (Figures 21.24a–21.24d). Whole-body radiographs were also obtained (Figures 21.27a–21.27c)	Upon presentation, the 755 g turtle appeared bright, alert, and responsive (Figure 21.21). There was a small defect along the plastron. Otherwise, the turtle appeared healthy and exhibited no neurologic disorders. Only enough blood was collected to create a blood film (Figures 21.25a–21.25d). Whole-body radiographs (Figures 21.28a–21.28d) and coelomic ultrasound imaging were performed to evaluate the coelomic cavity (Figure 21.29).

(a) (b)

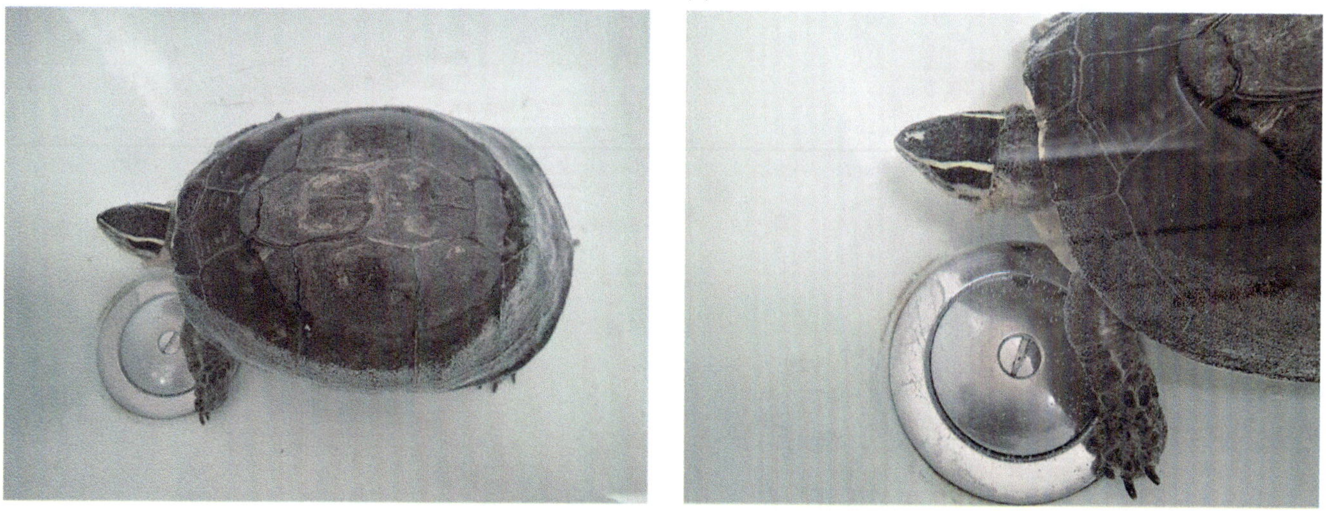

Fig. 21.20. (a) The Malayan box turtle in a tub of shallow water. (b) Skin sloughing on the neck of the Malayan box turtle.

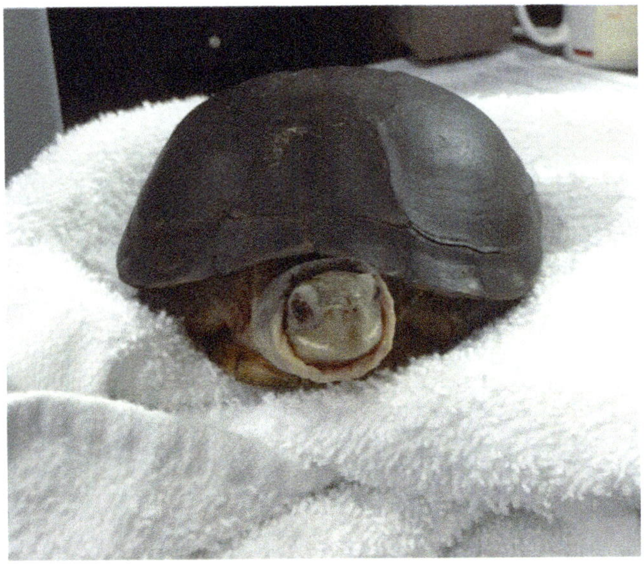

Fig. 21.21. Yellow pond turtle on physical exam.

Table 21.8. Turtle 1: Malayan box turtle hematology results (Case 4).

		Reference[a] (*Cuora flavomarginata*)
PCV (%)	20.0	(23–44)
Leukocytes		
WBC (×10³/μL)	8.1	(0.60–10.4)
Heterophils (×10³/μL)	5.9	(0.58–7.17)
(%)	73	—
Lymphocytes (×10³/μL)	1.9	(0–3.11)
(%)	23	—
Monocytes (×10³/μL)	0	(0–0.76)
(%)	0	—
Eosinophils (×10³/μL)	0	(0–0.43)
(%)	0	—
Basophils (×10³/μL)	0.3	(0–1.82)
(%)	4	—
Thrombocytes		
Adequate thrombocytes	—	
Plasma protein (refractometry)		
(g/dL)	4.3	—
Notes		
Many very immature nRBCs present on slide		

[a]Gibbons et al. (2019, pp. 344–345).

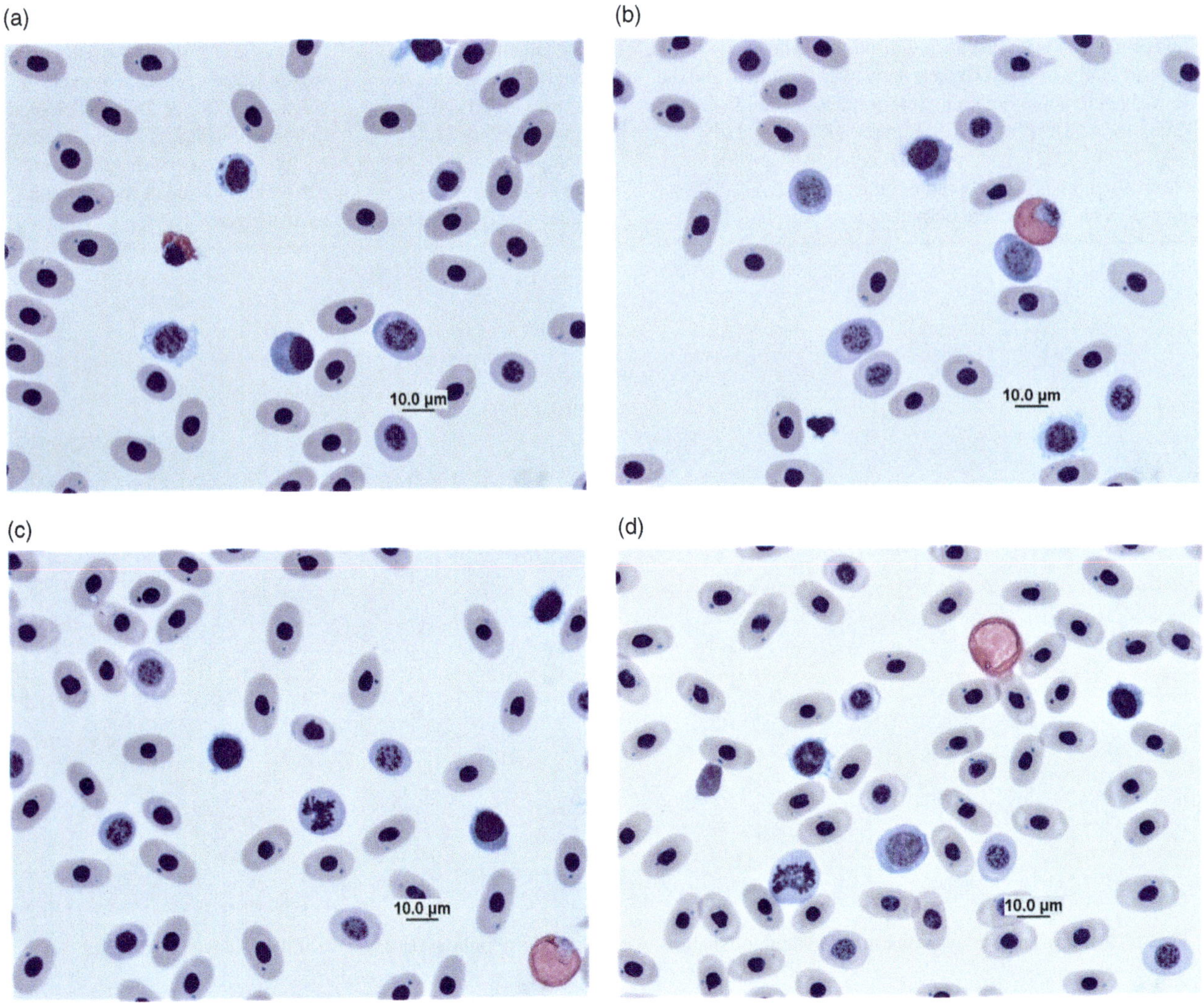

Fig. 21.22. (a)–(d) Blood films (Wright–Giemsa stain, 100× oil).

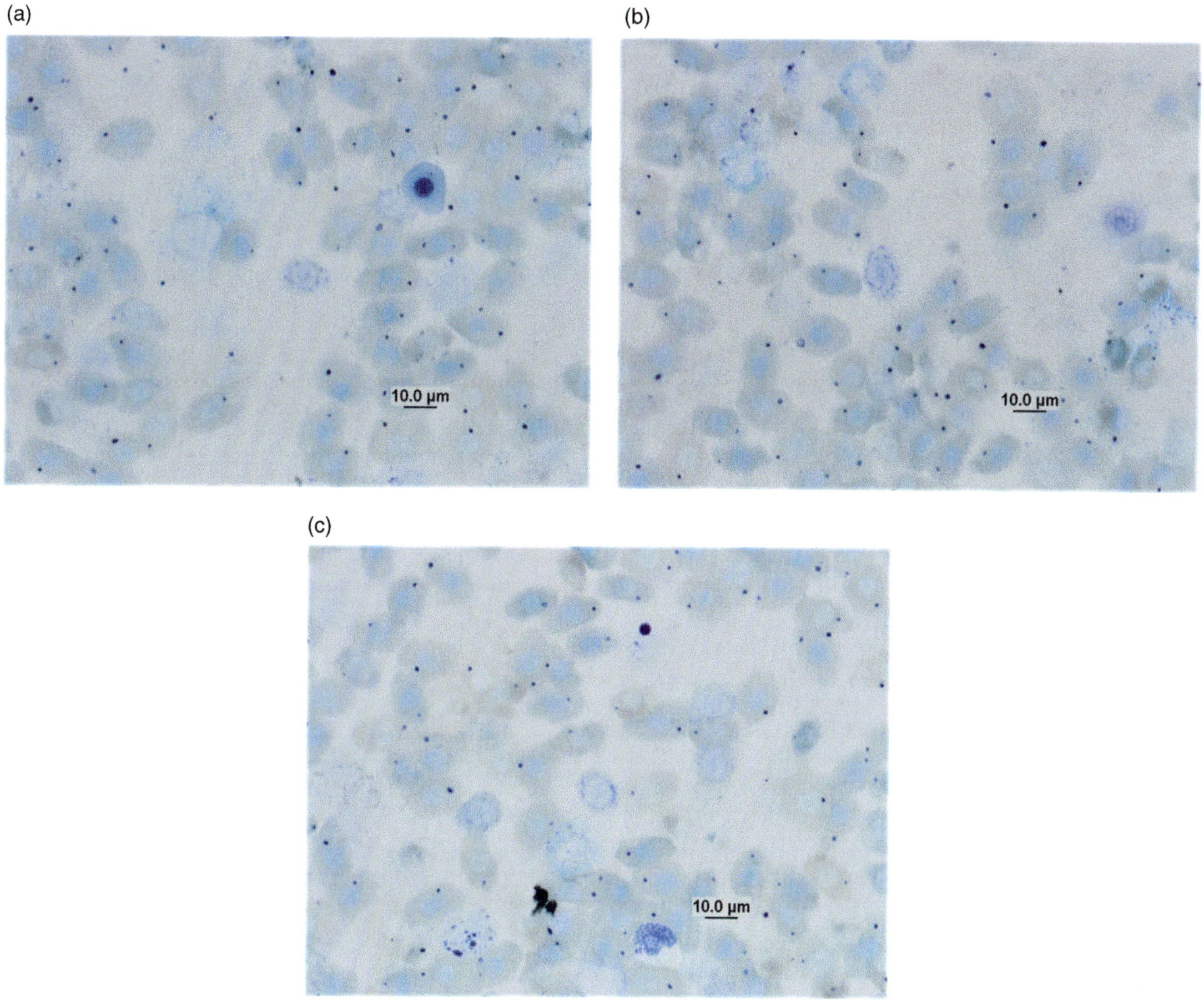

Fig. 21.23. (a)–(c) Blood films (New methylene blue stain, 100× oil).

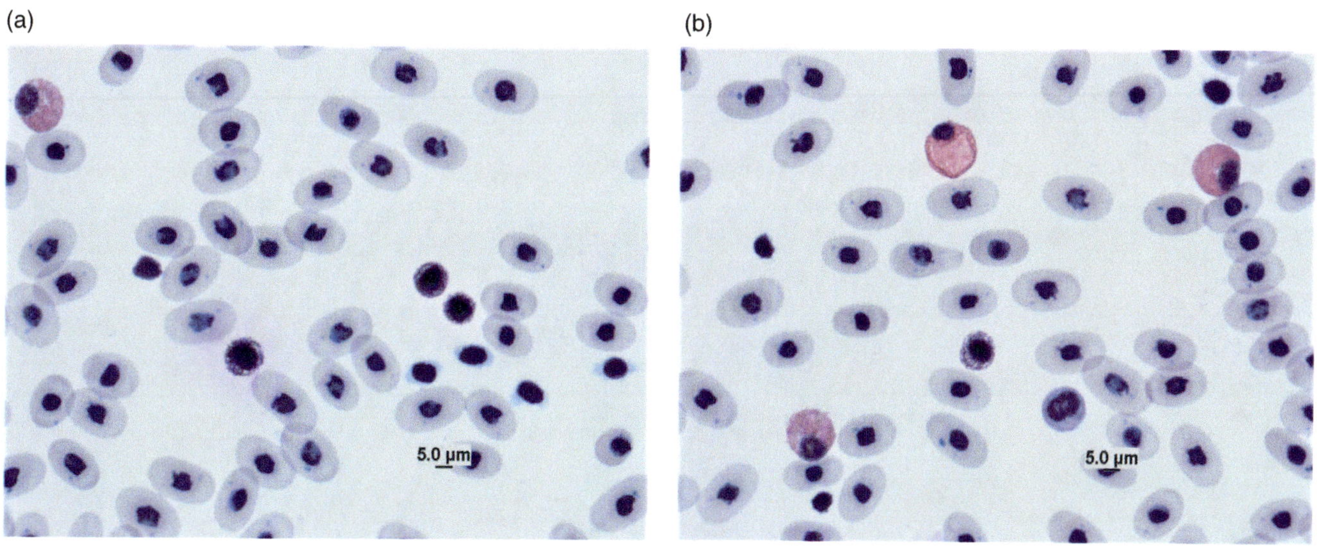

Fig. 21.24. (a)–(d) Blood films (Wright–Giemsa stain, 100× oil).

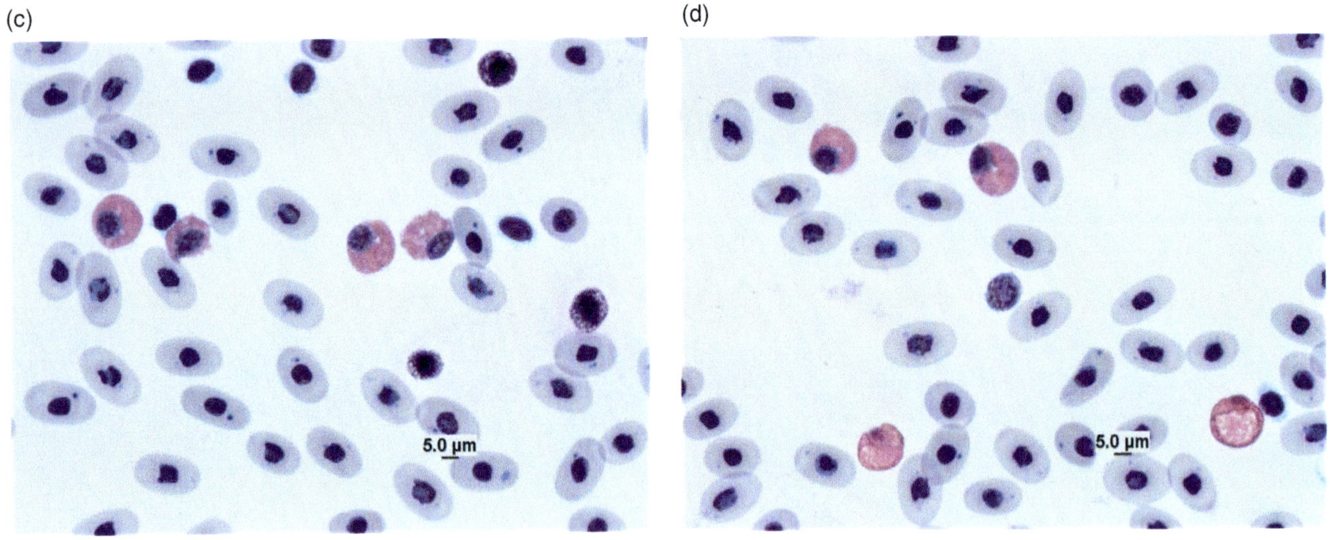

Fig. 21.24. *(Continued)*

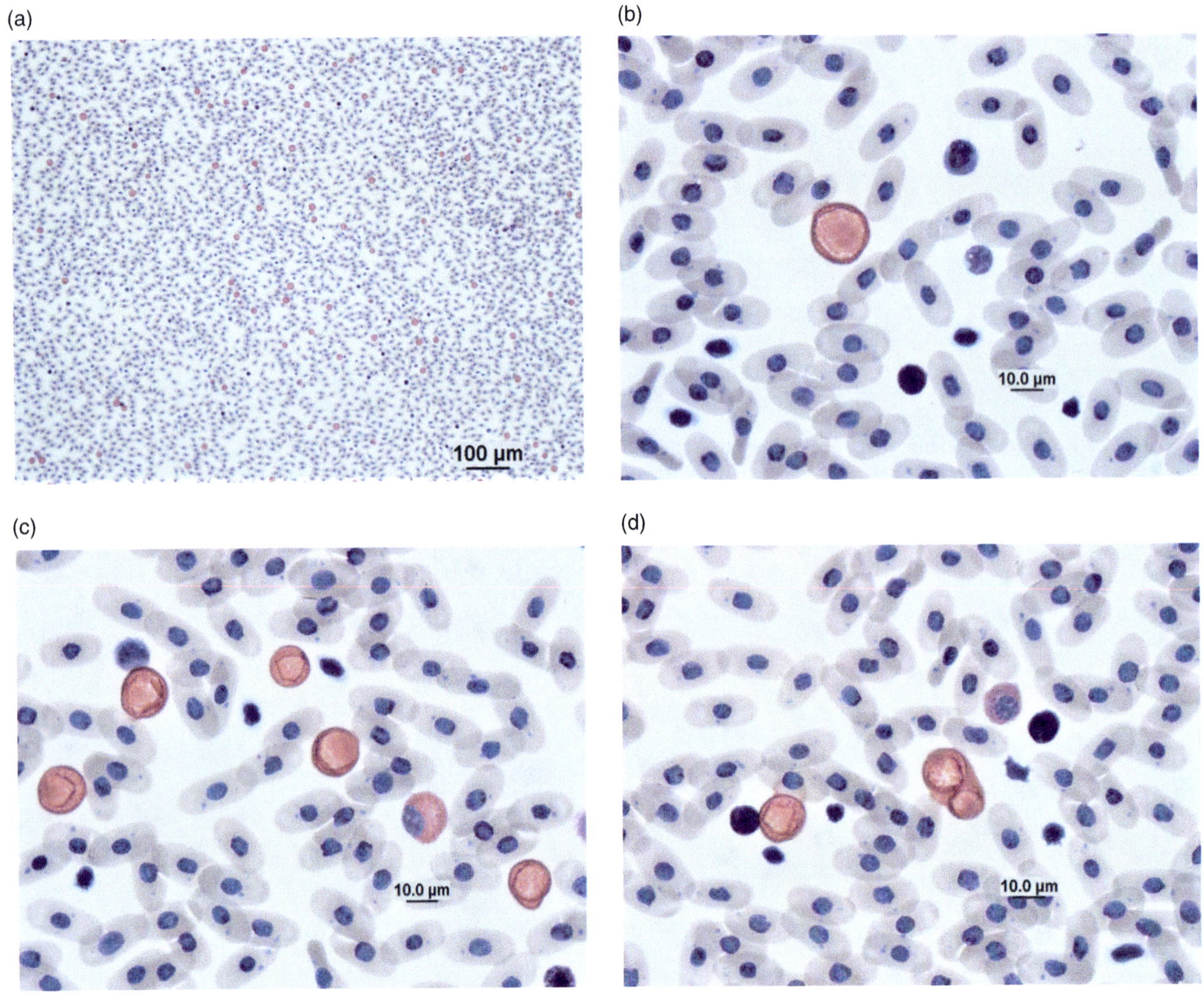

Fig. 21.25. (a) Blood film (Wright–Giemsa stain, 10×); (b–d) blood films (Wright–Giemsa stain, 100× oil).

Table 21.9. Turtle 1: Malayan box turtle plasma biochemical results (Case 4).

		Reference[a] (*Cuora flavomarginata*)
Glucose (mg/dL)	18	28–182
BUN (mg/dL)	75	2–48
Phosphorus (mg/dL)	4.7	1.8–12.3
Calcium (mg/dL)	8.0	8.9–29.9
Uric acid (mg/dL)	18.1	0.4–3.1
Total protein (biuret) (g/dL)	4.1	3.9–9.1
Albumin (g/dL)	1.0	1.3–3.2
Globulin (g/dL)	3.1	—
Cholesterol (mg/dL)	207	48–420
Creatine kinase (IU/L)	2920	61–2156
Aspartate aminotransferase (IU/L)	429	46–299
Sodium (mEq/L)	98	—
Potassium (mEq/L)	8.0	—
Chloride (mEq/L)	62	—

[a] Gibbons et al. (2019, p. 345).

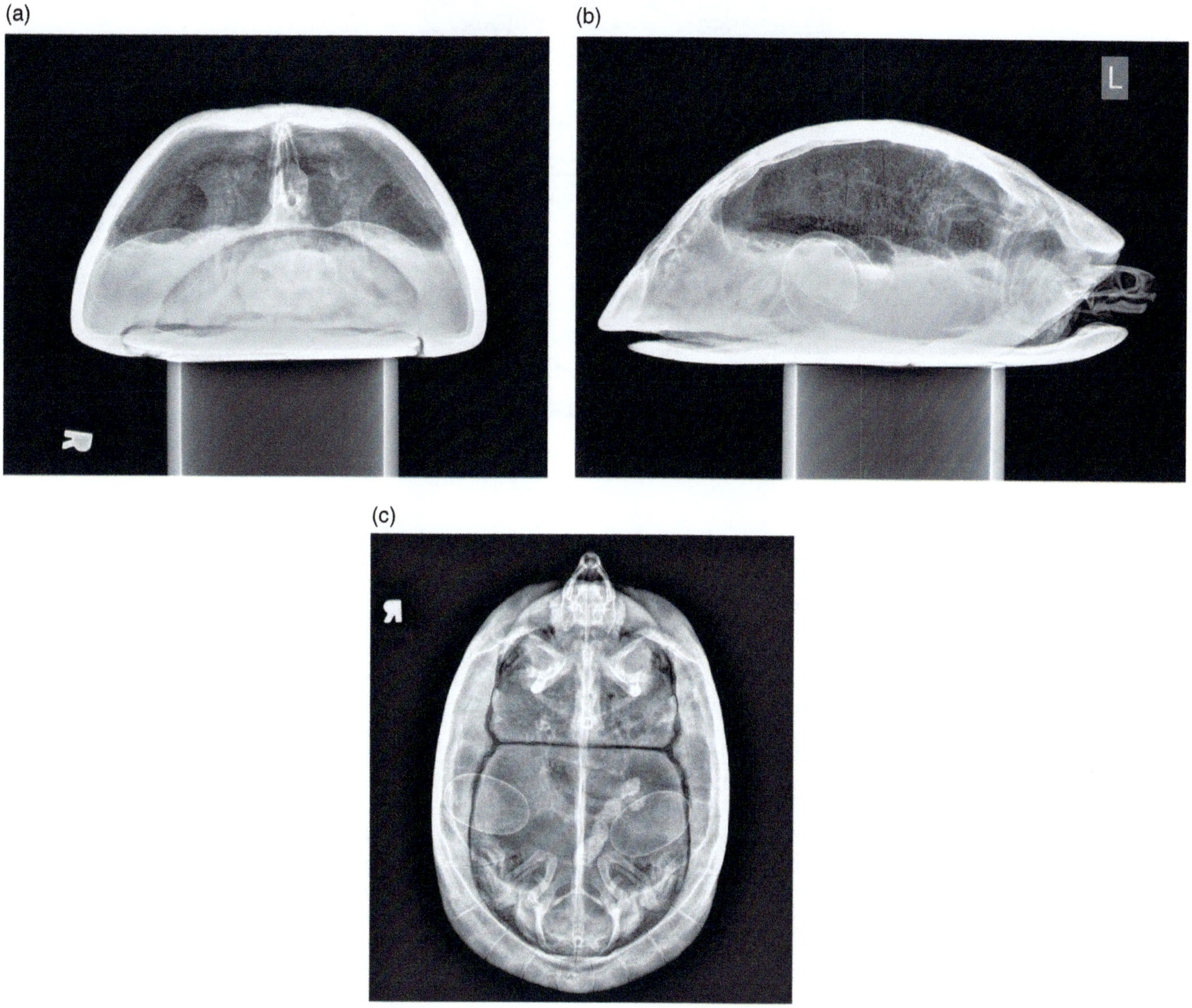

Fig. 21.26. (a)–(c) Radiographs showing cranial-caudal, lateral, and dorsoventral views.

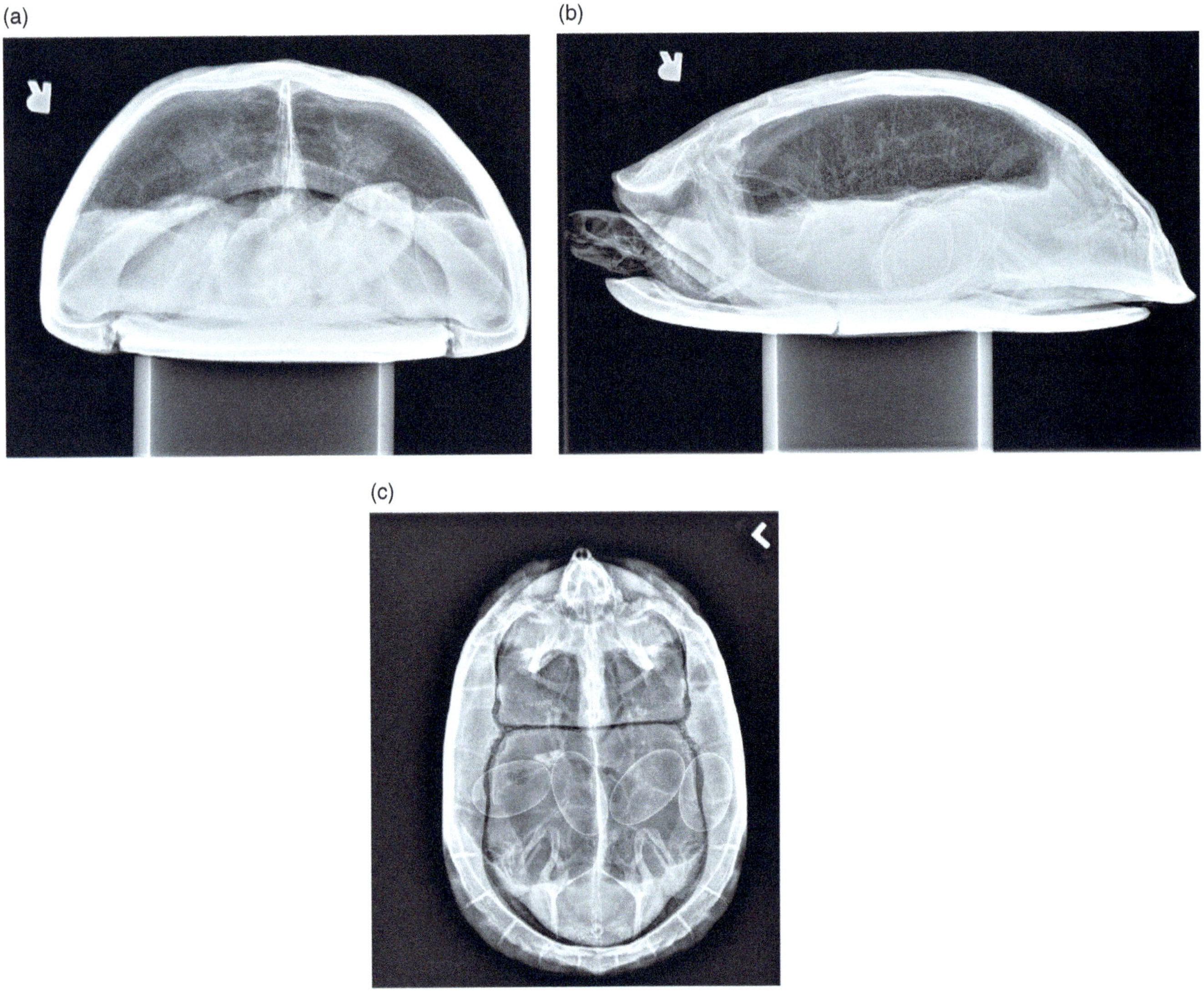

Fig. 21.27. (a)–(c) Radiographs showing cranial-caudal, lateral, and dorsoventral views.

Interpretive Discussion

Turtle 1	Turtle 2	Turtle 3
Blood was drawn from the subcarapacial sinus for CBC and chemistry. Figures 21.22a and 21.22b each show an immature erythrocyte, a heterophil, a monocyte, a thrombocyte, and a lymphocyte. Figures 21.22c and 21.22d each show a cell with a mitotic figure among immature erythrocytes, one heterophil, and one lymphocyte. Figures 21.23a–21.23c each reveal a cell in the center of the image with a ring of aggregated reticulum encircling the nucleus.	A blood film revealed increased inflammatory cells (heterophils, basophils, lymphocytes, and monocytes) and immature red blood cells. Figure 21.24a reveals three basophils, one heterophil, one lymphocyte, and four thrombocytes. Figure 21.24b reveals three normal heterophils, one basophil, one monocyte, and three lymphocytes. Figure 21.24c reveals four normal heterophils, three basophils, and four thrombocytes. Figure 21.24d reveals four normal heterophils, one lymphocyte, and one thrombocyte.	The results of the blood film indicated an inflammatory leukogram. The differential on the blood film revealed 56% nontoxic heterophils, 22% basophils, 14% lymphocytes, and 8% monocytes. Figure 21.25a shows the blood film viewed at 10× indicating the presence of numerous leukocytes and a significant leukocytosis. Figure 21.25b reveals one morphologically normal heterophil, one monocyte, one lymphocyte, one basophil, four thrombocytes, and no polychromasia. Figure 21.25c reveals six normal heterophils, one basophil, one monocyte, and three thrombocytes. Figure 21.25d reveals four normal heterophils, two basophils, four lymphocytes, and one thrombocyte.

Turtle 1	Turtle 2	Turtle 3
The hematology results showed a PCV of 20%, and many immature RBCs were visualized. The plasma chemistry revealed a glucose level of 18 mg/dL (likely false because the sample sat on cells for a long period of time). Although normal blood values for this species are not well documented (a similar genus was noted in the table), it indicated a regenerative anemia, renal and hepatic compromise, and electrolyte abnormalities. Whole-body three-view radiographs were performed (Figures 21.26a–21.26c), which revealed two eggs in the coelomic cavity, as well as a mineralized area likely in the colon.	Figure 21.27c reveals that within the mid to caudal coelomic cavity there were four mineralized, well-formed eggs, which were smaller than the pelvic inlet. Cranial to the eggs within the right aspect of the coelomic cavity there was a focal area of mineralization, likely within the colon. The remainder of the study was normal. The radiographic conclusion was that the turtle was gravid (four mineralized eggs) and likely had non-obstructive foreign material in her colon.	Whole-body radiographs included cranial-caudal, lateral, and dorsoventral views (Figures 21.28a–21.28c). Because the content of the coelomic cavity was obscured by either soft tissue or fluid, an additional ventrodorsal view with the turtle placed on right lateral recumbency (Figure 21.28d) was obtained. This view allowed any fluid to settle by gravity, thereby observing a "fluid line" on the image. No fluid line was observed suggesting that a mass or mass-like effect was compressing the lung space (decreasing the lung space). An ultrasound revealed multiple bilateral ovarian follicles (Figure 21.29) indicative of follicular stasis. It is not uncommon to see reproductive disease in captive chelonians. It is typical to see these animals suffer from anorexia, not able to pass feces, and/or collapse. However, they appear to maintain their body weight, which can be misleading to owners.

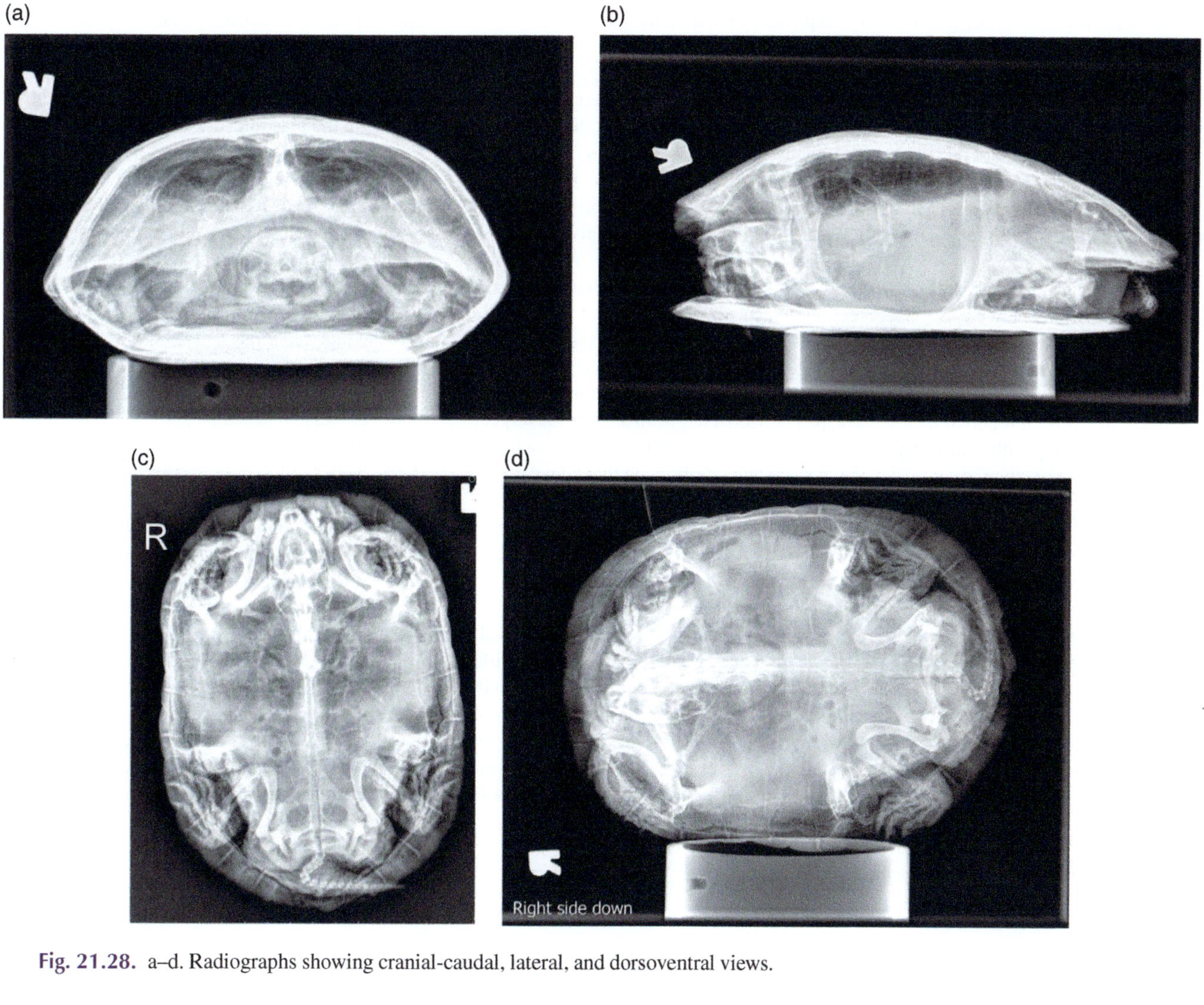

Fig. 21.28. a–d. Radiographs showing cranial-caudal, lateral, and dorsoventral views.

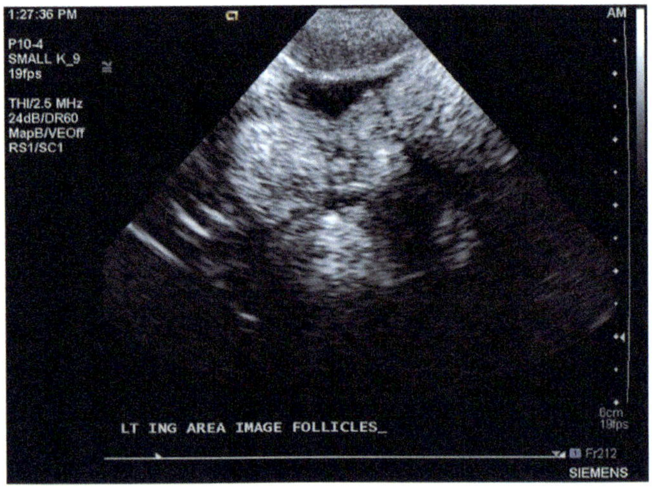

Fig. 21.29. Ultrasound image from the left inguinal region.

Summary

Turtle 1	Turtle 2	Turtle 3
The turtle was placed under general anesthesia for an ovariosalpingohysterectomy. Although a fibrotic and fragile reproductive tract was surgically removed, the turtle did not recover from the anesthesia. A necropsy revealed mineralization and necrosis involving multiple organs including the liver, kidney, pancreas, stomach, spleen, and heart. These results may be an indication of visceral gout (the histopathology was lost in follow-up). Visceral gout and pseudogout has been reported in Chelonia and is typically caused by renal failure, dehydration, or an overproduction of uric acid (Martinez-Silvestre A, 1995; Divers and Innis, 2019; Rodriguez et al., 2018). There was evidence of renal failure in this case. The regenerative anemia did not appear severe with a PVC of 20%; however, in the face of severe dehydration, the PCV was not accurately portraying either the degree of anemia or the dehydration.	An exploratory coeliotomy and ovariosalpingohysterectomy confirmed the presence of four mineralized eggs within the coelom. Additionally, there were many follicles on both ovaries. The entire reproductive tract was removed, as well as the eggs. The remainder of the coelom was unremarkable. Both the reproductive tract and a liver biopsy were submitted for histopathology analysis. The plastron was placed back into its anatomical location, and plumber's epoxy putty was used to secure each corner of the plastron incision. Bone wax was used to seal the cut surfaces. An esophageal feeding tube was used to administer carnivore critical care liquid diet until recovery. The patient recovered from anesthesia/surgery and was bright, alert, responsive, and swimming the next morning. Following three days of hospitalization, she was discharged with pain medication (Meloxicam 0.3 mg/kg intramuscularly every 24 hours for 5 days). Histopathology results revealed moderate, diffuse fatty degeneration in the liver; normal ovaries; mild and circumferential edema with patchy lymphoplasmacytic inflammation in the lamina propria and edema in the muscular tunic of the oviduct. There were no histologic lesions noted in the ovaries or oviducts suggesting the turtle was at risk for coelomitis at the time of surgery.	An exploratory coeliotomy and ovariosalpingohysterectomy revealed normal-appearing heart, liver, stomach, visible bowel, and urinary bladder. The incision was closed by replacing the plastron "door" that was created to enter the coelom and securing it in place using plumber's epoxy resin. She did well during surgery and recovered uneventfully. Her postoperative weight was 695 g. Postoperative medications included an antibiotic (ceftazidime, 20 mg/kg IM for seven treatments), meloxicam (0.5 mg/kg PO q24h for five days), and carnivore diet (syringe fed 3 mL daily). She was eating fish two days following surgery. Her discharge weight was 715 g. She was kept in "dry-dock" until her incision healed. Three weeks following surgery, a blood film revealed 43% heterophils, 30% basophils, 21% lymphocytes, and 5% monocytes with normal heterophil morphology. Three months following surgery, her weight was 778 g and she appeared to be doing and eating well. The plastron patch was red, but otherwise appeared to be healing (Figure 21.30a). The discoloration was suspected to be from blood pooling. The residue around the surgery site was from attempts to cover the incision for waterproofing bandages, which failed; therefore, the need for dry-docking. Six months after surgery, she was doing well in the exhibit (Figure 21.30b). The plastron patch healed.

(a) (b)

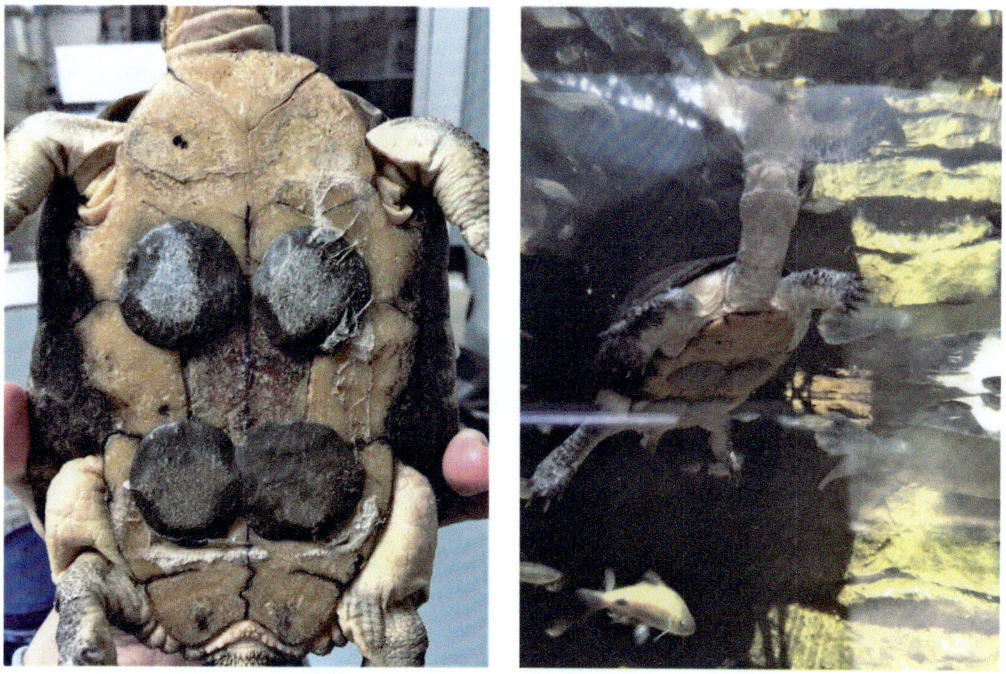

Fig. 21.30. (a) Three months post-op, the plastron patch is dark red but appeared to be healing. (b) Six months post-op, the plastron was intact and healing, and the turtle was introduced back into the exhibit.

Case 5: Lizard with Limb Lameness, Lethargy, and Anorexia

Signalment

2-year-old intact female bearded dragon (*Pogona vitticeps*)

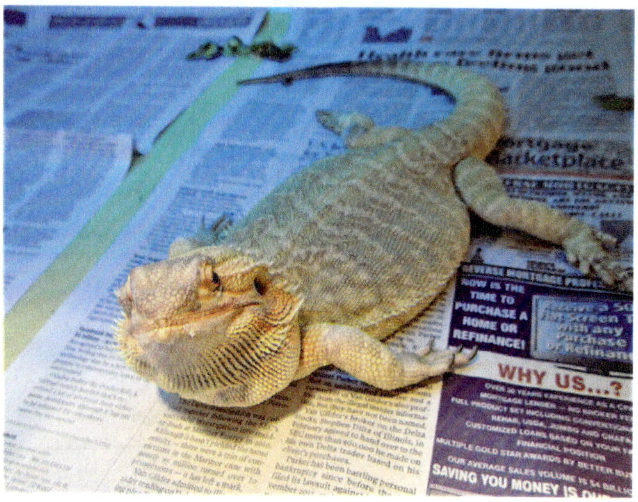

Fig. 21.31. Bearded dragon at presentation with limited use of all four limbs.

History

The bearded dragon developed lameness in all four limbs, lethargy, and anorexia and was evaluated by urgent care two days prior to presentation. The owner noticed that the lizard had not been eating well and regurgitated a cricket diet with mouse hair. The lizard struggled to walk and appeared more lame in the forelimbs. The bearded dragon was housed in a 40-gallon aquarium with ceramic tile flooring, a rock for basking, water bowl, and food bowl, but no hiding area. The lizard was fed mice, mealworms, and a variety of vegetables.

Physical Examination

Upon presentation, the 560 g bearded dragon appeared lethargic and exhibited diarrhea. She was able to move all four limbs and tail when stimulated, but had an abnormal stance when resting (put less amount of weight on forelimbs) (Figure 21.31).

Radiographic images provided by the referring veterinarian revealed ovarian follicular development and gas in the intestines; otherwise, they were unremarkable with normal osseous structures. Pre-ovulatory stasis was considered based on the radiographic findings. A fecal wet mount revealed an overgrowth of *Trichomonas*, and metronidazole treatment was initiated. Blood was collected for a CBC (Figures 21.32a– 21.32d) and plasma chemistry panel (Tables 21.10 and 21.11).

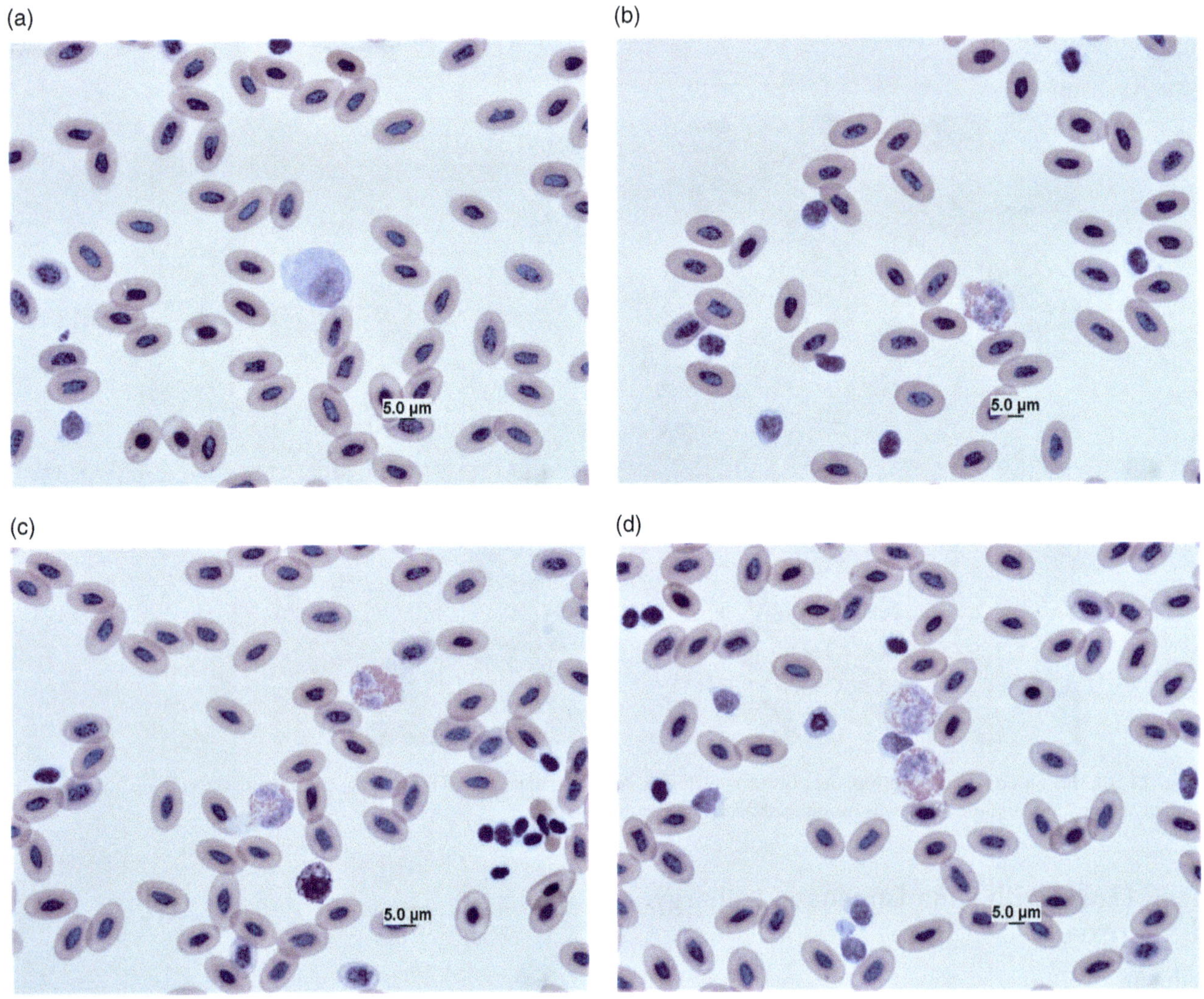

Fig. 21.32. (a)–(d) Blood films (Wright–Giemsa stain, 100× oil).

Table 21.10. Bearded dragon hematology results (Case 5).

	Day 1	Reference[a]
PCV (%)	29.0	30 (17–45)
Leukocytes		
WBC (×10³/μL)	15.4	6.21 (1.45–19.0)
Heterophils (×10³/μL)	6.3	2.09 (0.24–7.77)
(%)	41	27 (17–43)[b]
Lymphocytes (×10³/μL)	8.3	2.77 (0.29–11.3)
(%)	54	59 (47–69)[b]
Monocytes (×10³/μL)	0.5	0.25 (0.03–1.39)*
(%)	3	1 (0–4)[b]*
Eosinophils (×10³/μL)	0	0.12 (0.01–0.37)
(%)	0	—
Basophils (×10³/μL)	0.3	0.26 (0.04–1.28)
(%)	2	9 (2–18)[b]
Thrombocytes		
Adequate thrombocytes	Clumped	
Plasma protein (refractometry) (g/dL)	8.2	—
Notes		

[a]Gibbons et al. (2019, p. 338).
[b]Ellman (2019).
*Azurophils were reported separately.

Table 21.11. Bearded dragon plasma biochemical results (Case 5).

	Day 1	Day 3	Day 8	Reference[a]
Glucose (mg/dL)	177	—	—	202 (108–333)
BUN (mg/dL)	1	—	—	2 (1–5)
Phosphorus (mg/dl)	8.6	—	5.9	4.4 (2.1–10.6)
Calcium (mg/dL)	15.2	—	—	11.9 (8.6–18)
Uric acid (mg/dL)	55.7	36.4	8.3	3.1 (0.5–9.8)
Total protein (biuret) (g/dL)	7.5	—	—	5.0 (3.0–8.1)
Albumin (g/dL)	3.2	—	—	2.5 (1.2–4.0)
Globulin (g/dL)	4.3	—	—	2.5 (1.1–4.5)
Cholesterol (mg/dL)	327	—	—	271 (79–606)
Creatine kinase (IU/L)	563	—	—	563 (33–4042)
Aspartate aminotransferase (IU/L)	6	—	—	20 (2–90)
Sodium (mEq/L)	141	136	155	157 (140–179)
Potassium (mEq/L)	9.39	8.25	3.88	4.0 (2.5–7.1)
Chloride (mEq/L)	103.9	106.1	111.9	120 (94–149)

[a]Gibbons et al. (2019, pp. 338–339).

Interpretive Discussion

The results indicated an inflammatory leukogram based on the toxic changes in the heterophils. The values from the CBC were within available reference intervals (Table 21.10). Figure 21.31a shows a monocyte. Figure 21.31b shows one toxic heterophils and two lymphocytes. Figure 21.31c shows two heterophils with varying degrees of toxicity evident by the cytoplasmic vacuolization and basophilia and the varying morphology of granules, one basophil, clumped thrombocytes, and polychromatic erythrocytes. Figure 21.32d shows two heterophils with varying degrees of toxicity, four lymphocytes, and one cell with a mitotic figure. Comments on the laboratory report included moderate heterophil toxicity (a few of the toxic heterophils have vacuoles), and a moderate number of erythrocyte precursor cells are present.

The biochemical profile revealed a marked hyperkalemia and marked increase in uric acid (Table 21.11).

Summary

Based on the diagnostics results, the bearded dragon was diagnosed with trichomoniasis, renal disease, and pre-ovulatory stasis (follicular stasis). Trichomonads are not commonly pathogenic in bearded dragons; however, large numbers can cause or contribute to diarrhea and weight loss. Because trichomoniasis has been shown to resolve with one dose of metronidazole (Maas, 2014), this bearded dragon was treated with a single dose of metronidazole (40 mg/kg PO) during her hospitalization of nine days. Subcutaneous fluid therapy was given to rehydrate the patient and provide diuresis for possible renal disease. She was gavage fed a critical care diet for herbivores and soon became more active and alert. Although she remained relatively immobile and unwilling to move throughout her cage, she showed more mobility when handled. A limited diagnostic profile was repeated two days after presentation that showed mild improvements in her hyperkalemia and increased uric acid (Table 21.11, day 3). Peritoneal dialysis was offered; however, the owner opted to continue with the subcutaneous fluids. A fecal wet mount on day 3 revealed no evidence of *Trichomonas*. On day 5, the plasma chemistry values were within the reference interval, indicating that the azotemia had resolved. The lizard was discharged from the hospital with a plan to transition the carnivorous diet to a primary herbivorous diet for adult bearded dragons (although feeding crickets was acceptable in moderation and to eliminate feeding pinkie mice). The excess protein in the diet may have contributed to the change in renal values. An ovariosalpingohysterectomy was recommended once the lizard regained normal health.

References

Carpenter JW. (ed), 2018. *Exotic Animal Formulary*, 5th edn. St. Louis: Elsevier Saunders, p.117.

Chang L, Fu D, Stenglein MD, Hernandez JA, DeRisi JL, Jacobson ER. 2016. Detection and prevalence of boid inclusion body disease in collections of boas and pythons using immunological assays. *Vet J* 218:13–18.

Chang L, Fu A, Wozniak E, et al. 2013. Immunohistochemical detection of a unique protein within cells of snakes having inclusion body disease, a world-wide disease seen in members of the families boidae and pythonidae. *PLOS One* 8(12):e82916.

Divers SJ, Innis CJ. 2019. Urology. In: Divers SJ, Stahl SJ (eds), *Mader's Reptile and Amphibian Medicine and Surgery*, 3rd edn. St. Louis, MO: Elsevier, pp. 624–648.

Ellman MM. 2019. Hematology and plasma chemistry of the inland bearded dragon, *Pogona vitticeps*. *ARAV* 7(4):10–12.

Gibbons PM, Whitaker BR, Carpenter JW, et al. 2019. Hematology and biochemistry tables. In: Divers SJ, Stahl SJ (eds), *Mader's Reptile and Amphibian Medicine and Surgery*, 3rd edn. St. Louis, MO: Elsevier, pp. 333–350.

Heckers KO, Aupperle H, Schmidt V, Pees M. 2012. Melanophoromas and iridophoromas in Reptiles. *J Comp Pathol* 146:258–268.

Knotek Z, Divers SJ. 2019. Pulmonology. In: Divers SJ, Stahl SJ (eds), *Mader's Reptile and Amphibian Medicine and Surgery*, 3rd edn. St. Louis, MO: Elsevier, pp. 786–804.

Marschang RE. 2019. Virology. In: Divers SJ, Stahl SJ (eds), *Mader's Reptile and Amphibian Medicine and Surgery*, 3rd edn. St. Louis, MO: Elsevier, pp. 247–269.

Martinez-Silvestre A. 1995. Treatment with allopurinol and probenecid for visceral gout in a Greek tortoise, *Testudo graeca*. *ARAV*, 7(4):4–5.

Maas AK. 2014. Considerations and conditions involving protozoal inhabitation of the reptilian gastrointestinal tract. *Vet Clin Exot Anim* 17:263–297.

McNulty E, Hoffman R. 1995. Fibrosarcoma in a corn snake, *Elaphe guttata*. *ARAV*, 5(3):7–8.

Munoz-Gutierrez F, Garner MM, Kiupel M. 2016. Cutaneous chromatophoromas in captive snakes. *Vet Pathol* 53(6):1213–1219.

Ramsay EC, Munson L, Lowenstine L, Fowler ME. 1996. A retrospective study of neopasia in a collection of captive snakes. *J Zoo Wildl Med* 27(1):28–34.

Rodriguez CE, Duque AMH, Steinberg J, Woodburn DB. 2018. Chelonia. In: Terio KA, McAloose D, St. Leger J (eds), *Pathology of Wildlife and Zoo* Animals. London, UK: Academic Press, pp. 819–847.

22 Sample Collection for Herptile Cytodiagnosis

It will be helpful to review cytology sampling and evaluation techniques for mammals in Chapter 6 and avian patients in Chapter 14 before reading this chapter.

Sample Locations

Alimentary Tract

Cytological examination of smears made from a swab or scraping of a lesion in the oral cavity will often prove the presumptive or definitive diagnosis (Figure 22.1). Masses found in the oral cavity can be aspirated or excised to obtain a cytological sample (Figure 22.2). An oral speculum should be used in animals capable of biting and breaking the swab.

A cytological sample of the esophagus can be obtained by passing a sterile cotton swab through the oral cavity into the esophageal lumen (an oral speculum should be used in animals capable of biting and breaking the swab). A cytological sample can also be obtained by a touch imprint of a biopsy sample or a brush cytological preparation.

Sampling of the reptile stomach for cytological evaluation can be obtained by inserting a swab, such as an equine uterine culture swab, into the stomach (Bogan, 2019). Cytological evaluation of the stomach and intestines is complicated by the presence of many bacteria and much cell debris. Samples are also obtained via gastric washes, endoscopy, or exploratory surgery (Figures 22.3a and 22.3b).

Cloacal cytology and microbiology are often a part of the routine physical examination of the reptilian patient. Cloacal samples are easily obtained by inserting

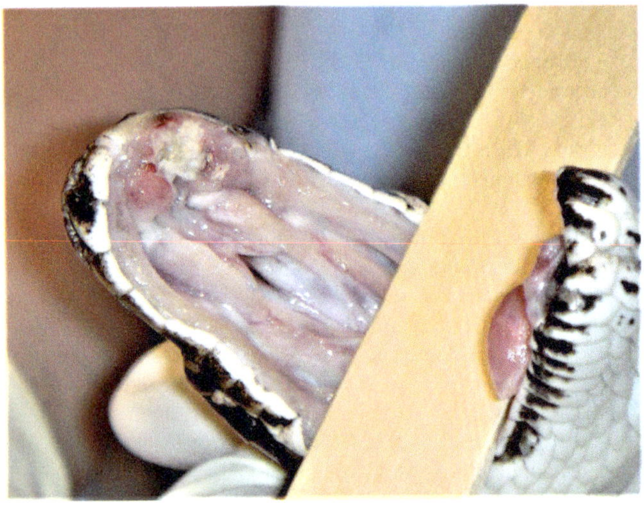

Fig. 22.1. Samples for cytological examination of lesions in the oral cavity can be obtained from a swab or scraping.

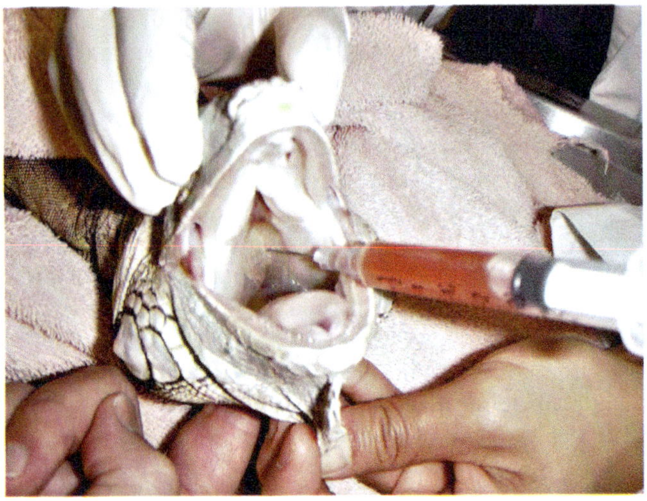

Fig. 22.2. Aspiration of a pharyngeal cyst in a green iguana (*Iguana iguana*) for cytological examination.

Exotic Animal Hematology and Cytology, Fifth Edition. Terry W. Campbell and Krystan R. Grant.

Companion website: www.wiley.com/go/campbell/exotic

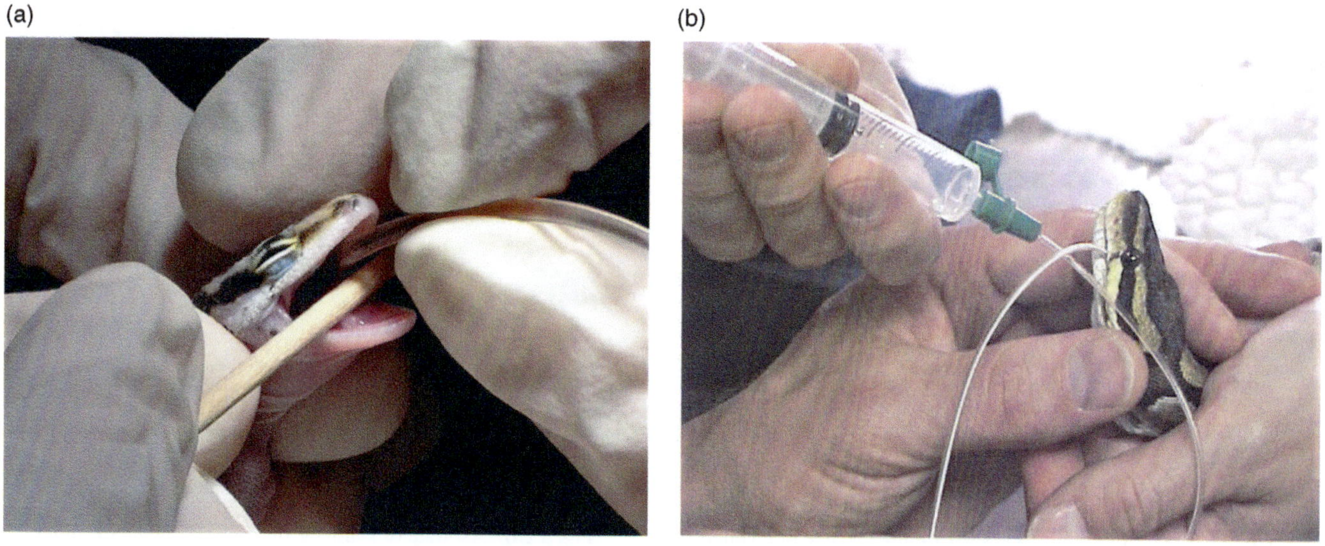

Fig. 22.3. (a) Gastric wash in a lizard for cytological evaluation of the stomach content. (b) Gastric wash in a snake for cytological evaluation of the stomach content.

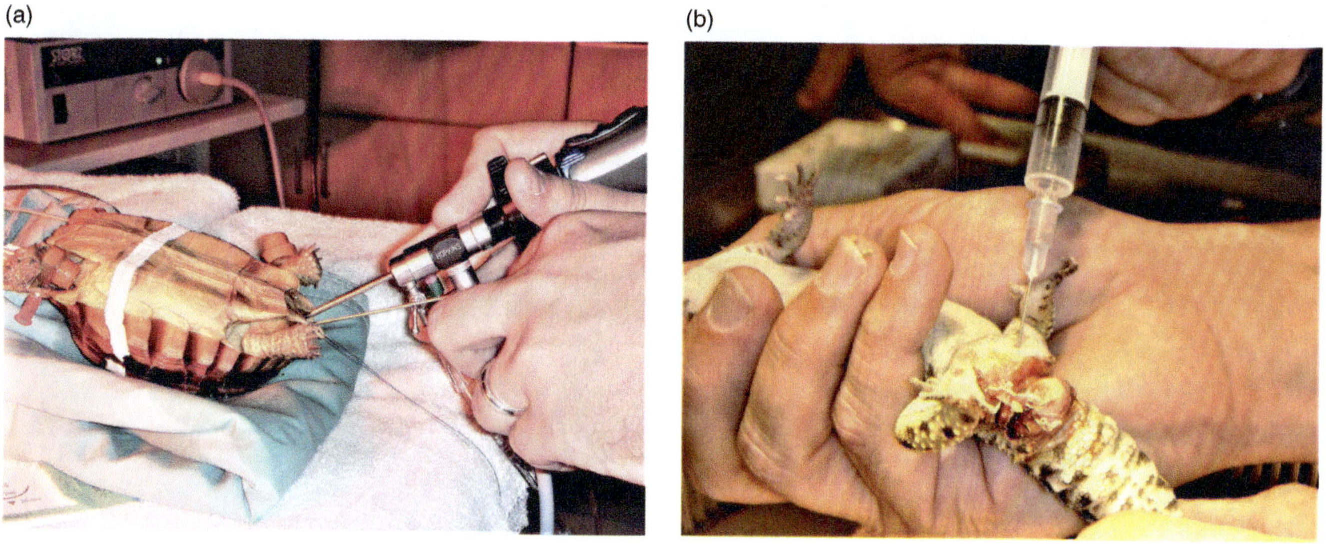

Fig. 22.4. (a) Use of a rigid endoscope to visual a cloacal mass and biopsy forceps to obtain a sample for cytologic examination in a chelonian. (b) Fine-needle aspiration biopsy of a cloacal mass in a lizard for cytologic examination.

a sterile, saline-moistened, cotton-tipped swab into the cloaca. Fine-needle aspiration biopsy of solid masses or contact films made from excised masses often provide useful cytological samples (Figures 22.4a and 22.4b).

Respiratory Tract

A choanal swab is used as a sampling technique in the cytological diagnosis of upper respiratory disease in herptiles. The mouth of some reptiles with powerful biting capability is held open using an oral speculum, taking care not to damage the teeth and gingiva. A cotton-tip applicator is used to swab the nasopharynx dorsal to the choanal slit, taking care not to touch other areas of the oral cavity. The swab is rolled onto a glass slide. Often, cells from the oral cavity contaminate the sample. The nasal or sinus flush technique described for an avian patient can also be used to sample the choanal area of a reptile.

Respiratory tract infections in reptiles are often diagnosed from tracheal wash samples using techniques described for the avian patient. Lung washes and aspirates are commonly performed on reptile patients, especially snakes, with lung disease. The procedure is performed in the same manner as a tracheal wash, except that the tube is advanced into the lung.

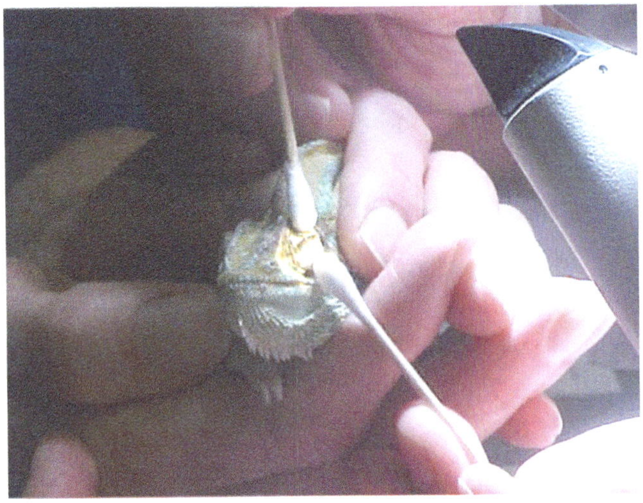

Fig. 22.5. Use of cotton swabs to examine the eye of a veiled chameleon (*Chamaeleo calyptratus*). An ophthalmic swab can be used to collect material for cytologic examination.

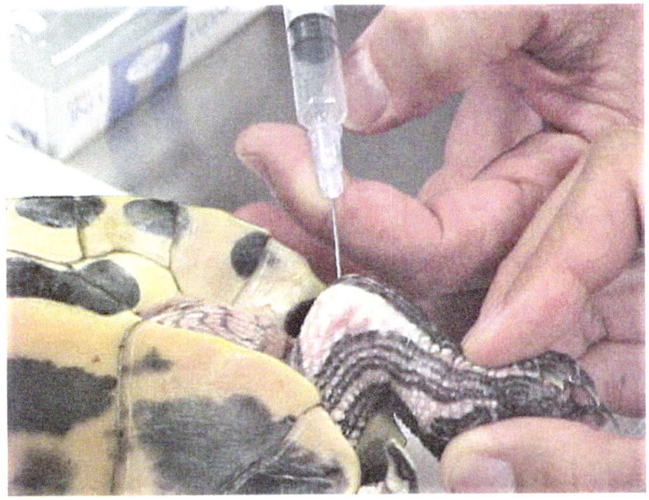

Fig. 22.6. Aspirate of synovial fluid for cytologic examination in a chelonian.

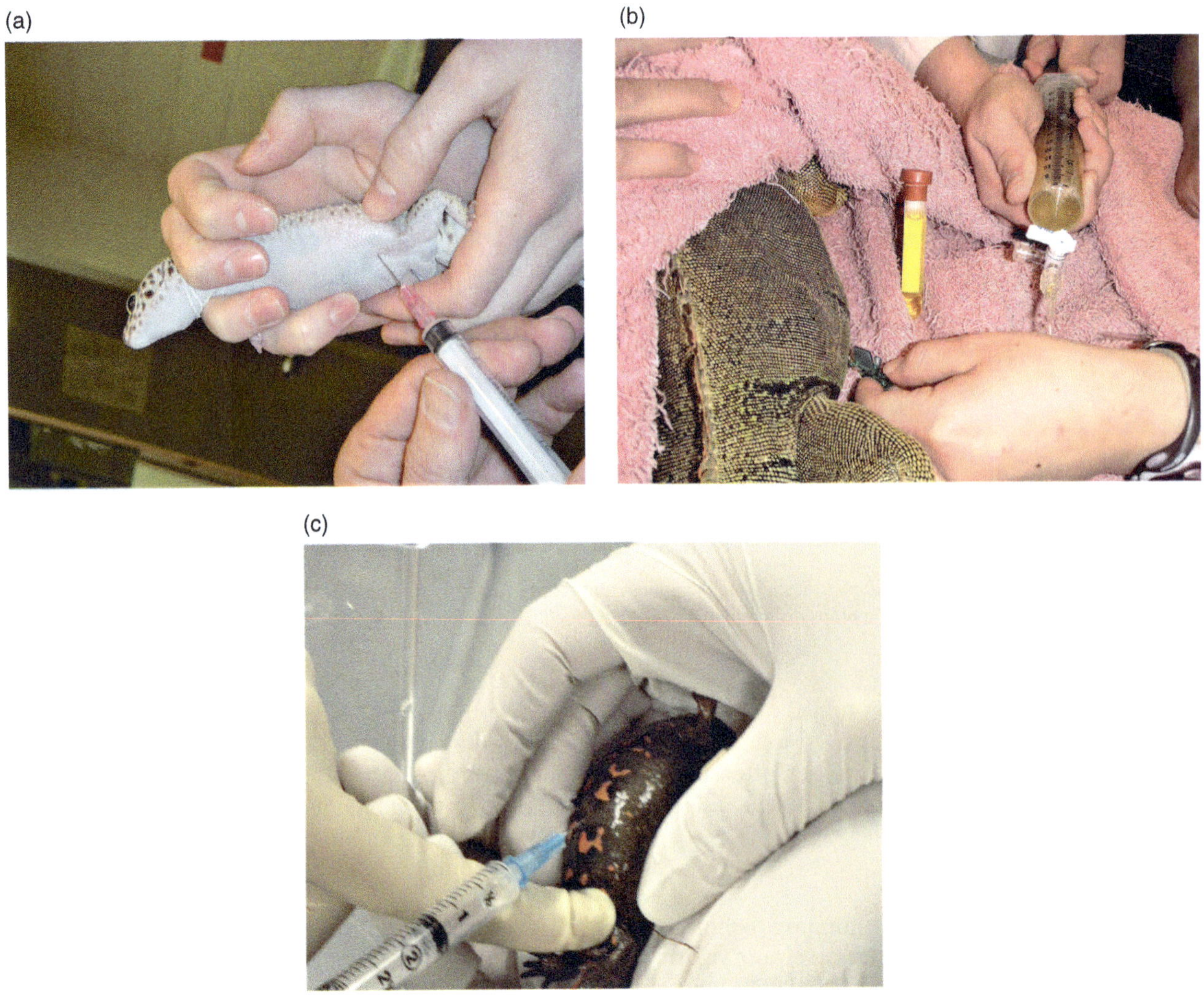

Fig. 22.7. (a) Celiocentesis in a leopard gecko (*Eublepharis macularius*); note the paramedian approach to avoid the abdominal vein that lies along the ventral midline. (b) Celiocentesis in a green iguana (*Iguana iguana*) using extension tubing to keep the needle stable while aspiration a large volume of fluid. (c) Celiocentesis in a fire belly newt (*Cynops pyrrhogaster*).

Conjunctiva and Cornea

Cytological samples of the conjunctiva of herptiles can be obtained using identical procedures used in domestic mammal and avian medicine. Corneal cytology is indicated in superficial erosions and progressive ulceration associated with infiltrations of inflammatory cells. To obtain a sample for cytology, a topical anesthetic is instilled (1 or 2 drops), and after 60 s the sample is taken by gentle scraping or use of an ophthalmic swab (Figure 22.5). It is important to remember that a topical anesthetic may cause systemic toxicity and even general anesthesia in some herptile patients.

Synovial Fluid

Normally, the joints of reptiles and amphibians contain a fluid volume that is too small for sampling or proper evaluation; however, fluid distension of a joint may occur with certain arthropathies, allowing for collection of enough synovial fluid for evaluation. To collect synovial fluid, the skin over the joint at the sampling site is prepared using aseptic techniques as one would use for surgery. A 22-gauge (or smaller) needle and syringe (usually a 3-cc syringe) is used to aspirate the synovial fluid sample (Figure 22.6). Identification of the best site for needle insertion is made by palpation and flexion of the joint. The needle is inserted through the joint capsule, and fluid is withdrawn into the syringe once the joint cavity has been entered. Negative pressure in the syringe should be removed by releasing the plunger before removing the needle from the joint. The sample is then used to prepare direct films using glass microscope slides for microscopic evaluation and fluid analysis if enough sample is obtained, as described in Chapter 6.

Coelomic Fluid

Fluid in the coelomic cavity of reptiles and amphibians can be simply aspirated by inserting the needle through the skin and body wall along the ventral aspect of the animal. A paramedian approach should be made to avoid the abdominal vein that lies along the ventral midline (Figures 22.7a–22.7c). Fluid in the peritoneal cavity of chelonians can be sampled by inserting the needle through the body wall in the inguinal area just in front of a hind leg.

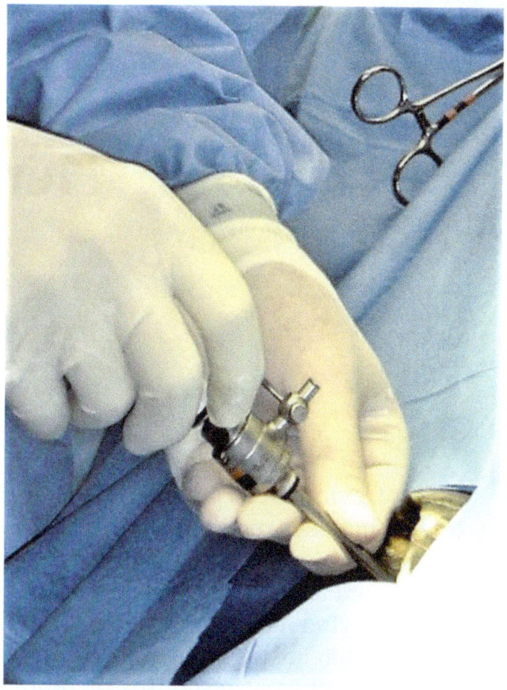

Fig. 22.8. Biopsy samples for cytologic examination of internal organs can be obtained endoscopically.

Coelomic Organs

In reptiles, biopsy samples for cytological and histologic examination of internal organs, such as the liver, spleen, and kidneys are routinely collected either surgically or endoscopically using fine-diameter (1–2.7 mm) rigid endoscopes (Figure 22.8). Visual assessment of coelomic organs is currently considered more successful than transcutaneous blind techniques due to the increased risk of iatrogenic trauma and hemorrhage associated with these procedures; however, a coelomic ultrasound-guided manual biopsy device can be used for sample collection (Nardini et al., 2016).

References

Bogan JE. 2019. An alternative technique for gastric sampling in snakes. *JHMS* 29(1–2):13–16.

Nardini G, Origgi FC, Leopardi S, et al. 2016. Preliminary evaluation of Spirotome® device for liver biopsy in Green iguanas (*Iguana iguana*): a pilot study. *J Zoo Wildl Med* 47(2):508–513.

23 Herptile Cytodiagnosis

Interpretation of cytological preparations from herptiles (a term that includes reptiles (of orders Testudines or Chelonia, Squamata, and Crocodilia) and amphibians (of orders Anura and Caudata)) is like that of birds; therefore, avian cytodiagnosis is a useful guideline for herptile cytodiagnosis. As with mammals and birds, the basic cytological responses of reptiles and amphibians can be classified as inflammation, tissue hyperplasia/benign neoplasia, malignant neoplasia, or normal cellularity. The inflammatory lesions can be classified as heterophilic, mixed cell (pyogranulomatous), macrophagic, or, rarely, eosinophilic based upon the predominant types of inflammatory cells in the sample.

Normal Cytology

The Digestive Tract

Normal exfoliation of the superficial cells of the epithelium lining the upper alimentary tract reveals normal, mature squamous epithelial cells (superficial and intermediate epithelial cells) (Figures 23.1a and 23.1b). These cells often exfoliate singly, are angular, polygonal in shape, contain a condensed pyknotic nucleus, and demonstrate varying degrees of cornification. The cells that are highly cornified typically possess angular or folded cytoplasmic margins and are typically anucleated.

The esophagus of reptiles contains ciliated cells and goblet cells. Intermediate squamous epithelial cells are

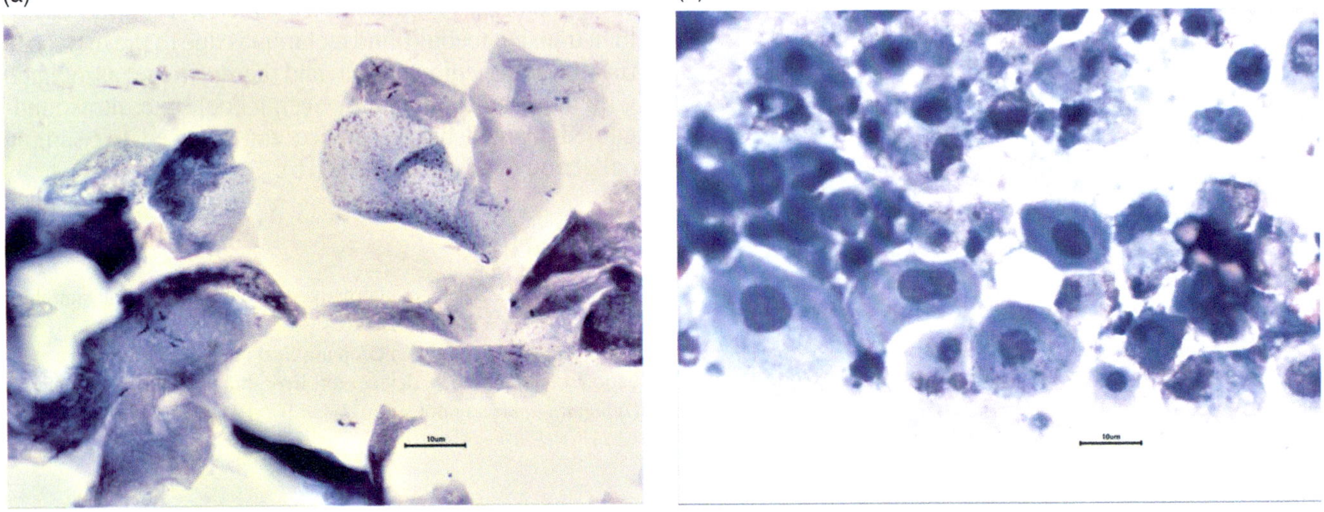

Fig. 23.1. (a) Mature cornified squamous epithelial cells from an oral cavity swab specimen from a water dragon (*Intellagama lesueurii*), Wright–Giemsa stain (100× oil). (b) Intermediate squamous epithelial cells from an oral cavity swab specimen from an emerald tree boa (*Corallus caninus*), Wright–Giemsa stain (100× oil).

Exotic Animal Hematology and Cytology, Fifth Edition. Terry W. Campbell and Krystan R. Grant.

Companion website: www.wiley.com/go/campbell/exotic

common in normal esophageal specimens. Intermediate squamous epithelial cells often occur in sheets and are oval to polygonal in shape, have a low N:C ratio, and possess an oval, centrally located vesicular nucleus with a finely granular chromatin (Figures 23.1b and 23.2). These cells typically do not have folded cytoplasmic margins. Basal cells may be seen in normal cytology samples if traumatic exfoliation occurs during sample collection. Basal cells are the cells that are normally found adjacent to the basement membrane and are smaller in size than intermediate cells. These cells are typically round and contain a deeply basophilic cytoplasm, eccentric nuclei, and a high N:C ratio.

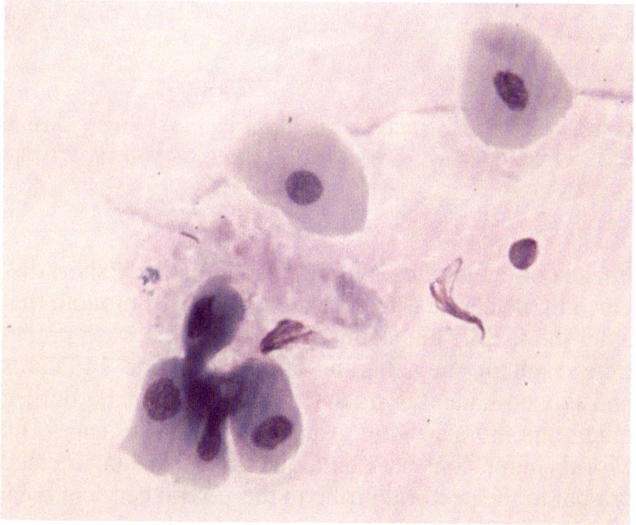

Fig. 23.2. Intermediate squamous epithelial cells from an esophageal swab specimen from a bearded dragon (*Pogona vitticeps*), Wright–Giemsa stain (100× oil).

Extracellular bacteria made up of a variety of morphological types are often associated with squamous epithelial cells in normal cytological samples from the upper alimentary tract. Additionally, a moderate amount of background debris and foreign material (e.g., plant fibers and other material entering the mouth) is often present in the samples obtained from the alimentary tract of animals.

The mucosa of the stomach is lined with columnar epithelial cells containing moderate amounts of lightly basophilic or eosinophilic cytoplasm and oval to round nuclei with dispersed chromatin (Figures 23.3a and 23.3b). Columnar epithelial cells tend to exfoliate in clusters of uniform-appearing cells.

The reptilian cloaca consists of three compartments: the coprodeum (the distal opening of the intestinal tract), the urodeum (the distal opening of the urinary and reproductive tracts), and the proctodeum (the common opening of the coprodeum and urodeum, which terminates at the vent). In birds, the cloacal bursa also opens into the proctodeum. The cloaca is lined by simple columnar epithelium and lymphoid tissue, and the vent is lined by cornified, stratified squamous epithelium (Figures 23.4a and 23.4b). If cells are present, there is a predominance of epithelial cells. Most of the epithelial cells from normal cloacal tissue appear as noncornified squamous or columnar epithelial cells with a centrally or eccentrically positioned vesicular nucleus. Basal epithelial cells may be seen on the films obtained by traumatic exfoliation. A variable quantity of bacteria made up of a wide variety of morphological types, rare flagellate protozoa and yeast, and background debris are also present in normal specimens. Urate crystals are commonly seen in normal cloacal and fecal samples as well (Figure 23.5).

(a) (b)

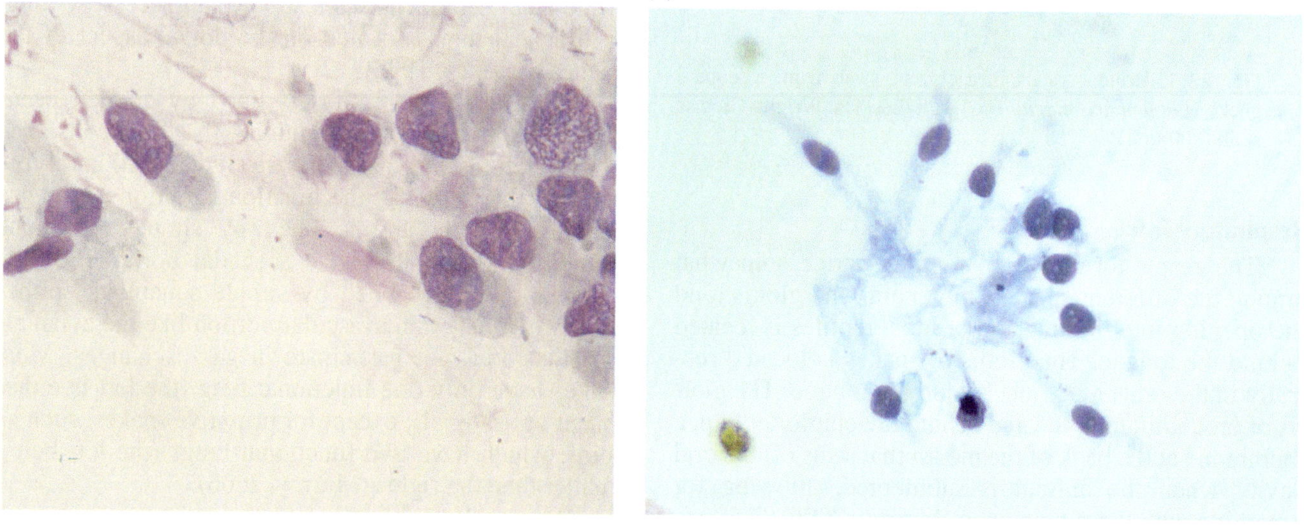

Fig. 23.3. (a) Gastric epithelial cells in a stomach wash specimen from a Common boa constrictor (*Boa constrictor*), Wright–Giemsa stain (100× oil). (b) Gastric epithelial cells in a stomach wash specimen from a Ball python (*Python regius*), Wright–Giemsa stain (100× oil).

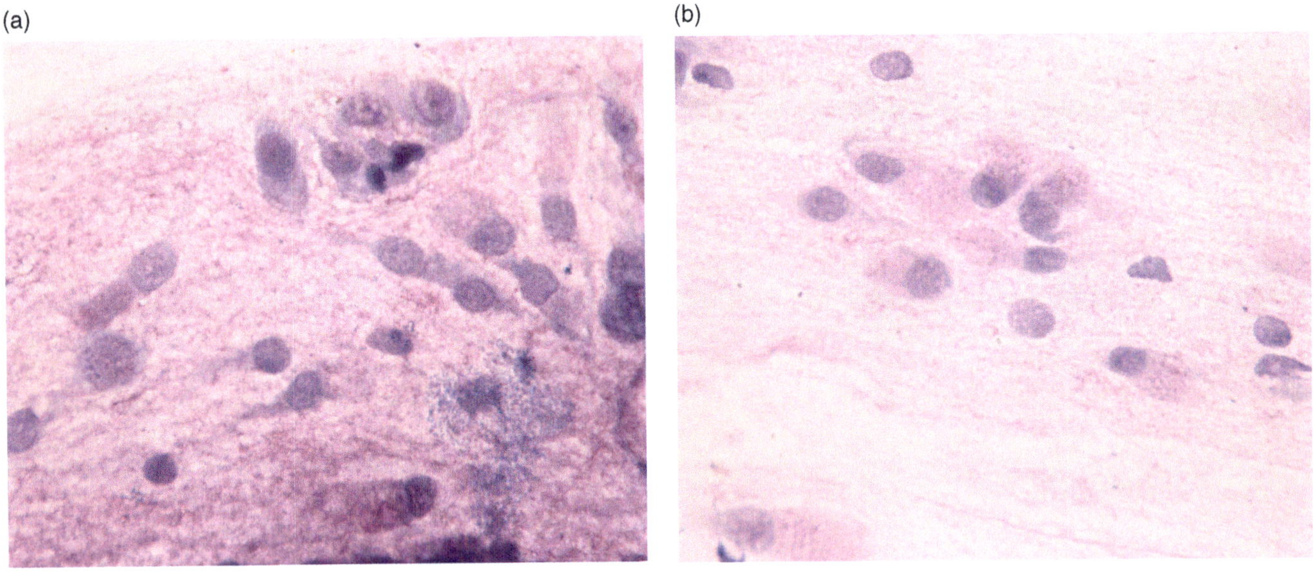

Fig. 23.4. (a) Columnar epithelial cells in a colon swab specimen from a veiled chameleon (*Chamaeleo calyptratus*), Wright–Giemsa stain (100× oil). (b) Columnar epithelial cells in a cloacal wash specimen from a Jackson's chameleon (*Trioceros jacksonii*), Wright–Giemsa stain (100× oil).

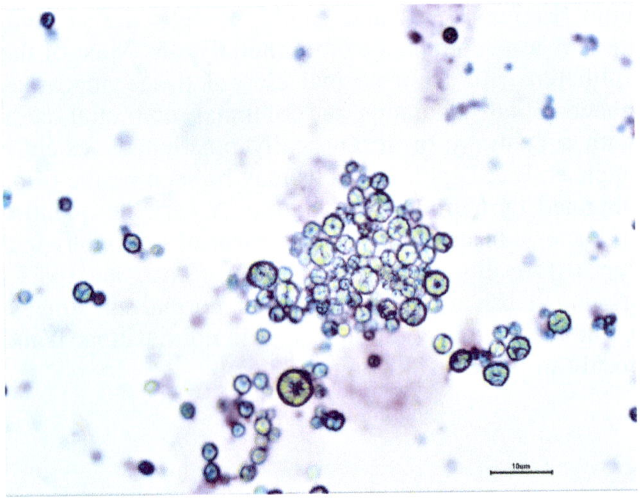

Fig. 23.5. Urate crystals in a cloacal swab from a leopard gecko (*Eublepharis macularius*) with diarrhea, Wright–Giemsa stain (100× oil).

Respiratory Tract

The respiratory tract of reptiles varies somewhat among the different species. In general, the glottis (and the opening into the trachea) of most reptiles is located behind the tongue. The glottis of snakes is located rostrally in the oral cavity just behind the tongue. The glottis of crocodilians is located behind the epiglottal flap, a membrane at the back of the mouth that seals off the oral cavity when the animal is submerged, allowing for breathing with the mouth open (Murray, 2006). The epiglottal flap must be pushed back to expose the glottis for tracheal or lung wash sampling in crocodilians. The trachea of chelonians bifurcates at a relatively short distance in the cervical region, creating paired bronchi that enter the saclike lungs; therefore, a tracheal wash procedure results in the sampling of only one side. In lizards and crocodilians, the trachea does not bifurcate until it enters the thoracic inlet near the base of the heart. Old World chameleons have a unique accessory lung located cranial to the pectoral girdle in the ventral cervical area. This accessory lung can be distended with inflammatory exudates that can be collected either by a tracheal wash, by an aspiration method with a tube entering near or in the accessory lung, or by direct aspiration by passing a needle through the overlying skin and into the accessory lung. The trachea of snakes enters the lung near the base of the heart. Some snakes also have an accessory lung, or "tracheal lung," located on the dorsal aspect of the trachea (Stoakes, 1992).

The trachea of reptiles is lined by ciliated pseudostratified columnar epithelium with goblet cells. The lungs of lizards and snakes have a cranial portion (alveolar lung) that serves as the functional portion where gas exchange occurs and is lined by simple squamous epithelium. They also have a caudal portion (saclike membranous lung) lined by simple squamous epithelium, which is a thin avascular portion like the avian air sacs that does not participate in gas exchanges. Most snakes have only one functional lung (the left is either absent or vestigial); except for primitive snakes, such as boids, which have two functional lungs (the left being smaller than the right) (Murray, 2006).

The samples collected from the respiratory system of normal healthy animals tend to be poorly cellular; however, when present, normal respiratory cells typically

cellular sample consisting of nonkeratinized squamous epithelial cells with central vesicular nuclei. Sampling of the cornea is not possible without removing part of the spectacle, a transparent membrane composed of the stratum corneum of the epidermis, in snakes and some lizards (Underwood, 1970). A section of the spectacle can be removed surgically to gain access to the cornea (Hernandez-Divers, 2006).

Other Tissues

The normal cytology of other tissues from reptiles resembles that described for birds. For example, the spleen is one of the largest single masses of lymphoid tissue in the body (Figure 23.9).

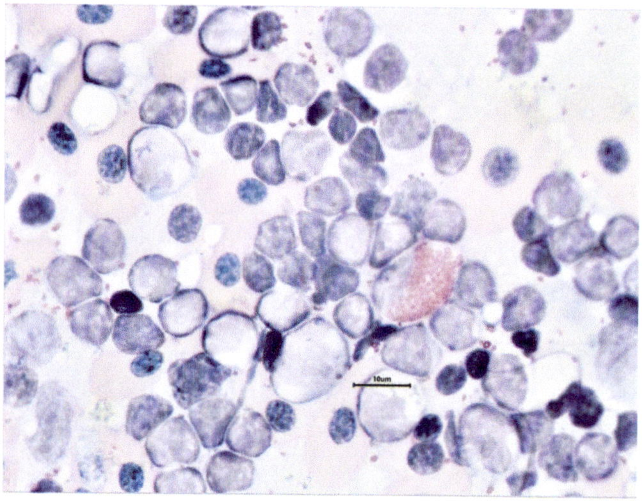

Fig. 23.9. Splenic imprint from a common snapping turtle (*Chelydra serpentina*) showing a predominance of small mature lymphocytes with medium and large lymphocytes, Wright–Giemsa stain (100× oil).

Inflammation

Inflammation occurs with the release of chemotactic factors commonly created by microbes and their toxins, physical and chemical trauma, death of cells from circulatory insufficiency, and immune reactions. The rate of the inflammatory response is temperature dependent in poikilotherms, such as reptiles and amphibians; whereas, the rate of response in endotherms, such as mammals and birds, is more consistent and predictable.

Heterophilic/Neutrophilic Inflammation

Heterophilic inflammation of reptiles is represented by a predominance of heterophils (greater than 80% of the inflammatory cells) in the cytological sample (Figure 23.10). Heterophil granules in cytological specimens tend to lose their normal rod-shaped appearance and either appear more rounded or degranulated (Campbell and Grant, 2010). As with birds, a heterophilic inflammation likely indicates an acute phase of the inflammatory response in the reptile.

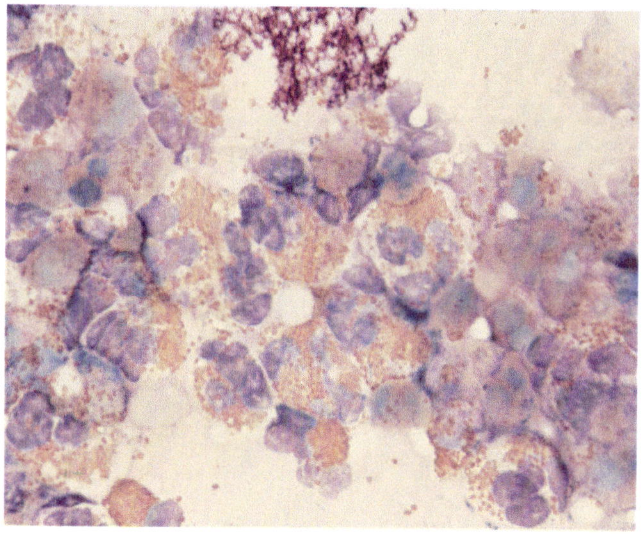

Fig. 23.10. Heterophilic inflammation in a green iguana (*Iguana iguana*), Wright–Giemsa stain (100× oil).

Amphibians with circulating neutrophils instead of heterophils will demonstrate a neutrophilic inflammation instead of a heterophilic inflammation as seen in reptiles.

Heterophilic or neutrophilic inflammation is classified by the presence or absence of degeneration of these granulocytes. Degenerate heterophils, as with degenerate mammalian neutrophils or degenerate avian heterophils, likely represent rapid cell death and suggest the presence of toxins, such as bacterial toxins, in the microenvironment (Figure 23.11a and 23.11b). Close examination of the heterophils for infectious agents should be made when this type of inflammation is present. Septic lesions caused by pathogenic bacteria are often responsible for heterophilic inflammation; however, fungal agents may also cause heterophilic granulomas associated with degenerate and nondegenerate heterophils (Figures 23.12–23.15). Heterophilic inflammation can also be associated with noninfectious agents, such as foreign material.

Mixed-Cell Inflammation

Mixed-cell inflammation is the most commonly encountered type of inflammatory response of herptiles and indicates an established, active inflammatory lesion (originally known as chronic active inflammation). Mixed-cell inflammation is typically represented by a predominance of heterophils or neutrophils (greater than 50% of the inflammatory cells) with an increased number of mononuclear leukocytes (Figures 23.16a–23.16e).

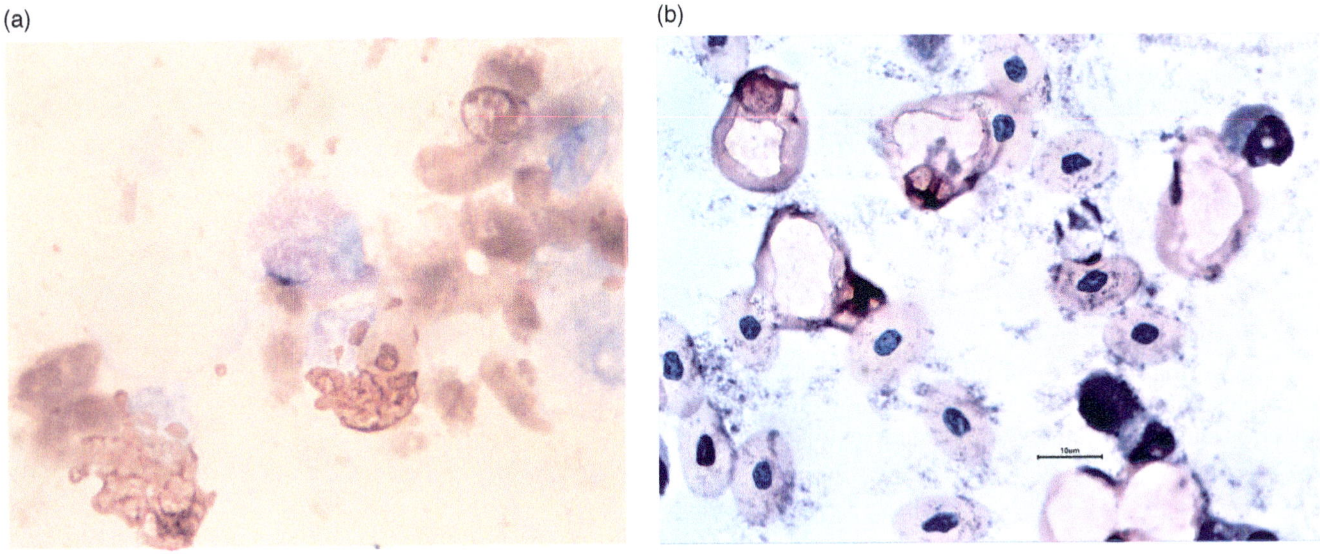

Fig. 23.11. (a) Degenerate heterophils from an abscess in a leopard gecko (*Eublepharis macularius*), Wright–Giemsa stain (100× oil). (b) Degenerate heterophils from an abscess in a hognose snake (*Heterodon platirhinos*), Wright–Giemsa stain (100× oil).

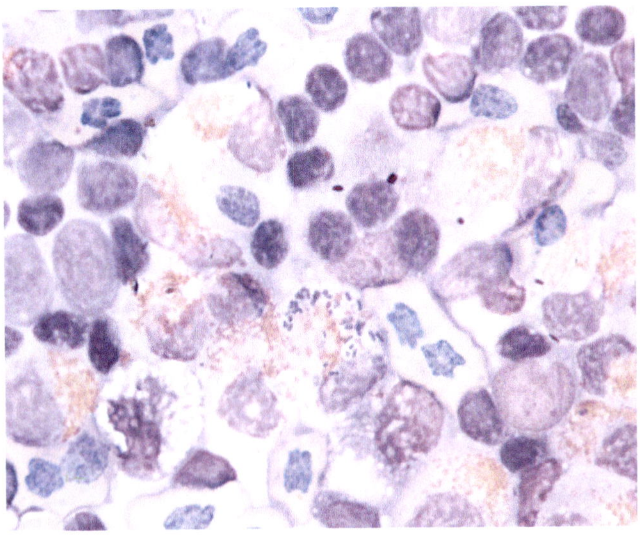

Fig. 23.12. Septic heterophilic inflammation in a splenic imprint from a green iguana (*Iguana iguana*), Wright–Giemsa stain (100× oil).

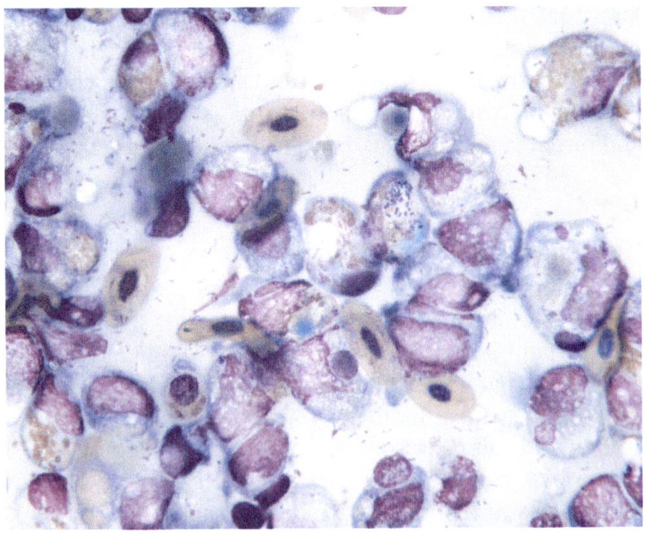

Fig. 23.13. Septic heterophilic inflammation in a leopard gecko (*Eublepharis macularius*), Wright–Giemsa stain (100× oil).

Heterophils and neutrophils in mixed-cell inflammatory lesions are usually normal and nondegenerate in appearance. Lymphocytes and plasma cells are often associated with acute neutrophilic/heterophilic granulomas, whereas the presence of epithelioid cells (macrophages that contain no vacuoles or phagocytized material) and connective tissue cells (i.e., fibroblasts) suggests chronic granulomas. Frequently, the epithelial and mesenchymal cells adjacent to inflammatory lesions proliferate, resulting in the presence of these cell type demonstrating features of tissue hyperplasia (Figures 23.17a and 23.17b). This type of inflammatory response is commonly observed with a variety of infectious (i.e., bacterial and fungal) and noninfectious (i.e., traumatic and foreign body) etiologies.

Lymphocytic and plasmacytic infiltration is indicated by increased numbers of lymphocytes and plasma cells in the cellular response (Figures 23.18a, 23.18b and 23.19). Conditions that are often associated with this type of cellular response include early viral infections, immune-mediated disorders, and chronic inflammation. Infection with *Mycoplasma* spp. is often associated with lymphoplasmacytic inflammation. The lymphocyte population is composed of small and intermediate-sized mature lymphocytes and plasma cells.

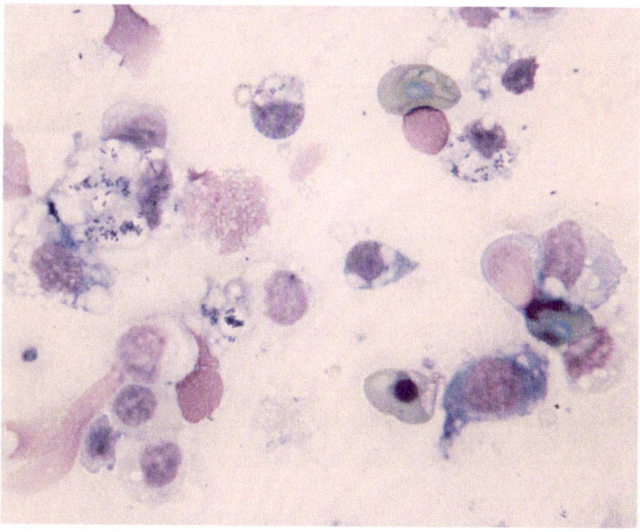

Fig. 23.14. Septic inflammation in a White's tree frog (*Litoria caerulea*), Wright–Giemsa stain (100× oil).

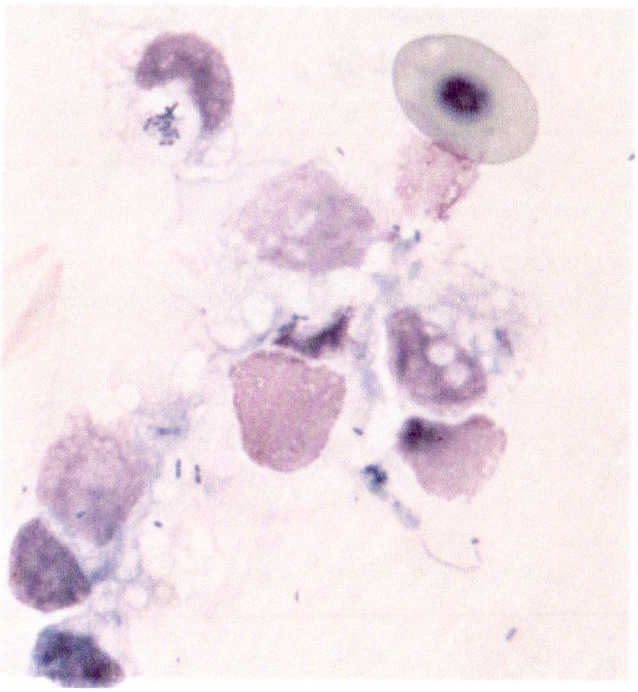

Fig. 23.15. Septic inflammation in a Woodhouse toad (*Bufo woodhousii*), Wright–Giemsa stain (100× oil).

Macrophagic Inflammation

Macrophagic (histiocytic or granulomatous) inflammation consists primarily of macrophages with multinucleated giant cells and lesser numbers of other inflammatory cells (Figures 23.20a and 23.20b). This type of inflammation can be associated with chronic inflammatory disease or certain diseases, such as infections caused by mycobacteria and tissue-invading metazoan parasites. Multinucleated giant cells are often associated with macrophagic inflammation in reptiles and can appear within hours of the onset of certain inflammatory diseases, and therefore their presence does not necessarily imply chronicity (Figure 23.21a and 23.21b).

Melanomacrophages are melanin-synthesizing mononuclear phagocytes that can be seen in cytological preparations of the liver, spleen, kidney, and sites of chronic inflammation in reptiles and amphibians (Pessier, 2007; Stacy and Pessier, 2007; Stacy et al., 2007) (Figures 23.22a and 23.22b). They are also found in peripheral blood films, where they are reported as macrophages because not only do they contain intracytoplasmic melanin pigment granules, but also sometimes debris, infectious agents, or hemosiderin (Origgi, 2007; Stacy et al., 2017). Healthy chelonians exhibit greater numbers of melanomacrophages in their tissues compared to other reptiles, and these aggregates of melanomacrophages (termed melanomacrophage centers) become hyperplastic with chronic inflammation, infection, and other chronic conditions, such as cachexia or stress (Stacy et al., 2017). Their numbers also exhibit seasonal variation.

Melanomacrophages are derived from hematopoietic cells progenitors, whereas melanocytes originate from the neural crest (Colombo et al., 2011). Melanin present in several types of cells is the final product of the prophenoloxidase activation system and plays a central role in the main defense system of insects and invertebrates against microorganisms (Mackintosh, 2001).

In general, macrophages, including melanomacrophages, participate in cell turnover by removing apoptotic cells from the cellular environment through phagocytosis (clearance), and by secreting growth factors (Geissmann et al., 2010). Melanomacrophages play a role in the control of circulating basophils (promelanogenic cells), the turnover of liver collagen stroma, and the clearance of senescent erythrocytes (Wynn and Barron, 2010). Basophil engulfment has the added benefit of preventing unwanted inflammations in the liver, limiting melanogenesis, and providing protect against the development of allergic diseases and systemic anaphylaxis (Gutierre et al., 2018).

Cells and microorganisms phagocytized by melanomacrophages are neutralized by free radicals and antimicrobial compounds (Stacy and Pessier, 2007). Because melanomacrophages can contain a variety of pigments, additional special stains are often needed to identify the cytoplasmic inclusions in the microscopic evaluation (Stacy et al., 2017).

Inflammatory Lesions of the Alimentary Tract

Inflammatory lesions involving the upper alimentary tract (i.e., stomatitis and esophagitis) can be caused by traumatic injury, foreign bodies, chemical irritation, and infectious agents. The cytology reveals an increased

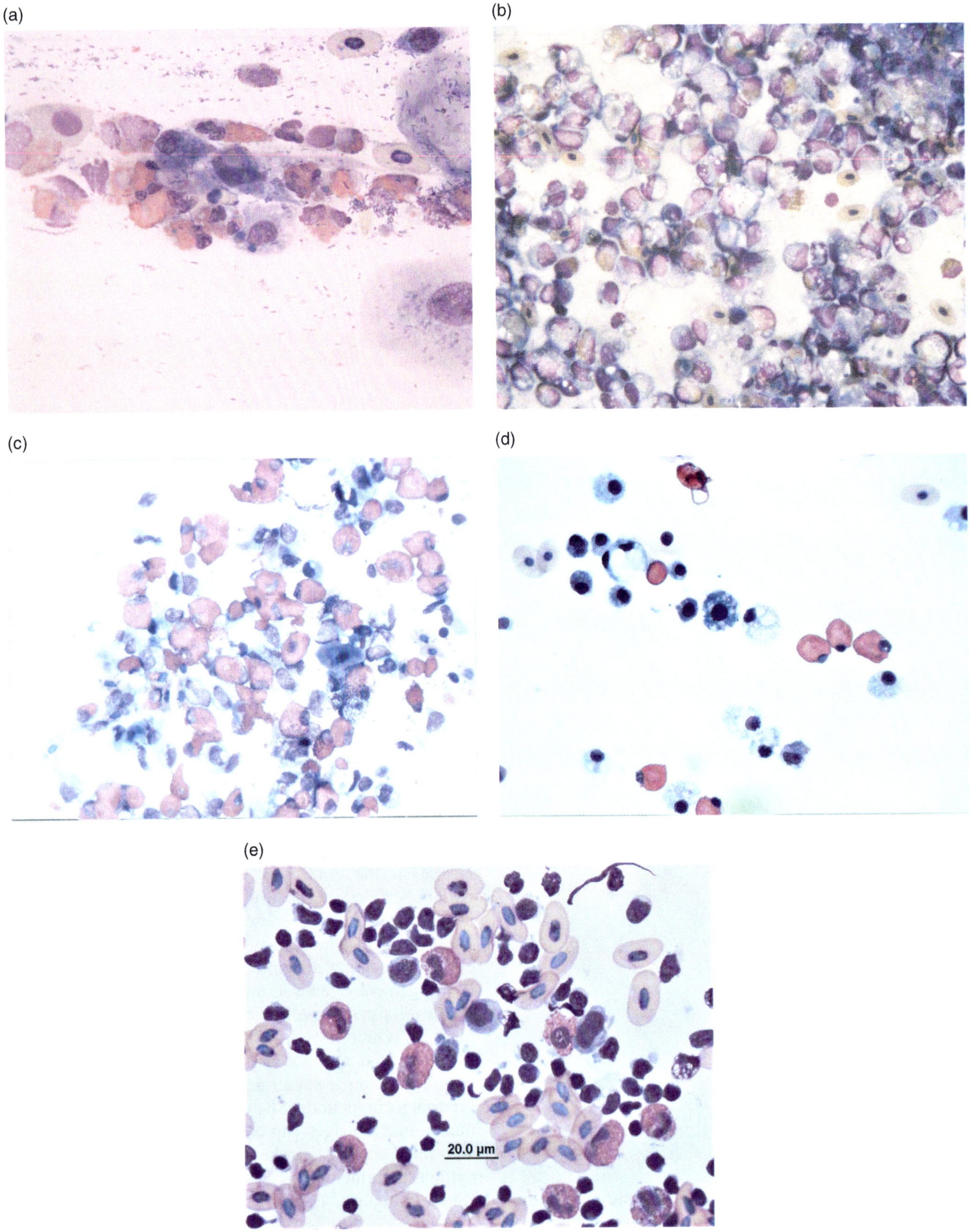

Fig. 23.16. (a) Mixed-cell inflammation in the oral cavity of a water dragon (*Intellagama lesueurii*), Wright–Giemsa stain (100× oil). (b) Septic mixed-cell inflammation in fine-needle aspiration biopsy of a vent abscess from a leopard gecko (*Eublepharis macularius*), Wright–Giemsa stain (40×). (c) Mixed-cell inflammation in a ball python (*Python regius*) with dermatitis, Wright–Giemsa stain (100× oil). (d) Mixed-cell inflammation in an oral swab from a common boa constrictor (*Boa constrictor*) with stomatitis, Wright–Giemsa stain (100× oil). (e) Mixed-cell inflammation in fine-needle aspiration biopsy of a mandibular mass from a bearded dragon (*Pogona vitticeps*) with a protozoan granuloma, Wright–Giemsa stain (100× oil).

(a) (b)

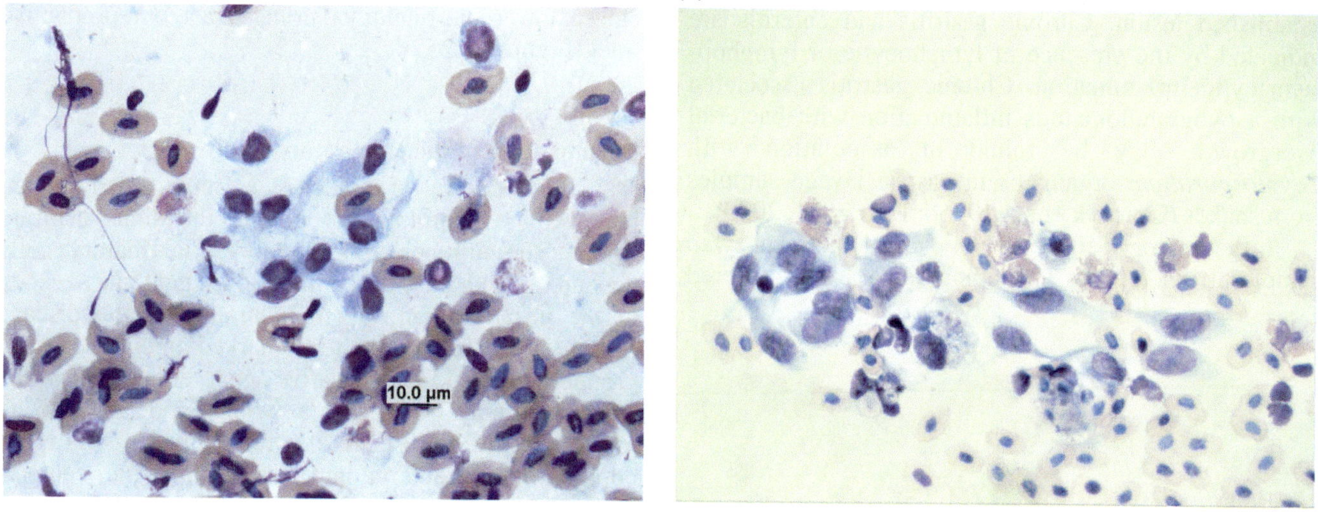

Fig. 23.17. (a) Fibroblasts in the aspirate from a protozoan granuloma from a bearded dragon (*Pogona vitticeps*), Wright–Giemsa stain (100× oil). (b) Fibroblasts in the aspirate from an inflammatory polyp in the oral cavity of green iguana (*Iguana iguana*), Wright–Giemsa stain (100× oil).

(a) (b)

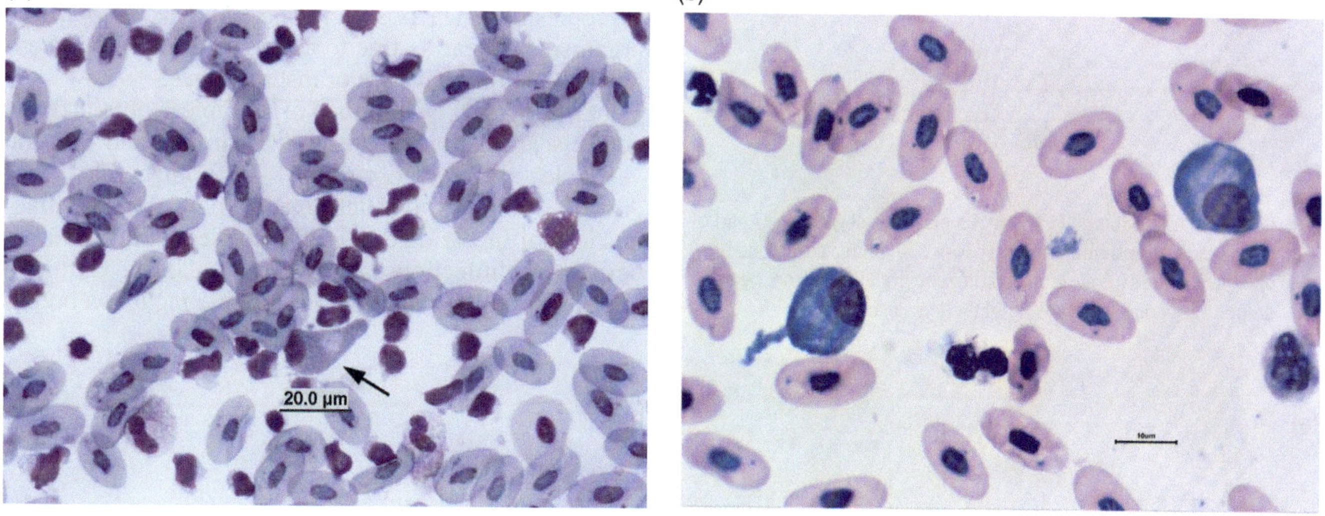

Fig. 23.18. (a) A plasma cell (arrow) as part of the mixed-cell inflammatory response containing numerous lymphocytes in the aspirate from a protozoan granuloma from a bearded dragon (*Pogona vitticeps*), Wright–Giemsa stain (100× oil). (b) Plasma cells in a lung imprint from a Burmese python (*Python bivittatus*) with pneumonia, Wright–Giemsa stain (100× oil).

number of inflammatory cells and a variable number of squamous epithelial cells. Septic lesions reveal inflammatory cells (heterophilic or mixed-cell inflammation) containing intracytoplasmic bacteria (either primary or secondary pathogens) and may contain degenerate leukocytes (primarily neutrophils/heterophils).

Caseous lesions are also found in the oropharynx of reptiles and are usually associated with bacterial infections; however, the other etiologies described in avian cytodiagnosis may be involved as well. Cytology can be useful in the differentiation of these diseases. Infectious stomatitis is a common disorder of reptiles, especially snakes, and is often associated with a mixed infection of bacteria (Figures 23.23a–23.23c and 23.24a–23.24c). Fungal pathogens can also be a cause of stomatitis in reptiles (Cheatwood et al., 2003).

Branchial cysts are rare congenital anomalies in reptiles, but should be included in the differential diagnoses for neck masses (Cloup et. al., 2019). An inflammatory response may occur due to leakage of fluid from the cyst lumen, and cytological examination may reveal squamous to non-ciliated columnar epithelial cells, inflammatory cells, and bacteria.

Gastritis and enteritis are indicated by the presence of inflammatory cells along with bacteria and cell debris. Acute inflammatory lesions exhibit primarily heterophils. A mixed-cell inflammation indicates an established lesion. Chronic gastritis and enteritis are indicated by the presence of lymphocytic or lymphoplasmacytic inflammation. Chronic gastritis associated with a pyogranulomatous inflammation with bacterial overgrowth may be found in association with *Cryptosporidium* organisms in gastric lavage samples from snakes (Graczyk et al., 1996b; Harr et al., 2000).

Inflammatory cells found on cloacal and fecal swab samples from reptiles and amphibians are considered abnormal and reflect an inflammatory lesion involving the cloaca, lower intestinal tract, urinary tract, or reproductive tract (Figure 23.25).

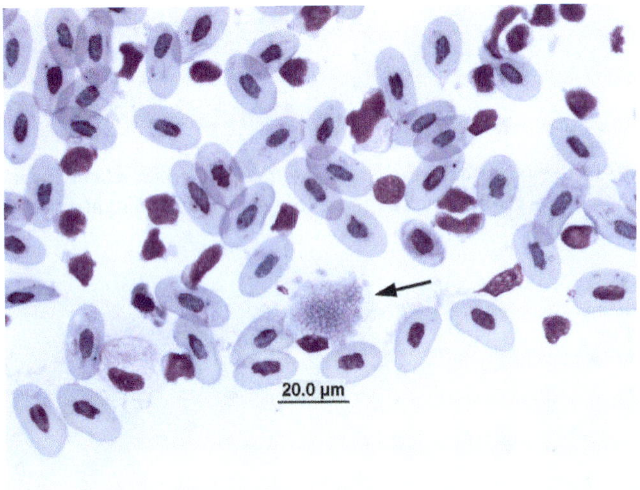

Fig. 23.19. A Mott cell variant of a plasma cell (arrow) as part of the mixed-cell inflammatory response containing numerous lymphocytes in the aspirate from a protozoan granuloma from bearded dragon (*Pogona vitticeps*), Wright–Giemsa stain (100× oil).

Inflammation of the Respiratory Tract

The cytology of sinusitis is represented by an increase in inflammatory cells in the sinus aspirate smear. The number and type of inflammatory cells depend on the nature of the infectious agent, the severity of the inflammation, and the duration of the disease (Figure 23.26). A moderate to marked amount of background debris and the causative agent, either primary or secondary, may be present as well. Septic sinusitis is indicated by the presence of a relatively monomorphic population of bacteria and intracytoplasmic bacteria within leukocytes (typically neutrophils or heterophils). Bacterial sinusitis may not reveal the microorganisms on the cytology specimen; however, a positive culture would support the diagnosis.

Heterophilic inflammation is commonly found in the exudates from the nasal passages of tortoises with mycoplasmosis (Jacobson et al., 1991). The *Mycoplasma* organisms appear as fine to aggregated basophilic bodies within epithelial cells or macrophages.

Cytological evaluation of samples obtained by gentle scarification of the lingual surface and the oral vestibule using cytobrushing (Cytobrush Plus GT, Alcyon, France) was determined to be a valuable diagnostic tool in the detection of tortoises with testudinid herpesvirus infections (Vetere et al., 2021). Cytology samples reveal intranuclear acidophilic inclusion bodies

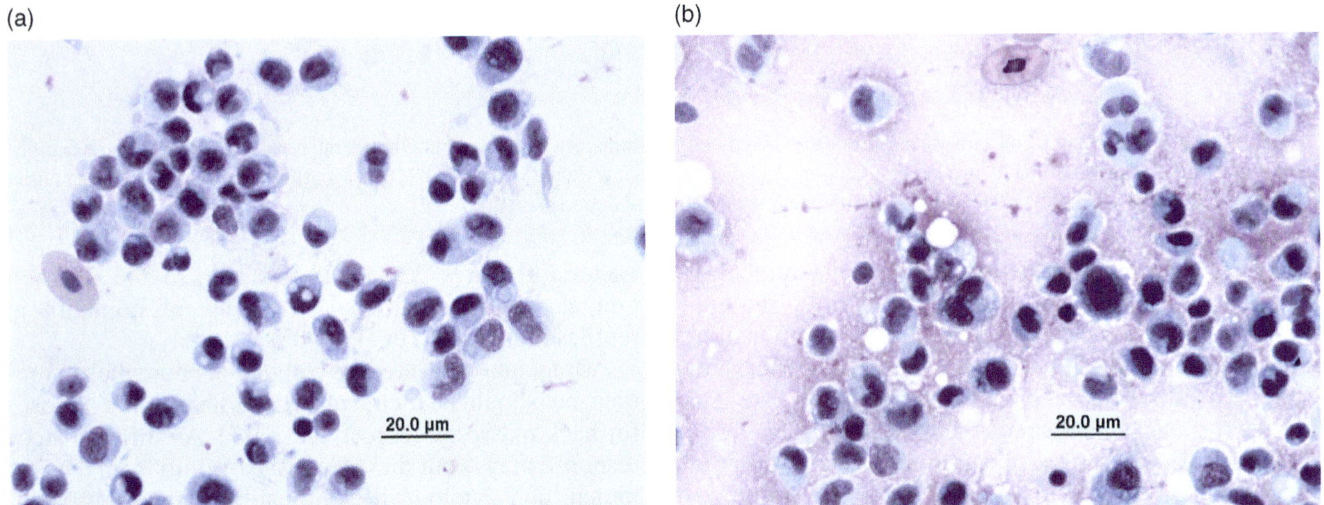

Fig. 23.20. (a) Macrophagic inflammation in an imprint from an ovary from a Ramsay's (or Woma) python (*Aspidites ramsayi*) with granulomatous oophoritis, Wright–Giemsa stain (100× oil). (b) Macrophagic inflammation in an ovary from a Ramsay's (or Woma) python (*Aspidites ramsayi*) with granulomatous oophoritis. The heavy eosinophilic background is associated with yolk material. Wright–Giemsa stain (100× oil).

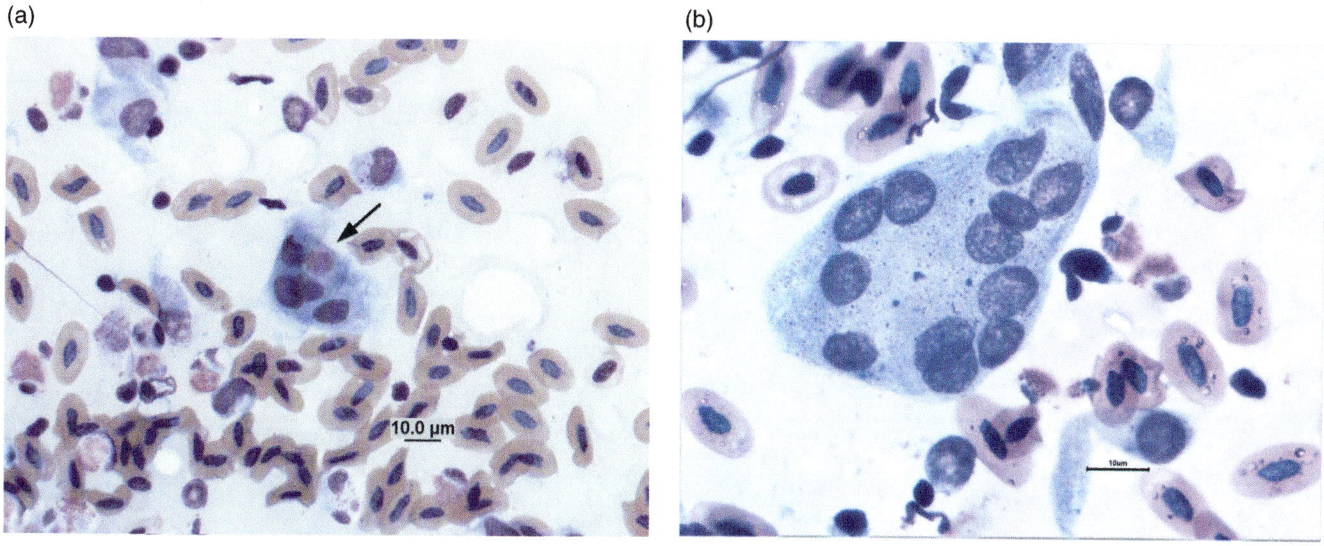

Fig. 23.21. (a) Multinucleated giant cell exhibiting leukophagocytosis (arrow) as part of the inflammatory response in a bearded dragon (*Pogona vitticeps*), Wright–Giemsa stain (100× oil). (b) Multinucleated giant cell in an imprint of a skin lesion associated with fungal dermatitis in a bearded dragon (*Pogona vitticeps*), Wright–Giemsa stain (100× oil).

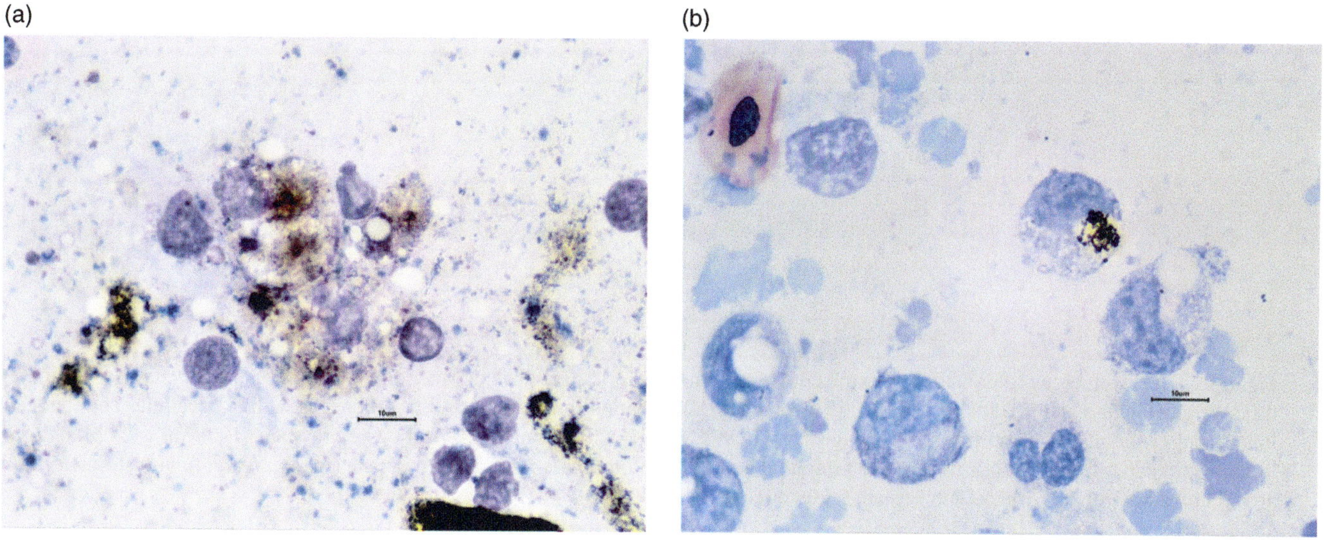

Fig. 23.22. (a) Melanomacrophages in a liver imprint from a green iguana (*Iguana iguana*), Wright–Giemsa stain (100× oil). (b) Melanomacrophage in an aspirate of an abscess in a poison dart frog (family Dendrobatidae), Wright–Giemsa stain (100× oil).

in the epithelial acantholytic cells, multinucleate cellular syncytia with chromatin margination, numerous bacteria (originating from the oral cavity), and heterophilic inflammation.

Along with the inflammatory response, severe infections of the respiratory tract may reveal degenerate ciliated respiratory epithelial cells. These cells exhibit losses of cilia, cytoplasmic vacuolation, cell lysis, and karyolysis (Figure 23.27). Septic lesions are confirmed by the presence of leukocyte phagocytosis of bacteria. Ulcerative lesions may show an increase in erythrocytes and cellular debris.

Lung washes of reptiles that exhibit many heterophils and macrophages, increased numbers of goblet cells, and increased mucin in the background indicate a tracheobronchitis or pneumonia. Heterophils are more predominant in acute lesions. When chronic inflammation is present, increased numbers of macrophages, lymphocytes, and plasma cells are present. Macrophages associated with chronic inflammation of

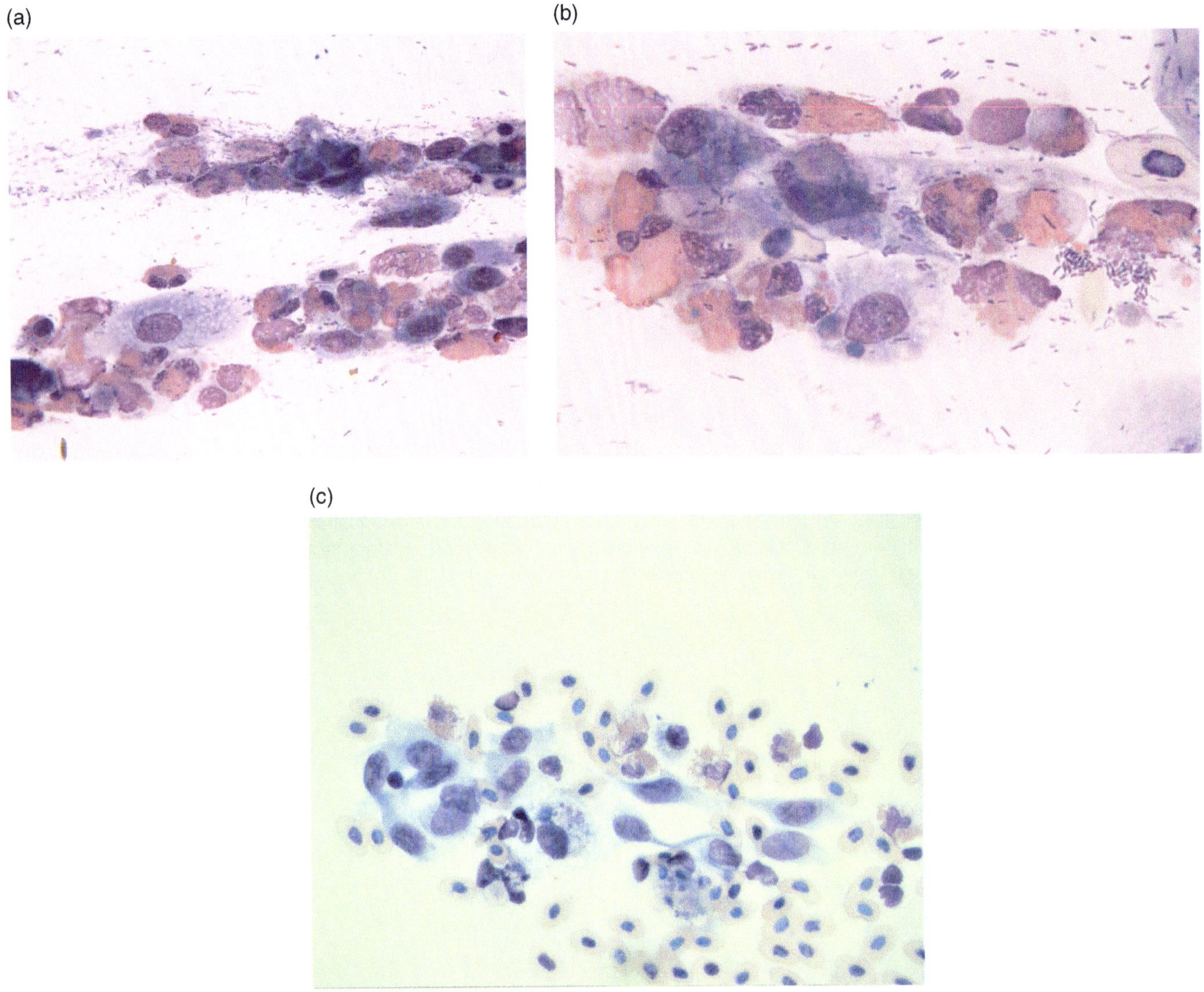

Fig. 23.23. (a) Numerous heterophils and extracellular bacteria in an oral swab from a water dragon (*Intellagama lesueurii*) with stomatitis, Wright–Giemsa stain (100× oil). (b) Septic mixed-cell inflammation (heterophils and macrophages with extracellular and intracellular bacteria) in an oral swab from a green iguana (*Iguana iguana*) with stomatitis, Wright–Giemsa stain (100× oil). (c) Mixed-cell inflammation and fibroblasts in a fine-needle aspiration biopsy of an oral mass from a green iguana (*Iguana iguana*) with stomatitis and an inflammatory polyp, Wright–Giemsa stain (100× oil).

lower respiratory tract are often large and multinucleated (Figure 23.28). Heterophilic inflammation in reptiles is associated with a suppurative inflammatory process that is often associated with infectious agents, especially when these leukocytes are degenerate (Figures 23.29a and 23.29b).

Inflammation of Skin

Lesions involving the skin and subcutis can be classified using the basic categories of cytodiagnosis: inflammatory, hyperplasic, and neoplastic. Inflammatory lesions can have an infectious or a noninfectious etiology (Figures 23.30a–23.30c). Suppurative inflammation of the skin and subcutaneous tissue is common because bacterial infections of the skin and subcutaneous usually result in this type of inflammation where intracellular bacteria are often easy to find and the neutrophils/heterophils often appear degenerate. Thus, bacterial infections are characterized cytologically by numerous degenerate neutrophils/heterophils, cellular debris, and bacteria. Septic inflammation is indicated by the presence of intracellular bacteria. Granulomas in the skin are represented cytologically by the presence of a macrophagic inflammation with epithelioid cells (epithelial macrophages) and giant cells (Figure 23.31). Granulomas are often caused by noninfectious agents, such as foreign bodies, or infectious agents, such as fungi or

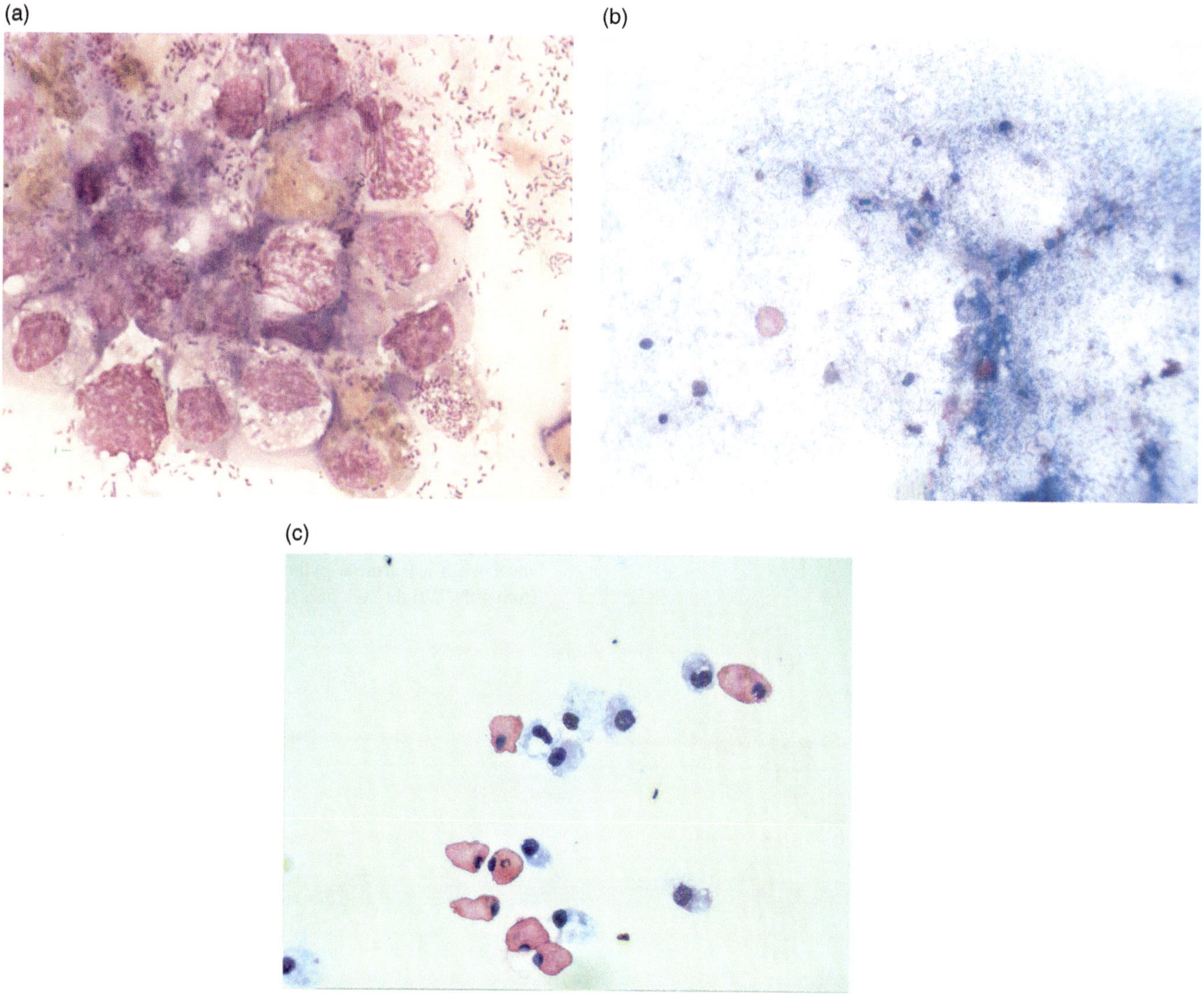

Fig. 23.24. (a) Septic inflammation (extracellular and intracellular bacteria) in an oral swab from a common boa constrictor (*Boa constrictor*) with stomatitis, Wright–Giemsa stain (100× oil). (b) Heterophil and erythrocytes with a marked number of extracellular bacteria suggesting an overwhelming bacterial infection in an oral swab from a short-tailed boa (*Boa constrictor amarali*) with stomatitis, Wright–Giemsa stain (100× oil). (c) Mixed-cell inflammation in an oral swab from a common boa constrictor (*Boa constrictor*) with stomatitis, Wright–Giemsa stain (100× oil).

Mycobacterium (Figures 23.31–23.33). Exfoliation of striated skeletal muscles cells may rarely be found in cytological samples obtained from ulcerative lesions in the skin (Figure 23.34).

Inflammation of Synovial Joints

Inflammatory joint disease can be caused by infectious agents such as bacteria, fungi, parasites, mycoplasma, and viruses or by noninfectious etiologies such as gout and immune-mediated disease. The cytology of inflammatory joint disease reveals an increase in neutrophils/heterophils, abnormal color and clarity, and reduced viscosity and mucin quality. The background of the smears made from synovial fluid with poor mucin quality lacks the granular appearance of normal joint fluid. Synovial lining cells (synoviocytes), large mononuclear cells with eccentric nuclei, and abundant vacuolated cytoplasm that often contains pink-staining granules may be seen (Figure 23.35a). The presence of multinucleated osteoclasts or spindle-shaped fibroblasts indicates erosion of the articular cartilage, exposing underlying bone, or erosion into the fibrous layer of the articular capsule.

Septic arthritis is indicated by a high cell count and the presence of large numbers of neutrophils/heterophils. Extracellular bacteria are suggestive of bacterial involvement, and bacterial phagocytosis is considered

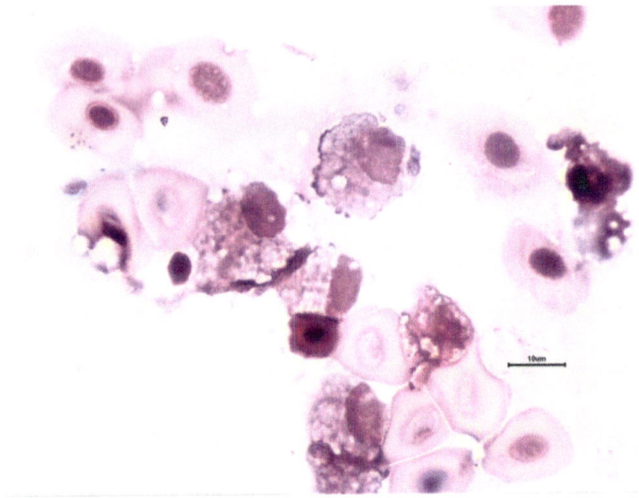

Fig. 23.25. Degenerate inflammatory cells in a cloacal swab sample from a leopard gecko (*Eublepharis macularius*) with enteritis, Wright–Giemsa stain (100× oil).

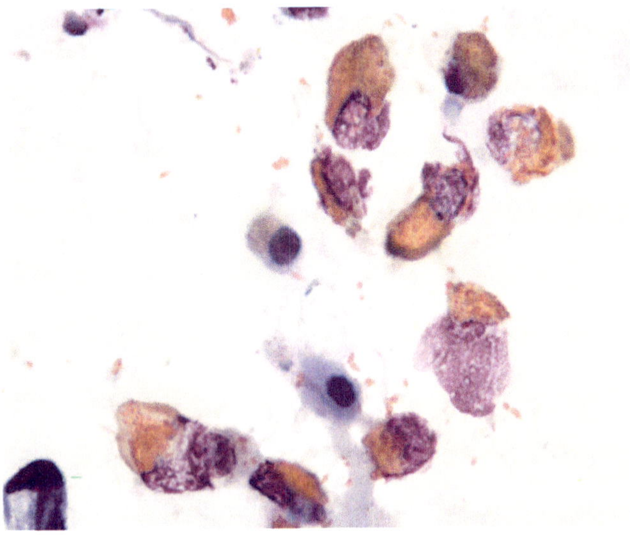

Fig. 23.26. Heterophilic inflammation in leopard tortoise (*Stigmochelys pardalis*) with sinusitis, Wright–Giemsa stain (100× oil)

diagnostic for septic joint disease. Bacteria often are not inherently obvious on the slide; however, the presence of degenerative neutrophils/heterophils is suggestive of a septic lesion (Figure 23.35b).

Traumatic injury to the joint (traumatic arthritis) may reveal an increase in the number of inflammatory leukocytes, primarily neutrophils/heterophils in cases of acute trauma. Depending upon the degree of joint injury, synoviocytes and mesenchymal cells representing exfoliation of cells from the underlying cartilage may be present. Cartilage fragments may also be found. These are represented by the presence of amorphous material with variable staining characteristics on the Romanowsky-stained smear. The mucin clot test and viscosity of synovial fluid

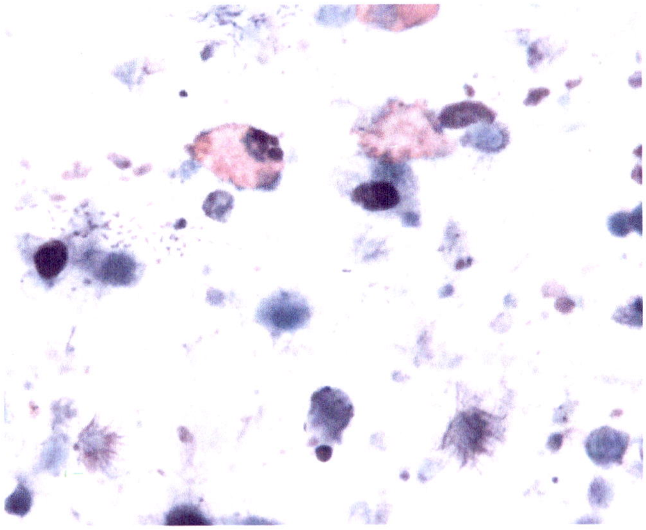

Fig. 23.27. Degenerate ciliated respiratory epithelial cells with cell fragments containing tufts of cilia and heterophils in a tracheal wash a Burmese python snake (*Python bivittatus*) with stomatitis, Wright– Giemsa stain (100× oil).

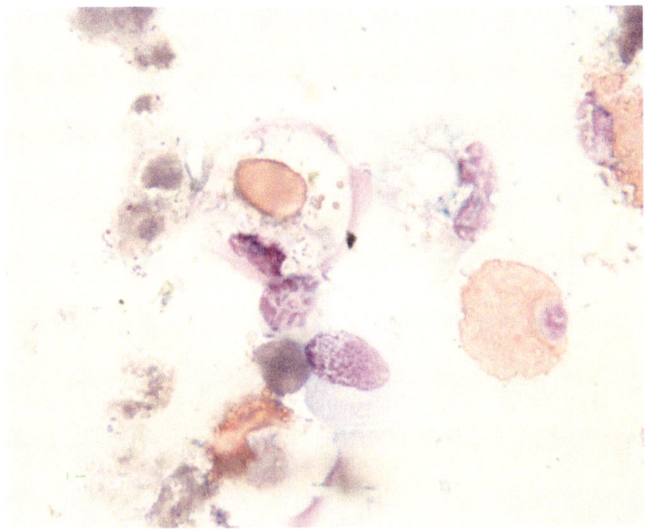

Fig. 23.28. Large macrophages exhibiting leukophagocytosis and bacterial phagocytosis in a tracheal wash from a common boa constrictor (*Boa constrictor*), Wright–Giemsa stain (100× oil).

associated with acute traumatic arthritis are typically normal if hemarthrosis is not involved (Figure 23.36).

Articular gout is the most common and best-characterized cause of nodular deposits of crystalline material in and around the joints of reptiles. The synovial fluid of joints affected by gout appears thick, chalky white, and opaque with a grainy consistency. Gouty tophi are composed of monosodium urate crystals surrounded by a granulomatous inflammatory response. However, nodular periarticular deposits of crystalline material other than urates (termed pseudogout, false gout, and hydroxyapatite deposition disease) also occur

(a)

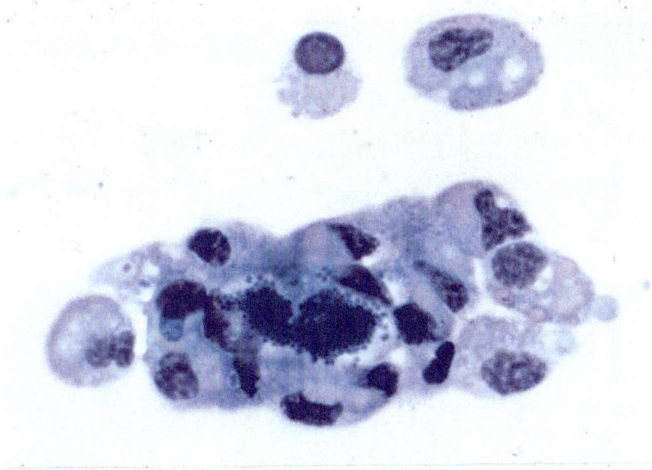

(b)

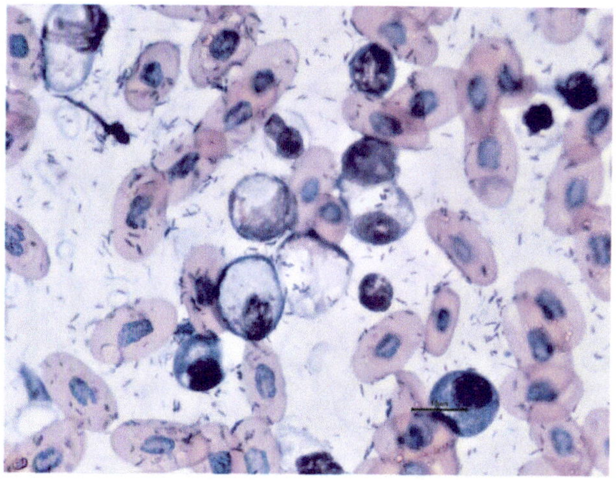

Fig. 23.29. (a) Heterophilic inflammation with degenerate heterophils, some exhibiting bacterial phagocytosis, indicative of an acute septic tracheitis in a tracheal wash sample from a green iguana (*Iguana iguana*), Diff–Quik stain (100×, oil). (b) Mixed-cell inflammation with macrophages, plasma cells, and degenerate heterophil exhibiting bacterial phagocytosis and a marked number of erythrocytes and extracellular bacteria in a lung wash sample from a green tree python (*Morelia viridis*) with septic pneumonia, Wright–Giemsa stain (100× oil).

(a)

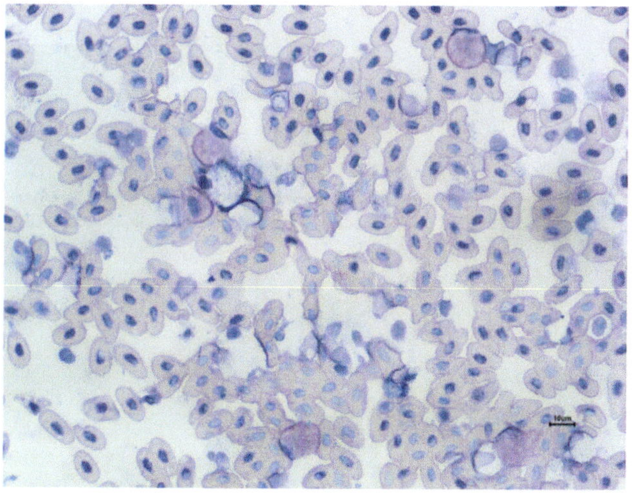

(b)

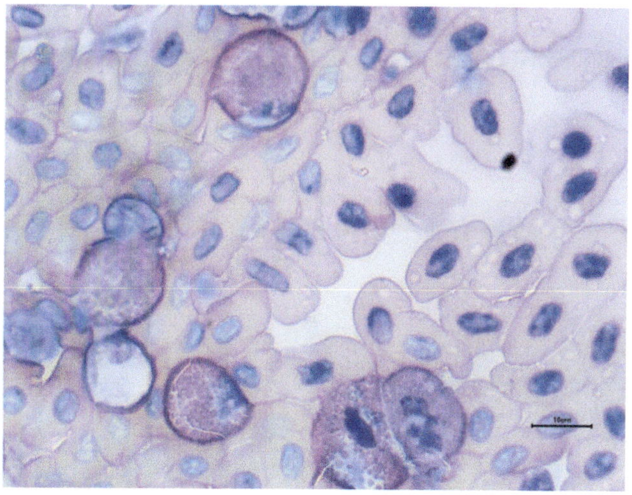

(c)

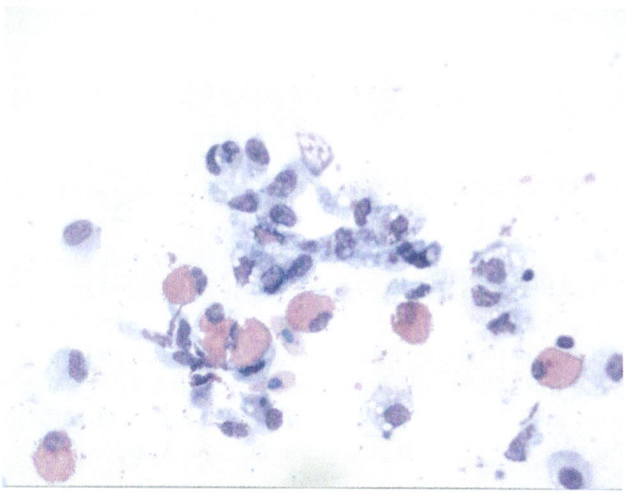

Fig. 23.30. (a) Mixed-cell inflammation in a skin scrapping from an Argentine horned frog (*Ceratophrys ornate*) with dermosepticemia, Wright–Giemsa stain (40×). (b) Mixed-cell inflammation in a skin scrapping from an Argentine horned frog (*Ceratophrys ornate*) with dermosepticemia, Wright–Giemsa stain (100× oil). (c) Mixed-cell inflammation in a skin scrapping from a hognose snake (*Heterodon platirhinos*), Wright–Giemsa stain (100× oil).

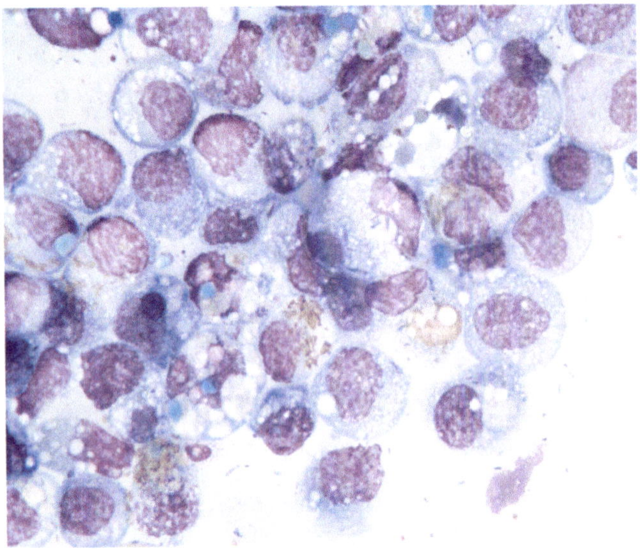

Fig. 23.31. Macrophagic inflammation in an aspiration biopsy of a cutaneous mass in a leopard gecko (*Eublepharis macularius*), Wright–Giemsa stain (100× oil). Source: Image from Campbell and Grant (2010, p. 287).

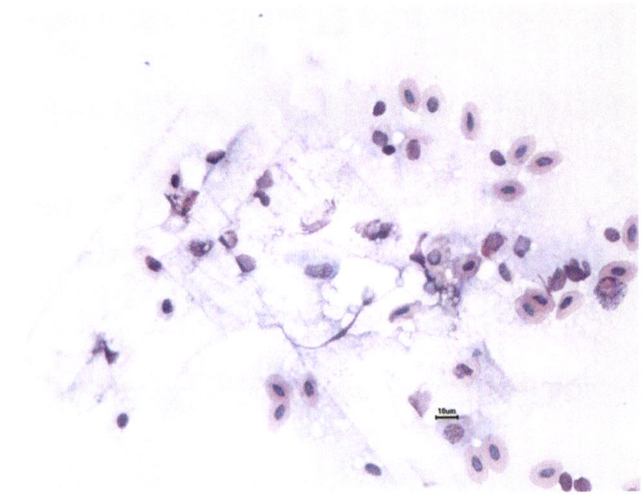

Fig. 23.32. Cholesterol crystals in a biopsy imprint of a xanthomatosis lesion in skin of a leopard gecko (*Eublepharis macularius*). Cholesterol crystals induce a macrophagic inflammatory response, Wright–Giemsa stain (40×).

in reptiles and must be clinically differentiated from gout. Primary gout is related to overproduction of uric acid, and secondary gout occurs when hyperuricemia is a result of other diseases or administration of drugs that affect the excretion of uric acid (Mader, 2006; Neogi, 2011). Increased uric acid production can be the result of excessive intake of inappropriate protein diets, such as a herbivorous reptile consuming a diet high in animal protein (Wellehan et al., 2004a).

Cytological evaluation of synovial fluid can be used as a quick and definitive tool to diagnose gout in reptiles.

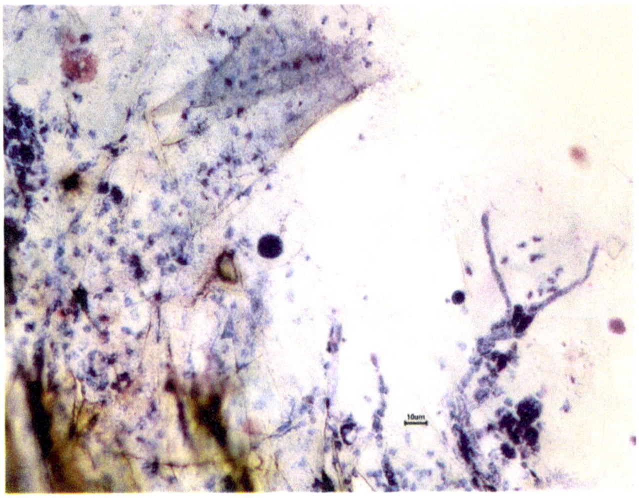

Fig. 23.33. Fungal hyphae in a skin scrapping of a cutaneous lesion in a spiny soft-shelled turtle (*Apalone spinifera*), Wright–Giemsa stain (40×).

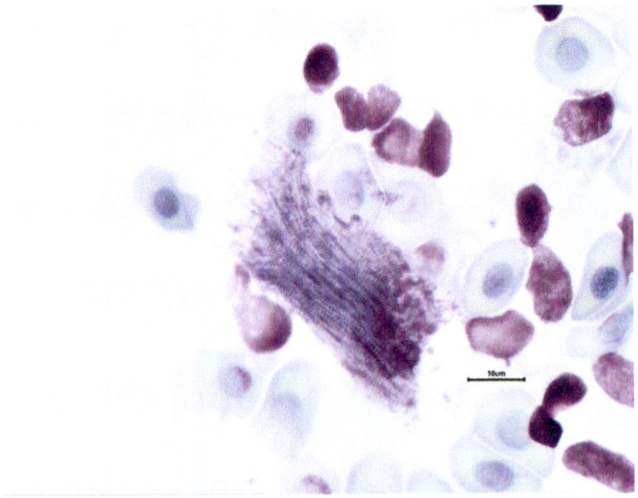

Fig. 23.34. Striated muscle cells from a swab of an ulcerated lesion on the leg of an African clawed frog (*Xenopus laevis*), Wright–Giemsa stain (100× oil).

Microscopically, the fluid often contains variable numbers of spindle cells, macrophages, lysed cells, and erythrocytes within a pale blue background that contains irregular, refractile, gray, brown, to black, amorphous, and needle-like crystalline material (Figures 23.37a and 23.37b). Multinucleated giant cells containing the needle-like crystals may also be seen. Polarization is used to identify the needle-shaped, highly birefringent crystals scattered throughout the preparations as uric acid. The differentiation between articular gout and pseudogout is based on birefringence under polarized light and concurrent hyperuricemia and normal plasma calcium concentration (Jones and Fitzgerald, 2009; Lee et al., 2011; Johnson III et al., 2014; Drzewiecka et al., 2016).

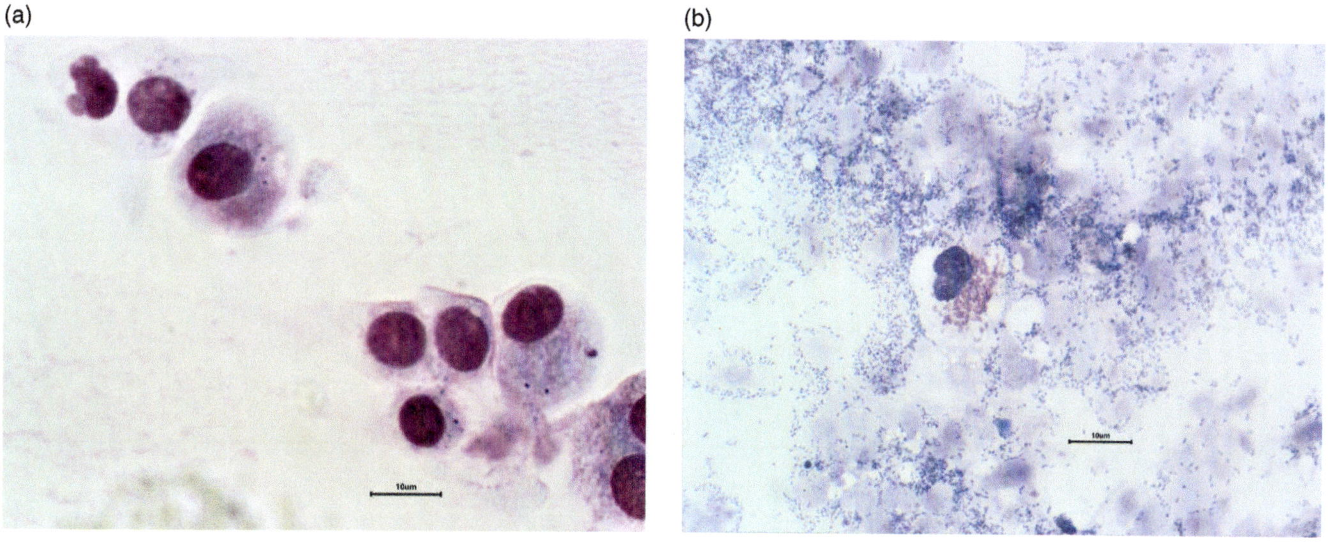

Fig. 23.35. (a) Synoviocytes in a joint aspirate from a spiny-tailed lizard (*Uromastyx* sp.), Wright–Giemsa stain (100× oil). (b) An overwhelming number of extracellular bacteria and a degenerate heterophil in a joint aspirate from a green iguana (*Iguana iguana*) with a joint abscess, Wright–Giemsa stain (100× oil).

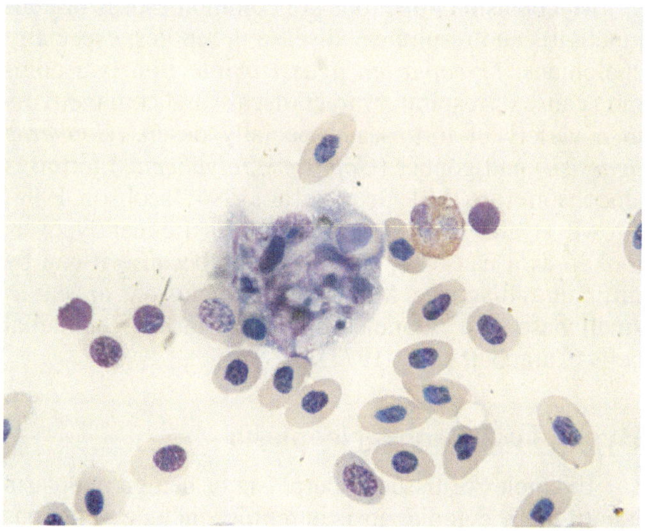

Fig. 23.36. A multinucleated giant cell exhibiting erythrophagocytosis with erythrocytes and a heterophil in a joint fluid aspirate from a green iguana (*Iguana iguana*) with hemarthrosis, Wright–Giemsa stain (100× oil).

Polarized light microscopy is used to identify the birefringence of urate crystals by positioning a polarizer filter beneath the specimen stage and placing an analyzer (second polarizer filter) above the specimen. When the analyzer and polarizer filters are positioned perpendicular to each other, a dark view field is present. Monosodium urate crystals are anisotropic and have optical properties that vary with the orientation of incident light with the crystallographic axes (Pennick et al., 2017). They also have a range of refractive indices and act as beam splitters by dividing light rays into two orthogonal components. When light enters the monosodium urate crystals, light is refracted into two rays that are perpendicular to one another (this is termed *double refraction* or *birefringence*). Polarized microscopy reunites the split light rays along the same optical path, thereby revealing the birefringent crystals.

Inflammation of the Liver

Hepatocytes are large (25–30 μm), slightly oval to polygonal cells with distinct cell margins that occur singly or in sheets and clusters (Figure 23.38). The cytoplasm is abundant and lightly basophilic, and fine eosinophilic granulation may be seen occasionally with Wright's stain. The nuclei are round to oval, uniform in appearance, and are slightly eccentric in location within the cells. The nuclei contain coarse chromatin and one or two prominent nucleoli. Binucleation is occasionally seen.

Heterophilic inflammation in reptiles may be differentiated from hepatic heterophil granulocytopoiesis by the presence of a predominance of mature heterophils and an absence of immature, developing heterophils. Septic inflammation is indicated by the presence of bacteria within leukocytes. Extracellular bacteria must be differentiated from "cadaver" bacteria or bacterial contamination of the sample when the sample is obtained during necropsy.

Mixed-cell or macrophagic inflammation of the liver can be associated with mycotic, parasitic, or mycobacterial infections. Granulomatous lesions reveal macrophages that are often vacuolated and multinucleated giant cells. Melanomacrophages are pigmented phagocytic cells found in most ectotherms (fish, amphibians, and reptiles) that phagocytize microorganisms. These macrophagic cells are recognized by the presence of

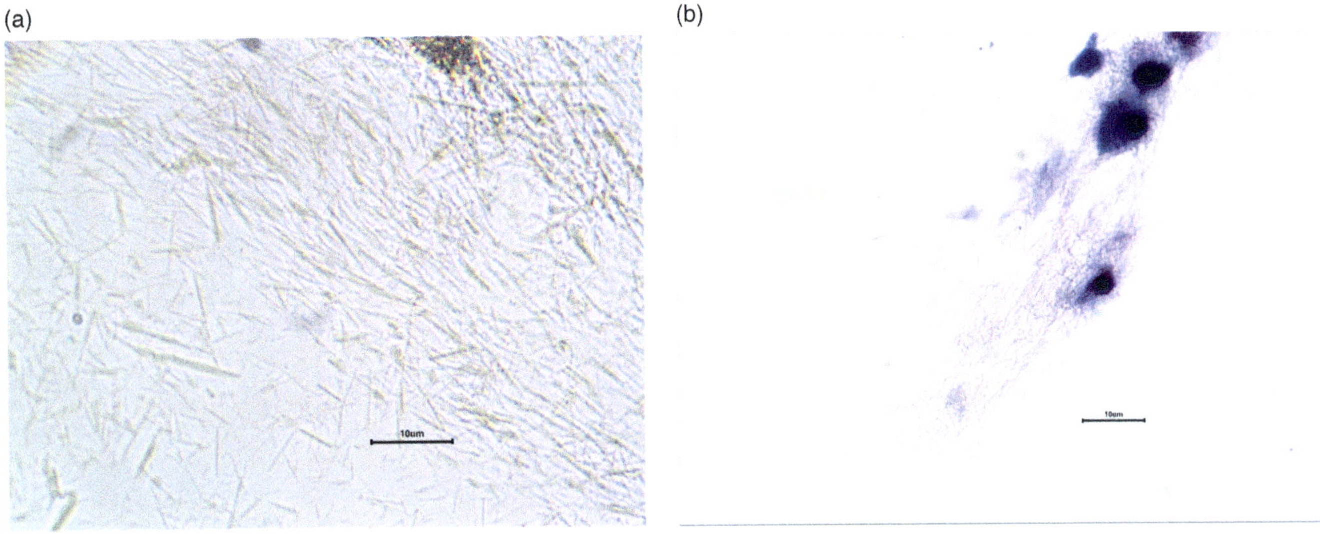

Fig. 23.37. (a) Golden needle-shaped uric acid crystals in the joint fluid from a spiny-tailed lizard (*Uromastyx* sp.) with articular gout, Wright–Giemsa stain (100× oil). (b) Golden needle-shaped uric acid crystals in the joint fluid from a leopard gecko (*Eublepharis macularius*) with articular gout, Wright–Giemsa stain (100× oil).

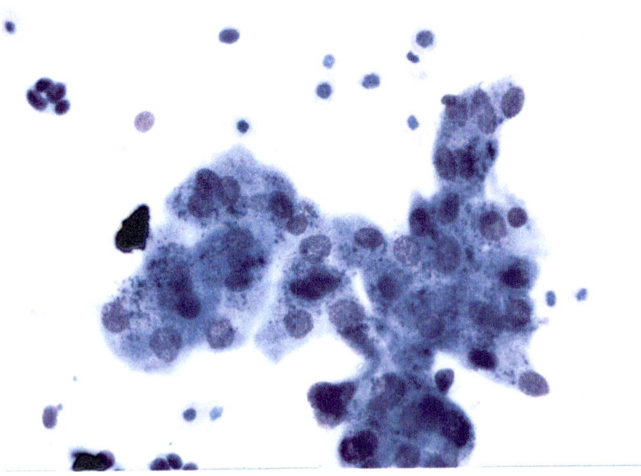

Fig. 23.38. Hepatocytes in an imprint from a liver biopsy from green iguana (*Iguana iguana*) with liver failure, Wright–Giemsa stain (100× oil).

golden-brown melanin pigment in the cytoplasm (Figures 23.39a and 23.39b). Granulomas made of melanomacrophages are often found in the liver of these animals.

Ophthalmic Inflammation

Conjunctivitis is a common cause for sampling the conjunctiva for cytological examination and is recognized by the presence of many inflammatory cells (Figures 23.40a–23.40d). Neutrophilic/heterophilic inflammation of the conjunctiva can be caused by bacteria, viruses, or noninfectious agents, such as trauma, foreign bodies, and environmental irritants.

Mycoplasma infections are common causes of conjunctivitis and respiratory disease in reptiles, especially chelonians. *Mycoplasma agassizii* infection is a common cause of respiratory tract disease and conjunctivitis in a variety of tortoises, especially desert (*Gopherus agassizii*) and gopher (*Gopherus polyphemus*) tortoises (Jacobson et al., 1991; Brown et al., 1994; Jacobson, 1994; Brown et al., 1999). Mycoplasma is frequently overlooked as a cause for conjunctivitis because it can be difficult to diagnose. Mycoplasmal inclusions appear as small basophilic granules on the surface of epithelial cells (Campbell et al., 1973).

Hyperplasia/Benign Neoplasia

Examples of tissue hyperplasia or benign neoplasia identified by cytodiagnosis in reptiles include squamous cell hyperplasia or metaplasia associated with hypovitaminosis A, lipomas, and hepatic lipidosis.

Adipose

Lipomas are uncommon benign mesenchymal cell tumors of normal-appearing adipocytes of the skin of reptiles. Lipomas and liposarcomas have been reported in the integument of lizards and snakes (Machotka, 1984; Done, 1996).

Corneal Lipidosis

Captive amphibians exhibit a lipid storage disorder resulting from hyperlipidemia with cholesterol deposits in the corneal tissue referred to as corneal lipidosis or xanthomatosis (Wright, 2014).

(a) (b)

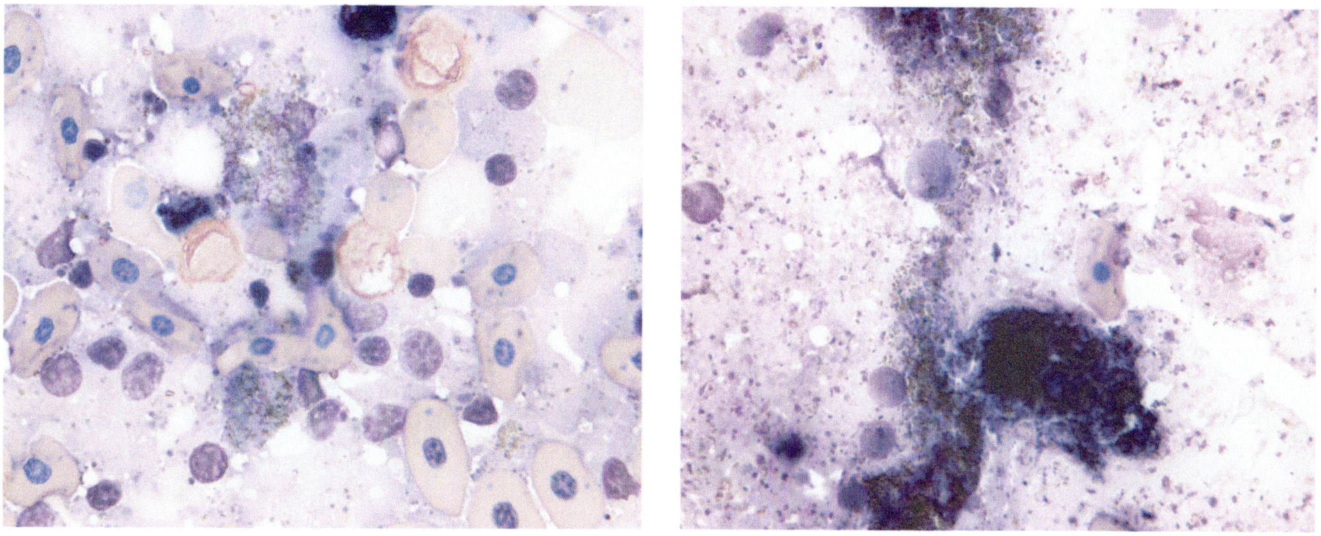

Fig. 23.39. (a) An imprint of a liver biopsy reveals heterophils, erythrocytes, and melanomacrophages containing golden-brown ovoid melanin granules from a loggerhead sea turtle (*Caretta caretta*) with hepatitis, Wright–Giemsa stain (100× oil). (b) An imprint of a liver biopsy reveals numerous golden-brown ovoid melanin granules from ruptured melanomacrophages from a loggerhead sea turtle (*Caretta caretta*) with hepatitis, Wright–Giemsa stain (100× oil).

Hepatic Lipidosis

Hepatic lipidosis (fatty liver syndrome or steatosis) is represented by the appearance of hepatocytes with many small or large clear cytoplasmic vacuoles, which represent lipid that has dissolved during the staining process (Figures 23.41a–23.41d). Unstained smears made from livers with fatty change may appear "greasy" on gross inspection of the slide.

Squamous Hyperplasia/Metaplasia

Hypovitaminosis A is the most common cause of conjunctivitis in reptiles, especially semiaquatic chelonians and box turtles. Hypovitaminosis A causes dyskeratotic changes of the Harderian gland; cytological findings reveal numerous keratinocytes and inflammatory cells (Figure 23.42a and 23.42b) (McArthur, 2004).

The cornea may respond to irritation with hyperplasia of the nonkeratinized epithelial cells (Figure 23.43).

Malignant Neoplasia

Lymphoma/Lymphocytic Leukemia

Although rarely reported in reptiles, hematopoietic neoplasia is more commonly seen in lizards (Hernandez-Divers and Garner, 2003). A severe leukocytosis associated with high numbers of atypical blast cells leads to a cytological diagnosis of leukemia. Medium- to large- sized blast cells with round to pleomorphic nuclei, slightly clumped chromatin, indistinct nucleoli, and scant moderate-to-dark blue cytoplasm with occasional red-to-purple cytoplasmic granulation are indicative of lymphoid leukemia (Georoff et al., 2009; Bezjian et al., 2013). Cytochemical and immunohistochemical staining allow for further evaluation and differentiation of the neoplastic cell populations and a definitive diagnosis, such as either a T-cell or B-cell lymphoid leukemia.

Chronic myelogenous leukemia (CML) is a rare disease in herptiles. Myelogenous leukemia is a neoplastic disorder of the multipotent stem cell characterized by the purposeless production or accumulation of differentiated hematopoietic precursors or both (Figures 23.44a and 23.44b).

Sarcoma

Mesenchymal neoplasia in snakes is associated with a rate (up to 90%) of malignancy (Sharpe et al., 2013) (Figures 23.45a and 23.45b).

Chondrosarcoma are common in colubrid snakes, where they arise from vertebral articulations and are invasive, but tend not to be metastatic (Webb et al., 2015). Cytological preparations of chondrosarcomas in snakes may reveal clusters of large, round to slightly polygonal cells with a distinct border and a large, round nucleus, coarse chromatin a single prominent round, blue nucleolus, and abundant eosinophilic cytoplasm (that may occasionally have a glassy appearance) embedded in amorphous to streaming homogenous magenta material (Webb et al., 2015) (Figures 23.46a and 23.46b). The cells exhibited marked anisocytosis and anisokaryosis, and multinucleation and mitotic figures are occasionally seen.

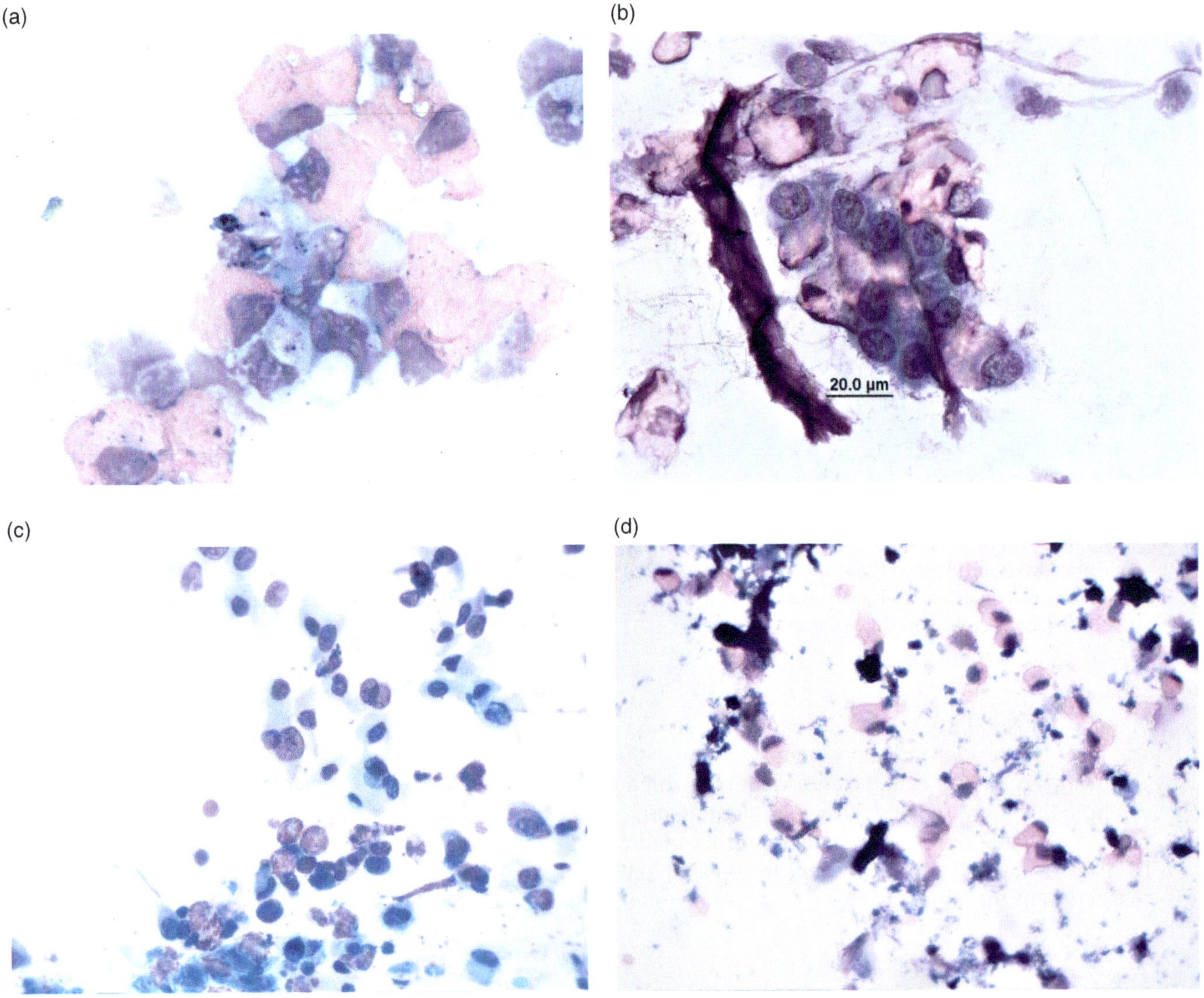

Fig. 23.40. (a) Mixed-cell inflammation with heterophils and macrophages in a conjunctival swab from a sulcata tortoise (*Chelonoidis sulcata*) with conjunctivitis, Wright–Giemsa stain (100× oil). (b) Heterophils and epithelial cells in a conjunctival swab from a Burmese mountain tortoise (*Manouria emys*) with conjunctivitis (note the presence of uric acid crystals, which should prompt an evaluation of the plasma uric acid concentration in this patient for the possibility of renal failure and visceral gout), Wright–Giemsa stain (100× oil). (c) Heterophils and epithelial cells in a conjunctival swab from a tegu (*Salvator merianae*) with conjunctivitis, Wright–Giemsa stain (100× oil). (d) Heterophils and debris with possible melanin pigment in a conjunctival swab from a three-toed box turtle (*Terrapene carolina triunguis*) with conjunctivitis, Wright–Giemsa stain (100× oil).

Neoplasia of the Gastrointestinal Tract

Neoplasia, such as a fibrosarcoma and squamous cell carcinoma, can occur in the oral cavity of reptiles (Salinas, et al., 2013; Steeil, et al., 2013). Gastrointestinal neoplasia can also occur in herptiles (Figures 23.47a–23.47d). Reviews have revealed that gastric carcinomas are more common than sarcomas in reptiles (Done, 1996; Lamglait B, Lemberger K. 2017). Although a variety of neoplasms involving the gastrointestinal tract of reptiles have been reported, lymphoid neoplasia (lymphoma and lymphosarcoma) appears to be the most common type (Harshbarger, 1976; Duncan et al., 2002). Gastrointestinal neoplasia, such as intestinal adenocarcinoma, has seldom been reported in the literature (Stilwell et al., 2020, Santos et al., 2021).

Cytological examination of a fine-needle aspiration biopsy of the stomach, liver, or other areas of the gastrointestinal tract provides a valuable diagnostic tool for the evaluation of masses involving these internal structures. Cytological examination of fine-needle aspiration biopsies can be used to detect and characterize neoplasia. Besides sarcomas and carcinomas, endocrine and neuroendocrine neoplasia can be identified by the presence of small, cuboidal epithelial cells that are uniform in

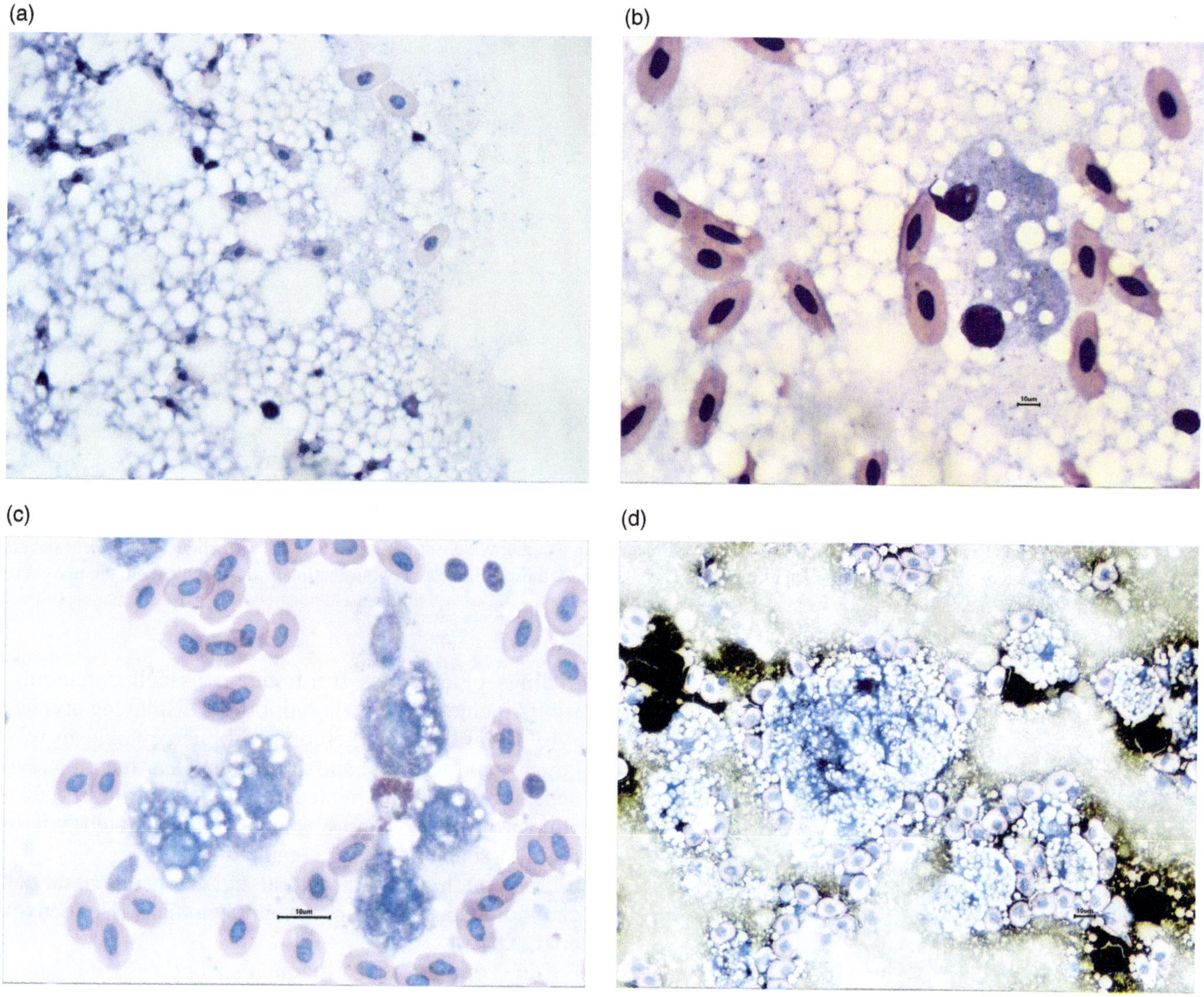

Fig. 23.41. (a) Erythrocytes among many small and large clear vacuoles, which represent lipid that has dissolved during the staining process in an imprint of a liver biopsy from a red-footed tortoise (*Chelonoidis carbonaria*) with hepatic lipidosis, Wright–Giemsa stain (100× oil). (b) Hepatocytes with intracytoplasmic round vacuoles among many small and large clear round vacuoles, which represent lipid that has dissolved during the staining process in an imprint of a liver biopsy from a bearded dragon (*Pogona vitticeps*) with hepatic lipidosis, Wright–Giemsa stain (100× oil). (c) Hepatocytes with intracytoplasmic round vacuoles either representing lipid and associated with background lipid vacuoles and hepatic lipidosis or degenerative changes in the cells in an imprint from a liver biopsy from a green tree python (*Morelia viridis*), Wright–Giemsa stain (100× oil). (d) Hepatocytes with intracytoplasmic round vacuoles among many small and large clear round vacuoles, which represent lipid that has dissolved during the staining process in an imprint of a liver biopsy from a Cuban tree frog (*Osteopilus septentrionalis*) with hepatic lipidosis. Note the melanin pigment likely associated with melanomacrophages in the liver. Wright–Giemsa stain (100× oil).

appearance and associated with bare nuclei in the cytological sample (Figures 23.48a and 23.48b) (Anderson, et al., 2019).

Neoplasia of the Respiratory Tract

Chondromas are seen most commonly in ball pythons (*Python regius*). They appear as glistening white masses within the trachea. Cytological examination of the tissue reveals mesenchymal cells showing moderate anisocytosis embedded in an eosinophilic background material (Campbell and Grant, 2010) (Figures 23.46a and 23.46b). The cytoplasm of the cells contains fine eosinophilic granules. The nucleus to cytoplasm ratio of the cells tends to vary, and the nucleus often appears near one edge of the cell and contains coarsely granular chromatin. Nucleoli are often prominent.

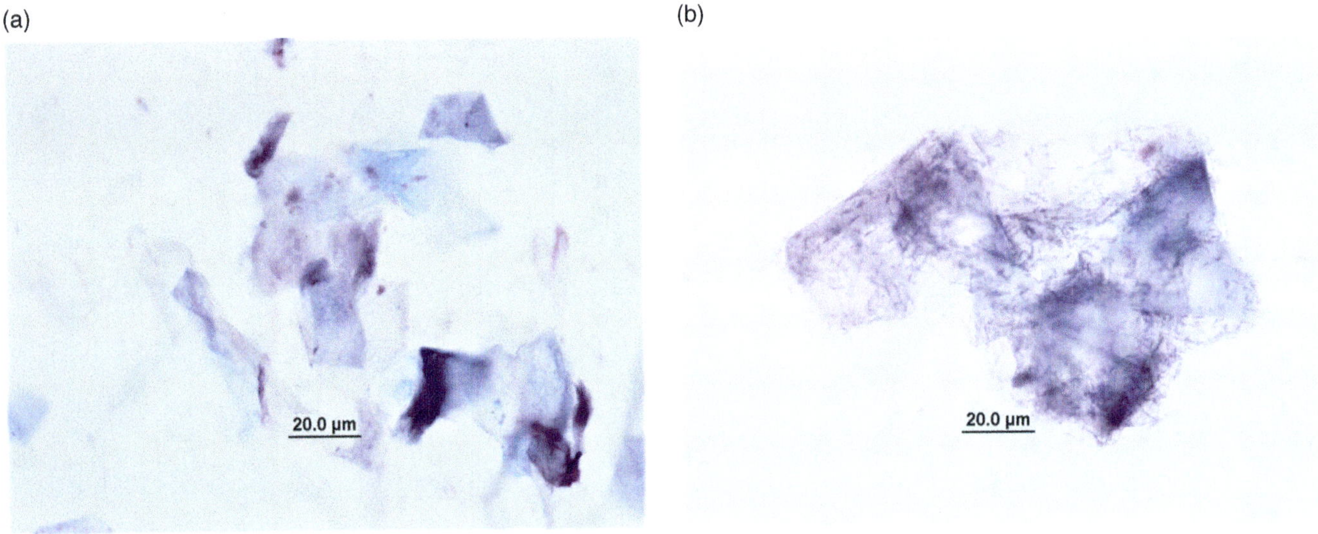

Fig. 23.42. (a) Keratinocytes in a conjunctival scraping from a water dragon (*Intellagama lesueurii*) with hypovitaminosis A, Wright–Giemsa stain (100× oil). (b) Keratinocytes with associated bacteria in a conjunctival scraping from a red-eared slider (*Trachemys scripta elegans*) suspected of suffering from hypovitaminosis A. It is also likely these cells were contamination of the sample from the margin of the eyelid. Wright–Giemsa stain (100× oil).

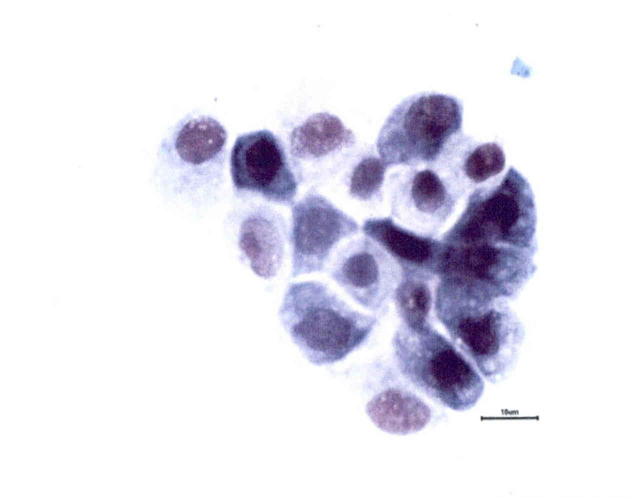

Fig. 23.43. Nonkeratinized epithelial cells in a scraping from a corneal lesion in a Cuban tree frog (*Osteopilus septentrionalis*), Wright–Giemsa stain (100× oil).

Cutaneous Neoplasms

Although neoplasia of the skin is rarely reported in reptiles, it can occur (Cowan, 1968; Done, 1996; Dietz et al., 2016). Squamous cell carcinoma is also an uncommon neoplasm of reptiles, although it has been reported in chelonians, lizards, and snakes (Done, 1996; Campbell and Grant, 2010; Brenner et al., 2020; Hall et al., 2020; Andersson et al., 2021) (Figures 23.49a–23.49e). In a review of neoplasia in reptiles, chelonians had an overall incidence of 2.7%, with squamous cell carcinoma being the second most common tumor type behind fibropapillomas (Ferris and Quesenberry, 2020). Expected cytological findings of aspirates from squamous cell carcinomas would include isolated keratinocytes displaying atypical cytological features (keratinized bluish cytoplasm with large, round nucleus) and atypical nuclear features (evident nucleoli in the nucleus of some keratinized cells) along with other features, such as degenerated heterophils and bacteria (Vetere et al., 2020).

Although uncommon, oral and cutaneous basal cell carcinoma has been reported in chelonians (Hellebuyck et al., 2016).

In contrast with mammals, lipomas are rarely reported in snakes, though they are overrepresented in corn snakes (Marrinhas et al., 2019; Crews et al., 2020). Evaluation of cytological preparations generally reveals adipocytes and free lipid material in the background (Burkert et al., 2002). Oil Red O staining can be used to highlight free lipid material in the background derived from disrupted adipocytes and intact adipocytes (Marrinhas et al., 2019). Cytologically, infiltrative lipomas look like cutaneous lipomas (Haag et al., 2008; Marrinhas et al., 2019).

Papillomas have been reported in reptiles, and although they usually appear as solitary lesions, they can occur in multiple places anywhere on the skin (Done, 1996; Gull, 2012). Fibropapillomas caused by a virus are commonly reported in free-ranging green sea turtles (*Chelonia mydas*), and papillomas have also been reported in crocodilians and lizards (Jacobson et al., 1991; Done, 1996; Schumacher, 1996). Papillomaviruses have been associated with papillomas or fibropapillomas in reptiles (Eleni et al., 2017).

Reptile fibromas and fibrosarcomas are primarily observed in the skin and oral cavity of snakes, lizards,

(a) (b)

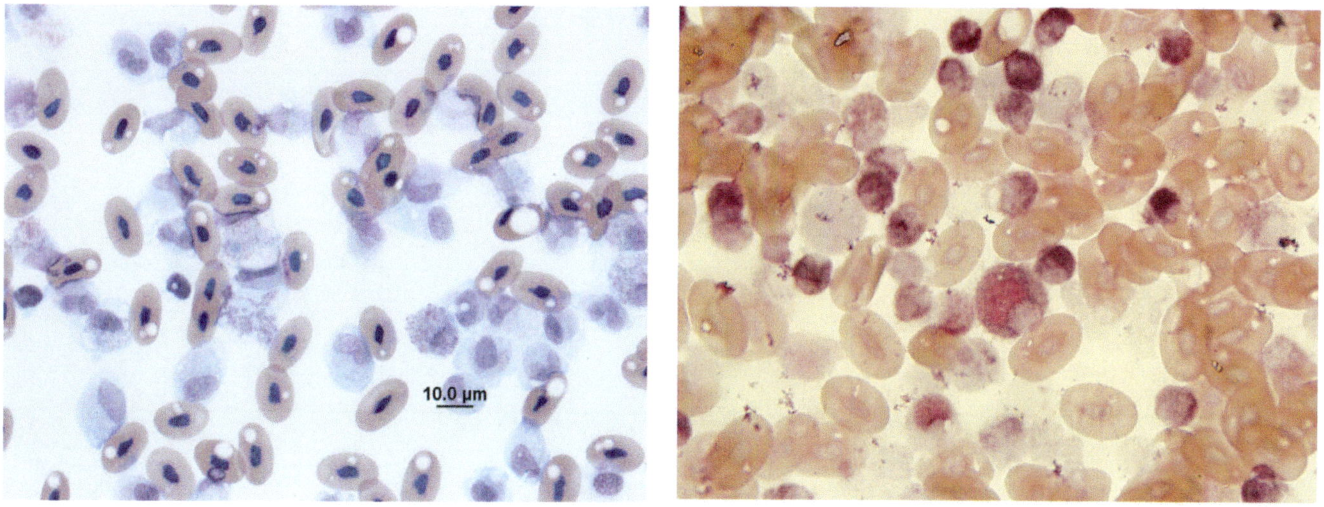

Fig. 23.44. (a) A predominance of monocytic leukocytes (absolute monocyte count of 2897/µL) in the peripheral blood of a bearded dragon (*Pogona vitticeps*) with myelomonocytic leukemia, Wright–Giemsa stain (100× oil). (b) Positive alkaline phosphatase staining of the monocytic leukocytes in the peripheral blood of a bearded dragon (*Pogona vitticeps*) with myelomonocytic leukemia, alkaline phosphatase stain (100× oil).

(a) (b)

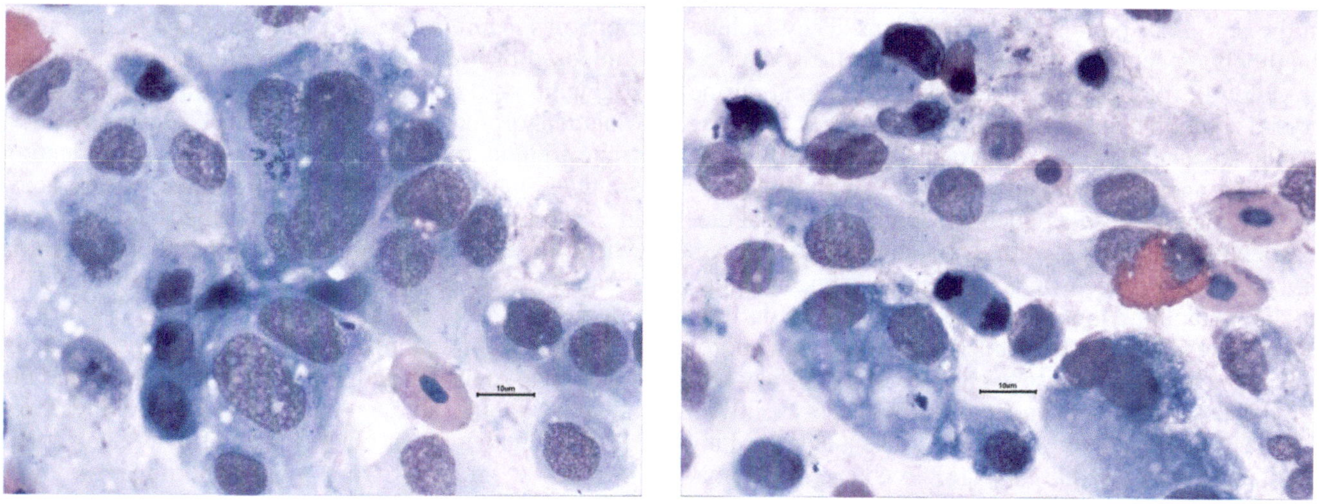

Fig. 23.45. (a) Imprint of an excised sarcoma lesion in the mouth of a jungle carpet python (*Morelia spilota cheynei*), Wright–Giemsa stain (100× oil). (b) Same imprint of an excised sarcoma lesion in the mouth of a jungle carpet python (*Morelia spilota cheynei*) as in Figure 23.45a, Wright–Giemsa stain (100× oil).

and crocodiles (Orós et al., 2009). Although tumors are reported uncommonly in chelonians, cutaneous fibroma has been reported in freshwater turtles, where the cytological preparations demonstrate spindle cells with mild anisocytosis and anisokaryosis surrounded by a collagenous stroma (Gonzales-Viera et al., 2012).

Cutaneous fibropapillomatosis is a well-documented neoplasm in green sea turtles (*Chelonia mydas*) and characterized by the presence of multiple cutaneous papillomas, fibromas, fibropapillomas and occasional visceral fibromas (Jacobson et al., 1989; Herbst et al., 1999). A herpesvirus along with other contributing factors, such as immunosuppression, pollutants, marine biotoxins, and water temperature, are considered predisposing causes for this disorder (Jacobson et al., 1991a; Aguirre and Lutz, 2004). In freshwater species, cutaneous fibroma has been described in snapping turtles (*Macrochelys temminckii* and *Chelydra serpentine*) (Frye, 1991; Gonzales-Viera, et al., 2012).

The reptilian epidermis contains melanocytes, and the dermal layer contains chromatophores, including melanophores, xanthophores, erythrophores, and iridophores.

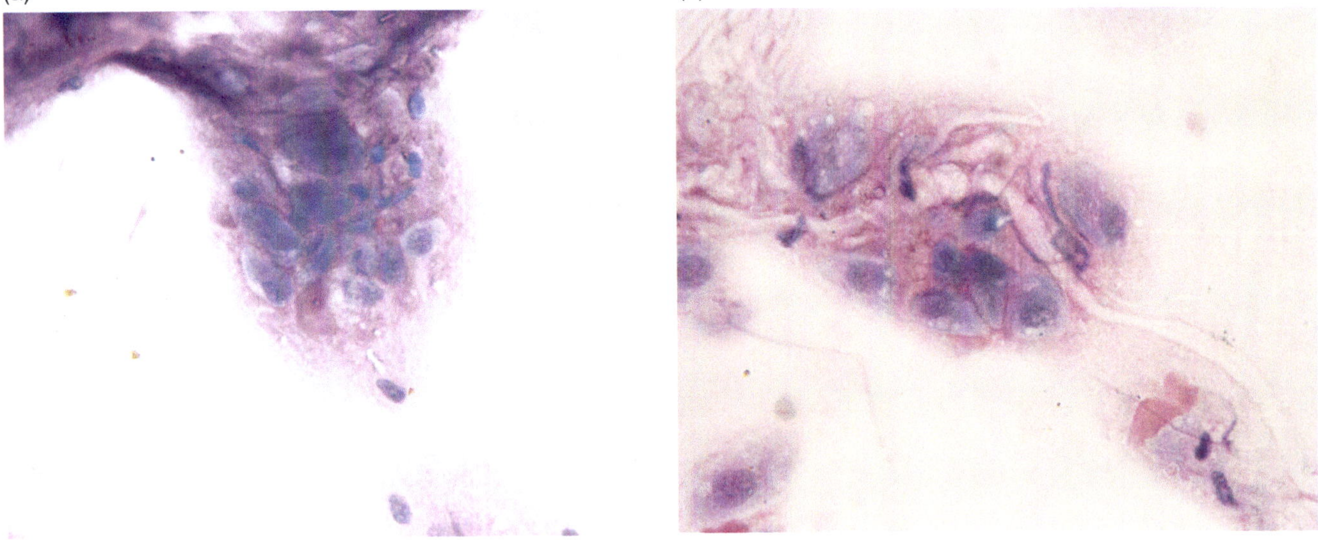

(a) (b)

Fig. 23.46. (a), (b) Large, plump mesenchymal cells within a pink, amorphous background substance in an imprint from a tracheal chondroma in a ball python (*Python regius*), Wright–Giemsa stain (100× oil).

Chromatophores are a group of pigment-bearing and light-reflecting cells, derived from the neural crest, in the dermis of reptiles and amphibians. They include xanthophores (containing carotenoids and pteridine (red or yellow)), iridophores (containing birefringent purine crystals (variable color)), and melanophores (containing melanosomes, the melanin-producing cells (black)). Chromatophores are organized in units within the dermis and contain vesicles filled with compounds that dictate coloration or as with iridophores that contain crystalline purine inclusions including guanine, adenine, and hypoxanthine, impart coloration by reflecting light (Rooney et al., 2020). In chameleon species, iridophores confer the animals' ability to change color and may also provide passive thermal protection (Teyssier et al., 2015). The reptilian epidermis contains melanocytes. Many reptilian species also have a large percentage of chromatophores in the coelomic cavity and lungs (Rivera et al., 2015).

Chromatophoromas (neoplasia of the chromatophores) are subclassified depending on the type of chromatophore affected. Chromatophoromas are common neoplasms of pigment-producing cells found in reptiles (primarily in lizards and snakes) and other lower vertebrates (Irizarry-Rovira et al., 2006; Suedmeyer et al., 2007; Heckers et al., 2012; Muñoz-Gutiérrez et al., 2016; Taggart et al., 2021). They commonly occur in the subcutis and dermis (Elkan, 1974; Ryan et al., 1981; Okihiro, 1988; Jacobson et al., 1989; Leach, et al., 1991; Gregory et al., 1997; Kusewitt et al., 1997; Mikaelian et al., 2000; Heckers et al., 2012). Chromatophoromas may be subclassified according to the type of chromatophore found in the tumor (Bagnara and Hadley, 1973; Lewis et al., 2015). For example, a tumor composed of melanophores is referred to as melanophoroma or melanoma; a tumor composed of xanthophores is referred to as xanthophoroma; and a tumor composed of iridophores is referred to as iridophoroma (Bagnara and Hadley, 1973; Bagnara et al., 1979). Melanophoromas appear grossly black or gray in color, while iridophoromas are white, and the light-reflecting granules (guanine, adenine, hypoxanthine, or uric acid) in iridophoromas reflect a white blue birefringence when viewed in polarized light, while melanophoroma granules do not (de Brot et al., 2015; Rivera et al., 2015; Tong et al., 2018) (Figure 23.50).

Cells from mammalian melanomas are typically spindled to round shaped and often pleomorphic, and the melanin granules may be punctate, slightly elongate, or spherical with a green-black, black, or blue-black color. In contrast, granules from melanophoromas of lower vertebrates, such as reptiles, tend to be larger and round to oval with a brown color (Irizarry-Rovira et al., 2006). In one study, chromatophoromas of reptiles generally arose from the skin of the body and head, and ranged in size from 0.2 to 2.0 cm in diameter (Heckers et al., 2012).

Discrete, pigmented, neoplastic cells consistent with melanin-producing neoplastic chromatophores called melanophoromas are uncommon neoplasms of reptiles and amphibians (Irizarry-Rovira et al., 2006; Martínez-Silvestre et al., 2011). Cytological findings most consistent with a melanocytic neoplasia include aggregates and individualized, pigmented, discrete, mononuclear neoplastic cells admixed with moderate numbers of erythrocytes, leukocytes (especially heterophils), and extracellular, brown-black or sometimes green-black pigment granules (round to slightly oval). The cells (20- to 25-μm) tend to be spindle- to stellate- shaped, but

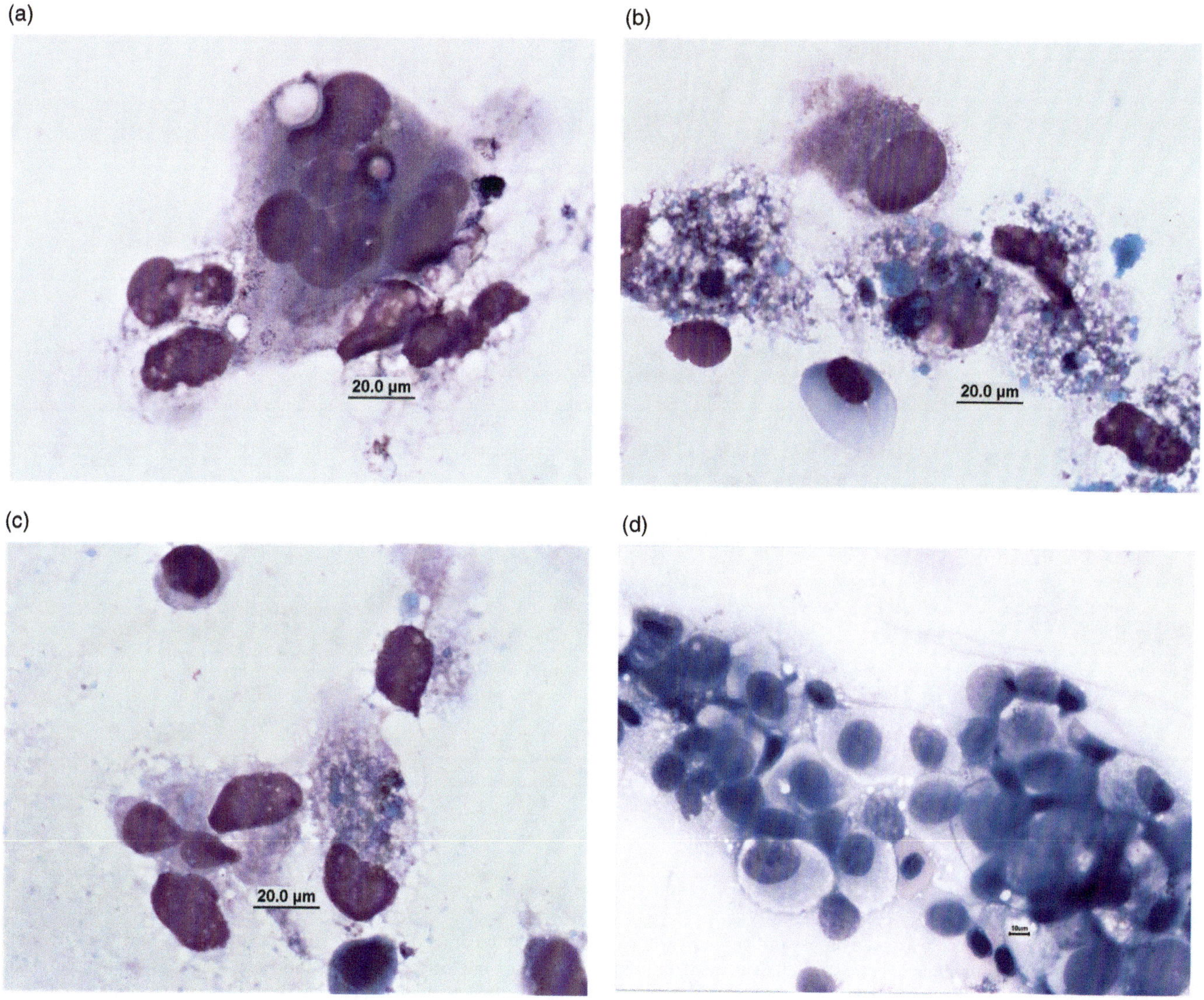

Fig. 23.47. (a) Multinucleated giant cell with pleomorphic nuclei in an impression smear from an intestinal mucinous adenocarcinoma from a tiger salamander (*Ambystoma tigrinum*), Wright–Giemsa stain (40×). (b) A large epithelial cell with indistinct margins and eosinophilic cytoplasm with degenerate cells and iron pigment in an impression smear from an intestinal mucinous adenocarcinoma from a tiger salamander (*Ambystoma tigrinum*), Wright–Giemsa stain (40×). (c) A large epithelial cell with indistinct margins and eosinophilic cytoplasm with degenerate cells and iron pigment in an impression smear from an intestinal mucinous adenocarcinoma from a tiger salamander (*Ambystoma tigrinum*). Spindled cells may be part of the fibrovascular stroma as described in the histopathology of the mass, Wright–Giemsa stain (40×). (d) Epithelial cells with distinct cytoplasmic margins and abundant cytoplasm from an impression smear of an intestinal adenocarcinoma from a different tiger salamander (*Ambystoma tigrinum*) than Figures 23.47a, b, c. Wright–Giemsa stain (100× oil).

round cells can be found (Bielli et al., 2015). Most of the cells have indistinct cytoplasmic borders with moderate amounts of colorless to pale blue cytoplasm that contains brown-black granules. The nuclei tend to be round to oval, with coarsely stippled chromatin and small single to multiple nucleoli. There is generally a mild anisokaryosis and anisocytosis.

Melanophoromas appear to be more common in snakes (Done, 1996; Muñoz-Gutiérrez et al., 2016). Although the exact etiology of these tumors is unknown, there is a suggestion that environmental contaminants may be at play when they occur in wild populations of amphibians (Martínez-Silvestre et al., 2011). One third of reptilian melanophoromas are classified as malignant (Heckers et al., 2012). In reptiles, melanomas usually occur in the thorax, are invasive, and have a poor prognosis for the patient (De Santi et al., 2020).

A fine-needle aspirate of an iridophoroma may reveal white- to cream-colored chalky material. The cytological preparation stained with Diff–Quik reveals

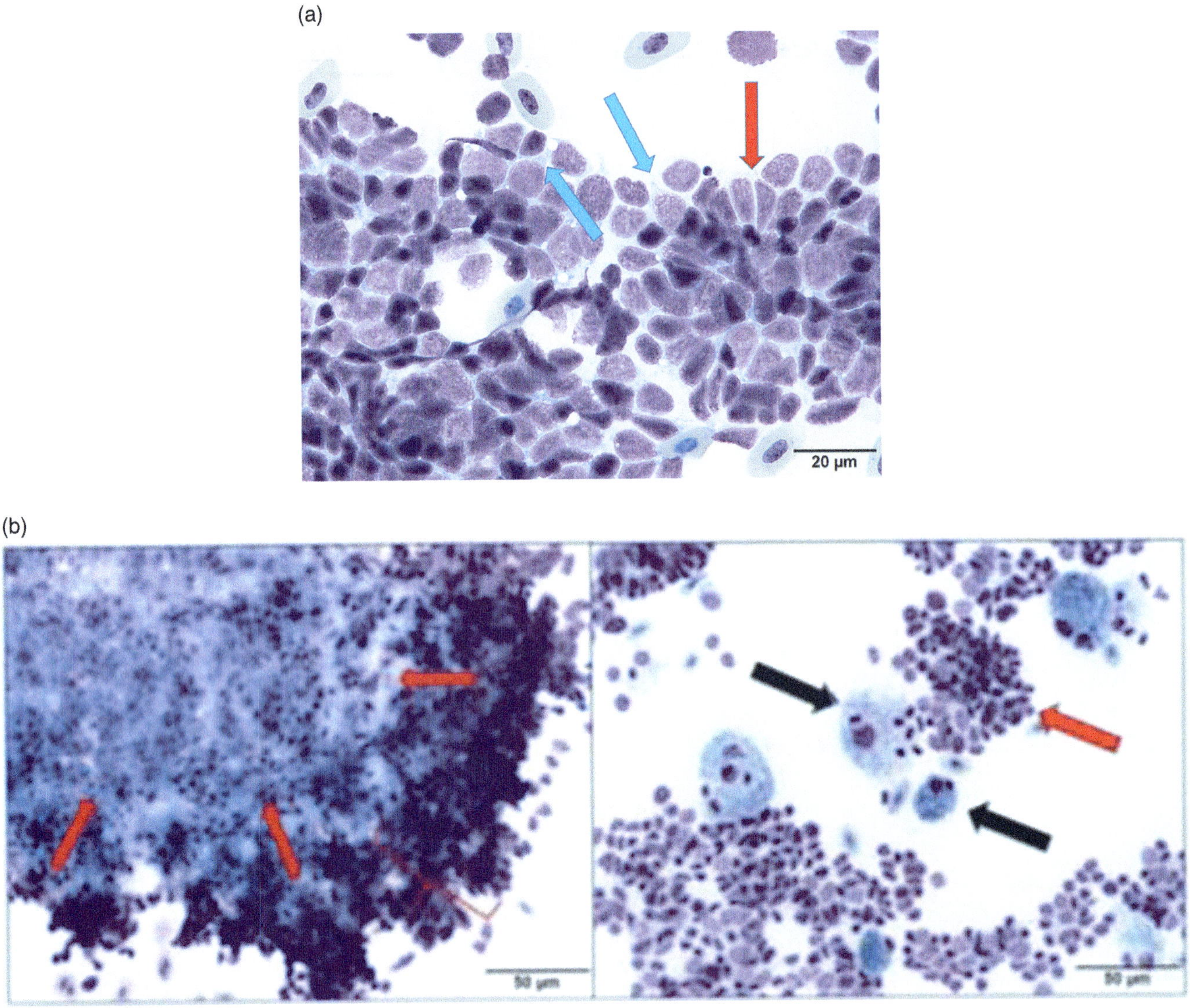

Fig. 23.48. (a) Fine-needle aspirate biopsy of liver mass from an inland bearded dragon (*Pogona vitticeps*) diagnosed with a gastric neuroendocrine carcinoma. Intact neoplastic cells are small, cuboidal with a high nuclear:cytoplasmic ratio and scant basophilic cytoplasm (blue arrows). Nuclei are generally round with stippled chromatin and lack visible nucleoli. Nuclei are densely crowded and often deform surrounding nuclei (red arrow). (Aqueous Romanowsky stain. 1000× original magnification). (b) Fine-needle aspirate biopsy of liver mass from an inland bearded dragon (*Pogona vitticeps*) diagnosed with a gastric neuroendocrine carcinoma. Left: In the middle of poorly spread-out clusters of cells, intact neoplastic cells are evident. Nuclei are spaced apart by light staining cytoplasm (red arrows). At the periphery of clusters are dense aggregates of bare nuclei (red bracket). Right: Well-spread-out areas of the slides consist predominantly of a diffuse background of intact, bare nuclei, often in dense aggregates (red arrow). Low numbers of intact macrophages, often containing hemosiderin, are present among the bare nuclei (black arrow). (Aqueous Romanowsky stain. 500× original magnification.) Source: Image from Anderson et al. (2019).

Fig. 23.49. (a) Marked number of heterophils, small spindle-shaped cells (fibrocytes), and squamous epithelial cells exhibiting dysmaturation of the nucleus and cytoplasm in an impression smear from a squamous cell carcinoma from a green iguana (*Iguana iguana*), Wright–Giemsa stain (50×). (b) A marked heterophilic inflammatory response associated with a pleomorphic population of squamous epithelial cells exhibiting features of malignancy in an impression smear from a squamous cell carcinoma from a green iguana (*Iguana iguana*), Wright–Giemsa stain (100× oil). (c) Highly pleomorphic population of squamous epithelial cells exhibiting features of malignancy (anisokaryosis, nuclear pleomorphism, multinucleation, nuclear chromatin clumping, and cytoplasmic basophilia) in an impression smear from a squamous cell carcinoma from a green iguana (*Iguana iguana*). A marked heterophilic inflammatory response is often associated with squamous cell carcinomas, Wright–Giemsa stain (100× oil). Source: Image from Campbell and Grant (2010, p. 291). (d) Highly pleomorphic population of squamous epithelial cells exhibiting features of malignancy (anisokaryosis, nuclear pleomorphism, multinucleation, nuclear chromatin clumping, and cytoplasmic basophilia) in an impression smear from a squamous cell carcinoma from a green iguana (*Iguana iguana*). A marked heterophilic inflammatory response is often associated with squamous cell carcinomas, Wright–Giemsa stain (100× oil). Source: Image from Campbell and Grant (2010, p. 291). (e) Squamous epithelial cells exhibiting dysmaturation of the nucleus and cytoplasm in an impression smear from a squamous cell carcinoma from a green iguana (*Iguana iguana*), Wright–Giemsa stain (100× oil).

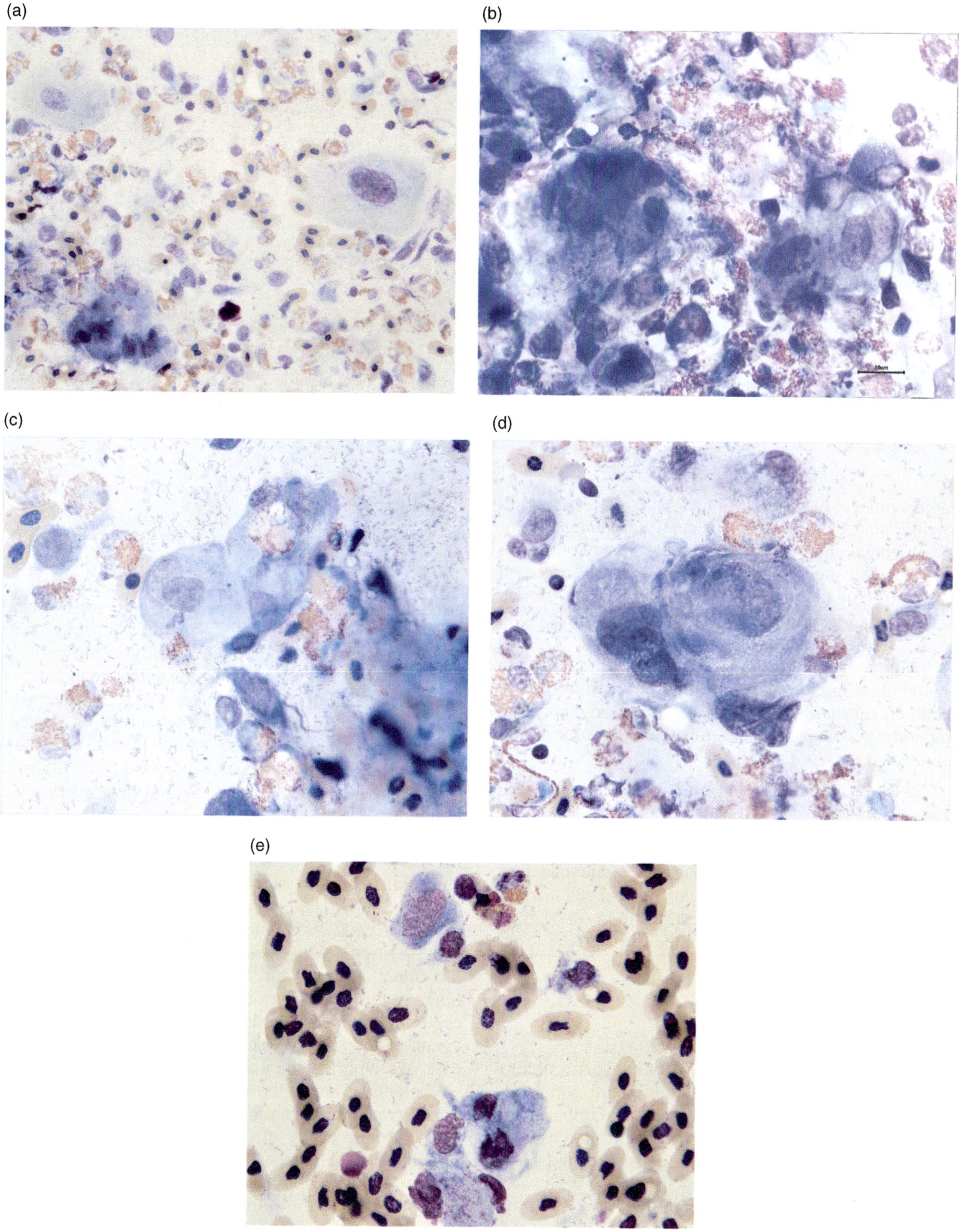
(a)
(b)
(c)
(d)
(e)

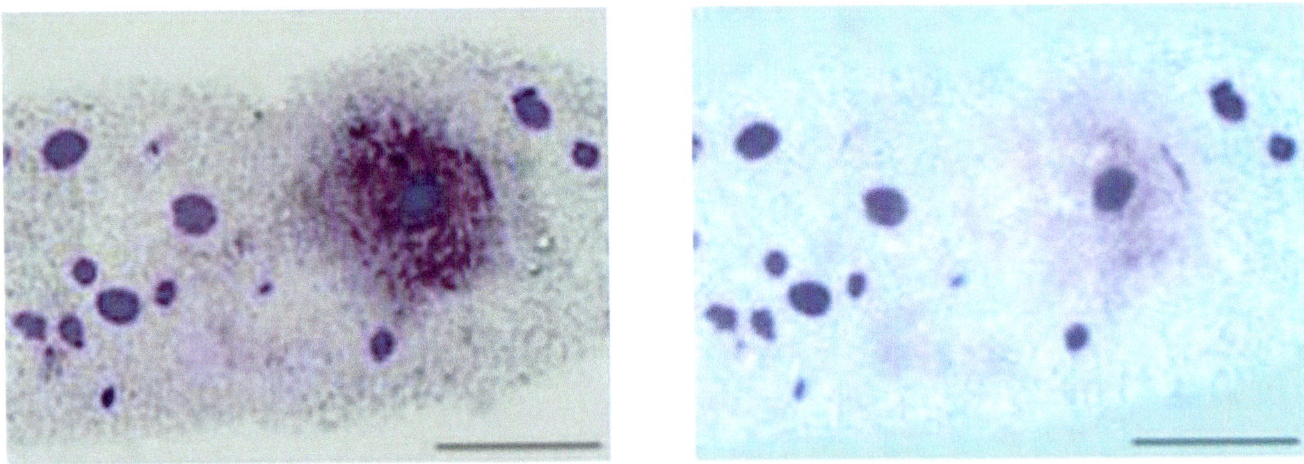

Fig. 23.50. (Left) Fine-needle aspirate of the dermal mass on the distal lateral brachium, composed of cells of indistinct shape with abundant cytoplasm containing copious refractile olive green pigment, and exhibiting mild anisokaryosis. (Right) Birefringence of granular pigments under polarized light. Diff–Quik. Bar, 50 mm. Source: Tong et al. (2018).

large, mildly pleomorphic mesenchymal cells with small, round, centrally located nuclei and abundant cytoplasm containing copious amounts of intracytoplasmic, refractile, olive green, fine granular pigment (iridescent purple to blue under polarized light) that is also found scattered throughout the noncellular background (Tong et al., 2018).

Although immunohistochemical studies used in mammalian species need validation for their use in reptilian diagnostics, S-100 and PNL-2 may be helpful for supporting a diagnosis of chromatophoroma for poorly pigmented cases (Thompson et al., 2015; Muñoz-Gutiérrez et al., 2016).

Mast cell tumors and systemic mastocytosis are rare in reptiles. When they do occur, the exfoliative cytological findings are consistent with neoplastic mast cells, and like those of domestic animals, reveal mononuclear, discrete, neoplastic round cells with distinct cell margins and numerous intracytoplasmic purple to magenta granules, which were also present in the extracellular space (Meinkoth and Cowell, 2002; Rovira et al., 2014).

Reproductive Tract Neoplasia

Ovarian cystadenocarcinomas and adenocarcinomas have been reported in reptiles, more commonly in the green iguana (*Iguana iguana*) (Gibbons and Schiller, 2000; Stacy et al., 2004). The cytology is characterized by neoplastic epithelial cells associated with cystic structures.

Granulosa cell tumors can also occur. One was described in a garter snake (*Thamnophis sirtalis*) that revealed neoplastic epithelial cells arranged in rosette-like structures (Onderka and Zwart, 1978).

Effusions

Because they lack the extensive air sac system of birds, the peritoneal cavity of many of the other lower vertebrates, such as reptiles, amphibians, and fish, is often a simple single cavity called the pleuroperitoneal cavity (Schildger et al., 1999). The only separate compartment of the pleuroperitoneal cavity is the pericardium, which lies on the ventral cranial thoracoabdominal area at the level of the pectoral girdle. Therefore, effusions in these animals occur throughout the entire coelomic cavity. Many lizards commonly seen in veterinary practices (e.g., green iguanas, *Iguana iguana*) and snakes have a coelomic cavity with a pleuroperitoneal design.

Reptiles that have additional compartments within the coelomic cavity include monitors (*Varanus* spp.), chelonians (turtles and tortoises), and crocodilians (Taylor, 2006). The pleural cavity is separated from the peritoneal cavity in monitors by a well-developed transverse post-pulmonary septum and completely occupies the cranial aspect of the thoracoabdominal cavity. The lungs of turtles and tortoises are located dorsally in the coelomic cavity, where they are partially attached to the carapace and are likewise separated from the peritoneal cavity by a post-pulmonary septum. However, the lungs of chelonians, unlike those of monitors, occupy only the dorsal-cranial aspect of the thoracoabdominal cavity. The coelomic cavity of crocodilians resembles that of monitors except that they have an additional post-hepatic septum (that functions somewhat like a mammalian diaphragm) that separates the liver from the caudal aspect of the peritoneal cavity (Schildger et al., 1999).

Fluid in the coelomic cavity of reptiles and amphibians can be simply aspirated by insertion of the needle

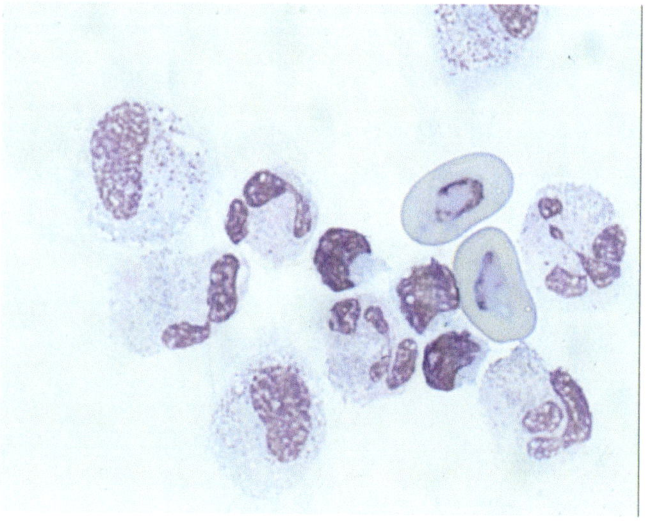

Fig. 23.51. Inflammatory cells (heterophils and macrophages) indicating an exudative effusion in the coelomic fluid from a lizard (*Chamaeleo calyptratus*), Wright–Giemsa stain (100× oil).

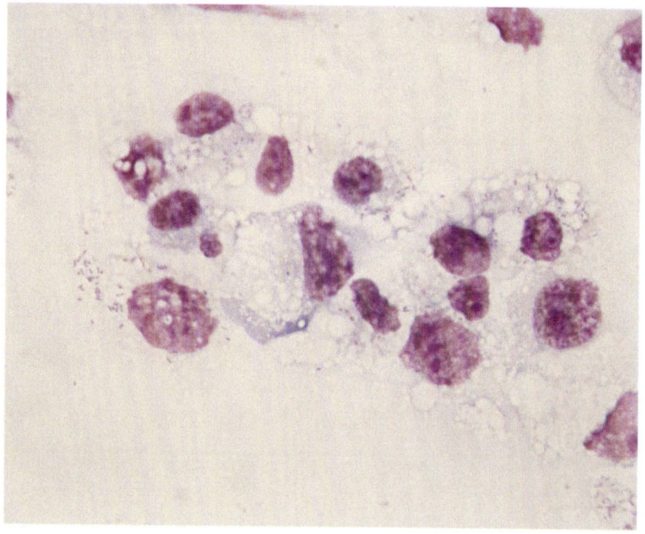

Fig. 23.52. A cytocentrifuge-concentrated coelomic fluid sample reveals inflammatory cells (predominately macrophages) indicating an exudative effusion in the coelomic fluid from a frog (*Litoria caerulea*). The leukocytes have phagocytized bacteria indicating a septic coelomitis, Wright–Giemsa stain (100× oil).

through the skin and body wall along the ventral aspect of the animal. A paramedian approach should be made to avoid the abdominal vein, which lies along the ventral midline. Fluid in the peritoneal cavity of chelonians can be sampled by inserting the needle through the body wall in the inguinal area just in front of a hind leg.

Coelomic effusions in herptiles are likely caused by many of the same conditions as described for birds and mammals. These include right heart failure, liver failure, mycobacteriosis, reproductive tract disorders (i.e., egg-related peritonitis and cystic ovary), and neoplastic diseases of other coelomic organs. These effusions are classified as transudates, modified transudates, exudates, hemorrhagic effusions, and malignant effusions (Figures 23.51– 23.53). The cytological appearances of these effusions resemble those found in birds. Egg-related coelomitis in reptiles has the same cytological characteristics as those described in birds. The inflammatory response is either a mixed-cell or macrophagic inflammation with a background that contains round fat droplets and large, blue "protein" bodies (Campbell and Grant, 2010) (Figures 23.54 and 23.55).

A coelomic effusion was reported in a frog associated with *Mycobacterium marinum* complex infection that revealed a mixed population of inflammatory cells (heterophils with a predominance of macrophages) that often contained intracytoplasmic, negatively stained, rod-shaped to filamentous organisms consistent with *Mycobacterium* sp. Ziehl–Neelsen stain revealed bright pink to red acid-fast organisms with a beaded appearance indicative of *M. marinum* complex (Tarigo et al., 2006).

Fluid accumulation disorders in amphibians are common. The etiology is often multifactorial and particular to amphibians' unique anatomy and physiology. Hydrocoelom (also called ascites and hydrops) refers to the accumulation of free fluid in the coelom; whereas lymphedema (also called anasarca) refers to the accumulation of fluid in the lymph sacs or other areas outside the coelom, especially the gular region and hind limbs. These disorders can occur separately or concurrently, and both may be generally referred to as bloat (Wright KM, 2001; Pessier AP, 2009).

The anuran kidney is mesonephric and lacks the ability to create hyperosmotic urine (Uchiyama and Yoshizawa, 2002). Terrestrial species can adjust water reabsorption in the distal segment of the nephron and via arginine vasotocin regulation of bladder epithelial permeability (Holz and Raidal, 2006; Raidal and Raidal, 2006). Terrestrial frogs are tolerant of dehydration, with high transcutaneous evaporative water loss, by absorbing water (approximately 80% of their total water intake) through a ventral "drink patch" lined with specialized electrolyte pumps and water transport aquaporins (Pessier, 2009). The specialized skin of anurans overlies large lymph sacs, which collect and store lymph to be returned to circulation by lymph hearts located in the pelvic region; therefore, any disturbance to the skin, lymphatics, or renal system could cause fluid accumulation in frogs.

Common causes of hydrocoelom and lymphedema include infections (commonly mycobacteriosis and

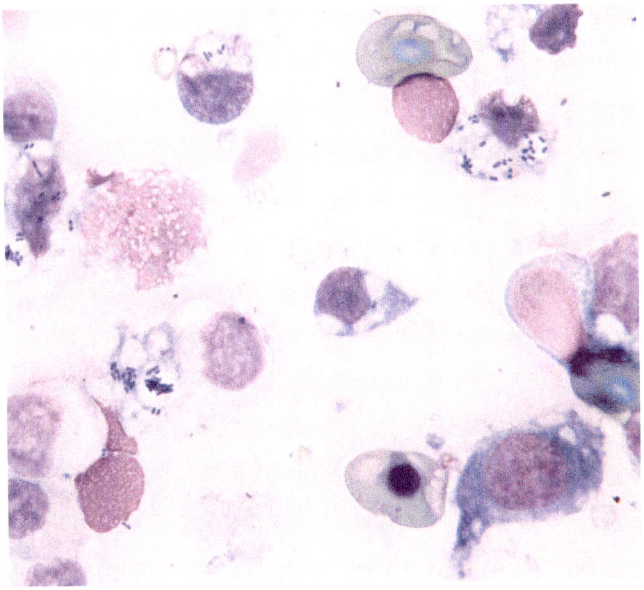

Fig. 23.53. A cytocentrifuge-concentrated coelomic fluid sample reveals inflammatory cells (predominately macrophages) indicating an exudative effusion in the coelomic fluid from a toad (*Bufo boreas boreas*). The leukocytes have phagocytized bacteria indicating a septic coelomitis, Wright–Giemsa stain (100× oil).

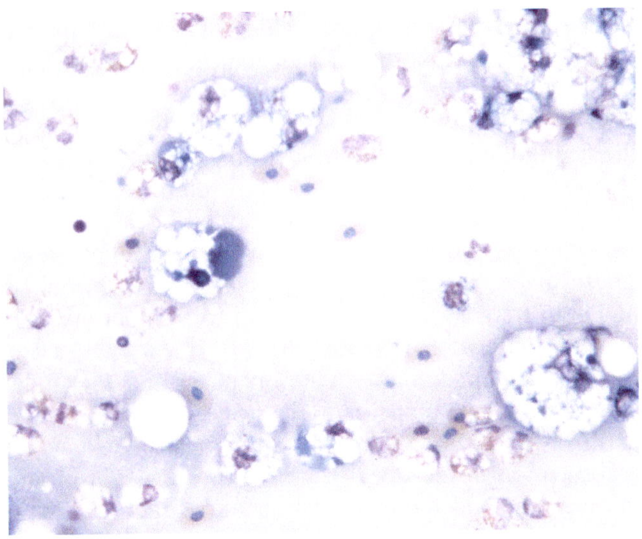

Fig. 23.54. Mixed-cell inflammation with numerous foamy macrophages and a background that contains round, fat droplets and large, basophilic globular material (presumed to be egg protein aggregates) are indicative of egg-related coelomitis in the coelomic fluid of a female lizard (*Chamaeleo calyptratus*), Wright–Giemsa stain (100× oil)

chytridiomycosis), gastrointestinal disease, and renal disease (Tarigo et al., 2006; Mangus et al., 2008; Freeman et al., 2008; Martinho and Heatley, 2012; Clancy et al., 2015). Gastrointestinal disease likely leads to protein loss and dysregulation of oncotic pressure and fluid homeostasis.

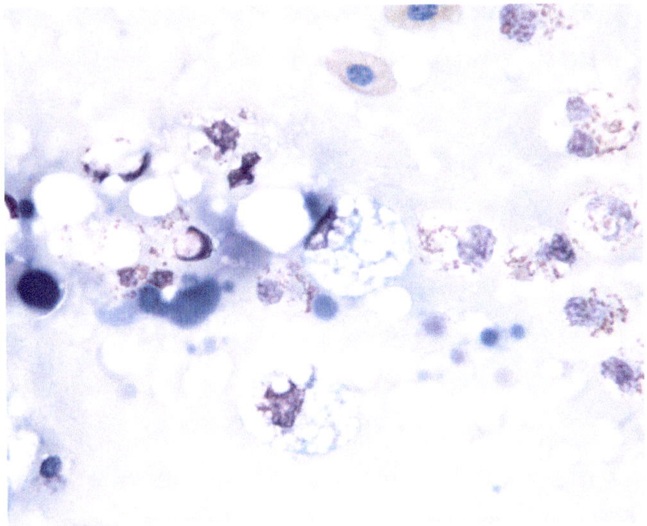

Fig. 23.55. Mixed-cell inflammation (heterophils and macrophages) with a background that contains round, fat droplets and large, basophilic globular material (presumed to be egg protein aggregates) are indicative of egg-related coelomitis in the coelomic fluid of a female lizard (*Iguana iguana*), Wright–Giemsa stain (100× oil).

Septic effusions exhibit intracellular bacteria observed on cytology preparations with the expected fluid specific gravity ranging between 1.005 to 1.020 and total solids measuring 1.06 g/dL to 3.4 g/dL (Clancy et al., 2015). Cytology of the fluid reveals erythrocytes, macrophages, heterophils, and lymphocytes.

Infectious Agents

Bacteria

Mycoplasmosis

Mycoplasmosis is the most important chronic infectious disease of wild and captive North American and European tortoises (Jacobson et al., 2014). The causative agents include *Mycoplasma agassizii* and *Mycoplasma testudineum*. Cytological preparations reveal varying degrees of epithelial hyperplasia and inflammatory infiltrates of lymphocytes, macrophages, and heterophils.

See Chapter 15 for a description of the organism.

Chlamydiosis

Chlamydial infections in reptiles and amphibians have been associated with granulomatous inflammation in internal organs (Ruegg et al., 2012). Chlamydia pneumoniae is frequently isolated from lesions as well as cloacal and choanal swab samples (Staub et al., 2018).

See Chapter 15 for a description of the organism.

Mycobacterium

Mycobacteriosis is an important cause of morbidity and mortality in amphibians, especially those in captivity. The most common isolates recovered from diseased amphibians are *Mycobacterium marinum*, *Mycobacterium fortuitum*, *Mycobacterium ulcerans*, and *Mycobacterium xenopi* (Milnes et al., 2020). The nontuberculous mycobacteria, especially *M. marinum*, are common in aquatic environments, and likely endemic in many zoo exhibits. *M. marinum* is an environmental opportunist rather than an obligate pathogen and is not closely related to or classified as part of the *M. tuberculosis* complex group (Milnes et al., 2020).

Nontuberculosis mycobacteria are variably gram-positive, often acid-fast, small rods that are ubiquitous in aquatic environments (Tarigo et al., 2006; Jarzembowski and Young, 2008). *Mycobacterium marinum* can cause chronic nonlethal granulomatous disease in immunocompetent frogs and acute lethal infections in immunosuppressed frogs (Ramakrishnan et al., 1997; Haridy et al., 2014). Mycobacteria granulomas in the skin and multiple internal organs of amphibians are often caused by a group of mycobacteria called mycolactone-producing mycobacteria (MPM) that contain a mycolactone-producing plasmid that causes immunosuppressive and cytotoxic toxin (mycolactone), which are considered to be important virulence factors in MPM infections (Li et al., 2017). Other species of nontuberculous *Mycobacterium* that have been isolated from frogs include *M. chelonae*, *M. gordonae*, *M. szulgai*, *M. xenopi*, *M. ulcerans*, and *M. liflandii* (Green et al., 2000; Trott et al., 2004; Fremont-Rahl, et al., 2011; Haridy et al., 2014; Fogelson et al., 2019). Mycobacteriosis should be considered in the differential diagnosis of coelomic effusion in amphibians.

Romanowsky-stained cytological preparations often reveal mixed-cell or macrophagic inflammation and varying numbers of negative-staining rod-shaped to filamentous organisms in the cytoplasm within the vacuoles of foamy macrophages (Figures 23.56a–23.56c). Acid-fast stains reveal large numbers of extracellular and intracellular bacteria that stain red.

Mycobacteria are well-recognized potential pathogens of reptiles and have been reported in various species, primarily in captive individuals. Mycobacterial infections have been described in different reptile species with granulomatous lesions, most often associated with *Mycobacterium marinum*, *Mycobacterium chelonae*, and *Mycobacterium thamnopheos*, but also sporadically with *Mycobacterium haemophilum*, *Mycobacterium kansasii*, *Mycobacterium agri*, *Mycobacterium confluentis*, *Mycobacterium hiberniae*, *Mycobacterium neoaurum*, and *Mycobacterium nonchromogenicum* (Muro et al., 2020).

Nontuberculous *Mycobacterium haemophilum* has been identified as the causative agent of disseminated mycobacteriosis in free-ranging sea turtles where the enteric swab cytology revealed marked mixed-cell inflammation with macrophages containing multiple negative-staining bacilli that were positive with Ziehl–Neelsen acid-fast stain (Donnelly et al., 2016).

Fungal Infections

Fungal agents are identified by the presence of yeast-like cells or hyphae (Figures 23.57 and 23.58). Some have special characteristics that aid in their identification.

Fungal dermatitis in reptiles is often related to compromised host immunity and involves infections with a variety of fungal organisms, such as *Aspergillus* spp., *Basidobolus* spp., *Geotrichum* spp., *Mucor* spp., *Saprolegnia* spp., *Candida* spp., and the *Chrysosporium* anamorph of *Nannizziopis vriesii* (Figures 23.33 and 23.58) (Bemis et al., 1999; Buenviaje et al., 2004; Cooper, 2006; Mitchell and Walden, 2013). Dermatophilosis is a contagious zoonotic skin infection caused by *Dermatophilus* spp. (i.e., *D. congolensis*) in a wide variety of animals; however, it is rare in free-ranging wild reptiles (Li et al., 2020).

Austwickia chelonae (basonym, *Dermatophilus chelonae*) thrives at lower temperatures, and as a result, it has lower pathogenicity for mammals compared with *Dermatophilus congolensis;* however, it may have host-adapted to poikilotherms, such as reptiles (Masters et al., 1995; Wellehan et al., 2004b). Cutaneous lesions appear as multiple, raised, encrusted nodules with proliferative or hyperkeratotic and heterophilic or granulomatous epidermatitis or dermatitis on histopathologic examination (Simmons et al., 1972; Tamukai et al., 2016). Impression smear preparations from the nodules may reveal numerous branching filaments composed of rows of coccoid to short rod-shaped organisms (Li et al., 2020).

Chytridiomycosis

Infections with the pathogenic keratinophilic chytrid fungus, *Batrachochytrium dendrobatidis* (chytridiomycosis), has been proved to cause massive amphibian declines worldwide (Berger, et al., 1998; Stuart et al., 2004; Lips et al., 2006; Skerratt et al., 2007; Wake and Vredenburg, 2008; Thien et al., 2013; Ruano-Fajardo et al., 2016; Talbott et al., 2018; Scheele et al., 2019; Latney and Klaphake, 2020). *Batrachochytrium dendrobatidis* is one of only two reportable amphibian pathogens (the other being ranavirus) that are listed by the World Animal Health Organization (Conradie et al., 2011). Unlike *Batrachochytrium dendrobatidis*, the species *Batrachochytrium salamandrivorans* is highly lethal to

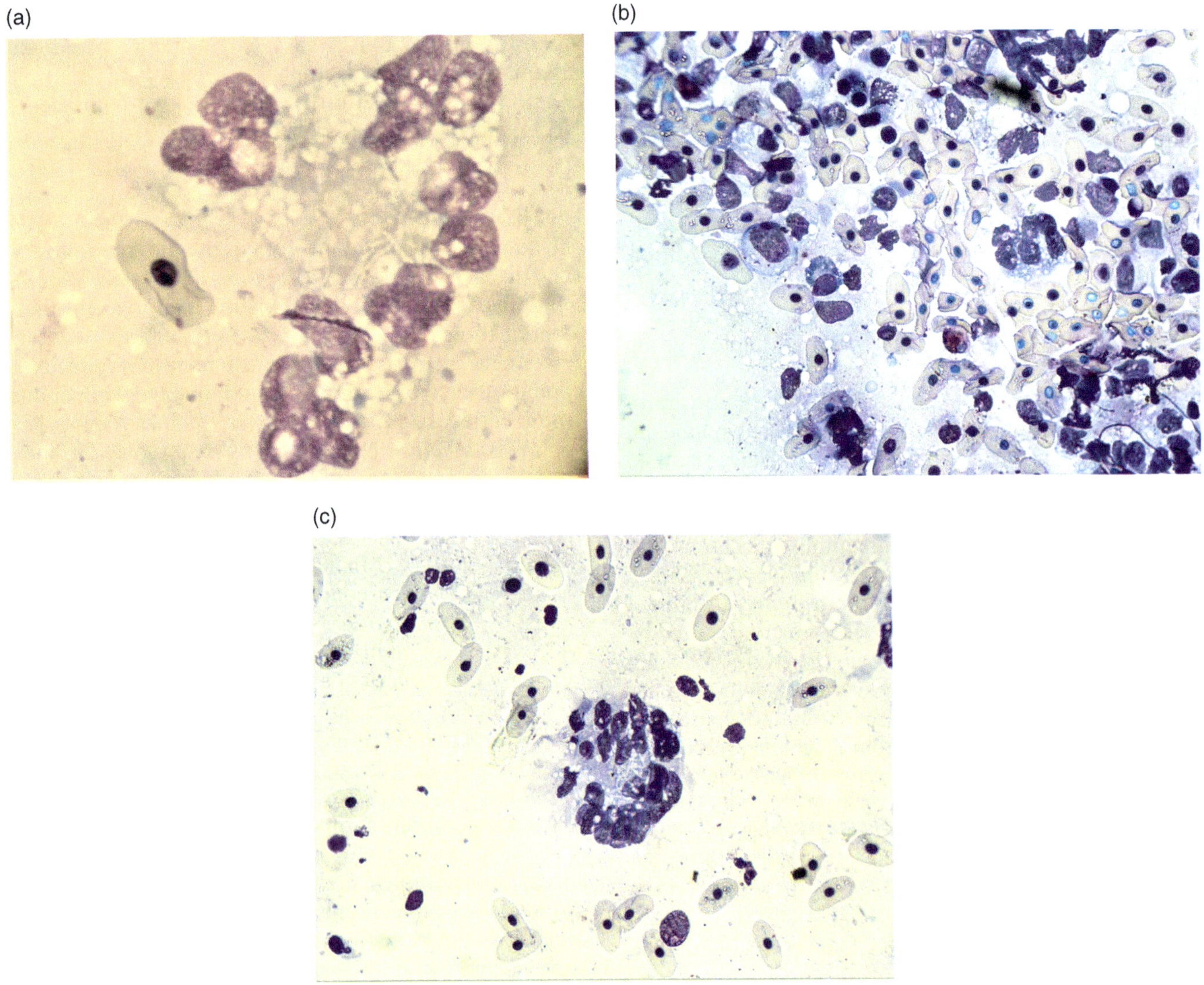

Fig. 23.56. (a) A multinucleated giant cell containing numerous bacterial rods that fail to stain (negative staining) in an imprint of a skin lesion associated with *Mycobacterium* sp. on a spectacled caiman (*Caiman crocodiles*), Wright–Giemsa stain (100× oil). (b) Macrophagic inflammation in an imprint of a skin lesion on an American alligator (*Alligator mississippiensis*) with multiple granulomas associated with *Mycobacterium* sp. on its digits, Wright–Giemsa stain (100× oil). (c) A multinucleated giant cell containing numerous bacterial rods that fail to stain (negative staining) in an imprint of a skin lesion on an American alligator (*Alligator mississippiensis*) with multiple granulomas associated with *Mycobacterium* sp. on its digits, Wright–Giemsa stain (100× oil).

many species of salamanders (Martel et al. 2014; Diaz et al., 2020; Hardman et al., 2020).

The disease is found in captive and wild populations of amphibians, including anurans, urodeles, and caecilians. B. *dendrobatidis* is one of the most common pathogens related to diseases in captive amphibian collections (Churgin et al., 2013; Tamukai et al., 2014; Mutschmann, 2015; Bauer et al., 2018).

Chytridiales are primitive fungi that lack hyphae and produce flagellated, movable zoospores. They are primarily found in aquatic or moist environments, where they infect algae, plants, protozoans, or invertebrates (Paulraj et al., 2016). *Batrachochytrium* is the only known genus that infects vertebrates, and is restricted to amphibians (Skerratt et al., 2011; Mutschmann, 2015).

Batrachochytrium dendrobatidis can infect all anurans and urodeles; however, the effects of the fungus on species range from subclinical infection to morbidity with mortality (Greenspan et al., 2012b; Martel et al., 2012; Kärvemo et al., 2019). For example, the bullfrog typically develops nonlethal infections and is considered a carrier of *B. dendrobatidis*. *B. salamandrivorans* is highly pathogenic to salamanders (Mutschmann, 2015; Talbott et al., 2018).

The flagellated motile zoospore is the infective stage. After the zoospore encysts on the surface of the

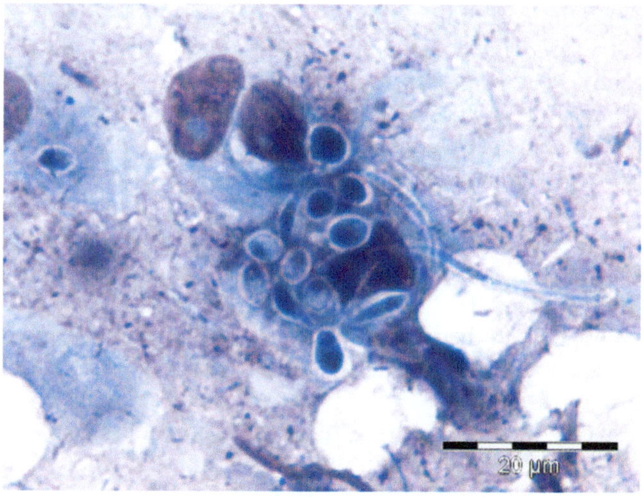

Fig. 23.57. Cytological smear of the tongue lesions from a veiled chameleon (*Chamaeleo calyptratus*) with yeast-like ovoid cells, short hyphae, and an epithelium cell, Diff–Quik stain (100× oil). Source: Schmidt (2015). Figure 7.

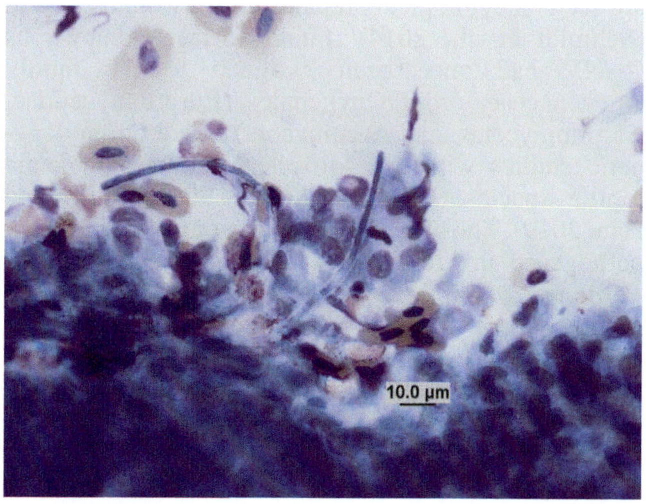

Fig. 23.58. Fungal hyphae in a scraping from a necrotic skin lesion in a bearded dragon (*Pogona vitticeps*), Wright–Giemsa stain (100× oil).

stratified keratinizing epithelial cells of amphibian's skin, the flagellum is resorbed, and a cell wall is formed. The cyst wall elongates to form a germination tube that penetrates a skin cell membrane within deeper cell layers beneath the stratum corneum (Greenspan et al., 2012; Van Rooij et al., 2012). The cytoplasm of the host cell is digested, allowing the contents of the encysted zoospore to migrate through the germ tube and develop into an intracellular thallus. The thallus, in turn, matures from sporangium to zoosporangium. The contents of the zoosporangium divide to form flagellated zoospores, and as it matures, the superficial stratum corneum cells shed more rapidly, allowing the infected cells to be brought to the skin surface (Berger et al., 2005; Greenspan et al., 2012). At this stage, the thallus forms a discharge papilla that extends through the skin cell surface, allowing the motile zoospores to exit and disperse once enough moisture is present for them to migrate. Established thalli can also directly infect deeper cells via projection of rhizoid-like structures that form new sporangia (Van Rooij et al., 2012).

Cytological diagnosis is made from samples obtained by gentle skin scrapings from the feet (particularly webbing) and ventral body or from shed skin fragments of infected amphibians. These can be examined either as a wet-mount preparation or routinely stained air-dried smear. Microscopic examination of skin scrapings stained with quick stains or lactophenol is a rapid method for detection of *B. dendrobatidis* on dead and living animals (Oevermann and Robert, 2004). Quantification of infections on frogs as zoospore equivalents can be made by using a swabbing approach combined with quantitative real-time polymerase chain reaction (Waddle et al., 2018).

Cytological preparations of skin lesions contain nucleated epidermal cells occasionally containing variable numbers of intracytoplasmic, round to oval fungal organisms (thalli) 3–10 μm long and 3–8 μm wide with a thin, non-staining exterior wall and numerous extracellular bacteria (Dusick et al., 2017) (Figures 23.59a and 23.59b). Important features that differentiate the thalli from the epithelial cells, soil debris, and yeast, algae, non-chytrid fungi, and protozoa normally found on the skin of amphibians include thalli-like structures that contain numerous 1 to 2 μm basophilic zoospores; empty thalli (ones that have previously discharged their zoospores); and colonial thalli, which exhibit evidence of internal septation (Pessier, 2007) (Figures 23.60a–23.60c). Congo red stain has been shown to delineate the chytrid zoosporangia from these non-chytrid structures and can be used as a rapid screening test for chytridiomycosis (Briggs and Burgin, 2003). These zoosporangia have average diameters that range from 10 to 45 μm and produce zoospores. After maturing, the zoospores are released through a "discharge tube." The ovoid or sometimes slightly elongated zoospores have average diameters that range from 0.7 and 6 μm (Mutschmann, 2015).

Amphibians infested with the organisms have thickened skin with hyperkeratosis with sloughing of the outer layers. Oval structures with distinct cell walls and multiple nuclei in the thickened or sloughed skin likely indicate the thalli or zoosporangia of the chytrid fungus, *Batrachochytrium dendrobatidis*, especially when they contain multiple discrete zoospores (Pessier et al., 1999; Campbell and Grant, 2010). In anurans, keratin is restricted to the mouthparts of tadpoles; *B. dendrobatidis* is gradually distributed to the skin during

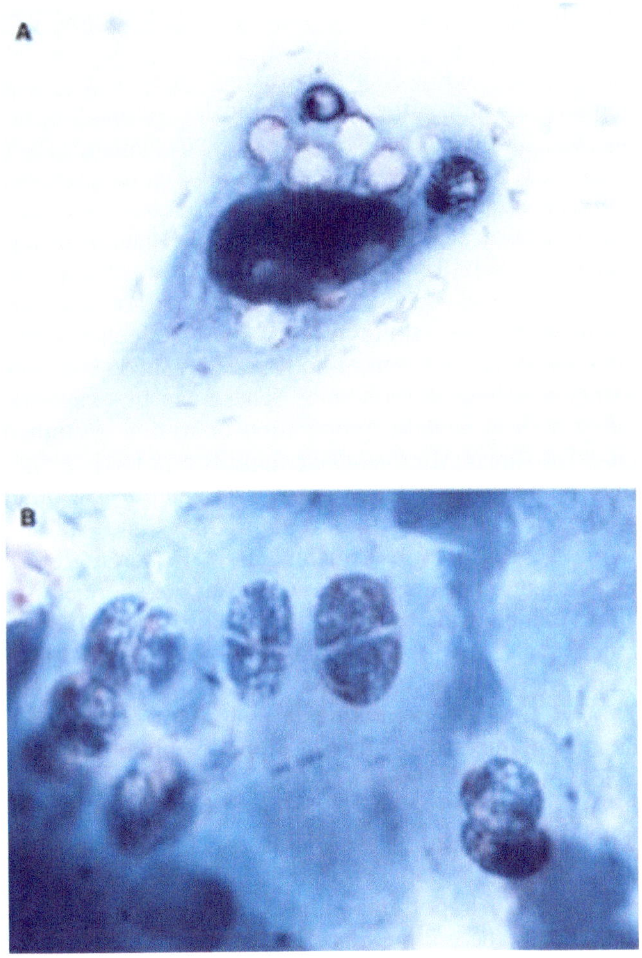

Fig. 23.59. Cytology of a postmortem skin scraping from a hellbender (*Cryptobranchus alleganiensis*). The sample consisted primarily of nucleated epidermal cells occasionally containing variable numbers of intracytoplasmic, round to oval fungal organisms (thalli) 3–10 μm long and 3–8 μm wide with a thin, non-staining exterior wall. Developing thalli were internally diffusely basophilic with or without a small amount of focal, magenta to purple stippling (containing developing zoospores). Empty thalli (after zoospore discharge) were primarily non-staining (Figure A). There were occasional colonial thalli characterized by a non-staining septal division (Figure B). There were numerous extracellular bacteria. Methanolic Wright's stain, 100× objective. Source: Image from Dusick et al. (2017).

metamorphosis and remains in the stratified epidermis post metamorphosis (Marantelli et al., 2004; Fernández-Beaskoetxea et al., 2016).

Onygenalean Dermatomycosis (*Chrysosporium*)

Many different filamentous fungi and yeasts can cause cutaneous and systemic infections in reptiles. *Chrysosporium* species constitute a large group of ubiquitous, primarily soil-borne and often keratinolytic anamorphic species, which are responsible for occasional opportunistic infections in humans, and different *Chrysosporium* species have been identified in multiple reptile species presenting with clinical signs of infection (Kahraman et al., 2015; Chandrakar et al., 2016).

Like the pathogenic chytrid fungus, *Batrachochytrium dendrobatidis*, *Chrysosporium* anamorph of *Nannizziopsis vriesii*, or CANV, is a keratinophilic fungus that causes severe and often fatal dermatitis in multiple reptile species (Paré et al., 2006; Bowman et al., 2007; Abarca et al., 2008; Toplon et al., 2012; Rhim and Han, 2019). It is especially pathogenic to the inland bearded dragon, where it causes a deep granulomatous dermatomycosis known as "yellow fungus disease."

CANV is a catch-all term that represents a group of closely related fungi, many of which have not been named; therefore, fungi causing skin infections in reptiles are commonly referred to as members of the CANV complex (Sigler et al., 2013; Paré, 2014). For example, *Devriesea agamarum* and *Chrysosporium guarroi* fungi, identified by PCR and culture, are responsible for causing a deep dermatitis in an inland bearded dragon where hyphal elements and bacteria are seen on cytological preparations of wound exudate (Schmidt et al., 2014). Fungi formerly known as CANV had once been assigned to the family Onygenaceae, order Onygenales (Eurotiomycetidae, Eurotiomycetes, and Ascomycota) based on phylogenetic studies with nine different known pathogenic reptile species (Paré and Sigler, 2016; Rhim and Han, 2019). The order Onygenales contains significant pathogens in reptiles, including *Ophidiomyces*, *Parananizziopsis*, *Emydomyces*, and *Nannizziopsis* species; all of which appear morphologically similar and produce aleurioconidia and fission arthroconidia (Pare´ et al., 2020). Within Onygenales, there is a trend in host specificity: Nannizziopsis includes nine species associated with chamaeleonid, gekkonid, cordylid, teiid, agamid, and iguanid lizards, crocodiles, and human hosts; Paranannizziopsis includes four species that infect squamates and tuataras; and there are two monotypic genera, *Ophidiomyces* (*O. ophiodiicola* [formerly *Chrysosporium ophiodiicola*]) is associated with terrestrial or semiaquatic snakes, and *Emydomyces* (*E. testavorans*) is associated with freshwater aquatic turtles (Pare and Sigler, 2016; Woodburn et al., 2019; Pare´ et al., 2020).

CANV-related dermatomycosis is found in lizards, terrestrial and aquatic snakes, and crocodiles worldwide (Sigler et al., 2013; Schmidt-Ukaj et al., 2016). Among them, Onygenalean dermatomycosis (formerly yellow fungus disease-associated pathogenic fungi) in bearded dragons include *N. guarroi*, *N. chlamydospora*, *N. draconii*, and *N. barbata* (Abarca et al., 2009; Johnson et al., 2011). *Nannizziopsis* spp. are pathogenic in lizards, whereas *Ophidiomyces* spp. are pathogenic to snakes (Rhim and Han, 2019). *N. guarroi* is the most

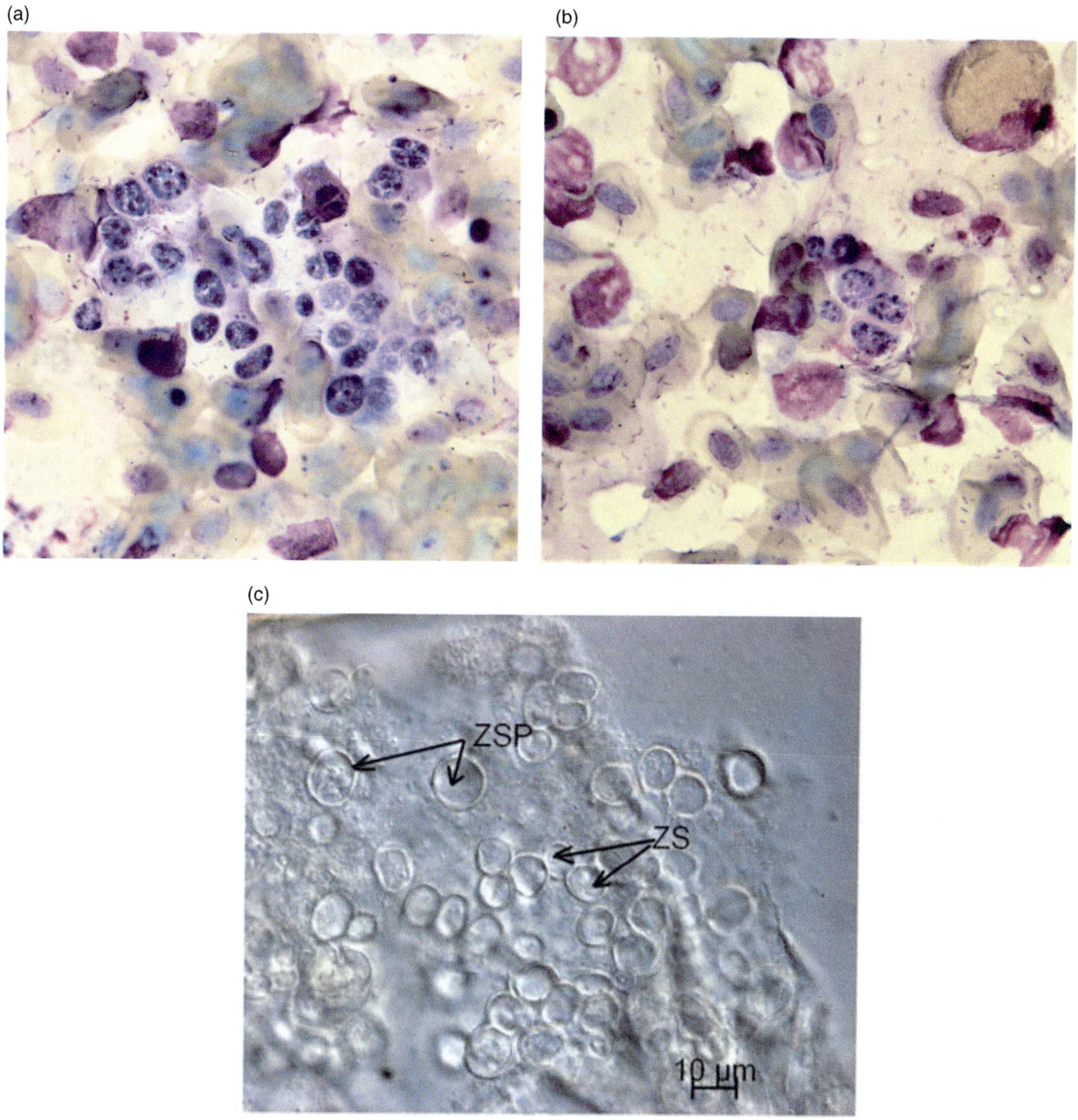

Fig. 23.60. (a) Zoosporangia or thalli, the round to oval structures with distinct cell walls and multiple nuclei, of the chytrid fungus, *Batrachochytrium dendrobatidis,* in the scraping of thickened skin on a poison dart frog (family Dendrobatidae), Wright–Giemsa stain (100× oil). Source: Image from Campbell and Grant (2010, p. 318). (b) Numerous erythrocytes and a heterophil with zoosporangia or thalli of the chytrid fungus, *Batrachochytrium dendrobatidis,* the round to oval structures with distinct cell walls and multiple nuclei in the center of the field, in the scraping of thickened skin on a poison dart frog (family Dendrobatidae), Wright–Giemsa stain (100× oil). Source: Image from Campbell and Grant (2010, p. 318). (c) Zoosporangia in pieces of sloughed skin of a marine toad (*Rhinella marina*). ZS: zoospore; ZSP: zoosporangia. Source: Mutschmann (2015).

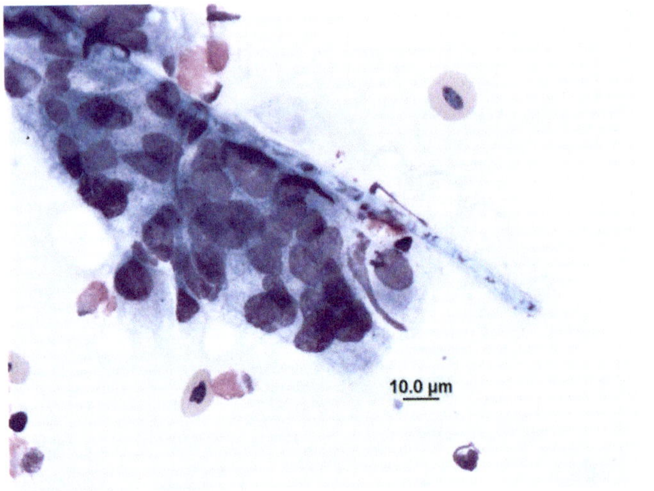

Fig. 23.61. Septate hyphae in a scraping from a necrotic skin lesion in a bearded dragon (*Pogona vitticeps*) with *Chrysosporium* anamorph of *Nannizziopsis vriesii* (CANV) fungal infection, Wright–Giemsa stain (100× oil)

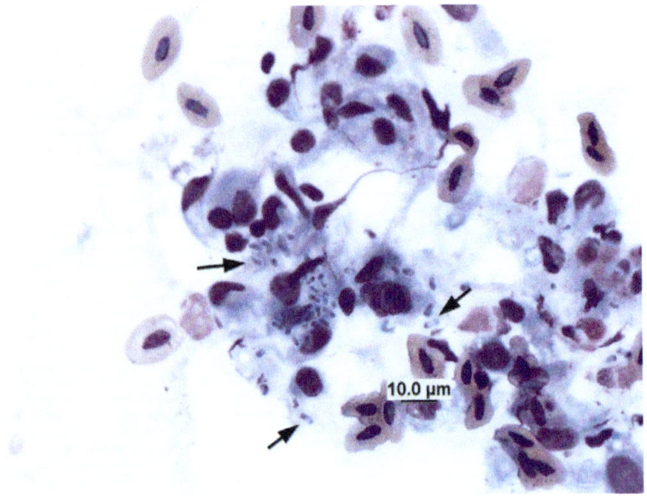

Fig. 23.62. Arthroconidia, rectangular spores with rounded ends (a few indicated by arrows), in a scraping from a necrotic skin lesion in a bearded dragon (*Pogona vitticeps*) with *Chrysosporium* anamorph of *Nannizziopsis vriesii* (CANV) fungal infection, Wright–Giemsa stain (100× oil).

important fungal organism responsible for causing dermatitis in commonly kept lizards; whereas, *O. ophiodiicola* causes fungal dermatitis in free-living and captive snakes (Rajeev et al., 2009; Rhim and Han, 2019; Pare´ et al., 2020).

Onygenalean dermatomycosis (CANV-complex dermatitis) should be suspected with any ulcerative or nodular skin lesion in a reptile. Cytological preparations of cutaneous lesions infected with this organism reveal mixed-cell inflammation with septate hyphae with the presence of conidia (aleurioconidia and arthroconidia) usually in aggregates and embedded within keratinaceous material (Figures 23.58, 23.61, and 23.62). The conidia appear as rectangular spores with rounded ends (ovoid- to club-shaped and occasionally budding and septate) scattered throughout the sample. The conidia measure approximately 2–3 × 3–7 µm and typically have a central purple nucleus and occasionally a thin clear capsule (Minard et al., 2016). Because onygenalean dermatomycosis is caused by a variety of fungal species, a definitive identification of the etiologic agent is based on sequence data and probe hybridization (Pare´ et al., 2020).

Ophidiomycosis

Ophidiomycosis (snake fungal disease) is caused by the fungus *Ophidiomyces ophiodiicola* and has been documented in captive and free-ranging snakes worldwide (McKenzie et al., 2020). Lesions cause by this fungus include facial swelling, granulomatous dermatitis, emaciation, and death. Fungal hyphae may be seen on cytological samples from granulomatous lesions.

Chamaeleomyces

Chamaeleomyces granulomatis has been associated with a disseminated systemic mycosis in captive veiled chameleons (Schmidt et al., 2012; Schmidt, 2015). C. *viridis*, formerly *Paecilomyces viridis*, is closely related to C. *granulomatis* and has caused disseminated systemic mycoses in carpet chameleons, panther chameleons, and bearded dragons (Sigler et al., 2010). Cytological preparations of lesions associated with these fungi reveal macrophages, lymphocytes, heterophils, yeast-like ovoid cells, and short hyphae indicative of fungal infection (Schmidt, 2015) (Figure 23.63).

Saprolegniasis

Saprolegniasis is a catch-all term for white, fuzzy mold growth on the skin of fish. Oomycetes, such as *Saprolegnia* and related genera, are common water molds that are frequently associated with skin infections on fish and amphibians, and rarely, reptiles (Noga, 2000). Although oomycetes produce hyphae and sporangia that release numerous zoospores into the environment, they are not classified as fungi, but rather as Stramenopiles within the kingdom Protista, a group that also includes brown algae and diatoms (Lau et. al., 2020). Oomycetes behave as fungi, thriving when moist and penetrating tissues with the turgor of its hyphal filaments to cause disease, and the term *saprolegniasis* refers specifically to the infectious process affecting freshwater fish and amphibians, usually by the genera *Saprolegnia*, *Aphanomyces*, *Achlya*, and *Branchiomyces*.

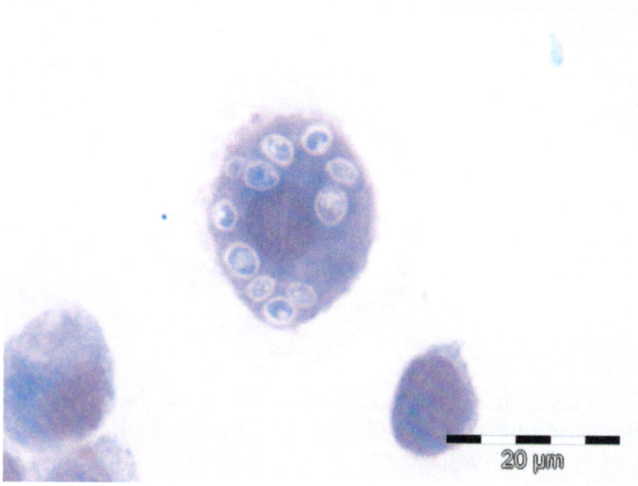

Fig. 23.63. Cytological smear of the pharynx lesions from a bearded dragon (*Pogona vitticeps*) with yeast-like ovoid cells inside the cytoplasm of erythrocytes, Diff–Quik stain (100× oil). Source: Schmidt (2015).

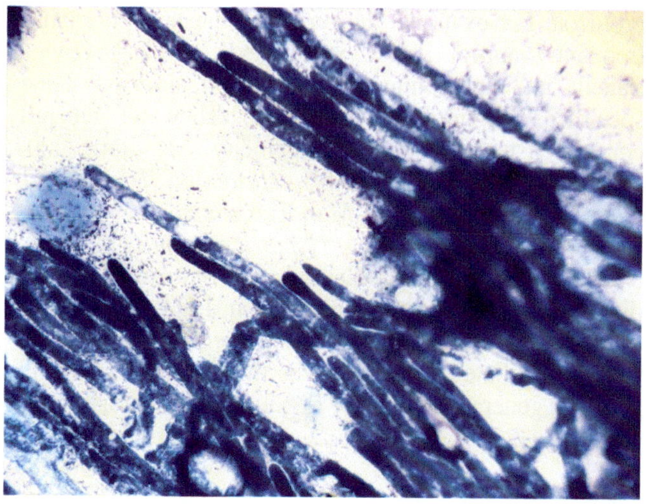

Fig. 23.64. Septate, non-branching fungal hyphae compatible with that of *Saprolegnia* in a scraping from a white patchy skin lesion in a rough-skinned newt (*Taricha granulosa*), Wright–Giemsa stain (100× oil). Source: From Campbell and Grant (2010, p. 315).

Gross lesions caused by these fungi appear as white, cotton-like growths on the skin and gills. Wet-mount preparations reveal wide (7–30 μm) aseptate- or septate-non-branching hyphae that are often associated with other pathogens, such as bacteria and protozoa (Figure 23.64).

Parasitic Infections

Cryptosporidiosis

Cryptosporidium spp. are a diverse group of obligate, coccidian parasites that can cause significant morbidity and mortality in a wide range of vertebrate species, including captive and free-ranging reptiles. *Cryptosporidium* spp. generally affect the gastrointestinal and respiratory tracts of reptiles; however, extra-enteric cryptosporidiosis can also occur (Cranfield and Graczyk, 1996; Xiao et al., 2004; Richter et al., 2012; Díaz et al., 2013; Rivas et al., 2018). Reptile patients with the gastrointestinal form of cryptosporidiosis present clinically with hypertrophic gastritis, or progressive enteritis with chronic diarrhea, lethargy, and wasting. *Cryptosporidium serpentis* and *C. varanii* are the predominant species found in reptiles with *C. ducismarci* also found in chelonians; however, *Cryptosporidium avium*, usually considered a pathogen of birds, can also infect reptiles (Lewis et al., 2020).

Carnivorous reptiles may pass nonpathogenic cryptosporidial organisms obtained from their rodent prey, causing a false-positive diagnosis of cryptosporidiosis (Cranfield and Graczyk, 1994). *Cryptosporidium* develop via a direct life cycle. Transmission occurs by the oral-fecal route or from exposure to contaminated food or water. Autoinfection can occur as well because the oocysts are passed fully sporulated. After ingestion, the oocyst encysts and four sporozoites are released. The sporozoites then invade the microvillus border of the gastric glands. Once an active infection is established, approximately 80% of the oocysts produced are thick-walled and pass in the feces to the environment. Twenty percent of the oocyst are thin-walled and rupture in the lumen of the gastrointestinal tract, releasing sporozoites resulting in autoinfection of the host (Georgi and Georgi, 1990).

Cryptosporidium serpentis has been associated with both high morbidity and mortality in captive collections of snakes (Cranfield and Graczyk, 2006; da Paixao et al., 2011; Richter et al., 2012). *Cryptosporidium saurophilum* is associated with lizards. Whereas *C. serpentis* is associated with the stomach, *C. saurophilum* is associated with the intestine. *Cryptosporidium varanii* occurs in lizards (also described in ophidian species) and tends to infect the mucous membrane of the small intestine and more rarely the stomach or large intestine (Richter et al., 2012). Specific gastric and intestinal *Cryptosporidium* are common in captive tortoise species, where the intestinal species, *Cryptosporidium ducismarci*, has been associated with clinical disease and pathological lesions (Brinkmeier et al., 2013).

Cryptosporidial organisms are typically identified on acid-fast (TB Quick Stain, Becton-Dickinson Microbiology Systems, Sparks, MD) stained fecal or regurgitated meal smears where they appear as round (4–6 μm diameter), bright pink organisms (Figure 23.65). When stained with Wright–Giemsa stain, *Cryptosporidium* spp. appear as round, clear to pale blue extracellular organisms approximately the size of mammalian erythrocytes that contain numerous dark blue internal structures when viewed under an oil-immersion objective (100×) (Harr et al., 2000) (Figures 23.66a and 23.66b). Faster and more sensitive detection methods include commercial immunofluorescent assays or immunoenzymatically assay kits, or PCR on feces or tissues (Graczyk et al., 1996a; Richter et al., 2012; Hallinger et al., 2018; Latney and Wellehan, 2020).

Coccidiosis

Coccidiosis is a major cause of morbidity and mortality in reptiles. Coccidia are identified by finding their oocyst in the feces in direct smears or by enrichment methods like centrifugation and flotation. *Eimeria* is the more commonly encountered genus; however, its clinical significance is unknown (Jacobson, 2007). *Isospora* spp. has been rarely reported in chelonians (Bardi et al., 2019). *Isospora amphiboluri* is of special concern to neonatal bearded dragons, causing stunted growth and death. The genus *Caryospora* has been described only in green sea turtles. *C. cheloniae* has been responsible for epizootic outbreaks in wild and captive green sea turtles with high mortality rate (Gordon et al., 1993).

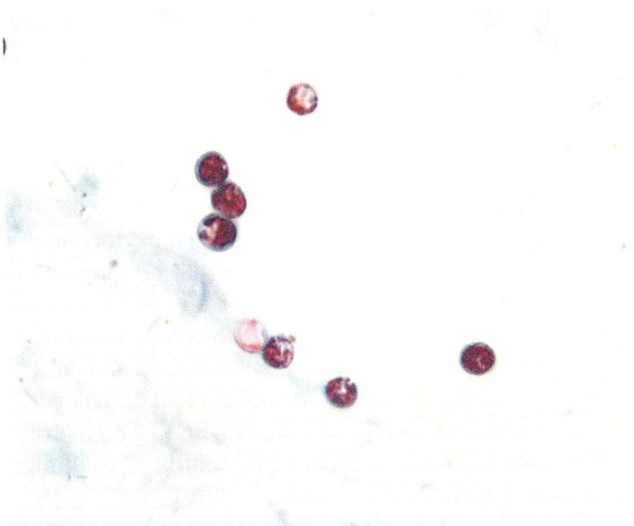

Fig. 23.65. Acid-fast positive *Cryptosporidium* in a fecal smear from a leopard gecko (*Eublepharis macularius*), acid-fast stain (100× oil).

Flagellated Protozoa

Flagellated protozoa are common in the digestive tract flora of reptiles and found on fecal cytology (Figures 23.67a and 23.67b). Wet-mount preparations are useful in the detection of the mobile trophozoites in fresh fecal smears. Staining the smear with a drop of methylene blue will kill protozoans and helps to identify trophozoites, and morphological identification is aided by staining air-dried fecal smears with quick stains (Bardi et al., 2019). Stained air-dried preparations often alter the appearance of the protozoa. For example, the piriform-shaped trichomonads frequently appear round, vacuolated, and lack obvious flagella and undulating membranes on air-dried stained specimens (Figures 23.68a–23.68d). They are generally considered to be of low pathogenicity (McArthur, 2004; Scullion and Scullion, 2009). *Hexamita, Trichomonas, Giardia, Leptomonas, Monocercomonas*, and, less frequently *Hexamastix, Hypotrichomonas, Tetratrichomonas*, and *Tritrichomonas* have been associated with disease in reptiles (Barnard and Upton, 1994). Of these, the trichomonad flagellate *Monocercomonas* and the diplomonad flagellate *Hexamita* appear to be the most frequently involved genera in reports of flagellate-induced/-associated

(a)

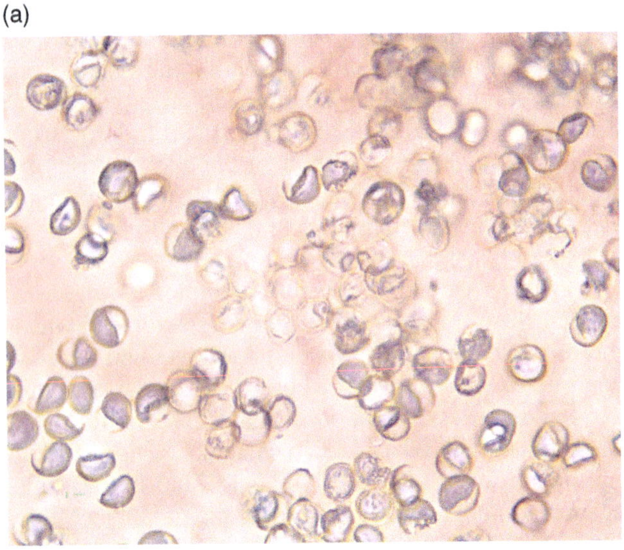

(b)

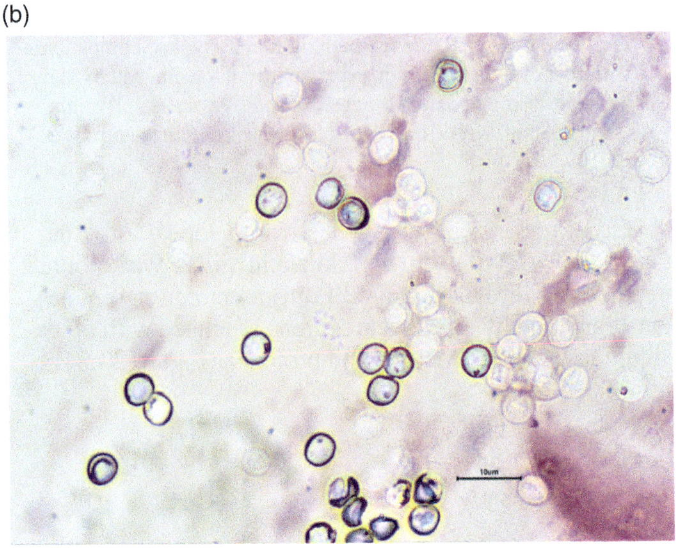

Fig. 23.66. (a) *Cryptosporidium* in a fecal smear from a leopard gecko (*Eublepharis macularius*), Wright–Giemsa stain (100× oil). (b) *Cryptosporidium serpentis* in a gastric lavage sample from a corn snake (*Elaphe* [*Pantherophis*] *guttata*), Wright–Giemsa stain (100× oil).

(a)

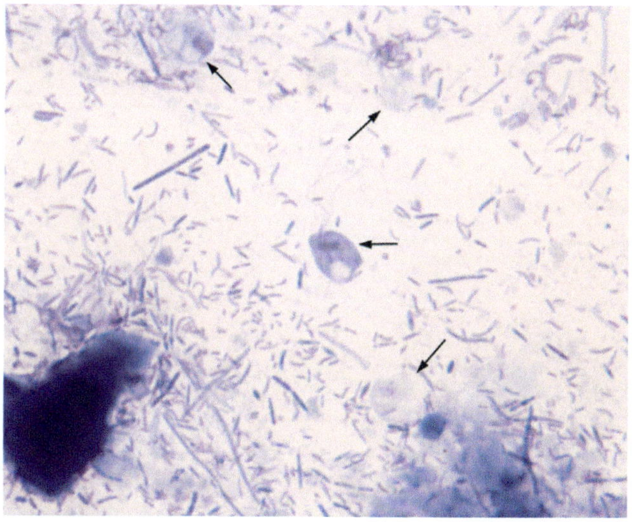

(b)

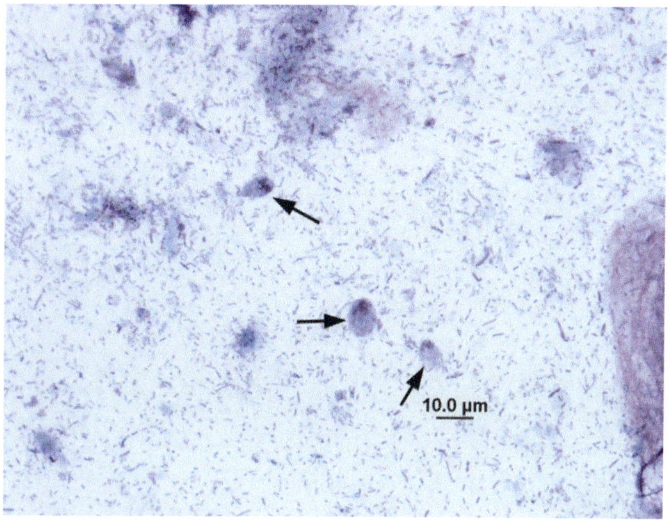

Fig. 23.67. (a) Stained piriform-shaped organisms (arrows, some are pale staining) in the feces that previously was examined as a wet-mount preparation that revealed numerous motile flagellate protozoa with undulating membranes that was supportive of a diagnosis of trichomoniasis in a leopard gecko (*Eublepharis macularius*), Wright–Giemsa stain (100× oil). (b) Stained piriform-shaped organisms (arrows) in the feces that previously was examined as a wet-mount preparation that revealed numerous motile flagellate protozoa with undulating membranes that was supportive of a diagnosis of trichomoniasis in a green tree python (*Morelia viridis*), Wright–Giemsa stain (100× oil).

disease (Zwart, 2006). *Hexamita* naturally inhabits the digestive tract of chelonians and snakes, and it has been associated with digestive, renal, and hepatic disease in chelonians. *Hexamita* spp. (especially *Hexamita parva*) is probably the most important flagellate in chelonians. Diagnosis of hexamitiasis by finding the mobile trophozoites in fecal or urinary samples is possible, but it is not always easy to differentiate *Hexamita* from other nonpathogenic flagellates. The egg-shaped Hexamita trophozoite (8×5 µm) has three pairs of flagella emerging from the cranial portion and one pair from the caudal portion. *Giardia* spp. are not pathogenic to reptile species (Bardi et al., 2019).

Renal disease caused by flagellate protozoa is rarely reported, but has been described with *Hexamita*, particularly in tortoises and turtles, where ascension from the cloaca to the lower urinary tract and later the kidneys is assumed to occur in reptiles with flagellate-associated disease (Juan-Sallés et al., 2014).

Tritrichomonas spp. and *Monocercomonas* spp are commonly found in the gastrointestinal tract of terrestrial chelonians without being associated with pathological conditions and are therefore generally considered symbiotic organisms: however, an overgrowth of these flagellates may be associated with enteritis (Bardi et al., 2019).

Ciliate Protozoa

Intestinal ciliate protozoa (phylum: Alveolata, subphylum: Ciliophora) are identified by the presence of hair-like cilia. Diagnosis of gastrointestinal ciliates is achieved by detection of the cysts in a fecal direct smear with saline or after flotation, or by finding the large, mobile trophozoites (>100 µm) in direct wet-mount preparations. These protozoans are generally considered to be symbiotic and play a role in cellulose digestion in herbivorous reptiles.

Balantidium spp. and *Nyctotherus* spp. are the most frequently encountered ciliates, especially in terrestrial tortoises (Scullion and Scullion, 2009; Hedley et al., 2013). *Balantidium* can have a facultative pathogenicity: during systemic or pre-existent gastroenteric condition, it can invade large intestine mucosa, causing necrotic-hemorrhagic colitis and even spread to the liver and biliary system causing hepatic abscesses (Bardi et al., 2019).

Specific Bacterial Infections

Spirochetes

Spiral-shaped bacteria or spirochetes have been found in the mucus of reptiles suffering from mild upper respiratory disease (Figure 23.69)

Helicobacter

Helicobacter has been associated with gastric ulcers, ulcerative colitis, cholangiohepatitis, cellulitis, and bacteremia in mammals and birds; however, the organism is rarely reported in reptiles. However, it can cause fatal septicemia chelonians (Stacy and Wellehan, 2010).

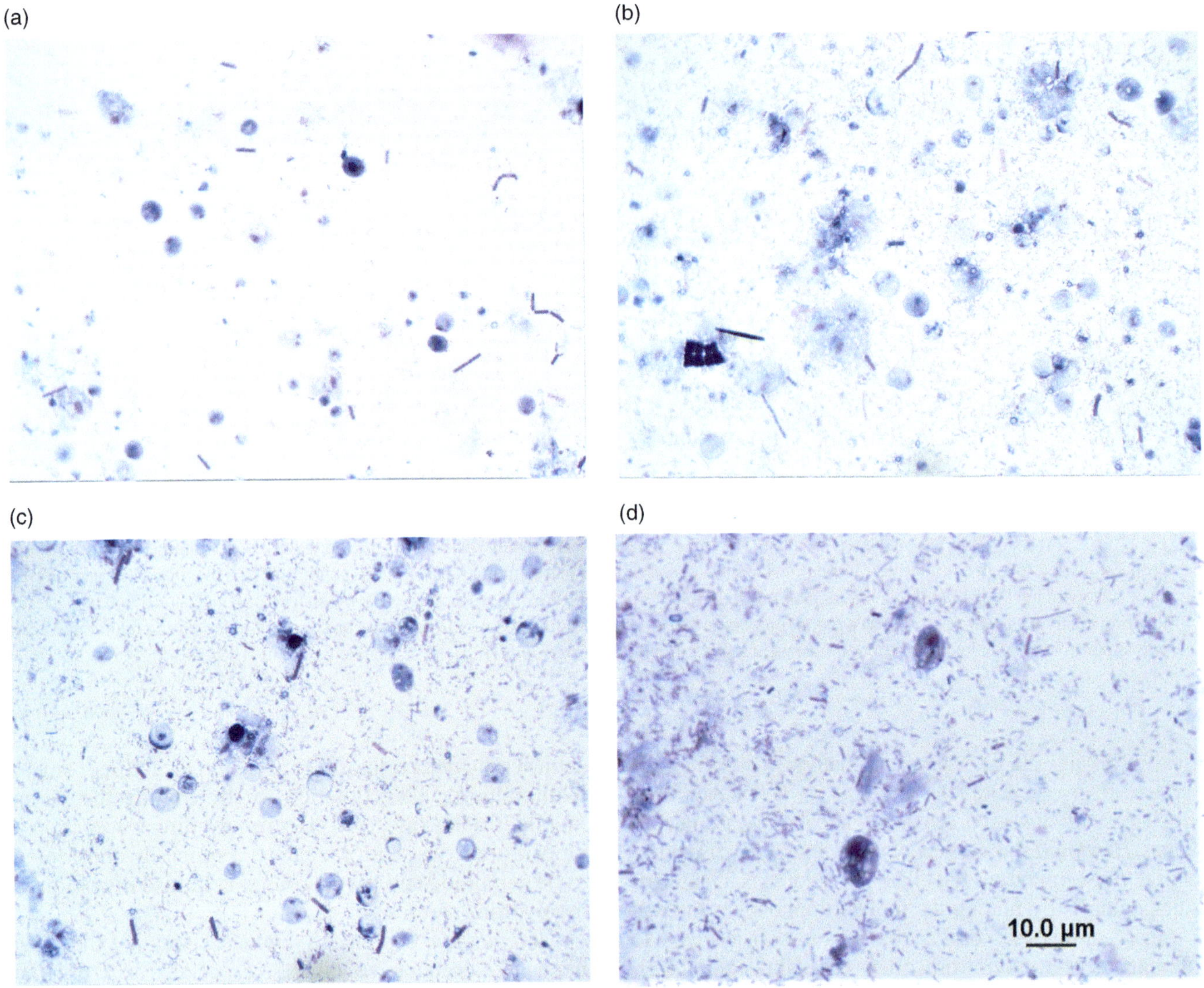

Fig. 23.68. (a) Variably stained, round trichomonad organisms that do not exhibit prominent flagella, undulating membrane, and axostyle in the feces that previously, on a wet-mount preparation, revealed numerous motile flagellate protozoa with undulating membranes that was supportive of a diagnosis of trichomoniasis in a red-footed tortoise (*Chelonoidis carbonaria*), Diff–Quik stain (100× oil). (b) Numerous variably stained, round trichomonad organisms that do not exhibit prominent flagella, undulating membrane, and axostyle in the feces that previously, on a wet-mount preparation, revealed numerous motile flagellate protozoa with undulating membranes that was supportive of a diagnosis of trichomoniasis in a red-footed tortoise (*Chelonoidis carbonaria*), Wright–Giemsa stain (100× oil). (c) Numerous variably stained, round, and vacuolated trichomonad organisms that do not exhibit prominent flagella, undulating membrane, and axostyle in the feces that previously, on a wet-mount preparation, revealed numerous motile flagellate protozoa with undulating membranes that was supportive of a diagnosis of trichomoniasis in a red-footed tortoise (*Chelonoidis carbonaria*), Wright–Giemsa stain (100× oil). (d) Stained piriform-shaped organisms lacking prominent flagella and undulating membranes in the feces that previously was examined as a wet-mount preparation that revealed numerous motile flagellate protozoa with undulating membranes that was supportive of a diagnosis of trichomoniasis in a hognose snake (*Heterodon platirhinos*), Wright–Giemsa stain (100× oil).

Viral Infections

Inclusion Body Disease of Boids

Inclusion body disease, a common and highly contagious disease seen worldwide in snakes of the families Boidae and Pythonidae, is caused by an arenavirus transmitted by the mite *Ophionyssus natricis* (Hetzel et al., 2013; Hepojoki et al., 2015; Tecilla and Roccabianca, 2018). Signs of infection range from mild to inapparent until the onset of central nervous system lesions that result in the snake's inability to feed (Tecilla and Roccabianca, 2018).

Diagnosis relies on finding the characteristic intracytoplasmic inclusions either in blood films or cytological preparations. The inclusions can be found in erythrocytes, lymphocytes, or heterophils. Inclusions

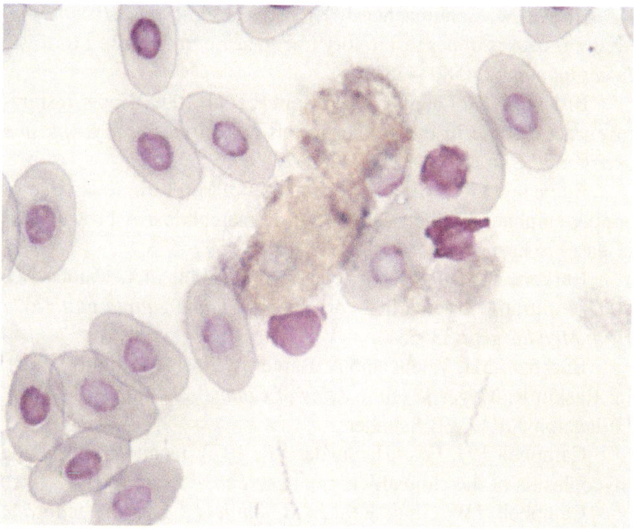

Fig. 23.69. Spiral-shaped bacteria or spirochetes and heterophils in a mucus swab from a three-toed box turtle (*Terrapene carolina triunguis*) suffering from mild upper respiratory disease.

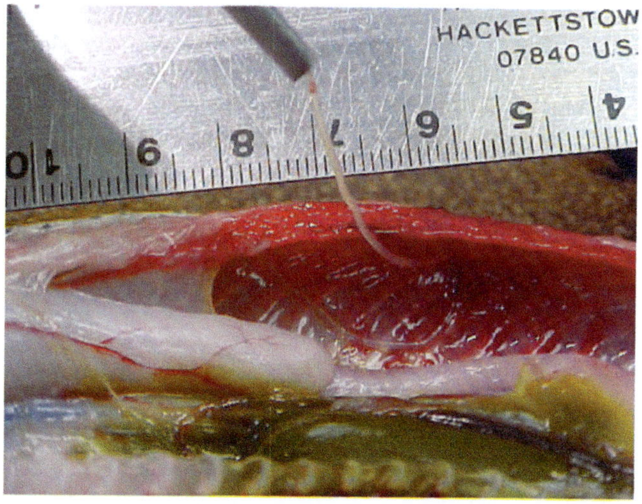

Fig. 23.70. An adult pentastomid in the air sac of a Guyana red-tailed boa (*Boa constrictor*).

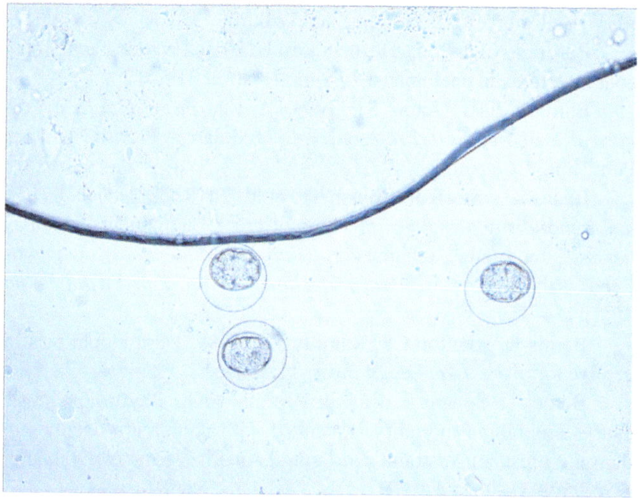

Fig. 23.71. Pentastomid ova found in a fecal sample from a Guyana red-tailed boa (*Boa constrictor*).

stained with Wright–Giemsa appear as lightly basophilic, homogenous, intracytoplasmic inclusions of varying size (2–6 μm in diameter) and shape (oval to elongate) that displaced the nucleus to the periphery of the cell (Banajee et al., 2012; Schilliger et al., 2014). Erythrocytic inclusions are distinct from the incidental basophilic punctate structures (believed to be degenerate organelles) commonly found in reptilian erythrocytes (Figures 19.9a and 19.9b in Chapter 19). Lymphocytosis is often present, presumably due to chronic antigenic stimulation from the infectious agent.

Herpesvirus

Although cheilitis in captive lizards is typically associated with onygenalean dermatomycosis caused by the CANV complex, other etiologic agents may also be responsible. For example, a novel herpesvirus (chamaeleonid herpesvirus 1) has been the cause of cheilitis with intracellular epidermal inclusions in chameleons (Hellebuyck et al., 2021).

Pentastomes

Pentastomes, crustacean endoparasites, are found as adults in the respiratory systems of reptiles, birds, and mammals (Figure 23.70). There, they lay eggs that pass out of the definitive host (Figure 23.71). The eggs are ingested by an intermediate host, commonly a fish or a small herbivorous mammal, where the larva hatches inside the intermediate host and breaks through the wall of the intestine (Woodyard et al., 2019). The larva then enters the tissues of its suitable host (Figure 31.33 in Chapter 31). The adults generally parasitize the respiratory systems of reptiles with little if any pathological tissue response, whereas, in accidental hosts, the response may be highly inflammatory.

References

Abarca ML, Martorell J, Castellá G, et al. 2008. Cutaneous hyalohyphomycosis caused by a *Chrysosporium* species related to *Nannizziopsis vriesii* in two green iguanas (*Iguana iguana*). *Med Mycol* 46:349–354.

Abarca ML, Martorell J, Castellá G, Ramis A, Cabañes FJ. 2009. Dermatomycosis in a pet inland bearded dragon (*Pogona vitticeps*) caused by a *Chrysosporium* species related to *Nannizziopsis vriesii*. *Vet Dermatol* 20:295–299.

Aguirre AA, Lutz PL. 2004. Marine turtles as sentinels of ecosystem health: is fibropapillomatosis an indicator? *Eco-Health* 1:275–283.

Anderson KB, Meinkoth J, Hallman M, Bailey L, Brandão J. 2019. Cytological diagnosis of gastric neuroendocrine carcinoma in a pet Inland bearded dragon (*Pogona vitticeps*). *J Exotic Pet Med* 29:188–193.

Andersson KE, Adamovicz L, Mumm LE, et al. 2021. Detection of a novel herpesvirus associated with squamous cell carcinoma in a free-ranging Blanding's turtle. *J Vet Diagn Invest* 33(2):348–351.

Baker R, Lumsden JH. 2000. Cytopathology techniques and interpretation. In: Baker R, Lumsden J (eds), *Color Atlas of the Dog and Cat*. St. Louis: Mosby.

Bagnara JT, Hadley ME. 1973. *Chromatophores and Color Change*. Englewood Cliffs, NJ: Prentice-Hall Inc., pp. 4–131.

Bagnara JT, Matsumoto J, Ferris W, et al. 1979. Common origin of pigment cells. *Science* 203(2):410–415.

Banajee KH, Chang L-W, Jacobson ER, Rich GA, Royal AB. 2012. What is your diagnosis? Blood film from a boa constrictor. *Vet Clin Pathol* 41(1):158–159.

Banks WJ. 1974. Histology and comparative organology. In: Banks, WJ (ed), *Histology and Comparative Organology: A Text Atlas*. Baltimore, MD: Williams and Wilkins.

Bardi E, Noviello E, Hofmannová L. 2019. Protozoa and protozoal infections in chelonians. *J Exotic Pet Med* 31:5–12.

Barnard SM, Upton SJ. 1994. *A Veterinary Guide to the Parasites of Reptiles: Protozoa, Vol. I*. Malabar, Florida, Krieger Publishing Company.

Bauer KL, Steeil JC, Walsh TF, et al. 2018. *Batrachochytrium dendrobatidis* in a captive collection of green salamanders (*Aneides aeneus*), long-tailed salamanders (*Eurycea longicauda*), and two-lined salamanders (*Eurycea bislineata*). *J Zoo Wildl Med* 49(2):454–459.

Bemis DA, Patton CS, Ramsay EC. 1999. Dermatophilosis in captive tortoises. *J Vet Diagn Invest* 11:553–557.

Berger L, Speare R, Daszak P, et al. 1998. Chytridiomycosis causes amphibian mortality associated with population declines in the rain forests of Australia and Central America. *Proc Nat Acad Sci USA* 95:9031–9036.

Berger L, Hyatt AD, Speare R, et al. 2005. Life cycle stages of the amphibian chytrid *Batrachochytrium dendrobatidis*. *Dis Aquat Organ* 68(1):51–63.

Bezjian M, Diep AN, de Matos R, Schaefer D. 2013. Case report: Chinese box turtle (*Cuora flavomarginata*) with lymphoid leukemia characterized by immunohistochemical and cytochemical phenotyping. *Vet Clin Pathol* 42(3):368–376.

Bielli M, Forlani A, Nardini G, Avallone G. 2015. Mucinous melanophoroma in a Northern red-bellied cooter (*Pseudemys rubriventris*). *J Exotic Pet Med* 24:71–75.

Bowman MR, Pare JA, Sigler L, et al. 2007. Deep fungal dermatitis in three inland bearded dragons (*Pogona vitticeps*) caused by the *Chrysosporium* anamorph of *Nannizziopsis vriesii*. *Med Mycol* 45(4):371–376.

Brenner EE, Sanchez CR, Garner MM. 2020. Squamous cell carcinoma in a group of Solomon island leaf frogs (*Ceratobatrachus guentheri*). *J Herpetol Med Surg* 30(4):242–247.

Briggs L, Burgin S. 2003. A rapid technique to detect chytrid infection in adult frogs. *Herpetol Rev* 34:124–126.

Brinkmeier BRM, Vrhovecy MG, Nedorost N, Pantchevy N. 2013. Cryptosporidial infections in captive tortoises. *ESVP/ECVP Proceedings*, p. 80.

Brown M, Schumacher J, Klein P, et al. 1994. *Mycoplasma agassizii* causes upper respiratory tract disease in the desert tortoise. *Infect Immun* 62:4580–4586.

Brown M, McLaughlin GL, Klein P, et al. 1999. Upper respiratory tract disease in the gopher tortoise is caused by *Mycoplasma agassizii*. *J Clin Microbiol* 37:2262–2269.

Buenviaje GN, Millan JM, Summers PM, et al. 2004. Use of copper sulphate for the treatment of dermatophilosis ('brown spot' disease) in farmed crocodiles. *Aust Vet J* 82:577–578.

Burkert, BA Tully TN, Nevarez J, Mitchell MA, Camus AC. 2002. Infiltrative lipoma in a corn snake (*Elaphe guttata guttata*). *J Herp Med Surg* 12:33–35.

Burkhard MJ, Valenciano A, Barger A. 2001. Respiratory tract. In: Raskin R, Meyer D (eds), *Atlas of Canine and Feline Cytology*. Philadelphia, PA: WB Saunders.

Campbell LH, Fos GJ, Snyder SB. 1973. Ocular bacteria and mycoplasma of the clinically normal cat. *Feline Pract* 1:10–12.

Campbell TW, Grant KR. 2010. *Clinical Cases in Avian and Exotic Animal Hematology and Cytology*. Ames: Wiley-Blackwell.

Chandrakar S, Dias M, Shetty P, Tiewsoh JBA, Guarro J. 2016. Isolation and characterization of an unknown *Chrysoporium* sp. producing subcutaneous mycosis in an immunocompromised patient. *Mycopahologia* 181(1–2):115–118.

Cheatwood JL, Jacobson ER, May PJ, et al. 2003. An outbreak of fungal dermatitis and stomatitis in a free-ranging population of pigmy rattlesnakes (*Sistrurus miliarius barbouri*) in Florida. *J Wild Dis* 39(2):329–337.

Churgin SM, Raphael BL, Pramuk JB, Trupkiewicz JG, West G. 2013. *Batrachochytrium dendrobatidis* in aquatic caecilians (*Typhlonectes natans*): a series of cases from two institutions. *J Zoo Wildl Med* 44(4):1002–1009.

Clancy MM, Clayton LA, Hadfield CA. 2015. Hydrocoelom and lymphedema in dendrobatid frogs at National Aquarium, Baltimore: 2003– 2011. *J Zoo Wildl Med* 46(1):18–26.

Cloup E, Thomas C, Cooper JE. 2019. A branchial cyst in a Diamond python (*Morelia spilota*) *J Comp Pathol* 173:92–95.

Colombo S, Berlim I, Delmas V, et al. 2011. Classical and non-classical melanocytes in vertebrates. In: Borovansky J, Riley PA (eds), *Melanins and Melanosomes: Biosynthesis, Biogenesis, Physiological and Pathological Functions*. Weinheim: Wiley-VCH, pp. 21–62.

Conradie W, Weldon C, Smith KG, Du Preez LH. 2011. Seasonal pattern of chytridiomycosis in common river frog (*Amietia angolensis*) tadpoles in South African Grassland Biome. *Afr Zool* 46(1):95–102.

Cooper JE. 2006. Dermatology. In: Mader DR (ed), *Reptile Medicine and Surgery*, 2nd edn. St Louis: WB Saunders, pp. 196–216.

Cowan DF. 1968. Diseases of captive reptiles. *J Am Vet Med Assoc* 153:848.

Cranfield MR, Graczyk TK. 1996. Cryptosporidiosis. In: Mader (ed), *Reptile Medicine and Surgery*. Philadelphia, PA: WB Saunders, pp. 359–363.

Cranfield MR, Graczyk TK. 1994. Experimental infection of elaphid snakes with *Cryptosporidium serptentis* (Apicomplexa: Cryptosporidiidae). *J Parasitol* 80:823–826.

Cranfield MR, Graczyk TK. 2006. Cryptosporidiosis. In: Mader DR (ed), *Reptile medicine and surgery*, 2nd edn. St. Louis, MO: Saunders Elsevier, pp. 756–762.

Crews J, Gendron K, Sladakovic I, et al. 2020. Liposarcoma of the fat body in a bearded dragon (*Pogona vitticeps*). *J Herpetol Med Surg* 30(4):232–236.

da Paixao A, Sercundes MK, Martins J, et al. 2011. Occurrence and molecular diagnosis of *Cryptosporidium serpentis* in captive snakes in Sao Paolo, Brazil. *J Zoo Wildl Med* 42:326–329.

de Brot S, Sydler T, Nufer L, Ruetten M. 2015. Histologic, immunohistochemical, and electron microscopic characterization of a malignant iridophoroma in a Dwarf bearded dragon (*Pogona henrylawsoni*). *J Zoo Wildl Med* 46(3):583–587.

De Santi M, Cruz N, Barranco G, et al. 2020. Cutaneous melanoma in a red-footed tortoise (*Chelonoidis carbonaria*). *J Exotic Pet Med* 34:44–47.

Díaz P, Rota S, Marchesi B, et al. 2013. Cryptosporidium in pet snakes from Italy: molecular characterization and zoonotic implications. *Vet Parasitol* 197(1–2):68–73.

Dietz, J, Heckers, KO, Aupperle, H, Pees, M. 2016. Cutaneous and subcutaneous soft tissue tumours in snakes: a retrospective study of 33 cases. *J Comp Pathol* 155:76- 87.

Diaz L, Hernandez-Gomez O, Unger SD. 2020. Prevalence of *Batrachochytrium dendrobatidis* in immature eastern hellbenders *Cryptobranchus alleganiensis* from North Carolina, USA. *Dis Aquat Organ* 140:73–78.

Done LB. 1996. Neoplasia. In: Mader D (ed), *Reptile Medicine and Surgery*. Philadelphia, PA: WB Saunders.

Donnelly K, Waltzek TB, Wellehan JFX, et al. 2016. *Mycobacterium haemophilum* infection in a juvenile leatherback sea turtle (*Dermochelys coriacea*). *J Vet Diagn Invest* 28(6):718–721.

Drzewiecka A, Kulec-Ploszczycay E, Terech-Majewskaz E, et al. 2016. Diathesis urica in terrestrial turtles. *J Comp Pathol* 154:96.

Duncan M, Dutton CJ, Junge RE. 2002. Lymphosarcoma in African spurred tortoises (*Geochelone sulcata*). *Proc Am Assoc Zoo Vet* 71–72.

Dusick A, Flatland B, Craig L, Ferguson S. 2017. What is your diagnosis? Skin scraping from a hellbender. *Vet Clin Pathol* 46(1):183–184.

Eleni C, Corteggio A, Altamura G, et al. 2017. Detection of papillomavirus DNA in cutaneous squamous cell carcinoma and multiple papillomas in captive reptiles. *J Comp Pathol* 157:23–26.

Elkan E. 1974. Malignant melanoma in a snake. *J Comp Pathol* 84:51–57.

Fernández-Beaskoetxea S, Bosch J, Bielby J. 2016. Infection and transmission heterogeneity of a multi-host pathogen (*Batrachochytrium dendrobatidis*) within an amphibian community. *Dis Aquat Org* 118:11–20.

Ferris RL, Quesenberry K. 2020. Treatment of multifocal cutaneous squamous cell carcinoma with strontium-90 and cryotherapy in a Midland painted turtle (*Chrysemys picta marginata*). *J Herpetol Med Surg* 30(1):3–8.

Fogelson SB, Camus AC, Lorenz WW, et al. 2019. Variation among human, veterinary and environmental *Mycobacterium chelonae-abscessus* complex isolates observed using core genome phylogenomic analysis, targeted gene comparison, and anti-microbial susceptibility patterns. PLoS ONE 14(3):1–20.

Freeman, K, Clayton L, Hadfield CA, Tuxbury K, Stoskopf M. 2008. Dissecting frog mortalities: filtering out the role of the kidneys. *Proc Assoc Reptil Amphib Vet*, p. 49.

Fremont-Rahl JJ, Ek C, Williamson HR, et al. 2011. *Mycobacterium liflandii* outbreak in a research colony of *Xenopus (Silurana) tropicalis* frogs. *Vet Pathol* 48:856–867.

Frye FL (ed). 1991. Common pathological lesions and disease processes: neoplasia. In: *Reptile Care: An Atlas of Diseases and Treatments, Vol. 2*. Neptune City, NJ: TFH Publishing.

Geissmann F, Manz MG, Jung S, et al. 2010. Development of monocytes, macrophages and dendritic cells. *Science* 327:656–661.

Georgi J, Georgi M (eds). 1990. Parasitology for veterinarians. In: *Parasitology for Veterinarians*, 5th edn. Philadelphia, PA: WB Saunders.

Georoff TA, Stacy NI, Newton AN, et al. 2009. Diagnosis and treatment of chronic T lymphocytic leukemia in a green tree monitor (*Varanus prasinus*). *J Herpetol Med Surg* 19:106–114.

Gibbons PM, Schiller CA. 2000. What's your diagnosis? Ovarian adenocarcinoma in a green iguana (*Iguana iguana*). *J Herpetop Med Surg* 10:34–38.

Gonzales-Viera O, Bauer G, Bauer A, et al. 2012. Cutaneous fibroma in a captive common snapping turtle (*Chelydra serpentina*). *J Comp Pathol* 147:574–576.

Gordon AN, Kelly WR, Lester RJG. 1993. Epozootic mortality of free-living green turtles, *Chelonia mydas*, due to coccidiosis. *J Wildl Dis* 29:490–494.

Graczyk TK, Owen R, Cranfield MR. 1996a. Diagnosis of subclinical cryptosporidiosis in captive snakes based on stomach lavage and cloacal sampling. *J Vet Parasitol* 67:143–151.

Graczyk TK, Cranfield MR, Fayer R. 1996b. Evaluation of commercial enzyme immunoassay (EIA) and immunofluorescent antibody (FA) test kits for detection of *Cryptosporidium* oocysts of species other than *Cryptosporidium parvum*. *Am J Trop Med Hyg* 54:274–279.

Green Sl, Lifland BD, Bouley DM, et al. 2000. Disease attributed to *Mycobacterium chelonae* in South African clawed frogs (*Xenopus laevis*). *Com Med* 50(6):675–679.

Greenspan SE, Longcore JE, Calhoun AJ. 2012. Host invasion by *Batrachochytrium dendrobatidis*: fungal and epidermal ultrastructure in model anurans. *Dis Aquat Organ* 100(3):201–210.

Greenspan SE, Calhoun AJK, Longcore JE, Levy MG. 2012b. Transmission of *Batrachochytrium dendrobatidis* to Wood frogs (*Lithobates sylvaticus*) via Bullfrog (L. *catesbeianus*) vector. *J Wildl Dis* 48(3):575–582.

Gregory CR, Harmon BG, Latimer KS, et al. 1997. Malignant chromatophoroma in a canebrake rattlesnake (*Crotalus horridus atricaudatus*). *J Zoo Wildl Med* 28(2):198–203.

Gull JM, Lange CE, Favrot C, Dorrestein GM, Hatt J-M. 2012. Multiple papillomas in a diamond python, *Morelia spilota spilota*. *J Zoo Wildl Med* 43(4):946–949.

Gutierre RC, Jared C, Antoniazzi MM, Coppi AA, Egami MI. 2018. Melanomacrophage functions in the liver of the caecilian *Siphonops annulatus*. *J Anat* 232:497–508.

Haag KM, Hernandez-Divers S, Latimer KS, et al. 2008. Infiltrative lipoma in a black rat snake, *Elaphe obsoleta*. *J Herp Med Surg* 17:129–131.

Hall J, Bender H, Parrish K, et al. 2020. Squamous cell carcinoma in two wild Bell's turtles (*Myuchelys bellii*). *J Wildl Dis* 56(4):937–940.

Hallinger MJ, Taubert A, Hermosilla C, et al. 2018. Occurrence of health-compromising protozoan and helminth infections in tortoises kept as pet animals in Germany. *Parasit Vectors* 11:352–364.

Hardman RH, Sutton WB, Irwin KJ, et al. 2020. Geographic and individual determinants of important amphibian pathogens in Hellbenders (*Cryptobranchus alleganiensis*) in Tennessee and Arkansas, USA. *J Zoo Wildl Dis* 56(4):803–814.

Haridy M, Tachikawa Y, Yoshidax S, et al. 2014. *Mycobacterium marinum* infection in Japanese forest green tree frogs (*Rhacophorus arboreus*). *J Comp Pathol* 151:277–289.

Harr KE, Henson KL, Raskin RE, et al. 2000. Gastric lavage from a Madagascar tree boa (*Sanzinia madagascarensis*). *Vet Clin Pathol* 29(3):93–96.

Harshbarger JC. 1976. *Activities Report Registry of Tumors in Lower Animals, 1975 Supplement.* Washington, DC: Smithsonian Institute Press.

Heckers KO, Aupperle H, Schmidt V, Pees M. 2012. Melanophoromas and iridophoromas in reptiles. *J Comp Pathol* 146:258–268.

Hedley J, Eatwell K, Shaw DJ. 2013. Gastrointestinal parasitic burdens in UK tortoises: a survey of tortoise owners and potential risk factors. *Vet Rec* 173:525–532.

Hellebuyck T,Ducatelle R, Bosseler L, et al. 2016. Basal cell carcinoma in two Hermann's tortoises (*Testudo hermanni*). *J Vet Diagn Invest* 28(6):750–754.

Hellebuyck T, Couck L, Ducatelle R, Van den Broeck W, Marschang RE. 2021. Cheilitis associated with a novel herpesvirus in two panther chameleons (*Furcifer pardalis*). *J Comp Pathol* 182:58–66.

Hepojoki J, Salmenperä P, Sironen T, et al. 2015. Arenavirus coinfections are common in snakes with boid inclusion body disease. *J Virol* 89(16):8657– 8660.

Herbst LH, Jacobson ER, Klein PA, et al. 1999. Comparative pathology and pathogenesis of spontaneous and experimentally induced fibropapillomas of green turtles (*Chelonia mydas*). *Vet Pathol* 36:551–564.

Hernandez-Divers S, Garner M. 2003. Neoplasia of reptiles with an emphasis on lizards. *Vet Clin N Am Exot Anim Pract* 6(1):251–273.

Hernandez-Divers SJ. 2006. Diagnostic techniques. In: Mader D (ed), *Reptile Medicine and Surgery*. St. Louis: Saunders Elsevier.

Hetzel U, Sironen T, Laurinmäki P, et al. 2013. Isolation, identification, and characterization of novel arenaviruses, the etiological agents of boid inclusion body disease. *J Virol* 87(20):10918–10935.

Holz PH, Raidal SR. 2006. Comparative renal anatomy of exotic species. *Vet Clin North Am Exot Anim Pract* 9:1–11.

Irizarry-Rovira AR, Wolf A, Ramos-Vara JA. 2006. Cutaneous melanophoroma in a green iguana (*Iguana iguana*) *Vet Clin Pathol* 35:101–105.

Jacobson ER, Ferris W, Bagnara JT, Iverson WO. 1989. Chromatophoromas in a pine snake. *Pigment Cell Res* 2:26–33.

Jacobson ER, Gaskin JM, Brown MB, et al. 1991. Chronic upper respiratory tract disease of free-ranging desert tortoises (*Xerobates agassizii*). *J Wild Dis* 27(2):296–316.

Jacobson ER, Burgelt C, Williams B, Harris RK. 1991a. Herpesvirus in cutaneous fibropapillomas of the green sea turtle (*Chelonia mydas*). *Dis Aquat Organ* 12:1.

Jacobson ER, 1994. The desert tortoise and upper respiratory tract disease. *Bull Assoc Rept Amphib Vet* 4(1):6.

Jacobson ER. 2007. Parasites and parasitic diseases of reptiles. In: Jacobson ER (ed), *Infectious Diseases and Pathology of Reptiles: Color Atlas and Text.* Boca Raton, FL: CRC Press, pp. 571–666.

Jacobson ER, Brown MB, Wendland LD, et al. 2014. Mycoplasmosis and upper respiratory tract disease of tortoises: a review and update. *Vet J* 201(3):257–264.

Jarzembowski J, Young M. 2008. Nontuberculous mycobacterial infections. *Arch Pathol Lab Med* 132:1333–1341.

Johnson III JG, Hulesch J, Schnelle A, et al. 2014. Diagnostic challenge. *J Exotic Pet Med* 23:113–116.

Johnson RS, Sangster CR, Sigler L, Hambletond S, Parée JA. 2011. Deep fungal dermatitis caused by the *Chrysosporium* anamorph of *Nannizziopsis vriesii* in captive coastal bearded dragons (*Pogona barbata*). *Aust Vet J* 89:515–519.

Jones YL, Fitzgerald SD. 2009. Articular gout and suspected pseudogout in a Basilisk lizard (*Basilicus plumifrons*). *J Zoo Wildl Med* 40(3):576–578.

Juan-Sallés C, Garner MM, Nordhausen RW, Valls X, Gallego M, Soto S. 2014. Renal flagellate infections in reptiles: 29 cases. *J Zoo Wildl Med* 45(1):100–109.

Kahraman BB, Sığırcı BD, Metiner K, et al. 2015. Isolation of *Chrysosporium guarroi* in a green iguana (*Iguana iguana*), in Turkey. *J Exotic Pet Med* 24:427–429.

Kärvemo S, Laurila A, Höglund J. 2019. Urban environment and reservoir host species are associated with *Batrachochytrium dendrobatidis* infection prevalence in the common toad. *Dis Aquat Org* 134:33–42.

Kusewitt DF, Reece RL, Miska KB. 1997. S-100 immunoreactivity in melanomas of two marsupials, a bird, and a reptile. *Vet Pathol* 34:615–618.

Lamglait B, Lemberger K. 2017. Colonic adenocarcinomas in a familial group of captive Amur rat snakes (*Elaphe schrencki*). *J Zoo Wildl Med* 48(2):491–496.

Lau CH, Snook ER, Swinford AK, Bryan LK. 2020. *Achlya* sp. dermatitis in an American alligator (*Alligator mississippiensis*). *J Comp Pathol* 175:1–4.

Latney LV, Klaphake E. 2020. Selected emerging infectious diseases of amphibians. *Vet Clin Exot Anim* 23:397–412.

Latney LV and Wellehan JFX. 2020. Selected emerging infectious diseases of squamata: an update. *Vet Clin Exot Anim* 23:353–371.

Leach MW, Nichols DK, Hartsell W, Torgerson RW. 1991. Radiation therapy of a malignant chromatophoroma in a yellow rat snake (*Elaphe obsolete quadrivittata*). *J Zoo Wildl Med* 22:241–244.

Lee S-Y, Kim J-W, Park H-M. 2011. Diagnosis and management of articular gout in Red-eared Slider (*Trachemys Scripta Elegans*). *J Korean Society of Vet Clin* 28(4):449–451.

Lewis N, Martinson S, Wadowska D, et al. 2015. Malignant mixed chromatophoroma with cutaneous, pulmonary and testicular metastases in a veiled chameleon (*Chamaeleo calyptratus*). *J Herpetol Med Surg* 25:16–20.

Lewis M, Bartley PM, Katzer F, et al. 2020. Conjunctival *Cryptosporidium avium* infection in a captive inland bearded dragon (*Pogona vitticeps*). *J Exotic Pet Med* 35:1–4.

Li W-T, Chang H-W, Pang VF, et al. 2017. Mycolactone-producing *Mycobacterium marinum* infection in captive Hong Kong warty newts and pathological evidence of impaired host immune function. *Dis Aquat Org* 123:239–249.

Li W-T, Tsai M-S; Chang H-W, Pang VF, Jeng C-R. 2020. Pathology in practice. *J Am Vet Med Assoc* 256(11):1233–1236.

Lips KR, Brem F, Brenes R, et al. 2006. Emerging infectious disease and the loss of biodiversity in a neotropical amphibian community. *Proc Nat Acad Sci USA* 103:3165–3170.

Mader DR. 2006. Gout. In: Mader DR (ed), *Reptile Medicine and Surgery*, 2nd edn. St. Louis, MO: Elsevier Saunders, pp. 793–800.

McArthur S. 2004. Problem-solving approach to common diseases of terrestrial and semiaquatic chelonians. In: McArthur S, Wilkinson S, Meyer J (eds), *Medicine and Surgery of Tortoises and Turtles*. Ames, Iowa: Wiley-Blackwell, pp. 309–377.

Machotka SV. 1984. Neoplasia in reptiles. In: Hoff GL, Frye FL, Jacobson ER (eds), *Diseases of Amphibians and Reptiles*. New York: Plenum Press.

Mackintosh JA. 2001. The antimicrobial properties of melanocytes, melanosomes and melanin and the evolution of black skin. *J Theor Biol* 211:101–113.

Mangus, LM, Montali, RJ, Clayton, LA, Bronson E. 2008. Renal disease in captive frogs: a retrospective study of amphibian histopathology. *Proc Assoc Reptil Amphib Vet*, p. 17.

Marantelli G, Berger L, Speare R, Keegan L. 2004. Distribution of the amphibian chytrid *Batrachochytrium dendrobatidis* and keratin during tadpole development. *Pac Conserv Biol* 10:173–179.

Marrinhas C, Santos J, Lopes, C, Marcos R. 2019. What is your diagnosis? Multiple masses in a Corn snake (*Pantherophis guttatus*). *Vet Clin Pathol* 48:134–136.

Martel A, Fard MS, Rooij PV, et al. 2012. Road-killed common toads (*Bufo bufo*) in Flanders (Belgium) reveal low prevalence of Ranaviruses and *Batrachochytrium dendrobatidis*. *J Wildl Dis* 48(3):835–839.

Martel A, Blooi M, Adriaensen C, et al. 2014. Recent introduction of a chytrid fungus endangers western palearctic salamanders. *Science* 346:630–631.

Martínez-Silvestre A, Amat F, Bargalló F, Carranza S. 2011. Incidence of pigmented skin tumors in a population of wild Montseny brook newt (*Calotriton arnoldi*). *J Wildl Dis* 47(2):410–414.

Martinho F, Heatley JJ. 2012. Amphibian mycobacteriosis. *Vet Clin North Am Exot Anim Pract* 15:113–119.

Masters AM, Ellis TM, Carson JM, et al. 1995. *Dermatophilus chelonae* sp. nov., isolated from chelonids in Australia. *Int J Syst Bacteriol* 45:50–56.

McKenzie CM, Oesterle PT, Stevens B, et al. s2020. Ophidiomycosis in red cornsnakes (*Pantherophis guttatus*): potential roles of brumation and temperature on pathogenesis and transmission. *Vet Pathol* 57(6):825–837.

Meinkoth JH, Cowell RL. 2002. Recognition of basic cell types and criteria of malignancy. *Veterinary Clinics of North America: Small Animal Practice* 32:1209–1235.

Mikaelian I, Lynch S, Harshbarger JC, Reavill DR. 2000. Malignant chromatophoroma in a day gecko. *Exot Pet Pract* 5(10):73–74.

Milnes EL, Delnatte P, Lentini A, et al. 2020. Mycobacteriosis in a zoo population of Chinese gliding frogs (*Rhacophorus dennysi*) due to *Mycobacterium marinum*. *J Herpetol Med Surg* 30(1):14–20.

Minard HM, Burrell C, Delgado JD, Rech RR, Nabity MB. 2016. What's your diagnosis? Skin impression smear from a bearded dragon. *Vet Clin Pathol* 45(3):505–506.

Mitchell MA, Walden MR. 2013. *Chrysosporium anamorph Nannizziopsis vriesii*: an emerging fungal pathogen of captive and wild reptiles. *Vet Clin North Am Exot Anim Pract* 16:659–668.

Muñoz-Gutiérrez JF, Garner MM, Kiupel M. 2016. Cutaneous chromatophoromas in captive snakes. *Vet Pathol* 53(6):1213–1219.

Muro J, Canturri A, Velarde R, et al. 2020. Atypical systemic mycobacteriosis in Hermann's tortoises (*Testudo hermanni*). *J Exotic Pet Med* 32:8–12.

Murray ML. 2006. Pneumonia and lower respiratory tract disease. In: Mader D (ed), *Reptile Medicine and Surgery*. St. Louis: Saunders Elsevier.

Mutschmann F. 2015. Chytridiomycosis in amphibians. *J Exotic Pet Med* 24:276–282.

Neogi T. 2011. Gout. *New Engl J Med* 364(5):443–452.

Noga EJ. 2000. Fish disease: diagnosis and treatment. In: Noga E (ed), *Fish Disease: Diagnosis and Treatment*. Ames, IA: Iowa State University Press.

Oevermann A, Robert N. 2004. Chytridiomycosis – an emerging and fatal infectious skin disease of amphibians. *Vet Dermatol* 15:70.

Okihiro MS. 1988. Chromatophoromas in two species of Hawaiian butterflyfish *Chaetodon multicinctus* and *C. miliaris*. *Vet Pathol* 25:422–431.

Onderka DK, Zwart P. 1978. Granulosa cell tumor in a garter snake (*Thamnophis sirtalis*). *J Wildl Dis* 14:218–221.

Origgi FG. 2007. Reptile immunology. In: Jacobson ER (ed), *Infectious Diseases and Pathology of Reptiles*. Boca, Raton: CRC Press, pp.131–157.

Orós J, Monagas P, Andrada M, Calabuig P, Pether J. 2009. Metastatic fibrosarcoma in a captive Saharan horned viper (*Cerastes cerastes*) with high hepatic levels of cadmium. *Vet Rec* 164:690– 692.

Paré JA, Coyle KA, Sigler L, et al. 2006. Pathogenicity of the *Chrysosporium* anamorph of *Nannizziopsis vriesii* for veiled chameleons (*Chamaeleo calyptratus*). *Med Mycol* 44:25–31.

Paré J. 2014. Update on fungal infections in reptiles. In: Mader DR, Divers SJ (eds), *Current Therapy in Reptile Medicine & Surgery*. St. Louis, MO: Elsevier Saunders, pp. 53–56.

Paré JA, Sigler L. 2016. An overview of reptile fungal pathogens in the genera *Nannizziopsis*, *Paranannizziopsis*, and *Ophidiomyces*. J Herp Med Surg 26(1–2):46–53.

Pare´ JA, Wellehan J, Perry SM, et al. 2020. Onygenalean dermatomycoses (formerly yellow fungus disease, snake fungal disease) in reptiles. *J Herpetol Med Surg* 30(4):198–209.

Paulraj A, Musthafa MS, Altaff K, et al. 2016. Chytrid *Batrachochytrium dendrobatidis* fungal infection in freshwater prawn, *Macrobrachium rosenbergii* (de Man) – a new report. *Aquac* 464:521–528.

Pennick KE, Holicky RA, Wilkerson MJ. 2017. What is your diagnosis? Joint and associated tissue aspirates from a bearded dragon (*Pogona vitticeps*). *Vet Clin Pathol* 46(2):363–364.

Pessier AP. 2009. Edematous frogs, urinary tract disease, and disorders of fluid balance in amphibians. *J Exotic Pet Med* 8:4–13.

Pessier A. 2007. Cytologic diagnosis of disease in amphibians. *Vet Clin North Am Exot Anim Pract* 10(1):187–206.

Pessier AP, Nichols DK, Longcore JE, Fuller MS. 1999. Cutaneous chytridiomycosis in poison dart frogs (*Dendrobates* spp.) and White's tree frogs (*Litoria caerulea*). *Vet Dian Invest* 11:194–199.

Raidal SR, Raidal SL. 2006. Comparative renal physiology of exotic species. *Vet Clin North Am Exot Anim Pract* 9:13–31.

Rajeev S, Sutton DA, Wickes BL, et al. 2009. Isolation and characterization of a new fungal species, *Chrysosporium ophiodiicola*, from a mycotic granuloma of a black rat snake (*Elaphe obsoleta obsoleta*). *J Clin Microbiol* 47:1265–1268.

Ramakrishnan L, Valdivia R, McKerrow J, Falkow S. 1997. *Mycobacterium marinum* causes both long-term subclinical infection and acute disease in the leopard frog (*Rana pipiens*). *Infect Immun* 65:767–773.

Rhim H, Han J-K. 2019. *Nannizziopsis chlamydospora* associated necrotizing dermatomycosis in a bearded dragon (*Pogona vitticeps*). *J Exotic Pet Med* 31:1–2.

Richter B, Rasim R, Vrhovec MG, Nedorost N, Pantchev N. 2012. Cryptosporidiosis outbreak in captive chelonians (*Testudo hermanni*) with identification of two *Cryptosporidium* genotypes. *J Vet Diagn Invest* 24(3):591–595.

Rivas AE, Boyer DM, Torregrosa K, Orrico WJ, Pare JA. 2018. Treatment of *Cryptosporidium serpentis* infection in a King cobra (*Ophiophagus hannah*). *J Zoo Wildl Med* 49(4):1061–1063.

Rivera S, Crane MM, McManamon R, Gregory CR. 2015. Surgical treatment of pulmonary melanophoroma in a Beaded lizard (*Heloderma horridum exasperatum*). *J Zoo Wildl Med* 46(2):397–399.

Rooney T, Eshar D, Njaa BL. 2020. Benign dermal iridophore aggregates in a crested gecko (*Correlophus ciliatus*). *J Exotic Pet Med* 35:17–19.

Rossi JV. 1996. Dermatology. In: Mader D (ed), *Reptile Medicine and Surgery*. Philadelphia, PA: WB Saunders.

Rovira ARI, Holzer TR, Credille KM. 2014. Systemic mastocytosis in an African fat-tail gecko (*Hemitheconyx caudicinctus*). *J Comp Pathol* 151:130–134.

Ruano-Fajardo G, Toledo LF, Mott T. 2016. Jumping into a trap: high prevalence of chytrid fungus in the preferred microhabitats of a bromeliad-specialist frog. *Dis Aquat Org* 121:223–232.

Ruegg S, Regenscheit N, Origgi FC, Borel N. 2012. *Chlamydia pneumoniae* in snakes: a case study. *ESVP/ECVP Proceedings* 2012, p. 54.

Ryan MJ, Hill DL, Whitney GD. 1981. Malignant chromatophoroma in a gopher snake. *Vet Pathol* 18(6):827–829.

Salinas EM, Arriaga BOA, Lezama JR, Bernal AM, Garrido SJL. 2013. Oral fibrosarcoma in a black iguana (*Ctenosaura pectinata*). *J Zoo Wildl Med* 44(2):513–516.

Santos IT, Carvalho AL, Henker LC, et al. 2021. Mucinous rectal adenocarcinoma in a Urutu snake (*Bothrops alternatus*). *J Comp Pathol* 184:56–59.

Scheele BC, Pasmans F, Skerratt LF, et al. 2019. Amphibian fungal panzootic causes catastrophic and ongoing loss of biodiversity. *Science* 363:1459–1463.

Schildger BJ, Häfeli W, Kuchling G, et al. 1999. Endoscopic examination of the pleuroperitoneal cavity in reptiles. *Semin Avian Exot Pet Med* 8(3):130–138.

Schilliger L, Rossfelder A, Bonwitt J, et al. 2014. Antemortem diagnosis of multicentric lymphoblastic lymphoma, lymphoid leukemia, and inclusion body disease in a Boa constrictor (*Boa constrictor imperator*). *J Herp Med Surg* 24(1):11–19.

Schmidt US, Loncaric I, Klang A, et al. 2014. Infection with *Devriesea agamarum* and *Chrysosporium guarroi* in an inland bearded dragon (*Pogona vitticeps*). *Vet Dermatol* 25(6):555.

Schmidt V. 2015. Fingal infections in reptiles – an emerging problem. *J Exotic Pet Med* 24:267–275.

Schmidt V, Plenz B, Pfaff M, et al. 2012. Disseminated systemic mycosis in veiled chameleons (*Chamaeleo calyptratus*) caused by *Chamaeleomyces granulomatis*. *Vet Microbiol* 161:145–152.

Schmidt-Ukaj S, Loncaric I, Spergser J, Richter B, Hochleithner M. 2016. Dermatomycosis in three central bearded dragons (*Pogona vitticeps*) associated with *Nannizziopsis* chlamydospore. *J Vet Diagn Invest* 28(3):319–322.

Schumacher J. 1996. Viral diseases. In: Mader D (ed), *Reptile Medicine and Surgery*. Philadelphia, PA: WB Saunders.

Scullion FT, Scullion MG. 2009. Gastrointestinal protozoal diseases in reptiles. *J Exotic Pet Med* 18:266–278.

Sharpe S, Lamm CG, Killick R. 2013. Intracoelomic anaplastic sarcoma in an intersex Madagascar tree boa (*Sanzinia madagascariensis*). *J Vet Diagn Invest* 25:153–157.

Sigler L, Gibas CF, Kokotovic B, et al. 2010. Disseminated mycosis in veiled chameleons (*Chamaeleo calyptratus*) caused by *Chamaeleomyces granulomatis*, a new fungus related to *Paecilomyces viridis*. *J Clin Microbiol* 48:3182–3192.

Sigler L, Hambleton S, Paré JA, et al. 2013. Molecular characterization of reptile pathogens currently known as members of the *Chrysosporium* anamorph of *Nannizziopsis vriesii* complex and relationship with some human-associated isolates. *J Clin Microbiol* 51:3338–3357.

Simmons GC, Sullivan ND, Green PE. 1972. Dermatophilosis in a lizard (*Amphibolurus barbatus*). *Aust Vet J* 48:465–466.

Skerratt LF, Berger L, Speare R, Cashins S, et al. 2007. Spread of chytridiomycosis has caused the rapid global decline and extinction of frogs. *EcoHealth* 4:125–134.

Skerratt LF, Mendez D, McDonald KR, et al. 2011. Validation of diagnostic tests in wildlife: the case of chytridomycosis in wild amphibians. *J Herpetol* 45(4):444–450.

Stacy B, Pessier AP. 2007. Host response to infectious agents and identification of pathogens in tissue section. In: Jacobson ER (ed), *Infectious Diseases and Pathology of Reptiles*. Boca, Raton: CRC Press, pp. 257–298.

Stacy BA, Vidal JD, Osofsky A, et al. 2004. Ovarian papillary adenocarcinomas in a green iguana (*Iguana iguana*). *J Comp Pathol* 130:223–228.

Stacy BA, Wellehan JFX. 2010. Fatal septicemia caused by *Helicobacter* infection in a pancake tortoise (*Malacochersus tornieri*). *J Vet Diagn Invest* 22:660–662.

Stacy NI, Ranly M, Pelton C. 2017. What is your diagnosis? Blood film from a green turtle (*Chelonia mydas*). *Vet Clin Pathol* 46(1):193–194.

Staub E, Marti H, Biondi R, et al. 2018. Novel species of *Chlamydia* isolated from snakes are temperature-sensitive and exhibit decreased susceptibility to Azithromycin. *J Comp Pathol* 158:114.

Steeil JC, Schumacher J, Hecht S, et al. 2013. Diagnosis and treatment of a pharyngeal squamous cell carcinoma in a Madagascar ground boa (*Boa madagascariensis*). *J Zoo Wildl Med* 44(1):144–151.

Stilwell JM, Boylan SM, Daniel W, et al. 2020. Intestinal adenocarcinoma with cloacal prolapse and reduction in a Northern leopard frog (*Lithobates pipiens*). *J Herpetol Med Surg* 30(4): 237–241.

Stoakes LC. 1992. Respiratory system. In: Benyon P, Lawton M, Cooper J (eds), *Manual of Reptiles*. Gloucestershire: British Small Animal Veterinary Association.

Stuart SN, Chanson JS, Cox NA, et al. 2004. Status and trends of amphibian declines and extinctions worldwide. *Science* 306:1783–1786.

Suedmeyer WK, Bryan JN, Johnson G, et al. 2007. Diagnosis and clinical management of multiple chromatophoromas in an eastern yellowbelly racer (*Coluber constrictor flaviventris*). *J Zoo Wildl Med* 38:127–130.

Taggart PL, Woolford L, Dunstan N, et al. 2021. Cutaneous chromatophoromas in four species of Australian elapid snake. *J Comp Pathol* 183:33–38.

Talbott K, Wolf TM, Sebastian P, et al. 2018. Factors influencing detection and co-detection of Ranavirus and *Batrachochytrium dendrobatidis* in Midwestern North American anuran populations. *Dis Aquat Org* 128:93–103.

Tamukai K, Une Y, Tominaga A, Suzuki K, Goka K. 2014. *Batrachochytrium dendrobatidis* prevalence and haplotypes in domestic and imported pet amphibians in Japan. *Dis Aquat Org* 109:165–175.

Tamukai K, Tokiwa T, Kobayashi H, et al. 2016. Ranavirus in an outbreak of dermatophilosis in captive inland bearded dragons (*Pogona vitticeps*). *Vet Dermatol* 27:99–105.

Tarigo J, Linder K, Neel J, et al. 2006. Reluctant to dive: coelomic effusion in a frog. What is your diagnosis? *Vet Clin Pathol* 35:341–344.

Taylor WM. 2006. Endoscopy. In: Mader D (ed), *Reptile Medicine and Surgery*, 2nd edn. St. Louis, MO: Saunders Elsevier.

Tecilla M, Roccabianca P. 2018. Inclusion body disease-associated necrotizing vascular lesions in a *Boa constrictor imperator*. *J Comp Pathol* 158:145.

Teyssier J, Saenko SV, van der Marel D, et al. 2015. Photonic crystals cause active colour change in chameleons. *Nat Commun* 6:6368.

Thien TN, Martel A, Brutyn M, et al. 2013. A survey for *Batrachochytrium dendrobatidis* in endangered and highly susceptible Vietnamese salamanders (*Tylototriton* spp.). *J Zoo Wildl Med* 44(3):627–633.

Thompson KA, Campbell M, Levens G, Agnew D. 2015. Bilaterally symmetrical oral amelonotic melanoma in a Boa constrictor (*Boa constrictor constrictor*). *J Zoo Wildl Med* 46(3):629–632.

Tong LJ, Ong W, Hulst F, et al. 2018. Clinical, diagnostic, and pathological features of 2 cases of metastatic iridophoroma in a Veiled chameleon (*Chamaeleo calyptratus*) and a red-barred dragon (*Ctenophorus vadnappa*) *J Exotic Pet Med* 27:53–60.

Toplon DE, Terrell SP, Sigler L, Jacobson ER. 2012. Dermatitis and cellulitis in Leopard geckos (*Eublepharis macularius*) caused by the *Chrysosporium* anamorph of *Nannizziopsis vriesii*. *Vet Pathol* 50(4) 585– 589.

Trott KA, Stacy BA, Lifland BD, et al. 2004. Characterization of a *Mycobacterium ulcerans*-like infection in a colony of African tropical clawed frogs (*Xenopus tropicalis*). *Com Med* 54(3):309–317.

Uchiyama M, Yoshizawa H. 2002. Nephron structure and immunohistochemical localization of ion pumps and aquaporins in the kidney of frogs inhabiting different environments. *Symp Soc Exp Biol* 54:109–128.

Underwood G. 1970. The eye. In: Gans C, Parsons T (eds), *Biology of Reptilia*, Vol. 2. London: Academic Press.

Van Rooij P, Martel A, D'Herde K, et al. 2012. Germ tube mediated invasion of *Batrachochytrium dendrobatidis* in amphibian skin is host dependent. *PLoS One* 7(7):e41481.

Vetere A, Simonini C, Casali S, et al. 2020. First report of oral squamous cell carcinoma in a green tree python (*Morelia viridis*). *J Exotic Pet Med* 35:1–2.

Vetere A, Bertocchi M, Pelizzone I, et al. 2021. Cytobrushing of the oral mucosa as a possible tool for early detection of testudinid herpesvirus in Horsfield's tortoises with nonspecific clinical signs. *Vet Diagn Invest* 33(1):116–119.

Waddle AW, Sai M, Levy JE, et al. 2018. Systematic approach to isolating *Batrachochytrium dendrobatidis*. *Dis Aquat Org* 127:243–247.

Wake DB, Vredenburg VT. 2008. Are we in the midst of the sixth mass extinction? a view from the world of amphibians. *Proc Natl Acad Sci USA* 105:11466–11473.

Webb KL, Grindem C, Dombrowski DS. 2015. What is your diagnosis? A soft tissue mass in a black rat snake. *Vet Clin Pathol* 44(4):611–612.

Wellehan JFX, Embury JE, Terrell SP, Raskin RE. 2004a. Synovial fluid from an African spur-thighed tortoise (*Geochelone sulcate*). *Vet Clin Pathol* 33(1):43–46.

Wellehan JF, Turenne C, Heard DJ, et al. 2004b. *Dermatophilus chelonae* in a king cobra (*Ophiophagus hannah*). *J Zoo Wildl Med* 35:553–556.

Woodburn DB, Miller AN, Allender MC, Maddox CW, Terio KA. 2019. *Emydomyces testavorans*, a new genus and species of onygenalean fungus isolated from shell lesions of freshwater aquatic turtles. *J Clin Microbiol* 57(2):1–11.

Woodyard ET, Baumgartner WA, Rosser TG, et al. 2019. Morphological, molecular, and histopathological data for *Sebekia mississippiensis* Overstreet, Self, and Vliet, 1985 (Pentastomida: Sebekidae) in the American alligator, *Alligator mississippiensis* Daudin, and the Spotted Gar, *Lepisosteus oculatus* Winchell. *J Parasitol* 105(2):283–298.

Wright K. 2014. Amphibian therapy. In: Mader DR, Divers SJ (eds), *Current Therapy in Reptile Medicine and Surgery*. St. Louis, MO: Elsevier Saunders, p. 287.

Wright KM, 2001.Amphibian hematology. In: Whitaker BM (ed), *Amphibian Medicine and Captive Husbandry*. Malabar, FL, Krieger Publishing, p. 570.

Wynn TA, Barron L. 2010. Macrophages: master regulators of inflammation and fibrosis. *Semin Liver Dis* 30(3):247–257.

Xiao L, Fayer R, Ryan U, Upton SJ. 2004. Cryptosporidium taxonomy: recent advances and implications for public health. *Clin Microbiol Rev* 17(1):72–97.

Zwart P. 2006. Renal pathology in reptiles. *Vet Clin North Am Exot Anim Pract* 9:129–159.

24 Herptile Cytology and Clinical Chemistry: Clinical Case Presentations

Case 1: Snake with a Bulging Right Eye

Signalment

11-year-old male jungle carpet python (*Morelia spilota cheynei*)

History

The snake presented for reevaluation of a bulging right eye (Figure 24.1a). The exophthalmos was first noticed 1 year ago when an ultrasound revealed no significant differences between the two eyes. At that time, no abnormalities were noted on oral examination. No improvement was noted following a 14-day course of antibiotics at that time. The eye and head mass did not appear to be bothering the snake, although he was slightly lethargic and had not been climbing as much as he had been, preferring to spend more time lying on the lower level of his enclosure. He was kept in a 75 gallon tank with heating lamps and a humidifier. His diet consisted of live rats, and his last meal was 3 weeks prior to presentation. Mites were noted in the snake's water bowl after he had been bathing in it. A total of 25 snakes were kept in the house.

Physical Examination

The 2.32 kg snake was bright, alert, and responsive on examination. Severe exophthalmos with scleral injection and mydriasis involving the right eye was noted. The left eye appeared normal. Examination of the oral cavity revealed a large soft-tissue swelling with small area of hemorrhage on the right maxilla (Figure 24.1b). There was moderate asymmetry of the cranium due to a 4 × 4 cm subcutaneous soft-tissue swelling in the retrobulbar space on the right side of the cranium. The mass on the maxilla appeared to be an extension of the mass within the head. Small black mites (*Ophionyssus natricis*) were observed on the snake's body and in the carrier.

The diagnostic plan included imaging that included radiographs and CT scan of the head, blood profile, and a fine-needle aspiration of the mass for cytodiagnosis (Tables 24.1, 24.2; Figures 24.2a–24.2c, 24.3a–24.3d).

Interpretive Discussion

The cell counts on the hemogram appeared normal; however, the leukophagocytosis whereby monocytes appeared to be phagocytizing heterophils was abnormal and likely indicative of an inflammatory response.

The plasma biochemical profile revealed hyperglobulinemia, which supports an inflammatory response or antigenic stimulation. The elevated creatinine kinase (CK) value likely was associated with skeletal muscle exertion or injury.

The aspirate sample of the mass on the head stained with Wright–Giemsa–Romanowsky stain revealed numerous mesenchymal cells with features of malignancy and a small number of inflammatory cells, predominately nondegenerate heterophils. A cytodiagnosis of a soft-tissue sarcoma was made; however, a histopathologic confirmation was required.

Exotic Animal Hematology and Cytology, Fifth Edition. Terry W. Campbell and Krystan R. Grant.

Companion website: www.wiley.com/go/campbell/exotic

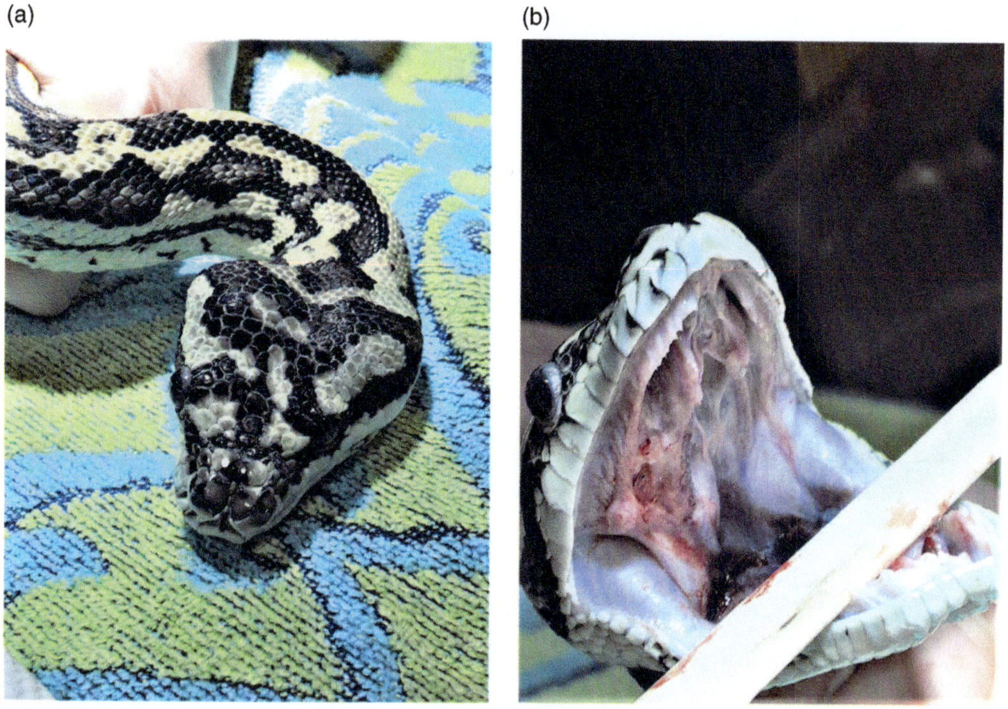

Fig. 24.1. (a) Snake with asymmetry of the head. (b) Oral examination.

Table 24.1. Python hematology results (Case 1).

		Reference[a]
PCV (%)	20	10–46
Leukocytes		
WBC (×10³/μL)	30.4	1.72–34.1
Heterophils (×10³/μL)*	8.2	0.29–11.3
(%)	27	—
Lymphocytes (×10³/μL)	11.8	0.6–19.9
(%)	39	—
Monocytes (×10³/μL)	10.3	0.15–26.8
(%)	34	—
Eosinophils (×10³/μL)	0	0.8–0.34
(%)	0	—
Basophils (×10³/μL)	0	0.05–1.76
(%)	0	—
Thrombocytes		
Estimated number	Adequate	1–5/1000× field
Morphology	Normal, clumped	
Plasma protein (refractometry) (g/dL)	10.5	

* Leukophagocytosis.
[a] Ranges for the jungle carpet python (*Morelia spilota cheynei*). Mader and Divers (2014).

Table 24.2. Python plasma biochemical results (Case 1).

		Reference[a]
Glucose (mg/dL)	64	9–55
BUN (mg/dL)	2	2–3
Uric acid (mg/dL)	4.1	—
Total protein (biuret) (g/dL)	9.4	15–15.8
Albumin (g/dL)	2.2	3.0
Globulin (g/dL)	7.2	0.19–3.39
Cholesterol (mg/dL)	223	264–386
Aspartate aminotransferase (IU/L)	50	5–46
Creatine kinase (IU/L)	3,775	27–1,350
Calcium (mg/dL)	16.5	12.8–16.5
Phosphorus (mg/dL)	2.8	2.8–33
Sodium (mEq/L)	154	—
Potassium (mEq/L)	5.5	4.2–5.5
Chloride (mEq/L)	110	109–123
Bicarbonate (mEq/L)	10.6	—
Anion gap (calculated)	39	—
Calculated osmolality	303	—

[a] Ranges for the jungle carpet python (*Morelia spilota cheynei*). Mader and Divers (2014).

Summary

An ill-defined soft-tissue opacity mass effect of the right orbital region causing mild right exophthalmos with diffuse soft-tissue thickening extending caudally to the level of the quadrate/compound articulation was noted on radiographs. Multiple dorsoventral (DV) views revealed mild widening of the space between the right compound bone and pterygoid/ectopterygoid bones in comparison to the left. Multiple DV and DV oblique views showed that the articulation between the right pterygoid and ectopterygoid bones was widened with mild lateral displacement of the caudal pterygoid bone.

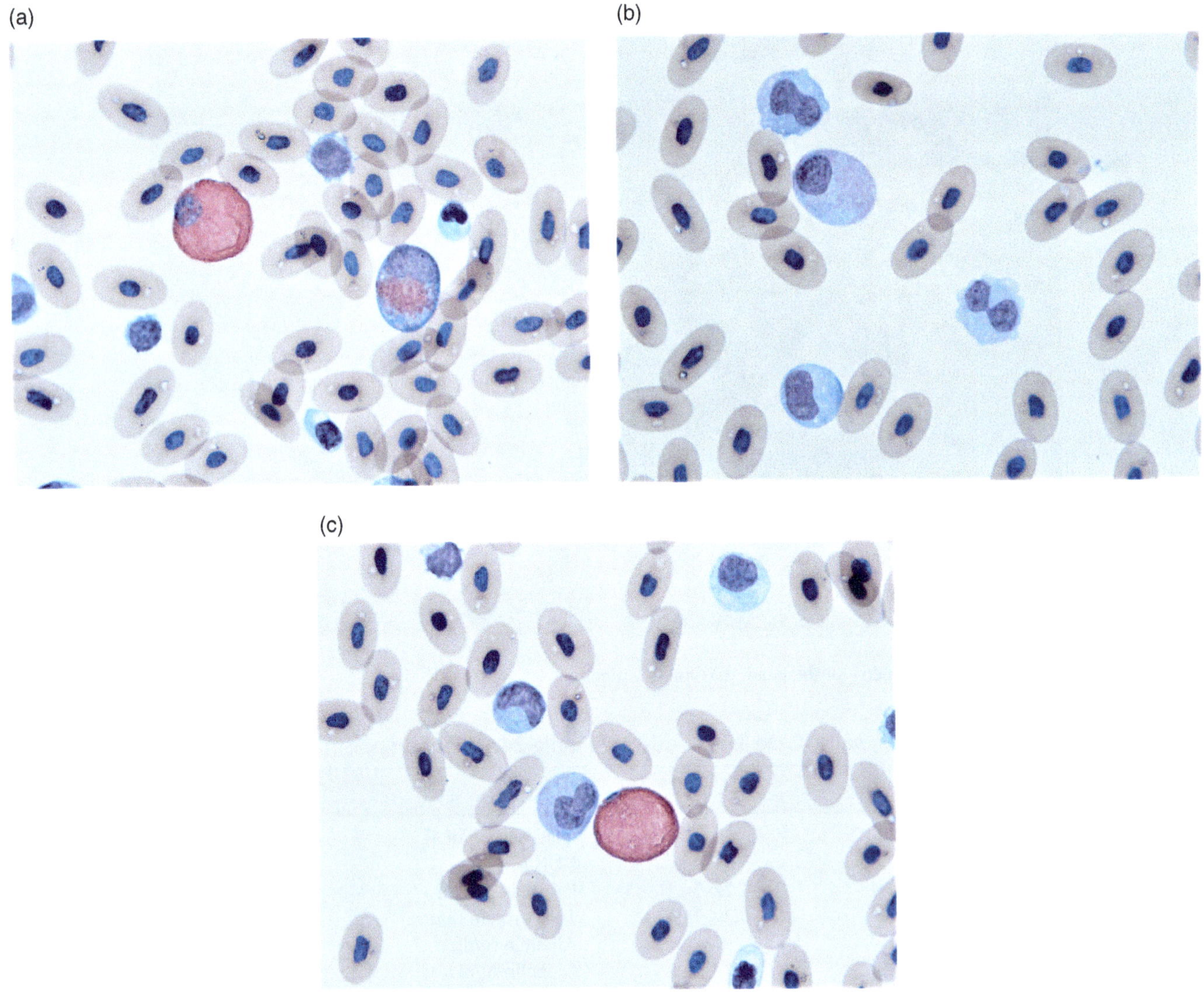

Fig. 24.2. (a)–(c) Blood film (Wright–Giemsa stain, 100× oil).

An undulating smooth lysis of the caudal distal margin of the right quadrate bone with mild widening of the supratemporal/quadrate and quadrate/compound bone articulations and rotation of the caudal articular aspect of the quadrate bone in comparison to the left was also noted. The axial margin of the right maxilla was undulating and ill-defined in comparison to the left on the DV views. The open mouth view highlighting the maxilla revealed that the axial margin of the soft-tissue mass of the right skull was well defined and extended across the midline at the level of the prefrontal sinuses and cranial margin of the cranial vault. There was increased soft-tissue opacity in the right prefrontal sinus when compared to the left side. A radiographic diagnosis concluded that a soft-tissue mass of the right retro-orbital space extended across the midline and caudally to the level of the articulations of the maxilla and compound bones and into the right prefrontal sinus. This was consistent with a soft-tissue sarcoma. Also, there was secondary luxation/subluxation of the right supratemporal/quadrate and quadrate/compound bones.

The CT scan revealed an ill-defined, expansile mildly heterogeneous soft-tissue-attenuating (32–65 HU) right retro-orbital mass. This mass extended cranially to the rostrolateral aspect of the right prefrontal bone, and caudally to the level of the right caudal pterygoid and quadrate bones.

This mass caused moderate exophthalmos and mild compression and deformation of the right orb, ventrolateral displacement of the right ectopterygoid and pterygoid bones, and dislocation of the supratemporal/quadrate bone joint and to a lesser extent the compound/quadrate/pterygoid joint. This mass caused near-complete lysis of the right axial orbital bone, moderate

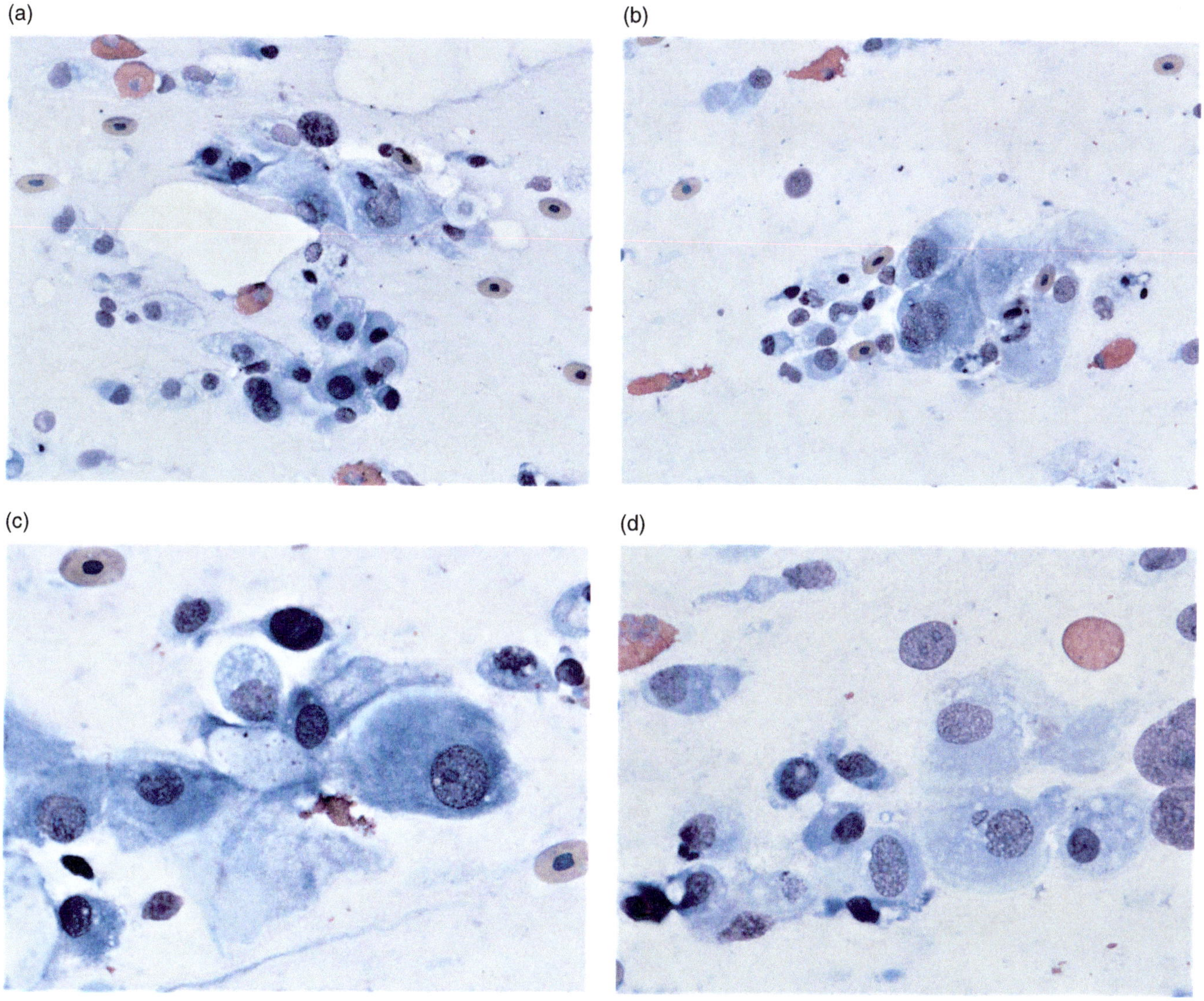

Fig. 24.3. (a), (b) Fine-needle aspirate of the mass (Wright–Giemsa stain, 50× oil). (c), (d) Fine-needle aspirate of the mass (Wright–Giemsa stain, 100× oil).

multifocal full thickness lysis of the postorbital bone, irregular lysis of the caudal aspect of the pterygoid bone, and smooth resorptive lysis of the axial margin of the proximal articular margin of the quadrate bone. The right frontal bone lateral margin was undulating although smooth, and there was moderate diffuse thickening of the maxillary bone adjacent to the mass. This mass displaced the maxilla and palatal tissues ventromedially and crossed the midline cranially at the level of the caudal prefrontal sinuses. The mass caused lysis of the left axial orbit with mild mass effect within the left mid to rostral retro-orbital tissues and mild left exophthalmos. There was moderate lysis of the left dorsal frontal bone and multifocal full thickness lysis of the right postorbital bone. There was a well-defined 3.5 mm length rectangular osseous fragment in the right dorsolateral aspect of the cranium at the level of the parietal bone adjacent to a full thickness lytic defect, possibly in the region of the optic nerve. The CT study concluded that a right retro-orbital soft-tissue mass with intracalvarial extension, prefrontal sinus invasion, and extension into the left retro-orbital space was supportive of a soft-tissue sarcoma.

The client elected to take the patient home and return for humane euthanasia when the snake stopped eating. The snake was treated for the mite infestation at home.

Case 2: Lizard with Lethargy and Neurologic Disorder

Signalment

8-year-old male bearded dragon (*Pogona vitticeps*)

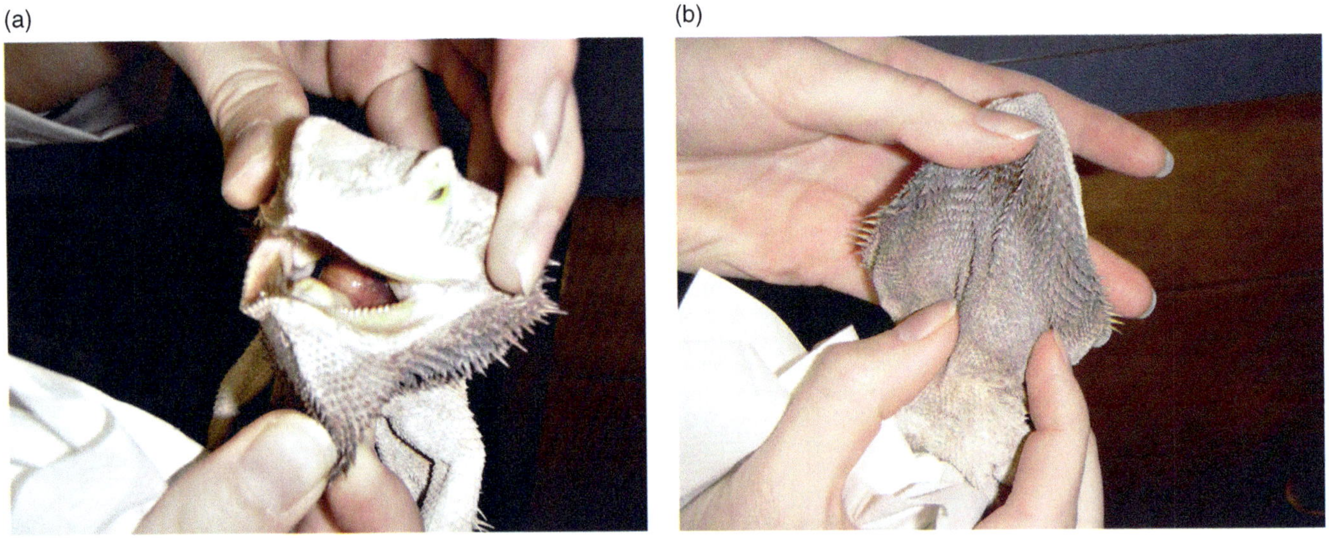

Fig. 24.4. (a) Examination of the oral cavity of the bearded dragon. (b) Palpation of the mass.

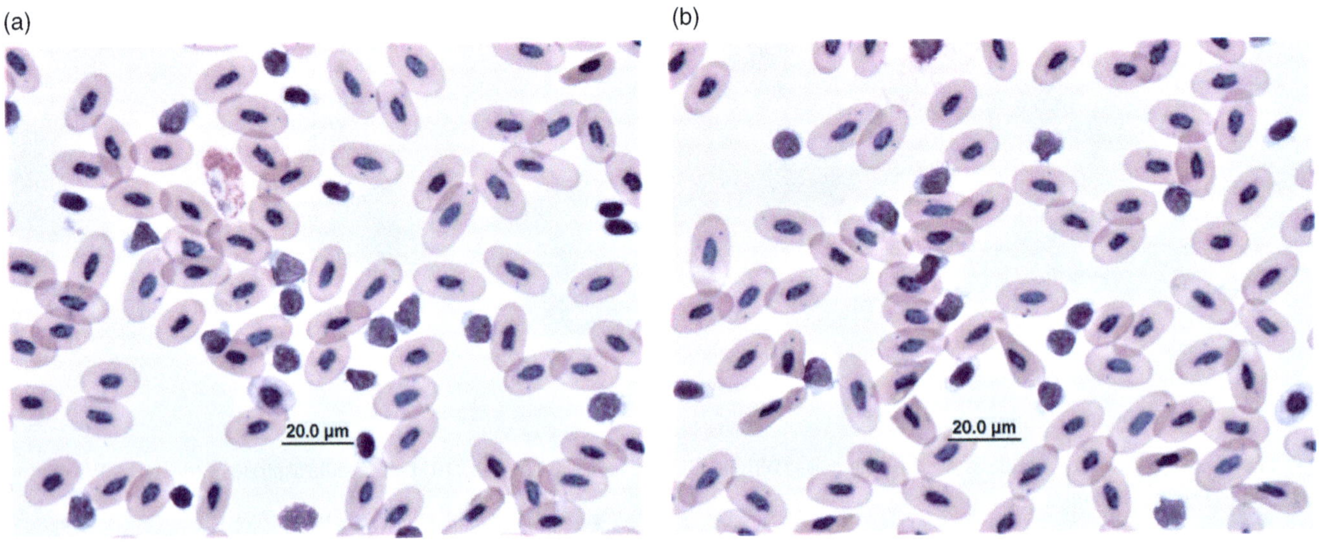

Fig. 24.5. (a), (b) Blood film (Wright–Giemsa stain, 100× oil).

History

The bearded dragon presented with a two-month history of lethargy, inappetence, and weight loss. The owner noticed possible neurologic symptoms, such as loss of muscle strength, vigorous lateral headshaking, and inability to grab onto perches.

Physical Examination

The lizard was thin, and loss of muscle and fat pad mass was evident. Examination of the oral cavity revealed a rounded attached mass at the back of the mouth, located more on the left side. The mass was not easily visualized, as his mouth was difficult to open. The mass was firm, highly vascularized, and measured 2 cm × 2 cm × 0.5 cm in size (Figures 24.4a and 24.4b).

A peripheral blood film and a fine-needle aspirate of the mass were obtained for cytodiagnosis (Figures 24.5a, 24.5b, 24.6a–24.6d).

Interpretive Discussion

The blood film stained with Wright–Giemsa–Romanowsky stain revealed a marked number of small, mature lymphocytes.

The aspirate sample of the mass stained with Wright–Giemsa–Romanowsky stain was highly cellular and consisted primarily of inflammatory cells. The

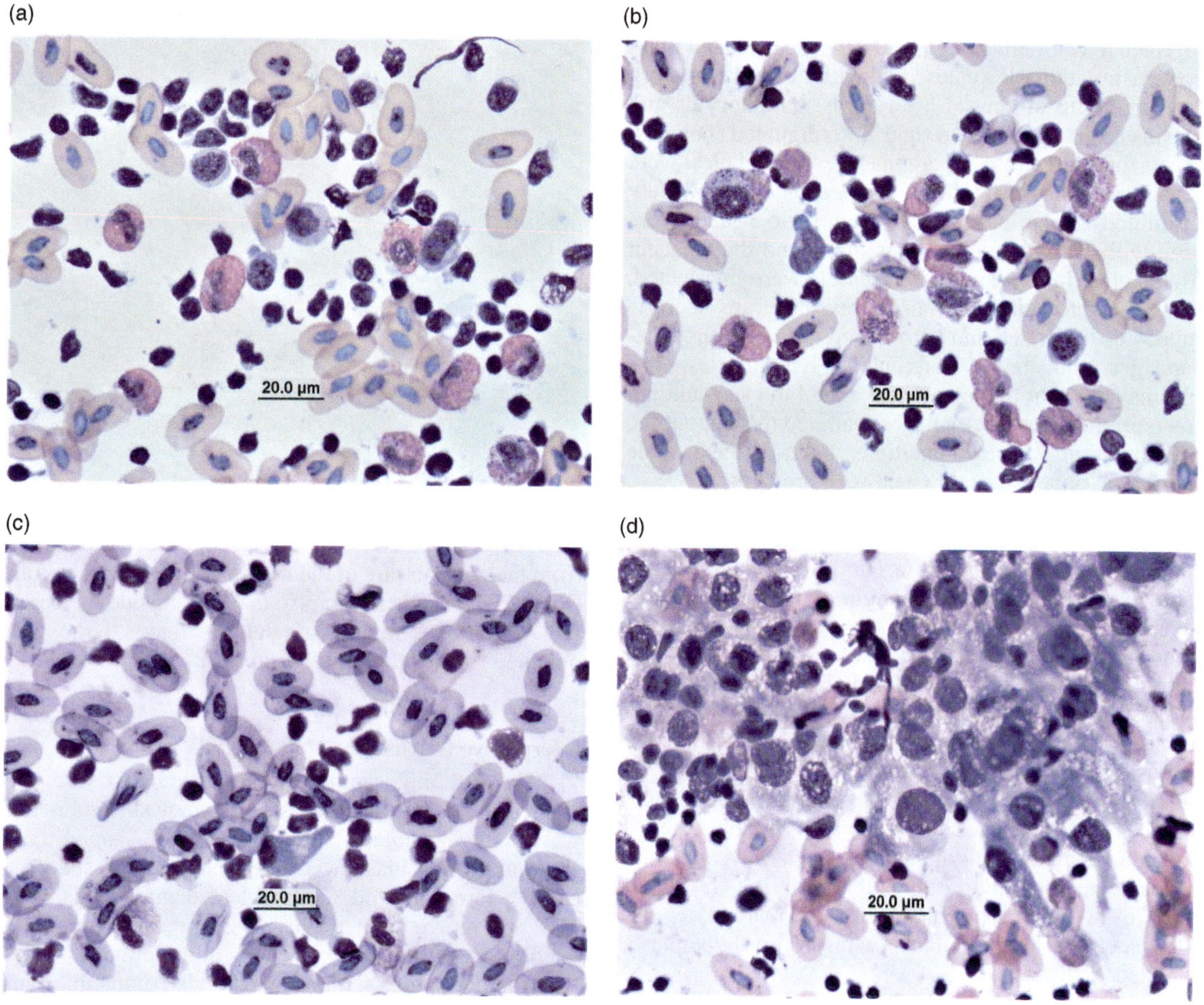

Fig. 24.6. (a)–(d) Fine-needle aspirate of the mass (Wright–Giemsa stain, 100× oil).

inflammatory cell population included numerous lymphocytes with plasma cells, heterophils, and macrophages. Clusters of epithelioid macrophages could be found. The cytodiagnosis was a mixed cell inflammation indicative of a granuloma.

Summary

Due to the poor prognosis associated with the poor body condition and mass in the oral cavity, the client opted for humane euthanasia and necropsy.

Gross necropsy findings revealed a bearded dragon in poor body condition with no gross autolysis. Behind the left mandible was a freely movable, 2-cm-diameter, tan, firm multilobulated mass surrounding a major vessel (Figure 24.7). The inguinal fat pads were diffusely small and dark.

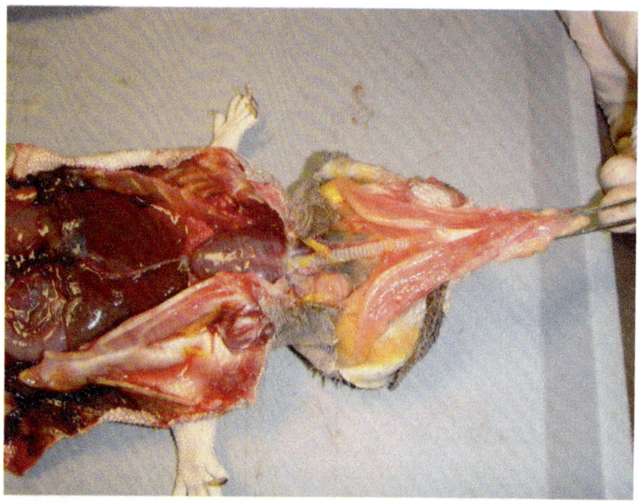

Fig. 24.7. Gross necropsy of the bearded dragon showing the mass near the left mandible.

Histopathology of the left retromandibular mass revealed a well-demarcated, partially encapsulated mass comprising multiple coalescing lobules of inflammatory cells made up of central heterophils, lymphocytes and plasma cells surrounded and interdigitated between sheets of epithelioid macrophages. The lobules were separated by abundant, dense collagenous tissue widely infiltrated by lymphocytes. No etiologic agents were seen within this granulomatous mass, and the adjacent esophagus, trachea and major vessels were unaffected. The associated skeletal muscle revealed rare necrotic myocytes infiltrated and surrounded by numerous macrophages with fewer heterophils, lymphocytes, and plasma cells that moderately expanded the surrounding interstitium. Rare macrophages scattered throughout the inflammation contained multiple, 1-µm-diameter, pale basophilic organisms consistent with protozoa.

No evidence of neoplasia was seen in the retromandibular mass. The intracellular organisms found within the retromandibular granuloma and the skeletal muscle were probably of protozoal origin and possibly microsporidia. There was marked widespread hepatic fibrosis and biliary hyperplasia that may be associated with chronic exposure to a hepatotoxin. The skeletal muscles of mastication and the inflammatory lesion may have prevented proper mastication and the ability to open the jaw on visible exam.

The final diagnosis was a granuloma with probable intracellular protozoa and an associated moderate, multifocal, histiocytic, and lymphoplasmacytic myositis with myocyte necrosis and rare possible protozoa. The diagnosis from the necropsy also included a marked, regionally extensive hepatic fibrosis with biliary hyperplasia and hepatic lipidosis.

Case 3: Lizard with Skin Lesion

Signalment

1.5-year-old female bearded dragon (*Pogona vitticeps*)

History

The lizard presented for dermatitis involving the skin on the left side of the face of 1-year duration. The lesion partially resolved with antibiotic treatment both systemically and topically; however, it never completely resolved, and during the past year stacked retained sheds developed in the area.

Physical Examination

The lizard was alert and active on physical examination. She was in good body condition. A scab was easily removed from a skin lesion on the left side of the face, revealing a severe ulcerative dermatitis that extended from the commissure of the mouth to the ear and beyond (Figure 24.8). The lesion also extended inside the ear.

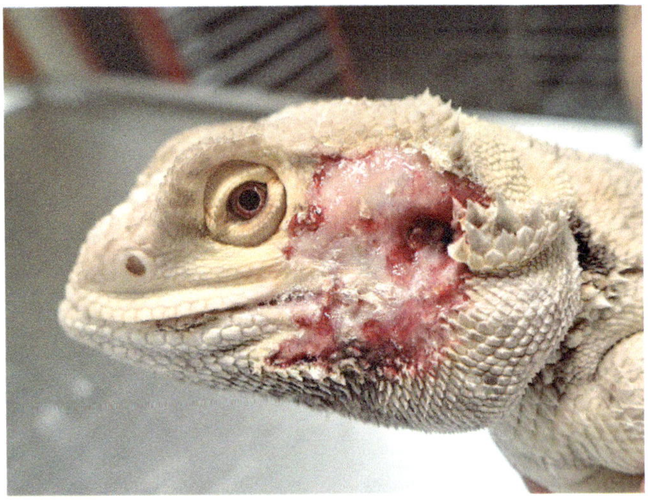

Fig. 24.8. Ulcerative dermatitis on head of lizard

A gentle scraping of the ulcerated tissue was obtained for cytodiagnosis (Figures 24.9a–24.9d).

Interpretive Discussion

The scraping sample of the ulcerated tissue was stained with Wright–Giemsa–Romanowsky stain and was highly cellular. Numerous spindle-shaped cells resembling fibroblasts were seen. Numerous nondegenerate heterophils and multinucleated giant cells were also present. Septate hyphae were present among the fibroblasts, inflammatory cells, and epithelial cells. Rectangular spores with rounded ends compatible with arthroconidia were seen scattered throughout the sample. The cytodiagnosis was compatible with a fungal dermatitis, onygenalean dermatomycosis, specifically *Nannizziopsis guarroi*.

Summary

The lizard was sent home with a guarded to favorable prognosis depending upon the response to the antimicrobial treatment (itraconazole and silver sulfadiazine cream for the fungal dermatitis).

Case 4: Thin Snake with Swollen Mouth

Signalment

5-year-old female ball python (*Python regius*)

History

The snake presented a history of anorexia and a swollen mouth.

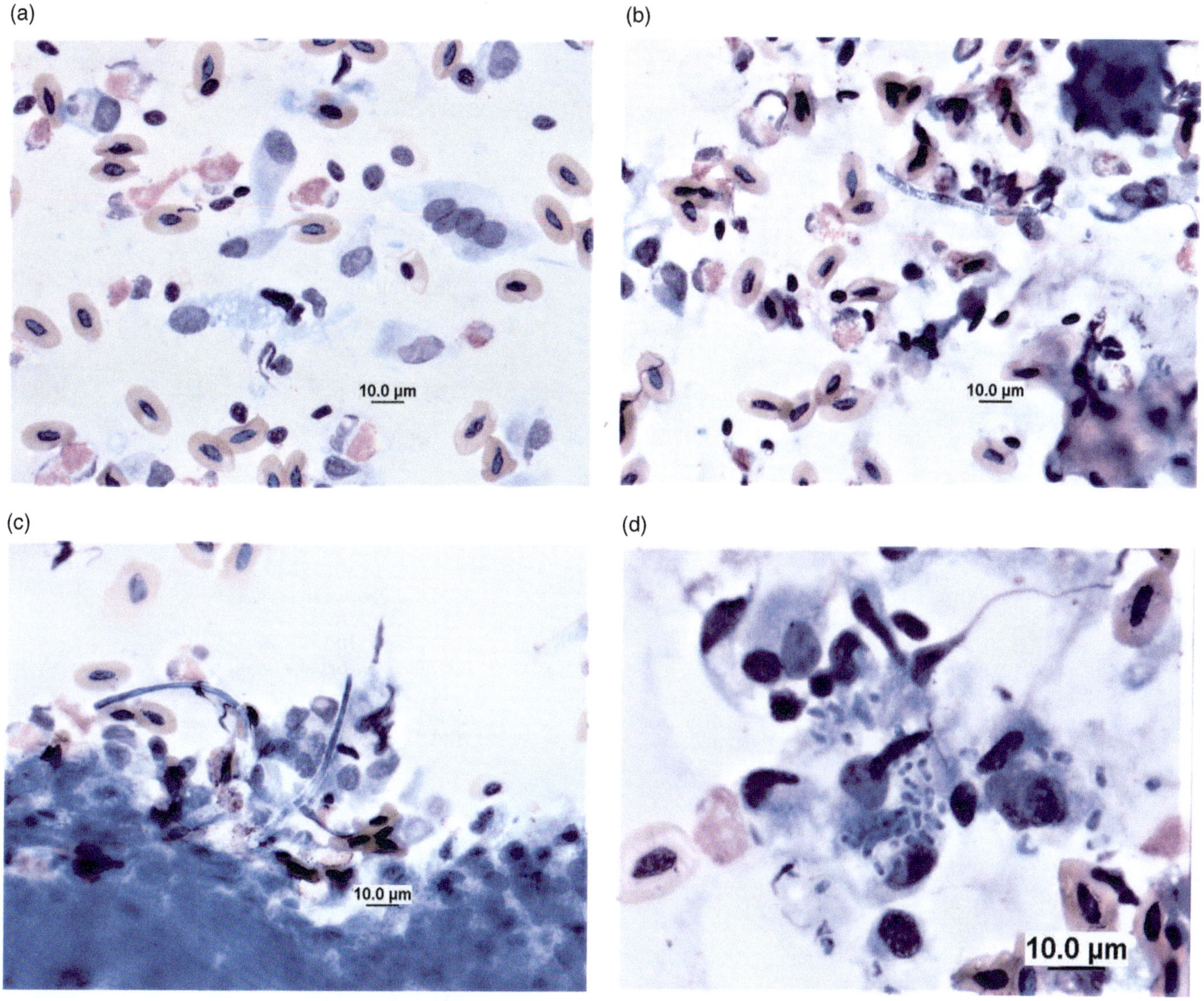

Fig. 24.9. (a)–(d) Imprint of scraping of skin lesion (Wright–Giemsa stain, 100× oil)

Physical Examination

The snake was lethargic on physical examination. She was in poor body condition based upon the loss of the epaxial muscle mass along the length of the body. There was marked mandibular gingiva and pharyngeal edema (Figure 24.10).

The client refused blood profiling, but did allow for a small blood sample for evaluation of the blood film (Figures 24.11a and 24.11b).

A gentle scraping of the gingival tissue was obtained for microbial culture and cytodiagnosis (Figures 24.12a and 24.12b).

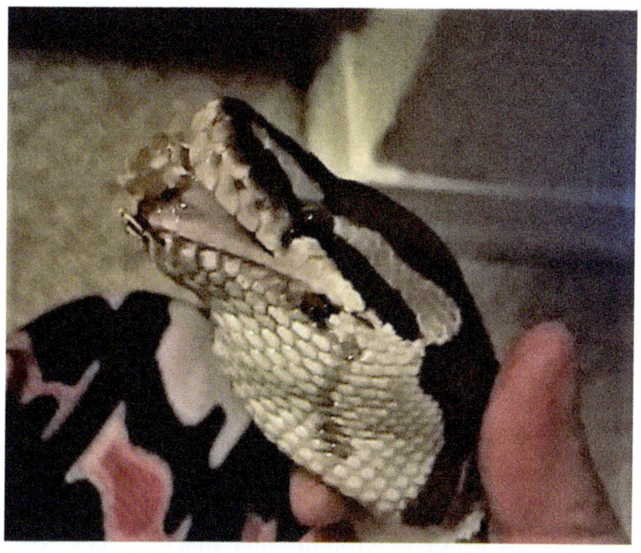

Fig. 24.10. Edematous tissue in the mouth of the snake.

Interpretive Discussion

The blood film stained with Wright–Giemsa–Romanowsky stain revealed a leukocyte differential of 36% heterophils, 18% lymphocytes, 42% monocytes, and

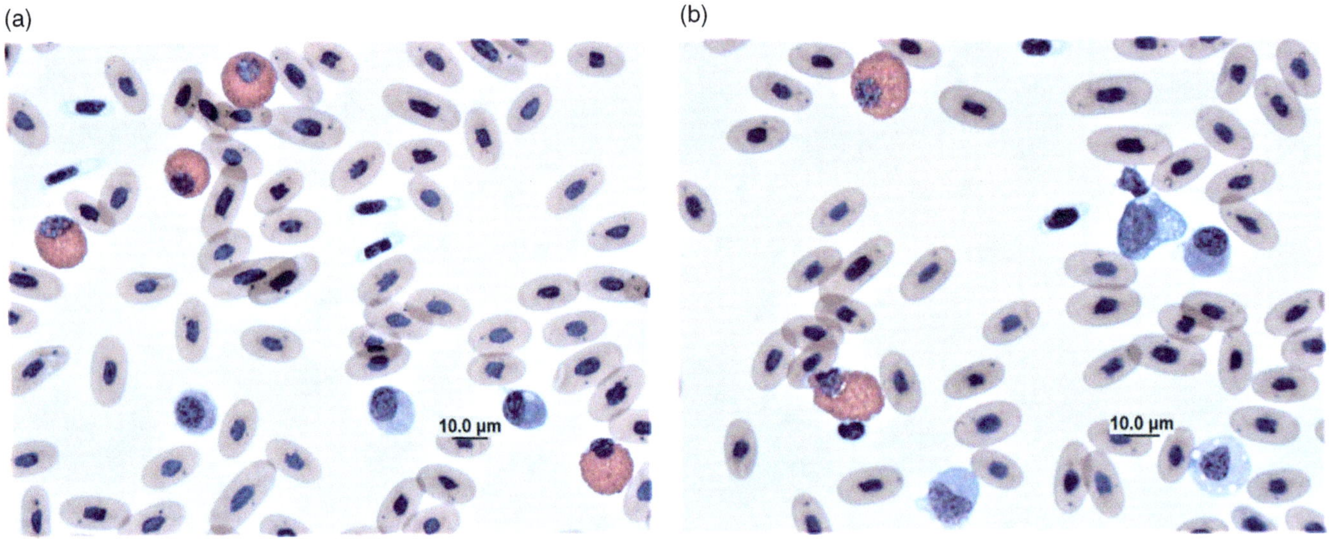

Fig. 24.11. (a), (b) Blood film (Wright–Giemsa stain, 100× oil).

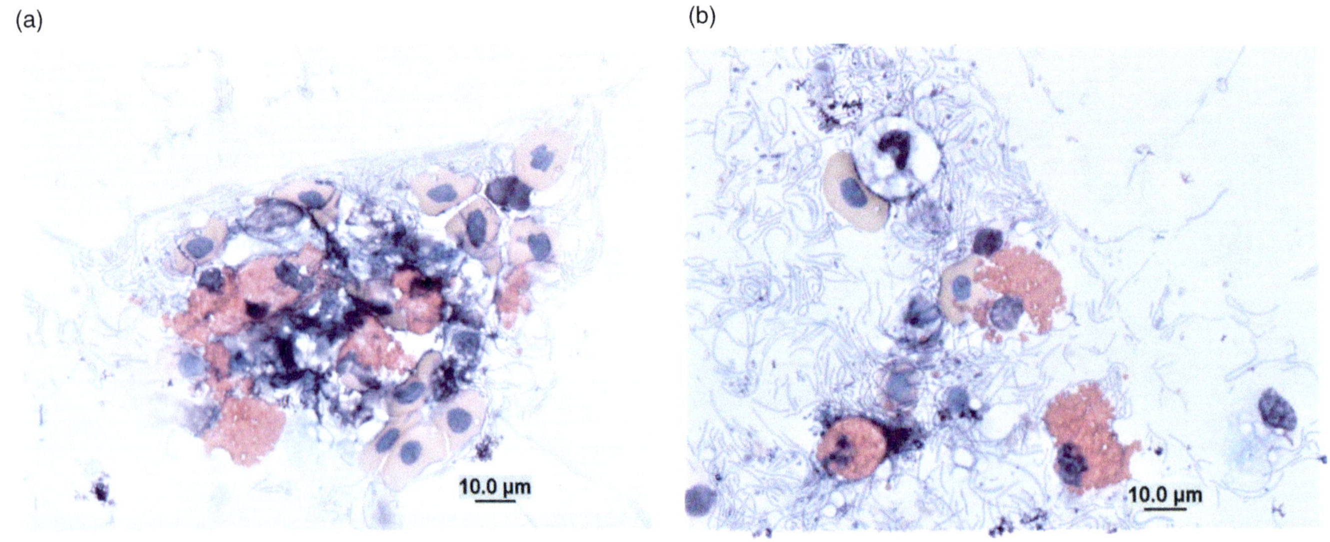

Fig. 24.12. (a), (b) Imprint of scraping of oral lesion (Wright–Giemsa stain, 100× oil).

4% basophils. There was an average of 6 heterophils, 7 monocytes, 3 lymphocytes, and 1 basophil per oil immersions field containing an average of 200 erythrocytes. The number of thrombocytes appeared to be adequate. Therefore, the blood film indicated leukocytosis, based upon the number of leukocytes per oil immersion field.

The impression smear made from the scraping of the gingival tissue and stained with Wright–Giemsa–Romanowsky stain revealed a marked number of filamentous bacteria in the background. The cellularity was low, but occasionally revealed clusters of inflammatory cells consisting of heterophils and macrophages. The cytology indicated a severe septic stomatitis.

Summary

Microbial culture revealed heavy growth of *Escherichia coli*, *Fusobacterium* sp., and *Klebsiella oxytoca*. The snake was treated with antibiotics based upon the culture and sensitivity tests; however, she died within 48 hours due to the severity of the infection and the likelihood of immunosuppression based upon poor husbandry.

Significant necropsy findings included severe, subacute to early chronic, necrotizing, and proliferative stomatitis with fibrinoid vasculitis, fibrin, thrombi, edema, granulation tissue, mild bone remodeling, and myriad intralesional mixed gram-negative bacteria.

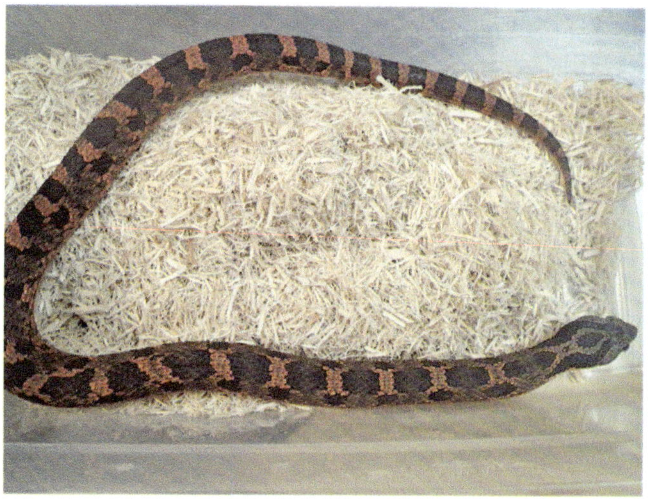

Fig. 24.13. Image of the snake.

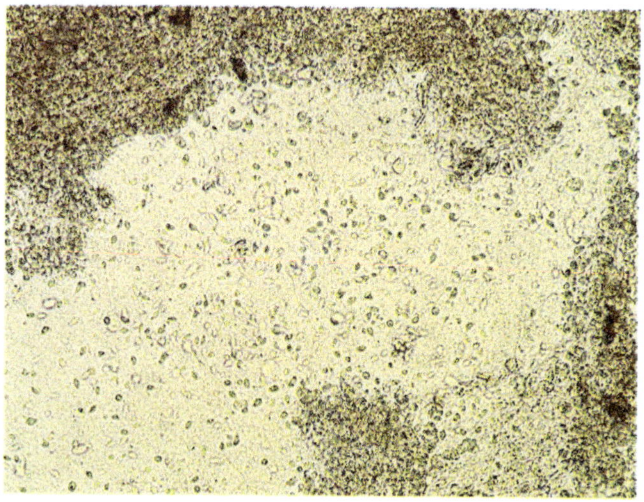

Fig. 24.14. Wet mount image of colonic wash sample (10×).

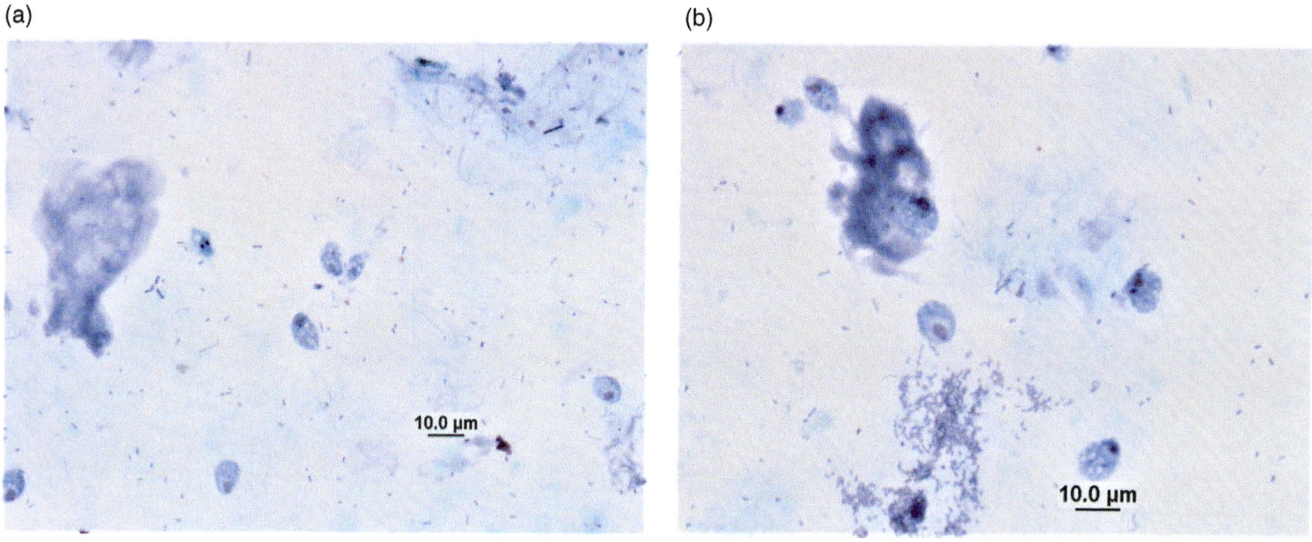

Fig. 24.15. (a), (b) Stained image of colonic wash sample (Wright–Giemsa stain, 100× oil).

Case 5: Snake with Diarrhea

Signalment

3-year-old male hognose snake (*Heterodon platirhinos*)

History

The snake presented a history of diarrhea.

Physical Examination

The snake was bright, alert, and active on physical examination. He was in good body condition based upon the amount of epaxial muscle mass along the length of the body (Figure 24.13).

A colonic wash sample was obtained for examination as a wet mount under the microscope and for cytodiagnosis (Figures 24.14, 24.15a, and 24.15b).

Interpretive Discussion

The wet mount sample was teeming with highly mobile, piriform-shaped organisms with visible flagella and undulating membrane.

The colonic wash sample stained with Wright–Giemsa–Romanowsky stain revealed a marked number of blue-staining, piriform-shaped organisms with flagella at the nuclear end of the cell. The moderately heavy background contained bacteria represented by a variety of morphological types.

Summary

Based upon the wet mount and cytology findings, the organisms were compatible with a *Trichomonas* sp. and a diagnosis of trichomoniasis.

References

Mader DR, Divers SJ (eds), 2014. *Current Therapy in Reptile Medicine & Surgery*. St. Louis, MO: Elsevier Saunders, p. 395.

SECTION IV

Fish

25 Blood Sample Collection and Preparation in Fish

Blood Sample Collection

General Considerations

In general, fish are often broadly referred to by taxonomic group, either Chondrichthyes (cartilaginous fish) or Osteichthyes (bony fish). The largest groups encompassing most species within each taxonomic group are elasmobranchs (within Chondrichthyes, subclass Elasmobranchii) and ray-finned bony fish (within Osteichthyes, class Actinopterygii). The largest group within the ray-finned bony fish group is from the infraclass Teleostei, known as teleosts. Throughout the fish section of this book, fish are differentiated broadly by cartilaginous and bony skeletal structure as either elasmobranchs or teleosts (excluding sturgeons, subclass Chondrostei), respectively.

Diagnostics to assess fish health are broadly desired due to their usefulness in aquaculture, conservation, and for pets. The standard practices and methods used for collecting, handling, and analyzing blood from mammals and birds can be misleading when they are applied to fish hematology. With over 34 000 known species, vastly different sizes, drastic environmental differences, and nutritional requirement variations, there are multiple physiologic responses impacting blood components to varying degrees. These variables coupled with additional factors associated with handling and diagnostic techniques, sample processing, and analytical methods make the establishment of reference intervals and the interpretation of hemogram results more challenging than for other vertebrates.

When establishing or using reference intervals, it is best to follow the American Society for Veterinary Clinical Pathology (ASVCP) guidelines (Friedrichs et al., 2012) and report or identify additional criteria specific for fish such as species, handling parameters (capture and handling technique, use of other equipment, length of capture and handling), environment (tank, pond, exhibit volume, season, photoperiod), life support system details (filter type, volume, maintenance), water quality parameters (dissolved oxygen, temperature, pH, ammonia, nitrite, nitrate, hardness, alkalinity, salinity), tank mates (stock density), reproductive status, diet, parasites (type and load), and venipuncture site (Table 25.1) (Cray, 2015).

This chapter will review common techniques for capture, handling, and restraint used to prepare for blood collection; the common anatomical sites on fish to obtain blood samples; and handling and processing the blood sample in preparation for evaluation.

Capture and Handling

The size of the fish and its environment will determine the approach for capture, handling, and restraint since the activities and duration of these events may influence the hemogram. The approach to safe capture and handling should include a strategy to minimize stress, such as minimizing the time of the capture event.

Capture and handling of fish for venipuncture or cardiocentesis can have a marked effect on the hemogram, resulting in a significant increase in the hematocrit by as much as 25% (Railo et al., 1985; Heming, 1989). The magnitude of this effect is directly related to the handling and analytical time. Handling of fish for as little as 20 s results in the release of catecholamines that tend to cause hemoconcentration and swelling of the erythrocytes. The increase in blood catecholamines also causes ion exchanges (Na^+/H^+ and Cl^-/HCO^-) across the erythrocyte membrane. Na^+ and Cl^- enter the erythrocyte and water follows osmotically, which causes the cell to swell (Railo et al., 1985). Therefore, the hematocrit increases but the

Exotic Animal Hematology and Cytology, Fifth Edition. Terry W. Campbell and Krystan R. Grant.

Companion website: www.wiley.com/go/campbell/exotic

Table 25.1. Summary of parameters that may influence the hemogram and should be considered when establishing or referring to reference intervals.

Environmental factors	Fish-specific factors	Sample collection factors	Analytical factors
Tank or pond volume	Species/subspecies	Fasting status	Blood film technique
Water quality parameters	Age	Capture technique	Blood film stain type
Seasonal conditions	Sex	Animal handling technique	Stain manufacturer
Photoperiod	Reproductive status	Animal transport conditions	Manual/automatic staining
Water temperature	Animal use	Length of capture/handling	Manual/automatic counts
Salinity	Health status	Length of animal transport	Equipment used
Diet	Concurrent disease	Time of day sample collected	Counting stain
Life support system details	Parasites (type/load)	Venipuncture site	Centrifuge settings
Tank/pond mates (type/#)	Captive/farmed/wild	Needle/syringe size	Technician consistency
Geographic location	Activity level	Geographic location of sample collection/environmental conditions	Analyzer details
		Anticoagulant	
		Sample storage	
		Time/date of sample collection	
		Sample transport	

Source: Adapted from Cray (2015).

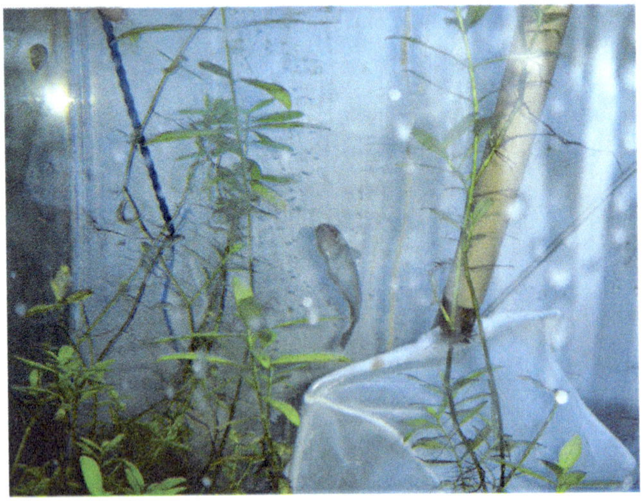

Fig. 25.1. Capture of a juvenile rainbow fish (*Melanotaenia boesemani*) using two nets. The small net (with the blue handle, left) is used to encourage the fish toward the larger net (right). Using two nets is often an efficient technique to reduce the time of the capture event.

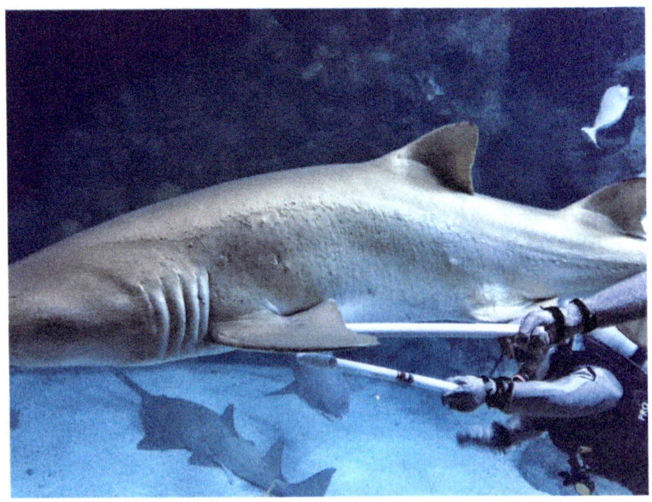

Fig. 25.2. Capture of an adult sand tiger shark (*Carcharias taurus*). Two divers used T-shaped PVC pipes as guides to encourage the shark to the examination staging area of the tank.

hemoglobin concentration remains the same, resulting in a decrease in the mean corpuscular hemoglobin concentration (Railo et al., 1985; Heming, 1989). Cannulation methods have been developed for use in research fish to minimize these effects; however, they are impractical in clinical studies (Railo et al., 1985).

Fish housed in a small aquarium are often captured using nets. To help capture a fish efficiently, two nets may be used to persuade the fish toward the sides or corner of the tank. One smaller net can be used to encourage the fish in the direction of the second larger net (Figure 25.1). The first net can then be used to cover the opening of the second net to ensure security during transfer. Large fish housed in an exhibit may benefit from operant conditioning training as part of their routine feeding to prepare them for safe and effective capture for examinations (Janssen et al., 2017). Training coupled with diver assistance works well to guide large fish to the examination staging area of the exhibit (Figure 25.2). When handling fish, powder-free latex or nitrile gloves should be worn to protect the fish and the handler from pathogen transmission and to avoid disrupting the mucous coat on the fish.

Restraint

The stress of capture and physical restraint has a significant effect on the hematologic indices of fish.

Therefore, it is generally recommended to use a general anesthetic to reduce the stress of handling during blood collection in active fish (Houston, 1990; Groff and Zinkl, 1999). Sedation or general anesthesia also reduces the chance of injury to the fish and those involved, and simplifies the procedure. If a general anesthetic is not used, the procedure of blood collection should take place in less than 30 s because fish held out of water for longer periods suffer from respiratory distress and electrolyte imbalance. In some circumstances, blood collection can be performed without completely removing the fish from the water. This can be performed while holding the fish, usually restrained in a net or stretcher, with the head and gills submerged in the water during blood collection. Some elasmobranchs undergo tonic immobility when placed in dorsal recumbency, allowing short and relatively non-invasive procedures like blood collection to be performed (Figure 25.3) (Henningsen, 1994; Grant, 2015; Williamson et al., 2018). As another example of allowing fish to remain in the water, a study introduced a blood collection technique where large elasmobranchs were sampled by veterinary staff swimming alongside the fish (Ueda et al., 2017).

In situations where sedation or general anesthesia is required, tricaine methanesulfonate (Tricaine, MS222, Sigma Chemical Co., Saint Louis, MO) in a concentration of 100–150 mg/L is commonly used. Special precautions should be given to the acidification of tricaine-treated water that is poorly buffered. The acidosis created by unbuffered tricaine can cause hemoconcentration and other hematologic alterations; therefore, it is recommended to use tricaine solutions that are neutralized to the pH of the water of the aquarium prior to exposing fish to the anesthetic (Smit et al., 1979; Groff and Zinkl, 1999). This is typically accomplished by adding sodium bicarbonate to the tricaine-water solution until the pH equilibrates to the aquarium water (Figures 25.4a and 25.4b). Generally, one to two parts of sodium bicarbonate to one part of tricaine can be safely used (Stamper, 2007; Grant, 2015; Lewbart and Yanong, 2018). In addition to inhalant sedation or general anesthesia, drugs delivered by other means, such as oral, intramuscular, intravenous, or intracoelomic, may be used. Options, doses, and delivery methods are described elsewhere (Neiffer, 2007; Stamper, 2007; Neiffer and Stamper, 2009; Penning et al., 2017; Lewbart and Yanong, 2018).

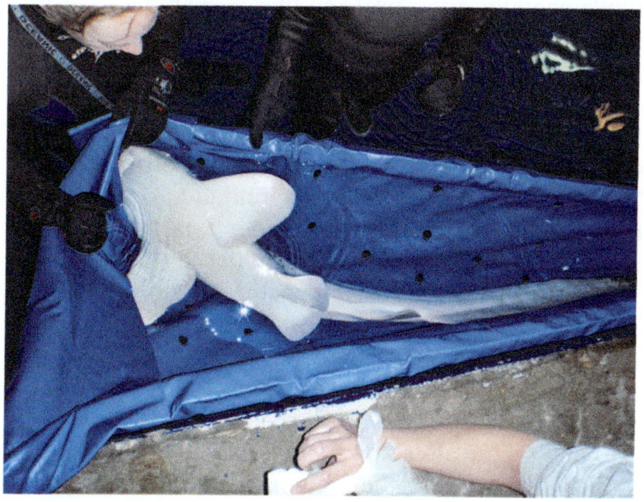

Fig. 25.3. A zebra shark (*Stegostoma fasciatum*) contained in a stretcher undergoing tonic immobility in preparation for physical and sonographic examination.

(a) (b)

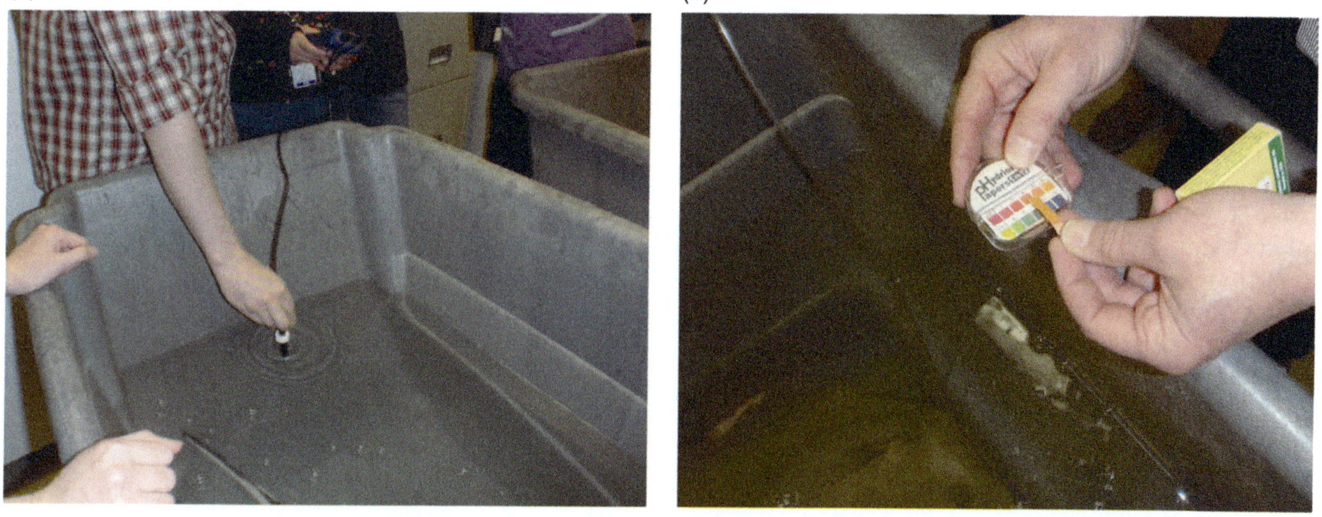

Fig. 25.4. (a) Checking the pH with a hand-held digital reader during induction with MS-222 and sodium bicarbonate. (b) Checking the pH with a paper tester during induction with MS-222 and sodium bicarbonate.

Blood Volume Collection

Cardiovascular and Lymphatic Systems

The primary circulatory system of fish is like the circulatory system of other vertebrates in that it is used to transport cells and substances (oxygen, nutrients, hormones, etc.). In mammals, the capillary blood (hydrostatic) pressure opposes an equal blood colloidal osmotic pressure across the capillary wall, whereas teleost fish have low arterial pressures, highly permeable capillaries, and a high protein concentration in the interstitial fluid, resulting in a much lower osmotic pressure across the capillary wall (Hargens et al., 1974). Due to these characteristics in teleosts, plasma runs freely through the capillary walls. This exchange and fluid balance are fundamentally different from that in mammals, so that large changes in plasma concentration can be tolerated (Roberts and Ellis, 2012).

Another unique feature of the circulatory system of teleost fish is the presence of a parallel secondary circulation that is a conduit for relatively cell-free blood. The function of the secondary circulation system is not clear; however, the plasma content, lack of oxygen transport, and the presence of it in tissues raised speculation of it being like a lymphatic system (Olson and Farrell, 2006). The lymphatic drainage system in fish is extensive owing to the high permeability of the capillaries, which results in a lymphatic fluid composition that is identical to that of blood plasma (Wardle, 1971). Although there are some morphological and molecular similarities between the mammalian lymphatic system and the teleost secondary circulatory system, there appear to be functional differences (Eliason and Stecyk, 2021). The proposed functions of the secondary circulatory system include retaining red blood cells to decrease the workload of the heart and erythrocyte production; assist with immune function, acid-base regulation, and epithelial ion transport; exchange gases through the skin; and transport nutrients and remove waste (Rummer et al., 2014). Most of the blood cells are directed through the primary circulatory system at a bifurcation of the two systems located at the major vessels of the gills and various surface areas such as skin and gut. Blood in the secondary circulation has a lower hematocrit and lower pressure, resulting in a circulatory time that occurs over hours rather than minutes, compared to the primary circulation (Steffensen and Lomholt, 1992; Iwama and Farrell, 1998).

Blood collected from major blood vessels generally represents blood in the primary circulation; however, lymphatic fluid dilution of the sample is possible, and careful observation of the color of the sample should be made during blood collection. Clear fluid mixing with the red blood is indicative of lymphatic contamination that will affect the results of hematologic evaluation.

Volume

Blood for diagnostic sampling can be collected safely from fish that are greater than 3 inches (8 cm) in length (Noga, 2010). Techniques for smaller fish exist, but are typically reserved for the research setting (Zang et al., 2013).

The blood volume of the primary circulation of teleost fish is small compared with other vertebrates. The estimated blood volume of these fish is approximately 5% of the body weight compared to 10% of the body weight of mammals (Gallaugher and Ferrell, 1998; Roberts and Ellis, 2012). Because of the fluid balance differences between fish and mammals, fish are more tolerant of acute blood loss compared to mammals; therefore, approximately 30–50% of the total blood volume can be safely collected from healthy fish (Groff and Zinkl, 1999).

Collection Sites

Caudal Vessel

Blood can be collected from fish by caudal venipuncture using the caudal vertebral vein or artery and can be accomplished with or without sedation or anesthesia. The caudal vertebral vein or artery can be approached ventrally or laterally. In teleost fish, the ventral approach involves insertion of the needle under a scale along the ventral midline near the base of the caudal peduncle (Figure 25.5a). The needle is directed toward the vertebral bodies, and after reaching the vertebral bodies, the needle is withdrawn slightly ventrally and laterally while negative pressure is applied to the syringe. Once the vessel has been entered, blood will enter the syringe. It may be necessary to rotate the needle slightly for proper positioning of the needle bevel in the vessel to facilitate blood collection. In elasmobranchs, the caudal vein and artery are located along the ventral aspect of the vertebral column, with the vein being more ventral (Figure 25.5b). The needle is inserted along ventral midline through the skin and cartilage to enter the vessel. Negative pressure from the syringe is applied to collect the blood (Figures 25.5c and 25.5d). Adjustment may be required if blood is not immediately seen in the hub of the needle.

A lateral approach to the caudal vertebral vessels is performed by inserting the needle a few millimeters below the lateral line near the base of the caudal peduncle in teleost fish (Figures 25.6a–d). The needle is directed toward the midline and under the vertebral bodies. Blood is aspirated into the syringe in the same manner as described for the ventral approach.

Cardiocentesis

Blood can be collected from the heart or bulbus arteriosus of teleosts using a ventral approach, although cardiocentesis has greater risk of damage to fish than the

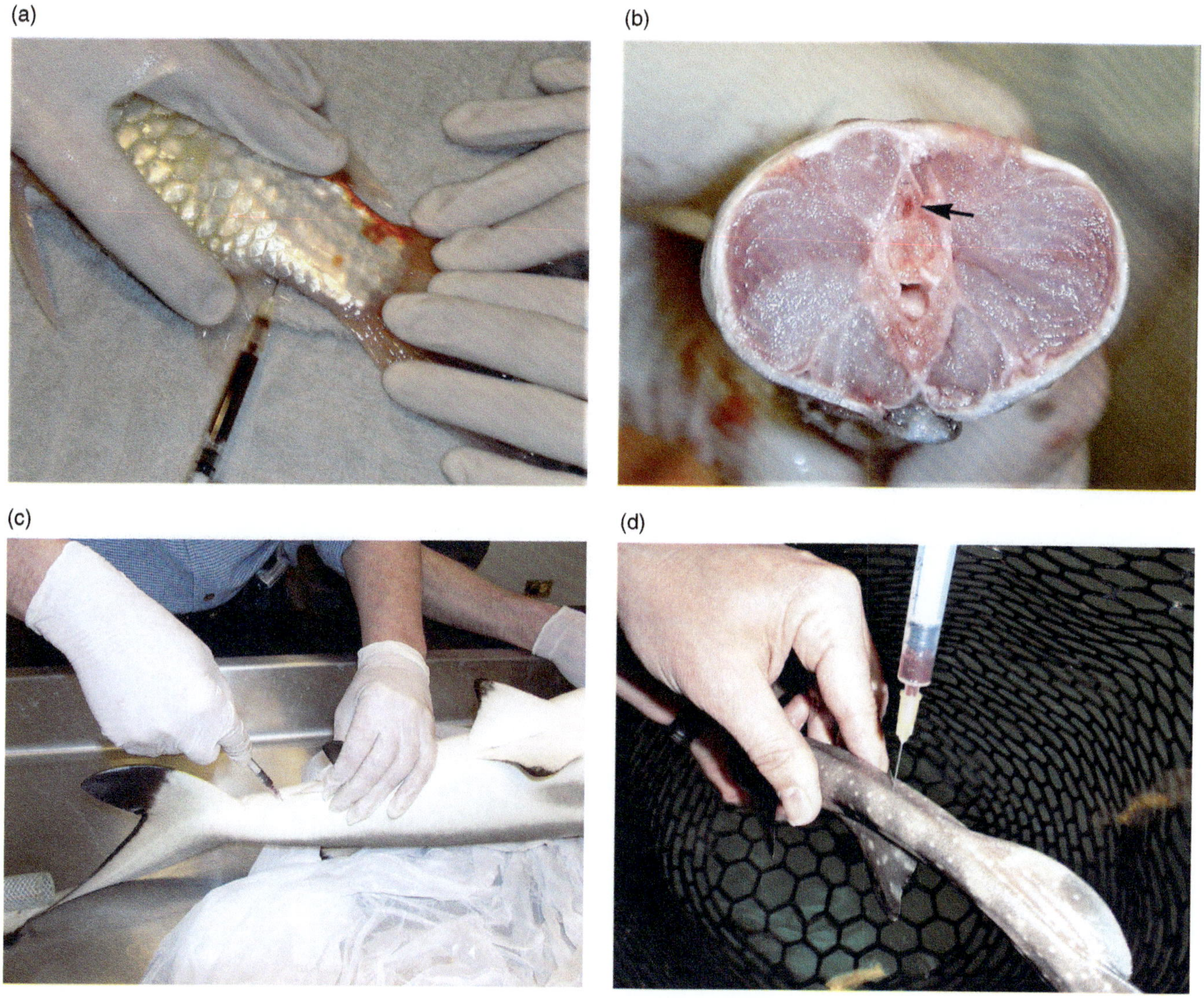

Fig. 25.5. (a) Blood collection from a goldfish (*Carassius auratus*) using the ventral approach to the tail vein. (b) Cross section of a southern stingray tail (*Hypanus americanus* formerly *Dasyatis americana*). The surface at the top of the image is the ventral aspect with the arrow pointing to the ventral artery/vein. Blood being collected using the ventral approach to the tail vein from a shark. (c) blacktip reef shark (*Carcharhinus melanopterus*). (d) whitespotted bamboo shark (*Chiloscyllium plagiosum*).

use of the caudal vertebral vessels for blood collection. To perform cardiocentesis, the needle is inserted slightly caudal to the apex of the V-shaped notch formed by the opercula (gill covers) and isthmus, and advanced toward the heart while applying a slight vacuum to the syringe. Blood will enter the syringe when the heart has been penetrated. Alternatively, an ultrasound may be used to locate the bulbus arteriosus of the heart and guide the needle and syringe for blood collection (Figures 25.7a and 25.7b).

Dorsal Sinus

Blood can be collected from elasmobranch fish (cartilaginous fish, such as sharks, rays, and skates) by caudal venipuncture as described previously or by using the vascular sinus located caudal and slightly ventral to the dorsal fins. To perform blood collection from the vascular sinus, first restrain the shark in ventral recumbency or in a protective sling with its back exposed and lift the dorsal fin dorsally. Insert a needle in a plane parallel to the back and slightly off the midline through the soft skin just under the caudal aspect of a dorsal fin (Figures 25.8a–c). A syringe or extension tube may be attached to the needle for blood collection. Use of an extension tube is often helpful in keeping the needle in position during blood collection should the shark move during the procedure. The advantage of using the vascular sinus as a site for blood collection instead of venipuncture of the caudal vertebral vessels in large elasmobranch fish is the relative ease of access to the sinus with proper restraint.

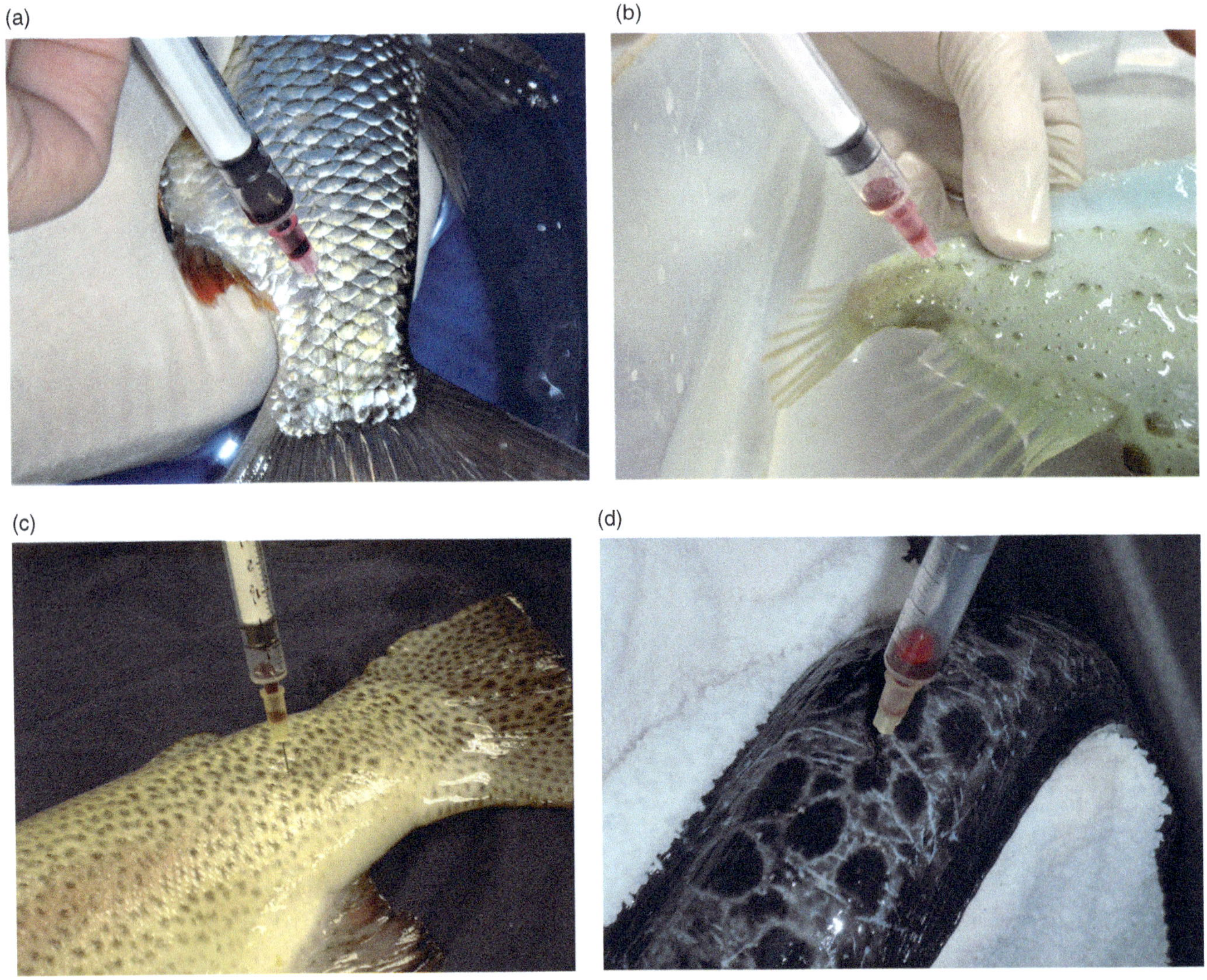

Fig. 25.6. The lateral approach to the tail vein for blood collection of a (a) tinfoil barb (*Barbus schwanenfeldi*), (b) lumpfish (*Cyclopterus lumpus*), (c) rainbow trout (*Oncorhynchus mykiss*), (d) wolf eel (*Anarrhichthys ocellatus*).

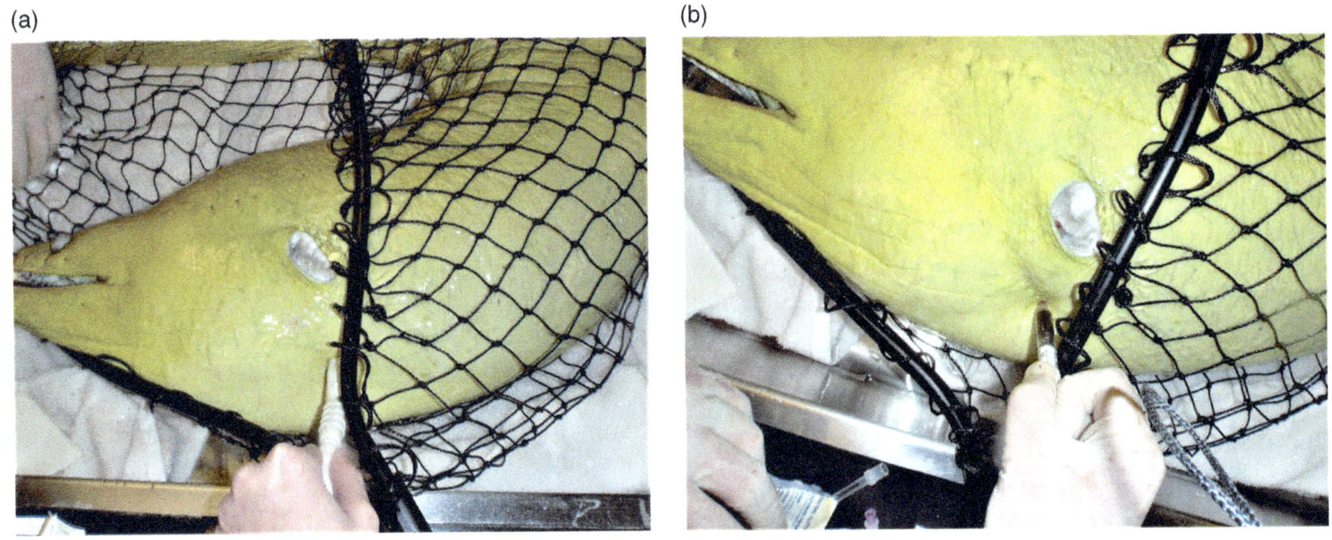

Fig. 25.7. (a) Using an ultrasound to locate the bulbus arteriosus in a green moray eel (*Gymnothorax funebris*) for (b) cardiocentesis.

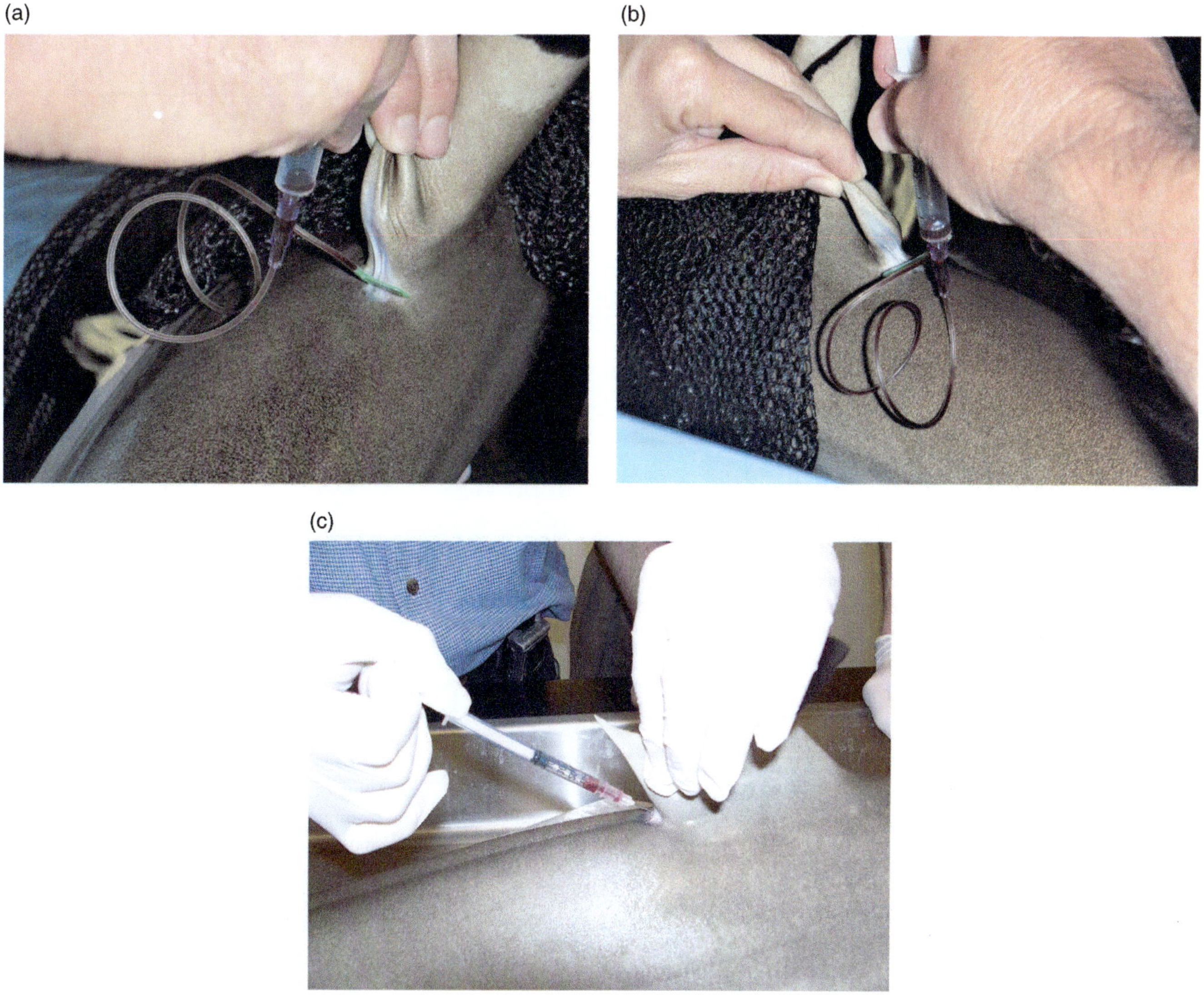

Fig. 25.8. (a–c) Collection of blood from a blacktip reef shark (*Carcharhinus melanopterus*) using the vascular sinus located caudal and slightly ventral to the dorsal fin.

Pectoral Vessels

The pectoral vasculature can be accessed for blood sample collection in stingrays. The stingray may be in either dorsal or ventral recumbency. The pectoral cartilaginous girdle can be palpated and, just distal and craniolateral from the margin, the ceratotrichia can be palpated along the wing. The needle is inserted at a 90° angle to the wing through the skin and between the ceratotrichia. Once the needle penetrates the skin, negative pressure is applied by the syringe (Phillips et al., 2016) (Figure 25.9). Another approach to pectoral vasculature is the mesopterygial vein (Westmoreland et al., 2019). With the stingray in dorsal recumbency, the metapterygium cartilage can be palpated. Insert an appropriately sized needle attached to a syringe, directing it medially toward the metapterygium cartilage at a 45° angle (Westmoreland et al., 2019) (Figures 25.10 and 25.11).

Other Sites

Other sites for collecting blood used in a laboratory, research, or field study, such as the dorsal aorta, are not used or recommended to be used in the clinical setting due to the high risk of mortality (Duman et al., 2019).

Blood Sampling Handling and Preparation

Anticoagulant

Blood collection is often performed using a needle or butterfly catheter and syringe with immediate transfer of the blood sample to a tube containing an anticoagulant. Common anticoagulants used for fish blood samples include heparin and ethylenediaminetetraacetic acid (EDTA). Lithium heparin is most commonly used for most fish species. Disadvantages of heparin as an anticoagulant include the tendency for the blood sample

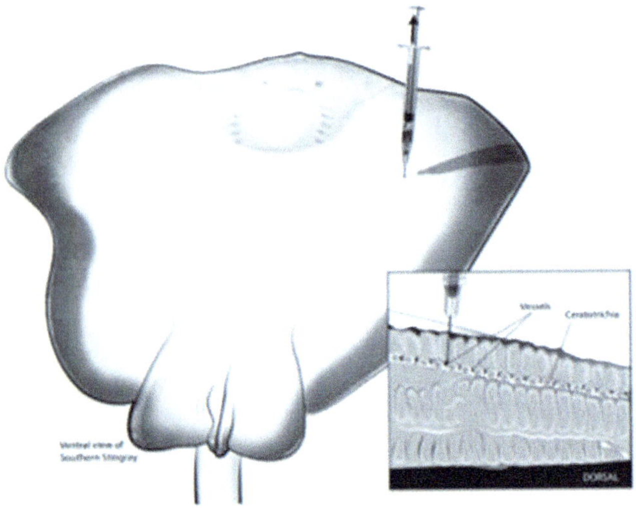

Fig. 25.9. Venipuncture technique for the pectoral vasculature site in a male southern stingray (*Hypanus americanus* formerly *Dasyatis americana*). The needle is inserted perpendicular to the pectoral fin between the lateral edge of the coelomic cavity and the lateral edge of the pectoral fin. The blood sample is obtained from the vessels that lie between the ceratotrichia. From the dorsal approach, there are additional vessels that may be encountered before reaching the ceratotrichia. Source: Phillips et al. (2016).

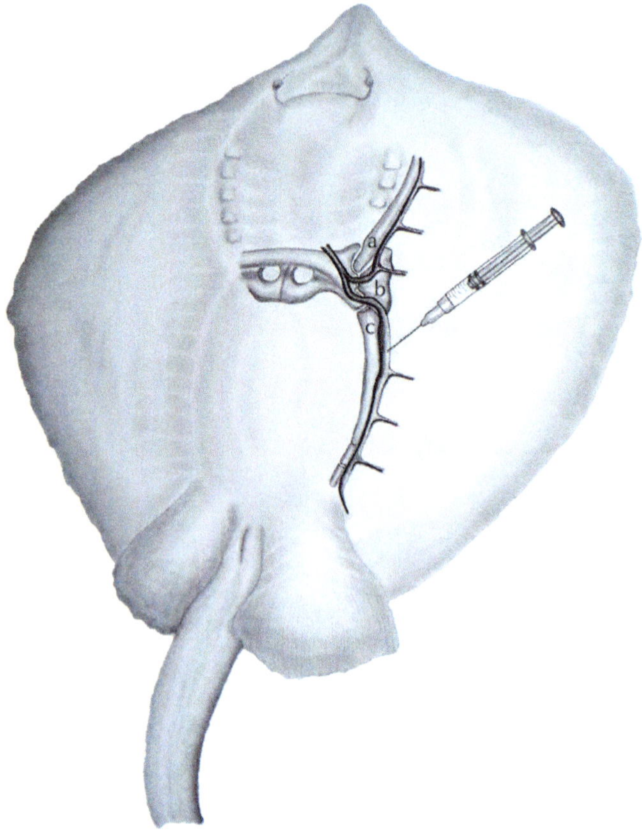

Fig. 25.10. Illustration of an Atlantic stingray (*Hypanus sabinus*) in dorsal recumbency with a needle placed in the cranial third of the mesopterygial vein that runs just ventrolateral to the metapterygium (C) cartilage. The figure shows the vasculature running along the propterygium (A), mesopterygium (B), and metapterygium (C) cartilages and ventral to the radial ceratotrichia. Source: Westmoreland et al. (2019).

to clot if a small clot is present in the sample and coagulation has started, the tendency for leukocytes and thrombocytes to clump, and the blue tinge imparted to blood films stained with Romanowsky stains. In some circumstances, it may be necessary to use an anticoagulant such as heparin to coat the syringe and needle before collecting blood from fish with blood that rapidly coagulates. This is often done in small fish, where the blood draw will be slow. EDTA is a commonly used anticoagulant of piscine hematologic studies; however, hemolysis may occur in blood collected from certain species of fish or fish anesthetized with tricaine and stored at temperatures above 4°C (39.2°F) or for long periods of time (Figure 25.12) (Korcock et al., 1988; Farias et al., 2016; Fazio et al., 2017). Cooling the blood sample to 4°C and rapidly preparing the film can minimize the hemolysis problem associated with tricaine (Noga, 2010).

Anticoagulants and diluents used for obtaining cell counts should be balanced for the osmolarity of the fish. The osmolarity of commonly used anticoagulants may be lower than that of the plasma osmolarity of some fish, especially cartilaginous fish (sharks and rays) resulting in hemolysis. The use of a solution that combines EDTA and heparin or of activated citrate dextrose solution has been recommended for this purpose (Walsh and Luer, 2004) (Appendix A).

Long-Term Storage

For longer term storage, preserving whole blood in formalin may be useful when leukocyte counts may be delayed (Arnold et al., 2014; Whitehead et al., 2019). If using formalin to preserve whole blood, samples should remain separated from blood films as formalin can alter the morphology of blood cells, which may complicate interpretation.

Blood Film Techniques and Stain

The techniques and stain described in Chapter 9 can be applied to fish. When creating blood films from fish blood, allowing them to air-dry in an arid environment is recommended. Depending on the situation, areas containing large volumes of water may create a contained humid environment. Air-drying blood films in a humid environment prolongs the process and may create artifacts.

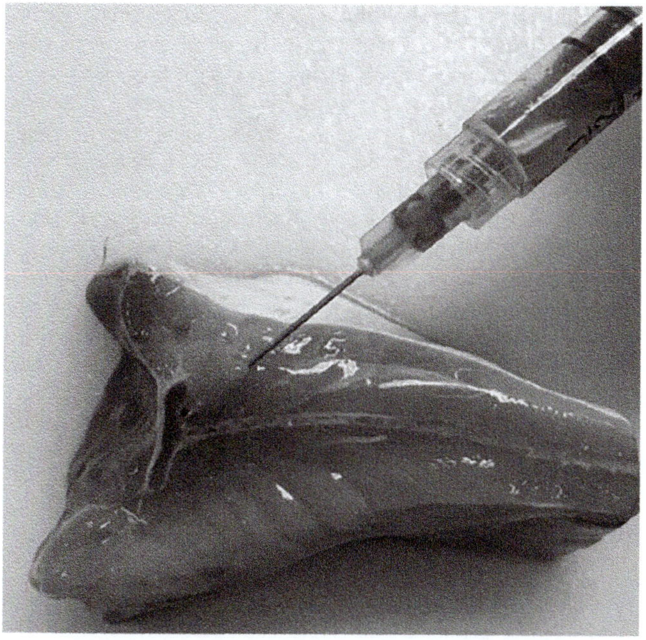

Fig. 25.11. Cross section of a juvenile cownose ray (*Rhinoptera bonasus*) pectoral fin oriented with the ventral surface upward and the wall of coelomic cavity to the left, with a 22-ga needle placed into the mesopterygial vein in the cranial third of the metapterygium cartilage. Source: Westmoreland et al. (2019).

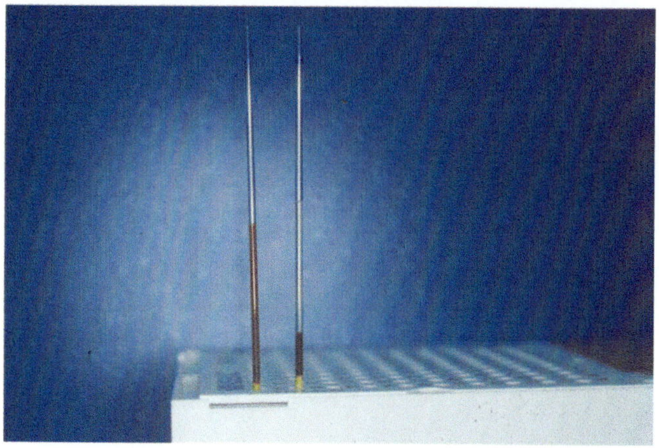

Fig. 25.12. Blood collected from a koi (*Cyprinus carpio*) and placed in microhematocrit tubes. The tube on the left showing hemolysis is from blood where EDTA was used as the anticoagulant. The tube on the right exhibits no hemolysis and is from blood where heparin was used as the anticoagulant.

Laboratory Submission

The recommendations described in Chapter 9 can be applied to fish samples.

References

Arnold JE, Matsche MA, Rosemary K. 2014. Preserving whole blood in formalin extends the specimen stability period for manual cell counts for fish. *Vet Clin Pathol* 43(4):613–620.

Cray C. 2015. Reference intervals in avian and exotic hematology. *Vet Clin Exot Anim* 18:105–116.

Duman M, Saticioglu IB, Suzer B, Altun S. 2019. Practices for drawing blood samples from teleost fish. *N Am J Aquac* 81:119–125.

Eliason EJ, Stecyk JAW. 2021. The cardiovascular system. In: Currie S, Evans DH (eds), *The Physiology of Fishes*, 5th edn. Boca Raton, FL: Taylor & Francis Group.

Farias THV, Pereira NL, de Padua SB, de Oliveira Alves L, Sakabe R, de Andrade Belo MA, Pilarski F. 2016. Na_2EDTA anticoagulant impaired blood samples from the teleost *Piaractus mesopotamicus*. *Pesq Vet Bras* 36(5):431–435.

Fazio F, Ferrantelli V, Saoca C, Giangrosso G, Piccione G. 2017. Stability of haematological parameters in stored blood samples of rainbow trout *Oncorhynchus mykiss* (Walbaum, 1792). *Vet Med* 62(7):401–405.

Friedrichs KR, Harr KE, Freeman KP, Szladovits B, Walton RM, Barnhart KF, Blanco-Chavez J. 2012. ASVCP reference interval guidelines: determination of de novo reference intervals in veterinary species and other related topics. *Vet Clin Pathol* 41(4):441–453.

Gallaugher P, Ferrell AP. 1998. Hematocrit and blood oxygen-carrying capacity. In: Perry S, Tufts B (eds), *Fish Physiol*, Vol. 17. San Diego, CA: Academic Press.

Grant KG. 2015. Fish hematology and associated disorders. In: Campbell TW (ed), *Vet Clin North Am: Exotic Animal Practice* 18(1):83–103.

Groff JM, Zinkl JG. 1999. Hematology and clinical chemistry of cyprinid fish. *Vet Clin North Am (Exotic Anim Pract)* 2(3):741–776.

Hargens AR, Millard RW, Johansen K. 1974. High capillary permeability in fishes. *Comp Biochem Physiol A Comp Physiol* 48:675–680.

Heming TA. 1989. Clinical studies of fish blood: importance of sample collection and measurement techniques. *Am J Vet Res* 50(1):93–97.

Henningsen AD. 1994. Tonic immobility in 12 elasmobranchs: use as an aid in captive husbandry. *Zoo Biol* 13(4):325–332.

Houston AH. 1990. Blood and circulation. In: Schreck C, Moyle P (eds), *Methods in Fish Biology*. Bethesda, MD: American Fisheries Society.

Iwama GK, Farrell AP. 1998. Disorders of the cardiovascular and respiratory system. In: Leatherland J, Woo P (eds), *Fish Diseases and Disorders*, 3rd edn. London: CABI Press.

Janssen JD, Kidd A, Ferreira A, Snowden S. 2017. Training and conditioning of elasmobranchs in aquaria. In: Smith M, Warmolts D, Thoney D, Hueter R, Murray M, Ezcurra J (eds), *The Elasmobranch Husbandry Manual II: Recent Advances in the Care of Sharks, Rays and their Relatives*. Columbus, OH: Ohio Biological Survey, Inc.

Korcock DE, Houston AH, Gray JD. 1988. Effects of sampling conditions on selected blood variables of rainbow trout (*Salmo gairdneri*) Richardson. *J Fish Biol* 33(3):19–330.

Lewbart GA, Yanong RPE. 2018. Fish. In: Carpenter JW (ed), *Exotic Animal Formulary*, 5th edn. St. Louis, MO: Elsevier, pp. 16–52.

Neiffer DL. 2007. Boney fish (lungfish, sturgeons, and teleosts). In: West G, Heard D, Caulkett N (eds), *Zoo Animal and Wildlife Immobilization and Anesthesia*. Ames, IA: Blackwell Publishing.

Noga EJ. 2010. Fish disease, diagnosis and treatment. In: Noga E (ed), *Fish Disease, Diagnosis and Treatment*. St. Louis, MO: Mosby.

Olson KR, Farrell AP. 2006. The cardiovascular system. In: Evans DH, Claiborne JB. (eds), *The Physiology of Fishes*, 3rd edn. Boca Raton, FL: Taylor & Francis Group.

Penning MR, Vaughan DB, Fivaz K, McEwan T. 2017. Chemical immobilization of elasmobranchs at uShaka Sea World, Durban, South Africa. In: Smith M, Warmolts D, Thoney D, et al. (eds), *The Elasmobranch Husbandry Manual II: Recent Advances in the Care of Sharks, Rays and their Relatives*. Columbus, OH: Ohio Biological Survey, Inc.

Phillips BE, Christiansen EF, Stoskopf MK, Broadhurst H, George R, Harms CA. 2016. Comparison of hematology, plasma biochemistry, and blood gas variables between 2 venipuncture sites in Southern Stingrays (*Dasyatis americana*). *Vet Clin Pathol* 45(4):627–633.

Railo E, Nikinmaa M, Soivio A. 1985. Effects of sampling of blood parameters in the rainbow trout, *Salmo gairdneri* Richardson. *J Fish Biol* 26:725–732.

Roberts RJ, Ellis AE. 2012. The anatomy and physiology of teleosts. In: Roberts R (ed), *Fish Pathology*, 4th edn. Philadelphia, PA. WB Saunders.

Rummer JL, Wang S, Steffensen JF, Randall DJ. 2014. Function and control of the fish secondary vascular system, a contrast to mammalian lymphatic systems. *J Exp Biol* 217:751–757. DOI: 10.1242/jeb.086348.

Smit GL, Hattingh J, Burger AP. 1979. Haematological assessment of the effects of the anaesthetic MS-222 in natural and neutralized form in three freshwater fish species: interspecies differences. *J Fish Biol* 15:633–653.

Stamper MA. 2007. Elasmobranchs (sharks, rays, and skates). In: West G, Heard D, Caulkett N (eds), *Zoo Animal and Wildlife Immobilization and Anesthesia*. Ames, IA: Blackwell Publishing.

Stamper MA, Neiffer DL. 2009. Fish sedation, anesthesia, analgesia, and euthanasia: considerations, methods, and types of drugs. *ILAR Journal* 50(4):343–360.

Steffensen JF, Lomholt JP. 1992. The secondary circulation. In: Hoar J, Randall J, Farrell A (eds), *Fish Physiology: The Cardiovascular System*, Vol. XII. New York: Academic Press.

Ueda K, Yanagisawa M, Murakumo K, Matsumoto Y, Sato K, Uchida S. 2017. Physical examination, blood sampling, and sedation of large elasmobranchs. In: Smith M, Warmolts D, Thoney D, et al. (eds), *The Elasmobranch Husbandry Manual II: Recent Advances in the Care of Sharks, Rays and their Relatives*. Columbus, OH: Ohio Biological Survey, Inc.

Walsh CJ, Luer CA. 2004. Elasmobranch hematology: identification of cell types and practical applications. In: Smith M, Warmolts D, Thoney D, Hueter R (eds), *The Elasmobranch Husbandry Manual: Captive Care of Sharks, Rays, and Their Relatives*. Columbus, OH: Ohio Biological Survey, Inc.

Wardle CS. 1971. New observations on the lymph system of the plaice (*Pleuronectes platessa*) and other teleosts. *J Mar Biol Ass UK* 51:977–990.

Westmoreland LSH, Archibald KE, Christiansen EF, Broadhurst HJ, Stoskopf MK. 2019. The mesopterygial vein: a reliable venipuncture site for intravascular access in batoids. *J Zoo Wildl* 50(2):369–374.

Whitehead MC, Vanetten CL, Zheng Y, Lewbart GA. 2019. Hematological parameters in largemouth bass (*Micropterus salmoides*) with formalin-preservation: comparison between wild tournament-caught and captive raised fish. *PeerJ* 7:e6669 http://doi.org/10.7717/peerj.6669.

Williamson MJ, Dudgeon C, Slade R. 2018. Tonic immobility in the zebra shark, *Stegostoma fasciatum*, and its use for capture methodology. *Environ Biol Fish* 101:741–748.

Zang L, Shimada Y, Nichimura Y, Tanaka T, Nishimura N. 2013. A novel, reliable method for repeated blood collection from aquarium fish. *Zebrafish* 10(3):425–432.

26 Hematologic Techniques for Quantitative Assessment in Fish

The in-house veterinary laboratory evaluation of the blood sample of fish involves the same routine procedures used in mammalian hematology with a few modifications. Like mammalian and avian hematology, hematologic evaluation of fish blood samples begins after the sample is prepared with preferred stains and solutions with the use of a centrifuge, microhematocrit tube, refractometer, hemacytometer, and slides. The systematic approach to evaluating the fish hemogram involves an assessment of cell and plasma parameters, morphologic features of the cells, and intra- and extracellular parasites. This chapter focuses on obtaining the sample parameter counts or concentrations, with some interpretation of the fish hemogram. Chapter 27 will continue with procedures on the fish hemogram with a focus on evaluating the blood film by identifying the morphologic features of the cells and parasites as well as the interpretation of findings.

Erythrocyte and Plasma Parameters

The same basic, primary hematologic procedures used for mammals and birds can be applied to fish. They include a packed cell volume (PCV) by centrifugation (or hematocrit by calculation), a plasma total protein estimation by refractometry, determination of hemoglobin concentration by spectrophotometry or hemoglobinometer, erythrocyte concentration by Natt and Herrick's solution dilution and use of a hemacytometer, and stained blood film evaluation. Erythrocytes of fish are larger compared to mammals and birds; therefore, the parameters and indices are relatively reflective of the difference. The blood collection site may also affect the erythrocyte numbers in fish. For example, hematocrit values have been shown to be significantly lower in blood samples collected from the cranial dorsal fin sinus of sharks when compared to the values from the samples collected from the caudal tail artery (Mylniczenko et al., 2006). In general, the PCV of fish is lower than that of mammals and birds (Campbell, 1988). Appendix B, Table B.11 provides guidelines for evaluating fish erythrocytes.

PCV

The PCV provides the percentage of whole blood that is composed of erythrocytes. Determination of the PCV via the microhematocrit method is the most-used method for evaluating the red cell mass of fish. The total erythrocyte count (TRBC) or erythrocyte concentration value, described later in the chapter, is commonly reported as well, but it is not as useful for clinical interpretation and generally parallels the PCV and hemoglobin concentration (Weiser, 2012). The TRBC may be useful in calculating red cell indices or for calculating the hematocrit (HCT) when instrument determinations are used.

Preparation of the microhematocrit tube with the blood sample can be done as described for mammals (Weiser, 2012). It is determined using the standard manual technique that employs microhematocrit tubes, tube sealant, a microhematocrit centrifuge (12 000 *g* for 5 min), and a tube-reading card or device. The three distinct layers observed in the spun microhematocrit tube of mammals are also present in blood samples from fish. The plasma column is located at the top of the tube, and the packed erythrocytes are located at the

Exotic Animal Hematology and Cytology, Fifth Edition. Terry W. Campbell and Krystan R. Grant.

Companion website: www.wiley.com/go/campbell/exotic

bottom. The buffy coat appears as a small white band located just above the erythrocyte column, and consists of leukocytes and thrombocytes. The buffy coat typically increases in size when the leukocyte concentration increases.

Much as in mammals and other lower vertebrates, the PCV of fish is affected by the number and size of the erythrocytes, as well as changes in the plasma volume that do not affect the total cell mass. These changes include increased plasma volume (hemodilution), decreased plasma volume (hemoconcentration), improper blood sampling (hemodilution), and epinephrine administration and hypothermia, which may result in hemoconcentration. The normal PCV of many species of fish ranges between 20% and 45% (see Appendix B for PCV ranges of selected species), but intrinsic and extrinsic factors may impact several values. In general, fish with a PCV greater than 45% are usually considered to be dehydrated, particularly when increased serum osmolality, sodium, chloride, and total protein are present. A diagnosis of anemia in fish is generally based on a marked reduction of the PCV and hemoglobin concentration. Anemic fish typically have low PCV values (less than 20%); however, normal PCV values for some species of fish, such as the Port Jackson shark (*Heterodontus portusjacksoni*) may be as low as 20% (Campbell, 1988). Anemia is described in more detail in Chapter 27.

Erythrocyte Sedimentation Rate (ESR)

The ESR is the time in which erythrocytes settle from the plasma, usually measured as millimeters per hour. The ESR is commonly used in human medicine, as well as in a limited way in marine mammal medicine, as an indirect marker to identify or monitor inflammatory conditions (Bossart et al., 2001; Tishkowski and Gupta, 2020). Inflammatory processes increase the amount of protein in the blood, thereby promoting erythrocyte aggregation and faster settling times (Tishkowski and Gupta, 2020). In addition to an increase of proteins (fibrinogen, haptoglobin, immunoglobulins, etc.) in the blood, other factors that may affect ESR include erythrocyte number, size, or shape; leukocyte count; or viscosity, which may be affected by anticoagulant. Measuring ESR in fish can be done using the Westergen or Wintrobe tube method (Gupta and Nigar, 2020). Commercial kits are available but, due to the volume required for the Westergren (2 mL) or Wintrobe (1 mL) tubes, they are not suitable for many smaller species. Adaptions of these methods using a microhematocrit tube have been used in apparently healthy fish (Blaxhill and Daisley, 1973). In one study, ESR was higher in spotted snakeheads, *Channa punctata*, acclimated to cold water temperatures compared to warm water temperatures (Jagtap and Mali, 2012).

Hemoglobin

Most teleost fishes have hemoglobin in their erythrocytes; however, oxygen can also be carried in simple solution via the plasma because the blood temperatures of fish are often low. For this reason, certain polar fish have no hemoglobin at all. There is considerable variation in the hemoglobins of fish, and up to four different types of hemoglobin, each with its own characteristics, can occur within an individual fish (Stoskopf, 1993; Roberts and Ellis, 2012). Modification of these hemoglobin isoforms allows fish to adapt to differing oxygen tensions, pH, and temperatures within the aquatic habitat (Roberts and Ellis, 2012). The environmental changes can affect the oxygen binding affinity to hemoglobin to allow for changes in demand during maintenance or activity (Sanyal et al., 2013). Hemoglobin concentration in fish has been measured using a variety of methods, but is measured most consistently using the cyanmethemoglobin method (using alkaline Drabkin's solution) in the same procedure as for birds and reptiles (Larsen and Snieszko, 1961; Hrubec and Smith, 2010). The cyanmethemoglobin method estimates hemoglobin from methemoglobin with a spectrophotometer. Another option to measure hemoglobin in fish is with a hemoglobinometer that estimates hemoglobin from azidemethemoglobin (Clark et al., 2008; Andrewartha et al., 2016). Obtaining the total hemoglobin concentration for fish using the standard cyanmethemoglobin method is similar to that used for mammals with one modification: the cyanmethemoglobin reagent–blood mixture should be centrifuged prior to analysis. The free nuclei from lysed erythrocytes are removed before obtaining the optical density value, to avoid an overestimation of the hemoglobin concentration. Using a hemoglobinometer, such as the HemoCue® (HemoCue America, Brea, CA), allows the blood to be mixed with a dry reagent within a cuvette before insertion into the device, which reads the sample with a built-in photometer. The use of the HemoCue system has been calibrated for several teleosts, including several salmon species (*Oncorhynchus nerka*, *Onchorhynus tshawytscha*, *Salmo salar*), the Pacific bluefin tuna (*Thunnus orientalis*), and the chub mackerel (*Scomber japonicus*). It has also been validated in several elasmobranch species including blacktip reef shark (*Carcharhinus melanopterus*), sicklefin lemon shark (*Negaprion acutidens*), and epaulette shark (*Hemiscyllium ocellatum*). In all studies, values from the HemoCue overestimated the hemoglobin concentration compared to the Drabkin's method and therefore required correction (Clark et al., 2008; Andrewartha et al., 2016; Schwieterman et al., 2019). Published hemoglobin concentration values for fish are usually low, 5–10 g/dL, compared to those for mammals (Hrubec and Smith, 2010).

Total Erythrocyte Concentration

The total erythrocyte concentration in fish can be determined using the same automated or manual methods used for the determination of total erythrocyte counts in mammalian blood. Electronic impedance cell counters provide a rapid, reliable method for obtaining total red blood cell concentrations. Erythrocyte counts with electronic cell counters are slightly inflated by the inclusion of leukocytes and thrombocytes in the count; however, these additional cells are not significant in most samples, as they make up approximately 0.1% of the peripheral blood cell population. Analyzers for automated cell counting have been used for fish, mostly because timely health evaluation of farmed fish and labor reduction in aquaculture confer an economic advantage in that industry. The use of analyzers and methodologies has been reviewed in several studies (Fazio et al., 2012; Fazio, 2019).

Previously, the two manual methods for obtaining total red blood cell counts in fish were the erythrocyte Unopette (Unopette, Becton-Dickinson, Rutherford, NJ) method used in mammalian hematology and Natt and Herrick's method, which involves the preparation of Natt and Herrick's solution to be used as a stain and diluent (Natt and Herrick, 1952) (see Appendix A). In 2009, the erythrocyte Unopette system was discontinued, but a similar kit is available for manual red cell counts in mammals (Erythro-pette™, Exotic Animal Solutions, Inc. Hueytown, AL), which has been used for counting avian red blood cells (Ferreyra et al., 2015). Natt and Herrick's solution is commercially available as a stain (Vetlab Supply, Palmetto Bay, FL) or within a kit (Natt-pette™, Exotic Animal Solutions, Inc. Hueytown, AL).

Manual red cell counts using Natt and Herrick's method involves making a 1:200 dilution of the blood using Natt and Herrick's solution and red-blood-cell-diluting pipettes. Alternatively, use of commercially prepared Natt and Herrick's solution kits provides an easy method for obtaining accurate dilutions for the total erythrocyte determination because dilutions are made using a provided capillary tube and not a diluting pipette. After mixing, the diluted blood is discharged into a hemacytometer counting chamber (Figure 26.1), and the cells are allowed to settle for 5 min to the ruled surface before counting (Figure 26.2). Erythrocytes located in the four corner squares and the central square within the large center square of the Neubauer-ruled hemacytometer chamber are counted when using any of the manual methods (Figures 10.3a and 10.3b). Using the 40× objective, the cells can be identified for counting (Figures 26.3). Cells on the borders of the squares should be counted on the top and left but not counted on the bottom and right borders, to avoid redundancy. Both sides of the hemacytometer should be counted separately. If the count totals from each side are within 10% of each other, then the total red blood cell count can be calculated. The number obtained from either side, or an average of the two sides, is multiplied by 10 000 to calculate the total red blood cell count per cubic millimeter (mm^3) or microliter (μL) of blood:

$$\text{RBC/mm}^3 = (\text{Average count from both sides of chamber}) \times 10\,000$$

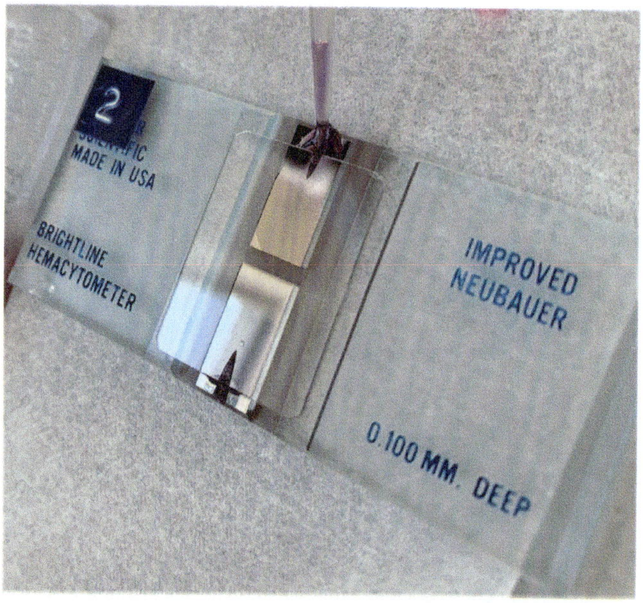

Fig. 26.1. This image shows the diluted blood with Natt–Herrick's solution being discharged into a Neubauer hemacytometer.

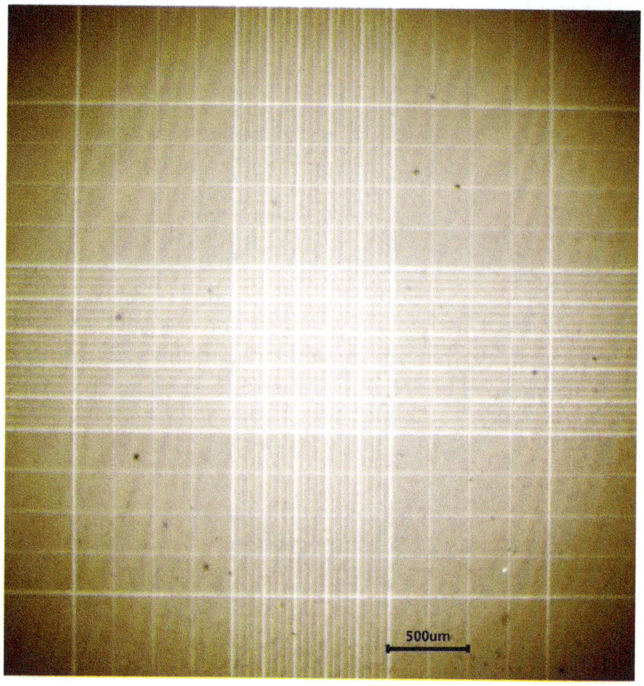

Fig. 26.2. The appearance of erythrocytes in a Neubauer-ruled hemacytometer using Natt and Herrick's method (Natt and Herrick's solution, 4×).

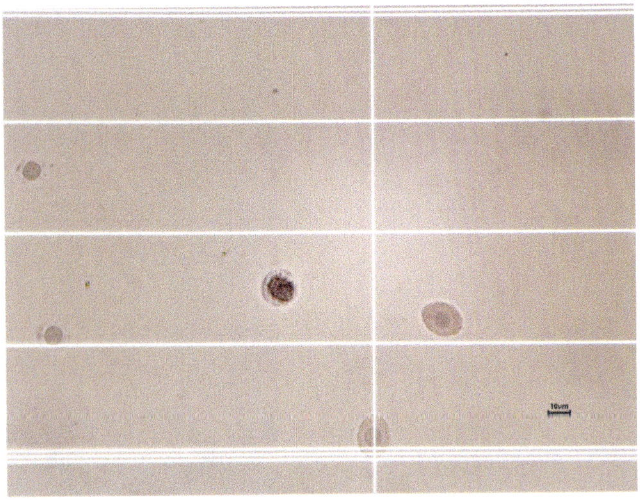

Fig. 26.3. The cells in the hemacytometer can be easily identified for counting using the 40× objective. The granular-appearing cell is a leukocyte (Natt and Herrick's solution, 40×).

This method, as with all manual counting methods, may have an inherent error of 10%; however, it is commonly used in clinical practice. Erythrocyte numbers of fish usually lie in the range 1.0–3.0 × $10^6/mm^3$, but are variably affected by species, activity, stress, and environmental temperatures (Hrubec et al., 1996; Hrubec and Smith, 2010; Roberts and Ellis, 2012; Witeska, 2013) (Appendix B, Table B.11). For example, the TRBC count in less active teleost species ranges from 0.5 to 1.5 × $10^6/\mu L$ compared to 3.0 to 4.2 × $10^6/\mu L$ in more active species (Witeska, 2013).

The TRBC of fish can also be determined using the modified Dacie's solution (Dacie and Lewis, 1968; Blaxhill and Daisley, 1973; Haley and Weiser, 1985) in the same way that the manual red-blood-cell-diluting pipettes are used in Natt and Herrick's method.

Erythrocyte Indices

After the primary hematologic parameters (PCV, erythrocyte count, and hemoglobin concentration) have been determined, the erythrocyte indices can be calculated. These include the mean cell volume (MCV) or mean erythrocyte volume (MEV), mean cell hemoglobin (MCH) or mean erythrocyte hemoglobin (MEH), and mean cell hemoglobin concentration (MCHC) or mean erythrocyte hemoglobin concentration (MEHC). The MCV is an index of red cell volume and is calculated similarly to mammalian MCV (Grant, 2015):

$$\text{MCV}(\text{fL}) = (\text{PCV}(\%) \times 10)/\text{TRBC}$$

The direct electronic measurement of MCV appears to be more sensitive in detecting erythrocyte size differences in fish and is more reproducible than using the calculated MCV (Haley and Weiser, 1985).

The MCH is an index of hemoglobin content in an average red blood cell and is calculated similarly to mammalian MCH, although it is not commonly used (Grant, 2015; Weiser, 2012).

$$\text{MCH}(\text{pg}) = (\text{Hb}(\text{g/dL}) \times 10)/\text{TRBC}$$

The MCHC is an index denoting the proportion of hemoglobin present in an average erythrocyte and is calculated as follows (Grant, 2015; Weiser, 2012):

$$\text{MCHC}(\text{g/dL or }\%) = (\text{Hgb}(\text{g/dL}) \times 100)/\text{PCV}(\%)$$

Erythrocyte parameters for selected fish species can be found in Appendix B (Table B.11).

Published MCV values for teleost fish generally range between 150 and 350 fL (femtoliters, μm^3). Published MCH and MCHC values typically range between 30 and 100 pg and between 18 and 30% (g/dL), respectively (Hrubec and Smith, 2010). Although published references are available for the erythrocyte indices of fish, the assessment of abnormal values has not been properly evaluated in these species.

Plasma Appearance and Protein

The color and clarity of the plasma column above the packed erythrocytes should be noted. Normal plasma is typically colorless; however, in some fish, it may appear blue or green (Fang and Bada, 1990; Fang, 1990). In some cases, colored plasma may be an indication of disease, such as hepatobiliary disease. The color of plasma may be due to bile pigment. Some of these animals lack the biliverdin reductase enzyme needed to reduce biliverdin (which is green) to bilirubin (which is yellow). Green plasma is suggestive of biliverdinemia (excess biliverdin bile pigment in blood); yellow plasma is suggestive of bilirubinemia, and typically is indicative of a poor prognosis for survival. Biliverdinemia or bilirubinemia may be an indication of hepatic failure or renal failure, because the kidney is normally very efficient at clearing bile pigments from the blood. Currently, biochemical tests exist to confirm the presence of biliverdin, but are not commercially available (Divers, 2019). Lipemia and hemolysis may be noted in some samples. Hemolysis usually results from lysis of erythrocytes during blood collection or sample handling. Intravascular hemolysis may also cause hemolysis of the sample in some instances. If the PCV is normal, then the presence of the hemolysis is probably associated with artifactual lysis of erythrocytes.

The biuret method of determining plasma proteins is preferred but obtained during biochemical analysis. Plasma protein concentration is typically determined using handheld refractometers, which have been the standard instruments for determining protein concentration in plasma and body cavity fluid samples since the 1960s (George and O'Neill, 2001). Major discrepancies found between biuret and refractometric results may be due to differences in the brand of refractometers used in the study, changes in the alteration of the chemical composition of the biuret reagent, use of different standards, or changes in reaction conditions (George and O'Neill, 2001). Sample-related causes of error in protein determination by refractometric methods include increased nonprotein solids, such as cholesterol, urea, lipoproteins, and glucose (George and O'Neill, 2001). These compounds can increase the refractometric protein measurements by 0.5–1.0 g/dL (5–10 g/L) (George and O'Neill, 2001). Female southern stingrays (*Hypanus americanus*) exhibited good correlation between plasma protein measured by refractometry and biuret methods (Grant and Campbell, 2020).

Leukocyte Parameters

As with methods for obtaining erythrocyte parameters, methods used for leukocyte counts in avian blood samples are applied to other lower vertebrates. Leukocyte counts may be obtained using manual and automated methods. However, significant differences may occur between the manual absolute and relative microscopic leukocyte differential count and the automated absolute and relative leukocyte count techniques (Post et al., 2003). Manual methods for the determination of a leukocyte differential exhibit greater variability compared to automated methods (Russo et al., 1986).

The presence of nucleated erythrocytes and thrombocytes in the blood of lower vertebrates presents a challenge when attempting to apply the automated counting methods used for obtaining mammalian white blood cell counts. The fact that these animals have an erythrocyte that is similar in size to many of the leukocytes, small lymphocytes, and thrombocytes presents an additional challenge. Direct and semidirect manual methods for obtaining absolute (total) leukocyte concentrations in animals with nucleated erythrocytes and thrombocytes have been developed.

Semidirect Method for Manual Leukocyte Concentration

A commonly used semidirect method involves staining heterophils and eosinophils using phloxine B (a specific stain for mammalian eosinophils) as the diluent. The procedure was simplified utilizing the Eosinophil Unopette 5877 System (Becton-Dickinson, Rutherford, NJ), which was developed for determining total eosinophil concentrations in mammalian blood but was discontinued in 2007. When it was available, the blood sample was diluted 1:32 with the phloxine B solution in the Unopette vial using the 25 μL pipette provided. The Eopette™ Test Kit (Exotic

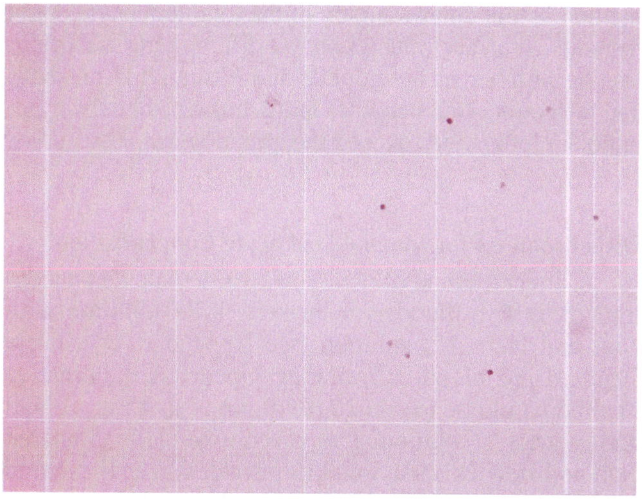

Fig. 26.4. Heterophils and eosinophils appear as round, refractile, eosinophilic cells in the Neubauer-ruled hemacytometer with Eopette™ method of counting leukocytes (Phloxine B, 10×).

Animal Solutions, Hueytown, AL) is now available as a substitute for the Eosinophil Unopette 5877 System to eliminate the need for a manual pipette to make the dilutions.

After a Neubauer-ruled hemacytometer chamber has been properly loaded with the blood–phloxine mixture and allowed to stand in a humid chamber for a minimum of 5 min, the eosin-stained heterophils and eosinophils are counted in both sides of the chamber (18 large squares) using the 10× (Figure 26.4) or 40× objective. It is important to load the hemacytometer immediately following proper mixing of the blood and phloxine diluent, because red blood cells may also stain following prolonged exposure. Next, the total leukocyte concentration (TWBC/mm^3) is calculated after completing a leukocyte differential to obtain the percent heterophils and eosinophils on the stained blood film using the following equation:

$$\text{WBC/mm}^3 = \frac{(\text{Total count in both sides of hemacytometer}) \times 1.1 \times 16 \times 100}{\%\ \text{Heterophils} + \%\ \text{Eosinophils from differential}}$$

For example, if the total number of eosin-stained cells counted in the nine large squares on both sides of a Neubauer-ruled hemacytometer chamber (total of 18 squares) is 73, and the differential leukocyte count revealed 16% heterophils and 2% eosinophils, then using the above formula, the TWBC/mm^3 is calculated to be 7138/mm^3 when rounded to the nearest whole number.

The phloxine B semidirect method is relatively easy to perform and has been shown to be more precise for hemacytometer counting than Natt and Herrick's method (next section) (Dein et al., 1994). A disadvantage of this method is that determination of the total leukocyte count depends on an accurate leukocyte differential (in particular, the number of heterophils and eosinophils present), and the count often becomes less accurate when the mononuclear leukocytes exceed the granulocytes.

Direct Method for Manual Leukocyte Concentration

A direct method of obtaining total leukocyte concentrations in fish blood is to make a 1:200 dilution with Natt and Herrick's solution (see Appendix A) using a standard red blood-cell diluting pipette. An alternative method would be to add 20 μL of blood to 4 mL of Natt and Herrick's solution. Use of commercially prepared Natt and Herrick's solution kits provides an easy method for obtaining accurate dilutions for the total erythrocyte determination because dilutions are made using a provided capillary tube and not a diluting pipette. The leukocytes in the sample will stain dark blue (Figure 26.5). The total leukocyte concentration is obtained by counting all the leukocytes (dark blue cells) in the nine large squares in the ruled area of the Neubauer-ruled hemacytometer chamber (Figure 26.2) using the following equation:

$$\text{TWBC/mm}^3 = \left(\text{total cells in nine large squares} + 10\ \%\right) \times 200$$

The advantage of using this method is that a total erythrocyte and thrombocyte count can also be obtained using the same charged hemacytometer. A disadvantage is that it is often difficult to differentiate thrombocytes from small lymphocytes, thus creating errors in the counts. It has been recommended that staining the blood sample for 60 min in Natt and Herrick's solution improves the differentiation between small lymphocytes and thrombocytes (Robertson and Maxwell, 1990). An alternative approach to the problem of differentiating lymphocytes and thrombocytes using this method is to include thrombocytes in the leukocyte differential and subtract the absolute thrombocyte count from the total count to obtain the total leukocyte count.

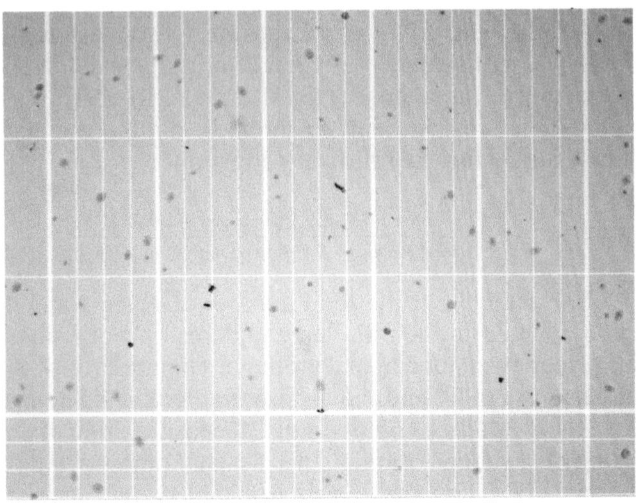

Fig. 26.5. This image shows the appearance of erythrocytes and leukocytes (the darker blue cells) from an elasmobranch fish (*Chiloscyllium plagiosum*) blood sample in a Neubauer-ruled hemacytometer using Natt and Herrick's method (Natt and Herrick's solution, 10×).

Leukocyte Differential

The differential leukocyte count and leukocyte morphology are obtained by microscopic evaluation of stained blood films. A variety of hematologic stains are available (Appendix A). Rapid stains (i.e., Diff–Quik, Dade Diagnostics, Aguada, Puerto Rico) or Hemacolor (Miles Laboratories, Inc., Elkhart, IN) have a shorter staining time, but do not always provide adequate differentiation between the various leukocytes. Stains such as Wright's and May–Grünwald–Giemsa stains are more time consuming, but provide better differentiation of the leukocytes, thrombocytes, and immature erythrocytes (Alleman et al., 1992; Muro et al., 1998).

The leukocyte differential is performed during the microscopic evaluation of Romanowsky-stained blood films. Blood samples collected into heparin make it necessary to prepare the blood films immediately following sample collection in order to decrease the incidence of cell clumping. Whenever possible, blood films should be prepared using blood containing no anticoagulant. The differential leukocyte count is performed by counting a minimum of 100 leukocytes in a monocellular area in the blood film. The cells counted are those consecutively encountered as one moves from one counting field to the next. Granulocyte classification differs between teleosts and elasmobranchs. The cells for teleosts are classified as neutrophils (Figure 27.8), eosinophils (Figure 27.9), basophils (Appendix C, plate C.20), lymphocytes (Figure 27.15), and monocytes (Figure 27.17). The cells for elasmobranchs are classified as G_1, heterophils, or fine eosinophilic granulocytes (FEGs) (Figures 27.10a–27.10d); G_2 or neutrophils (Figure 27.11); G_3, eosinophils, or coarse eosinophilic granulocytes (CEGs) (Figure 27.12); basophils (Figure 27.14); lymphocytes (Figure 27.15c); and monocytes (Figure 27.17). The number of each cell type becomes a fraction of the total or a percentage of the leukocyte population. Absolute numbers of each cell type are obtained by multiplying the total leukocyte concentration by the percentage of that type of leukocyte from the differential count.

Thrombocyte Parameters

The concentrations of thrombocytes in the blood of lower vertebrates vary. Using a fluorescent antibody technique, the ratio of thrombocytes to lymphocytes was found to be 1.4 to 1.0 which is approximately a concentration of 60 000 to 70 000/mm^3 (Roberts and Ellis, 2012). The actual thrombocyte concentration is difficult to determine because thrombocytes tend to clump; therefore, thrombocyte concentration is often reported as normal, increased, or decreased, based upon estimates from peripheral blood films.

Blood films may be used to assess thrombocyte numbers. In general, approximately 1–5 thrombocytes can be seen in a monolayer 1000× (oil-immersion) field in a blood film from normal fish, unless the thrombocytes clump excessively during preparation.

The absolute thrombocyte concentration can be obtained using the same hemacytometer used for obtaining total leukocyte and erythrocyte counts with Natt and Herrick's method. The number of thrombocytes counted in the central large square on both sides of the Neubauer-ruled hemacytometer is multiplied by 1000 to obtain the number of thrombocytes per microliter of blood (Figure 10.7).

$$\text{Thrombocytes/mm}^3 = (\text{total \# of thrombocytes in center large square on both sides}) \times 1000$$

Thrombocytopenia is suggested by thrombocyte numbers less than one per monolayer 1000× field. Thrombocytosis is suggested by numbers greater than five in an average monolayer 1000× field.

Whole Blood Preservatives

The use of whole blood preservatives may be useful when there is a delay between blood collection and the determination of the PCV, complete blood cell count, and assessment of hemic cell morphology. Freshly collected blood samples for delayed analysis are prepared by adding 100 μL of well-mixed heparinized whole blood to 400 μL of 10% neutral buffered formalin for a 1:5 dilution and thoroughly mixed (via multiple manual tube inversions) and stored at 4°C (Arnold et al., 2014). Dilution of the blood with Natt–Herrick diluent is adjusted to account for the added neutral buffered formalin to the sample to reach a final dilution of 1:100. Heparinized whole blood preservation with 10% neutral buffered formalin for hematologic evaluation of fish via manual hemocytometer can provide sample stability for up to 3.5 months with no evidence of adverse effects (Whitehead et al., 2019).

References

Alleman AR, Jacobson ER, Raskin RE. 1992. Morphologic and cytochemical characteristics of blood cells from the desert tortoise (*Gopherus agassizii*). *Am J Vet Res* 53:1645–1651.

Andrewartha SJ, Munns SL, Edwards A. 2016. Calibration of the HemoCue point-of-care analyser for determining haemoglobin concentration in a lizard and a fish. *Conserv Physiol* 4:10.1093/conphys/cow006.

Arnold JE, Matsche MA, Rosemary K. 2014. Preserving whole blood in formalin extends the specimen stability period for manual cell counts for fish. *Vet Clin Pathol* 43(4):613–620.

Blaxhill PC, Daisley KW. 1973. Routine haematological methods for use with fish blood. *J Fish Biol* 5:771–781.

Bossart GD, Reidarson TH, Dierauf LA, Duffield DA. 2001. Clinical pathology. In: Dierauf LA, Gulland FMD (eds), *CRC Handbook of Marine Mammal Medicine*, 2nd edn. CRC Press LLC.

Campbell TW. 1988. Fish cytology and hematology. *Vet Clin North Am: Sm Anim Pract* 18(2):349–364.

Clark TD, Eliason EJ, Sandblom E, Hinch SG, Farrell AP. 2008. Calibration of a hand-held haemoglobin analyser for use on fish blood. *J Fish Biol* 73(10):2587–2595.

Dacie JV, Lewis K. 1968. *Practical Hematology*, 4th edn. London: Churchill Livingstone.

Dein FJ, Wilson BA, Fischer MT. 1994. Avian leucocyte counting using the hemocytometer. *J Zoo Wildl Med* 25:432–437.

Divers SJ. 2019. Hepatology. In: Divers SJ, Stahl SJ (eds), *Mader's Reptile and Amphibian Medicine and Surgery*, 3rd edn. St. Louis, MO: Elsevier.

Fang LS. 1990. The identification of the blue-green pigment in the blood plasma of the cottid, *Clinocottus analis*. *Marine Nature* 3:53–60.

Fang LS, Bada JL. 1990. The blue-green blood plasma of marine fish. *Comp Biochem Physiol* 97B(1):37–45.

Fazio F. 2019. Fish hematology analysis as an important tool of aquaculture: a review. *Aquaculture* 500:237–242.

Fazio F, Filiciotto F, Marafioti S, et al. 2012. Automatic analysis to assess haematological parameters in farmed gilthead sea bream (*Sparu aurata* Linnaeus, 1758). *Marine and Freshwater Behaviour and Physiology* 45(1):63–73.

Ferreyra H, Beldomenico PM, Marchese K, et al. 2015. Lead exposure affects health indices in free-ranging ducks in Argentina. *Exotoxicology* DOI:10.1007/s10646-015-1419-7.

George JW, O'Neill SL. 2001. Comparison of refractometer and biuret methods for total protein measurement in body cavity fluids. *Vet Clin Pathol* 30:16–18.

Grant KR. 2015. Fish hematology and associated disorders. *Vet Clin Exot Anim* 18:83–103.

Grant KR, Campbell TW. 2020. Hematology and plasma biochemistry value differences between acclimated and recently captive female southern stingrays (*Dasyatis americana*). *JZAR* 8(1) DOI:10.19227/jzar.v8i1.254.

Gupta N, Nigar S. 2020. Detection of blood parasites and estimation of hematological indices in fish. In: Gupta N and Gupta V (eds), *Experimental Protocols in Biotechnology*. New York, NY: Humana Press.

Haley PJ, Weiser MG. 1985. Erythrocyte volume distribution in rainbow trout. *Am J Vet Res* 46:2210–2211.

Hrubec TC, Smith SA. 2010. Hematology of fishes. In: Weiss DJ, Wardrop KJ (eds), *Schalm's Veterinary Hematology*, 6th edn. Ames, IA: Wiley-Blackwell.

Hrubec TC, Smith SA, Robertson JL, et al. 1996. Comparison of hematologic reverence intervals between culture system and type of hybrid striped bass. *Am J Vet Res* 57:618–623.

Jagtap AR, Mali RP. 2012. Alterations in the erythrocyte sedimentation rate of freshwater fish, *Channa punctatus* on exposure to temperature stress form Godavari River, Nanded. *Int J Biomed & Adv Res* 3(12):870–873.

Larsen HN, Snieszko SF. 1961. Comparison of various methods of determination of hemoglobin in trout blood. *Prog Fish Cult* 23:8–17.

Muro J, Cuenca R, Pastor J, Vinas L, Lavin S. 1998. Effects of lithium heparin and tripotassium EDTA on hematologic values of Hermann's tortoises (*Testudo hermanni*). *J Zoo Wildl Med* 29:40–44.

Mylniczenko ND, Curtis EW, Wilborn RE, Young FA. 2006. Differences in hematocrit of blood samples obtained from two venipuncture sites in sharks. *Am J Vet Res* 67(11):1861–1864.

Natt MP, Herrick CA. 1952. A new blood diluent for counting erythrocytes and leucocytes of the chicken. *Poultry Sci* 31:735–738.

Post J, Rebel JMJ, ter Huurne AAHM. 2003. Automated blood cell count: a sensitive and reliable method to study corticosterone related stress in broilers. *Poultry Sci* 82:591–595.

Roberts RJ, Ellis AE. 2012. The anatomy and physiology of teleosts. In: Roberts R (ed), *Fish Pathology*, 4th edn. Philadelphia, PA: WB Saunders.

Robertson GW, Maxwell MH. 1990. Modified staining techniques for avian blood cells. *Br Poultry Sci* 31:881–886.

Russo EA, McEntee L, Applegate I, Baker JS. 1986. Comparison of two methods for determination of white blood cell counts in macaws. *J Am Vet Med Assoc* 189:1013–1016.

Sanyal M, Patil P, Jaiswal E, Deshmukh A. 2013. Structural and functional diversity of haemoglobin molecule properties amongst different classes and species of animals. *Acta Biologica Indica* 2(2):381–387.

Schwieterman GD, Bouyoucos IA, Potgieter K, et al. 2019. Analysing tropical elasmobranch blood samples in the field: blood stability during storage and validation of the HemoCue® haemoglobin analyser. *Conserv Physiol* 7(1): coz081; doi:10.1093/conphys/coz081.

Stoskopf MK. 1993. Clinical pathology. In: Stoskopf M (ed), *Fish Medicine*. Philadelphia, PA: WB Saunders.

Tishkowski K, Gupta V. 2020. Erythrocyte sedimentation rate. In: StatPearls [Internet]. Treasure Island (FL): StatPearls Publishing, Available from: https://www.ncbi.nlm.nih.gov/books/NBK557485/

Weiser G. 2012. Laboratory technology for veterinary medicine. In: Thrall M, Weiser G, Allison RW, Campbell T (eds), *Veterinary Hematology and Clinical Chemistry*, 2nd edn. Ames, IA: Wiley-Blackwell, pp. 3–33.

Whitehead MC, Vanetten CL, Zheng Y, Lewbart GA. 2019. Hematological parameters in largemouth bass (*Micropterus salmoides*) with formalin-preservation: comparison between wild tournament-caught and captive-raised fish. *PeerJ* DOI:10.7717/peerj.6669.

Witeska M. 2013. Erythrocytes in teleost fish: a review. *Zool Ecol* 23(4):275–181.

27 Evaluation and Interpretation of the Peripheral Blood of Fish

Hematologic evaluation of fish can be useful in the detection of diseases affecting the cellular components of blood. Certain diseases of fish can result in anemia, leukopenia, leukocytosis, thrombocytopenia, and other abnormal changes of the blood cells. Evaluation of the hemogram may also be useful in following the progression of the disease or response to therapy. Hematologic data are often not used in fish medicine due to the difficulty in obtaining blood samples, the challenges involved in obtaining cell counts, and the lack of meaningful reference intervals. Hematologic evaluation can be used to monitor the health status of fish if the interpretation accounts for the intrinsic and extrinsic factors that may influence the hematology values. However, many published reference intervals for fish do not include information involving intrinsic (i.e., sex and age) and extrinsic (i.e., water chemistry parameters and temperature) factors.

This chapter continues with the procedures of assessing the piscine hemogram with blood film evaluation. The information from the blood film, coupled with the results from the counts and red blood cell indices, allows for complete evaluation of the piscine hemogram.

Representative hemic cells found in fish blood films can be found in Appendix C.

Fish Erythrocytes

Morphology and Color

The erythrocytes of teleost fishes are similar in appearance and ultrastructure to those of birds and reptiles (Figures 27.1a–27.1c). The mature erythrocytes of elasmobranch fishes are also similar in appearance to avian and reptilian erythrocytes, but are much larger and rounded (Rowley, 1988) (Figures 27.2a–27.2c). Normal mature erythrocytes of fish are oval to ellipsoidal with abundant pale eosinophilic cytoplasm and centrally positioned oval to ellipsoidal nuclei in Romanowsky-stained blood films. The nuclei of fish erythrocytes can be large and may occupy as much as one-fourth the cell volume or greater. The long axis of the nucleus is parallel to the long axis of the cell, except in a few species of fish that have round erythrocyte nuclei. The nuclear chromatin is densely clumped and stains dark purple. The cytoplasm is typically homogeneous but may contain variable amounts of rarefied or pale-staining areas or vacuoles that are associated with degeneration of organelles, such as mitochondria (Stokes and Firkin, 1971; Walsh and Luer, 2004) (Figures 27.1a–27.1c, 27.2a–27.2c). Mature erythrocytes of some fish are biconvex with a central swelling that corresponds to the position of the nucleus, while other species have flattened biconcave erythrocytes. The size and number of erythrocytes vary between and within species depending upon the physiological conditions present (Hibiya, 1985).

A slight to moderate amount of anisocytosis and polychromasia (2–5% of the erythrocyte population) is normal in many species of fish. Polychromatic erythrocytes have a pale blue cytoplasm, may appear more rounded, and have nuclear chromatin that is less condensed compared to mature erythrocytes.

Immature Erythrocytes

Teleosts

Immature erythrocytes (1% of the red cell population) may be noted in normal blood films of teleost fish because erythropoiesis occurs in the peripheral blood

Exotic Animal Hematology and Cytology, Fifth Edition. Terry W. Campbell and Krystan R. Grant.

Companion website: www.wiley.com/go/campbell/exotic

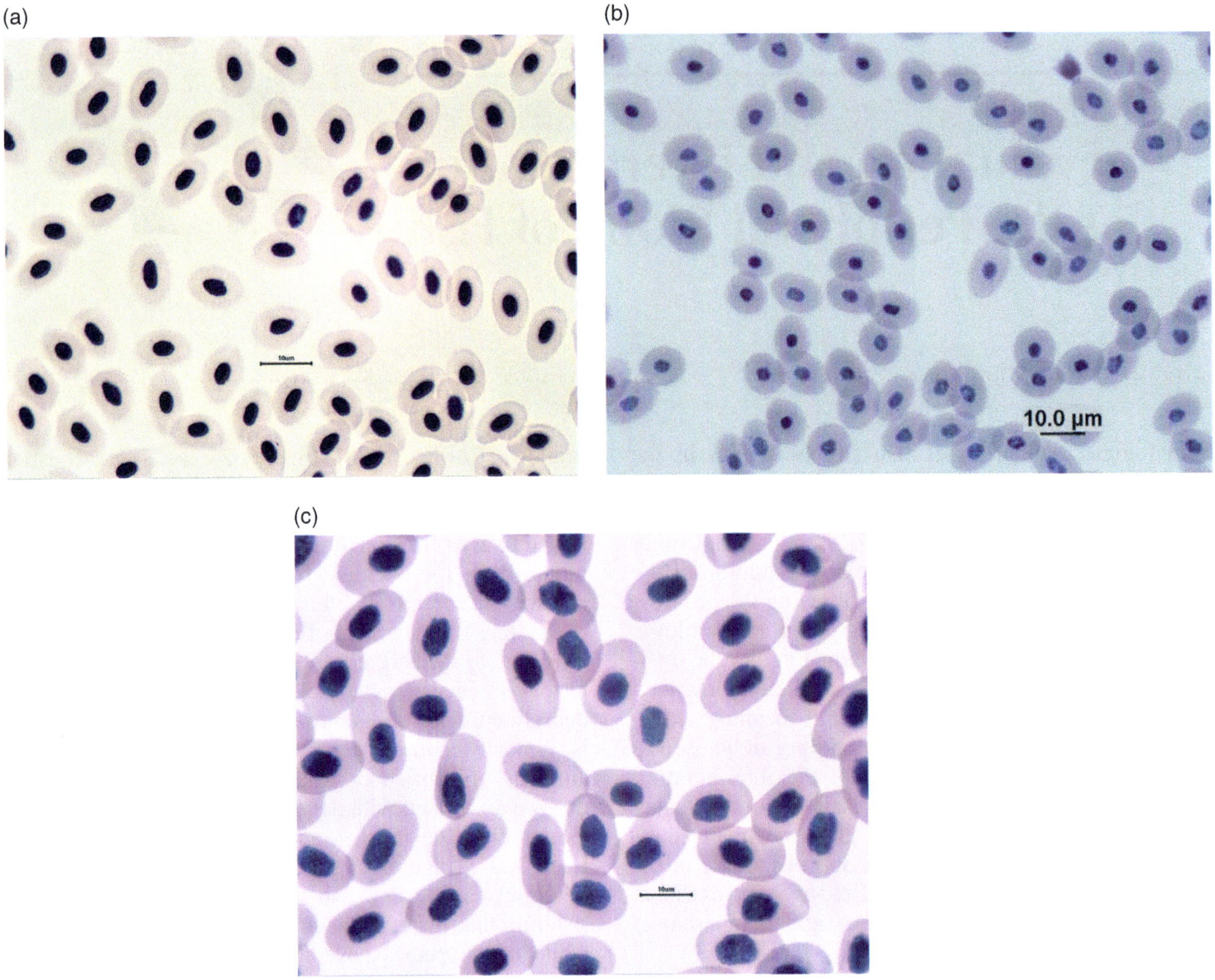

Fig. 27.1. (a) Normal erythrocytes in the blood film of a koi (*Cyprinus carpio*), Wright–Giemsa stain. (b) Normal erythrocytes in the blood film of a striped catfish (*Pangasianodon hypophthalmus*), Wright–Giemsa stain. (c) Normal erythrocytes in the blood film of a white sturgeon (*Acipenser transmontanus*), Wright–Giemsa stain.

(Stokes and Firkin, 1971; Rowley, 1988; Stoskopf, 1993; Roberts and Ellis, 2012). Immature erythrocytes (rubriblasts, prorubricytes, and rubricytes) appear as round cells containing less cytoplasm than mature erythrocytes (Figure 27.3a). Depending upon the stage of development, the cytoplasmic volume does vary in amount and in the intensity of basophilic staining with Romanowsky stains (Appendix C, Plates C.20 and C.21).

The nucleus of the immature erythrocyte is larger than the nucleus of the mature cell and is round, centrally positioned, and comparatively less condensed (Figures 27.3a and 27.3b). Ultrastructurally, the cytoplasm of immature fish erythrocytes contains mitochondria, Golgi apparatus, and small vacuoles, whereas the cytoplasm of mature erythrocytes is finely granular and contains no inclusions (Hyder et al., 1983). Erythroid cells demonstrating mitosis may also be present in peripheral blood films of normal teleost fish.

Elasmobranchs

Immature erythrocytes, including erythroblasts and proerythrocytes, are occasionally identified in peripheral blood films of healthy elasmobranch fishes. Immature erythrocytes appear as round cells with a high N:C ratio and basophilic cytoplasm much as described for the teleost fishes (Figures 27.4a–27.4c). Erythrocyte replication appears to occur in the peripheral blood of these fishes as well, as evidenced by the presence of erythrocyte mitotic activity (Stokes and Firkin, 1971; Kendall et al., 1992; Walsh and Luer, 2004) (Figure 27.4c). Maturation of erythrocytes involves an increase in cell size and hemoglobin content in some species, such as the carp (*Cyprinus carpio*), where the mature cells exhibit higher mean corpuscular volume (MCV) and mean corpuscular hemoglobin concentration (MCHC) values (Speckner et al., 1989).

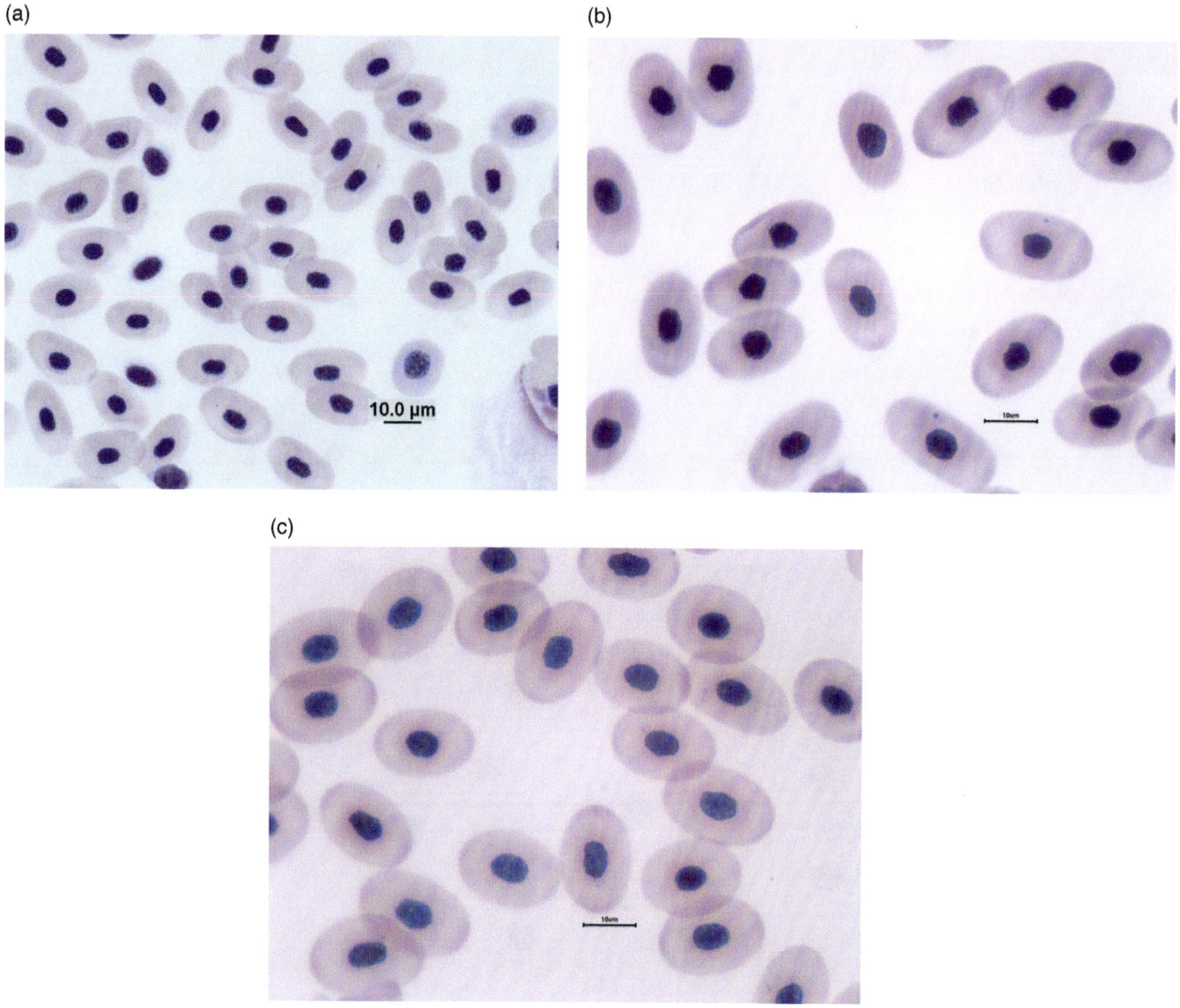

Fig. 27.2. (a) Normal erythrocytes in the blood film of a southern stingray (*Hypanus americanus*), Wright–Giemsa stain. (b) Normal erythrocytes in the blood film of a nurse shark (*Ginglymostoma cirratum*), Wright–Giemsa stain. (c) Normal erythrocytes in the blood film of a white-blotched river stingray (*Potamotrygon leopoldi*), Wright–Giemsa stain.

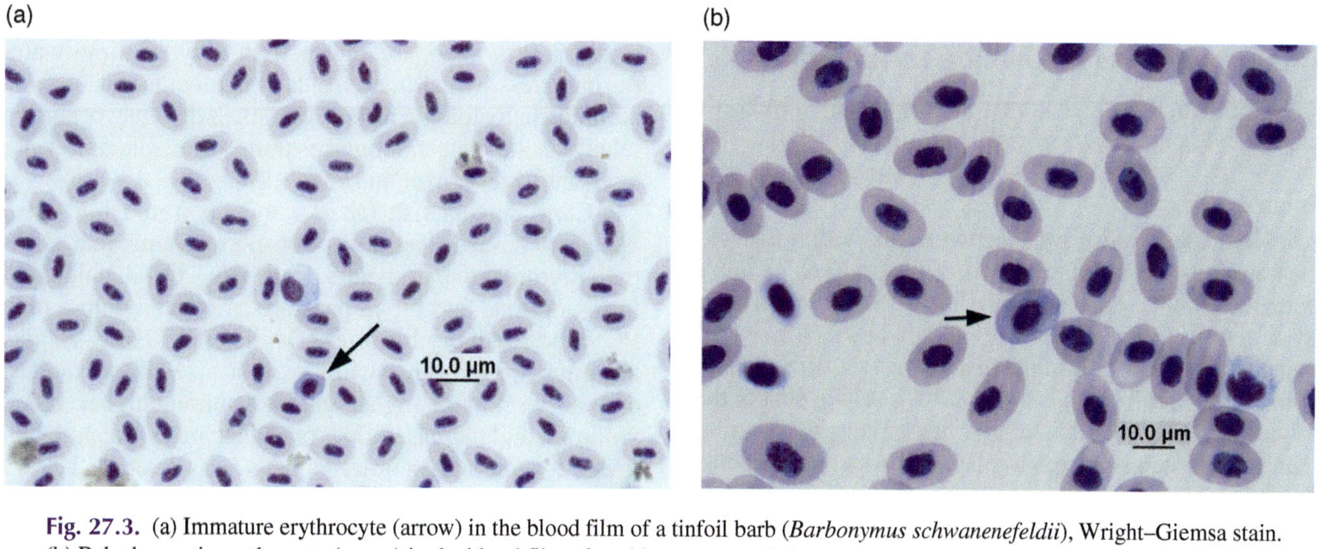

Fig. 27.3. (a) Immature erythrocyte (arrow) in the blood film of a tinfoil barb (*Barbonymus schwanenefeldii*), Wright–Giemsa stain. (b) Polychromatic erythrocyte (arrow) in the blood film of a white sturgeon (*Acipenser transmontanus*), Wright–Giemsa stain.

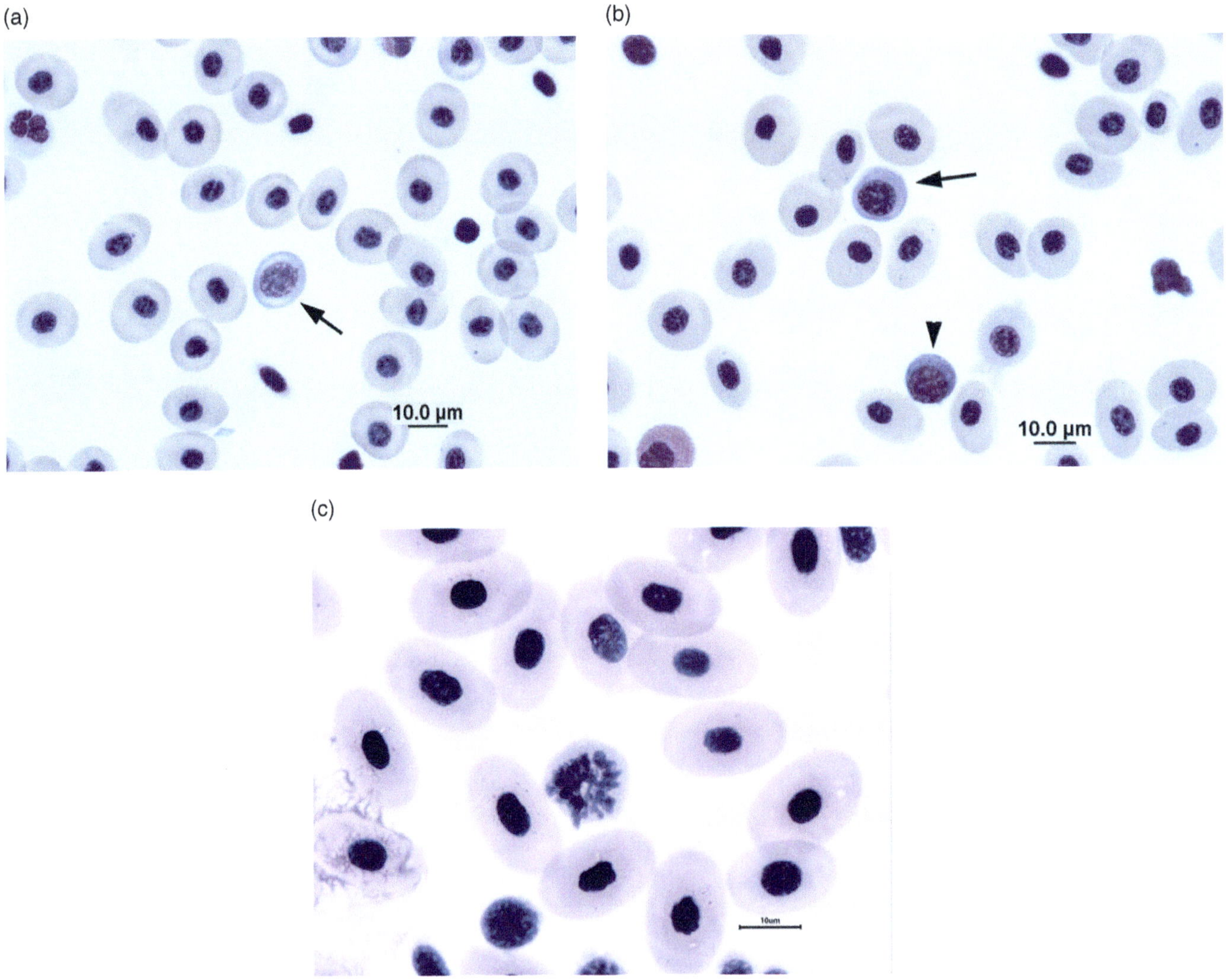

Fig. 27.4. (a) Polychromatic erythrocyte (arrow) in the blood film of a blacktip reef shark (*Carcharhinus melanopterus*), Wright–Giemsa stain. (b) Immature erythrocytes – early polychromatic rubricyte (arrowhead) and late polychromatic rubricyte (arrow) in the blood film of a blacktip reef shark (*Carcharhinus melanopterus*), Wright–Giemsa stain. (c) A mitotic figure likely associated with the erythrocyte cell line in the blood film of a southern stingray (*Hypanus americanus*), Wright–Giemsa stain.

Factors Affecting the Piscine Erythrogram

A summary of factors that reportedly affect the erythrocyte parameters of fish is presented in Table 27.1.

Species

Hematocrit values vary between and within fish species and can be affected by many factors. For example, hematocrit values appear to correlate with the normal activity of the fish; less active fish generally have a lower PCV than active, fast swimming fish (Rowley, 1988; Danilo et al., 1992; Hrubec and Smith, 2010). Active sharks that rely on aerobic metabolism have higher hematocrit values than more sedate, anaerobic-tolerant sharks (Mylniczenko et al., 2006). Also, freshwater fish may swallow water during stress, which may result in hemodilution. Another common hematologic response to stress that may occur is a relative hemoconcentration resulting from splenic release of erythrocytes (Groff and Zinkl, 1999).

Cartilaginous fish (sharks and rays) and bony fish appear to have different gas transport systems that affect their erythrocyte parameters. Bony fish exhibit a high cardiac workload and blood pressure associated with a high PCV and small erythrocytes (Danilo et al., 1992). Sharks and rays, on the other hand, exhibit a relatively modest cardiac workload, higher cardiac output, higher blood volumes, and increased flow rates that are associated with lower concentrations of larger cells (Danilo et al., 1992).

Table 27.1. Summary of factors that reportedly affect the erythrocyte parameters of fish.

Parameter	Increased	Decreased
PCV	Stress – splenic contraction	Stress – increased water intake
	Capture stress – RBC swelling[a]	Viral hemorrhagic septicemia (VHS) in trout[k]
	Inappropriate anesthesia - RBC swelling[a]	Trout juvenile < adults[l,r]
	Male > female smooth dogfish[b]	Starvation in traira[i]
	Endothermic > ectothermic sharks[c]	Dietary *Fusarium moniliforme*[m]
	Teleosts > sharks > rays[d,e,q]	Stingray - tourist sites (diet/parasites/crowding)[n]
	Active > Sedentary[a,d,e]	Sea louse infection in trout[o]
	Exposure to herbicide[f]	*Aeromonas* infection in carp[p]
	Dactylogyrid monogenean infestation[g]	Carp hibernation[t]
	Coccidiosis in carp[h]	Trout fed yeast[v]
	Atlantic salmon pre-spawning[s]	
	Small > Large fish in high temps[u]	
Hemoglobin	Endothermic > ectothermic sharks[c]	VHS in trout[k]
	Induced starvation[i]	Trout juvenile < adults[l,r]
	Elasmobranchs vs. teleosts[e]	*Aeromonas* infection in carp[p]
	Small > Large fish in high temps[u]	Carp hibernation[t]
TRBC	Coccidiosis in carp[h]	VHS in trout[k]
	Summer seasons in trout[j]	Dietary *Fusarium moniliforme*[m]
		Sea louse infection in trout[o]
		Aeromonas infection in carp[p]
		Induced starvation[i]
MCV	Induced starvation[i]	VHS in trout[k]
		Trout Juvenile < Adults[l,r]
		Trout fed yeast[v]
MCHC	Induced starvation[i]	VHS in trout[k]
		Trout Juvenile < Adults[l,r]
		Carp hibernation[t]
		Trout fed yeast[v]

[a]Hrubec and Smith, 2010; [b]Anderson et al., 2010; [c]Emery, 1986; [d]Walsh and Luer, 2004; [e]Filho et al., 1992; [f]Modesto and Martinez, 2010; [g] Del Rio-Zaragoza, 2011; [h] Steinhagen et al., 1997; [i]Rios et al., 2005; [j]Morgan et al., 2008; [k]Rehulka, 2003; [l]Hrubec et al., 2001; [m]Lumlertdacha et al., 1995; [n]Semeniuk et al., 2009; [o]Ruane et al., 2000; [p]Harikrishnan et al., 2003; [q]Danilo et al., 1992; [r] McCarthy et al, 1975; [s]Rowley, 1988; [t]Svetina et al., 2002; [u]Groff and Zinkl, 1999; [v]Sanchez-Muiz et al., 1982.

Age and Sex

Age and sex may also influence the PCV (Sano, 1960; Summerfelt, 1967; Lane, 1979; Matsche et al., 2017; Ahmed et al., 2020). For example, the PCV vof male fish of some species is so high that two reference intervals are required for evaluation. In rainbow trout (*Salmo gairdneri*) and hybrid striped bass (*Morone chrysops* × *Morone saxatilis*), the PCV, hemoglobin concentration, MCV, and MCHC are lower in juvenile fish compared to adults (McCarthy et al., 1975; Hrubec et al., 2001).

Season and Environment

Hematocrit and hemoglobin values may also vary during the life cycle of fish. Seasonal variations in these values are associated with changes in water temperature, dissolved oxygen concentration, population densities, photoperiod, and the reproductive status of the individual fish (Haws and Goodnight, 1962; Kamra, 1966; van Vuren and Hattingh, 1978; Burton and Murray, 1979; Munkittrick and Leatherland, 1983; Ram-Bhaskar and Srinivasa-Rao, 1989; Hrubec et al., 1997; Groff and Zinkl, 1999; Ahmed et al., 2020). For example, during prespawning conditions, Atlantic salmon (*Salmo salar*) have high hematocrits. During spawning, the hematocrits are comparatively lower (Rowley, 1988). During hibernation, a significant decrease in the hematocrit and hemoglobin concentration and an increase in the MCHC occur in carp (Svetina et al., 2002).

Water temperature influences the red cell indices by its effect on metabolism and oxygen requirements. Hematocrit and hemoglobin concentrations increase in smaller fish exposed to higher water temperatures compared to larger fish (Smeda and Houston, 1979; Chudzik and Houston, 1983; Groff and Zinkl, 1999).

Erythrocyte Response to Disease

The use of the "classic" hematologic indices typically used to evaluate the health status of animals remains controversial for fish because of the normal physiology of fish, the effect of the various intrinsic and extrinsic variables on the hematologic indices, and lack of well-defined reference values for fish (Lane, 1979; Houston, 1997; Groff and Zinkl, 1999) (Appendix B, Table B.11). For example, mild to moderate hypoxia does not always result in significant increases in the erythrocyte indices in fish, as would be predicted (Groff and Zinkl, 1999). As a result of these factors, general statements concerning the interpretation of the hemogram of fish rather than specific statements are typically made.

In general, fish with a PCV greater than 45% are usually considered to be dehydrated, particularly when increased serum osmolality, sodium, chloride, and total protein are present. A diagnosis of anemia in fish is generally based on a marked reduction of the PCV and hemoglobin concentration. Anemic fish typically have low PCV values (less than 20%); however, normal PCV values for some species of fish, such as the Port Jackson shark (*Heterodontus portusjacksoni*), may be as low as 20% (Campbell, 1988).

Anemia in Fish

Regenerative Anemias

Fish with regenerative anemia often have increased concentration of polychromatic and immature erythrocytes in their blood films (Figures 27.5a and 27.5b). Anemic fish that exhibit little to no polychromasia or immature erythrocytes have nonresponsive anemia. A microcytic normochromic anemia has been associated with environmental stresses, such as increased population densities (Burton and Murray, 1979; Murray and Burton, 1979). A microcytic hypochromic anemia with marked poikilocytosis has been reported in rainbow trout (*S. gairdneri*) fed diets containing yeast, which resulted in oxidative damage to the erythrocytes (Sanchez-Muiz et al., 1982). Oxidative damage to erythrocytes in fish exposed to crude oil can result in anemia as seen in other species, such as birds and mammals (Harr et al., 2018).

Anemias associated with conditions that interfere with splenic removal of senescent red blood cells from peripheral circulation are typified by erythrocytes with pyknotic nuclei, erythroplastids (erythrocytes without nuclei), and red blood cell fragmentation (Ellis, 1984) (Figure 27.6). Other causes of abnormal erythrocyte nuclei (i.e., amitosis, segmentation, and fragmentation) and the formation of erythroplastids may be related to nutritional disorders such as folic acid and vitamin E deficiency, or toxicosis from rancid oils and environmental pollutants (Eiras, 1983; Hibiya, 1985).

Microcytic anemia is often associated with marked hemorrhagic or hemolytic anemias because the regenerating immature erythrocytes make up the majority of the peripheral blood erythrocytes, and immature erythrocytes of fish are smaller than mature erythrocytes (Ferguson, 1989). An increase in the numbers of immature erythrocytes does not necessarily correlate with a regenerative response to an anemia in fish, however. An

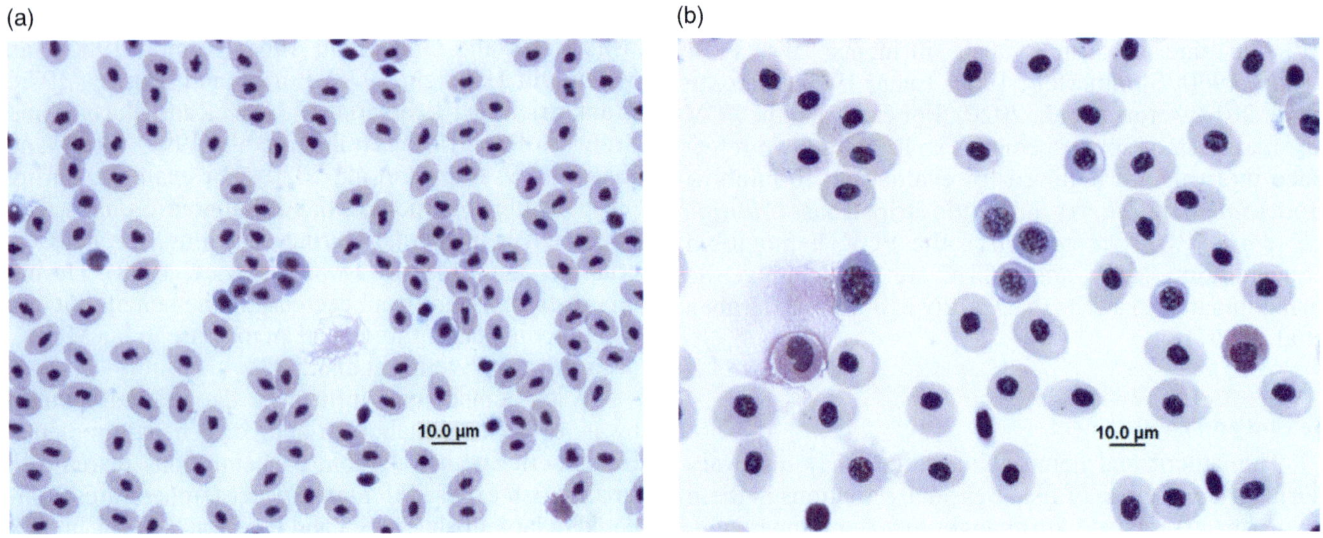

Fig. 27.5. (a) Increased polychromasia in the blood film of a green sunfish (*Lepomis cyanellus*), Wright–Giemsa stain. (b) Increased polychromasia in the blood film of a blacktip reef (*Carcharhinus melanopterus*), Wright–Giemsa stain.

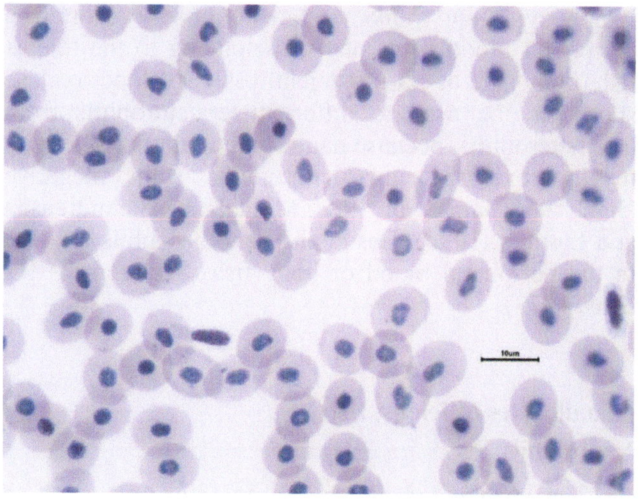

Fig. 27.6. An erythroplastid in the blood film of a striped catfish (*Pangasianodon hypophthalmus*), Wright–Giemsa stain.

increased number of immature erythrocytes has also been proposed as an indicator of nonspecific physiologic responses in fish to a variety of conditions that include anemia, hypoxia, stress, and temperature changes (Houston and Murad, 1991; Murad and Houston, 1992; Houston and Schrapp, 1994; Houston, 1997; Groff and Zinkl, 1999).

Hemorrhagic Anemia

Hemorrhagic anemia results from the loss of blood cells due to bleeding in excess of the rate at which they can be replaced. Increased production of immature erythrocyte stages in the circulating blood may occur in mild cases and represents a regenerative response. When severe blood loss occurs, the resulting net loss of iron may result in iron deficiency anemia. Hemorrhagic anemias of fish are frequently associated with trauma, cutaneous ulcerations, blood-sucking or burrowing parasites, nutritional deficiency, and septicemia (bacterial or viral).

Blood-sucking parasites that can cause hemorrhagic anemia in fish include leeches and lampreys. Fish infested with copepods, specifically *Lernaea cyprinacea*, have been reported with normocytic-normochromic anemia (Corrêa et al., 2016). Nutritional deficiencies in vitamin K, B vitamins (thiamin, riboflavin, pyridoxine, pantothenic acid, and niacin), inositol, and choline can cause coagulation defects that may result in hemorrhagic anemia (Groff and Zinkl, 1999). Bacterial infections associated with gram-negative bacteria, such as *Aeromonas* spp. and *Pseudomonas* spp., are common causes of septicemia and hemorrhagic anemia in freshwater fish (Groff and Zinkl, 1999). Enteric red mouth disease (yersiniosis) of marine fish results in a hemorrhagic septicemia with a hemogram characterized by a leukocytosis, low PCV, and reticulocytosis (Stokes and Firkin, 1971). Viral diseases causing hemorrhagic anemia in fish include viral hemorrhagic septicemia of rainbow trout, spring viremia of carp, and channel catfish virus disease.

Hemolytic Anemia

Hemolytic anemia of fish may be associated with toxins (bacterial or environmental), viral infections (i.e., erythrocytic necrosis virus), certain nutritional deficiencies, and hemoparasites (hematozoan parasites, such as trypanosomes, and hemogregarines) (Ferguson, 1989; Noga, 1996). The most common causes of hemolytic anemia are infectious and are associated with bacteria that produce hemolysins (*Vibrio anguillarum*) and protozoa (Roberts and Rodger, 2012). The presence of erythrophagocytosis in the peripheral blood is indicative of a hemolytic anemia (Campbell and Grant, 2010).

Toxins can affect the erythrocyte parameters in fish (Iwama et al., 1986). For example, nitrite poisoning (brown blood disease, new tank syndrome) of fish can result in a severe cyanosis and hemolytic anemia. Nitrite is readily absorbed from the gills and enters the blood, where it oxidizes hemoglobin to methemoglobin, gradually turning the blood from a red to a brown color. Methemoglobin is not able to bind oxygen because the iron component of the hemoglobin has been oxidized from the ferrous to the ferric state. Cyanosis occurs because of the reduced oxygen carrying capacity of the blood, and hemolytic anemia occurs when the damaged erythrocytes are removed from circulation, usually by macrophages in the spleen or liver.

Viral erythrocytic necrosis is a condition caused by an iridovirus that results in hemolytic anemia in marine fish. Blood films from affected fish may demonstrate basophilic inclusion bodies in the cytoplasm of erythrocytes (Smail and Egglestone, 1980). Hemolytic anemia develops as splenic macrophages remove the affected erythrocytes from circulation (Ellis, 1984).

Nonregenerative Anemia

Nonregenerative anemia resulting from red cell hypoplasia is caused by the failure of the hemopoietic tissue to produce adequate numbers of erythrocytes. Causes of nonregenerative anemia include nutritional deficiencies, toxins, and renal or splenic disease with

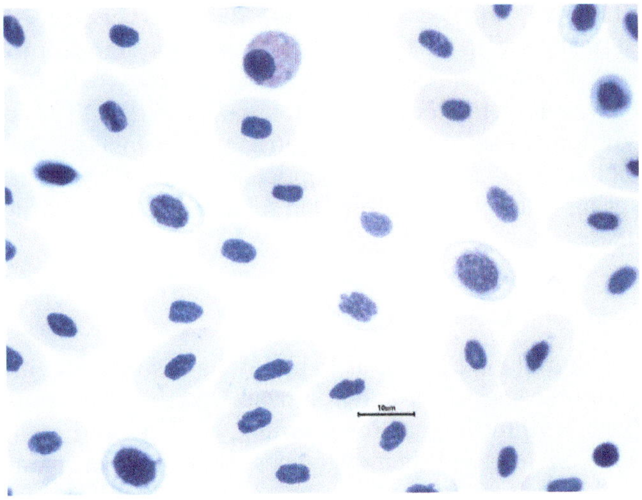

Fig. 27.7. Hypochromatic erythrocytes in the blood film of a green moray eel (*Gymnothorax funebris*), Wright–Giemsa stain.

either displacement of or destruction of erythropoietic tissues. Several anemias associated with nutritional deficiencies have been produced experimentally in fish. For example, folic acid deficiencies result in normochromic macrocytic anemias, and vitamin B_{12} deficiencies create hypochromic anemias (Figure 27.7) (Ferguson, 1989). Folate deficiency has also been suggested as a cause of a chronic hemolytic anemia that occurs in channel catfish (*Ictalurus punctatus*) (Plumb et al., 1991). Deficiencies of vitamin C, iron, or copper can cause a microcytic hypochromic anemia in fish (Groff and Zinkl, 1999). Toxicities that result in nonregenerative anemia in fish include ammonia and heavy metals such as lead, copper, and cadmium (Jensen et al., 1987; Jensen, 1990; Fänge, 1992; Noga, 1996).

Fish Leukocytes

There is a wide variation in the appearance of leukocytes, especially the granulocytes, among the various fish species. This has led to controversy and confusion when classifying piscine leukocytes and attempting to apply the nomenclature based on descriptions of leukocytes found in mammalian blood films (Galagarza et al., 2017). Evaluation of the cellular ultrastructure, differential cytochemical staining, immunofluorescence, and function testing of fish leukocytes have helped alleviate some of this controversy in some species (Ellis, 1977; Rowley, 1988; Fujimaki and Isoda, 1990; Houston, 1990; Zinkl et al., 1991). Reviews of the blood cells of fish are available in the literature (Yokote, 1982; Rowley, 1988; Walsh and Luer, 2004).

Cytochemical studies of piscine leukocytes appear to support the use of mammalian leukocyte terminology to classify them. In general, neutrophils or heterophils, lymphocytes, and monocytes are commonly reported in peripheral blood films of fish belonging to the teleost fish (bony fish, or class Osteichthyes). Myeloperoxidase stain may be used to differentiate neutrophils from true heterophils, because neutrophils stain positive with myeloperoxidase and heterophils stain negative (Jain, 1986; Jain et al., 1988; Montali, 1988; Andreasen and Latimer, 1990). Eosinophils and basophils are rare in the peripheral blood of bony fish (Saunders, 1966; Ellis, 1977).

Granulocytes of Teleost Fish

Neutrophils

The term *neutrophil* has been frequently used to describe the predominant granulocyte of teleost fish, even if the granules in the cells do not stain neutral, because overall the cells resemble mammalian neutrophils when stained with Romanowsky stains. Ultrastructural, cytochemical, and functional studies have demonstrated that the neutrophils of bony fish resemble mammalian neutrophils, although interspecies differences do exist (Ellis, 1975; Ferguson, 1975; Roberts and Ellis, 2012). Neutrophils generally make up 6–8% of the blood leukocyte population in teleost fishes. Absolute counts of $3–6 \times 10^3/mm^3$ are often considered normal (Roberts and Ellis, 2012).

The appearance of the neutrophil varies with the species of fish. The neutrophils of bony fish tend to be round to slightly oval cells with eccentric nuclei (Figures 27.8a–27.8c). The nucleus of mature neutrophils tends to be nonsegmented, but can vary in shape from round to oval, indented (metamyelocyte type), elongated (band cell type), and segmented (usually with two to three lobes). The nuclear chromatin is coarsely clumped and stains deeply basophilic in Romanowsky-stained blood films.

The cytoplasm of the mature neutrophil is typically abundant and colorless, grayish, or slightly acidophilic in color, whereas the cytoplasm of immature neutrophils stains gray or blue-gray. Small granules may be present within the cytoplasm. Staining of the cytoplasmic granules is variable and dependent on the species of fish or maturity of the cell. The granules do not stain at all in most fish species, but may stain pale red, blue, or violet in others (Zinkl et al., 1991).

Some species of fish, such as goldfish (*Carassius auratus*) and carp (*Cyprinus carpio*), have granulocytes with distinct, rod-shaped, slightly acidophilic cytoplasmic granules; colorless cytoplasm; and eccentric partially lobed nuclei with Romanowsky stains. These cells are often classified as heterophils rather than neutrophils although the cytochemical properties of these cells are like the neutrophils of other fish. These heterophils are peroxidase and Sudan black B

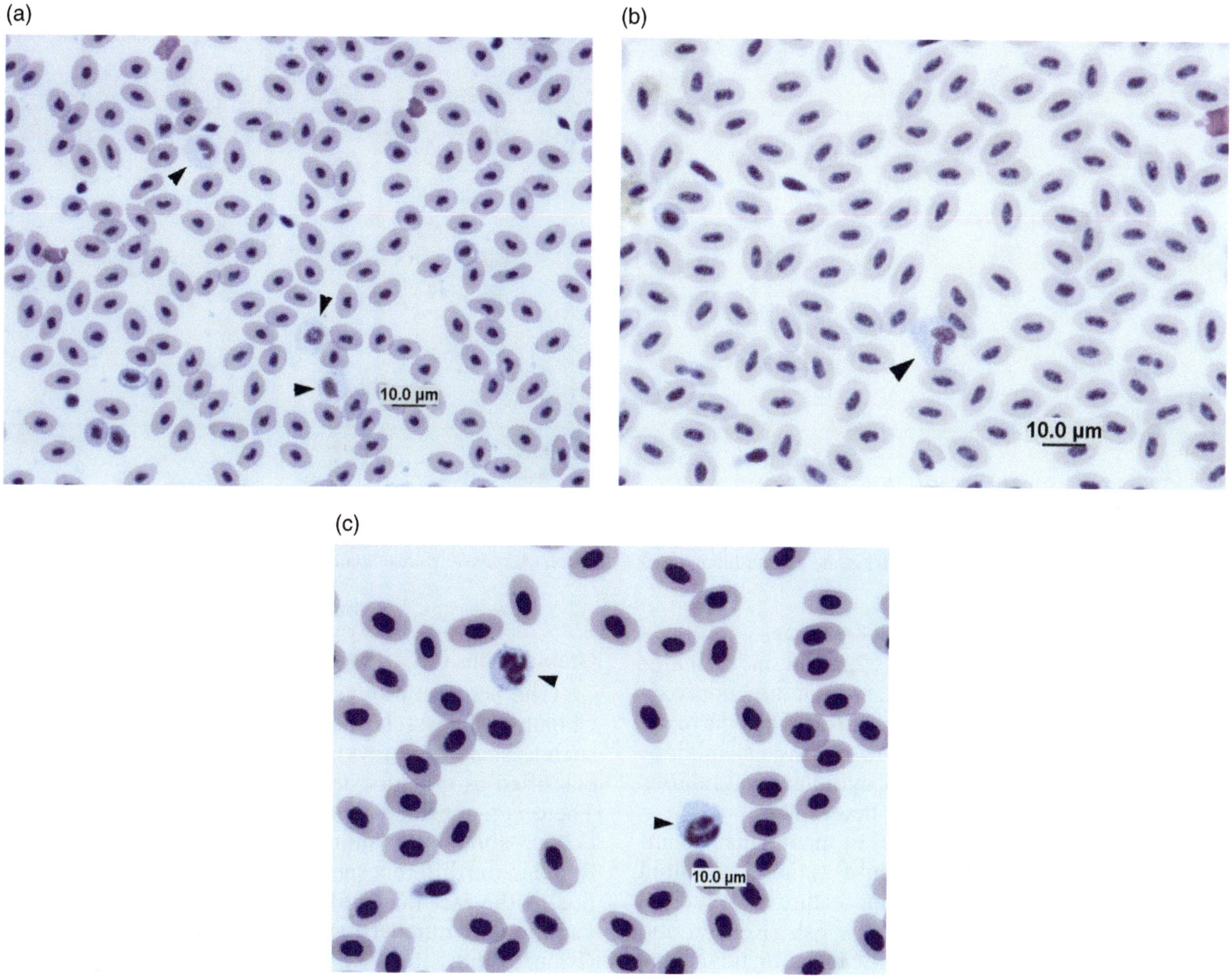

Fig. 27.8. (a) Neutrophils (arrowheads) in the blood film of a green sunfish (*Lepomis cyanellus*), Wright–Giemsa stain. (b) Neutrophil (arrowhead) in the blood film of a tinfoil barb (*Barbonymus schwanenefeldii*), Wright–Giemsa stain. (c) Neutrophils (arrowheads) in the blood film of a white sturgeon (*Acipenser transmontanus*), Wright–Giemsa stain.

positive when the granules are immature. but are peroxidase negative when the granules mature (Rowley, 1988). Neutrophils from channel catfish (*I. punctatus*) and certain species of eels may also contain prominent eosinophilic rod-shaped cytoplasmic granules. The granules of these cells are strongly peroxidase positive (Rowley, 1988). Similar cells have been identified in several other bony fish.

Eosinophils

There is much confusion concerning the presence and nature of eosinophils in fish in the literature. Eosinophils are rarely reported in blood films, and some authors doubt whether they exist at all; however, eosinophils have been reported in goldfish (*C. auratus*), white sturgeon (*Acipenser transmontanus*), and channel catfish (*I. punctatus*) (Catton, 1951; Weinreb, 1963; Williams and Warren, 1976; Ellis, 1977; Hyder et al., 1983; Zinkl et al., 1991). Others have found no eosinophils in channel catfish (*I. punctatus*) (Tavares-Dias and deMoraes, 2007). Some fish species possess blood granulocytes containing eosinophilic granules that morphologically resemble mammalian eosinophils; however, little biochemical work and no functional studies have been performed on these cells.

When present, eosinophils occur in low numbers and tend to be round, intermediate-sized granulocytes that can be differentiated from neutrophils or heterophils by the presence of numerous round- to rod-shaped eosinophilic staining cytoplasmic granules in films stained with Romanowsky stains (Figures 27.9a and 27.9b). The cytoplasm is pale blue, and the nucleus varies from round to lobed with dense chromatin. The granules will stain with acid dyes such as eosin in alkaline medium. The eosinophils of carp

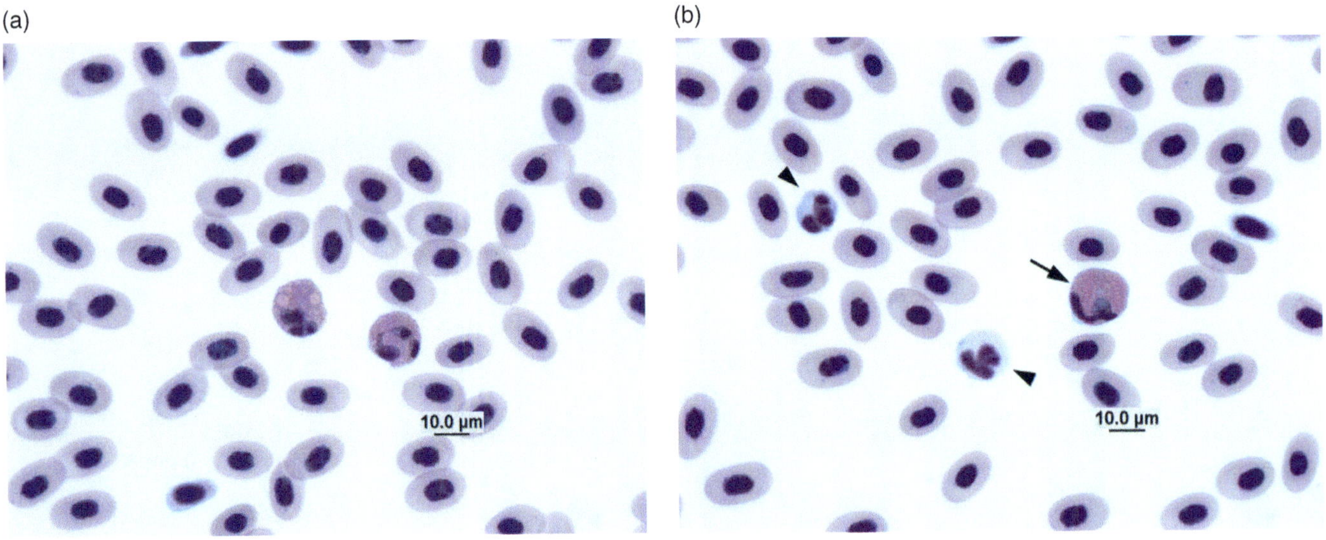

Fig. 27.9. (a) Eosinophils in the blood film of a white sturgeon (*Acipenser transmontanus*), Wright–Giemsa stain. (b) Eosinophil (arrow) and neutrophils (arrowheads) in the blood film of a white sturgeon (*Acipenser transmontanus*), Wright–Giemsa stain.

(*C. carpio*) are approximately 7.5 µm in diameter compared to their heterophils, which are approximately 10 µm in diameter. The eosinophils have an eccentric nucleus that is indented, sausage shaped, or partially lobed and eosinophilic cytoplasmic granules that are larger than those of the heterophils.

Ultrastructurally, the granules of mammalian eosinophils possess an electron-dense axial crystalloid that does not seem to be a constant feature of the eosinophils of other vertebrates, such as fish (Kelenyi and Nemeth, 1969). Fish eosinophils can be distinguished from neutrophils and heterophils based upon cytochemistry and ultrastructural findings, although the absence of crystalloids (used as a fingerprint for mammalian eosinophils) is often the rule with piscine eosinophils (Ellis, 1977).

Basophils

Basophils are rare in peripheral blood films of bony fish and have been reported in only a few fish species (Saunders, 1966; Ellis, 1977). When present, basophils occur in low numbers. Basophils are identified as round cells similar in appearance to mast cells that contain round, basophilic metachromatic cytoplasmic granules that often obscure the cell nucleus (Appendix C, Plate C.20). The nucleus is large, round, is eccentrically located within the cytoplasm, and contains homogeneous nuclear chromatin. The basophils of carp (*C. carpio*) measure between 10 and 20 µm and are larger than the heterophils (Rowley, 1988). Basophils are often affected by the staining process, and may appear as disrupted cells in the blood film, or as cells with partially dissolved cytoplasmic granules.

Granulocytes of Cartilaginous Fish (Sharks and Rays)

The peripheral blood of fish belonging to the class Chondrichthyes (elasmobranchs or cartilaginous fish, such as sharks and rays) contains leukocytes that can be classified as granulocytes, lymphocytes, or monocytes. There is a considerable amount of confusion in the literature about the naming of the various granulocytes found in the different species of elasmobranchs, partially due to the fact that the granulocytes exhibit a marked variation in numbers and types between the species (Fänge, 1968; Ellis, 1977; Mainwaring and Rowley, 1985; Hine and Wain, 1987a, 1987b, 1987c; Filho et al., 1992; Hine, 1992; Arnold, 2005; Carmezim and Marcos, 2020). The function and interrelationships of the granulocytes of cartilaginous fish are not known; however, they do appear to be separate cell types rather than intermediate stages of one cell type (Rowley, 1988). The granulocyte classification based upon ultrastructural and cytochemical studies performed in blood samples taken from the lesser spotted dogfish (*Scyliorhinus canicula*) has been used as a model for other cartilaginous fish, where the granulocytes are classified as G_1 (type I) granulocytes, heterophils, or fine eosinophilic granulocytes (FEGs); G_2 (type II) or neutrophils; or G_3 (type III) granulocytes, eosinophils, or coarse eosinophilic granulocytes (CEGs) (Rowley, 1988; Arnold, 2005). Not all species of cartilaginous fish exhibit all the granulocytes described for the lesser spotted dogfish (*S. canicula*). For example, only G_1 and G_3 granulocytes have been found in thornback rays (*Raja clavata*) and small-eyed rays (*Raja microcellata*) (Rowley, 1988).

An attempt to standardize and simplify the nomenclature involving elasmobranch granulocytes has also been offered using avian rather than mammalian terminology (Walsh and Luer, 2004). This system allows the granulocytes of elasmobranch fish to be classified as heterophils, eosinophils, and basophils using the descriptive criteria for those cells in avian hematology. This scheme works well for some species; however, other elasmobranchs exhibit granulocytes that possess neutral staining granules. These neutrophil-like granulocytes typically have an eccentric nonlobed nucleus. It is not known if these cells represent a fourth type of granulocyte or result from an artifact of the staining process (Walsh and Luer, 2004).

The G_1 (type I) granulocytes of elasmobranch fish are often the most common of the granulocytes and resemble avian heterophils (Campbell and Grant, 2010). These cells have colorless cytoplasm, an eccentric, irregular, nonlobed and lobed nucleus (depending on species and/or maturation of the cell), and round to oval eosinophilic cytoplasmic granules (Figures 27.10a–27.10d, 27.11a, 27.12c, and 27.13). This cell has also been called an FEG with nuclei described as nonsegmented or segmented (Arnold, 2005). The G_2 (type II) granulocytes resemble mammalian neutrophils and have a nonlobed or lobed nucleus and a colorless cytoplasm that lacks distinct granules (Campbell and Grant, 2010) (Figures 27.11a, 27.11b, and 27.13). The G_3 (type III) granulocytes resemble avian eosinophils and are characterized by a nonlobed or lobed nucleus (depending on the species and/or maturation of the cell), pale blue

(a) (b) (c) (d)

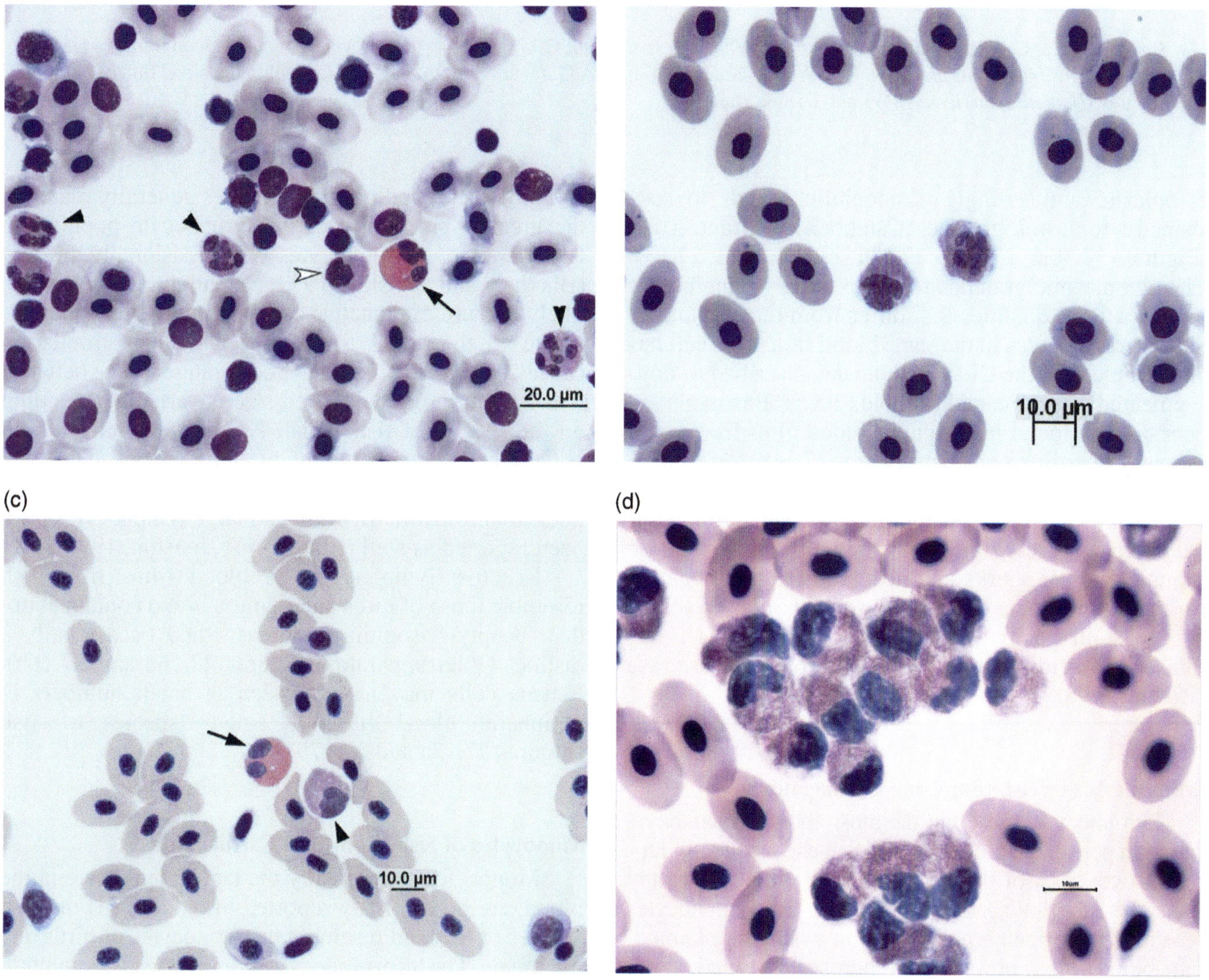

Fig. 27.10. (a) Segmented G_1 (heterophils/FEGs) granulocytes (solid arrowheads), a nonsegmented G_1 granulocyte (open arrowhead), and a segmented G_3 (eosinophil/CEG) granulocyte (arrow) in the blood film of a whitespotted bamboo shark (*Chiloscyllium plagiosum*), Wright–Giemsa stain. (b) G_1 (heterophils/FEGs) granulocytes in the blood film of a blacktip reef shark (*Carcharhinus melanopterus*), Wright–Giemsa stain. (c) A G_1 (heterophil/FEG) granulocyte (arrowhead) and a G_3 (eosinophil/CEG) granulocyte (arrow) in the blood film of a southern stingray (*Hypanus americanus*), Wright–Giemsa stain. (d) Clumping of G_1 (heterophils/FEGs) granulocytes as an artifact of sample preparation in the blood film of a whitespotted bamboo shark (*Chiloscyllium plagiosum*), Wright–Giemsa stain.

(a) (b)

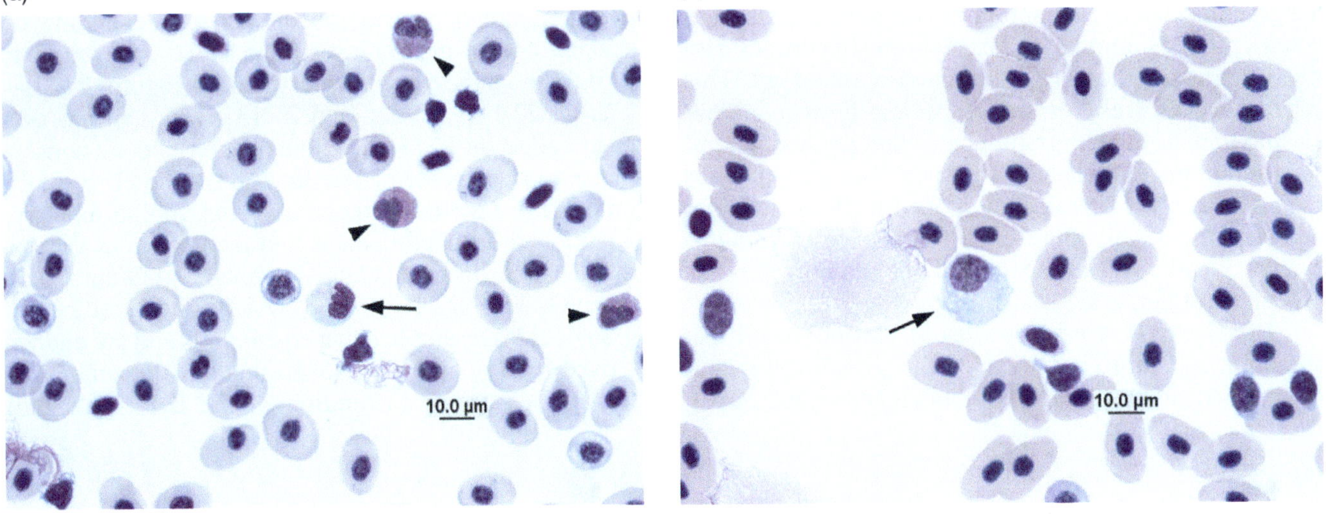

Fig. 27.11. (a) G_2 (neutrophil) granulocyte (arrow) and G_1 (heterophil/FEG) granulocytes (arrowheads) in the blood film of a blacktip reef shark (*Carcharhinus melanopterus*), Wright–Giemsa stain. (b) A G_2 (neutrophil) granulocyte (arrow) in the blood film of a southern stingray (*Hypanus americanus*), Wright–Giemsa stain.

cytoplasm, and strongly eosinophilic round- to rod-shaped cytoplasmic granules (Campbell and Grant, 2010) (Figures 27.10a, 27.10c, 27.12a–27.12c, and 27.13). The cytoplasmic granules found in the G_3 granulocytes have tinctorial qualities that differ from those found in the G_1 granulocytes in the same blood film. This cell has also been called the CEG, with nuclei described as non-segmented or segmented (Arnold, 2005). Basophils are occasionally found in peripheral blood films from some species of cartilaginous fish (Figure 27.14).

The eosinophilic granulocytes (G_1 and G_3) of the elasmobranchs share few morphologic and cytochemical characteristics with mammalian eosinophils. These granulocytes of sharks and rays tend to stain negative for peroxidase, beta glucuronidase, and Sudan black B, but do stain positive for acid phosphatase, aryl sulfatase, and acid naphthyl AS-D chloroacetate esterase (Rowley, 1988).

Lymphocytes of Fish (Bony and Cartilaginous)

Lymphocytes are often the most abundant leukocyte found in peripheral blood films of fish and frequently represent over 50% of the leukocyte differential in healthy fish. The morphology and function of fish lymphocytes resemble their counterparts found in avian and mammalian blood films; however, the number of lymphocytes present in blood is greater in fish than in mammals (Blaxhall and Daisley, 1973) (Figures 27.15a–27.15c). Piscine lymphocytes tend to be round, but may mold around adjacent cells in the blood film. The cytoplasm may exhibit azurophilic cytoplasmic granules or pseudopodia in some cases (Houston, 1990).

Small and medium lymphocytes generally make up the greatest proportion of the lymphocyte population; however, large lymphocytes are occasionally present (Blaxhall and Daisley, 1973). Small lymphocytes are likely to represent inactive undifferentiated cells that circulate in the small form until antigenic stimulation causes them to change. These cells range in size between 4 and 8 µm in diameter; cell size is variable depending on the species of fish. Small lymphocytes have a high N:C ratio, a scant amount of homogenous pale blue cytoplasm, and coarsely clumped, deeply basophilic nuclear chromatin. Medium and large lymphocytes have been reported as well (Ellis, 1977; Houston, 1990).

Reactive lymphocytes in blood films from fish resemble those of birds and mammals and contain abundant deeply basophilic cytoplasm and occasionally a distinct Golgi apparatus (Figures 27.16a and 27.16b). Plasma cells may also be seen in small numbers in peripheral blood films of many species of fish (Figures 27.17a and 27.17b).

Monocytes of Fish (Bony and Cartilaginous)

Monocytes are typically the largest leukocyte in the blood, are occasionally reported in blood films of most species of fish and resemble the monocytes of birds and mammals. The term *monocyte/macrophage* is frequently used to classify piscine monocytes, because cells resembling transformational forms between monocytes and macrophages are often found in peripheral blood films. However, the term *monocyte* is reserved for those cells found in peripheral blood, and *macrophage* for those cells found elsewhere. Monocytes in the blood are

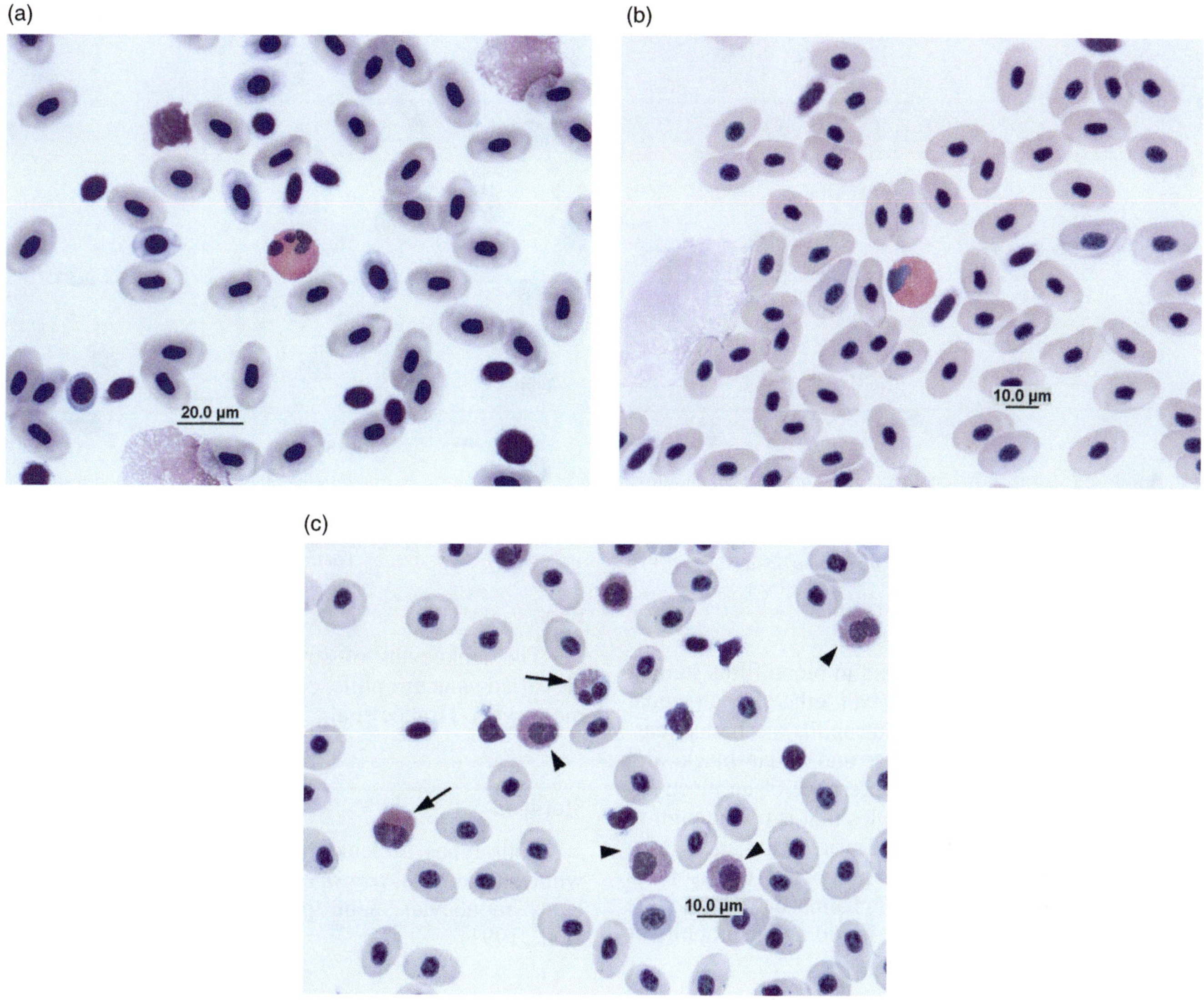

Fig. 27.12. (a) A G_3 (eosinophil/CEG) granulocyte in the blood film of a whitespotted bamboo shark (*Chiloscyllium plagiosum*), Wright–Giemsa stain. (b) A G_3 granulocyte (eosinophil/CEG) in the blood film of a southern stingray (*Hypanus americanus*), Wright–Giemsa stain. (c) A G_3 (eosinophil/CEG) granulocyte (arrow) and G_1 (heterophil/FEG) granulocytes (arrowheads) in the blood film of a blacktip reef shark (*Carcharhinus melanopterus*), Wright–Giemsa stain.

recruited to the sites of inflammation by kinetic activity to become macrophages in the tissues that are capable of giant cell formation, as observed in such conditions as foreign body reactions (Belo et al., 2005).

Fish monocytes are large, mononuclear leukocytes with abundant agranular gray to blue-gray cytoplasm in films stained with Romanowsky stains (Figures 27.17a and 27.17c–27.17f). The cytoplasmic margins may be indistinct or ragged owing to the presence of pseudopodia, and the cytoplasm may contain vacuoles. The nucleus varies in shape from kidney shaped to partially lobed and generally occupies less than 50% of the cytoplasmic volume. The nuclear chromatin of monocytes is generally more granular and less clumped when compared to the nuclear chromatin of the lymphocyte. Ultrastructural studies indicate that monocytes of all species of fish are similar to those of other vertebrates. Fish monocytes can be differentiated from immature granulocytes and lymphocytes by the positive nonspecific esterase reaction in monocytes (Tavares-Dias and deMoraes, 2007).

Leukocytes of Commonly Studied Bony Fish

Channel Catfish

Ultrastructural and cytochemical studies have identified the presence of heterophils, basophils, lymphocytes, and monocytes in the peripheral blood of channel catfish (*I. punctatus*) (Cannon et al., 1980; Ellsaesser et al., 1985; Rowley, 1988; Zinkl et al., 1991; Hanson and Ainsworth, 2000). These studies support the

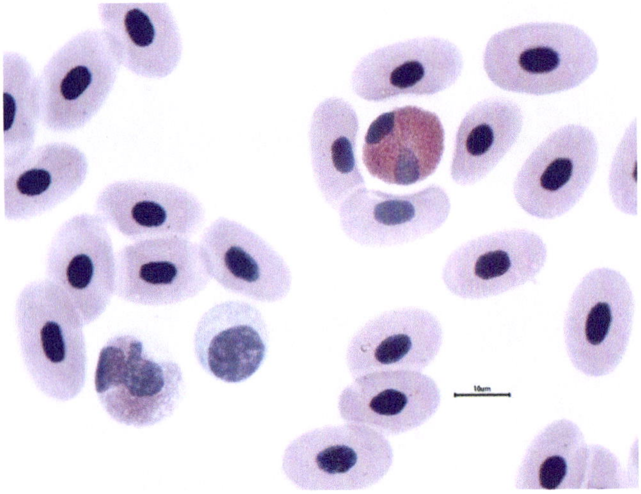

Fig. 27.13. A G_3 (eosinophil/CEG) granulocyte (cell on top); G_2 (neutrophil) granulocyte (cell left of center); and G_1 (heterophil/FEG) granulocyte (cell on bottom left) in the blood film from a southern stingray (*Hypanus americanus*), Wright–Giemsa stain.

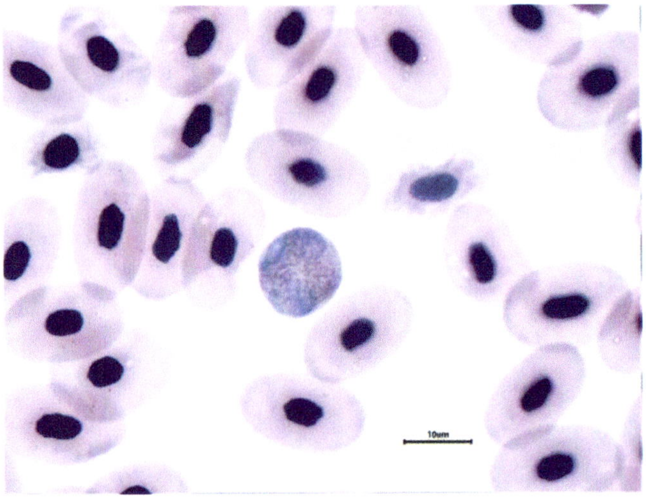

Fig. 27.14. A basophil in the blood film of a southern stingray (*Hypanus americanus*), Wright–Giemsa stain.

classification of these cells found in blood films stained with Romanowsky stains. However, other cytochemical studies have shown that the neutrophils of channel catfish stain positive for peroxidase and Sudan black, and their ultrastructure reveals the presence of an electron-dense structure inside the granules that is not enough to classify the cells as heterophils (Tavares-Dias and deMoraes, 2007). In other studies, no monocytes or basophils were found in the blood films of channel catfish (Grizzle and Rogers, 1985). Still others found no eosinophils or basophils (Lewis et al., 1979).

Goldfish, Koi, and Carp

Based upon electron microscopy and cytochemical analysis, the leukocytes found in the peripheral blood of goldfish (*C. auratus*) can be classified as heterophils or neutrophils, lymphocytes, monocytes, eosinophils, and rarely basophils (Weinreb, 1963; Ellis, 1977; Houston, 1990; Zinkl et al., 1991). An atypical, segmented granulocyte that does not appear to be analogous to any of the leukocytes found in mammals or birds has also been identified in blood films from goldfish (*C. auratus*) (Zinkl et al., 1991).

The leukocytes found in the peripheral blood of koi (*C. carpio*) are classified as neutrophils, eosinophils, basophils, lymphocytes, and monocytes (Tripathi et al., 2004). Lymphocytes predominate, and eosinophils are rare.

Salmonids (Trout and Salmon)

Salmonids appear to have lymphocytes, neutrophils, and monocytes present in the peripheral blood (McCarthy et al., 1975).

Bass

The leukocytes of striped bass (*M. saxatilis*) are classified as neutrophils, eosinophils, lymphocytes, and monocytes (Hrubec et al., 2001).

Sturgeon

Four types of leukocytes have been described in white sturgeon (*A. transmontanus*) and include lymphocytes, monocytes, neutrophils, and eosinophils (Zinkl et al., 1991).

Tilapia

The leukocytes of tilapia (*Oreochromis* spp.) are classified as neutrophils, eosinophils, lymphocytes, and monocytes (Hrubec and Smith, 2000).

Red Pacu

Six types of cells are classified as leukocytes in blood films from red pacu (*Colossoma brachypomum*) (Tocidlowski et al., 1997). The four common types are classified as heterophils, eosinophils, lymphocytes, and monocytes. Non-staining granulocytes are reported to occur in a frequency similar to that of eosinophils and are considered to be heterophils that failed to stain properly. The sixth cell type is referred to as a "granular-lymphocytoid cell" because it resembles a medium-sized lymphocyte containing one or more dull, fusiform eosinophilic granules. This cell type represents a significant population of the blood leukocytes of red pacu.

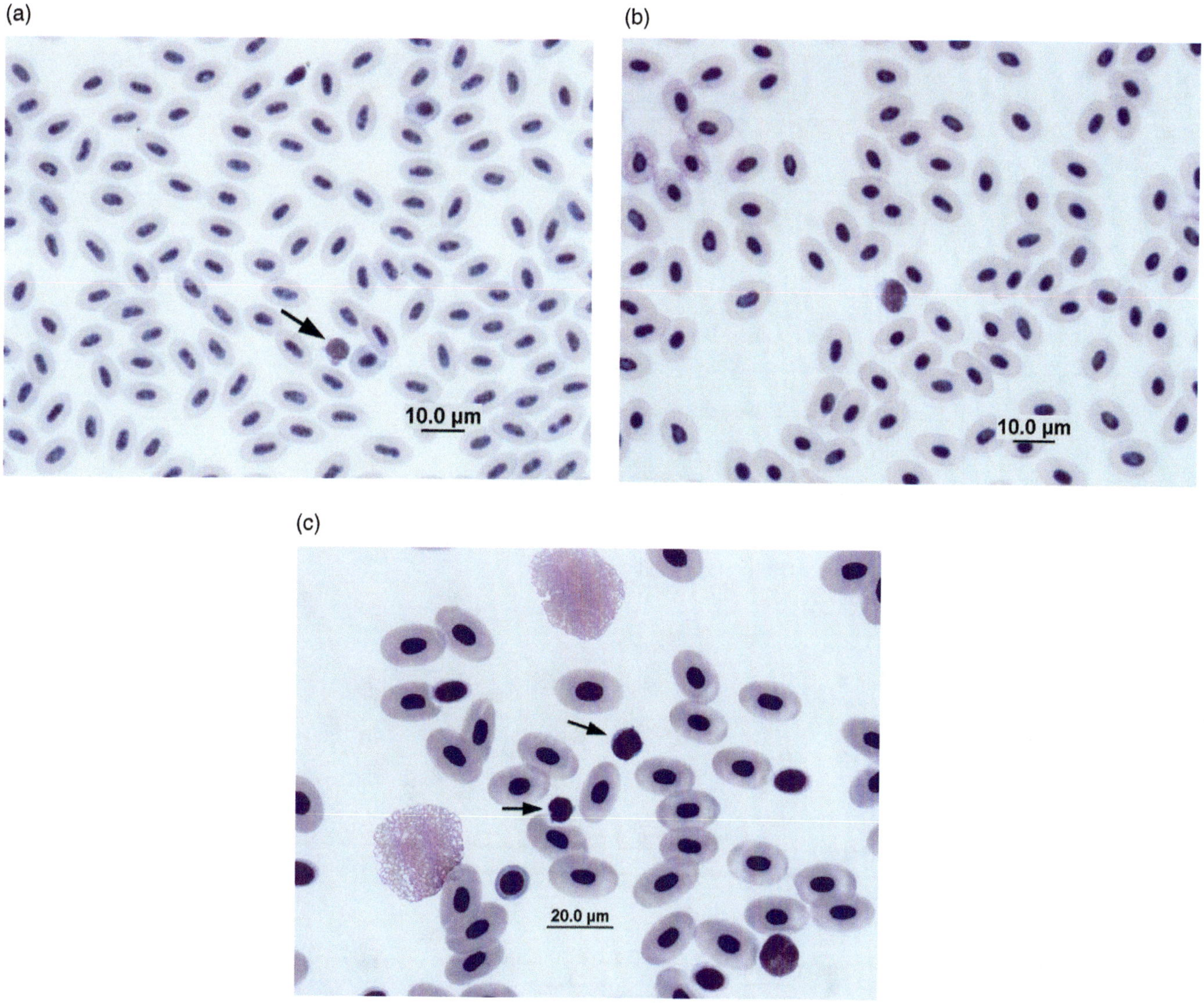

Fig. 27.15. (a) Small lymphocyte (arrow) in the blood film of a tinfoil barb (*Barbonymus schwanenefeldii*), Wright–Giemsa stain. (b) Medium lymphocyte in the blood film of a koi (*Cyprinus carpio*), Wright–Giemsa stain. (c) Small lymphocytes (arrows) in the blood film of a whitespotted bamboo shark (*Chiloscyllium plagiosum*), Wright–Giemsa stain.

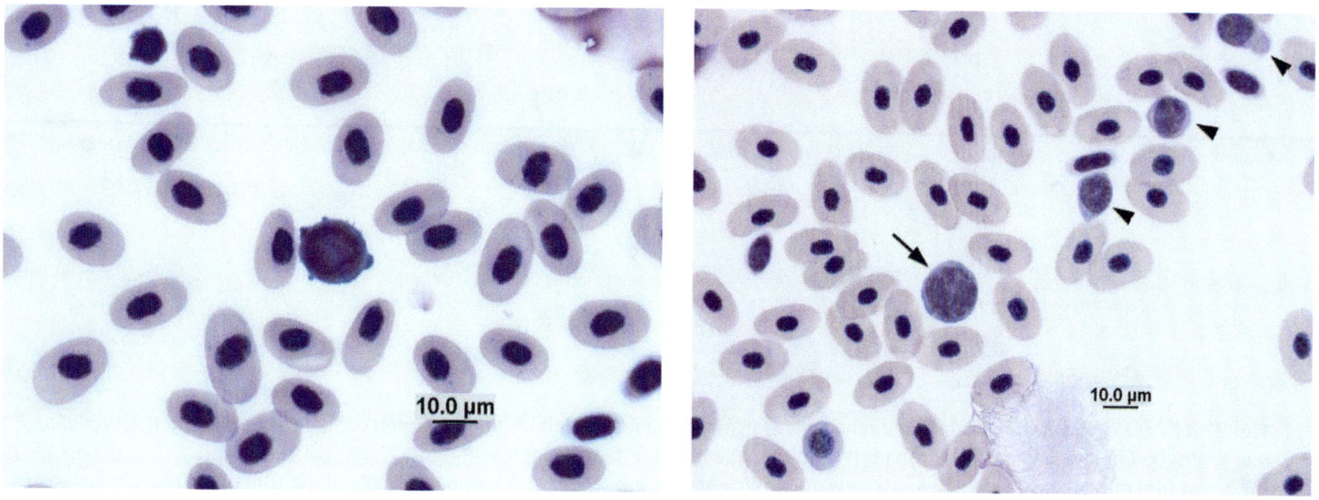

Fig. 27.16. (a) Reactive lymphocyte in the blood film of a white sturgeon (*Acipenser transmontanus*), Wright–Giemsa stain. (b) A large lymphocyte (arrow) and medium lymphocytes (arrowheads) in the blood film of a southern stingray (*Hypanus americanus*), Wright–Giemsa stain.

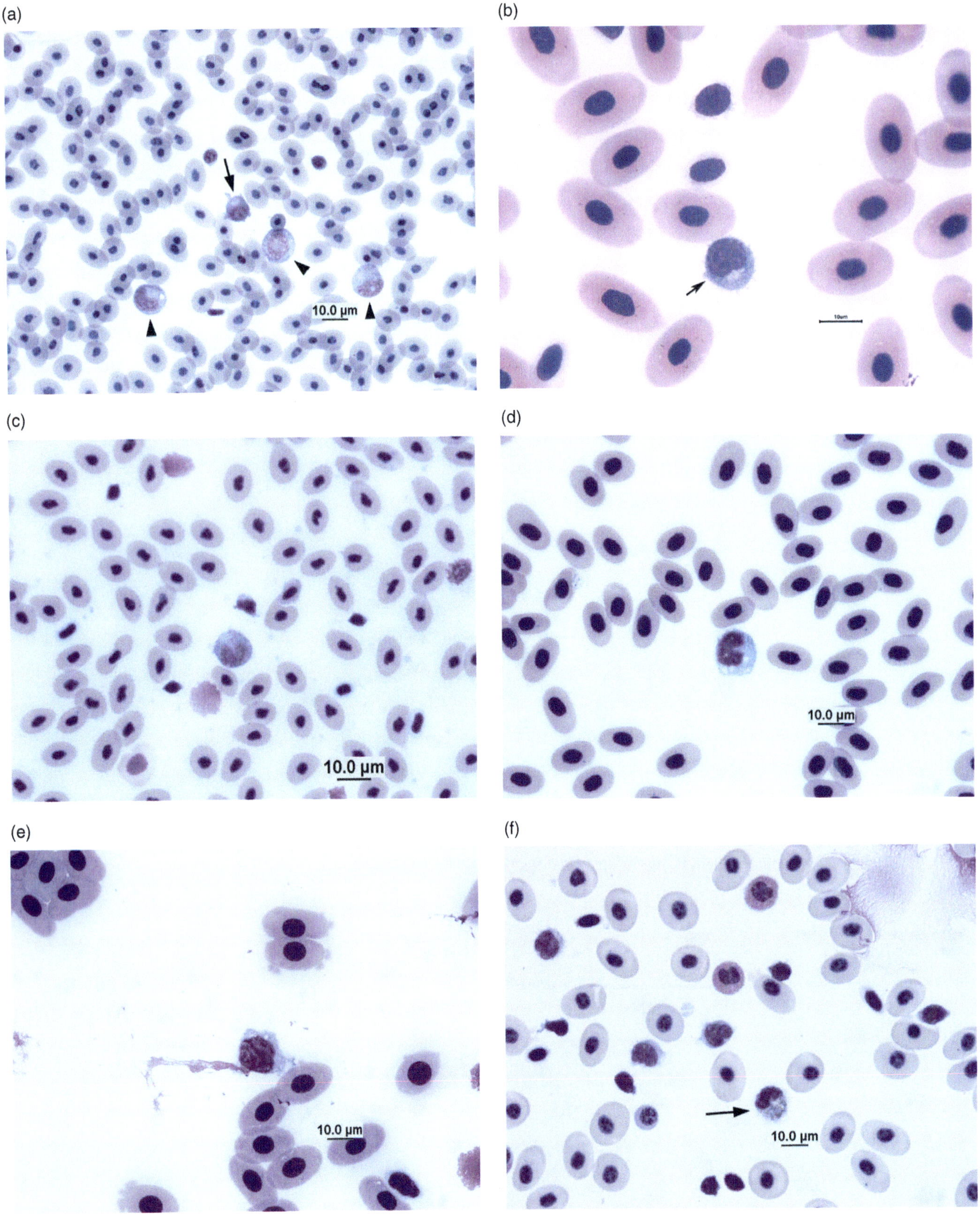

Fig. 27.17. (a) A plasma cell (arrow) and monocytes (arrowheads) in the blood film of a striped catfish (*Pangasianodon hypophthalmus*), Wright–Giemsa stain. (b) A plasma cell (arrow) in the blood film of a southern stingray (*Hypanus americanus*). (c) A monocyte in the blood film of a green sunfish (*Lepomis cyanellus*), Wright–Giemsa stain. (d) A monocyte in the blood film of a white sturgeon (*Acipenser transmontanus*), Wright–Giemsa stain. (e) A monocyte in the blood film of a whitespotted bamboo shark (*Chiloscyllium plagiosum*), Wright–Giemsa stain. (f) A cell (likely a monocyte or melanomacrophage) containing melanin granules (arrow) in the blood film of a blacktip reef shark (*Carcharhinus melanopterus*), Wright–Giemsa stain.

Variations in the Leukogram of Fish

The leukocyte response of fish is affected by stress, inflammatory and infectious diseases, and nutritional disorders as well as other intrinsic and extrinsic factors (Blaxhall and Daisley, 1973). Total leukocyte counts vary with species, physiological age, sex, season, and methods of rearing and nutrition (Grizzle and Rogers, 1985) (Appendix B, Table B.12). Normal physiological factors and various other stressors such as environmental factors and handling can cause leukocyte concentrations to range into or slightly above the upper limits of normal (Ferguson, 1989; Tocidlowski et al., 1997). Normal physiological factors include age, population densities, water quality, and other factors. For example, age-related changes in the total leukocyte and lymphocyte counts of fish are like those described in mammals. Juvenile fish have notably higher total leukocyte counts and lymphocyte concentrations compared to adults (Blaxhall, 1972; McCarthy et al., 1975; Hrubec et al., 2001). High total leukocyte counts and lymphocyte concentrations are also associated with fish kept in high-density production systems where there is constant exposure to high concentrations of bacteria in the water and poor water quality parameters (Hrubec et al., 2001).

Stress factors can cause a response like that of higher vertebrates in which a rapid increase in the release of catecholamines occurs followed by the release of corticosteroids (Mazeaud et al., 1977; Eddy, 1981; Schreck, 1981; Wedemeyer et al., 1990; Barton and Iwama, 1991; van Razij et al., 1996a, 1996b). In general, the effect of stress on the leukogram of fish is manifested as a leukopenia with a lymphopenia and a relative granulocytosis (heterophilia or neutrophilia), because lymphocytes are the predominate leukocyte in the peripheral blood of most fish (Wedemeyer et al., 1983; Wedemeyer et al., 1990; Stoskopf, 1993; Roberts and Ellis, 2001). Hematologic changes associated with stress may persist for several days after the removal of the stressor (Houston, 1990; Wedemeyer et al., 1990).

The leukogram of bony and cartilaginous fish can be used to follow the progress of the fish in the course of disease or response to therapy. For example, an initial increase in granulocyte concentration or decrease in lymphocyte concentration that has returned to a normal concentration indicates a favorable response to therapy and a good prognosis.

Granulocytes and Inflammation

Interpretation of changes in granulocyte concentrations in the peripheral blood of fish can be difficult. Piscine neutrophils and heterophils participate in inflammatory responses; however, it would be inappropriate to view them as homologous to the granulocytes of higher vertebrates because the exact function of fish granulocytes is not known. Fish granulocytes are not always phagocytic, and little is known about their methods of intracellular killing, digestion of phagocytized organisms, and other functions. Until further studies are performed that determine the function and responses of piscine granulocytes to disease, only broad generalizations about changes in the leukocyte counts of fish can be made.

Neutrophils/Heterophils

In general, increases in the concentration of fish neutrophils or heterophils are often associated with inflammatory diseases, especially those associated with infectious agents (Ellsaesser et al., 1985; Brenden and Huizinga, 1986; Groff and Zinkl, 1999). Fish neutrophils migrate to inflammatory sites to kill bacteria by producing a series of reactive oxygen species where the respiratory burst and the peroxidase contained in the neutrophils contribute to microbial killing activity during phagocytosis (Palic et al., 2005). Granulocytosis (neutrophilia) can also occur with inflammation associated with parasitic and viral diseases (Hines and Spira, 1973; Groff and Zinkl, 1999).

Toxic Change

Fish granulocytes exhibit toxic change in association with inflammatory responses. The same criteria used to describe toxic change in mammalian neutrophils and the heterophils of birds and reptiles also apply to the granulocytes of fish. Toxic neutrophils of teleost fish exhibit cytoplasmic basophilia, vacuolation, and the presence of Döhle bodies (Figures 27.18a–27.18c). Döhle bodies are aggregates of endoplasmic reticulum that appear as blue-gray cytoplasmic precipitates. Toxic change signals accelerated the production of the granulocytes that occurs with an inflammatory response.

Inflammatory Response in Elasmobranchs

The granulocytes of cartilaginous fish do appear to participate in inflammatory responses. It is important to note that because the granulocytes make up 20–30% of the total leukocyte population in sharks and rays, the normal granulocyte to lymphocyte (G:L) ratio is typically low (i.e., less than 0.5). An increase in granulocyte concentration is indicative of an inflammatory response. A decrease in the lymphocyte concentration typically results from the conditions that reduce the number of circulating lymphocytes, such as stress responses, for example. In sharks, increases in granulocyte concentrations and decreases in lymphocyte concentrations can be associated with bacterial septicemias. The presence of toxicity in the granulocytes as indicated by increased

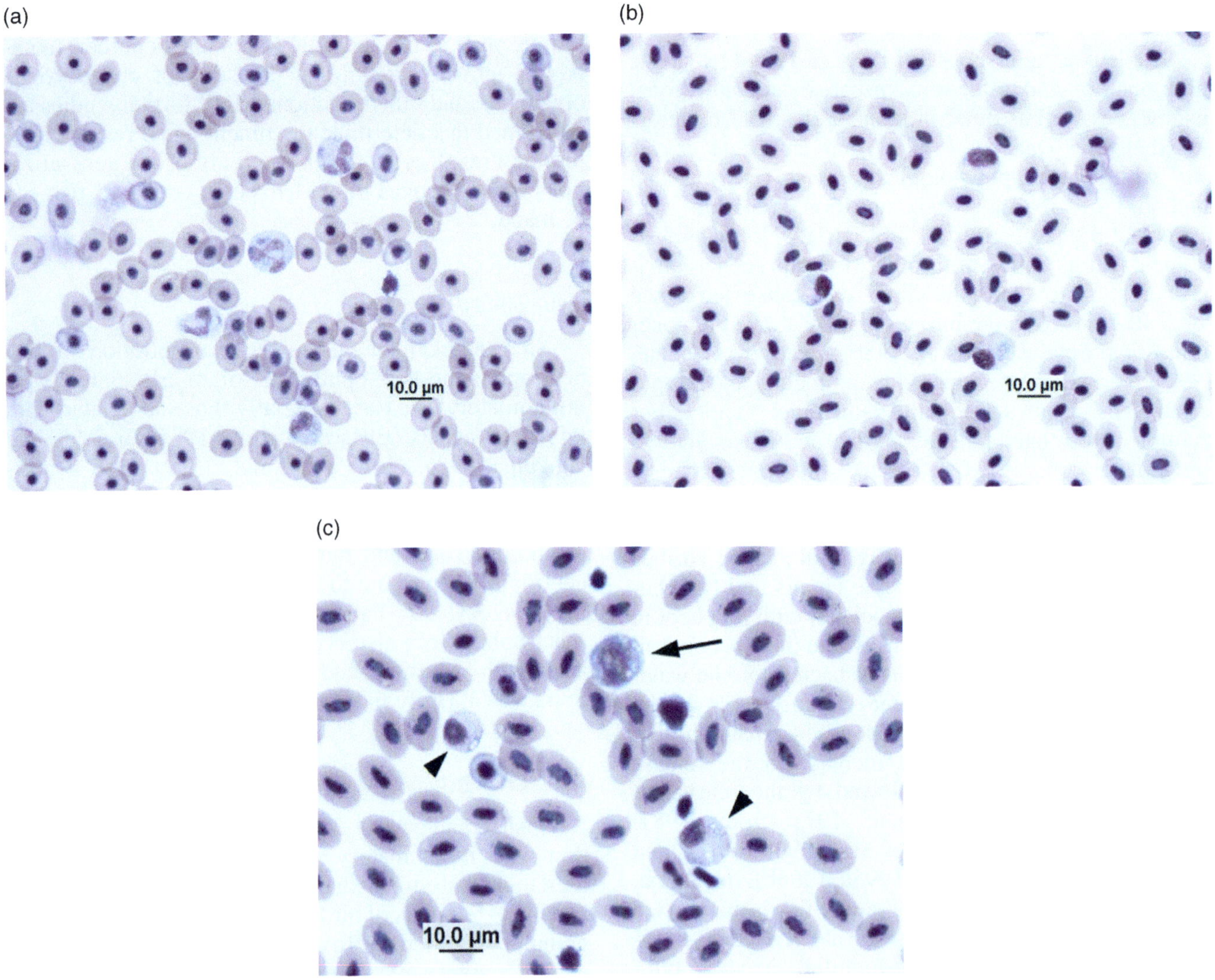

Fig. 27.18. (a) Neutrophils exhibiting toxic change (cytoplasmic basophilia and Döhle bodies) in the blood film of a knifefish (*Chitala chitala*), Wright–Giemsa stain. (b) Neutrophils exhibiting toxic change (cytoplasmic basophilia and Döhle bodies) in the blood film of a koi (*Cyprinus carpio*), Wright–Giemsa stain. (c) Neutrophils (arrowheads) exhibiting toxic change (cytoplasmic basophilia and Döhle bodies) and a reactive monocyte (arrow) in the blood film of a roundtail chub (*Gila robusta*), Wright–Giemsa stain.

cytoplasmic basophilia and vacuolation is indicative of a severe inflammatory leukogram regardless of the cell count (Campbell and Grant, 2010) (Figure 27.19).

Eosinophils

Eosinophils are usually found in low concentrations (i.e., 0–3% of the leukocyte differential) in the peripheral blood of normal fish. Some reports indicate that fish eosinophils participate in inflammatory responses along with neutrophils (heterophils) and macrophages, and appear to have limited phagocytic capability (Rowley, 1988; Roberts and Ellis, 2001). Apparently piscine eosinophils are involved in the control of metazoan parasite infections and participate in immune responses to antigenic stimulation (Stoskopf, 1993). Therefore, an increase in eosinophil concentration in peripheral blood of fish is suggestive of an inflammatory response associated with parasitic infections or antigenic stimulation.

Basophils

The presence of basophils in fishes is controversial. Some studies support the presence of basophils in piscine blood, and others dispute it (Ellis, 1975). It is interesting to note that the presence of the basophil in fish blood has not been associated with any recognized disease process, making the function of the fish basophil unclear even though these cells have cytochemical properties (5-hydroxy-tryptamine or 5HT) like mast cells. It is of interest to note that fish basophils and mast cells

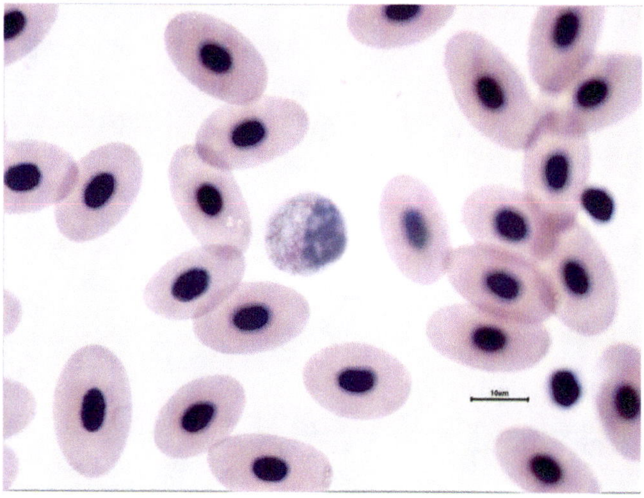

Fig. 27.19. A G_1 granulocyte (heterophil/FEG) exhibiting toxic change (cytoplasmic basophilia and vacuolation) in the blood film of a whitespotted bamboo shark (*Chiloscyllium plagiosum*), Wright–Giemsa stain.

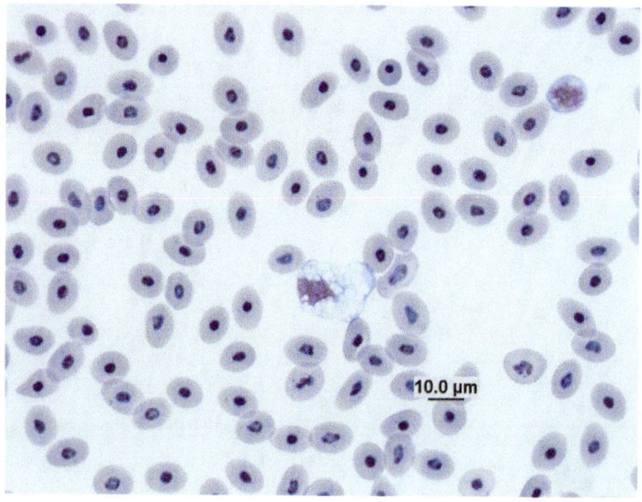

Fig. 27.20. A reactive monocyte resembling a macrophage in the blood film of a striped catfish (*Pangasianodon hypophthalmus*), Wright–Giemsa stain.

lack histamine, which is commonly the main vasoactive component of avian and mammalian mast cells (Roberts and Ellis, 2001).

Lymphocytosis and Lymphopenia

Lymphocytes play a major role in the humoral and cell-mediated immunity of fish (Clem et al., 1991; Evans and Jaso-Friedmann, 1992). Lymphocytosis is suggestive of immunogenic stimulation or perhaps lymphoid leukemia, and lymphopenia is suggestive of immunosuppressive conditions, such as stress or excessive exogenous glucocorticosteroids (McLeay, 1973; Ellsaesser and Clem, 1986). Bacterial septicemias commonly affect fish and can also result in marked leukopenia and lymphopenia (Brenden and Huizinga, 1986). Lymphoid leukemia has been reported in fish and is usually a neoplastic condition indicated by a leukocytosis associated with a lymphocytosis and lymphocytes with features of either degeneration, immaturity, or malignancy (Ferguson and Roberts, 1975; Mulcahy, 1976; Eaton and Kent, 1992).

Monocytes

Monocytes occur in low numbers (i.e., less than 5%) in the leukocyte differential of normal bony and cartilaginous fish. Piscine monocytes are actively phagocytic cells and participate in acute inflammatory responses (Rowley, 1988). Morphologic, cytochemical, and functional studies indicate that teleost monocytes resemble those of mammals. Monocytes and macrophages appear to be the primary phagocytic cells of fish (Figure 27.20) (Ellis, 1977; Blazer, 1991). Fish monocytes can also phagocytize melanosomes when released, suggesting a relationship with melanomacrophages (Figure 27.17f). A monocytosis is suggestive of an inflammatory response in fish, perhaps associated with an infectious agent, although monocyte numbers will also increase following the injections of foreign material (Roberts and Ellis, 2001).

Nutritional Disorders

Nutritional disorders may also affect the leukogram of fish. For example, a leukopenia may be caused by pyridoxine and vitamin C deficiencies, and a leukocytosis has been reported with biotin deficiency in cyprinid fishes (Groff and Zinkl, 1999).

Fish Thrombocytes and Hemostasis

Thrombocytes

Fish thrombocytes are nucleated cells that are smaller than erythrocytes and vary in shape. The cell shape may vary with the stage of maturity or degree of reactivity and can be round, elongate, or spindle shaped. Immature thrombocytes are round in some species of fish, and the oval and elongated forms tend to be nonreactive mature thrombocytes. Spindle-shaped thrombocytes appear to be reactive forms and generally appear as elongated cells with one pole of the cell often drawn out into a point. Because these cells readily participate in the formation of clots, they often appear as clusters of small, densely staining nuclei surrounded by a small amount of cytoplasm (Figures 27.21a–27.21c).

The cytoplasm of the piscine thrombocyte is colorless to faint blue and contains an intensely basophilic condensed nucleus that follows the shape of the cell and contains heavily clumped chromatin. The cytoplasm

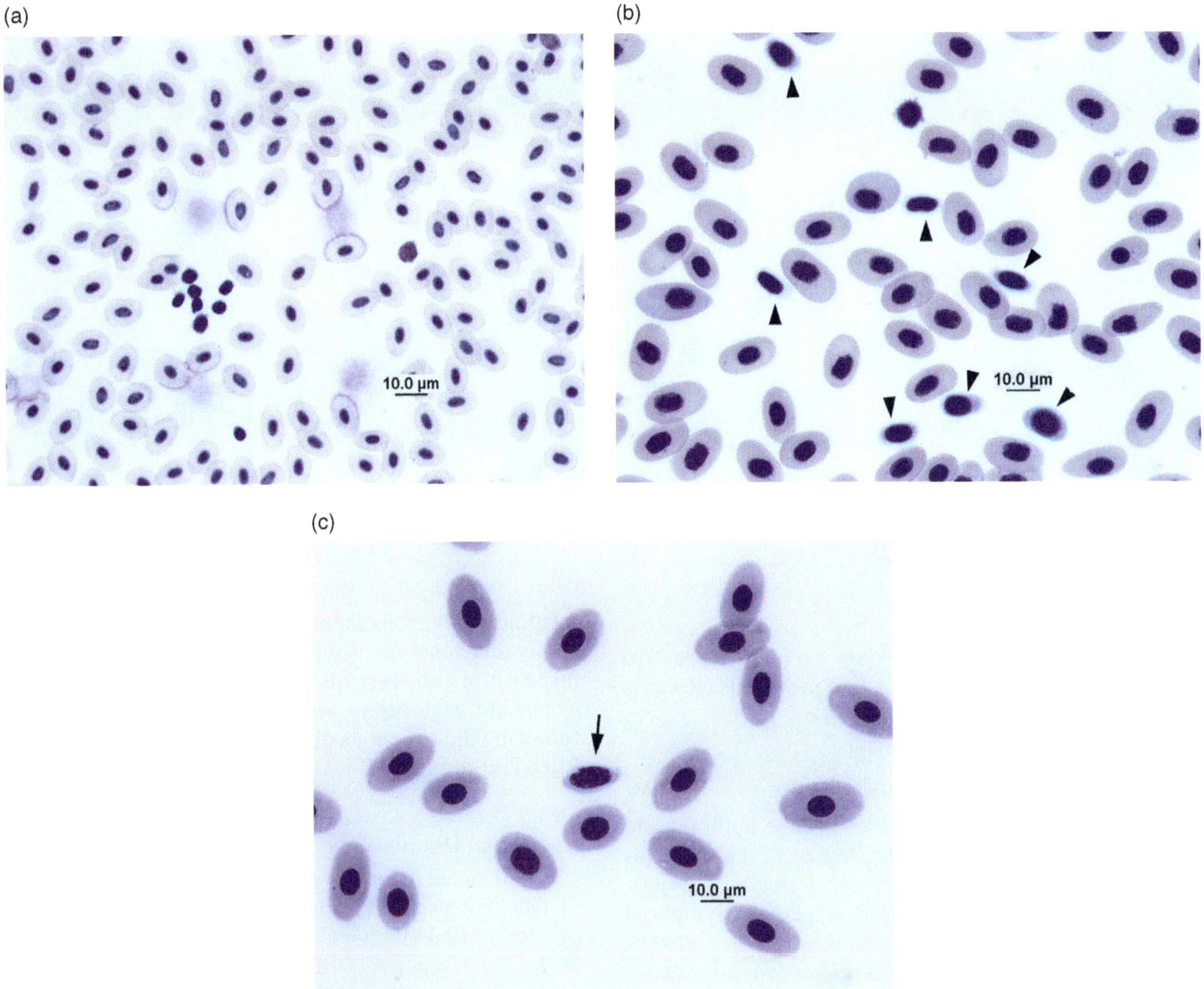

Fig. 27.21. (a) An aggregate of thrombocytes in the blood film of a koi (*Cyprinus carpio*), Wright–Giemsa stain. (b) Thrombocytes (arrowheads) in the blood film of a white sturgeon (*Acipenser transmontanus*), Wright–Giemsa stain. (c) A thrombocyte (arrow) in the blood film of a whitespotted bamboo shark (*Chiloscyllium plagiosum*), Wright–Giemsa stain.

often contains vacuoles or vesicles and a variable number of very small eosinophilic granules. Ultrastructural studies have demonstrated that the cytoplasm of teleost thrombocytes is like that of mammalian platelets (Ferguson, 1975). Cytochemical studies have shown that fish thrombocytes usually stain weakly positive with periodic acid-Schiff (PAS) and positive for acid phosphatase (Zinkl et al., 1991).

Thrombocyte numbers in the peripheral blood of fish range from 60 000 to 70 000/mm^3 (Roberts and Ellis, 2001). Fish thrombocytes can be easily confused with small, mature lymphocytes; however, by comparison, lymphocytes have slightly more abundant, mildly basophilic cytoplasm, and the nucleus of the lymphocyte is usually larger and less condensed (Figures 27.22a and 27.22b). The ratio of thrombocytes to lymphocytes in some teleost fish is estimated to be 1:4 to 1:1 (Roberts and Ellis, 2001).

Hemostasis

Hemostasis in fish is similar to that of mammals, but with some cellular and chemical differences. Thrombocytes instead of platelets are responsible for blood clotting and control of fluid loss from a surface injury in fish.

Fish blood will clot in response to injury; however, the speed and effectiveness is variable. The blood of teleost fish clots much faster compared to sharks and rays. Clot formation in bony fish usually occurs within 5 min,

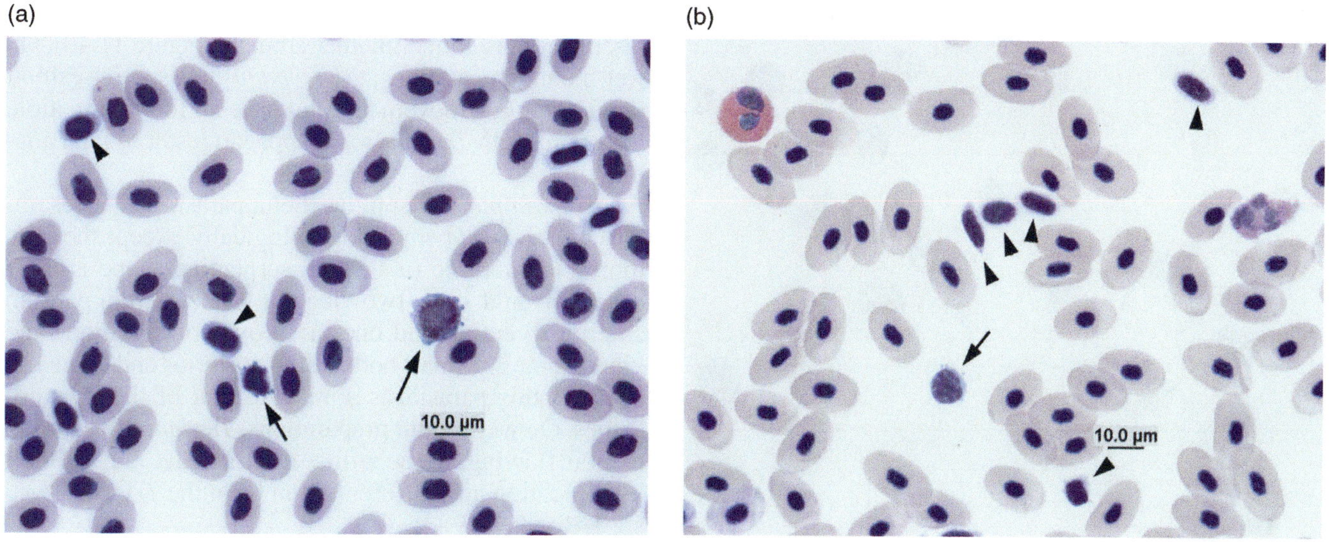

Fig. 27.22. (a) Thrombocytes (arrowheads) are seen with a small and medium lymphocyte (arrows) in the blood film of a white sturgeon (*Acipenser transmontanus*), Wright–Giemsa stain. (b) A lymphocyte (arrow) and thrombocytes (arrowheads) in the blood film of a southern stingray (*Hypanus americanus*), Wright–Giemsa stain.

whereas clotting of blood samples taken from sharks and rays can take 20 min or longer. Fish appear to rely primarily on extrinsic pathways of coagulation, because the addition of skin, high calcium solutions, sea water, or other extrinsic factors enhances clotting (Rowley, 1988).

As with mammalian hemostasis, clot formation in fish occurs with fibrinopeptides that are formed following the cleavage of fibrinogen, which is under the control of thrombin; however, fish fibrinopeptides differ chemically from those produced by mammals. The basic structure of piscine fibrin in fish is the same as in mammals, although the piscine fibrin molecule is much larger than its mammalian counterpart.

The aggregation of fish thrombocytes occurs differently from mammalian platelet aggregation. For example, fish thrombocytes convert arachidonic acid to prostaglandins with little, if any, thromboxane formation, whereas thromboxane is a potent inducer of platelet aggregation in mammals (Rowley, 1988). The control and outcome of thrombocyte aggregation also appears to differ from that in mammals. For example, thrombocyte aggregation in sharks is temperature reversible, a feature that is not seen with mammalian platelet aggregation (Rowley, 1988). Shark thrombocyte aggregation is also independent of thrombin.

Thrombocyte concentration and clotting time appear to be negatively affected by glucocorticoid excess in fish. Excessive levels of glucocorticoid tend to decrease the total thrombocyte count and increase the clotting time (Campbell, 1988). Prolonged clotting times also occur with vitamin K deficiency.

Thrombocytes of other lower vertebrates, such as birds, have demonstrated phagocytic function. Unlike avian thrombocytes, active phagocytosis does not likely occur with teleost thrombocytes (Roberts and Ellis, 2001).

Fish Blood Parasites

Intracellular Parasites

Hemogregarina

Little is known about the life cycle of fish hemogregarines. These hemoparasites are found most frequently in wild-caught fish and probably require a blood-feeding intermediate host such as leeches, copepods, and isopods. *Hemogregarina* is often considered to be an incidental finding; however, some species can cause anemia, a leukocytosis with a marked left shift, and large granulomas in internal organs (Stokes and Firkin, 1971; Ferguson and Roberts, 1975; Roberts, 2001).

The *Hemogregarina* spp. affecting fish may be identified by the presence of the characteristic gametocytes in the cytoplasm of erythrocytes and resemble those described in blood films of reptiles (Figure 27.23). *Hemogregarina* gametocytes lack refractile pigment granules and may create a bulge in the cytoplasmic membrane.

Piroplasmids

The piroplasmid parasites described in fish include *Babesiosoma*, *Haemohormidium*, *Haematractidium*, and *Mesnilium* (Cheung, 1993). Little is known of the life cycles of these parasites, which most likely require a blood-feeding intermediate host. The piroplasmids may be identified by their intracytoplasmic inclusions in

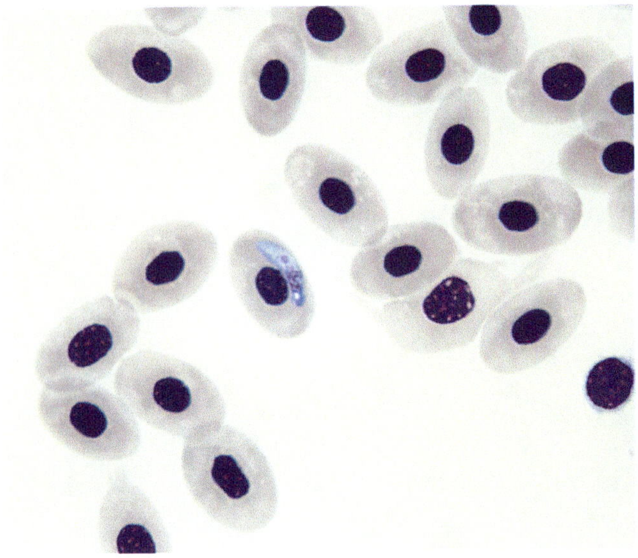

Fig. 27.23. Hemogregarine gametocyte within an erythrocyte in the blood film of a southern stingray (*Hypanus americanus*), Wright–Giemsa stain (100× oil).

circulating erythrocytes, which can vary from small ring-like forms to anaplasma-like inclusions. Piroplasmids may cause hemolytic anemia in fish.

Microsporidians

Enterocytozoon salmonis is an intranuclear microsporidium that primarily infects the hematopoietic cells of salmonid fish. Cells infected by this parasite exhibit intranuclear inclusion. This organism was once thought to be the causative agent of plasmacytoid leukemia of Chinook salmon (*Oncorhynchus tshawytscha*). However, the presence of high reverse transcriptase activity in affected tissues from infected fish suggests that an oncogenic retrovirus may be the etiologic agent for that disease (Hedrick et al., 1990; Newbound, 1993).

Extracellular Parasites

Trypanosomes and Trypanoplasms

Trypanosomes (*Trypanosoma* spp.) and trypanoplasms (*Trypanoplasma* spp.) may be occasionally found in blood films from fish, especially wild-caught cold-water fish species. Leeches serve as the intermediate host and pass the infective trypomastigotes to the fish host when the leech takes a blood meal. *Trypanosoma* spp. can occur in high concentrations (i.e., as much as 1 000 000/mL blood) and are especially prevalent in cytology imprints of renal tissue (Rowley, 1988). These are extracellular blood parasites found among the cells and not within them. *Trypanosoma* is identified by its slender serpentine shape, single anterior flagellum, prominent undulating membrane, nucleus, and kinetoplast that resemble those found in other animals (Figure 11.40). On wet-mount preparations, the *Trypanosoma* species exhibit rapid wriggling movements, but have no forward motion. Infections with *Trypanosoma* spp. can result in fatal anemias in fish.

Trypanoplasma spp. are hemoparasites that resemble *Trypanosoma* spp. morphologically except they are more pleomorphic (a slender, serpentine shape is most common) and have two flagella (one extending in an anterior direction and one in a posterior direction) and kinetosomes (a small body at the posterior end). The life cycle of this parasite is similar to that of the trypanosomes. On wet-mount preparations, *Trypanoplasma* spp. exhibit flowing, amoeba-like motility that aids in their identification and differentiation from the *Trypanosoma* spp. (Rowley, 1988).

Once the *Trypanoplasma* spp. has infected the fish host, a prepatent period occurs followed by parasitemia (cryptobiosis), which then results in clinical disease and either the death of the fish or the disappearance of the parasite from the blood (Rowley, 1988). Clinical signs in freshwater salmonids infected with *T. salmositica* include anemia, exophthalmia, ascites, and splenomegaly. *T. bullocki* infects marine fish, especially flatfish species along the western Atlantic and Gulf of Mexico (Rowley, 1988). *Trypanoplasma borreli* causes sleeping sickness of cyprinids (i.e., koi, goldfish, and carp) and causes a severe anemia (Rowley, 1988).

Viral Inclusions

Intracytoplasmic inclusions occur in the erythrocytes of fish with viral erythrocytic necrosis (piscine erythrocytic necrosis), erythrocytic inclusion body syndrome of young salmonids, and infectious salmon anemia (Coho anemia). Viral erythrocytic necrosis occurs in a variety of marine fish, including salmon, cod, and herring. The disease is characterized by marked poikilocytosis, karyolysis of the red blood cell nuclei, and a single intracytoplasmic inclusion (0.3–4.0 μm) (Stokes and Firkin, 1971).

Erythrocytic inclusion body syndrome of young salmonids is characterized by a severe, progressive anemia caused by a viral agent that creates 0.8–3.0 μm intracytoplasmic inclusions within the erythrocytes (Stokes and Firkin, 1971). The intracytoplasmic inclusions are best seen using a Giemsa stain, where they appear as single purple, round inclusions in erythrocytes (Noga, 2000). The probable causative agent is piscine orthoreovirus-2 (PRV-2), and recovered fish appear to acquire immunity (Takano et al., 2016).

Infectious salmon anemia is a viral disease of seawater-reared Coho salmon (*Oncorhynchus kisutch*) that causes anemia. Intracytoplasmic inclusions that are often rod shaped and range in size from 1.0 to 2.0 μm are found within the erythrocytes, especially in Giemsa-stained blood films (Stokes and Firkin, 1971).

References

Ahmed I, Reshi QM, Fazio F. 2020. The influence of the endogenous and exogenous factors on hematological parameters in different fish species: a review. *Aquaculture International* 28:869–899.

Anderson ET, Stoskopf MK, Morris Jr. JA, Clarke EO, Harms CA. 2010. Hematology, plasma biochemistry, and tissue enzyme activities of invasive red lionfish captured off North Carolina, USA. *J Aquat Anim Health* 22(4):266–273.

Andreasen CB, Latimer KS. 1990. Cytochemical staining characteristics of chicken heterophils and eosinophils. *Vet Clin Pathol* 19:51–54.

Arnold J. 2005. Hematology of the sandbar shark, *Carcharhinus plumbeus*: standardization of complete blood count techniques for elasmobranchs. *Vet Clin Pathol* 34(2):115–123.

Barton BA, Iwama Gk. 1991. Physiological changes in fish from stress in aquaculture with emphasis on the response and effects of corticosteroids. *Ann Rev Fish Dis* 1:3–26.

Belo MAA, Schalch SHC, Moraes FR, et al. 2005. Effect of dietary supplementation with vitamin E and stocking density on macrophage recruitment and giant cell formation in the teleost fish, *Piaractus mesopotamicus*. *J Comp Pathol* 133(2–3):146–154.

Blaxhall PC. 1972. The haematological assessment of the health of freshwater fish, a review of selected literature. *J Fish Biol* 4:593–604.

Blaxhall PC, Daisley KW. 1973. Routine hematological methods for use with fish blood. *J Fish Biol* 5:771–781.

Blazer VS. 1991. Piscine macrophage function and nutritional influences: a review. *J Aquat Anim Health* 3:77–86.

Brenden RA, Huizinga HW. 1986. Pathophysiology of experimental *Aeromonas hydrophila* infection in goldfish, *Carassius auratus* (L). *J Fish Dis* 9:163–167.

Burton CB, Murray SA. 1979. Effects of density on goldfish blood-I. *Hematology Comp Biochem Physiol* 62A:555–558.

Campbell TW. 1988. Tropical fish medicine. *Fish cytology and hematology. Vet Clin North Am (Sm Anim Pract)* 18(2):347–364.

Campbell TW, Grant KR. 2010. *Clinical Cases in Avian and Exotic Animal Hematology and Cytology*. Ames: Wiley-Blackwell.

Cannon MS, Mollernhauer HH, Eurell TE, et al. 1980. An ultrastructural study of the leukocytes of the channel catfish, *Ictalurus punctatus*. *J Morphol* 164:1–23.

Carmezim HS, Marcos R. 2020. There is plenty more fish nomenclature in the sea: the elasmobranch granulocytes. *Vet Clin Pathol* 49(2):196–197.

Catton WT. 1951. Blood cell formation of certain teleost fishes. *Blood* 6:39–60.

Cheung P. 1993. Parasitic diseases of marine tropical fishes. In: Stoskopf M (ed), *Fish Medicine*. Philadelphia, PA: WB Saunders.

Chudzik J, Houston AH. 1983. Temperature and erythropoiesis in goldfish. *Can J Zool* 61:1322–1325.

Clem LW, Miller NW, Bly JE. 1991. Evolution of lymphocyte subpopulations, their interactions, and temperature sensitivities. In: Cohen N, Warr G (eds), *The Phylogeny of Immune Functions*. Boca Raton, FL: CRC Press.

Corrêa LL, Tavares-Dias M, Ceccarelli PS, Adriano EA. 2016. Hematological alterations in *Astyanax altiparanae* (Characidade) caused by *Lernaea cyprinacea* (Copepoda: Lernaeidae). *Dis Aquat Organisms* 120:77–81.

Danilo WF, et al. 1992. Comparative hematology in marine fish. *Comp Biochem Physiol* 102A(2):311–321.

Del Rio-Zaragoza OB, Fajer-Ávila EJ, Almazán-Rueda P, Abdo de la Parra MI. 2011. Hematological characteristics of the spotted rose snapper *Lutjanus guttatus* (Steindachner, 1869) healthy and naturally infected by dactylogyrid monogeneans. *Tissue and Cell* 43(3):137–142.

Eaton WD, Kent MI. 1992. A retrovirus in Chinook salmon (*Oncorhynchus tshawytscha*) with plasmacytoid leukemia and evidence for the etiology of the disease. *Cancer Res* 52:6496–6500.

Eddy FB. 1981. Effects of stress on osmotic and ionic regulation in fish. In: Pickering A (ed), *Stress and Fish*. London: Academic Press.

Eiras JC. 1983. Erythrocyte degeneration in the European eel, *Anguilla anguilla*. *Bull Eur Assoc Fish Pathol* 3:8–10.

Ellis AE. 1975. Leucocytes and related cells in the plaice (*Pleuronectes platessa*). *J Fish Biol* 8:143–156.

Ellis AE. 1977. The leukocytes of fish: a review. *J Fish Biol* 11:453–491.

Ellis AE. 1984. Bizarre forms of erythrocytes in a specimen of plaice, *Pleuronectes platessa* L. *J Fish Dis* 7:411–414.

Ellsaesser CF, Clem LW. 1986. Hematological and immunological changes in channel catfish stressed by handling and transport. *J Fish Biol* 28:511–521.

Ellsaesser CF, Miller NW, Cuchens MA, Lobb CJ, Clem W. 1985. Analysis of channel catfish peripheral blood leucocytes by bright-field microscopy and flow cytometry. *Trans Amer Fish Soc* 114:279–285.

Emery SH. 1986. Hematological comparisons of endothermic vs ectothermic elasmobranch fishes. *Copeia* 700–705.

Evans DL, Jaso-Friedmann L. 1992. Nonspecific cytotoxic cells as effectors of immunity in fish. *Ann Rev Fish Dis* 2:109–121.

Fänge R. 1968. The formation of eosinophilic granulocytes in the oesophageal lymphomyeloid tissue of the elasmobranch. *Acta Zool* 49:155–161.

Fänge R. 1992 Fish blood cells. In: Hoar W, Randall D, Farrell A (eds), *Fish Physiology, vol. XIIB*. San Diego: Academic Press.

Ferguson HW. 1975. The ultrastructure of plaice (*Pleuronectes platessa*) leukocytes. *J Fish Biol* 8:139–142.

Ferguson HW, 1989. Systemic pathology of fish. In: Ferguson H (ed), *Systemic Pathology of Fish*. Ames: Iowa State University Press.

Ferguson HW, Roberts RJ. 1975. Myeloid leucosis associated with sporozoan infection in cultured turbot (*Scophthalmus maximus* L.). *J Comp Pathol* 85:317–326.

Filho DW, Eble GJ, Kassner G, et al. 1992. Comparative hematology in marine fish. *Comp Biochem Physiol* 102A:311–321.

Fujimaki Y, Isoda M. 1990. Fine-structural study of leucocytes in the goldfish, *Carassius auratus*. *J Fish Biol* 36:821–831.

Galagarza OA, Kuhn DD, Smith SA, Hrubec TC. 2017. Hematologic and plasma chemistry RIs for cultured striped catfish (*Pangasius hypophthalmus*) in recirculating aquaculture systems. *Vet Clin Pathol* 46(3):457–465.

Grizzle JM, Rogers WA. 1985. *Anatomy and Histology of the Channel Catfish*. Auburn, AL: Alabama University Press, pp. 1–94.

Groff JM, Zinkl JG. 1999. Hematology and clinical chemistry of cyprinid fish. *Vet Clin North Am (Exotic Anim Pract)* 2(3):741–776.

Hanson LP, Ainsworth AJ. 2000. Differential cytochemical staining characteristics of channel catfish leukocytes identify cell populations in lymphoid organs. *Vet Immunol Immunopathol* 73:129–144.

Harikrishnan R, Nisha Rani M, Balasundaram C. 2003. Hematological and biochemical parameters in common carp, *Cyprinus carpio*, following herbal treatment for *Aeromonas hydrophila* infection. *Aquac* 221(1):41–50.

Harr KE, Deak K, Murawski SA, Reavill DR, Takeshita RA. 2018. Generation of red drum *(Sciaenops ocellatus)* hematology reference intervals with a focus on identified outliers. *Vet Clin Pathol 47*(1):22–28.

Haws GT, Goodnight CJ. 1962. Some aspects of the hematology of two species of catfish in relation to their habitats. *Physiol Zool* 35(1):8017.

Hedrick RP, Groff JM, McDowell TS. 1990. Hematopoietic intranuclear microsporidian infections with features of leukemia in chinook salmon (*Oncorhynchus tschawytscha*). *Dis Aqua Organ* 8:189–197.

Hibiya T. 1985. An atlas of fish histology, normal and pathological features. In: Hibiya T (ed), *An Atlas of Fish Histology, Normal and Pathological Features*. Tokyo: Kodansha Ltd.

Hine PM. 1992. The granulocytes of fish. *Fish Shellfish Immunol* 2:79–98.

Hine PM, Wain LM. 1987a. Composition and ultrastructure of elasmobranch granulocytes. I. Dogfishes (Squaliformes). *J Fish Biol* 30:547–556.

Hine PM, Wain LM. 1987b. Composition and ultrastructure of elasmobranch granulocytes. II. Rays (Rajiformes). *J Fish Biol* 30:557–565.

Hine PM, Wain LM. 1987c. Composition and ultrastructure of elasmobranch granulocytes. III. Sharks (Lamniformes). *J Fish Biol* 30:567–576.

Hines R, Spira DT. 1973. Ichthyophthiriasis in the mirror carp. III. Leukocyte response. *J Fish Biol* 5:527–534.

Houston AH. 1990. Blood and circulation. In: Schreck C, Moyle P (eds), *Methods in Fish Biology*. Bethesda, MD: American Fisheries Society.

Houston AH. 1997. Review: are the classical hematological variables acceptable indicators of fish health? *Trans Am Fish Soc* 126:879–894.

Houston AH, Murad A. 1991. Hematological characterization of goldfish (*Carassius auratus* L) by image analysis. Effects of thermal acclimation and heat shock. *Can J Zool* 69:2041–2047.

Houston AH, Schrapp MP. 1994. Thermoacclimatory hematological response: have we been using appropriate conditions and assessment methods? *Can J Zool* 72:1238–1242.

Hrubec TC, Robertson JL, Smith SA. 1997. Effects of temperature on hematologic and serum biochemistry profiles of hybrid striped bass (*Morone chrysops* × *Morone saxatilis*). *Am J Vet Res* 58:126–130.

Hrubec TC, Smith SA. 2000. Hematology of fish. In: Feldman B, Zinkl J, Jain N (eds), *Schalm's Veterinary Hematology*, 5th edn. Baltimore, MD: Lippincott Williams & Wilkins.

Hrubec TC, Smith SA. 2010. Hematology of Fishes. In: Weiss DJ, Wardrop KJ (eds), *Schalm's Veterinary Hematology*, 6th edn. Ames, IA: Wiley-Blackwell.

Hrubec TC, Smith SA, Robertson JL. 2001. Age-related changes in hematology and plasma chemistry values in hybrid striped bass (*Morone chrysops* × *Morone saxatilis*). *Vet Clin Pathol* 30(1):8–15.

Hyder SL, Cayer ML, Pettey CL. 1983. Cell types in peripheral blood of the nurse shark: an approach to structure and function. *Tissue Cell* 15(3):437–455.

Iwama GK, Greer GL, Randall DJ. 1986. Changes in selected haemotological parameters in juvenile Chinook salmon subjected to a bacterial challenge and a toxicant. *J Fish Biol* 28:563–572.

Jain NC. 1986. Veterinary hematology. In: Jain N (ed), *Schalm's Veterinary Hematology*, 4th edn. Philadelphia, PA: Lea & Febiger.

Jain NC, et al. 1988. A comparison of cytochemical techniques to demonstrate peroxidase activity in canine leukocyes. *Vet Clin Pathol* 17:87–89.

Jensen FB. 1990. Nitrite and red cell function in carp. control factors for nitrite entry, membrane potassium ion permeation, oxygen affinity and methaemoglobin formation. *J Exp Biol* 152:149–166.

Jensen FB, Andersen NA, Heisler N. 1987. Effects of nitrite exposure on blood respiratory properties, acid-base and electrolyte regulation in the carp (*Cyprinus carpio*). *J Comp Physiol(B)* 157: 533–541.

Kamra SK. 1966. Effect of starvation and refeeding on some liver and blood constituents of Atlantic cod. *J Fish Res Board Can* 23(7):975–982.

Kelenyi G, Nemeth A. 1969. Comparative histochemistry and electron microscopy of the eosinophil leucocytes of vertebrates. *Acta Biol Acad Sci H* 20:405–422.

Kendall C, Valentino S, Bodine AB, Luer CA. 1992. Flow cytometric DNA analysis of nurse shark, *Ginglymostoma cirratum* (Bonaterre) and clearnose skate, *Raja eglanteria* (Bosc) peripheral red blood cells. *J Fish Biol* 41:123–129.

Lane HC. 1979. Progressive changes in hematology and tissue water of sexually mature trout, *Samo gairdneri* Richardson during the autumn and winter. *J Fish Biol* 15:425–436.

Lewis DH, Eurell TE, Cannon MS, Grumbles LC. 1979. T and B cell analogues from peripheral blood of immune channel catfish, *Ictalurus punctatus*. *J Fish Biol* 14:31–37.

Lumlertdacha S, Lovell RT, Shelby RA, Lenz SD, Kemppainen BW. 1995. Growth, hematology, and histopathology of channel catfish, *Ictalurus punctatus*, fed toxins from *Fusarium moniliforme*. *Aquac* 130(2):201–218.

Mainwaring G, Rowley AF. 1985. Studies on granulocyte heterogenicity in elasmobranchs. In: Mainwaring G, Rowley A (eds), *Fish Immunology*. New York: Academic Press.

Matsche MA, Rosemary K, Stence CP. 2017. A comparison of hematology, plasma chemistry, and injuries in Hickory shad (*Alosa mediocris*) captured by electrofishing or angling during a spawning run. *Vet Clin Pathol* 46(3):471–482.

Mazeaud MM, Mazeaud F, Donaldson EM. 1977. Primary and secondary effects of stress in fish. Some new data with a general review. *Trans Am Fish Soc* 106:201–212.

McCarthy DH, Stevenson JP, Roberts MS. 1975. Some blood parameters of the rainbow trout (*Salmo gairdneri* Richardson) II The Shasta variety. *J Fish Biol* 4:593–604.

McLeay DJ. 1973. Effects of cortisol and dexamethasone on the pituitary-interrenal axis and abundance of white blood cell types in juvenile Coho salmon, *Oncorhynchus kisutch*. *Gen Comp Endocrinol* 21:441–450.

Modesto KA, Martinez CB. 2010. Effects of roundup transorb on fish: hematology, antioxidant defenses and acetylcholinesterase activity. *Chemosphere* 81(6):781–787.

Montali RJ. 1988. Comparative pathology of inflammation in the higher vertebrates (reptiles, birds, and mammals). *J Comp Pathol* 99:1–26.

Morgan AL, Thompson KD, Auchinachie NA, Migaud H. 2008. The effect of seasonality on normal haematological and innate immune parameters of rainbow trout *Oncorhynchus mykiss* L. *Fish & shellfish immunology* 25(6):791–799.

Mulcahy ME. 1976. Epizootiological studies of lymphoma in northern pike in Ireland. *Prog Exp Tumour Res* 20:129–140.

Munkittrick KR, Leatherland JF. 1983. Haematocrit values in feral goldfish (*Carassius auratus* L) as indicators of the health of the population. *J Fish Biol* 23:153–161.

Murad A, Houston AH. 1992. Maturation of the goldfish (*Carassius auratus*) erythrocyte. *Comp Biochem Physiol* 102A:107–110.

Murray SA, Burton CB. 1979. Effects of density on goldfish blood-II. Cell morphology. *Comp Biochem Physiol* 62A:559–562.

Mylniczenko ND, Curtis EW, Wilborn RE, Young FA. 2006. Differences in hematocrit of blood samples obtained from two venipuncture sites in sharks. *Am J Vet Res* 67(11):1861–1864.

Newbound GC. 1993. Production of monoclonal antibodies specific for antigens derived from tissue of chinook salmon (*Oncorhynchus tshawytscha*) affected with plasmacytoid leukemia. *Am J Vet Res* 54(9):1426–1431.

Noga EJ. 1996. Fish disease, diagnosis and treatment. In: Noga E (ed), *Fish Disease, Diagnosis and Treatment*. St. Louis: Mosby.

Noga EJ. 2000. Fish disease: diagnosis and treatment. In: Noga E (ed), *Fish Disease, Diagnosis and Treatment*. Ames, IA: Iowa State University Press.

Palic D, Andreasen CB, Frank DE, Menzel BW, Roth JA. 2005. Gradient separation and cytochemical characterization of neutrophils from kidney of fathead minnow (*Pimephales promelas* Rafinesque, 1820). *Fish Shellfish Immunol* 18:263–267.

Plumb JA, Liu PR, Butterworth CE. 1991. Folate-degrading bacteria in channel catfish feeds. *J Appl Aguacult* 1:33–43.

Ram-Bhaskar B, Srinivasa-Rao K. 1989. Influence of environmental variables on hematology, and compendium of normal hematological ranges of milkfish, *Chanos chanos* (Forskal) in brackish culture. *Aquac* 83:123–136.

Rehulka J. 2003. Haematological analyses in rainbow trout *Oncorhynchus mykiss* affected by viral haemorrhagic septicaemia (VHS). *Dis Aquat Org* 56(3):185–193.

Rios FS, Oba ET, Fernandes MN, Kalinin AL, Rantin FT. 2005. Erythrocyte senescence and haematological changes induced by starvation in the neotropical fish traíra, *Hoplias malabaricus* (Characiformes, Erythrinidae). *Comparative Biochemistry and Physiology Part A: Molecular & Integrative Physiology* 140(3):281–287.

Roberts RJ. 2001. The parasitology of teleosts. In: Robers R (ed), *Fish Pathology*. London: WB Saunders.

Roberts RJ, Ellis AE. 2001. The anatomy and physiology of teleosts. In: Roberts R (ed), *Fish Pathology*. Philadelphia, PA: WB Saunders.

Roberts RJ, Ellis AE. 2012. The anatomy and physiology of teleosts. In: Roberts R (ed), *Fish Pathology*, 4th edn. Philadelphia, PA: WB Saunders.

Roberts RJ, Rodger HD. 2012. The pathophysiology and systematic pathology of teleosts. In: Roberts R (ed), *Fish Pathology*, 4th edn. Philadelphia, PA: WB Saunders.

Rowley AF. 1988. Fish. In: Rowley A, Ratcliffe N (eds), *Vertebrate Blood Cells*. Cambridge: Cambridge University Press.

Ruane NM, Nolan DT, Rotllant J, Costelloe J, Wendelaar Bonga SE. 2000. Experimental exposure of rainbow trout *Oncorhynchus mykiss* (Walbaum) to the infective stages of the sea louse *Lepeophtheirus salmonis* (Krøyer) influences the physiological response to an acute stressor. *Fish & Shellfish Immunology* 10(5)451–463.

Sanchez-Muiz FJ, De La Higuera M, Varela G. 1982. Alterations of erythrocytes of the rainbow trout *Salmo gairdneri* by the use of *Hansenula anomola* yeast as sole protein source. *Comp Biochem Physiol* 72A:693–696.

Sano T. 1960. Hematological studies of the culture fishes in Japan. *J Tokyo Univ Fish* 46:68–87.

Saunders DC. 1966. Differential blood cell counts of 121 species of marine fishes of Puerto Rico. *Trans Am Microsc Soc* 85:427–499.

Schreck CB. 1981. Stress and compensation in teleostean fishes. Response to social and physical factors. In: Pickering A (ed), *Stress and Fish*. London: Academic Press.

Semeniuk CA, Bourgeon S, Smith SL, Rothley KD. 2009. Hematological differences between stingrays at tourist and non-visited sites suggest physiological costs of wildlife tourism. *Biol Conserv* 142(8):1818–1829.

Smail DA, Egglestone SI. 1980. Viral infections of marine fish erythrocytes: prevalence of piscine erythrocytic necrosis in cod, *Gadus morhua*, and blenny, *Blennius pholis* L., in coastal and offshore waters of the United Kingdom. *J Fish Dis* 3:41–46.

Smeda JS, Houston AH. 1979. Evidence of weight-dependent differential hematological response to increased environmental temperature by carp (*Cyprinus carpio*). *Environ Biol Fish* 4:89–92.

Speckner W, Schindler JF, Albers C. 1989. Age-dependent changes in volume and hemoglobin content of erythrocytes in the carp (*Cyprinus carpio* L.). *J Exp Biol* 141:133–149.

Steinhagen D, Oesterreich B, Körting W. 1997. Carp coccidiosis: clinical and hematological observations of carp infected with *Goussia carpelli*. *Dis Aquat Org* 30:137–143.

Stokes EE, Firkin BG. 1971. Studies of the peripheral blood of the Port Jackson shark (*Heterodontus portusjacksoni*) with particular reference to the thrombocyte. *Br J Hematol* 20:427–435.

Stoskopf MK 1993. Clinical pathology. In: Stoskopf M (ed), *Fish Medicine*. Philadelphia, PA: WB Saunders.

Summerfelt RC. 1967. Measurement of some hematological characteristics of goldfish. *Prog Fish Cult* 29(10):13–20.

Svetina A, Matasin Z, Tofant A, et al. 2002. Haematology and some blood chemical parameters of young carp till the age of three years. *Acta Vet Hung* 50(4):459–467.

Takano T, Nawata A, Sakai T, et al. 2016. Full-genome sequencing and confirmation of the causative agent of erythrocytic inclusion body syndrome in coho salmon identifies a new type of piscine Orthoreovirus. *PLoS one* 11(10):e0165424. DOI:10.1371/journal.pone.0165424

Tavares-Dias M, deMoraes FR. 2007. Leukocyte and thrombocyte reference values for channel catfish (*Ictalurus punctatus* Raf), with an assessment of morphologic, cytochemical, and ultrastructural features. *Vet Clin Pathol* 36:49–54.

Tocidlowski ME, Lewbart GA, Stoskopf MK. 1997. Hematologic study of red pacu (*Colossoma brachypomum*). *Vet Clin Pathol* 26(3):119–125.

Tripathi NK, Latimer KS, Burnley VV. 2004. Hematologic reference intervals for koi (*Cyprinus carpio*), including blood cell morphology, cytochemistry, and ultrastructure. *Vet Clin Pathol* 33(2):74–83.

van Razij MTM, van den Thillart GEEJM, Vianen GJ, et al. 1996a. Substrate mobilization and hormonal changes in rainbow trout (*Onchorhynchus mykiss*, L) and common carp (*Cyprinus carpio*, L) during deep hypoxia and subsequent recovery. *J Comp Physiol B* 166:443–452.

van Razij MTM, van den Thillart GEEJM, Vianen GJ, et al. 1996b. Blood gas parameters and the responses of erythrocytes in carp exposed to deep hypoxia and subsequent recovery. *J Comp Physiol B* 166:453–460.

van Vuren JHJ, Hattingh J. 1978. A seasonal study of the haematology of wild freshwater fish. *J Fish Biol* 13:305–313.

Walsh CJ, Luer CA. 2004. Elasmobranch hematology: identification of cell types and practical applications. In: Smith M, Warmolts D, Thoney D, Hueter R (eds), *The Elasmobranch Husbandry*

Manual: Captive Care of Sharks, Rays, and their Relatives. Columbus: Ohio Biological Survey, Inc.

Wedemeyer GA, Gould RW, Yasutake WT. 1983. Some potentials and limits of the leucocrit test as a fish health assessment method. *J Fish Biol* 23:711–716.

Wedemeyer GA, Barton BA, McLeay DJ. 1990. Stress and acclimation. In: Schreck C, Moyle P (eds), *Methods in Fish Biology*. Bethesda, MD: American Fisheries Society.

Weinreb EL. 1963. Studies on the fine structure of teleost blood cells in peripheral blood. *Anat Rec* 147:219–238.

Williams RW, Warren MC. 1976. Some observations on the stained blood cellular elements of channel catfish, *Ictalurus punctatus*. *J Fish Biol* 9:491–496.

Yokote M. 1982. Blood cells. In: Hibiya T (ed), *An Atlas of Fish Histology*. Tokyo: Kodausha.

Zinkl JG, Cox WT, Kono CS. 1991. Morphology and cytochemistry in leucocytes and thrombocytes of six species of fish. *Comp Haemat Inter* 1:187–195.

28 Piscine Hematopoiesis

Because the primary location of hemopoiesis of fish occurs in the internal organs, cytological evaluation is rarely, if ever, used to assess unexplained abnormalities found in the peripheral blood as is done by the examination of bone marrow aspirates of mammals and birds (and sometimes lizards). The primary hemopoietic tissue of teleost fish is found in the interstitial stroma of the kidney and spleen. Minor hemopoietic components are found in the liver, intestines, and thymus as well (Fänge, 1992; Roberts and Ellis, 2001). The pronephric (anterior or head) and opisthonephric (main or trunk) kidneys are sites of hematopoiesis in these fish. The pronephric kidney is almost exclusively hemopoietic, functioning as the principal site of erythrocyte, granulocyte, lymphocyte, monocyte, and possibly thrombocyte development and differentiation, whereas the opisthonephric kidney also functions as an excretory organ (Rowley, 1988; Liu et al., 2017).

Erythropoiesis occurs in the major hematopoietic organs and progresses from erythroblasts to mature erythrocytes in the same manner as described for other vertebrates (Fijan, 2002). Fish do differ from mammals in that a small amount of erythropoiesis occurs in the peripheral blood as well (Fänge, 1992; Glomski et al., 1992). It is not uncommon to find mitotic activity and various stages of erythroid maturation in peripheral blood films of fish, although the numbers of erythroblasts present are low.

The erythrocyte maturation follows the same pattern described for other lower vertebrates that have nucleated mature erythrocytes. The typical progression occurs in which the round immature erythrocytes exhibit a progression in cellular and nuclear size until they finally mature as elliptical, flattened, nucleated cells (Fänge, 1992; Glomski et al., 1992; Houston and Murad, 1991; Houston and Murad, 1992; Murad and Houston, 1992). A progressive decrease in cytoplasmic basophilia with a corresponding increase in acidophilia occurs as the hemoglobin content increases. The nuclear chromatin also progresses from less condensed to more condensed as the erythrocyte matures. An occasional anucleated erythrocyte or erythroplastid may be noted in the blood film. These cells are thought to form due to erythrocyte deformation during transit through a capillary, or as a maturation defect (Watson et al., 1963).

The developmental stages of the erythroid series, from immature to mature, are rubriblast (proerythroblast), prorubricyte (basophilic erythroblast), rubricyte (polychromatic erythroblast), metarubricyte (orthochromatic erythroblast), polychromatic erythrocyte (reticulocyte), and mature erythrocyte (Liu et al., 2017)

Piscine erythrocytes in the peripheral circulation may also undergo amitotic proliferation. These red cells appear elongated and may possess cytoplasmic projections at one pole of the cell (Houston and Murad, 1992; Murad et al., 1993). Senescent or degenerative erythrocytes are occasionally found in peripheral blood films as well and appear as swollen erythrocytes with round cellular and nuclear profiles (Groff and Zinkl, 1999).

The typical stages of granulocyte development described for mammals have been identified for each type of granulocyte that develops in the kidney of bony fish. Thus, impression smears of teleost kidneys reveal granuloblasts like mammalian myeloblasts and myelocytes (Roberts and Ellis, 2001).

The developmental stages of the granulocyte (myeloid) series, from immature to mature, are myeloblast

Exotic Animal Hematology and Cytology, Fifth Edition. Terry W. Campbell and Krystan R. Grant.

Companion website: www.wiley.com/go/campbell/exotic

(granuloblast), promyelocyte (progranulocyte), myelocyte, metamyelocyte (metagranulocyte), and mature granulocyte. Differentiation between the granulocytes (neutrophil, eosinophil, and basophil) begins at the myelocyte stage (Liu et al., 2017).

The developmental stages of the monocyte series from immature to mature are monoblast, promonocyte, and monocyte (which develops into the macrophage) (Liu et al., 2017). Monoblasts are large cells, often with irregular shapes and cytoplasmic pseudopodia and prominent nucleoli. Promonocytes resemble monoblasts, but lack nucleoli and their cytoplasm has a "ground glass" appearance.

Melanomacrophage centers are found in the hematopoietic tissue of teleost fish and contain melanomacrophages, which are macrophages that contain melanosomes within lysosomes. Melanomacrophages of ectotherms appear to be specialized phagocytic cells that are adapted to hypothermic conditions (Pxytycz and Jozkowicz, 1994; Johnson et al., 1999). The melanin present in fish melanomacrophages is considered to originate from melanocytes; however, it has been demonstrated that reptilian and amphibian melanomacrophages can synthesize their own melanin (Agius, 1985; Scalia et al., 1988; Ellis, 2001). The dark brown to black pigment of melanomacrophages has the chemical properties of melanin. The role of the melanin is not known, but may play a role in bactericidal mechanisms or may function as a modulator of bactericidal mechanisms that involve the production of free radicals by phagocytic cells (Gyimesi and Howerth, 2004). Circulating monocytes and perhaps macrophages that contain phagocytized material congregate in the melanomacrophage centers for processing (Roberts and Ellis, 2001). This is one mechanism by which fish remove and destroy harmful foreign agents that find their way into the peripheral blood.

Teleost fishes (bony fishes) do not have lymph nodes, and their bones rarely contain a medullary cavity. The thymus is the first lymphoid organ to develop, and it seeds the spleen and kidney with lymphocytes. When present, the thymus is a paired organ situated subcutaneously in the dorsal commissure of the operculum. This organ involutes in lower teleosts before sexual maturity, but may persist for years in higher teleosts. The spleen is the only primary lymphopoietic tissue and lymph node-like organ in most mature teleost fish, and typically has a secondary role in hematopoiesis, except in some species where it is the only hematopoietic organ as well (Rowley, 1988).

The developmental stages of the lymphoid series from immature to mature are lymphoblasts, prolymphocytes, and small and large mature lymphocytes (Liu et al., 2017). The mature lymphocytes become reactive and develop into plasma cells (or the Mott cell variant).

Elasmobranch fishes lack bone marrow and lymph nodes, but have a lymphoid thymus, spleen, and other lymphomyeloid tissues, which include the epigonal organ, Leydig organ, and isolated lymphoid aggregates in the intestines (Walsh and Luer, 2004). The Leydig organ is in the submucosa of the alimentary tract and is the major site for granulopoiesis in most, but not all, cartilaginous fish species (Rowley, 1988). The epigonal organ is located caudal to the gonad and is the site for both lymphopoiesis and granulopoiesis (Zapata, 1980). Histologically, the epigonal organ resembles mammalian bone marrow without the fat (Walsh and Luer, 2004). Myeloblasts, progranulocytes, myelocytes, metamyelocytes, and mature granulocytes have all been described in the epigonal and Leydig organs.

The primary hematopoietic tissues of elasmobranch fishes are the epigonal organ and Leydig organ (Zapata, 1980; Mattisson and Fänge, 1982; Lloyd-Evans, 1993; Zapata et al., 1996). Significant hematopoietic activity also occurs in the sinusoids of the red pulp area of the spleen, where development of erythrocytes, thrombocytes, and lymphocytes occurs (there is little evidence that granulopoiesis occurs in the spleen) (Rowley, 1988). Erythrocyte development appears to occur in the same manner described for mammals. The peripheral blood may be an important component of erythropoiesis as well, since several stages of erythrocyte development can be found in routine blood films from cartilaginous fish.

References

Agius C. 1985. The melanomacrophage cells of fishes: a review. In: Manning M, Tatner M (eds), *Fish Immunology*. London: Academic Press.

Ellis AE. 2001. The immunology of teleosts. In: Roberts R (ed), *Fish Pathology*. Philadelphia, PA: WB Saunders.

Fänge R. 1992. Fish blood cells. In: Hoar W, Randall D, Farrell A (eds), *Fish Physiology, vol. XIIB*. San Diego: Academic Press.

Fijan N. 2002. Morphogenesis of blood cell lineages in channel catfish. *J Fish Biol* 60(4):999–1014.

Glomski CA, Tamburlin J, Chainani M. 1992. The phylogenetic odyssey of the erythrocyte. III. Fish, the lower vertebrate experience. *Histol Histopathol* 7:501–528.

Groff JM, Zinkl JG. 1999. Hematology and clinical chemistry of cyprinid fish. *Vet Clin North Am (Exotic Anim Pract)* 2(3):741–776.

Gyimesi ZS, Howerth EW. 2004. Severe melanomacrophage hyperplasia in a crocodile lizard, *Shinisaurus crocodilurus*: a review of melanomacrophages in ectotherms. *J Herpetolog Med Surg* 14(1):19–23.

Houston AH, Murad A. 1991. Hematological characterization of goldfish (*Carassius auratus* L) by image analysis. Effects of thermal acclimation and heat shock. *Can J Zool* 69:2041–2047.

Houston AH, Murad A. 1992. Erythrodynamics in goldfish (*Carassius auratus* L). Temperature effects. *Physiol Zool* 65:55–76.

Johnson JC, Schwiesow T, Ekwall AK, Christiansen JL. 1999. Reptilian melanomacrophages function under conditions of hypothermia: observations on phagocytic behavior. *Pigment Cell Res* 12:376–382.

Liu Y, Xiao Q, Yang S, et al. 2017. Characterization of hematopoiesis in Dabry's sturgeon (*Acipenser dabryanus*). *Aquaculture and Fisheries* 2(6):262–268.

Lloyd-Evans P. 1993. Development of the lymphomyeloid system in the dogfish, Scyliorhinus *canicula. Dev Comp Immunol* 17:501–514.

Mattisson A, Fänge R. 1982. The cellular structure of the Leydig organ in the shark, *Etmopterus spinax* (L.). *Biological Bulletin* 162:182–194.

Murad A, Houston AH. 1992. Maturation of the goldfish (*Carassius auratus*) erythrocyte. *Comp Biochem Physiol* 102A: 107–110.

Murad A, Everill SP, Houston AH. 1993. Division of goldfish erythrocytes in circulation. *Can J Zool* 71:2190–2198.

Pxytycz B, Jozkowicz A. 1994. Differential effects of temperature on macrophages of ectothermic vertebrates. *J Leukoc Biol* 56:729–731.

Roberts RJ, Ellis AE. 2001. The anatomy and physiology of teleosts. In: Roberts R (ed), *Fish Pathology*. Philadelphia, PA: WB Saunders.

Rowley AF. 1988. Fish. In: Rowley A, Ratcliffe N (eds), *Vertebrate Blood Cells*. Cambridge: Cambridge University Press.

Scalia M, Geremia E, Corsaro C, et al. 1988. The extracutaneous pigmentary system: evidence for the melanosynthesis in Amphibia and Reptilia. *Comp Biochem Physiol* 89B:715–717.

Walsh CJ, Luer CA. 2004. Elasmobranch hematology: identification of cell types and practical applications. In: Smith M, Warmolts D, Thoney D, Hueter R (eds), *The Elasmobranch Husbandry Manual: Captive Care of Sharks, Rays, and their Relatives*. Columbus: Ohio Biological Survey, Inc.

Watson LJ, Schechmeister IL, Jackson LL. 1963. The haematology of goldfish (*Carassius auratus*). *Cytologia* 28:118–130.

Zapata A. 1980. Ultrastructure of elasmobranch lympoid tissue. II. Leydig's and epigonal organs. *Dev Comp Immunol* 5:43–52.

Zapata AG, Torroba M, Sacedon R, Varas A, Vicente A. 1996. Structure of the lymphoid organs of elasmobranches. *J Exp Zool* 275:125–143.

29 Piscine Hematology and Clinical Chemistry: Clinical Case Presentations

Case 1: Nurse Shark with Excessive Gilling

Signalment

Adult male nurse shark (*Ginglymostoma cirratum*)

History

The nurse shark, along with two other adult male nurse sharks – a shovelnose guitarfish (*Rhinobatos productus*), a bat ray (*Myliobatis californica*), and a reticulate whipray (*Himantura uarnak*) – arrived at a public aquarium approximately three weeks prior to the initial presentation. Two weeks after arrival, one of the nurse sharks died. Upon gross necropsy, the only significant finding was a hemorrhagic spiral intestine. Histopathology revealed mild multifocal lymphoplasmacytic meningitis, segmental epithelial hyperplasia of the gills, and mild to moderate lymphoplasmacytic hepatitis. Because of marked autolysis, it was difficult to identify lesions on many of the organs submitted. Eight days later, the second nurse shark was observed with increased gilling, and blood was seen flowing from the vent. The second nurse was isolated from other fish, but died shortly after clinical signs were seen. Histopathology revealed a large liver cyst with several unidentified fungal organisms, necrotizing enteritis, and rhabdomyolysis. The presenting shark was observed with excessive gilling the same day that the second shark died.

Physical Examination

Upon physical examination, the shark was resting at the bottom of the quarantine tank with an increased respiratory rate and effort. He was pulled to the surface to obtain a blood sample from the dorsal venous sinus. The hematology and plasma biochemistry results are shown in Tables 29.1 and 29.2, Day 1, and representative samples of the blood film are shown in Figures 29.1a and 29.1b.

Interpretive Discussion

The hematology results in Table 29.1 and review of the blood film were indicative of an inflammatory leukogram, although the total leukocyte count was slightly elevated when compared to other elasmobranchs in captivity at the same aquarium (Parkinson et al., 2017; Grant and Campbell, 2020). Figure 29.1a revealed three mildly toxic heterophils (or G_1, type I granulocyte, or fine eosinophilic granulocyte) and one toxic neutrophil (or G_2, type II granulocyte). There is also one lymphocyte as well as four thrombocytes, three of which have a fine eosinophilic dusting of granules within the cytoplasm, and one is more spindle-shaped, indicating the reactive form. Figure 29.1b revealed five mildly toxic heterophils, three lymphocytes, and three thrombocytes. The toxicity in the heterophils is evidenced by the increased cytoplasmic basophilia. In addition to the presence of toxic heterophils, other determining factors of an inflammatory leukogram included the heterophilia and the increased heterophil:lymphocyte ratio. There were no significant findings on the plasma biochemistry profile (Table 29.2). The inflammatory leukogram with the presence of toxic heterophils and neutrophils was presumed to be due to an infection.

Summary

The shark was prescribed Nuflor® (florfenicol) at 20 mg/kg IM once every five days. Follow-up and recheck visits occurred 10 days, 25 days, and 39 days

Exotic Animal Hematology and Cytology, Fifth Edition. Terry W. Campbell and Krystan R. Grant.

Companion website: www.wiley.com/go/campbell/exotic

Table 29.1. Nurse shark hematology results (Case 1).

	Day 1	Day 10	Day 25	Day 39	Reference[a]
PCV (%)	25	20	16	10	24.7 (17–30)
Leukocytes					
WBC (×10³/μL)	18.6	7.2	6.4	3.5	—
Heterophils (×10³/μL)	14.9	3.7	3.9	1.6	—
(%)	80	51	61	46	24.5 (11–38)
Lymphocytes (×10³/μL)	2.0	3.2	1.0	1.8	—
(%)	11	44	15	51	73.3 (62–87)
Monocytes (×10³/μL)	0.7	0.4	0.1	0.1	—
(%)	4	5	1	1	2.2 (0–4)
Eosinophils (×10³/μL)	0.9	0	0	0	—
(%)	5	0	0	0	—
Basophils (×10³/μL)	0	0	1.5	0.1	—
(%)	0	0	23	1	—
Thrombocytes					
Adequate thrombocytes	Exist				
Plasma protein (refractometry)					
(g/dL)	7.2	5.6	6.1	4.8	—
Notes					
		Occasional plasmacytoid cell was seen.			

[a]Walsh and Luer (2004).

Table 29.2. Nurse shark plasma biochemical results (Case 1).

	Day 1	Day 10	Day 25	Reference[a]
Glucose (mg/dL)	85	19	20	43.14 (30.31–62.67)
BUN (mg/dL)	712	657	694	—
Phosphorus (mg/dL)	5.9	3.0	3.4	—
Calcium (mg/dL)	15.6	13.3	15.3	14.28 (13.03–15.61)
Uric acid (mg/dL)	0.3	0	0	0.15 (0.02–0.31)
Total protein (biuret) (g/dL)	4.7	3.4	3.4	4.41 (2.65–5.13)
Albumin (g/dL)	0.6	0.7	0.4	0.44 (0.35–0.60)
Globulin (g/dL)	4.1	2.7	3.0	—
Cholesterol (mg/dL)	46	35	44	—
Creatine kinase (IU/L)	50347	396	186	—
Aspartate aminotransferase (IU/L)	118	38	16	—
Sodium (mEq/L)	252	228	264	—
Potassium (mEq/L)	4.01	3.8	4.4	—
Chloride (mEq/L)	255	223	270	—

[a]Ferraz, et al. (2014).

after initial presentation. The shark exhibited gradual improvement, clinically, evidenced by eating and being more active, although his gills were pale. Blood was collected during subsequent visits, and complete blood counts (CBCs) and plasma biochemistry profiles were evaluated (apart from a plasma biochemistry profile on day 39). The results of these diagnostics are shown in Tables 29.1 and 29.2. Blood films were also evaluated at each visit, and representative images are shown in Figures 29.2 and 29.3 from the visits on days 25 and 39, respectively. The heterophils and neutrophils by day 39 appeared slightly toxic, indicating improvement along with the leukocyte count and relative heterophilia and H:L ratio. However, the PCV was decreasing with each visit, and the developing anemia likely was the cause for the pale gills. The anemia and decreasing plasma protein were suggestive of hemorrhage. The persistence of the toxic heterophils and neutrophils indicated accelerated production that is often related to bacterial infections or other inflammatory conditions. Because the two other nurse sharks died from hemorrhagic and necrotic enteritis, ultrasound imaging was planned; however, the shark died before the imaging could be performed. The gross necropsy revealed hemorrhagic enteritis.

Two days after the death of this shark, the shovelnose guitarfish died, and nine days later, the bat ray died. The

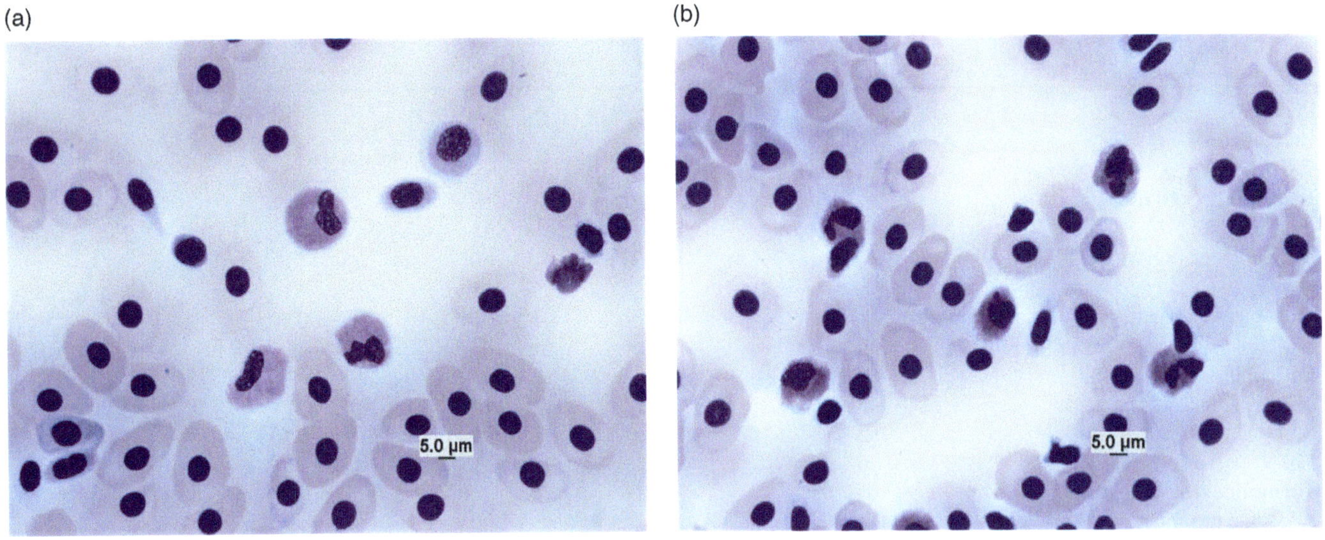

Fig. 29.1. (a), (b) Blood film from an adult male nurse shark (*Ginglymostoma cirratum* (Wright–Giemsa stain, 100× oil).

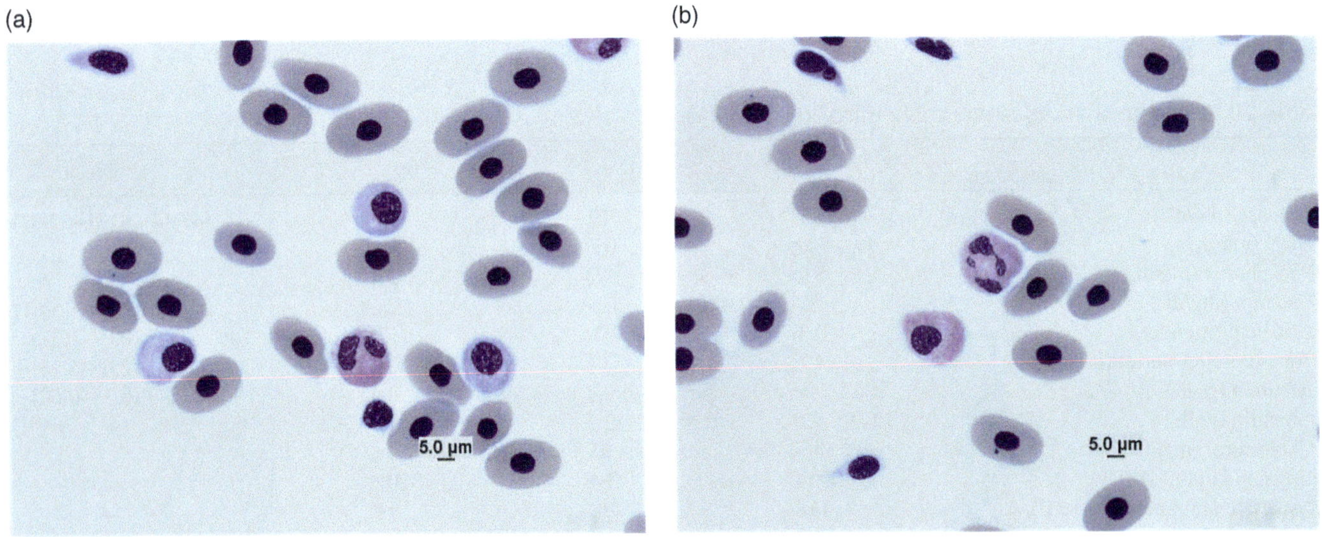

Fig. 29.2. (a) Blood film from an adult male nurse shark (*Ginglymostoma cirratum*) with three mildly toxic neutrophils, one mildly toxic heterophil, one lymphocyte, and one thrombocyte (Wright–Giemsa stain, 100× oil). (b) Blood film from an adult male nurse shark (*Ginglymostoma cirratum*) with two mildly toxic heterophils (one with a segmented nucleus and one with a non-segmented nucleus) and three spindle-shaped thrombocytes (Wright–Giemsa stain, 100× oil).

guitarfish histopathology revealed an enteritis, pigment accumulation in the liver, and chronic perivascular myocarditis. The bat ray histopathology revealed a severe hemorrhagic enteritis, coelomitis, pigment accumulation in the liver, and edema in the heart, kidney, and epigonal organ. Upon further investigation of these mortalities, it was identified that these fish were subjected to fenbendazole treatments prior to being shipped. The pathology observed involving the gastrointestinal tract, liver, and hematopoietic organs was likely the result of fenbendazole toxicity. Fenbendazole overdoses as well as therapeutic doses have been identified as resulting in toxicities in elasmobranchs and therefore should be avoided or used with extreme caution (Garner, 2013; Hadfield and Clayton, 2017; Stedman and Garner, 2018). Additional treatment in this case could have included a blood transfusion from a healthy nurse shark. This type of treatment has not been performed in this species, but has been used in cownose rays with some success (McDermott Delaune et al., 2017). As a precaution, the reticulate whipray was treated with enrofloxacin at a dose of 5 mg/kg orally once every 48 h for two weeks (see Case 2 in this chapter).

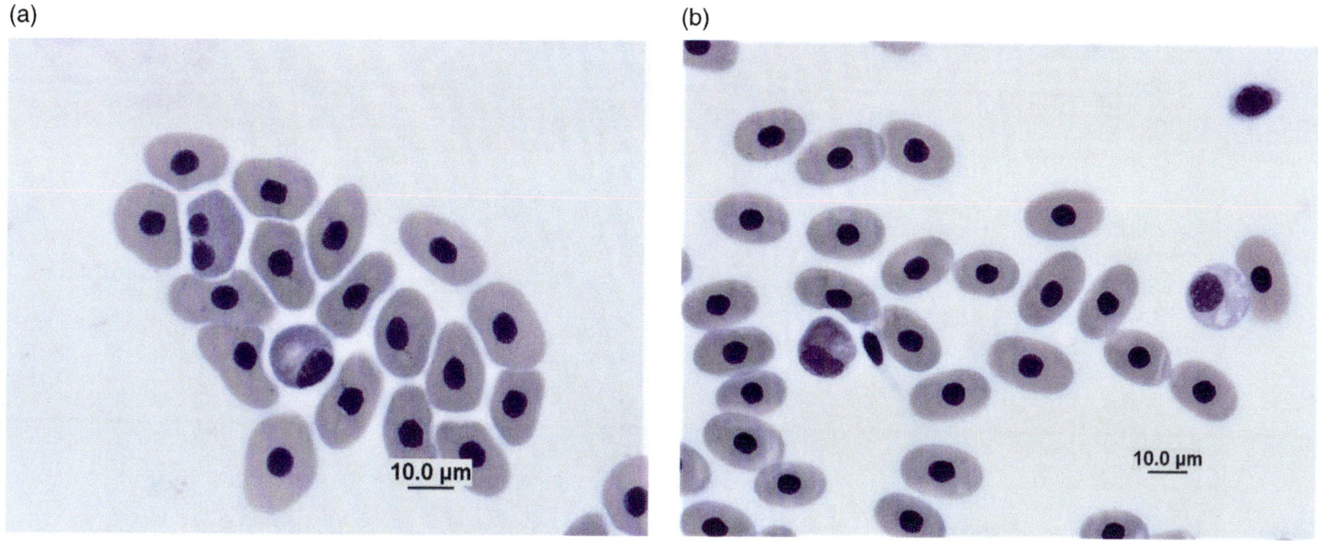

Fig. 29.3. (a) Blood film from an adult male nurse shark (*Ginglymostoma cirratum*) with one eosinophil (or G_3, type III granulocyte) and one heterophil with a non-segmented nucleus (Wright–Giemsa stain, 100× oil). (b) Blood film from an adult male nurse shark (*Ginglymostoma cirratum*) with a heterophil, neutrophil, and two thrombocytes (Wright–Giemsa stain, 100× oil).

Case 2: Reticulated Stingray with Bite Wounds

Signalment

An adult reticulate whipray (*Himantura uarnak*)

History

This reticulate whipray was among a group of elasmobranchs – including three nurse sharks (*Ginglymostoma cirratum*), a shovelnose guitarfish (*Rhinobatos productus*), and a bat ray (*Myliobatis californica*) – that recently arrived at a public aquarium after being transferred from another commercial facility. The nurse sharks, guitarfish, and bat ray all died within two-and-a-half months of arrival. Their deaths were attributed to fenbendazole toxicity; they were treated with fenbendazole before being shipped. The reticulate whipray was also exposed to the treatment, but did not show clinical signs (hemorrhagic enteritis with resulting anemia) upon, or shortly after, arrival. Once fenbendazole toxicity was suspected, the reticulate whipray was treated with enrofloxacin for two weeks as a precaution. The ray was moved to an appropriate exhibit following treatment with no issues; however, it was shortly removed and placed back into quarantine because of bite wounds, presumably from other stingrays.

Physical Examination

For the physical examination, the reticulate whipray was moved into a large rolling bin (Figures 29.4a and 29.4b). Superficial wounds were noted along the edge of the wings and on the tail; otherwise the physical exam was unremarkable. Blood was collected via caudal venipuncture prior to an ultrasound examination. A CBC and plasma biochemistry profile were performed (Tables 29.3 and 29.4 and Figures 29.5a–29.5d). No abnormal findings were noted on sonography.

Interpretive Discussion

Because reference intervals for this species were unavailable, the laboratory results were compared to known reference intervals from the southern stingray at the aquarium. The CBC and plasma biochemistry profile findings were unremarkable. The hemic cells in the blood film appeared normal. Figure 29.5a revealed one eosinophil, one heterophil, two small lymphocytes, and one medium lymphocyte. Figure 29.5b revealed one heterophil and two lymphocytes. Figure 29.5c revealed two heterophils, one lymphocyte, and one thrombocyte. Figure 29.5d revealed two heterophils, one eosinophil, two small lymphocytes, and two medium lymphocytes.

Summary

The ray recovered from the bite wounds and was returned to the exhibit approximately seven weeks later, but quickly returned to quarantine after being bitten by an eel. He was later moved to a larger shark quarantine tank to recover, where his left clasper was amputated by another shark. Antibiotics were administered (Nuflor® 600mg IM once every five days for seven treatments), and he recovered and was eventually moved to a large exhibit after five months in quarantine from both traumatic events.

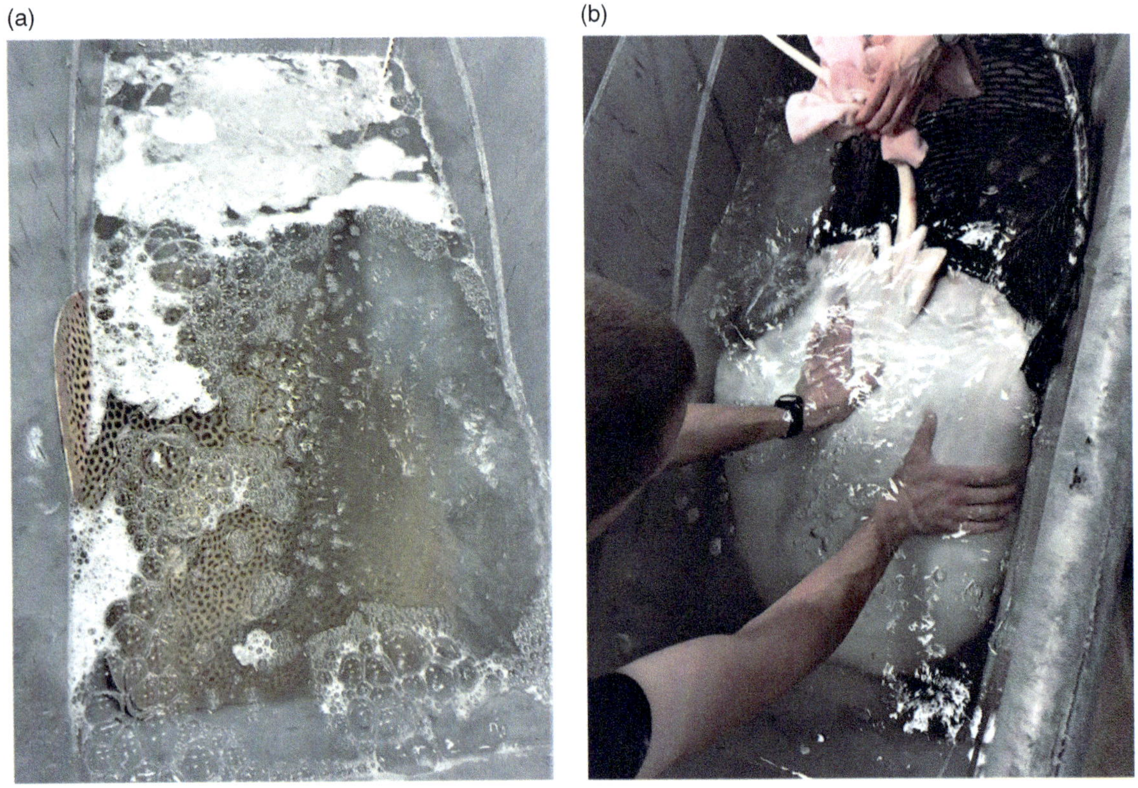

Fig. 29.4. (a), (b) The whipray in preparation for the physical examination.

Table 29.3. Reticulate whipray hematology results (Case 2).

		Reference[a] (*Hypanus americanus*)
PCV (%)	23	24 (21–31)
Leukocytes		
WBC (×10³/μL)	10.0	18 (3.8–40.2)
Heterophils (×10³/μL)	4.3	3.9 (1.0–8.8)
(%)	43	—
Lymphocytes (×10³/μL)	4.5	8.9 (2.5–30.1)
(%)	45	—
Monocytes (×10³/μL)	0.3	0.2 (0.1–0.8)
(%)	3	—
Eosinophils (×10³/μL)	0.9	0.7 (0.1–2.1)
(%)	9	—
Basophils (×10³/μL)	0	0 (0.0–0.1)
(%)	0	—
Thrombocytes		
Adequate thrombocytes	—	
Plasma protein (refractometry) (g/dL)	6.3	5.6 (5.4–6.2)
Notes		

[a] Grant and Campbell (2020).

Table 29.4. Reticulate whipray plasma biochemical results (Case 2).

		Reference[a] (*Hypanus americanus*)
Glucose (mg/dL)	—	38 (27–45)
BUN (mg/dL)	775	1110 (780–1330)
Phosphorus (mg/dL)	5.4	4.0 (3.1–7.1)
Calcium (mg/dL)	16.2	15.5 (14.6–17.2)
Uric acid (mg/dL)	—	—
Total protein (biuret) (g/dL)	—	2.5 (2.3–2.8)
Albumin (g/dL)	—	—
Globulin (g/dL)	—	—
Cholesterol (mg/dL)	—	122 (23–176)
Creatine kinase (IU/L)	—	371 (114–784)
Aspartate aminotransferase (IU/L)	7	11 (6–16)
Sodium (mEq/L)	—	277 (258–292)
Potassium (mEq/L)	—	3.7 (2.1–5.8)
Chloride (mEq/L)	—	285 (259–313)

[a] Grant and Campbell (2020).

Case 3: Southern Stingray with Anorexia

Signalment

Adult female southern stingray (*Hypanus americanus/Dasyatis americana*)

History

This stingray was housed in a large dining exhibit in a public aquarium with several other aquatic animals, including other elasmobranch and teleost fish. She was recently acquired from another public aquarium and transferred to this aquarium approximately three months prior to presentation. This stingray was moved into

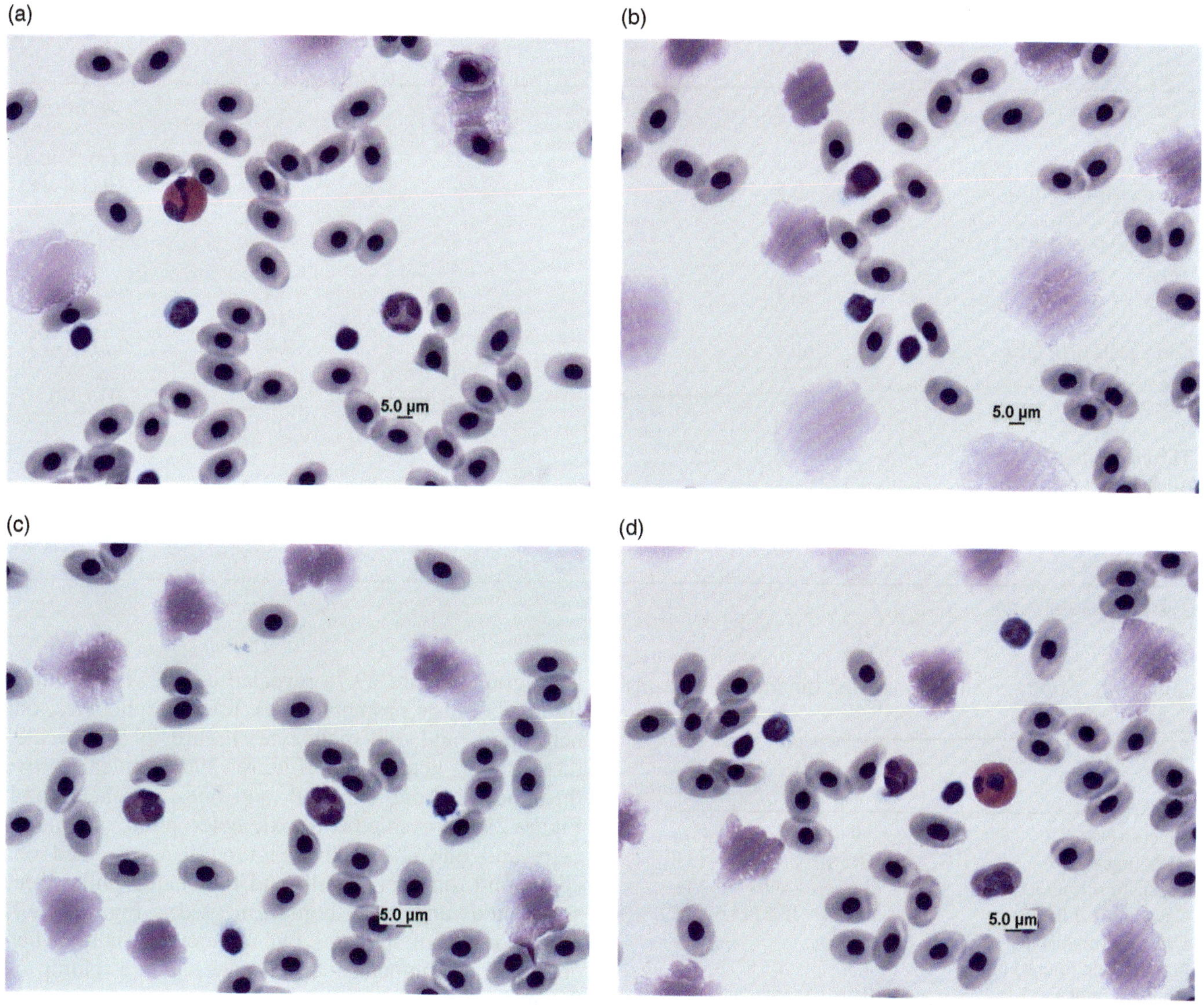

Fig. 29.5. (a)–(d) Blood film from an adult reticulate whipray (*Himantura uarnak*) (Wright–Giemsa stain, 100× oil).

quarantine from its exhibit because she was not eating. She also had red patches on the underside of her wings, and the wings were curled. She, along with two other female southern stingrays, were removed from the exhibit and placed in a quarantine tank together. The other two stingrays had similar lesions on their wings. All three stingrays had been in quarantine and were eating while in quarantine for approximately two weeks prior to examination.

Physical Examination

Upon physical examination, the stingray's disc width was approximately 65 cm. She was bright, alert, and responsive, and there were several superficial skin lesions along the margins of her wings (Figure 29.6). An ultrasound examination revealed the liver to be half the expected length, indicating she was in poor condition,

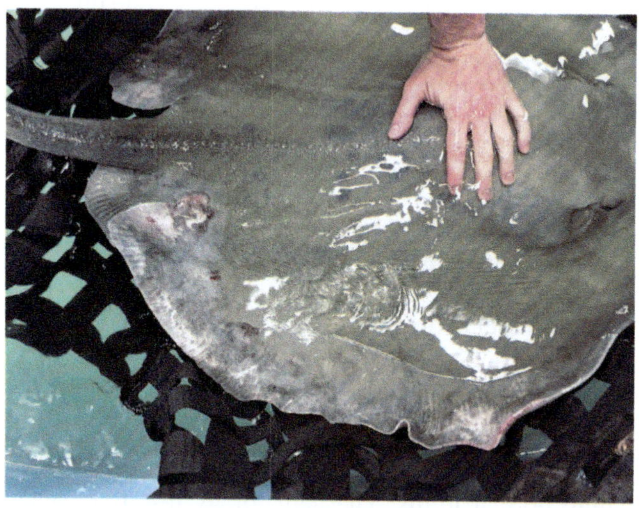

Fig. 29.6. Female southern stingray during physical examination.

Table 29.5. Southern stingray hematology results (Case 3).

	Day 1	Day 15	Day 29	Day 56	Reference[a]
PCV (%)	47	30	28	—	24 (21–31)
Leukocytes					
WBC (×10³/μL)	5.6	11.5	22.0	21.3	18 (3.8–40.2)
Heterophils (×10³/μL)	3.5	4.0	9.7	12.2	3.9 (1.0–8.8)
(%)	63	35	44	57	—
Lymphocytes (×10³/μL)	1.4	4.7	9.2	4.1	8.9 (2.5–30.1)
(%)	25	41	42	19	—
Monocytes (×10³/μL)	0.3	0.1	0.9	3.4	0.2 (0.1–0.8)
(%)	5	1	4	16	—
Eosinophils (×10³/μL)	0.4	2.6	2.4	1.7	0.7 (0.1–2.1)
(%)	7	23	11	8	—
Basophils (×10³/μL)	0	0	0	0	0 (0.0–0.1)
(%)	0	0	0	0	—
Thrombocytes					
Adequate thrombocytes					
Plasma protein (refractometry)	Exist				
(g/dL)	4.5	5.5	5.0	—	5.6 (5.4–6.2)
Notes					

[a]Grant and Campbell (2020).

Table 29.6. Southern stingray plasma biochemical results (Case 3).

		Reference[a] (*Hypanus americanus*)
Glucose (mg/dL)	39	38 (27–45)
BUN (mg/dL)	1045	1110 (780–1330)
Phosphorus (mg/dL)	3.6	4.0 (3.1–7.1)
Calcium (mg/dL)	13.6	15.5 (14.6–17.2)
Uric acid (mg/dL)	0	—
Total protein (biuret) (g/dL)	2.3	2.5 (2.3–2.8)
Ablumin (g/dL)	0.5	—
Globulin (g/dL)	1.8	—
Cholesterol (mg/dL)	106	122 (23–176)
Creatine kinase (IU/L)	1351	371 (114–784)
Aspartate aminotransferase (IU/L)	36	11 (6–16)
Sodium (mEq/L)	265	277 (258–292)
Potassium (mEq/L)	3.7	3.7 (2.1–5.8)
Chloride (mEq/L)	273	285 (259–313)

[a]Grant and Campbell (2020).

and had a distended uterus filled with material and fluid. Blood was collected for a CBC and plasma biochemistry profile (Tables 29.5 and 29.6). Blood films were made to evaluate the leukocyte morphology (Figures 29.7a–29.7f).

Interpretive Discussion

The plasma biochemistry profile parameters were within normal limits. The hematology results revealed an elevated PCV with a low plasma protein, an increased H:L, and toxic heterophils indicating an inflammatory leukogram. Figure 29.7a revealed a cell with a mitotic figure (possibly prometaphase), four lymphocytes, one heterophil, and one monocyte. Figure 29.7b revealed three toxic heterophils. Figure 29.7c revealed two thrombocytes, one basophil, and one toxic heterophil. Figure 29.7d revealed two toxic heterophils, one monocyte, and one eosinophil. Figure 29.7e revealed one eosinophil, one neutrophil, and four heterophils (three segmented and one non-segmented). Figure 29.7f revealed two lymphocytes, two monocytes, six toxic heterophils, an immature erythrocyte, and a clump of thrombocytes.

Summary

Based on the initial findings on CBC and sonography, a female southern stingray reproductive disease was suspected. Female southern stingrays at this aquarium were well studied due to the reproductive changes observed in the captive population. The reproductive changes have been noted at other facilities as well and include findings such as multiple mature follicles in an enlarged left ovary, cystic follicles, a large uterus often with trephonemata (spatulated projections of the uterine mucosa that increase the surface area to deliver histotroph) filled with histotroph (uterine milk secretions) (Grant, 2016; Stedman and Garner, 2018). The ovarian findings appear somewhat like those seen in oviparous animals undergoing follicular stasis. Southern stingray reproduction is described as aplacental viviparous (ovoviviparous) as the egg capsules are fertilized and hatched within the female ray. The trephonemata and histotroph serve as the nutrient delivery system as the pup

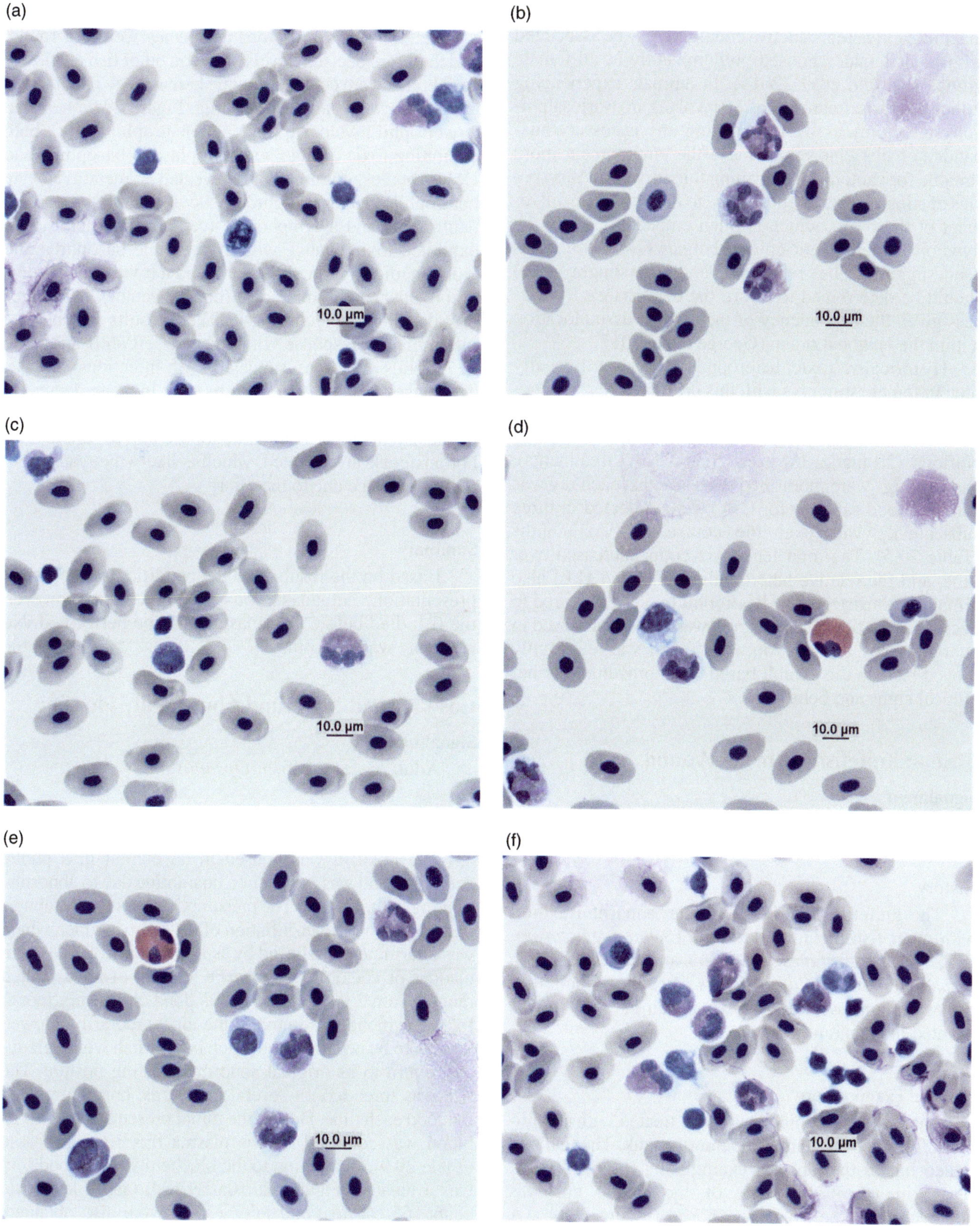

Fig. 29.7. (a)–(f) Blood film from an adult southern stingray (*Hypanus americanus*) on Day 1.

transitions from the yolk sac. It has also been speculated that this captive reproductive condition may be associated with adult females housed predominantly in all-female groups (Penfold et al., 2014). In animals experiencing follicular stasis, treatment often involves an ovariosalpingohysterectomy as well as making any necessary husbandry or diet changes to make the environment more suitable for captivity. Performing this surgery in this species of stingray is challenging due to the intimate involvement of the ovary, which is often embedded within the dynamic hematopoietic epigonal organ. Ovariectomy has been suggested, but reproductive status (stingray size) should be determined to afford the best chance for success given the dependency of the ovarian tissue location within the epigonal organ (George et al., 2017).

Historically, toxic heterophils were not typically seen in female stingrays with this presumptive reproductive condition; therefore, a concurrent infection was suspected. The stingray was maintained in quarantine on Nuflor® (20 mg/kg IM every 5 days for 7 treatments), and feedings were monitored to ensure that each ray was eating. Blood samples for CBC were collected in three subsequent visits over the course of two months (Table 29.5). The total leukocyte count increased over time, and the relative heterophilia (increased H:L) also remained consistent. The heterophil toxicity appeared to decrease over time. The stingray was closely observed in quarantine by the aquarium staff and was eventually moved back to the exhibit based on improvement of her clinical signs and behavior.

Case 4: Knifefish with Tail Wound

Signalment

Adult knifefish (*Chitala chitala*)

History

The knifefish was housed in an aquarium exhibit with other fish including arowana (*Scleropages formosus*), barramundi (*Lates calcarifer*), arapaima (*Arapaima gigas*), and turtles (*Carettochelys insculpta*). The knifefish was found with a large wound on its tail and was isolated in a quarantine tank.

Physical Examination

The knifefish, which was being treated with an antibiotic, was observed in the quarantine tank. The fish was pulled out of the tank for examination (Figure 29.8a). Approximately two inches of the caudal tail was degloved with the fin rays exposed (Figure 29.8b). A blood sample was collected (Figure 29.8c) for CBC, plasma biochemistry profile (Tables 29.7 and 29.8), and to evaluate blood films (Figures 29.9a–29.9d), but the fish was given a poor prognosis.

Interpretive Discussion

Reference intervals for this species were not found, and therefore decision levels based on other fish and lower vertebrates were considered. The hematology results indicate leukocytosis and neutrophilia. Figure 29.9a revealed a neutrophil myelocyte (left) and neutrophil (right), both exhibiting toxic change with cytoplasmic basophilia and Döhle bodies. Figure 29.9b revealed a metamyelocyte neutrophil (center). Figure 29.9c revealed three toxic neutrophils and a lymphocyte (center). The neutrophils exhibited toxic change with cytoplasmic basophilia and Döhle bodies. Figure 29.9d revealed a toxic band neutrophil (center) and lymphocyte (bottom center). All figures revealed slight polychromasia. These results indicated an inflammatory response with a severe left shift and toxic neutrophils therefore suggestive of infectious disease. The plasma biochemistry results may indicate decreased glucose and protein, which may be a result of the lack of dietary intake. The creatine kinase and aspartate aminotransferase are elevated, which is likely the result from muscle damage due to the injury.

Summary

Based on the results and the condition of the fish at presentation, euthanasia was recommended; however, the fish died before euthanasia could be performed. No necropsy was performed.

Case 5: Toadfish Found Abnormally Floating

Signalment

Adult oyster toadfish (*Opsanus tau*)

History

The toadfish was housed in an exhibit in a public aquarium, and was moved into quarantine due to abnormal floating in the exhibit. The presumptive cause of the abnormal floating was over-inflation of the swim bladder, which was intermittently relieved by aspirating air from the swim bladder or coelomic cavity. The amount of air aspirated ranged from 2 to 12 mL and was done once every month for three months. Removing the air temporarily allowed the fish to be negatively buoyant, but the fish would gradually return to its original abnormal floating posture. The fish was force-fed on several occasions, but regurgitated the food each time. During the initial presentation (Day 1), blood was collected for the plasma biochemical profile (Table 29.9). In addition to the biochemistry, a blood film was evaluated (Figures 29.10a–29.10d), and a leukocyte count (55 600/μL) and PCV (26%) were also obtained. Empirical treatment with antibiotics (Nuflor® 30 mg/kg IM) resulted in no improvement; therefore, two months later, the fish presented for a recheck and diagnostic work-up.

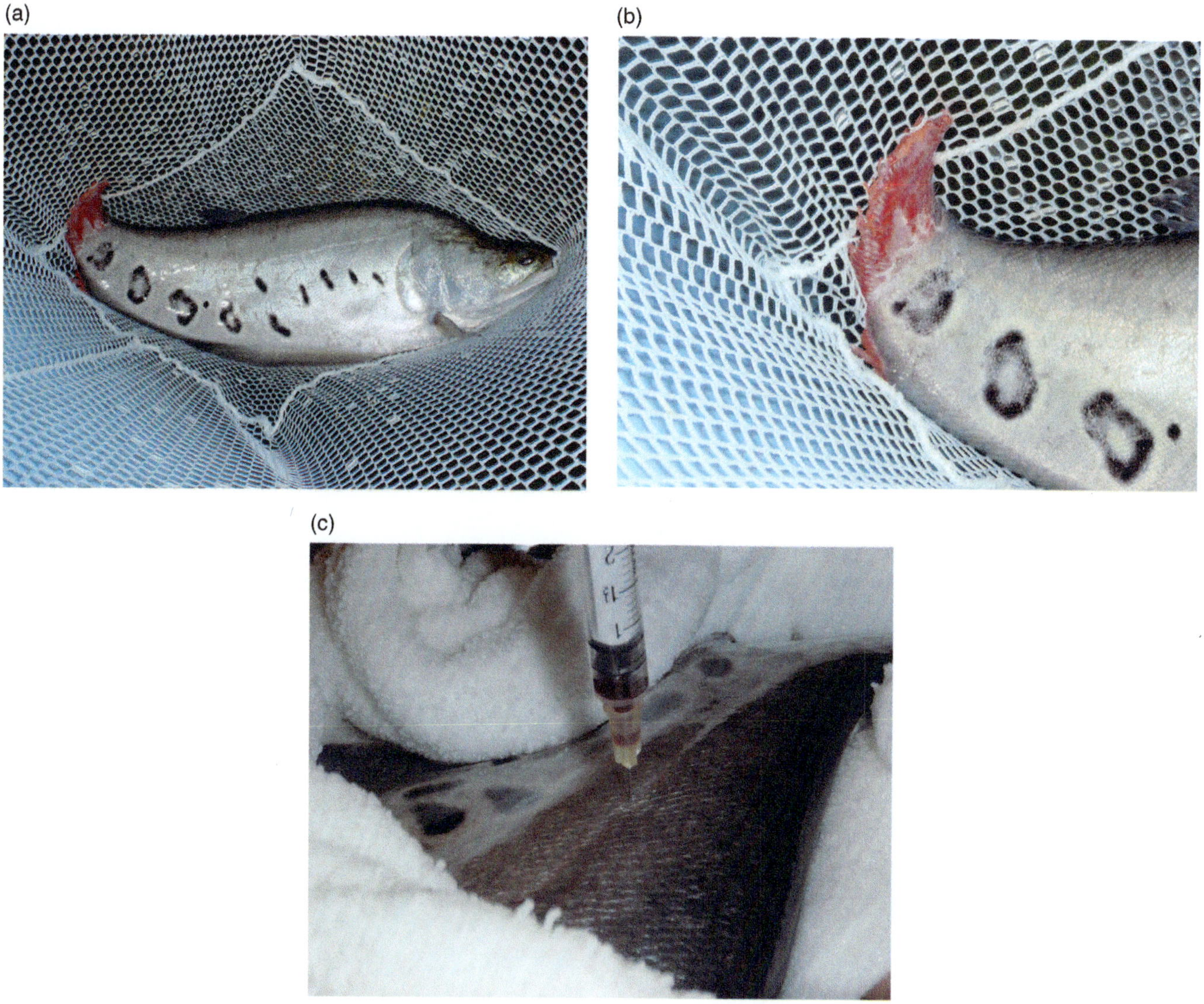

Fig. 29.8. (a) Knifefish during physical examination. (b) A close-up of the knifefish tail wound with bone exposure. (c) The lateral approach to collecting blood from the caudal vessels in a knifefish.

Physical Examination

Upon physical examination, the 240 g toadfish was observed as positively buoyant in the transport tank. The fish was easily handled for the exam (Figure 29.11a). An ulcerative skin lesion was noted around the vent (Figure 29.11b). Blood was collected from the tail vein using a ventral approach to recheck the plasma biochemistry profile and blood film (Table 29.9 and Figures 29.12a–29.12d). Radiographs were also taken (Figures 29.13a and 29.13b).

Interpretive Discussion

The plasma biochemistry profile was unremarkable except for the high BUN on the initial screening; however, this later dropped to within normal range. The initial elevated BUN could indicate the fish had difficulty excreting urea through the gill epithelium (Campbell, 2012).

Review of the blood film revealed the presence of toxic neutrophils based upon increased cytoplasmic basophilia. Figure 29.12a shows a marked increase in polychromatic erythrocytes and monocyte. Figure 29.12b shows two thrombocytes, a degenerate lymphocyte, and numerous polychromatic erythrocytes. Figure 29.12c shows a toxic neutrophil and three thrombocytes as well as a marked increase in erythrocyte polychromasia. Figure 29.12d shows three toxic neutrophils, a thrombocyte, and marked polychromasia. The toxic neutrophils are indicated by the increased basophilia. These findings support the presence of an inflammatory leukogram and a marked erythrocyte regenerative response.

The dorsoventral radiographic image (Figure 29.13a) reveals the heart-shaped swim bladder located in the

Table 29.7. Knifefish hematology results (Case 4).

PCV (%)	22
Leukocytes	
WBC (×10³/μL)	22.3
Myelocytes (×10³/μL)	0.4
%	2
Metamyelocytes (×10³/μL)	0.4
%	2
Bands (×10³/μL)	1.3
%	6
Neutrophils (×10³/μL)	13.6
(%)	61
Lymphocytes (×10³/μL)	6.2
(%)	28
Monocytes (×10³/μL)	0.2
(%)	1
Eosinophils (×10³/μL)	0
(%)	0
Basophils (×10³/μL)	0
(%)	0
Thrombocytes	
Adequate thrombocytes	Clumped
Plasma protein (refractometry)	
(g/dL)	2.1

Table 29.8. Knifefish plasma biochemical results (Case 4).

Glucose (mg/dL)	26
BUN (mg/dL)	2
Phosphorus (mg/dL)	2.6
Calcium (mg/dL)	7.8
Uric acid (mg/dL)	0.2
Total protein (biuret) (g/dL)	1.8
Albumin (g/dL)	0.7
Globulin (g/dL)	1.1
Cholesterol (mg/dL)	49
Creatine kinase (IU/L)	13 081
Aspartate aminotransferase (IU/L)	297
Sodium (mEq/L)	129
Potassium (mEq/L)	2.0
Chloride (mEq/L)	98

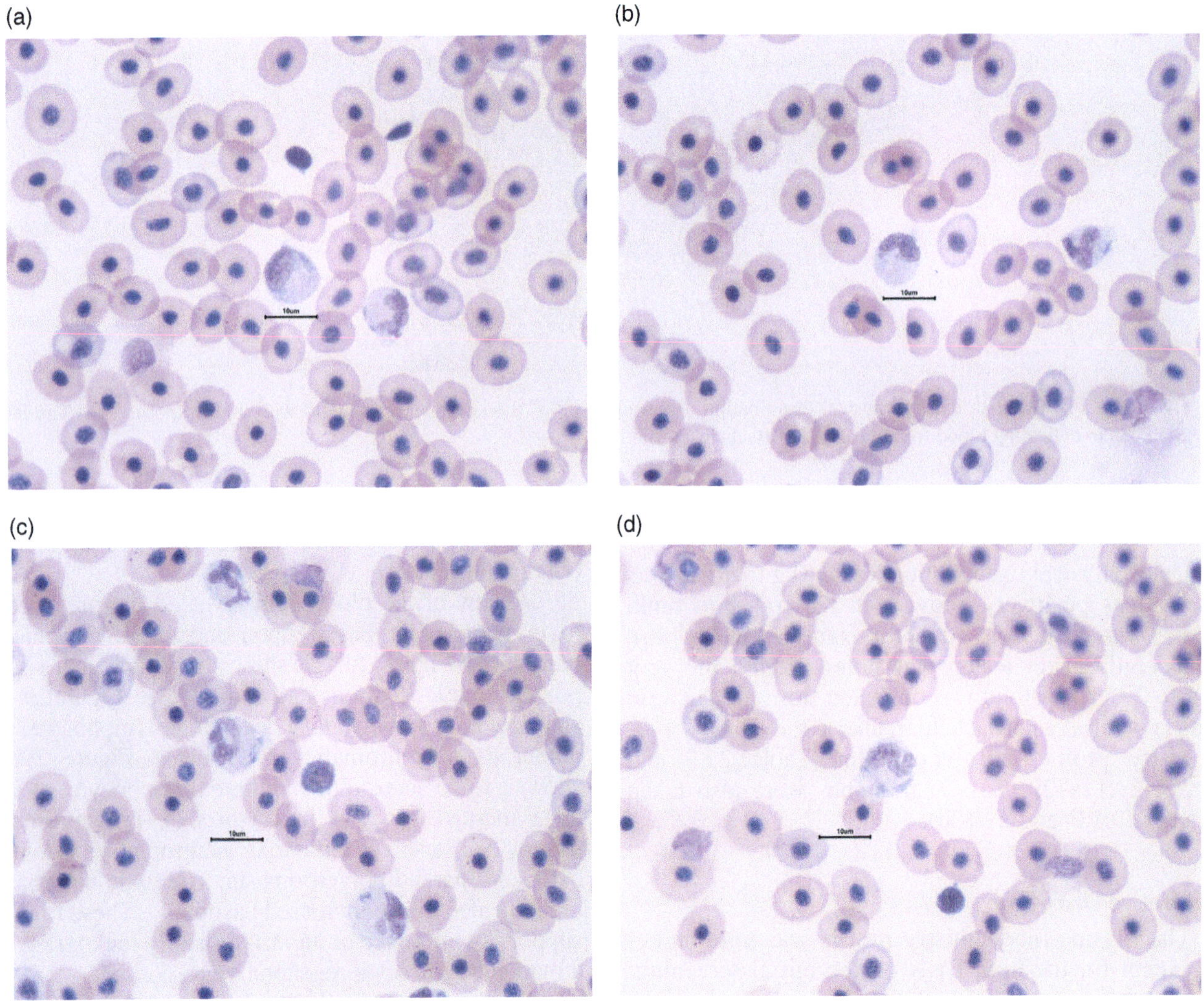

Fig. 29.9. (a)–(d) Blood film from an adult knifefish (*Chitala chitala*) (Wright–Giemsa stain, 100× oil).

Table 29.9. Toadfish plasma biochemical results (Case 5).

	Day 1	Day 64	Reference[a]
Glucose (mg/dL)	21	17	25 (19–34)
BUN (mg/dL)	71	9	12 (1.3–29.2)
Phosphorus (mg/dL)	4.7	4.5	—
Calcium (mg/dL)	9.7	9.8	9.2 (8.4–10.1)
Uric acid (mg/dL)	0.1	0	1.3 (1.1–1.4)
Total protein (biuret) (g/dL)	4.1	4.5	4.9 (4.0–5.4)
Albumin (g/dL)	0.9	1.3	—
Globulin (g/dL)	3.2	3.2	—
Cholesterol (mg/dL)	163	194	124 (87–183)
Creatine kinase (IU/L)	1123	259	—
Aspartate aminotransferase (IU/L)	11	3	—
Sodium (mEq/L)	166	160	—
Potassium (mEq/L)	3.9	3.5	—
Chloride (mEq/L)	148	140	—

[a] Mensinger (2005).

cranial aspect of the coelomic cavity. The heart shape is the normal shape of this species (Barimo and Fine, 1998). Although a standard technique for assessing the size of the swim bladder has yet to be established, upon comparison with published normal images (presumptive), the swim bladder appeared to be hyperinflated based on the number of vertebrae to which it extended (Barimo and Fine, 1998; Edds-Walton et al., 2015). It is worth noting that this fish was likely underconditioned, which may contribute to the subjective assessment of the swim bladder being hyperinflated. The lateral radiographic image (Figure 29.13b) revealed that the swim bladder extended almost the entire depth of the coelomic cavity. The swim bladder was somewhat masked by the overlay of the pectoral fins, but the compartmentalization of the swim bladder was appreciated as it was in the dorsal view. Just caudal

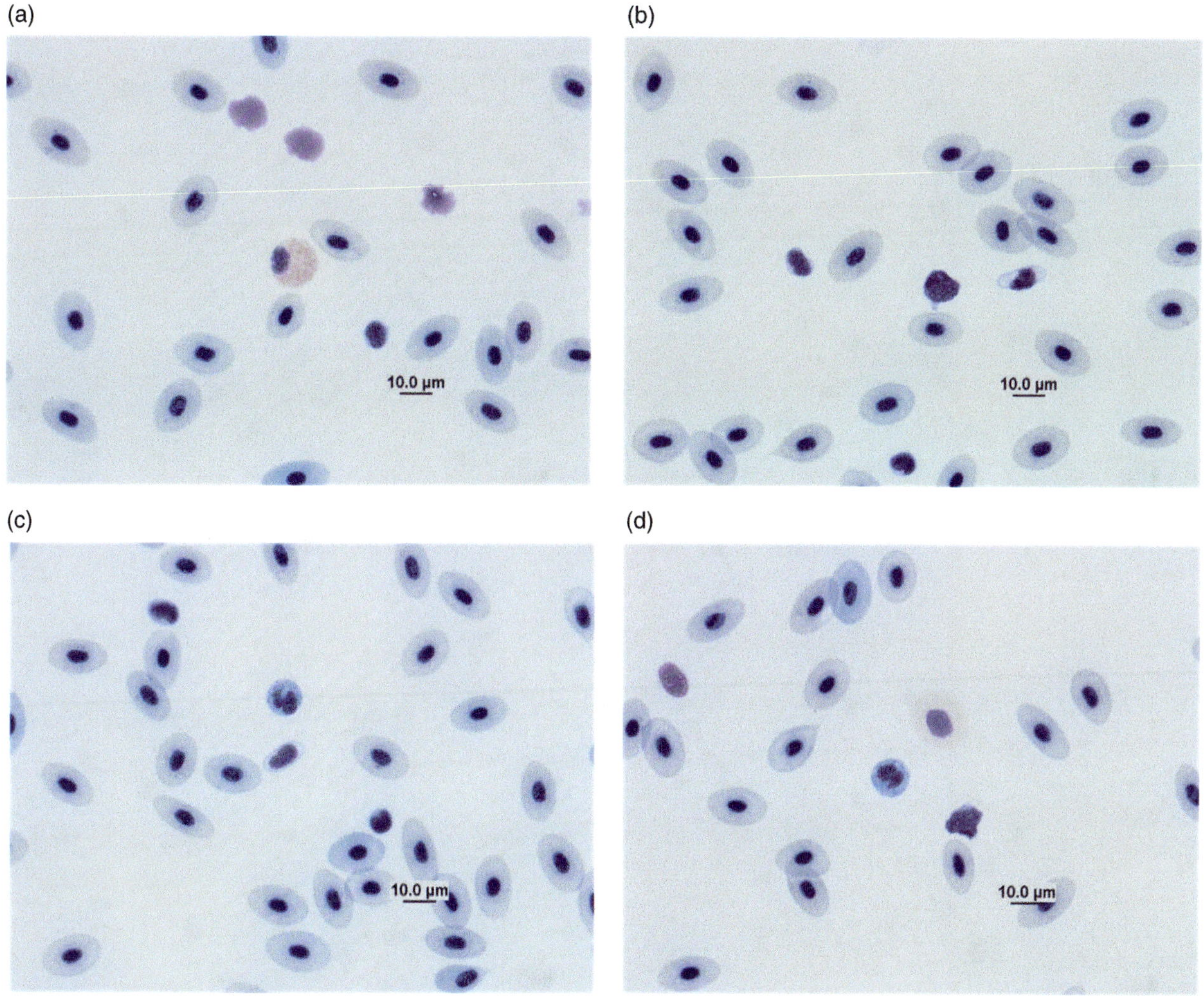

Fig. 29.10. (a) Day 1 Blood film from an oyster toadfish (*Opsanus tau*) showing an eosinophil and thrombocyte (Wright–Giemsa stain, 100× oil). (b) Day 1 Blood film from an oyster toadfish (*Opsanus tau*) showing a lymphocyte and two thrombocytes (Wright–Giemsa stain, 100× oil). (c) Day 1 Blood film from an oyster toadfish (*Opsanus tau*) showing a toxic neutrophil and three thrombocytes (Wright–Giemsa stain, 100× oil). (d) Day 1 Blood film from an oyster toadfish (*Opsanus tau*) showing a toxic neutrophil, a lymphocyte, and mild polychromasia (Wright–Giemsa stain, 100× oil).

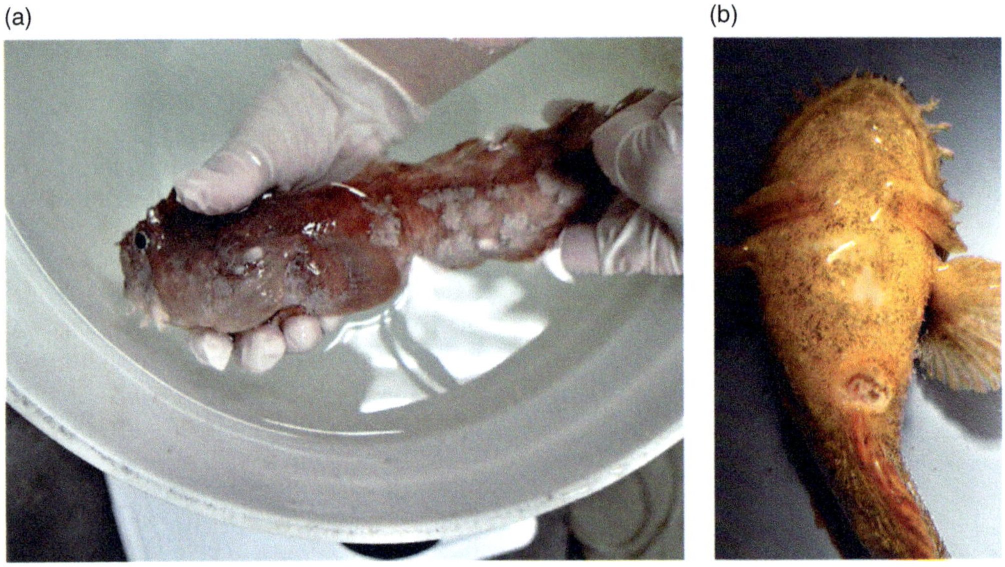

Fig. 29.11. (a) Oyster toadfish during physical examination. (b) Ventral view of toadfish showing inflammation and ulceration around the vent.

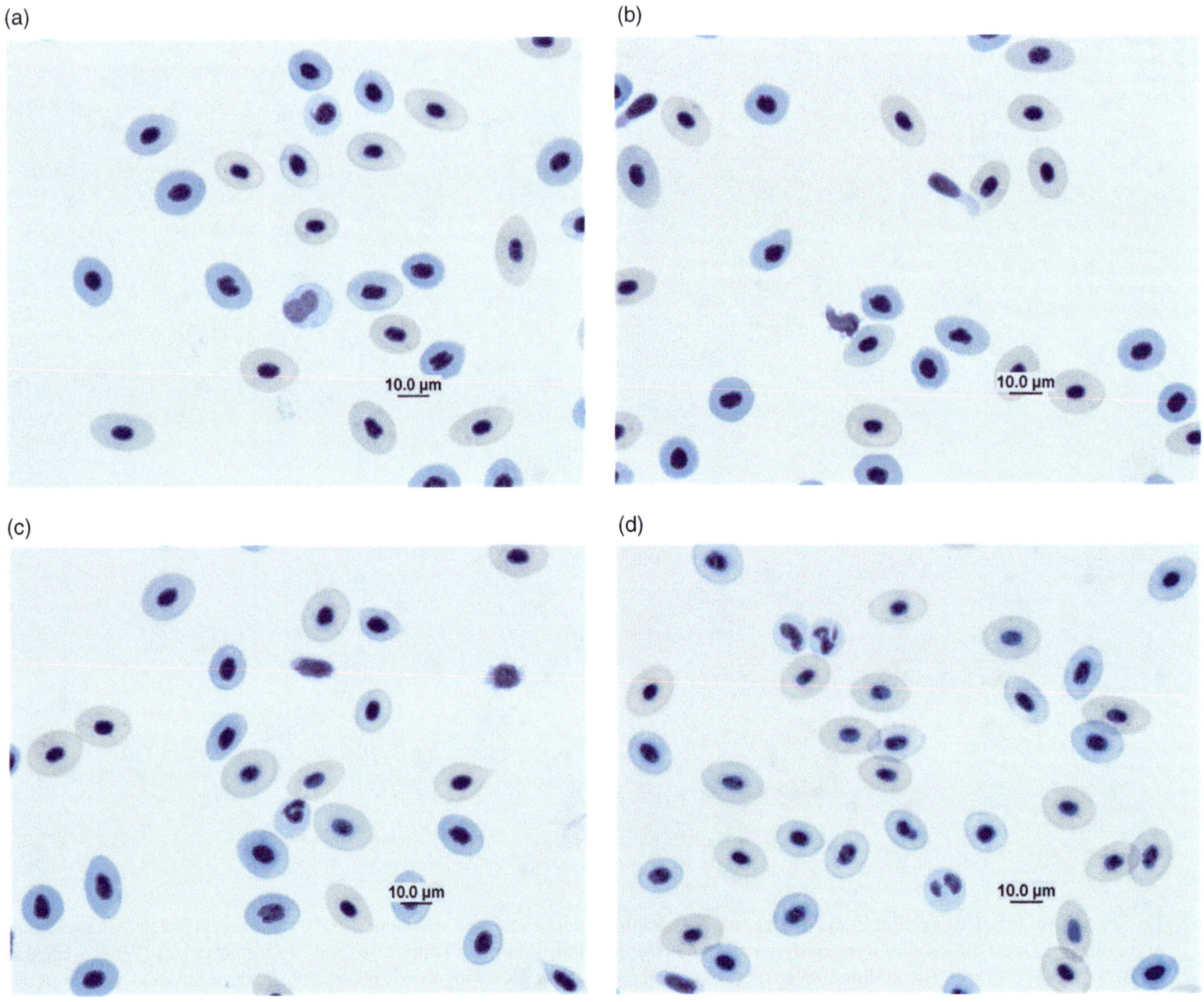

Fig. 29.12. (a)–(d) Blood film from an oyster toadfish (*Opsanus tau*) (Wright–Giemsa stain, 100× oil).

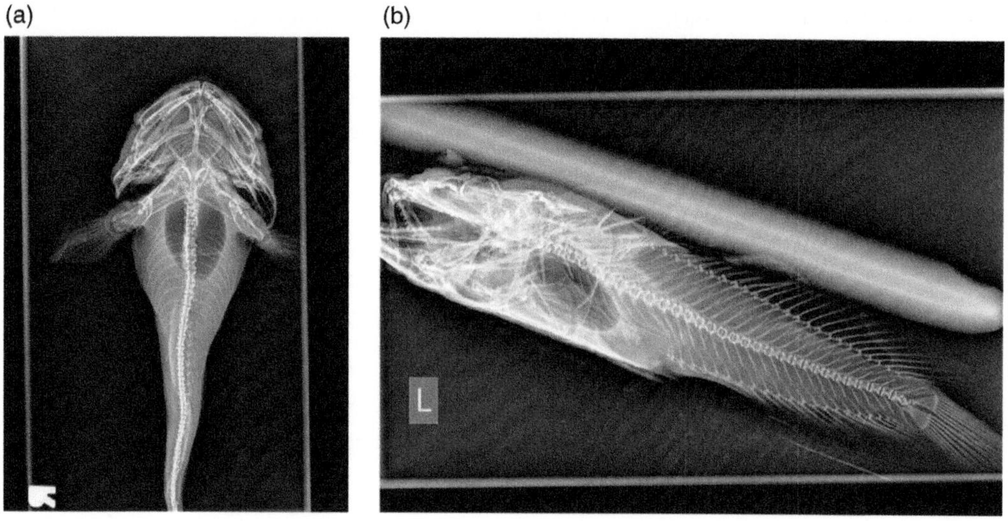

Fig. 29.13. (a) Radiograph of toadfish, dorsoventral view. (b) Radiograph of toadfish, lateral view.

to the swim bladder appeared to be a mineral opacity, perhaps in the gastrointestinal tract. An exploratory surgery was scheduled.

Summary

The toadfish was induced and maintained for anesthesia with MS-222. An exploratory coeliotomy revealed the only significant findings of an enlarged swim bladder. The toadfish recovered uneventfully. Although antibiotic treatment continued for possible bacterial infection, the toadfish showed no improvement and was euthanized five weeks later. Histopathology revealed mild to moderate, lymphocytic and granulocytic aerocystitis; moderate myeloid hyperplasia of the kidney; suspected intra-tubular myxosporidiosis of the kidney; and intestinal myxosporidiosis with mild lymphohistiocytic serositis. *Aeromonas hydrophila*, *Citrobacter freundii*, and *Corynebacterium* spp. were cultured from the swim bladder. The histologic findings in the swim bladder were most consistent with a bacterial aerocystitis, most likely from *Aeromonas hydrophila,* which was presumably the cause of the observed buoyancy problems and inflammatory leukogram. It was suspected that the myxosporidiosis was not clinically significant. It was likely this fish did not respond to treatment because of the poor blood supply to the swim bladder, making it difficult for the antibiotic to reach the source of infection.

References

Barimo JF, Fine ML. 1998. Relationship of swim-bladder shape to the directionality pattern of underwater sound in the oyster toadfish. *Can J Zoo* 76:134–143.

Campbell TW. 2012. Clinical chemistry of fish and amphibians. In: Thrall MA, Weiser G, Allison RW, Campbell TW (eds), *Veterinary Hematology and Clinical Chemistry*, 2nd edn. pp. 607–614.

Edds-Walton PL, Arruda J, Fay RR, Ketten DR. 2015. Computerized tomography of the otic capsule and otoliths in the oyster toadfish, *Opsanus tau*. *J Morph* 276:228–240.

Ferraz MC, Bezerra N, Cavalcanti E, et al. 2014. Bioquímica plasmática del tiburón-gata (ginglymostoma cirratum) capturado en la costa de pernambuco. Brasil, Medellin.

Garner MM. 2013. A retrospective study of disease in elasmobranchs. *Vet Pathol* 50(3):377–389.

George RH, Steeil J, Baine K. 2017. Diagnosis and treatment of common reproductive problems in elasmobranch. In: Smith M, Warmolts D, Thoney D, et al. (eds), *Elasmobranch Husbandry Manual II: Recent Advances in the care of Sharks, Rays and their Relatives*. Columbus, OH: Ohio Biological Survey, Inc., pp. 357–362.

Grant KR. 2016. The process for determining the risk factors involved with the morbidity and mortality of the southern stingray, *Dasyatis americana* at an aquarium. Ann Arbor, MI: ProQuest, LLC.

Grant KR, Campbell TW. 2020. Hematology and plasma biochemistry value differences between acclimated and recently captive female southern stingrays (*Dasyatis americana*). *JZAR* 8(1):1–7.

Hadfield CA, Clayton LA. 2017. Elasmobranch quarantine. In: Smith M, Warmolts D, Thoney D, et al. (eds), *Elasmobranch Husbandry Manual II: Recent Advances in the care of Sharks, Rays and their Relatives*. Columbus, OH: Ohio Biological Survey, Inc., pp. 113–133.

McDermott Delaune AJ, Field CL, Clauss TM. 2017. Whole blood transfusions to treat severe anemia in seven cownose rays (*Rhinoptera bonasus*) and one short-tail stingray (*Dasyatis brevicaudata*). *J Zoo Wild Med* 48(4):1172–1180.

Mensinger AF, Walsh PJ, Hanlon RT. 2005. Blood biochemistry of the oyster toadfish. *J Aq Anim* 17:170–176.

Parkinson LA, Alexander AB, Campbell TW. 2017. Variability in hematology of white-spotted bamboo sharks (*Chiloscyllium plagiosum*) in different living environments. *Zoo Bio* 36:284–288.

Penfold LM, Powell D, Traylor-Holzer K, Asa CS. 2014. "Use it or Lose it": characterization, implications, and mitigation of female infertility in captive wildlife. *Zoo Bio* 33:20–28.

Stedman NL, Garner MM. 2018. Chondrichthyes. In: Terio KA, McAloose D, St. Leger J (eds), *Pathology of Wildlife and Zoo Animals.*, pp. 995–1010.

Walsh CJ, Luer CA. 2004. Elasmobranch hematology: identification of cell types and practical applications. In: Smith M, Warmolts D, Thoney D, Hueter R (eds), Elasmobranch Husbandry Manual: Captive Care of Sharks, Rays, and their Relatives. Columbus, OH: Ohio Biological Survey, Inc., p. 319.

30 Sample Collection for Wet Mounts and Cytodiagnosis in Fish

Whereas diagnostic cytology plays a major role in the diagnosis and management of diseases affecting mammals, birds, and reptiles, diagnostic microscopy using wet-mount techniques plays a major role in the diagnosis and management of fish and amphibian diseases. Diseases readily diagnosed using wet-mount preparations include ectoparasites infestations, lymphocystis, fungal infections, and certain bacterial infections, such as columnaris disease (*Flexibacter columnaris*).

Sampling Techniques for Wet Mounts

Common samples used for wet-mount preparations in the evaluation of fish and amphibian patients include the mucus smear (skin scraping), fin biopsy (fin clip), gill biopsy (gill clip), and fecal specimen. Fluid samples, such as coelomic fluid, are also collected and evaluated in the same manner as fluid evaluation in other species, and not as wet-mount preparations. Blood collection has been discussed in Chapter 25.

Fish and aquatic amphibians should be handled quickly (less than 1 min) and safely during an examination and for sample collection. These animals tend to writhe violently when handled, which predisposes them to traumatic injury. Also, the mucus layer covering the skin makes the skin slippery and proper restraint difficult and unsafe. Safe handling may require sedation or general anesthesia to prevent excessive stress and trauma to the patient. Tricaine methanesulfonate (MS222 Sigma Chemical Co., Saint Louis, MO) in a concentration of 100–150 mg/L is commonly used for fish anesthesia. Higher concentrations are generally required for amphibians (500 mg/L to 3 g/L) (Wright, 2006). Special precautions should be taken regarding the acidification of tricaine-treated water that is poorly buffered. The acidosis created by unbuffered tricaine can cause potentially harmful metabolic changes in the patient (Smit et al., 1979; Groff and Zinkl, 1999). Sodium bicarbonate is often used at equal to two parts of tricaine, or until neutral pH, to buffer the solution (Grant, 2015; Lewbart and Yanong, 2018; Whitaker and McDermott, 2018).

Latex or nitrile surgical gloves without powder should be used when handling these animals to protect their delicate skin from the trauma. Fish and amphibian skin is sensitive to human handling, and the natural oils, soaps, lotions, alcohol, and other chemicals on the handler's skin will damage the skin of these animals. The mucus layer that covers the skin of aquatic animals is a protective surface that should be preserved during handling. Using dry paper or cloth towels, cotton gloves, or bare hands during handling will remove an excessive amount of the mucus coating and damage the skin. Latex or nitrile gloves should be rinsed with water, either from the fish tank or with distilled water, before handling a fish or aquatic amphibian. It should be noted that some salamanders have tail autotomy sites that result in the loss of the tail with improper handling (Wright, 2006). Additional information for capture, handling, and restraint has been discussed in Chapter 25.

An examination includes visual evaluation of the overall body condition, skin, and external structures. The fins are spread for a thorough examination. The oral cavity should be evaluated by carefully opening the mouth. The gills of fish are examined by lifting the opercular covering. The external gills of some aquatic amphibians are examined by direct visualization.

Mucus Smear

The mucus smear is the most commonly used and useful sampling method for evaluation of the fish patient. Because the skin is the first line of defense against

Exotic Animal Hematology and Cytology, Fifth Edition. Terry W. Campbell and Krystan R. Grant.

Companion website: www.wiley.com/go/campbell/exotic

infectious agents, cutaneous lesions are common. Suspected cutaneous bacterial or fungal infections and infestations with ectoparasites are common indications for the evaluation of a mucus smear. Ectoparasites irritate or damage the skin, causing epithelial hyperplasia and increased mucus production, which causes the skin to appear thickened and cloudy.

The procedure is simple; a sample of the mucus covering the surface of the skin is obtained by either pressing the surface of a clean microscope slide onto a skin lesion or gently scraping a small sample of mucus from the skin surface. A scraping can be obtained by using a dull scalpel blade, the blunt edge of a scalpel blade, a spatula, or the edge of a microscope slide or coverslip. The scraping motion should be performed in a cranial to caudal direction with the normal lay of the scales (Figures 30.1a and 30.1b). A light scraping using gentle pressure should be emphasized, as this technique is not analogous to a mammalian skin scraping but rather a method of harvesting a small mucus sample. Excessive pressure applied during the process will damage the skin. After the mucus sample has been transferred to the surface of a microscope slide, a drop of the tank water is added before the coverslip is mounted. The sample is examined under the microscope as a wet-mount preparation. Wet-mount preparations should be examined immediately following sample collection because many of the pathogenic protozoal parasites die quickly under the microscope. A drop of methylcellulose solution (Carolina Biological Supply Company, Burlington, NC) can be added to the sample to slow fast-moving protozoa to aid in their identification. Wet-mount preparations are used to identify ectoparasites, fungi, and bacteria and are more useful in fish diagnostics than air-dried smears stained with Romanowsky stains. If there is a delay in the evaluation of the sample, then the slide should be stored in a humid chamber, such as a plastic container containing moist gauze or towels, to prevent drying.

Fin Biopsy

A fin biopsy or fin clip is performed when visual lesions are observed involving the fin or a mucus smear has failed to identify the cause of a generalized skin disorder involving a fish or amphibian patient. The fin biopsy is a simple procedure. While the fin is spread, a fine-tipped scissor is used to cut a small triangular wedge from the fin tissue (Figures 30.2a–30.2d). The small biopsy wound will heal, as traumatic injury to the fins of fish is a common natural occurrence. The fin biopsy sample is placed onto the surface of a microscope slide, a drop of tank water is added, and a coverslip is mounted to prepare the sample for microscopic examination (Figure 30.3). If part of a fin ray is sampled, it may be difficult to properly seat the coverslip on top of the biopsy, making the evaluation more difficult. Because fin biopsy samples are examined as wet-mount preparations, they should be examined immediately.

Gill Biopsy

The gill biopsy is a useful diagnostic tool in the assessment of a fish patient, especially one exhibiting clinical signs of respiratory disease, such as piping (gulping air at the water air interface) and coughing

(a) (b)

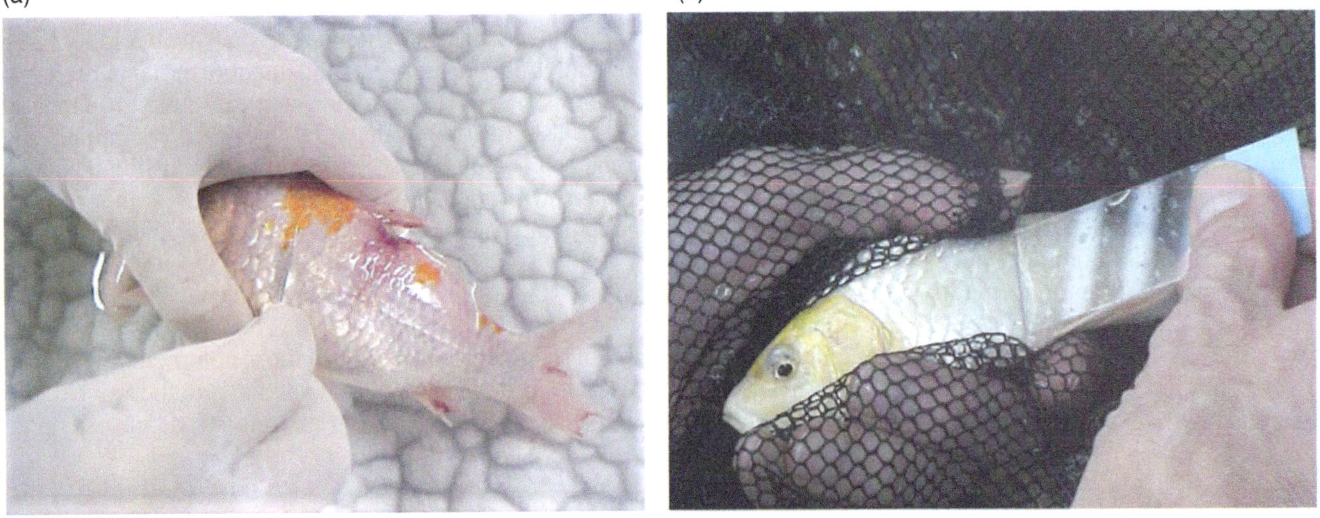

Fig. 30.1. (a) Obtaining a sample for a mucus smear from a koi (*Cyprinus carpio*) using a scalpel blade. (b) Obtaining a sample for a mucus smear from a goldfish (*Carassius auratus*) using the edge of a microscope slide.

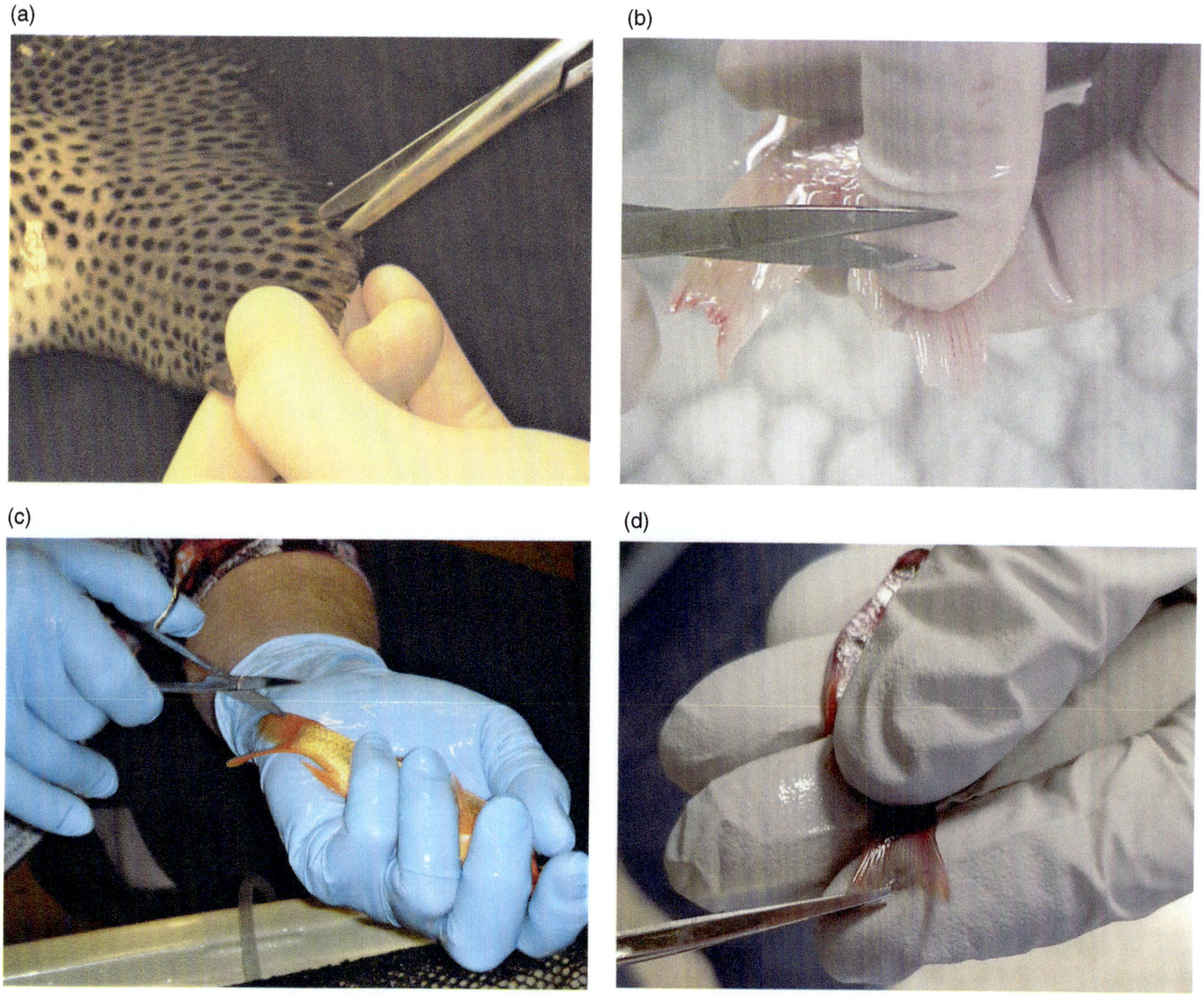

Fig. 30.2. (a) Obtaining a fin biopsy from a rainbow trout (*Oncorhynchus mykiss*). (b) Obtaining a fin biopsy from a koi (*Cyprinus carpio*). (c) Obtaining a fin biopsy from a goldfish (*Carassius auratus*). (d) Obtaining a fin biopsy from a tiger barb (*Puntigrus tetrazona*).

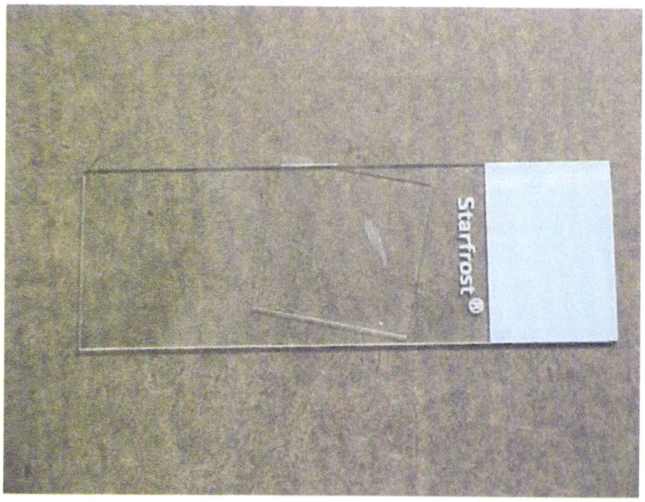

Fig. 30.3. A fin biopsy sample as a wet-mount preparation ready for examination under the microscope.

(flaring of the operculum followed by rapid closure in an attempt to dislodge an irritant from the gills) behavior.

Before obtaining a biopsy, the gills should be examined grossly for signs of gill disease. Normal healthy gills are uniformly bright red. Pale gills are suggestive of anemia, and slightly tan gills suggest methemoglobinemia (Noga, 2000). Gills with areas of discoloration, ulcerations, and missing lamellae should be noted.

A gill biopsy is performed by inserting the tip of a pair of fine-tipped scissors into the gill chamber under the operculum. The tips of a few primary lamellae are cut and removed using the tips of the scissors (Figures 30.4a–30.4d). Bleeding is expected to be minimal if just the outer tips of the primary gill lamellae are sampled. The small gill biopsy is transferred to the surface of a microscope slide. A drop of water from the fish's environment is placed on

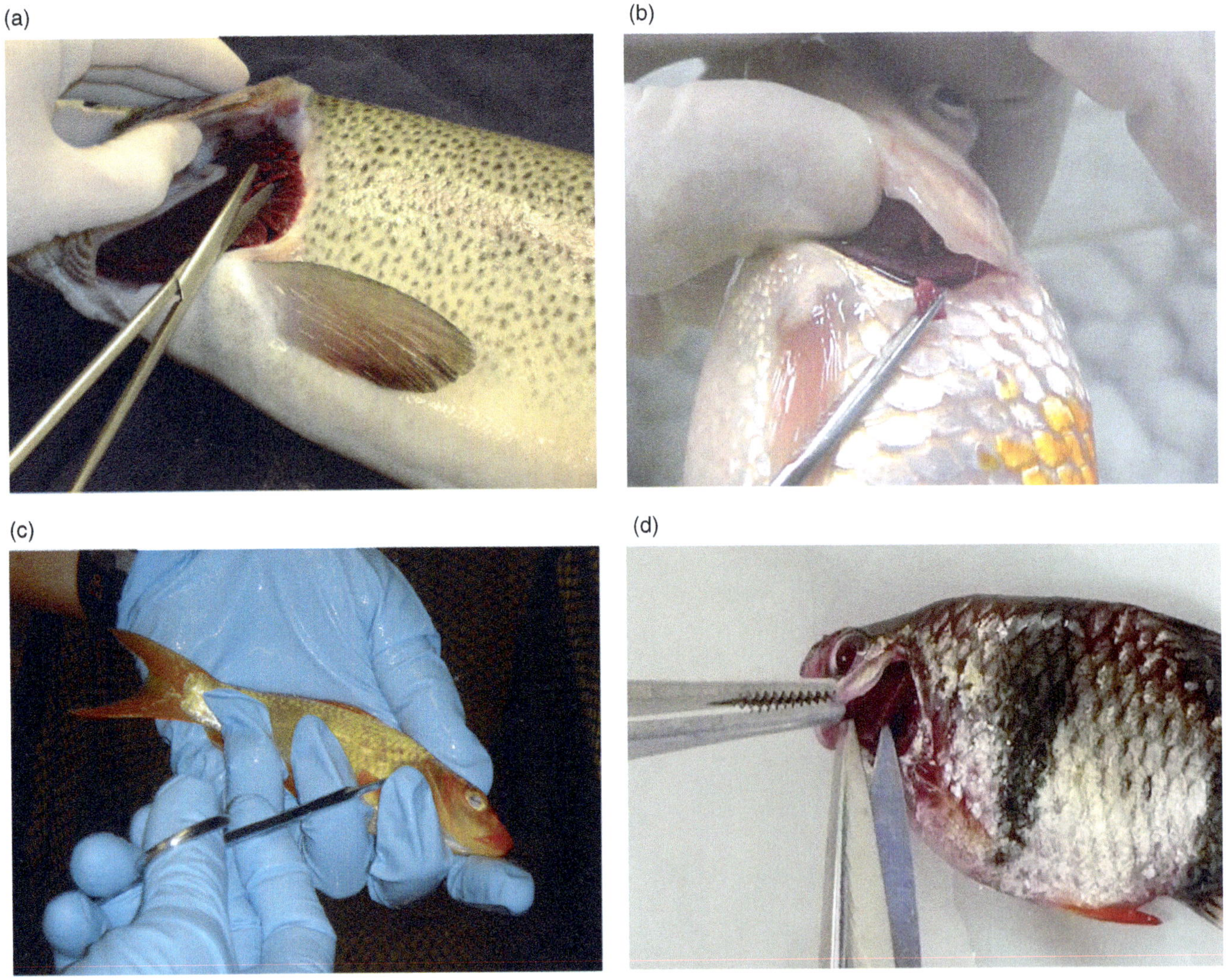

Fig. 30.4. (a) Obtaining a gill biopsy from a rainbow trout (*Oncorhynchus mykiss*). (b) Obtaining a gill biopsy from a koi (*Cyprinus carpio*). (c) Obtaining a gill biopsy from a goldfish (*Carassius auratus*). (d) Obtaining a gill biopsy from a tiger barb (*Puntigrus tetrazona*).

the sample before covering it with a coverslip (Figure 30.5). The sample is examined as a wet-mount preparation under the microscope.

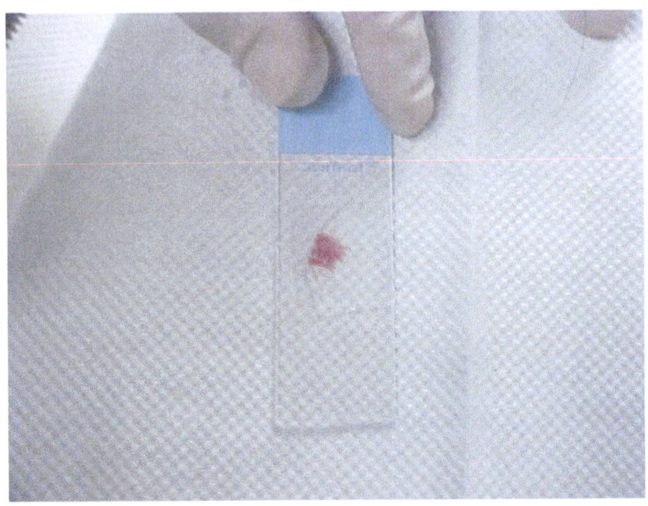

Fig. 30.5. A gill biopsy sample as a wet-mount preparation ready for examination under the microscope.

Fecal Sample

A fecal sample is obtained by inserting a swab or small loop through the vent and into the intestine or by collecting feces as it is passed from the fish. This is also examined as a wet mount.

Sampling Techniques for Cytodiagnosis

Review of cytology sampling and evaluation techniques for mammals in Chapter 6, avian patients in Chapter 14, and reptile and amphibian patients in Chapter 22 will be helpful in collection and evaluation of samples obtained from fish. The safe handling techniques for fish described in the "Sampling Techniques for Wet Mounts" section should be followed when collecting samples for cytodiagnosis.

The Integument

Examination of the skin is the most common aspect of the physical examination of the piscine patient. Lesions on the skin of a fish, such as papules, nodules, vesicles, pustules, or ulcers can be evaluated cytologically from samples obtained from smears made from swabbing or scraping of the lesion. Masses found in or under the skin can be aspirated or excised to obtain a cytological sample (Figures 30.6–30.8). A touch imprint of a biopsy sample can also provide a cytological sample (Figure 30.9).

Alimentary Tract

Cytological examination of smears made from a swab or scraping of a lesion in the oral cavity is often useful in providing a presumptive or definitive diagnosis (Figure 30.10). Sampling of the stomach for cytological evaluation can be obtained by inserting a swab, such as an equine uterine culture swab, into the stomach. In larger fish, stomach samples for cytodiagnosis can also be obtained via gastric washes or endoscopy (Figure 30.11). Vent samples are easily obtained by inserting a sterile, saline-moistened, cotton-tipped swab into the vent.

Respiratory Tract

The gill biopsy as described for wet-mount preparations can be used as an air-dried imprint on a microscope slide that is stained for cytological examination.

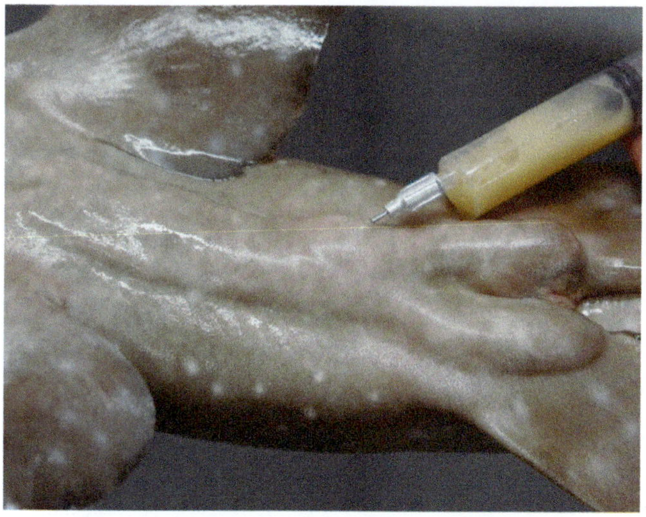

Fig. 30.6. Aspiration of a fluid-filled cyst in the skin of a white-spotted bamboo shark (*Chiloscyllium plagiosum*) for cytological examination.

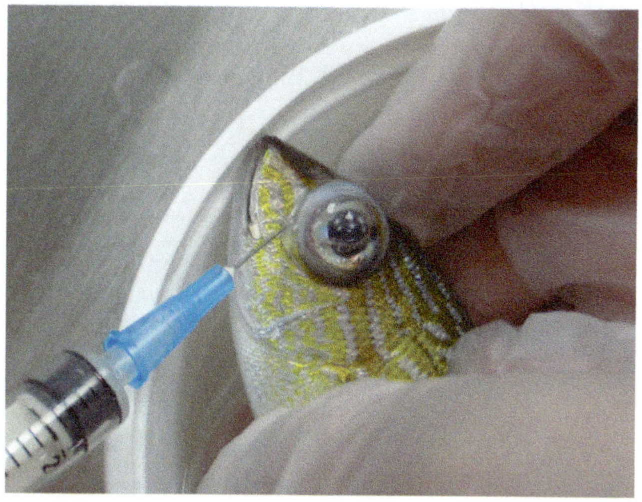

Fig. 30.8. Aspiration of a periocular mass in a French grunt (*Haemulon flavolineatum*) for cytological examination.

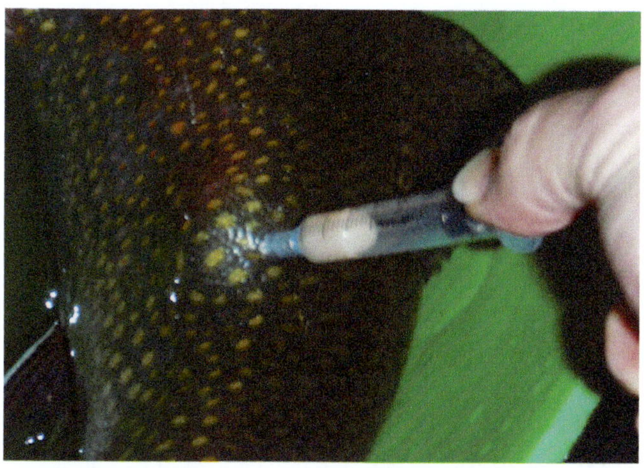

Fig. 30.7. Aspiration of a cutaneous pustule in the skin of a brook trout (*Salvelinus fontinalis*) for cytologic examination.

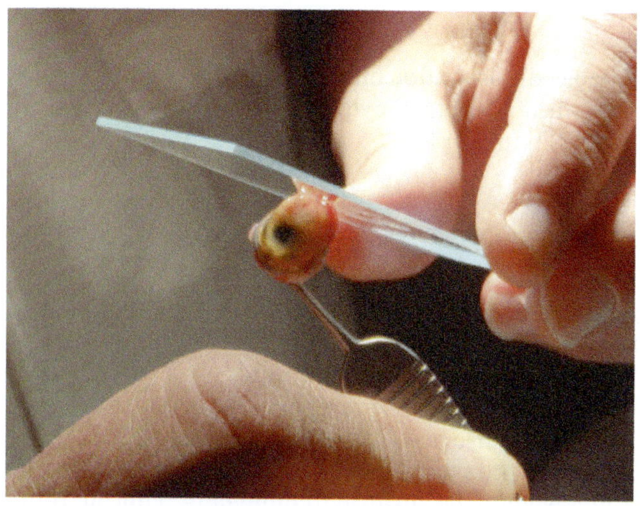

Fig. 30.9. Imprint of an excised mass from a fish for cytological examination.

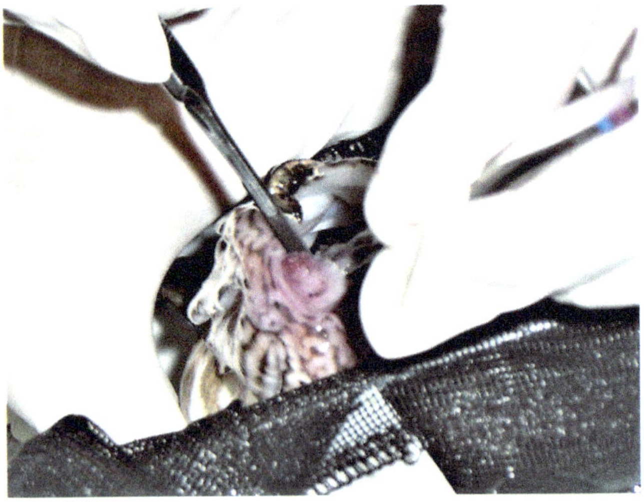

Fig. 30.10. Scraping of a lesion in the mouth of a lionfish (*Pterois volitans/miles*) for cytological examination.

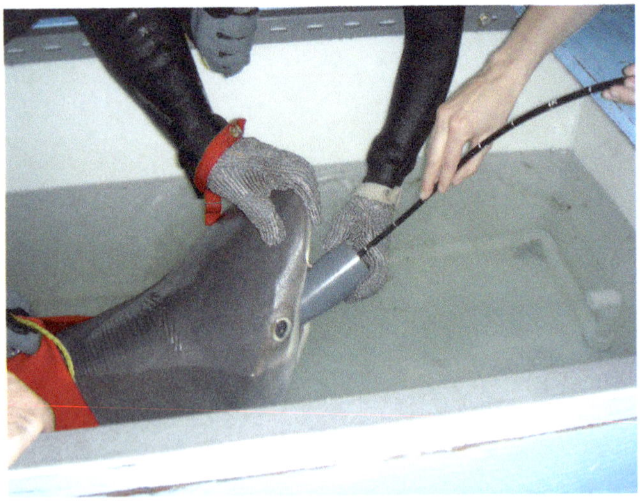

Fig. 30.11. Endoscopy examination in a shark (*Carcharhinus plumbeus*).

Fine-needle aspiration biopsy and fluid collection can be performed to obtain cytological specimens from gill lesion (Figure 30.12).

Coelomic fluid

Fluid in the coelomic cavity of fish can be simply aspirated by insertion of the needle through the skin and body wall, usually along the ventral aspect of the animal; however, the sampling location may vary depending upon the handling circumstances (Figure 30.13).

Fresh air-dried smears are adequate for the Romanowsky stains (i.e., Giemsa and Wright's stains). Slides should be air-dried completely, kept at room temperature, protected from formalin fumes, and stained within three days to prevent cell deterioration

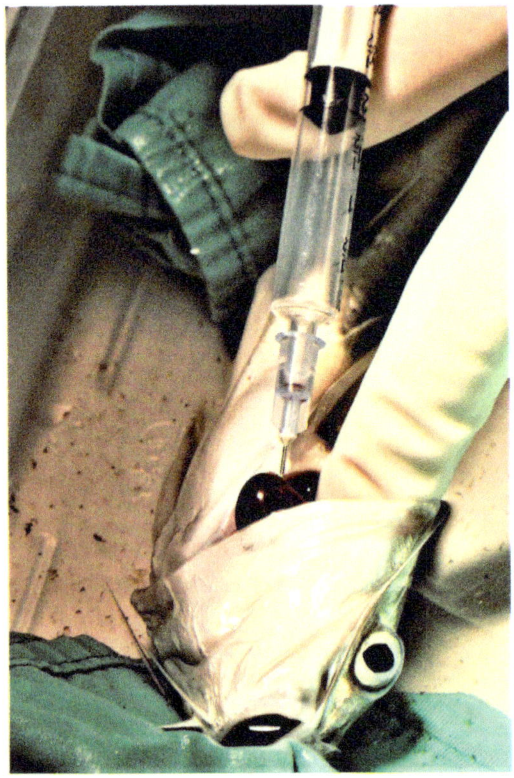

Fig. 30.12. Aspiration of a mass in the gill of a channel catfish (*Ictalurus punctatus*) for cytologic examination.

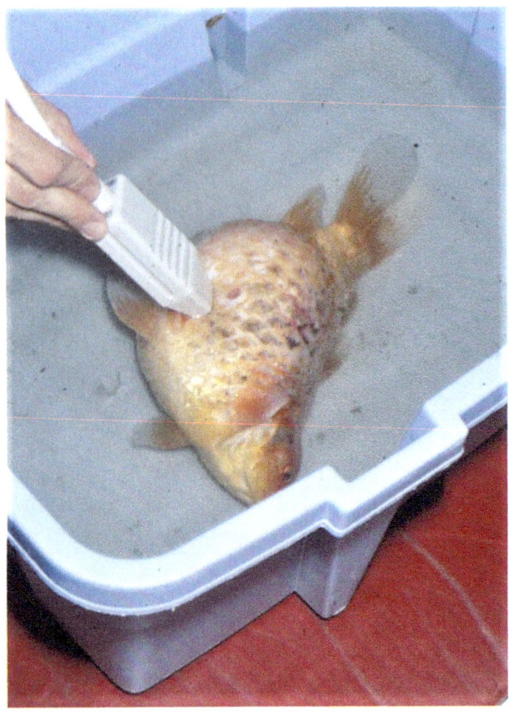

Fig. 30.13. Ultrasound can be used to guide the needle into the coelomic cavity for aspiration of coelomic fluid or an intracoelomic mass for cytological examination.

and staining artifacts (Allison, 2022). Slides should also be protected from salt water when handling marine fish.

References

Allison RW. 2022. Inflammation and infectious agents. In: Thrall MA (ed), *Veterinary Hematology, Clinical Chemistry, and Cytology*, 3rd edn. Ames, IA: Wiley-Blackwell, in press.

Grant KG. 2015. Fish hematology and associated disorders. In: Campbell TW (ed), *Vet Clin North Am: Exotic Anim Pract* 18(1):83–103.

Groff JM, Zinkl JG. 1999. Hematology and clinical chemistry of cyprinid fish. *Vet Clin North Am (Exotic Anim Pract)* 2(3):741–776.

Lewbart GA, Yanong RPE. 2018. Fish. In: Carpenter JW (ed), *Exotic Animal Formulary*, 5th edn. St. Louis, MO: Elsevier, pp. 16–52.

Noga EJ. 2000. Fish disease, diagnosis and treatment. In: Noga E (ed), *Fish Disease, Diagnosis and Treatment*. Ames, IA: Iowa State University Press.

Smit GL, Hattingh J, Burger AP. 1979. Haematological assessment of the effects of the anaesthetic MS-222 in natural and neutralized form in three freshwater fish species: intraspecies differences. *J Fish Biol* 15:633–653.

Whitaker BR, McDermott CT. 2018. Amphibians. In: Carpenter JW (ed), *Exotic Animal Formulary*, 5th edn. St. Louis, MO: Elsevier, pp. 16–52.

Wright KM. 2006. Overview of amphibian medicine. In: Mader D (ed), *Reptile Medicine and Surgery*, 2nd edn. St. Louis: Saunders Elsevier.

31 Wet-Mount Microscopy in Fish

During a disease outbreak in ornamental, aquaculture, or natural populations, the identification of the causative agent(s) is challenging because the piscine patient may be infected with multiple pathogens, which may contribute to the observed pathology (Mizuno et al., 2017; Adamek et al., 2019).

Sample Evaluation

Gill Biopsies

Because gills play a major role in their physiology, gill diseases seriously affect the health of fish. Microscopic examination of gill biopsies, therefore, becomes an important diagnostic tool in fish medicine.

Each gill arch has rows of macroscopic finger-like primary lamellae. Each primary lamella has rows of microscopic secondary lamellae. Each secondary lamella contains blood vessels that move blood countercurrent to the water flow to facilitate gas and nitrogenous waste exchange (Ellis et al., 1978; Rummer and Brauner, 2021). Normal gill filaments as viewed in a wet-mount preparation under the microscope have slender, triangular, smooth-surfaced lamellae, and interlamellar water channels are approximately equal in size (Figure 31.1).

Abnormal gill filaments are thick, have a ragged surface, and are coated with a layer of hyperplastic epithelium and mucus (Figures 31.2a–31.2c). Hyperplasia and hypertrophy of epithelial cells indicate gill damage and can lead to fusion of adjacent secondary lamellae. Hyperplastic lesions lead to death of the fish owing to a reduction or blocking of the respiratory water flow over the lamellar epithelium, thus reducing the exchange of gases and ions across the lamellar epithelium (Bullard et al., 2001).

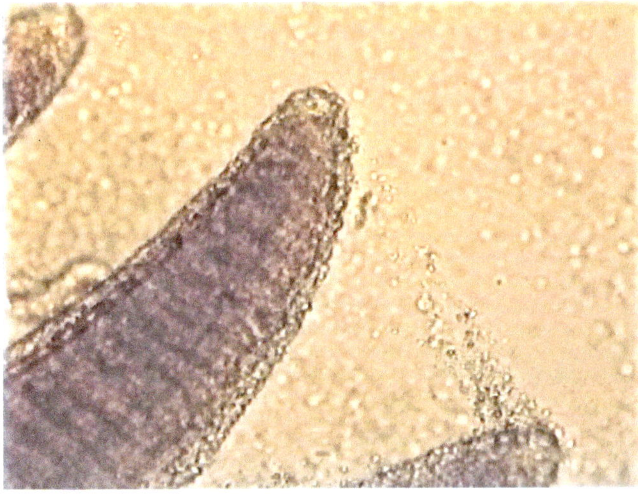

Fig. 31.1. This gill biopsy wet-mount preparation reveals a gill lamella with a slight irregularity to the margins suggestive of mild cellular and mucus coating. The normal gill biopsy should reveal slender, triangular, smooth-surfaced primary lamellae with interlamellar water channels of approximately equal size (10×).

Although many opportunistic pathogens may be present in low numbers on gills without causing disease, increased numbers often result in gill disease. Most infectious agents that involve the skin also infect the gills. Gill damage from bacteria, parasites, and poor water quality causes epithelial proliferation and thickened gill filaments (Figure 31.3). Severe gill damage results in telangiectasis or necrosis of the gill filaments. Telangiectasis occurs with gill infections or environmental toxins and is indicated by dilatation of groups of small blood vessels in the secondary lamellae (Figure 31.4). Severe necrosis of gill tissue is characterized by the

Exotic Animal Hematology and Cytology, Fifth Edition. Terry W. Campbell and Krystan R. Grant.

Companion website: www.wiley.com/go/campbell/exotic

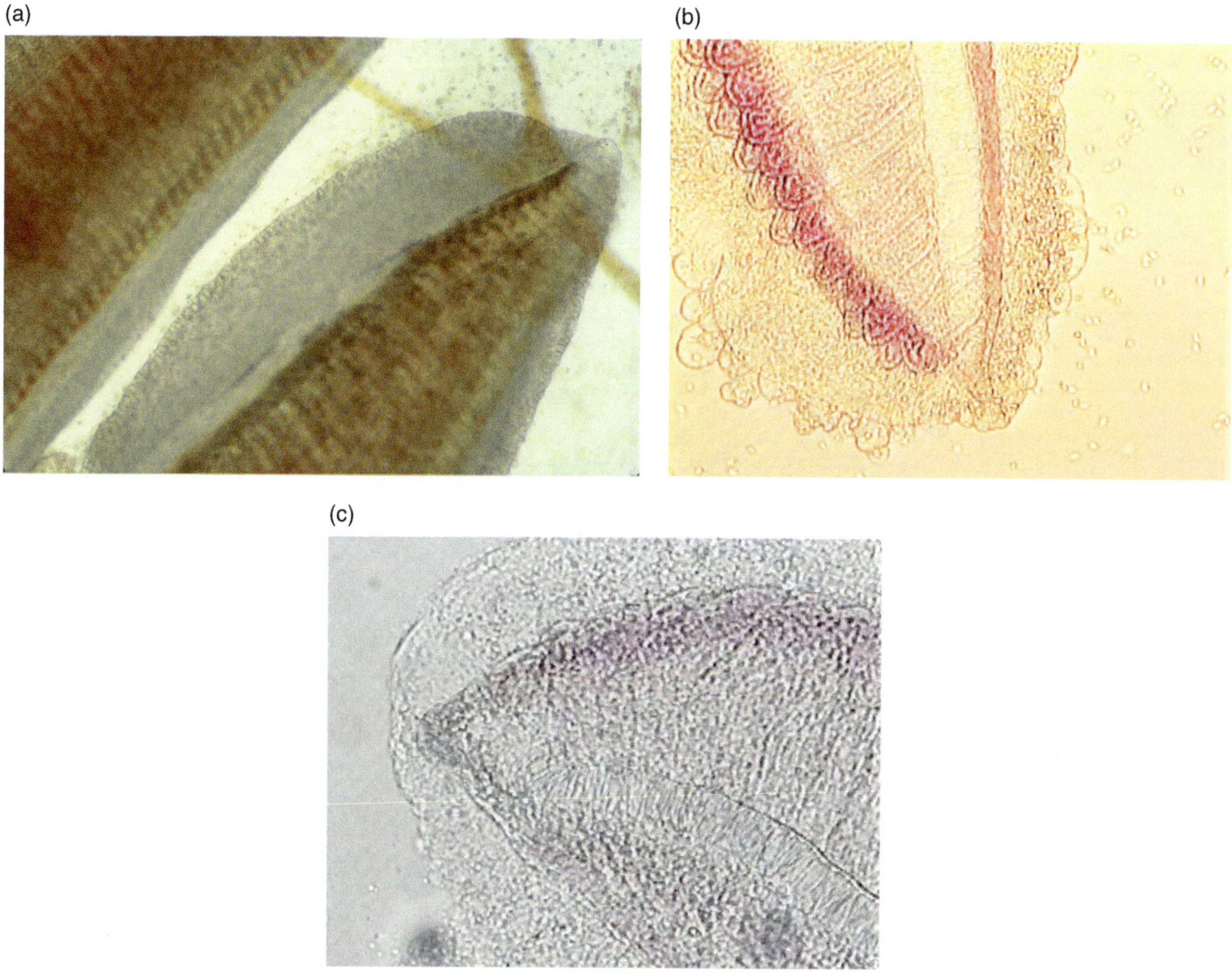

Fig. 31.2. (a) This gill biopsy wet-mount preparation indicates a heavy mucus and cellular coating over the primary lamellae (10×). (b) This gill biopsy wet-mount preparation indicates a heavy mucus and cellular coating over the primary lamellae (20×). (c) This gill biopsy wet-mount preparation indicates a heavy mucus and cellular coating over the primary lamellae, which appears thickened (20×).

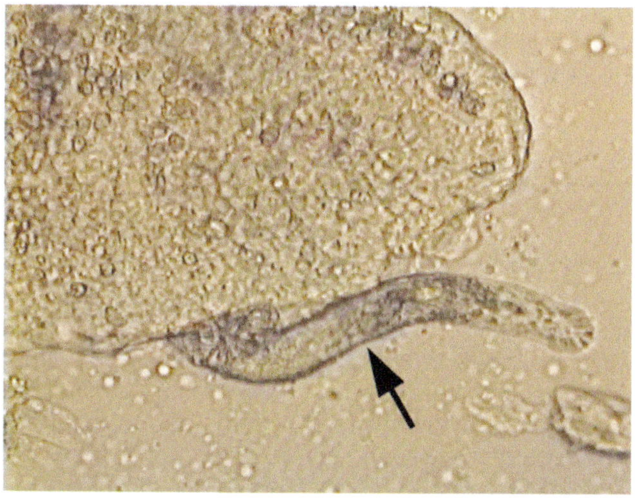

Fig. 31.3. The tip of a primary gill lamella from a wet-mount preparation of a gill biopsy reveals a heavy mucoid and cellular coating of the gill, most likely associated with the trauma to the gill tissue by a monogenean (arrow) infestation (40×).

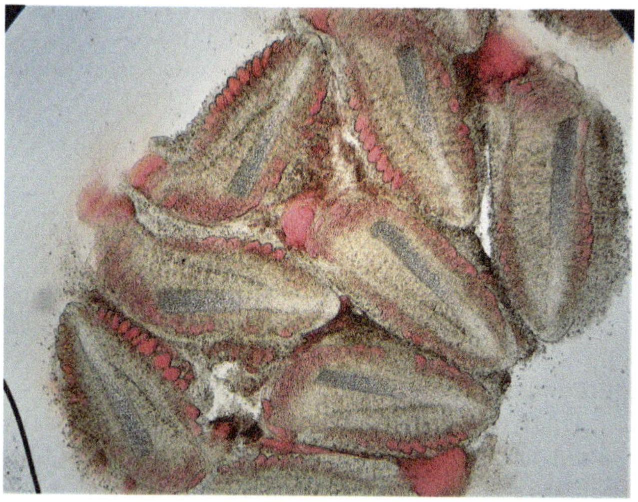

Fig. 31.4. This wet-mount preparation of a gill biopsy reveals the dilatation of groups of small blood vessels in the secondary lamellae (telangiectasis), which occurs with gill infections or environmental toxins, from a koi (*Cyprinus carpio*). (4×). Image courtesy of Steve Schultz.

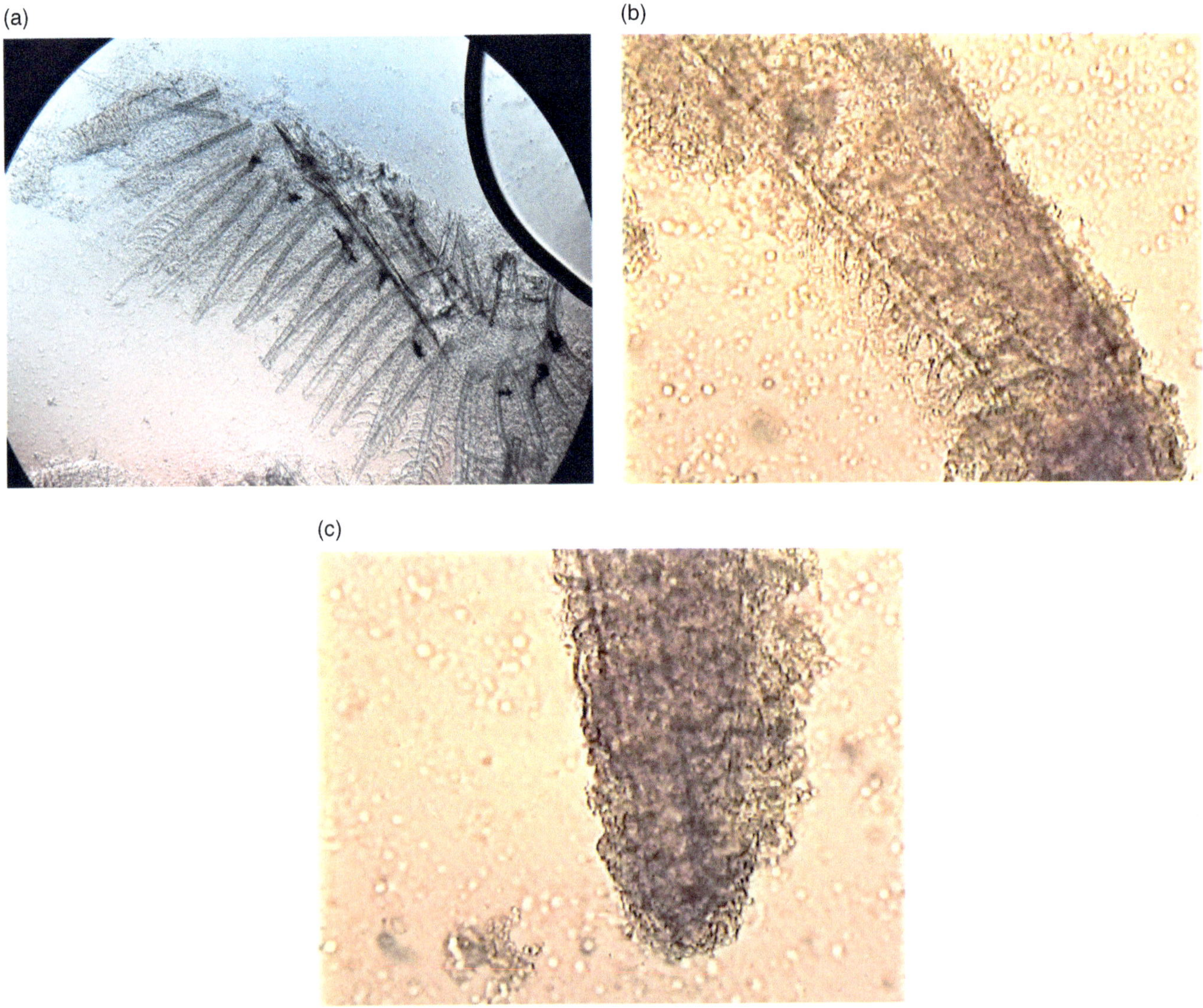

Fig. 31.5. (a) This wet-mount preparation of a gill biopsy reveals necrosis of the primary lamella from a neon tetra (*Paracheirodon innesi*) (4×). Image courtesy of Steve Schultz. (b) This wet-mount preparation of a gill biopsy reveals severe necrosis of the primary lamella with exposure of the underlying cartilaginous skeleton (20×). (c) Necrosis of the primary lamella in a wet-mount preparation of a gill biopsy (20×).

destruction of secondary lamellae with the loss of the epithelium and exposure of the underlying cartilaginous skeleton of the primary lamellae (Figures 31.5a–31.5c).

Mucus Smears and Fin Biopsies

Although the skin of fish is not keratinized, it does contain the layers seen in mammalian skin (Noga, 2000). The dermis contains scales and pigmented cells. The scales are embedded in connective tissue and overlap one another. Some species lack scales, and others have very small scales. The epidermis, which is made of stratified squamous epithelium with goblet cells, also covers the scales. The epidermis is covered by the cuticle, a thin layer of mucus produced by goblet cells and sloughed epithelial cells.

Normal wet-mount preparations from mucus smears and fin biopsies reveal mucus strands, a few superficial squamous epithelial cells, and an occasional scale that may contain normal pigment. Bacteria and ectoparasites can occur in low numbers in healthy fish. Many of the protozoan parasites are commensals that utilize the integument and gills as a substrate and only become harmful (usually in immunocompromised fish or amphibians) when their increased numbers interfere with skin or gill function (Roberts, 2001). Others are obligate parasites of skin and gill epithelium that cause disease and death. Large numbers of ectoparasites, such as numbers greater than two per low-power (40× to 100× magnifications) field, and numerous bacteria and fungi are considered abnormal.

Nonparasitic Pathogens

Bacteria

The significance of the number of bacteria present on a wet-mount preparation is usually the subjective opinion of the cytologist, as no guideline is available for the assessment of bacterial numbers (Figure 31.6). However, the presence of inflammatory cells associated with increased numbers of bacteria is suggestive of bacterial involvement. Stained air-dried smears made by allowing the wet-mount preparation to dry following the removal of the coverslip are often helpful in the assessment of bacterial involvement (Figures 31.7a and 31.7b). Septic lesions are identified by the presence of bacterial phagocytosis by leukocytes.

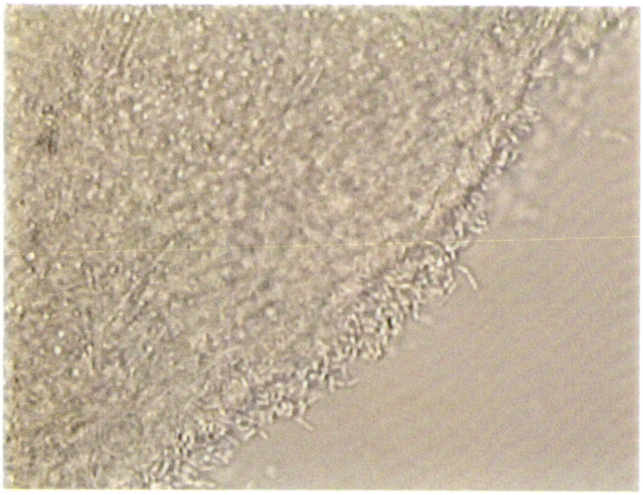

Fig. 31.6. A wet-mount preparation of a mucus smear from a freshwater fish reveals numerous bacteria (100×).

Columnaris disease is an acute to chronic bacterial infection that affects a variety of freshwater and marine fish and is of commercial importance worldwide, especially to channel catfish farming (Mohammed and Arias, 2014). *Flavobacterium columnare*, the causal agent of freshwater columnaris disease and *Flexibacter maritimus*, the causal agent of the disease in marine fish, are gram-negative bacteria, ubiquitous in aquatic environments (Noga, 2000). This disease is also commonly known as saddleback disease, cotton wool disease, cotton mouth disease, and fin rot (Tripathi et al., 2005). Lesions associated with these bacteria include cutaneous ulcers, fin necrosis (fin rot), and gill necrosis. Wet-mount preparations of the lesions reveal a homogeneous population of long, thin, gliding bacterial rods (0.5–1.0 μm wide and 4–10 μm long) that form moving mounds or columns that resemble haystacks. Bacteria on the outer edges of the specimen exhibit a characteristic gliding or flexing motion (Figures 31.8a and 31.8b).

Fungus

Fungal infections are another major cause of disease in fish and are usually the result of immunosuppression associated with poor water quality, chronic stress, and coexisting diseases. Prolonged treatment with antibiotics may also predispose fish to fungal infections. Fungal disease of fish by water mold is widespread in fresh water and is responsible for the most important and extensive commercial losses by reducing both quality and yield in fish production (Mousavi et al., 2009; Zoller et al., 2017).

(a) (b)

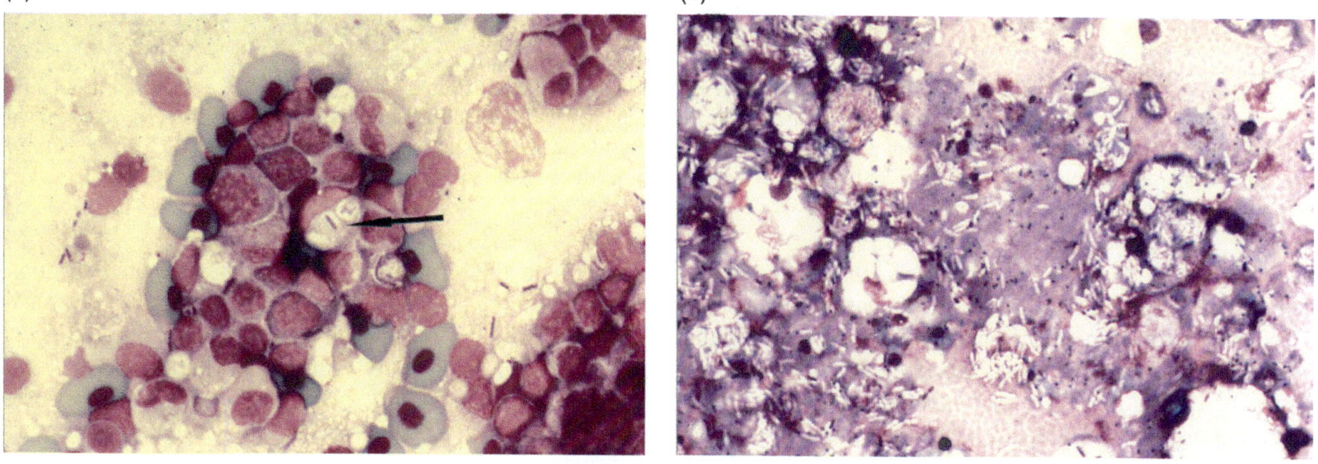

Fig. 31.7. (a) Imprint from a lesion found on a gill biopsy from a freshwater fish reveals bacterial phagocytosis (arrow) indicating a septic inflammatory lesion. Wright–Giemsa stain (100× oil). (b) Imprint of a cutaneous lesion on a dwarf gourami (*Trichogaster lalius*) reveals a macrophagic inflammation and negative staining bacteria suggesting mycobacteriosis. Wright–Giemsa stain (100× oil).

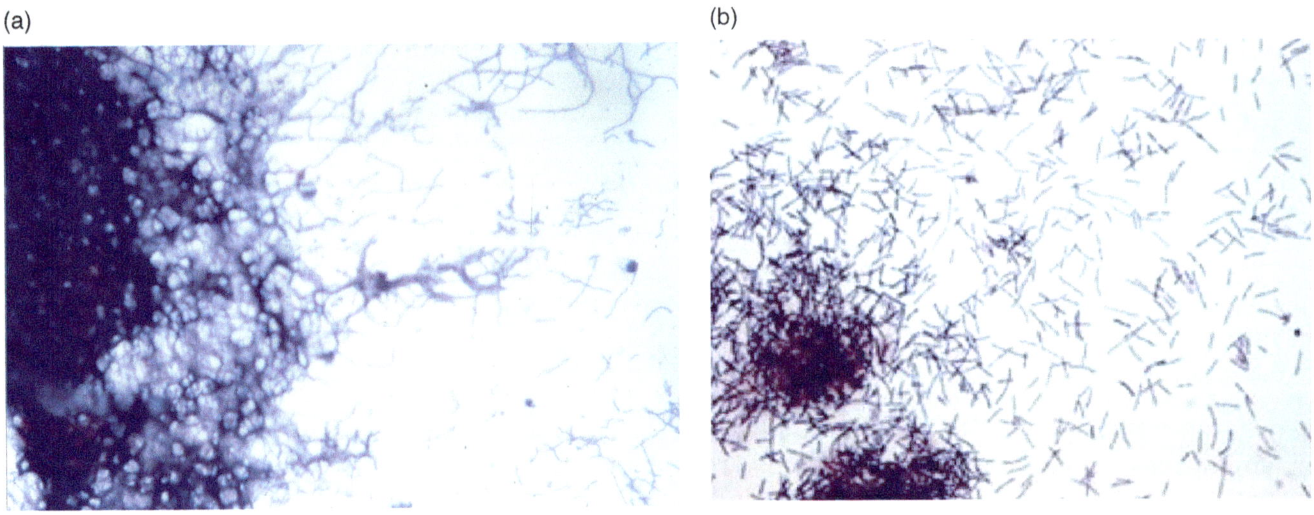

Fig. 31.8. (a) Stained imprint of a skin lesion near the mouth of an Atlantic spadefish (*Chaetodipterus faber*) reveals numerous long, thin, bacterial rods. The bacteria in the wet-mount preparation exhibited a gliding movement indicative of *Flexibacter maritimus*. Wright–Giemsa stain (100× oil). (b) *Flavobacterium columnare* appear as a uniform population of long, thin bacilli (0.5–10 μm) in a Wright–Leishman-stained cytological preparation from a cutaneous ulcer on a koi (*Cyprinus carpio*). Source: Image from Tripathi et al. (2005).

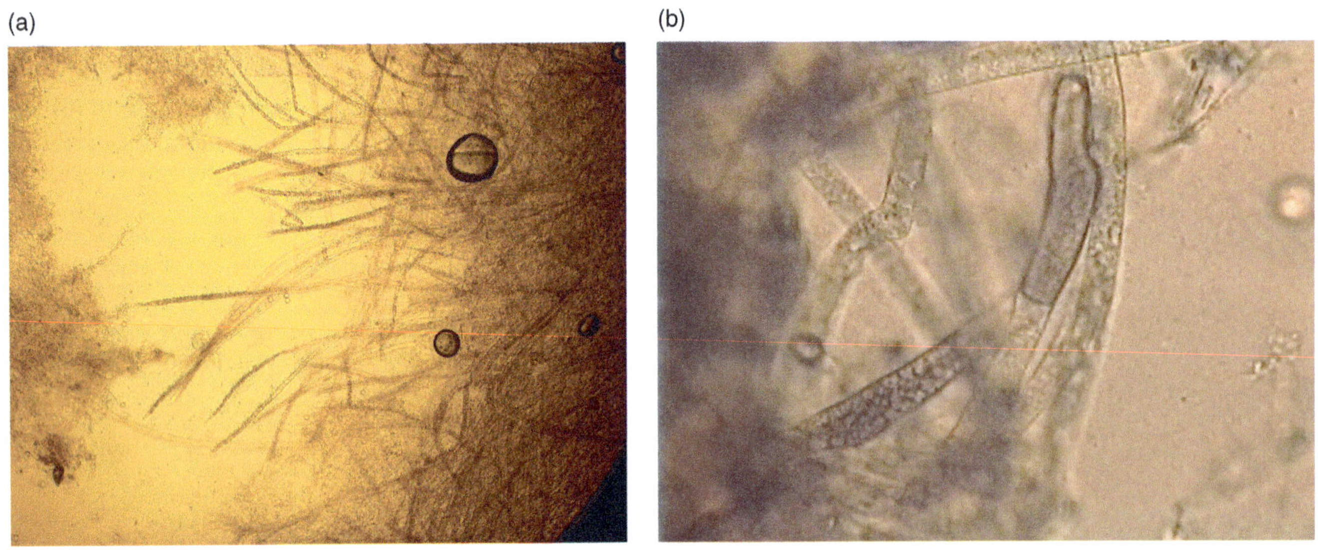

Fig. 31.9. (a) Fungal hyphae in a wet-mount preparation from a mucus smear taken from a cotton-like lesion from the skin from a koi (*Cyprinus carpio*). Saprolegniasis is a commonly used term for the diagnosis of fungal infections on the skin of fish (10×). (b) Fungal hyphae in a wet-mount preparation from a mucus smear taken from a cotton-like lesion from the skin from a koi (*Cyprinus carpio*). Saprolegniasis is a commonly used term for the diagnosis of fungal infections on the skin of fish (40×).

Oomycetes fungi, such as *Saprolegnia* and related genera, are common freshwater molds that are frequently associated with skin infections on fish and amphibians (Noga, 2000). Saprolegniasis caused by *Saprolegnia* spp. is one of the major water mold diseases in aquaculture (Munir et al., 2017). Ulcers or other vulnerable regions on the skin of immunocompromised fish provide a point of entry for the fungal infection to proliferate, and are therefore often considered a secondary infection. Saprolegniasis is a catch-all term for superficial, cottony-like, white growth on the skin and gills of fish, and on fish eggs. Lesions on the skin of fish may also appear in a crescent-shape colony with radiating extensions forming adjacent growths. The hyphae are typically limited to the skin and superficial musculature; however, they may infect into deeper cutaneous tissue, resulting in edema or respiratory compromise (Smith et al., 2019). Wet-mount preparations reveal wide (7–30 μm) aseptate hyphae that are often associated with other pathogens, such as bacteria and protozoa (Gieseker et al., 2006) (Figures 31.9a and 31.9b).

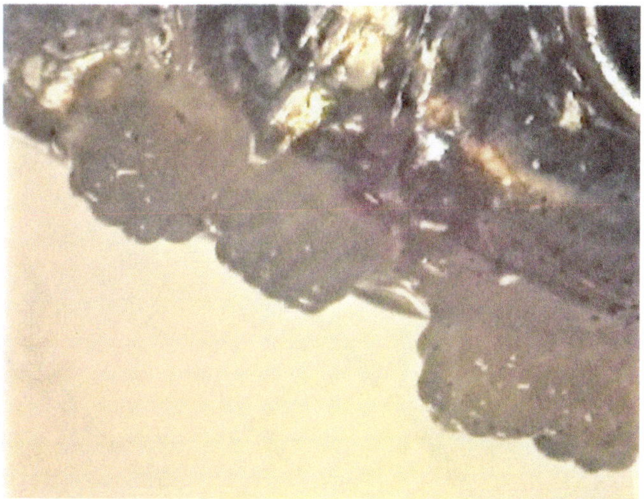

Fig. 31.10. Close-up image of a wart-like lesion on the skin of a fish with a lymphocystis infection. Viewed through a dissecting microscope.

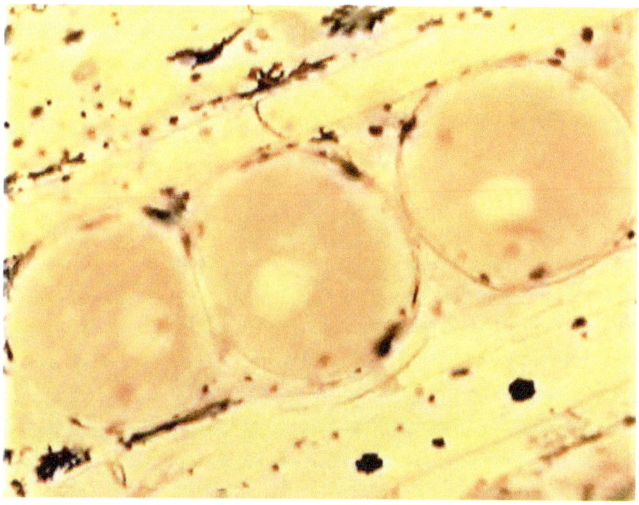

Fig. 31.11. Large, round cells associated with a scale in this image of a mucus/skin scraping wet mount from a fish are the enlarged dermal fibroblasts associated with a lymphocystis infection (50×).

Lymphocystis

Lymphocystis disease virus (LCDV) is the causative agent of lymphocystis disease, which affects over 140 different wild and cultured freshwater and marine fish species worldwide (Wu et al., 2015). The virus is a DNA iridovirus that causes a marked hypertrophy of the infected cells (dermal fibroblasts) and forms tumor-like nodules on the skin, fins, mouth, gills, and internal organs (Alonso et al., 2005; Hine et al., 2016). Infected cells can be up to 100 000 times their normal size; therefore, they are visible without magnification. Advanced lesions exhibit large wart-like tumorous growths on the skin and fins (Figure 31.10).

Histopathologic preparations of lymphocystis disease are characterized by cytomegaly of dermal fibroblasts and only rarely, systemic involvement; therefore, it has been regarded as mesotheliotropic (Gibson-Kueh et al., 2003). Extremely large hypertrophied cells with aberrant nuclei and intracytoplasmic inclusions are seen on histopathology samples (Weber, 2013). The disease is transmitted by direct contact and is typically self-limiting, unless growths around the mouth cause starvation.

Microscopic examination of wet-mount preparations from lymphocystis lesions reveals extremely enlarged dermal fibroblasts. These cells appear round rather than spindle-shaped and occur in clusters (Figure 31.11). Each of these large, round cells has a small centrally positioned nucleus.

Cutaneous Fish Parasites

Important cutaneous fish parasites capable of causing serious harm to their host include numerous protozoan and metazoan parasites. These organisms are detected either by direct observation of the parasite on the fish or from wet-mount preparations of mucus scrapings, gill-clip biopsy, or fin-clip biopsy using the microscope.

External protozoans induce injury primarily by impairing individual cell metabolism or irreversibly damaging a cell, with subsequent cell death; however, actual cell death is rarely observed by the fish disease diagnostician (MacMillan, 1991). More commonly, they cause epithelial hyperplasia in the gills and skin. A critical factor and probably the most important virulence factor is the protozoan's mode of feeding and attachment to the host.

In the gills, an inflammatory response tends to increased secondary lamellae cellularity, resulting in impaired blood circulation, increased lamellar thickness, and impaired gas exchange (MacMillan, 1991). Increased mucus production may be one consequence of an inflammatory response.

Ciliate Protozoa

Most of the ciliate protozoa found on fish are commensals, and most are harmless. However, a few are notoriously pathogenic. For example, *Ichthyophthirius* of freshwater fish and *Cryptocaryon* of marine fish are highly pathogenic ectoparasites that feed on host cells. Because ciliate protozoa have a direct life cycle, they can occur in high numbers and create heavy infestations.

Ichthyophthirius multifiliis, a holotrich ciliate protozoan, is the etiologic agent of "white spot,"' also known as Ich, which is a commercially important disease of freshwater fish (Dickerson and Findly, 2014; Howell et al., 2019; Maceda-Veiga and Cable, 2019). It is cosmopolitan in distribution and with high virulence, affects most species of freshwater fish. This parasite can cause a sudden onset of a marked outbreak in

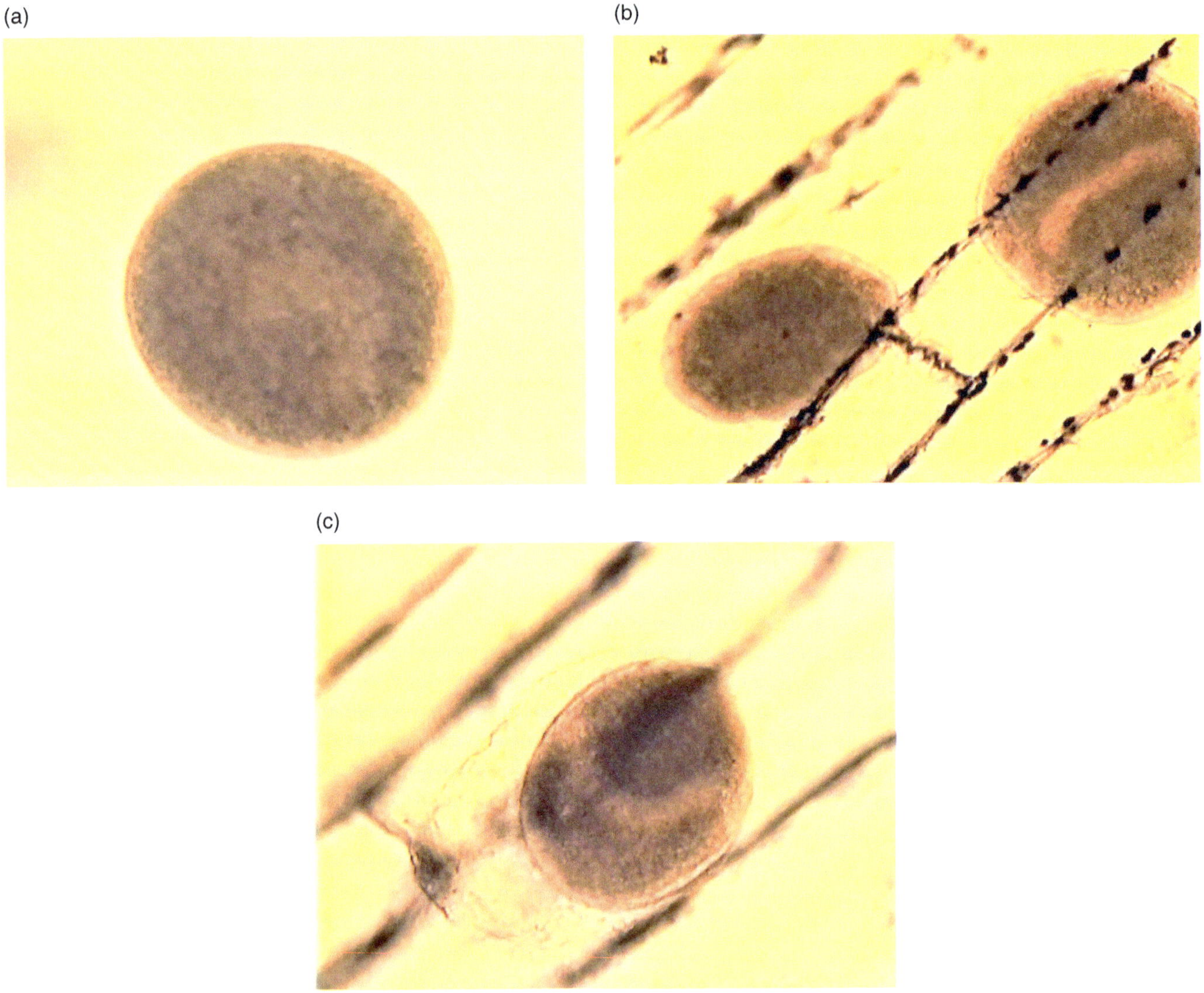

Fig. 31.12. (a) This wet mount of a mucus scraping from a freshwater fish exhibiting a heavy mucus coating of the skin reveals a characteristic trophont of *Ichthyophthirius multifiliis*. The trophont has a characteristic horseshoe-shaped macronucleus. It exhibited a slow rolling movement when viewed in the wet-mount preparation (10×) (b) This wet mount of a mucus scraping from a freshwater fish exhibiting small, slightly raised white spots on the skin reveals the characteristic trophonts of *Ichthyophthirius multifiliis*. Trophonts have a characteristic horseshoe-shaped macronucleus. They exhibit a slow rolling movement when viewed in the wet-mount preparation (10×). (c) This wet mount of a mucus scraping from a freshwater fish exhibiting a heavy mucus coating of the skin reveals a characteristic trophont of *Ichthyophthirius multifiliis*. The trophont has a characteristic horseshoe-shaped macronucleus. It exhibits a slow rolling movement when viewed in the wet-mount preparation. (10×).

several warm and temperate freshwater fish and is common in aquarium fish. The three morphologically and functionally distinct stages of this organism consist of the infectious, free-swimming theronts; host-associated trophonts; and encysted tomonts that divide mitotically off the fish. Theronts burrow into the epithelial layers of the host and rapidly transform into trophonts that feed on host tissue. Trophonts grow to several hundred microns in diameter, becoming visible as the characteristic white spots associated with disease. After 7–10 days, trophonts mature, escape from the fish, and attach to a solid surface, becoming tomonts. Tomonts then secrete a gelatinous cyst wall and produce in the range of 100–1000 daughter cells by multiple rounds of asexual division. Within 20–24 h, theronts burst from the cyst and restart the infectious cycle (Matthews, 2005). The trophont stage causes numerous pathophysiological changes to the host due to its mechanical presence and enzymatic feeding mechanism (Abdel-Hafez et al., 2014). The *Ichthyophthirius* trophont is easily recognized in mucus scrapings or gill or fin biopsies by its size (up to 1 mm in diameter), characteristic horseshoe-shaped macronucleus, and slow rolling movement (Figures 31.12a–31.12c).

Cryptocaryon irritans is the marine counterpart of the freshwater *I. multifiliis*. This holotrich ciliate protozoan resembles its freshwater counterpart in appearance and movement. The macronucleus is typically not seen in wet-mount preparations because it is hidden by the granular cytoplasm (Figures 31.13a and 31.13b). *Cryptocaryon* and *Ichthyophthirius* are capable of penetrating into the epithelium of their fish host.

Chilodonella spp. are important holotrich ciliate protozoan parasites of tropical and subtropical freshwater fish. These parasites appear as flattened, ovoid-shaped protozoa that measure up to 80 μm in length and are covered by rows of cilia. They are identified by their shape and slow steady gliding movements in wet-mount preparations (Figures 31.14a and 31.14b). *Chilodonella* spp. actively feed on epithelial cells and may cause ulcerative skin lesions.

Brooklynella spp. are the marine counterpart to the freshwater *Chilodonella* spp. and are significant pathogens of the skin and gills of marine aquarium fish

(a) (b)

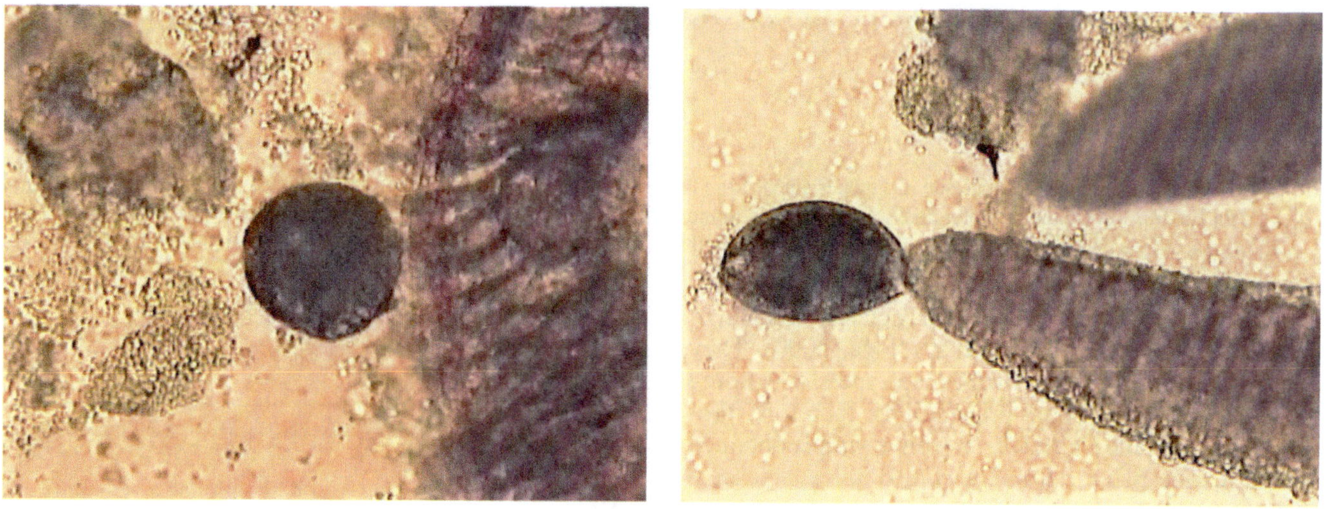

Fig. 31.13. (a) This gill biopsy from a marine fish exhibiting signs of rapid respirations and "coughing" behavior reveals a *Cryptocaryon irritans* trophont. This marine parasite is a holotrich ciliate protozoan with the rolling movements of its freshwater counterpart, *Ichthyophthirius multifiliis*. The macronucleus is typically not seen in wet-mount preparations owing to the granular cytoplasm (10×). (b) A *Cryptocaryon irritans* trophont in a gill biopsy from a marine fish exhibiting signs of rapid respirations and "coughing" behavior (10×).

(a) (b)

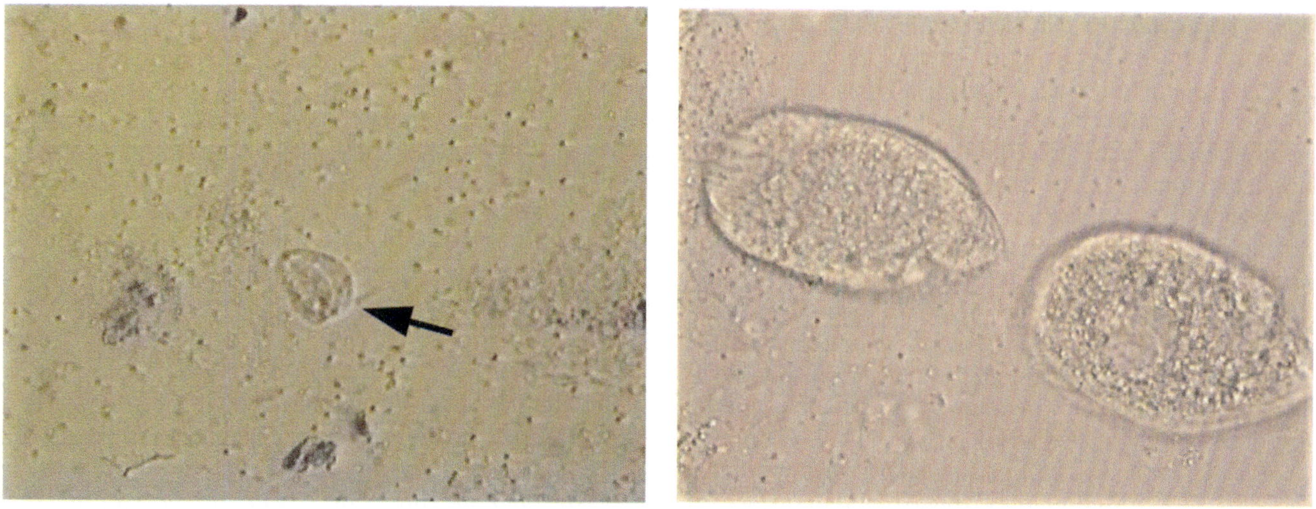

Fig. 31.14. (a) This wet mount of a mucus smear taken from a freshwater fish exhibiting a rough appearance to the slime coating of the skin reveals one of many flat, oval to heart-shaped ciliate protozoa (arrow). The shape and characteristic slow gliding movement with occasional turning in wide circles supports the diagnosis of chilodonellosis. (10×) (b) A higher magnification of the *Chilodonella* organisms found in Figure 31.14a (100×).

(a) (b)

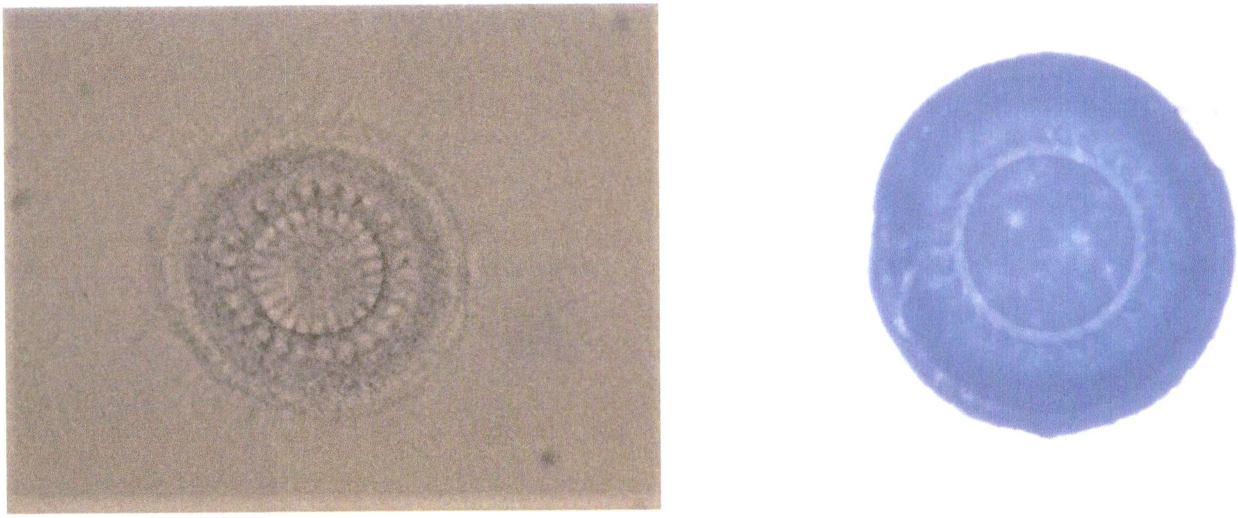

Fig. 31.15. (a) A trichodinid parasite in a mucus smear from the skin of a freshwater fish (10×). (b) A stained trichodinid parasite found in a mucus smear from the skin of a freshwater fish. This is one of few protozoal parasites that can be identified on a stained smear. Note the characteristic denticle rings of the trichodinid parasites in this image and in Figure 31.15a. Wright–Giemsa stain (100× oil).

(Lom, 1970). They have been associated with high mortalities in tropical marine fish (Noga, 2000). They are also identified by their ovoid shape and slow gliding movements on wet-mount preparations; therefore, protozoa that resemble *Chilodonella* from a sample obtained from a marine fish are *Brooklynella*. Both cause excessive mucus production and gill hemorrhage.

Peritrichous ciliates, such as *Trichodina*, *Epistylis*, and *Apisoma*, are primarily bactivorous, feeding on bacteria in the water or on mucous; thus, their mode of feeding is innocuous to the fish host.

Trichodina spp. of freshwater and marine fish are another pathogenic ciliate protozoon that can damage the gills and skin, especially when they occur in large numbers. *Trichodina* are peritrich ciliate protozoa that are easily recognized by a ring of internal denticles, which have a skeletal function (Figures 31.15a and 31.15b). They are generally considered to be part of the infusoria culture of the aquatic habitat, and their presence in large numbers indicates poor water quality or immunosuppression and can cause erosion of epithelial surfaces. Trichodinids may constitute a problem in rearing tanks with high densities. The adhesive discs of *Trichodina* attach to the epithelial surface of the fish, which results in cellular injury and increased mucous production by the host. This increases the amount of nutrients available to the organism and therefore allows for an increase in the size of its population (MacMillan, 1991).

Epistylis spp. are colonial stalked peritrich protozoal parasites that are commonly found on the surface of freshwater fish in ponds with high organic material (Roberts, 2001). The surface of the affected fish is used as a substrate for attachment, creating white tuft-like lesions on the surface of the skin or fins. They measure up to 100 µm in length, and they have buccal cilia at one end of a bell-shaped structure called a zooid, which can recoil and extend (Figure 31.16).

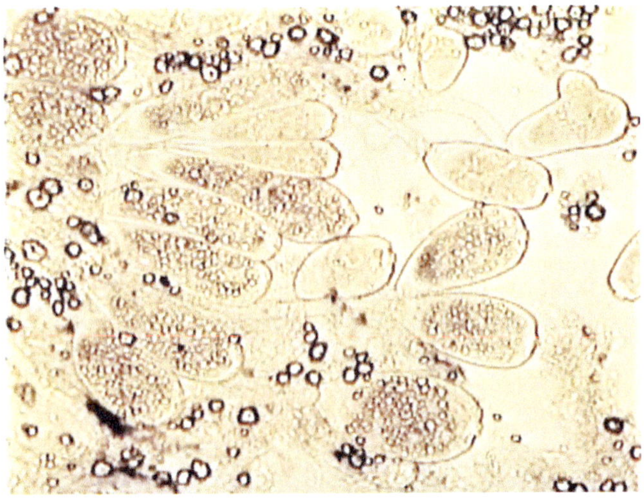

Fig. 31.16. A wet-mount preparation from a mucus smear of a cotton-like cutaneous lesion on a goldfish (*Carassius auratus*) living in a pond reveals the numerous stalked peritrich protozoa called *Epistylis*. These are colonial protozoal parasites that measure up to 100 µm in length. They have buccal cilia at one end of a bell-shaped structure called a zooid, which can recoil and extend (10×).

Apisoma sp. (previously *Gloassatella* sp.) are sessile ciliated protozoans that attach to the skin, gills, and fins of pond fish and are rarely seen in ornamental or marine fish. They appear as vase-shaped organisms under the microscope (Figure 31.17).

Tetrahymena spp. is a saprozoic ciliated protozoan of the phylum ciliophoran that is common in nature and appears to have no geographical limits where it feeds on organic matter and bacteria in natural habitats (Sharon et al., 2014). *Tetrahymena* spp. is the causative agent of tetrahymeniosis or "tet disease," also known as "guppy killer disease," in tropical aquarium fish, which causes severe economic losses in commercial guppy farms worldwide. The organisms can also infect a variety of other organisms, including dogs (Lynn et al., 2000; Lynn et al., 2018). The free-living, ciliated *Tetrahymena* spp. become secondary pathogens capable of becoming highly invasive and resulting in systemic infestations in freshwater fish. Conditions that allow such infestations are not known but are likely associated with severe immunosuppressive conditions, such as wounded fish or those weakened by high ammonia level, high organic load, extreme water temperature, non-optimal shipment conditions (e.g., high fish density) or a disease. The affected fish may exhibit pale cutaneous lesions surrounded by hemorrhage. Wet-mount preparations of gill clips or mucus smears reveal numerous actively motile, pear-shaped ciliate protozoa that measure 60 μm by 100 μm. The appearance and movement of this protozoan is like that of a spiraling football (Noga, 2000) (Figure 31.18).

Uronema marinum is the marine counterpart to *Tetrahymena*. This organism can be a serious pathogen in marine aquaria. It is identical to its freshwater counterpart in appearance and movement as well as the clinical disease that it causes (Figures 31.19a and 31.19b).

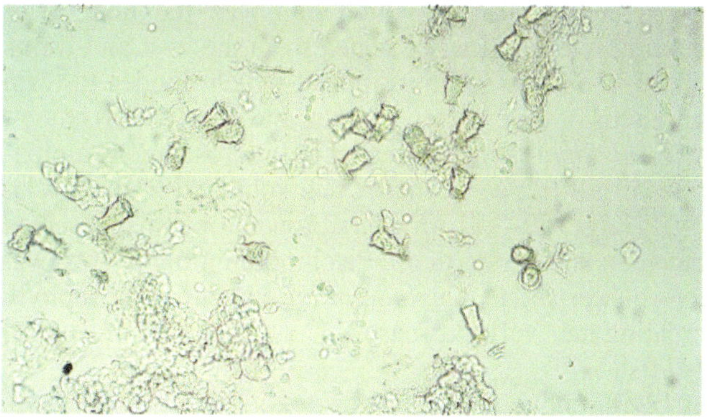

Fig. 31.17. *Apisoma* sp. in a mucus smear from a Siamese fighting fish (*Betta splendens*) (10×). Source: Image courtesy of Steve Schultz.

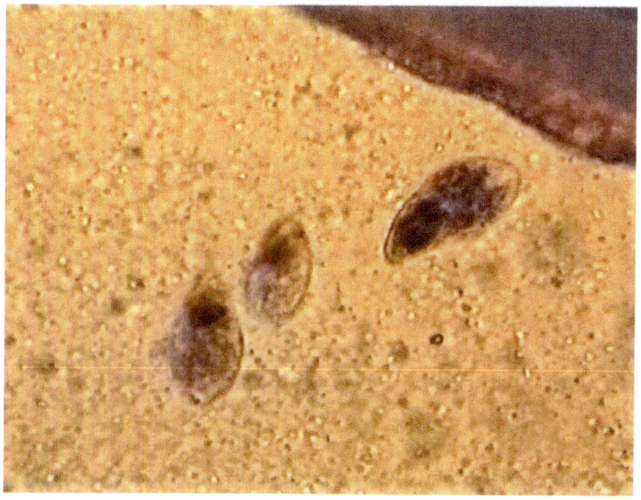

Fig. 31.18. A wet-mount preparation from a mucus smear from a freshwater fish reveals four actively motile, pear-shaped ciliate protozoa, *Tetrahymena*. The wet-mount preparation contained a marked number of these protozoans, which tended to move about the debris on the slide like bumper cars and often in a spiraling football manner (40×).

(a) (b)

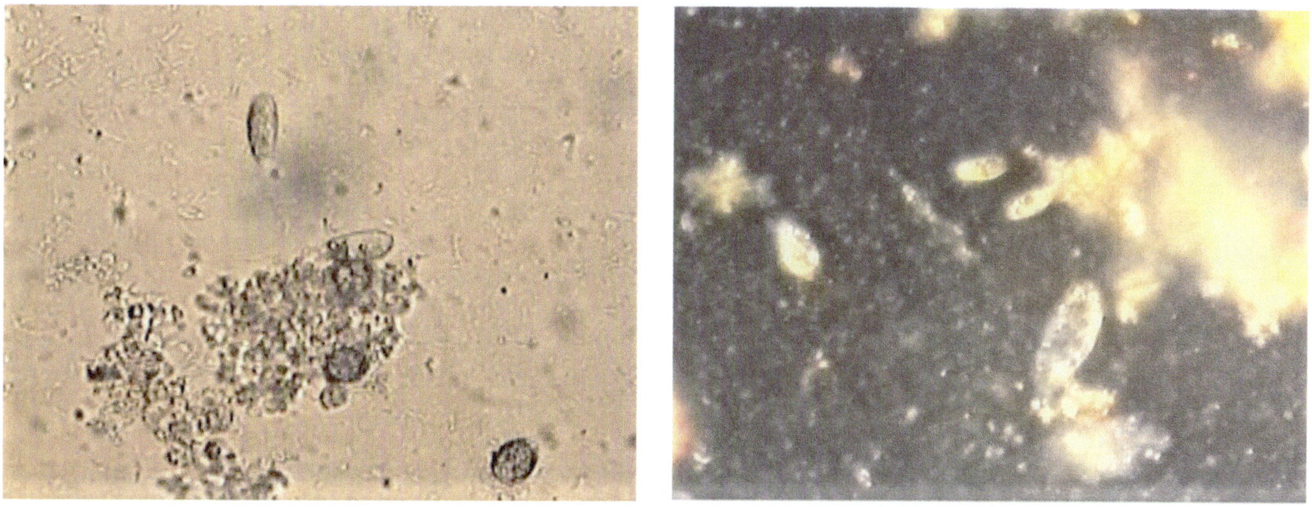

Fig. 31.19. (a) A wet-mount preparation from a mucus smear from a marine fish reveals pear-shaped ciliate protozoa that resemble *Tetrahymena*; however, these are the marine counterpart, *Uronema*. The wet-mount preparation contained many of these highly motile protozoans (40×). (b) The same *Uronema* protozoans in Figure 31.19a under phase contrast microscopy (40×).

Flagellate Protozoa

Flagellate protozoa are another common type of ectoparasite of fish. They often have direct life cycles, and some have resistant cyst stages. The hemoflagellates have indirect life cycles.

The best-known flagellate protozoan parasite of fish is *Ichthyobodo necator* (formerly *Costia necatrix*) which causes ichthyobodiasis in several fish species (Isaksen, 2013; Adamek et al., 2019). This parasite affects practically any freshwater fish and is cosmopolitan in distribution. Although it is highly pathogenic to freshwater fish (especially young fish and those with immunosuppression), *I. necator* can also cause disease and mortality in marine fish (Noga, 2000). The parasite attaches itself to the skin and gills of fish, where it feeds on its host's cells, causing hyperplasia of the epithelium and destruction of goblet cells.

Ichthyobodosis is commonly diagnosed by observation of *Ichthyobodo* in a wet-mount preparation of a mucus smear or gill biopsy. It is detected in its free-living stage, which is a small oval to kidney-bean-shaped protozoan, measuring 10–15 μm in length, about the size of many fish erythrocytes (Figure 31.20). It has two pairs of flagella of unequal length that are held in a groove over most of the length of the body. This causes the parasite to swim in a jerky spiral that exhibits a flickering or flashing image as it turns its crescent-shaped body in the light path of the microscope (Noga, 2000). When attached, it swims in a circular motion.

Dinoflagellates are found on the epithelial surfaces of marine and freshwater fish, usually in tropical or subtropical waters. The dinokaryotic dinoflagellate *Amyloodinium ocellatum* is a nonspecific marine fish ectoparasite that causes extensive economic losses in the aquaculture and aquarium industries (Gómez and Gast, 2018). This obligate parasite is responsible for amyloodiniosis, or "velvet disease" (owing to the dust-like sheen it creates on the skin of the infected fish), one of the most serious diseases of almost every species of marine fish of temperate and warm waters. Pathogenicity occurs when it attaches to the fish using rhizoids that embed deeply into epithelial cells of the gills and skin, causing hyperplasia, inflammation, hemorrhage, and necrosis. It causes severe epizootics with high mortality because it can reproduce quickly, especially fish in crowded conditions, such as in closed aquarium systems (Noga and Levy, 1995). It is one of the few fish parasites that can infest both teleost fish and elasmobranchs (Noga, 2000).

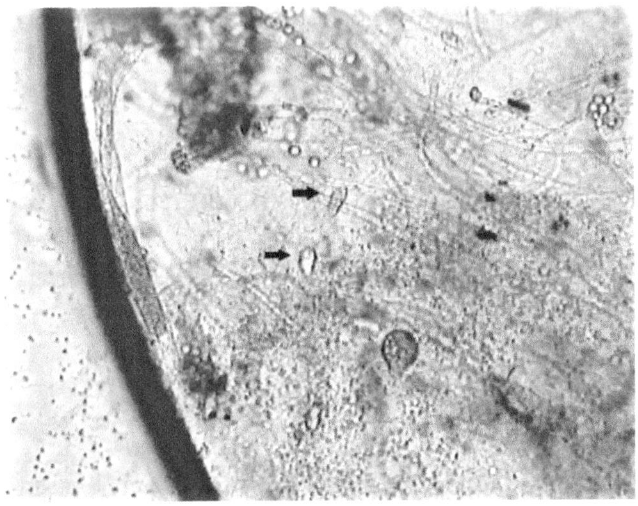

Fig. 31.20. A wet-mount preparation of a mucus smear from a freshwater fish reveals many fungal elements and the small, oval *Ichthyobodo* protozoan (arrows). *Ichthyobodo* measures 10–15 μm in length and swims in a jerky spiral manner that causes the protozoan to flicker as it turns its crescent-shaped body in the light path of the microscope. The attached protozoans have a circular motion (20×).

The life cycle comprises an infective stage (dinospore) that attaches to the host tissue, forming the feeding stage (trophont), which damages the host; after feeding, the trophont detaches from the host and forms the reproductive stage (tomont), which divides to form hundreds of dinospores (Gómez and Gast, 2018).

Amyloodinium is detected by microscopic examination of gill filaments that reveal spherical to oval, relatively large (50–350 μm), dark brown trophonts dispersed between and inside them. Piscinoodinium, the freshwater counterpart to *Amyloodinium*, contains chlorophyll, creating the "velvet disease" or "rust disease" of tropical pet fish.

Diplomonad flagellate protozoa (*Spironucleus* spp. and *Hexamita* spp.) are commonly encountered in the digestive tract of a wide variety of hosts, including fish, amphibians, rodents, and birds. They may also be found in the blood and internal organs. The impact of the infections ranges from minimal to significant morbidity and mortality. These are small, pleomorphic, very active flagellates that are typically 10–20 μm long, which makes their identification difficult using light microscopy alone. They have an anterior end with six flagella in two groups of three and a posterior end with two trailing flagella (Poynton, 2001). *Hexamita* and *Spironucleus* are flagellate protozoans in the gastrointestinal tract of freshwater and marine fish that can cause anorexia, lethargy, and death. Fish exhibiting scant, mucoid feces should be examined for a possible intestinal flagellate infestation. Massive systemic infections, especially with *Spironucleus*, are lethal (Figures 31.21a and 31.21b).

Trypanosome infections are usually asymptomatic, and the pathogenesis is unknown. They are found as incidental finding in blood films or imprints of tissues (i.e., kidneys). *Cryptobia* spp. are morphologically like *Trypanoplasma* spp. but are found in wet-mount preparations of the gills or possibly feces. *Cryptobia* spp. can be pathogenic to both freshwater and marine fishes.

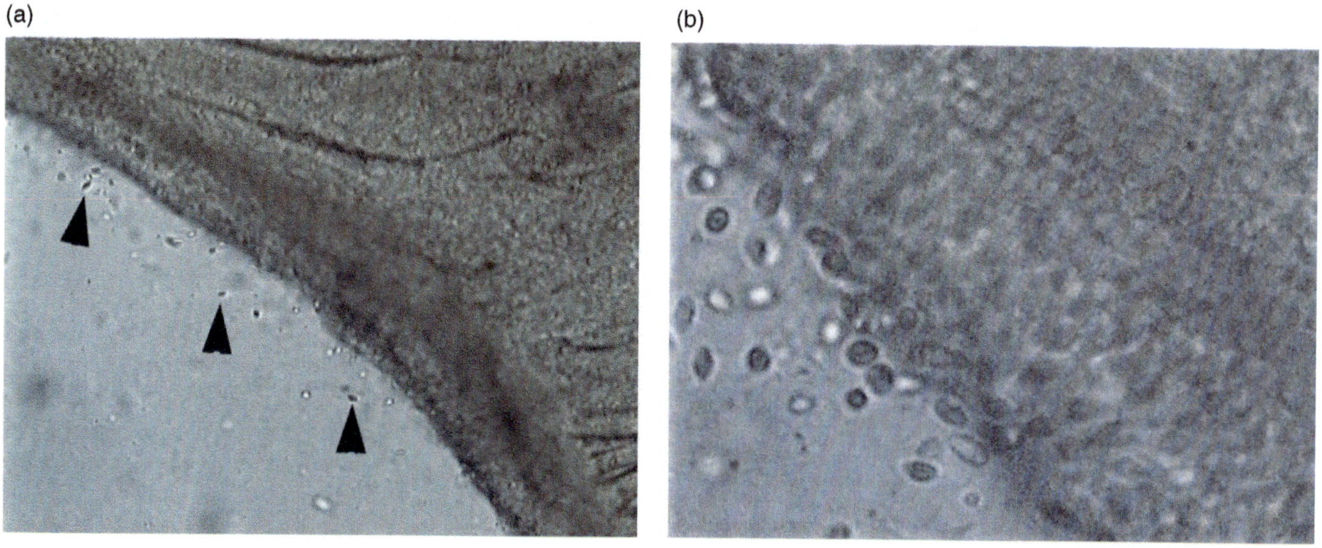

Fig. 31.21. (a) This low magnification of a wet mount of an intestinal sample obtained during necropsy of a freshwater angelfish (*Pterophyllum scalare*) that had died of emaciation shows a sample teeming with the actively motile flagellate protozoa *Hexamita* or *Spironucleus* (a few represented by arrowheads) (10×). (b) The same image shown in Figure 31.19a at a higher magnification reveals the oval shape of highly active flagellate *Hexamita* or *Spironucleus* organisms (100×).

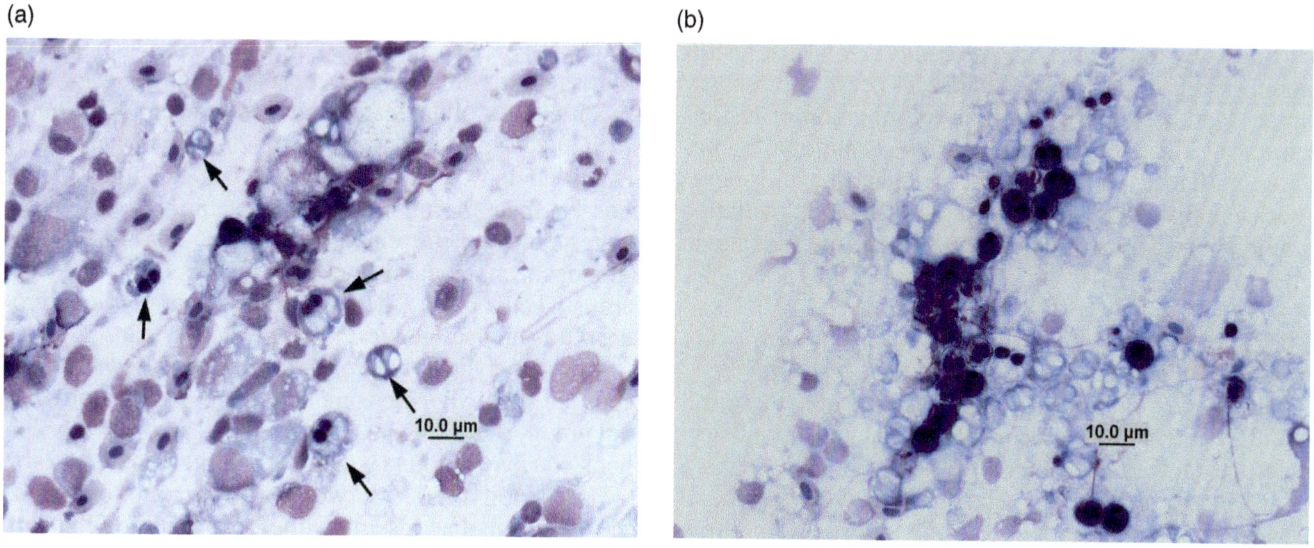

Fig. 31.22. (a) Mixed-cell inflammation associated with numerous spores (arrows) with two polar capsules characteristic of myxosporeans in a fine-needle aspiration biopsy of a gill mass from a koi (*Cyprinus carpio*). Wright–Giemsa stain. (b) Numerous spores (a few represented by arrowheads) with two polar capsules characteristic of myxosporeans in a fine-needle aspiration biopsy of a gill mass from a koi (*Cyprinus carpio*). Wright–Giemsa stain.

Myxozoa

Members of the phylum Myxozoa that infect fish are in the class Myxosporea, often known as myxosporeans or myxozoan parasites. Historically, myxozoans have been grouped based on spore morphology, host, or site fidelity and geographic location (Cavin et al., 2012). Myxozoans are an extensive group of aberrant parasitic cnidarians with more than 50 species and a complex lifecycle, including actinosporean and myxosporean development stages (Li et al., 2017; Sokolov et al., 2019). For the most part, the myxosporean stage is hosted by marine and freshwater fish. These organisms are characterized by their multicellular spores (usually measuring between 8 and 25 µm) that contains two polar capsules (Noga, 2000) (Figures 31.22a and 31.22b).

Myxosporidia are highly pathogenic, usually intracellular parasites that can involve all organs. Most of these parasites infect target organs, causing site-specific infestations, especially involving the gills and skin of marine and freshwater fish. Skin infections are less serious than those in gill tissue. Myxozoans most commonly infect gills in part due to rich blood supply, gaseous exchange, and ready access to the external environment for transmission. They form cream-colored plasmodia, which vary in size and location depending on the myxozoan species (Kaur and Katoch, 2016).

Henneguya infection is an example of a disease caused by a myxosporean parasite that causes serious gill damage in marine and freshwater fish with the formation of interlamellar cysts (Özer et al., 2016). *Henneguya* cysts appear as discrete nodules that contain hundreds of spores with spindle-shaped polar capsules that are identified microscopically from a ruptured nodule (Figures 31.23a–31.23e). The symmetrical oval, rounded, or fusiform spores in frontal view exhibit two caudal projections, two polar capsules, and binucleate sporoplasm (Sokolov et al., 2019). Each caudal projection of *Henneguya* spp. is a continuation of the shell in the direction opposite to the end of the spore with the polar capsules.

Myxobolus cyprinid, another myxozoan parasite, is the etiologic agent for pernicious anemia of carp and related species (Roberts, 2001). Whirling disease of trout is caused by infection of the cranial and vertebral cartilages by the spores of *Myxobolus cerebralis*, resulting in a skeletal deformity that causes nerve and sensory organ dysfunction. Microscopic examination of lesions caused by these organisms may reveal multiple aggregates of 10 to 13 µm, basophilic, circular to ovoid spores (occasionally with a darkly basophilic nucleus) with two similarly sized pyriform polar capsules at one end (Cavin et al., 2012).

Microsporidians

Microsporidia are highly specialized obligate intracellular (intracytoplasmic and/or intranuclear) eukaryotes that are closely related to the fungi. They have a relatively simple development, consisting of two general stages: merogony and sporogony. Meronts multiply inside the infected host cell, eventually forming sporonts and then spores, which are ultimately released from the host and transmit the infection. The host range extends from protists and invertebrates (especially insects and other arthropods) to vertebrates, particularly fish and mammals (Vergneau-Grosset and Larrat, 2015; Picard-Sanchez et al., 2020).

Microsporidians are parasites of the order Microsporidia that have smaller spores (usually less than 7 µm) than the myxosporeans, and their spores contain only one polar capsule. Fish-infecting microsporidia often cause the formation of xenomas, or spore-filled cysts, in their fish hosts. Xenomas are host cells that have undergone extreme hypertrophy as the parasite uses host resources to produce massive numbers of spores to infect new hosts (Ryan and Kohler, 2016). Spore production results in the eventual death of infected host cells, while the host itself suffers varying amounts of reduced fitness. Microsporidians, such as *Glugea*, can affect the skin and gills of fish where they create masses that resemble those caused by myxozoan parasites. These infections can result in epithelial hyperplasia and distortion of gill filaments (Roberts, 2001). *Pleistophora hyphessobryconis* is another microsporidian parasite that affects a broad range of freshwater fish species (Gratzek, 1988). Members of the genus *Glugea* have caused substantial mortality in both wild and farmed economically important fish (Kent et al., 2014; Ryan and Kohler, 2016). *Glugea* sp. infection causes the formation of xenomas associated with the body wall, fat body, gonads, and kidneys. Infections range from mild to very heavy, with variable xenoma numbers and sizes.

Monogeneans

Monogeneans are a group of parasites with a series of hooks that attach to the gills, skin, or fins of a fish, and these parasites lead to significant injury or death of the fish (Li et al., 2018).

Monogenean infestation occurs in both freshwater and marine fish. There are many different species of monogeneans, and most are host specific; however, their specificity is often lost in aquaculture and aquariums with mixed species of fish (Noga, 2000). They are easily identified on wet-mount preparations of the gills, skin, or fins by their morphology and stretching and recoiling (caterpillar-like) movements (Figures 31.24a and 31.24b). Monogeneans contain hooks or suckers. Most measure around 4 cm or less. The most important groups are gyrodactylid and dactylogyrid monopisthocotyleans.

Gyrodactylids, *Gyrodactylus* spp. and *Gyrodactyloides* spp., are small viviparous monogeneans that measure 0.3–1.0 µm in length (Figure 31.25a). Small embryos (or their hooklets) may be found within the parasite (Figure 31.25b).

Dactylogyrids, *Dactylogyrus* spp., are oviparous monogenean that resemble the gyrodactylids, but are slightly larger (up to 2 µm in length) and possess eye spots (Figures 31.26a–31.26c). These monogeneans possess a haptor (attachment organ), have a direct life cycle, and are ectoparasites that live on skin, gills, and fins. Dactylogyrus is an oviparous monogenean parasite that is often found in co-infections with other parasites, bacteria, fungi, or viruses, and causes serious damage to the hosts (Lu et al. 2013).

Eggs from monogeneans may be found without the presence of the adult. When numerous eggs are found on mucus smears, they represent either a heavy monogenean infestation or few (or possibly an individual) parasites that have been present on the fish for a long period of time (Figure 31.27).

Microcotyle sp. is a monogenean ectoparasites with larvae that attach to the gills of fish, where they develop

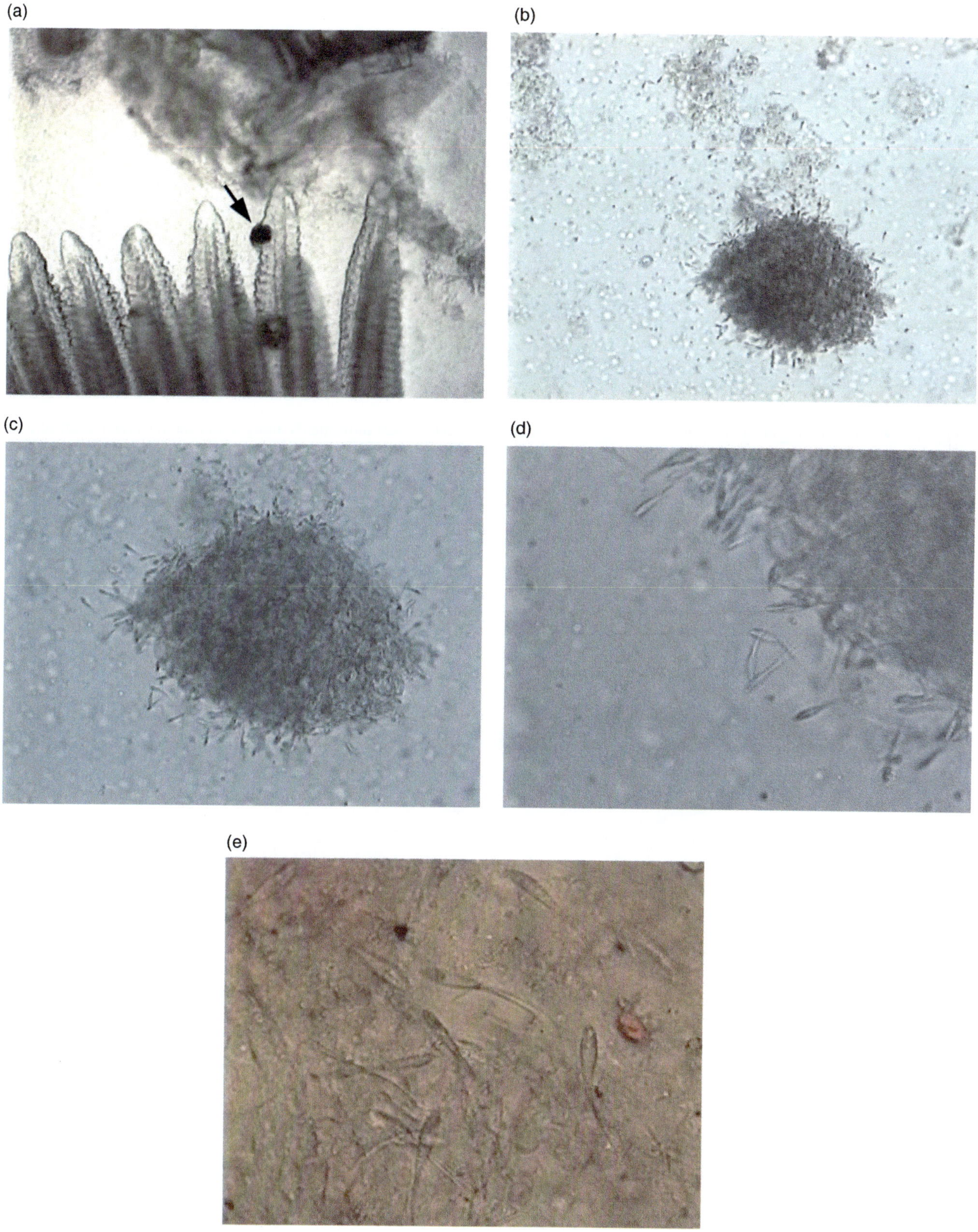

Fig. 31.23. (a) A wet mount of a gill biopsy from a freshwater fish reveals an enlarged secondary gill lamella associated with an intralamellar infection with the myxozoan parasite *Henneguya* (arrow) (4×). (b) A higher magnification (10×) of a *Henneguya* lesion similar to that seen in Figure 31.23a revealing the spores spilling out of the ruptured lesion. (c) A higher magnification (20×) of the image shown in Figure 31.23a. (d) A higher magnification (40×) of the image shown in Figure 31.23a. (e) A higher magnification (100× oil) of the image shown` in Figure 31.23a.

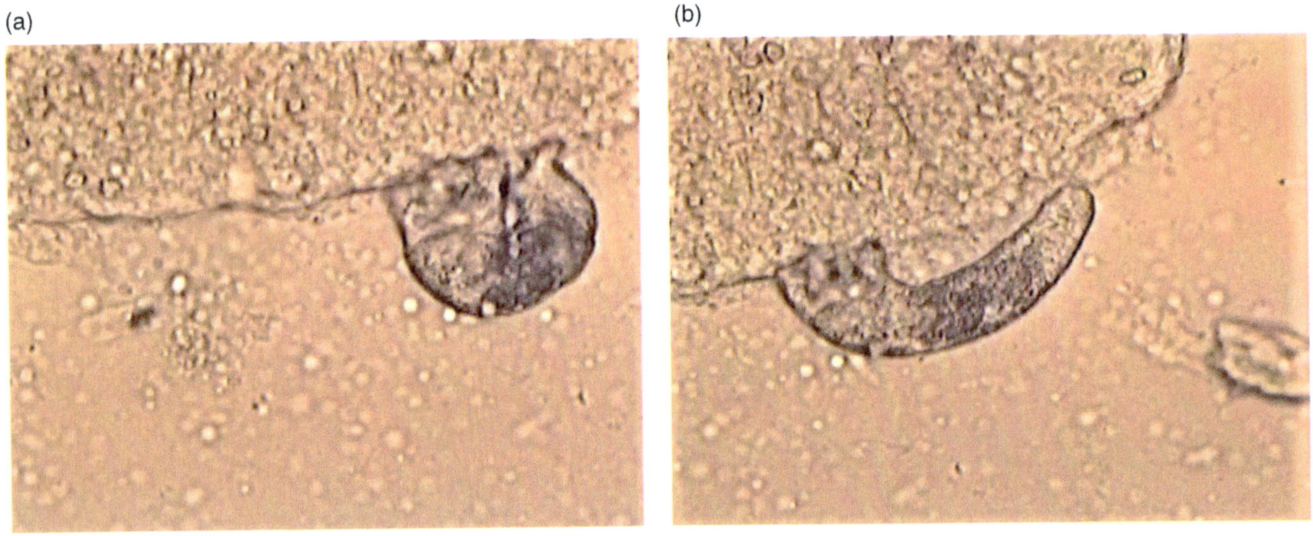

Fig. 31.24. (a) A monogenean parasite stretching and recoiling (caterpillar-like) movements along a wet-mount preparation of a gill biopsy (10×). (b) The same monogenean parasite as in Figure 31.24a stretching and recoiling (caterpillar-like) movements along a wet-mount preparation of a gill biopsy (10×).

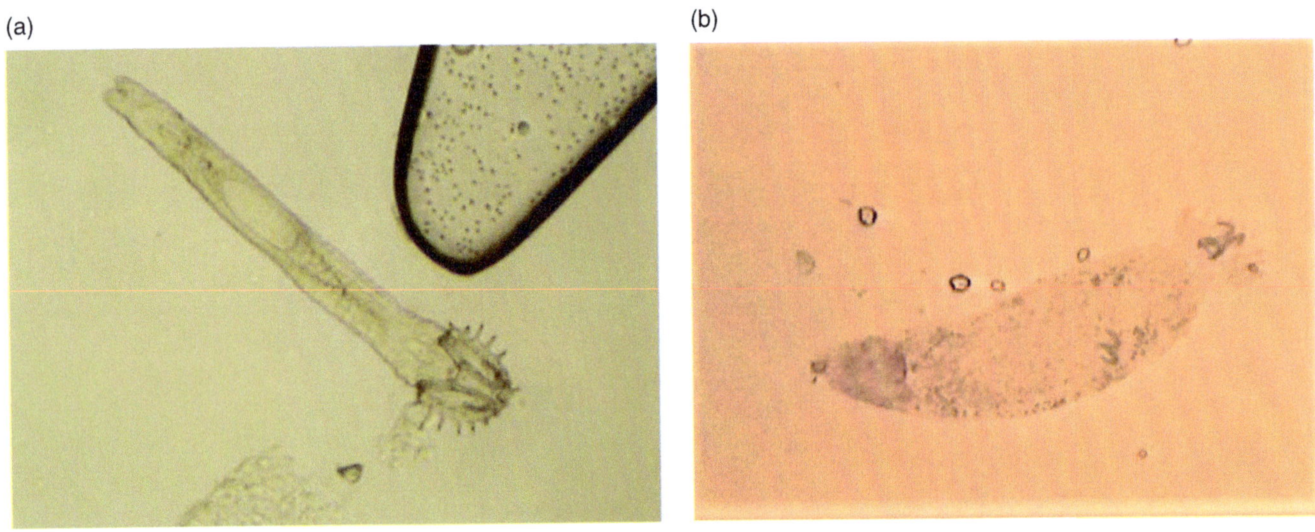

Fig. 31.25. (a) A monogenean parasite, *Gyrodactylus* sp., extending its body (40×). (b) A monogenean parasite, *Gyrodactylus* sp., found in a wet-mount preparation from a mucus scraping from a fish exhibiting flashing behavior (frequently rubbing on objects in its environment). Note the small hooklets of an embryo in the body of the parasite (40×).

into the adult stage (Kathorios et al., 2006). The larval stage (oncomiracidium) appears as free-swimming ciliates. The microcotylids have been reported on several hosts in wild and cultured marine fish.

Monogenean parasites in wild fish usually occur in low numbers presenting few, if any problems to the host. However, under culture conditions, they can cause serious problems to the host from severe anemia in the gills, reduced growth performance, loss of appetite, and mortalities (Kathorios et al., 2006). Because of their direct life cycle, monogeneans can occur in large numbers, especially when stressful conditions, such as poor water quality, occur. Clinical signs associated with monogenean infestation include flashing and skin disorders because of the injury to the skin. The principal pathological effects are from the feeding action of the parasite on the skin, gills, and fins. Injury to the host fish is also caused by the parasite's haptors, as the hooklets penetrate the epithelial cells.

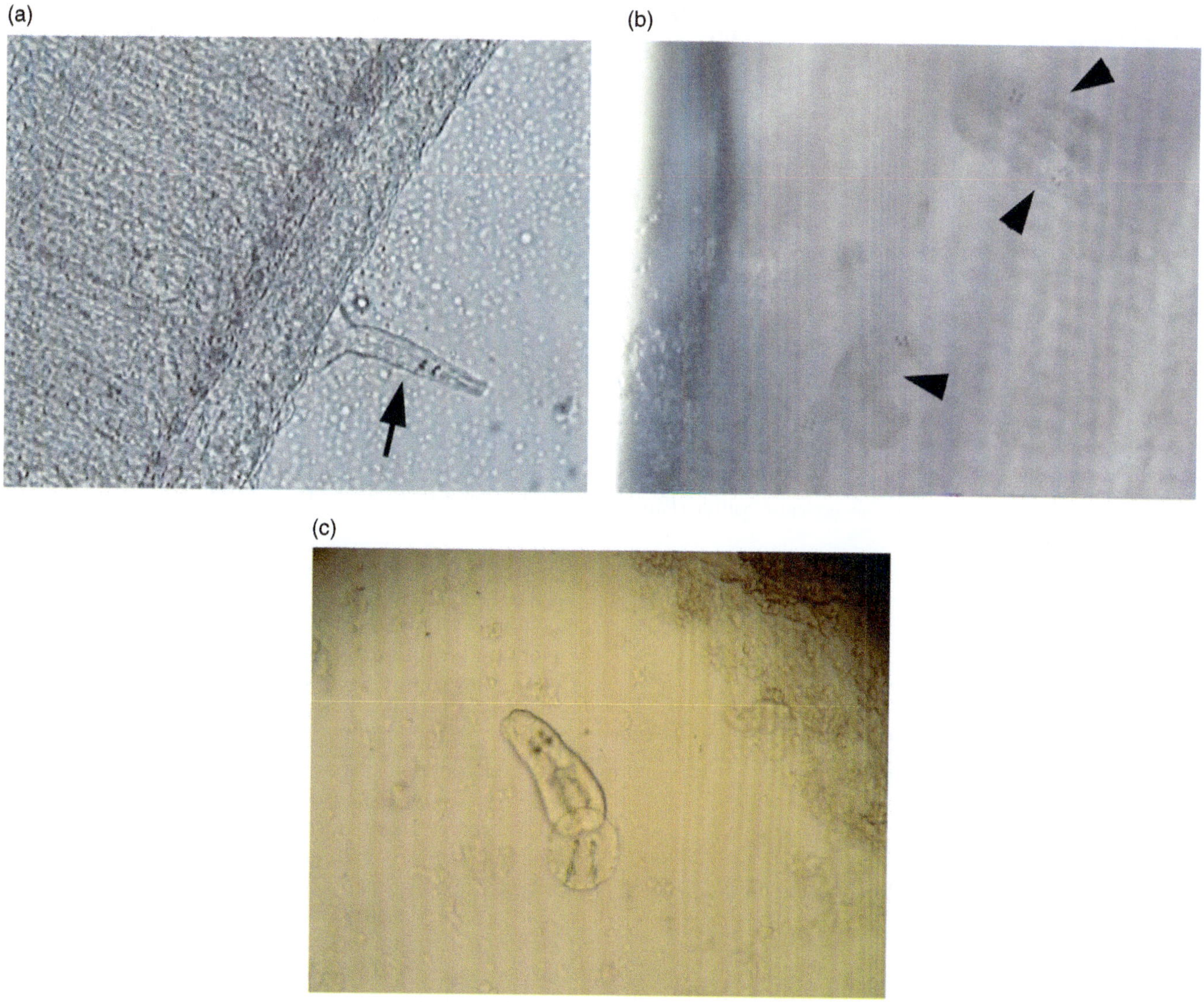

Fig. 31.26. (a) A monogenean, *Dactylogyrus* sp. (arrow), was taken from a wet-mount preparation of a gill biopsy from a freshwater fish with signs of respiratory distress (rapid gilling and coughing behavior). Note the eye spots. (10×). (b) Several dactylogyrids, *Dactylogyrus* sp. (arrowheads), taken from a wet-mount preparation of a gill biopsy from a freshwater fish with a heavy infestation of the parasite (10×). (c) A monogenean, *Dactylogyrus* sp., from a mucus smear preparation from a regal tang (*Paracanthurus hepatus*) with skin lesions (10×).

Digenean Trematodes

Digenean trematodes are endoparasites with an indirect life cycle. Digenean infestations are common in wild freshwater and marine fish. Adults live in the GI tract, have two suckers, and a Y-shaped gut. The larvae encyst throughout the host fish's body. The indirect life cycle of digenetic trematodes involves a definitive host, such as a piscivorous bird, a first intermediate host that is a snail, and a second intermediate host that is a fish. Diagnosis is based on the detection of the encysted metacercariae in wet-mount preparations of squash preparations, such as the skin, gill, fins, and internal organs (Figure 31.28). The encysted metacercariae have many of the characteristics of the adult digenean, such as suckers. Melanin pigment associated with the encysted digenean parasite results in "blackspot disease."

Turbellarians

Turbellarians are primarily free-living organisms that can be pathogenic to marine fish. Juvenile turbellarians feed on the skin and gills of the fish host during their growing phase (which lasts approximately 6 days). The turbellarian eventually drops off the host and continues to grow and develop numerous offspring in the detritus at the bottom of the aquatic habitat. The rapid life cycle of this parasite takes less than 2 weeks, resulting in high infestations in captive fish (Kent and Olson, 1986). High infestations can result in the death of the affected fish. Clinical signs for turbellarian infestations resemble those for other parasitic infestations, such as cryptocaryonosis and digenean metacercariae (Noga, 2000). Turbellarians are identified from mucus or gill biopsy wet-mount preparations. Turbellarians

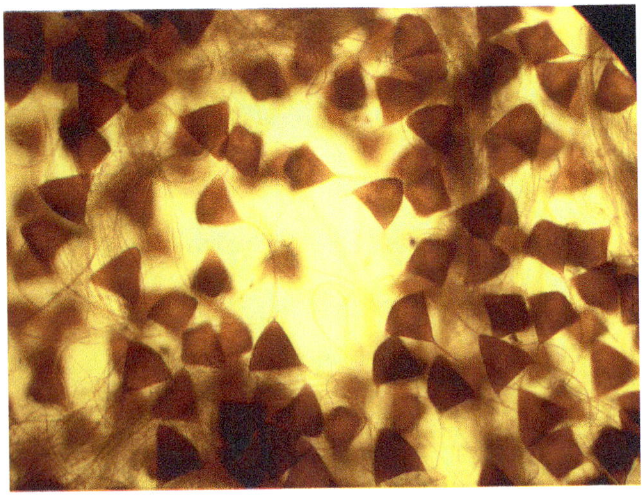

Fig. 31.27. Numerous golden capsulid monogenean eggs in a mucus smear preparation from an orbicular batfish (*Platax orbicularis*) (10×).

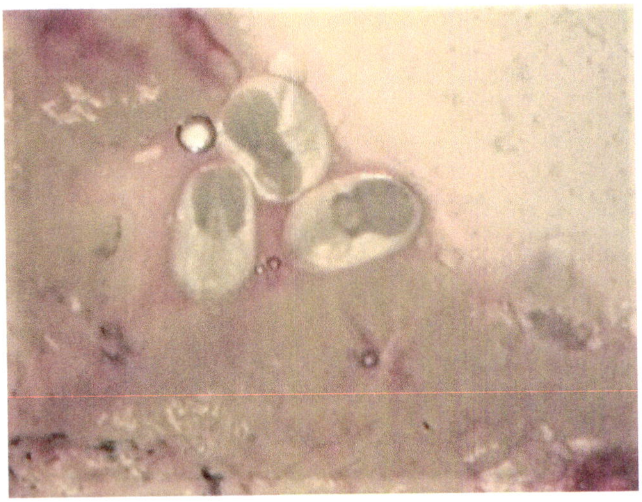

Fig. 31.28. A wet-mount preparation of a liver sample taken at necropsy of a freshwater fish reveals digenetic trematode larvae that have encysted in the liver (40×).

measure between 100 and 500 μm (Noga, 2000). This parasite is recognized by its oval shape, cilia, and two eyespots (Figure 31.29).

Crustaceans

Parasitic crustaceans cause serious gill and skin disease in freshwater and marine fish by their attachment or feeding processes. Crustacean parasites include the branchiurans and copepods. Branchiurans are ectoparasites with a dorsoventrally flattened body, measure over 1 cm in length, and possess prehensile suckers that attach to the body of freshwater fish. *Argulus* spp., often called the fish louse, is the best-known parasitic crustacean of the branchiurans group (Figures 31.30a and 31.30b). It

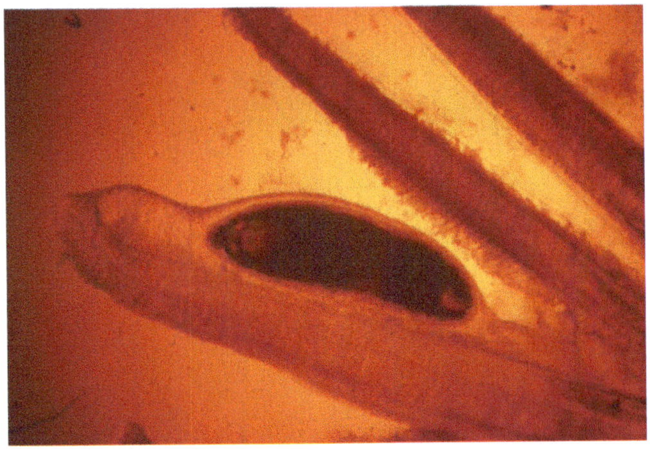

Fig. 31.29. This wet-mount preparation from a gill biopsy from a yellow tang (*Zebrasoma flavescens*) reveals a turbellarian parasite (*Paravortex*, or tang turbellarian). (10×).

has paired curved hooks and suckers as attachment organs. The direct life cycle of this parasite leads to heavy infestations in captive fish, resulting in cutaneous lesions and respiratory distress. *Argulus* is large enough (5–8 mm in length) to be seen with the naked eye.

Copepods have a diversity of body forms with variable appendages. Lernaeids are a species of highly modified copepods. These common copepod species of freshwater and marine fish are also known as the anchor worm because they possess anchorlike processes for attaching themselves directly to the host (Noga, 2010). There are approximately 110 species of cyclopoid copepods that are classified in the family Lernaeidae, with *Lamproglena* and *Lernaea* being the two largest genera. *Lernaea* spp., a parasite of freshwater fish and the best-known example of a parasitic copepod, are typically associated with high morbidity and low mortality, although they can have a high rate of mortality in small fish and affect fish growth. Members of the Lernaeidae have an antenna that is armed with a hook like terminal claw, a maxilla bearing two terminal claws, and the maxilliped carrying five terminal claws that contribute to their pathogenicity (Noga, 2010). Adult *Lernaea* spp. are visible macroscopically and can be identified on affected fish; however, developmental stages are only visible microscopically. The head of *Lernaea* spp. is a stellate anchor that embeds into the body musculature of the host fish. Females appear as Y-shaped parasites composed of an elongated trunk and two egg sacs hanging from the skin or fins of the affected fish (Figures 31.31a–31.31d). Microscopic examination of wet mounts of mucus scrapings, gill or fin biopsies, or mouth swabs may be useful in the identification of the various stages of the copepod. Scrapings may leave the head of the anchor worm embedded in fish.

Ergasilids (*Ergasilus* spp.) are another type of parasitic copepod of fish. They are commonly found on the

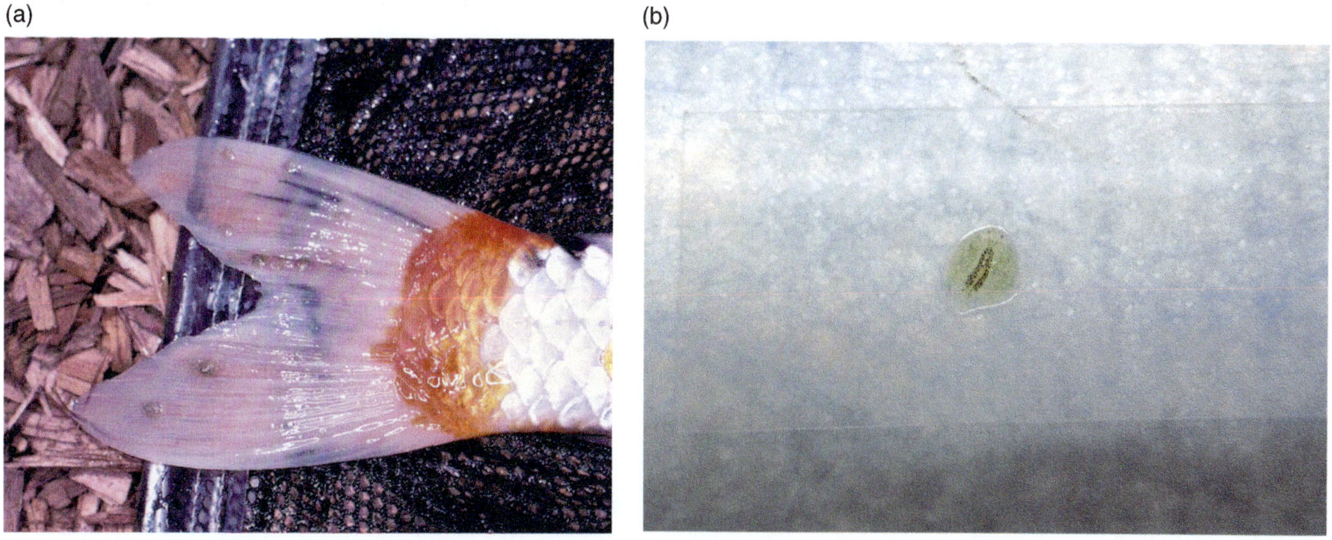

Fig. 31.30. (a) This image of the caudal fin of a koi (*Cyprinus carpio*) reveals copepod parasites of the genus *Argulus*, also known as the fish louse. (b) A copepod parasite, *Argulus*, from a freshwater aquarium fish (*Cyprinus carpio*).

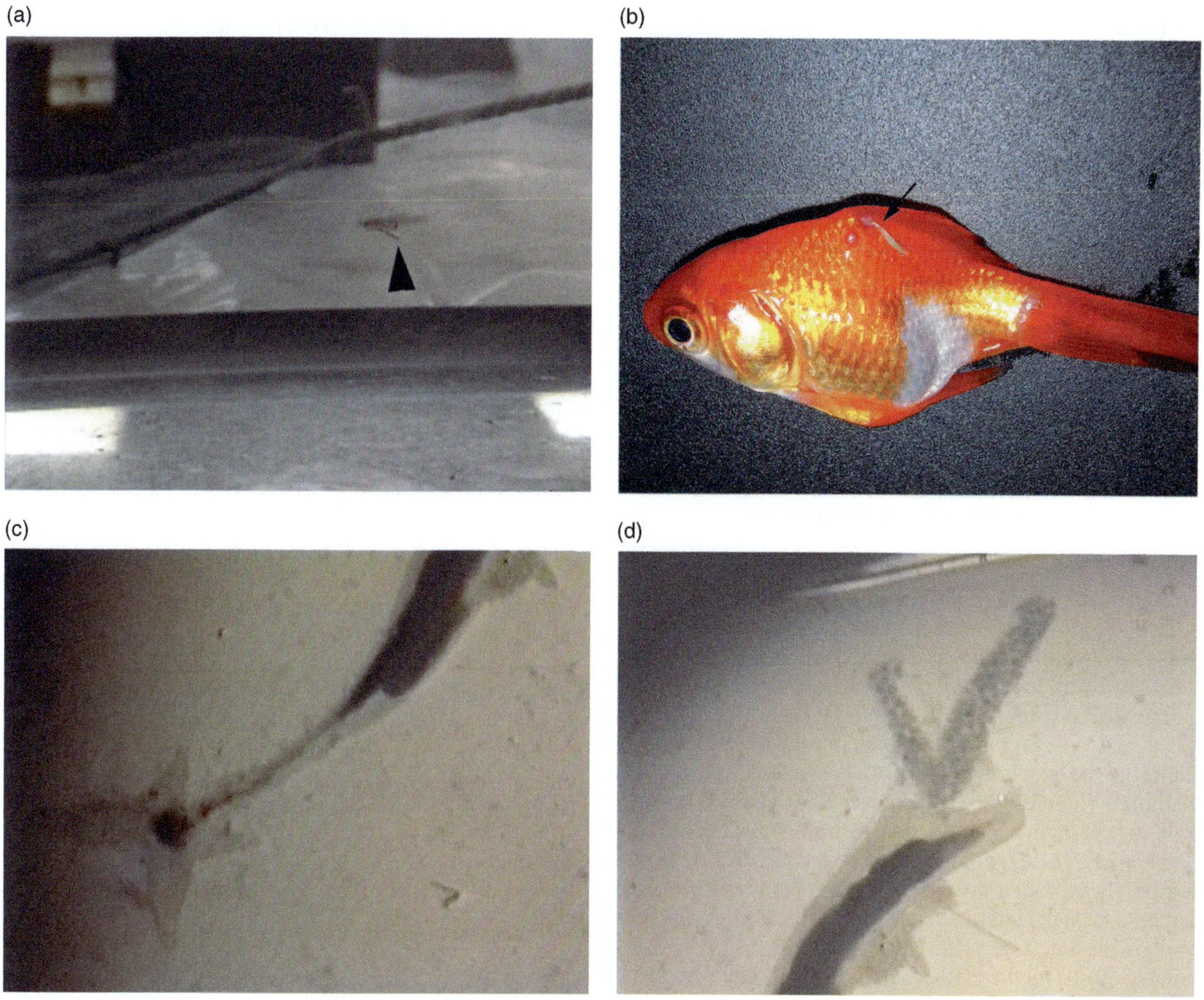

Fig. 31.31. (a) A freshwater fish (*Poecilia reticulate*) with an anchor worm (*Lernaea*) (arrowhead) attached to its skin. (b) A goldfish (*Carassius auratus*) with an anchor worm (*Lernaea*) (arrow) attached to its skin. (c) The attachment organ of the *Lernaea* seen in Figure 31.31b under a dissection microscope. (d) The attachment organ of the *Lernaea* seen in Figure 31.31b under a dissection microscope.

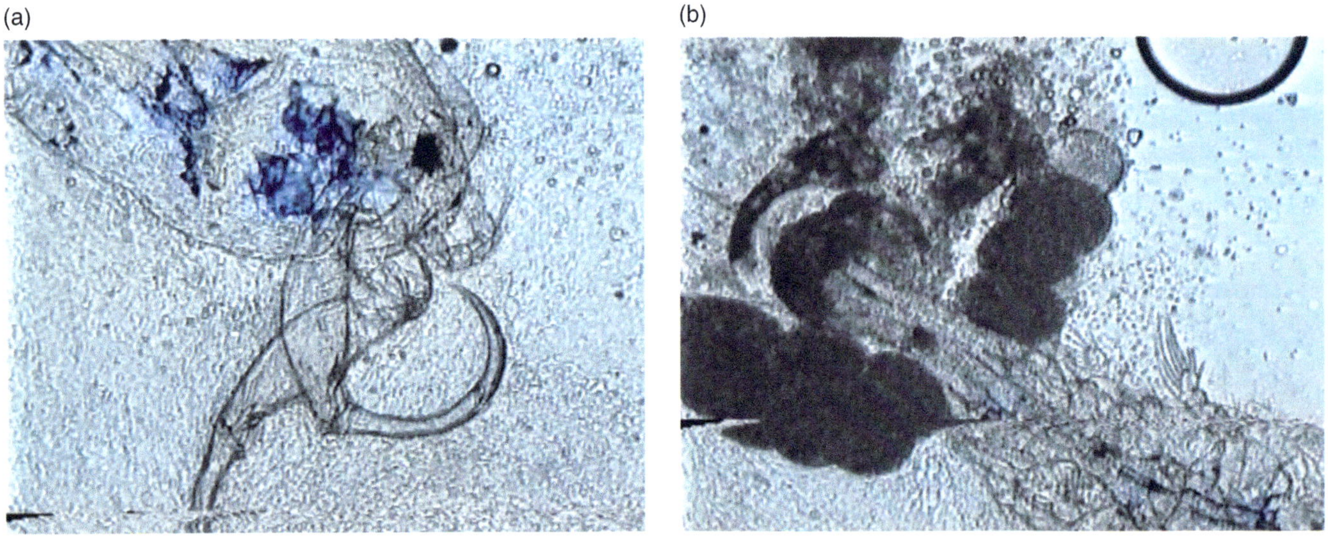

Fig. 31.32. (a) The head of the parasitic copepod, *Ergasilus* sp., of freshwater fish. Note the blue pigment associated with this parasite (20×). (b) The tail end of the same *Ergasilus* parasite shown in Figure 31.32a. Note the egg sacs of this parasite (20×).

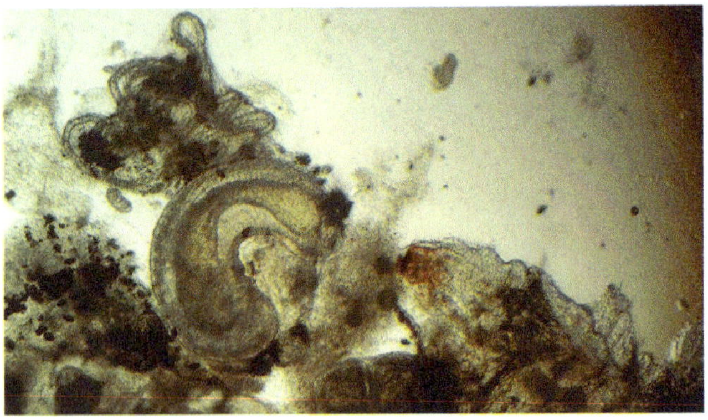

Fig. 31.33. The larva of a pentastomid in a wet-mount preparation from a swordtail fish (*Xiphophorous hellerii*).

gills of freshwater or brackish water fish, where they cause severe gill damage. These copepods are usually less than 2 mm long and have a conical, segmented body (Noga, 2000) (Figures 31.32a and 31.32b).

Pentastomes, crustacean endoparasites, are found as adults in the respiratory systems of reptiles, birds, and mammals (Figure 23.62 in Chapter 23). There, they lay eggs that pass out of the definitive host (Figure 23.63 in Chapter 23). The eggs are ingested by an intermediate host, commonly a fish or a small herbivorous mammal. The larva hatches inside the intermediate host and breaks through the wall of the intestine. The larva enters the tissues of its suitable host (Figure 31.33). It has two double hooked appendages, a penetration spine at the anterior end of the cephalothorax and in some, a long strongly hooked tail. Adult pentastomes do not resemble the larval form found in fish (Woodyard et al., 2019). Pentastomid infections can result in diseases associated with high morbidity and mortality in some species of fish, while causing no apparent ill effects in others.

Nematodes

Parasitic nematodes are typically found as internal parasites of the gastrointestinal tract of fish. Adult nematodes can be found during necropsy examination after opening the gastrointestinal tract of dead fish or protruding from the vent of living fish. Fish are often intermediate hosts for nematodes; therefore, larval forms can be found in other tissues, including the subcutis (Figures 31.34a–31.34c).

Coccidia

Coccidian oocyst are important features in differentiating the many genera and species of coccidia in fishes. Except for three genera, *Cryptosporidium, Octosporella,* and *Isospora,* fish coccidia have oocysts containing four sporocysts, each with two sporozoites (tetrasporocystic and dizoic). Fish coccidia, like those of other vertebrates, frequently develop in the gastrointestinal tract; therefore, are found in wet-mount preparations of intestinal content. Also, because fish coccidia frequently exhibit extra intestinal development, they may be found in cytologic preparations of other locations (Molnár and Székely, 2017).

Nonpathogenic Organisms

Nonpathogenic organisms are frequently found in wet-mount preparations from fish. For example, species of the genus *Euplotes* are widely distributed in marine

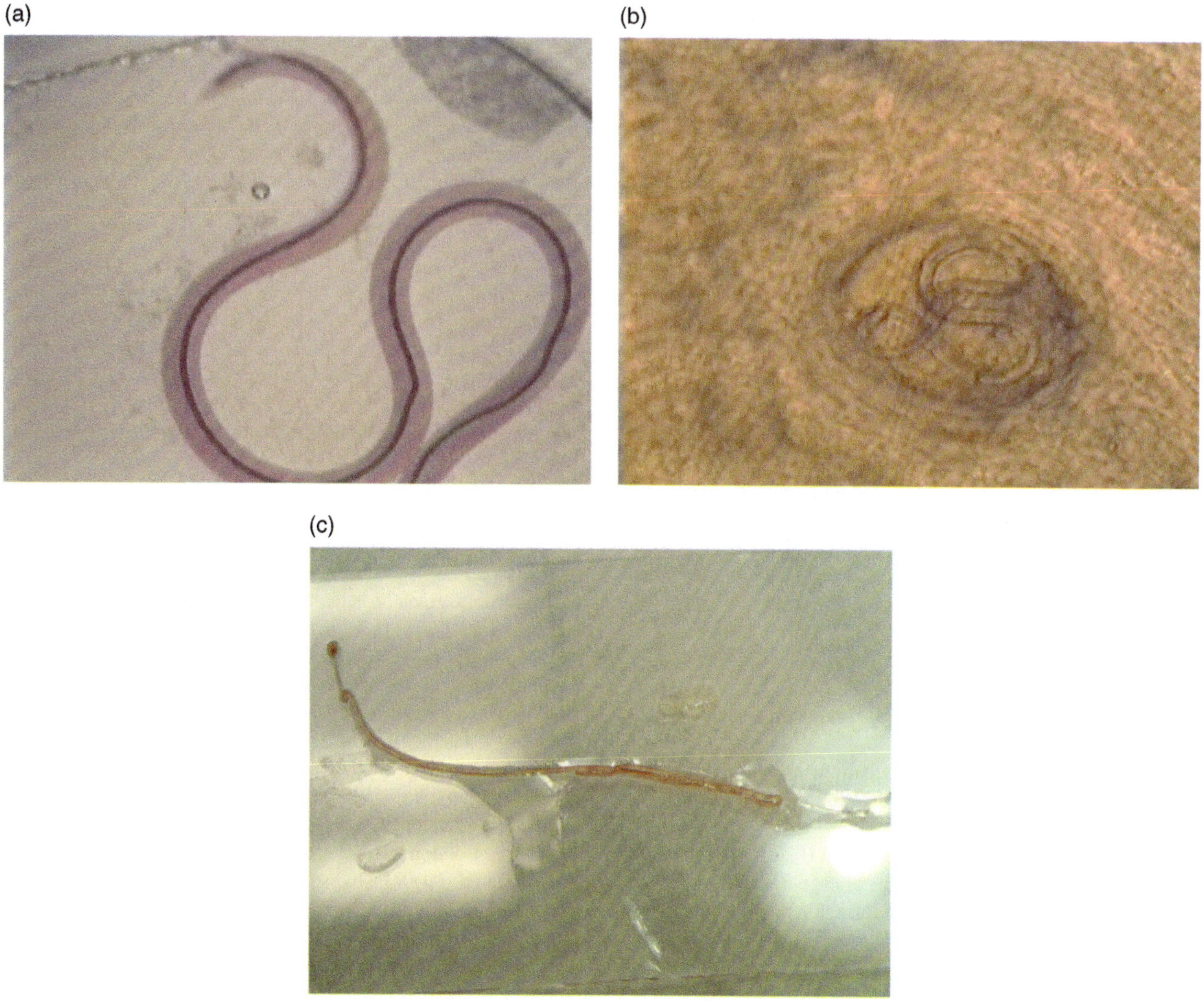

Fig. 31.34. (a) A small nematode found in the intestinal tract of a fish during a necropsy examination (40×). (b) A nematode encysted in the muscle of a fish was found during a necropsy examination (40×). (c) An 8-cm-long nematode removed from under the skin of an 8-cm-long sharpnose puffer (*Canthigaster* sp.).

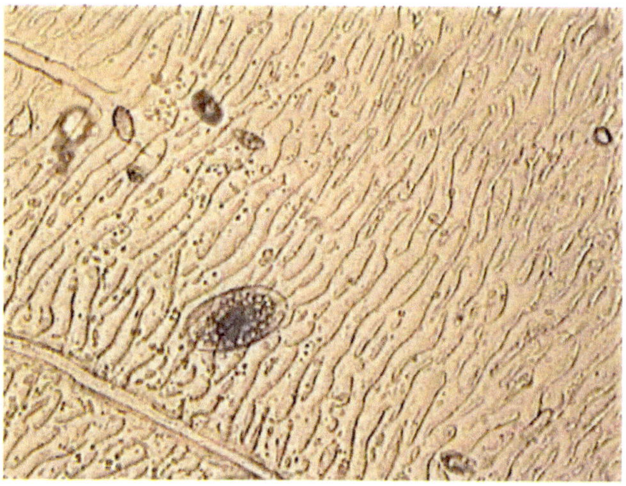

Fig. 31.35. A larger free-living, nonpathogenic *Euplotes* sp. is seen on a scale in this wet-mount preparation of a mucus smear along with pathogenic *Uronema* sp. (40×).

and freshwater environments (Figure 31.35). When seen, these free-living ciliates should be recognized as an incidental finding.

References

Adamek M, Teitge F, Steinhagen D. 2019. Quantitative diagnostics of gill diseases in common carp: Not as simple as it seems. *Dis Aquat Org* 134:197–207.

Abdel-Hafez G, Lahnsteiner F, Mansourx N, Licek E. 2014. Pathophysiology of *Ichthyophthirius multifiliis* infection in rainbow trout (*Oncorhynchus mykiss*) and chub (*Leuciscus cephalus*). *J Comp Pathol* 151:394–399.

Alonso MC, Cano I, Garcia-Rosado E, et al. 2005. Isolation of lymphocystis disease virus from sole, *Solea senegalensis* Kaup, and blackspot sea bream, *Pagellus bogaraveo* (Brunnich). *J Fish Dis* 28:221–228.

Bullard SA, Frasca S, Benz Gw. 2001. Gill lesions associated with *Erpocotyl tiburonis* (Monogenea: Hexabothriidae) on wild and aquarium-held bonnethead sharks (*Sphyrna tiburo*). *J Parasitol* 87(5):972–977.

Cavin JM, Donahoe SL, Frasca Jr S, et al. 2012. *Myxobolus albi* infection in cartilage of captive lumpfish (*Cyclopterus lumpus*). *J Vet Diagn Invest* 24(3):516–524.

Dickerson HW, Findly RC. 2014. Immunity to *Ichthyophthirius* infections in fish: a synopsis. *Dev Comp Immunol* 43:290–299.

Ellis AE, Roberts RJ, Tytler P. 1978. The anatomy and physiology of teleosts. In: Roberts R (ed), *Fish Pathology*. London: Bailliere-Tindall.

Gibson-Kueh S, Netto P, Ngoh-Lim GH, et al. 2003. The pathology of systemic iridoviral disease in fish. *J Comp Pathol* 129(2–3):111–119.

Gieseker CM, Serfling SG, Reimschuessel R. 2006. Formalin treatment to reduce mortality associated with *Saprolegnia parasitica* in rainbow trout, *Oncorhynchus mykiss*. *Aquac* 253:120–129.

Gómez F, Gast RJ. 2018. Dinoflagellates *Amyloodinium* and *Ichthyodinium* (Dinophyceae), parasites of marine fishes in the South Atlantic Ocean. *Dis Aquat Org* 131:29–37.

Gratzek JB. 1988. Parasites associated with ornamental fish. *Vet Clin North Am (Sm Anim Pract)* 18(2):375–399.

Hine PM, Wakefield StJ, Mackereth G, Morrison R. 2016. Ultrastructural morphogenesis of a virus associated with lymphocystis-like lesions in parore *Girella tricuspidata* (Kyphosidae: Perciformes). *Dis Aquat Org* 121:129–139.

Howell CK, Atkinson SD, Bartholomew JL, Hallett SL. 2019. Development and application of a qPCR assay targeting *Ichthyophthirius multifiliis* in environmental water samples. *Dis Aquat Org* 134:43–55.

Isaksen TE. 2013. Ichthyobodo infections on farmed and wild fish. Methods for detection and identification of *Ichthyobodo* spp. PhD thesis, University of Bergen.

Kathorios P, Papandroulakis N, Divanach P. 2006. Treatment of *Microcotyle* sp. (Monogenea) on the gills of cage-cultured red porgy, *Pagrus pagrus* following baths with formalin and mebendazole. *Aquac* 251:167–171.

Kaur H, Katoch A. 2016. Prevalence, site and tissue preference of myxozoan parasites infecting gills of cultured fish in Punjab (India). *Dis Aquat Org* 118:129–137.

Kent ML, Olson AC. 1986. Interrelationships of a parasitic turbellarian (*Paravortex* sp.) (Graffillidae, Rhabdocoela) and its marine fish hosts. *Fish Pathol* 21:65–72.

Kent ML, Shaw RW, Sanders JL. 2014. Microsporidia in fish. In: Weiss ML, Becnel JJ (eds), *Microsporidia: Pathogens of Opportunity*. Ames, IA: John Wiley & Sons, pp. 521–570.

Li D, Zhai Y, Gu Z, Liu Y. 2017. Development of a multiplex PCR method for the simultaneous detection of four myxosporeans infecting gibel carp *Carassius auratus gibelio*. *Dis Aquat Org* 124:31–39.

Li J-P, Fu1Y-W, Zhang Q-Z, et al. 2018. Grass carp which survive *Dactylogyrus ctenopharyngodonid* infection also gain partial immunity against *Ichthyophthirius multifiliis*. *Dis Aquat Org* 129:63–70.

Lom J. 1970. Protozoa causing diseases in marine fishes. In: Snieszko S (ed), *A Symposium on Diseases of Fishes and Shellfishes*. Special Publication No. 5. Washington, DC: American Fisheries Society.

Lu C, Ling F, Ji J, Kang YJ, Wang GX. 2013. Expression of immune-related genes in goldfish gills induced by *Dactylogyrus intermedius* infections. *Fish Shellfish Immunol* 34:372–377.

Lynn DH, Gransden SG, Wright ADG, Josephson G. 2000. Characterization of a new species of the ciliate *Tetrahymena* (Ciliophora: Oligohymenophorea) isolated from the urine of a dog: first report of *Tetrahymena* from a mammal. *Acta Protozool* 39:289–294.

Lynn DH, Doerder FP, Gillis PL, Prosser RS. 2018. *Tetrahymena glochidiophila* n. sp., a new species of *Tetrahymena* (Ciliophora) that causes mortality to glochidia larvae of freshwater mussels (Bivalvia). *Dis Aquat Org* 127:125–136.

Maceda-Veiga A, Cable J. 2019. Diseased fish in the freshwater trade: from retailers to private aquarists. *Dis Aquat Org* 132:157–162.

MacMillan JR. 1991. Biological factors impinging upon control of external protozoan fish parasites. *Annual Review of Fish Diseases*, pp. 119–131.

Matthews RA. 2005. *Ichthyophthirius multifiliis* fouquet and ichthyophthiriosis in freshwater teleosts. *Adv Parasitol* 59:159–241.

Mizuno S, Urawa S, Miyamoto M, et al. 2017. Epizootiology of the ectoparasitic protozoans *Ichthyobodo salmonis* and *Trichodina truttae* on wild chum salmon *Oncorhynchus keta*. *Dis Aquat Org* 126:99–109.

Mohammed HH, Arias CR. 2014. Epidemiology of columnaris disease affecting fishes within the same watershed. *Dis Aquat Org* 109:201–211.

Molnár K, Székely C. 2017. Epicellular coccidiosis in goldfish. *Dis Aquat Org* 125:1–5.

Mousavi SM, Mirzargar SS, Mousavi EZ, et al. 2009. Evaluation of antifungal activity of new combined essential oils in comparison with malachite green on hatching rate in rainbow trout (*Onchorhyncus mykiss*) eggs. *J Fish Aquat Sci* 4:103–110.

Munir E, Dewi RR, Yunasfi, Suryanto D. 2017. A study of potential control of water mold *Saprolegnia* sp. of Gouramy (*Osphonemus gouramy*) eggs by bacterial isolates. *J Pure Appl Microbio* 11(1):623–632.

Noga EJ, Levy MG. 1995. Dinoflagellida (Phylum Sarcomastigophona) in fish diseases and disorders. In: Woo P (ed), *Fish Diseases and Disorders*, Volume 1: Protozoan and Metazoan Infections. London: CABI.

Noga EJ. 2000. Fish disease: diagnosis and treatment. In: Noga E (ed), *Fish Disease: Diagnosis and Treatment*. Ames, IA: Iowa State University Press.

Noga EJ. 2010. *Fish Disease: Diagnosis and Treatment*, 2nd edn. Ames, IA: Wiley-Blackwell.

Özer A, Özkan H, Gürkanlı CT, Yurakhno V, Çiftçi' Y. 2016. Morphology, histology and phylogeny of *Henneguya sinova* sp. nov. (Myxobolidae: Myxozoa) infecting gills of *Parablennius tentacularis* in the Black Sea, Turkey. *Dis Aquat Org* 118:207–215.

Picard-Sanchez A, Piazzon MC, Ahmed NH, et al. 2020. *Enterospora nucleophila* (Microsporidia) in gilthead sea bream (*Sparus aurata*): pathological effects and cellular immune response in natural infections. *Vet Pathol* 57(4):565–576.

Poynton SL. 2001. Developments in diagnosis of diplomonad flagellate infections: *Spironucleus*, *Hexamita* and *Brugerolleia*. In: Proceedings of AAZV and IAAM. Joint Conference, pp. 213–214.

Roberts RJ. 2001. The parasitology of teleosts. In: Roberts RJ (ed), *Fish Pathology*. London: WB Saunders.

Rummer JL, Brauner CJ. 2021. Gas exchange. In: Currie S, Evans DH (eds), *The Physiology of Fishes*, 5th edn. Boca Raton, FL: CRC Press, pp. 33–45.

Ryan JA, Kohler SL. 2016. Distribution, prevalence, and pathology of a microsporidian infecting freshwater sculpins. *Dis Aquat Org* 118:195–206.

Sharon G, Leibowitz MP, Chettri JK, Isakovx N, Zilberg D. 2014. Comparative study of infection with tetrahymena of different ornamental fish species. *J Comp Pathol* 150:316–324.

Smith PA, Elliott DG, Bruno DW, Smith SA. 2019. Skin and fin diseases. In: Smith SA (ed), *Fish Diseases and Medicine*. Boca Raton, FL: CRC Press, Pp. 97–133.

Sokolov SG, Lebedeva DI, Murzina SA, et al. 2019. Morphology and phylogeny of *Henneguya oviperda* infecting oocytes of *Esox lucius*, with description of parasite-induced histopathology. *Dis Aquat Org* 133:91–98.

Tripathi NK, Latimer KS, Gregory CR, et al. 2005. Development and evaluation of an experimental model of cutaneous columnaris disease in koi *Cyprinus carpio*. *J Vet Diagn Invest* 17:45–54.

Vergneau-Grosset C, Larrat S. 2015. Microsporidiosis in vertebrate companion exotic animals. *J Fungi* 2(1):3–23.

Weber EPS. 2013. Itchy fish and viral dermatopathies: sampling, diagnosis, and management of common viral diseases. *Vet Clin Exot Anim* 16:687–703.

Woodyard ET, Baumgartner WA, Rosser TG, et al. 2019. Morphological, molecular, and histopathological data for *Sebekia mississippiensis* overstreet, self, and vliet, 1985 (Pentastomida: Sebekidae) in the American alligator, *Alligator mississippiensis* Daudin, and the spotted gar, *Lepisosteus oculatus* Winchell. *J Parasitol* 105(2):283–298.

Wu R-H, Tang X-Q, Sheng X-Z, Zhan W-B. 2015. Tissue distribution of the 27.8 kDa receptor and its dynamic expression in response to lymphocystis disease virus infection in Flounder (*Paralichthys olivaceus*). *J Comp Pathol* 153:324–332.

Zoller G, Santamaria-Bouvier A, De Lasalle J, et al. 2017. Total pneumocystectomy in a telescope goldfish (*Carassius auratus*) with fungal pneumocystitis. *J Exotic Pet Med* 26:19–28.

32 Wet-Mount Microscopy in Fish: Clinical Case Presentations

Case 1: Tiger Barb with Skin and Behavior Changes

Signalment

Tiger barb (*Puntigrus tetrazona*) in a freshwater aquarium

History

Fish from a recent shipment to a pet store were exhibiting skin and behavior changes.

Physical Examination

The fish exhibited slightly raised white spots on the fins (Figure 32.1). Some showed rapid respiration.

A mucus scraping over the white spots revealed numerous round protozoa moving about in a slow rolling motion across the wet-mount preparation (Figures 32.2a and 32.2b).

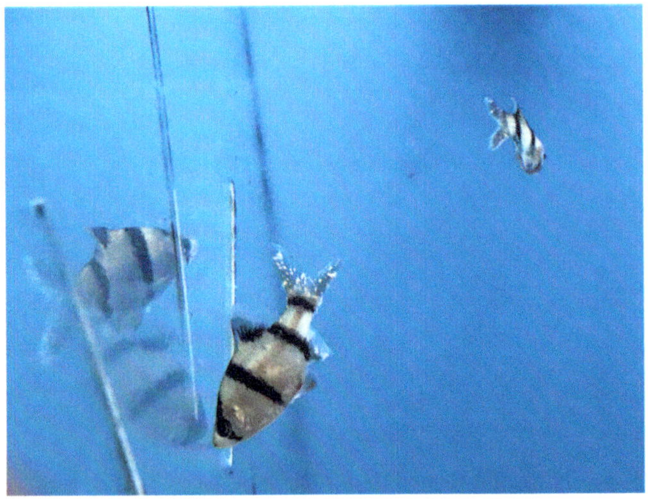

Fig. 32.1. Tiger barbs (*Puntigrus tetrazona*) exhibiting slightly raised white lesions on the fins.

Interpretive Discussion

The wet-mount preparation revealed motile round, but deformable (up to 1 mm in diameter) holotrich ciliate protozoan. The horseshoe-shaped macronucleus of these protozoa identifies them as *Ichthyophthirius multifiliis*.

Summary

A sudden onset of a marked outbreak of *Ichthyophthirius multifiliis* in warm and temperate freshwater fish is common in aquarium fishes. Incoming fish can be carriers of the parasite without showing clinical signs; however, the aquarium can also have a latent population of the parasite surviving on resistant fish. New fish additions are typically stressed and have lowered immune systems, making them more likely to become infected.

Case 2: Newly Arrived Goldfish

Signalment

Goldfish (*Carassius auratus*)

History

A new shipment of goldfish arrived at a pet store.

Exotic Animal Hematology and Cytology, Fifth Edition. Terry W. Campbell and Krystan R. Grant.

Companion website: www.wiley.com/go/campbell/exotic

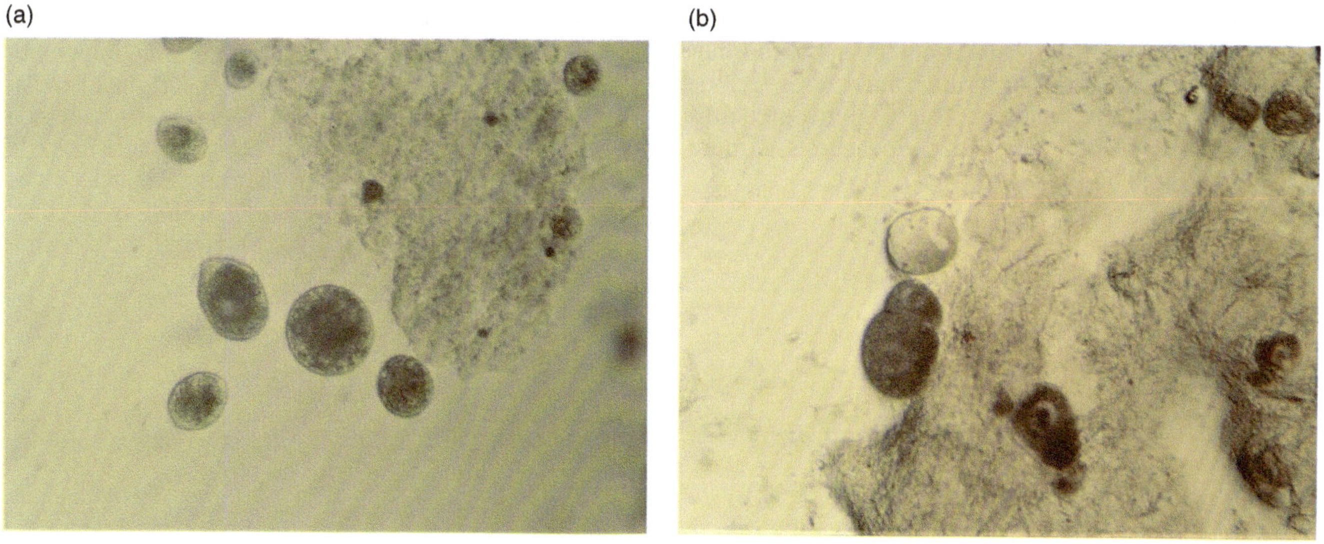

Fig. 32.2. (a), (b) Wet mount of white spot lesions on the fins (20×).

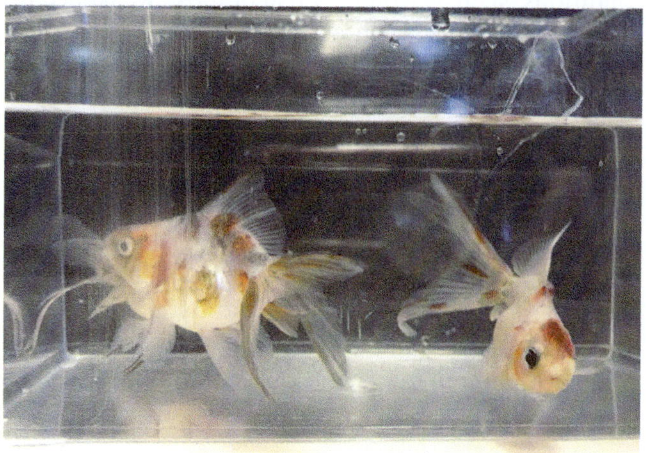

Fig. 32.3. Goldfish in a recent shipment to a pet store.

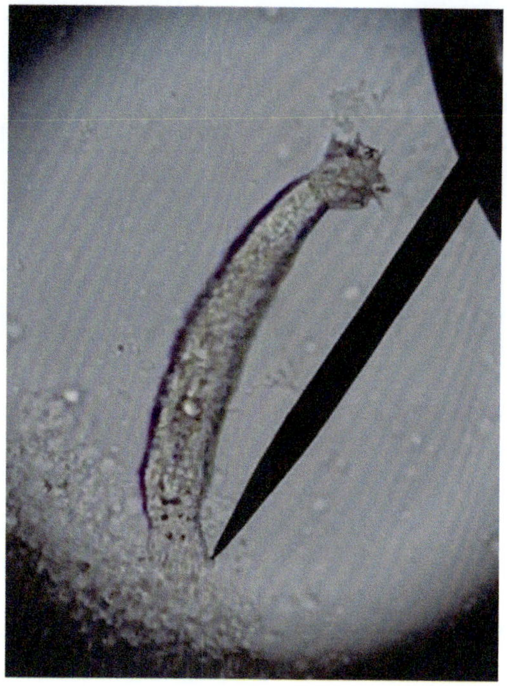

Fig. 32.4. View of the wet mount at 40× objective.

Physical Examination

The fish were netted for routine examination. They appeared healthy (Figure 32.3). A mucus smear was made from an area along the side of one of the fish and examined as a wet-mount preparation (Figure 32.4).

Interpretive Discussion

A monogenean, *Dactylogyrus*, on the skin.

Summary

Monogeneans are easily identified on wet-mount preparations of the gills, skin, or fins by their morphology and stretching and recoiling (caterpillar-like) movements. The gyrodactylids, *Gyrodactylus* spp. and *Gyrodactyloides* spp. are small viviparous monogeneans that measure 0.3–1.0 μm in length. Small embryos (or their hooklets) may be found within the parasite. The dactylogyrids, *Dactylogyrus* spp., are oviparous monogeneans that resemble the gyrodactylids, but are slightly larger (up to 2 μm in length) and possess eye spots. These monogeneans possess a haptor (attachment organ), have a direct life cycle, and are ectoparasites that live on skin, gills, and fins. The direct life cycle allows for heavy infestations in the confined space of the aquarium. Dactylogyrus is an oviparous monogenean parasite that is often found in co-infections with other parasites, bacteria, fungi, or viruses, and causes serious damage to the hosts. In general, Dactylogyrus predominantly affects the gills, whereas Gyrodactylus is more commonly found on the skin.

Case 3: Cichlid with a Missing Eye

Signalment

Cichlid (*Labidochromis caeruleus*)

History

This fish, kept in a home aquarium with other freshwater tropical fish, was presented with a missing eye.

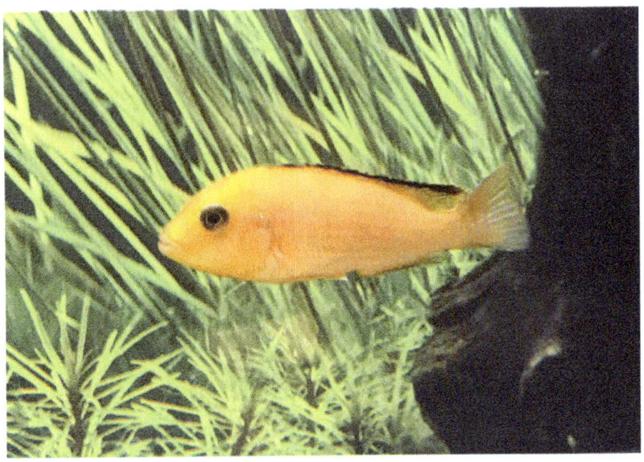

Fig. 32.5. Cichlid with missing right eye.

Physical Examination

The fish was netted for examination and appeared healthy except that it was missing the right eye. The skin below the eye appeared pale with a slight hemorrhage (Figure 32.5). A mucus smear was made from the area below the missing right eye and examined as a wet-mount preparation. A few motile, pear-shaped ciliate protozoa (60 µm by 100 µm) moving in a spiraling football-style movement were seen (Figures 32.6a and 32.6b).

Interpretive Discussion

Tetrahymena protozoa on the skin.

Summary

Conditions that allow for heavy *Tetrahymena* infestations are likely associated with immunosuppressive conditions, such as wounded fish or those weakened by poor water quality, such as high ammonia concentration, high organic content, extreme water temperature, high fish density, or a disease. *Tetrahymena* is commonly found living in organic debris at the bottom of an aquarium. When they occur on the body surface in low numbers (less than five organisms per low power field), they likely are an insignificant finding. They are commonly found on dead fish on the bottom of an aquarium and associated with high levels of organic material in the system. Therefore, the presence of *Tetrahymena* on dead fish on the bottom of the aquarium does not imply the parasite was the primary cause of death.

(a) (b)

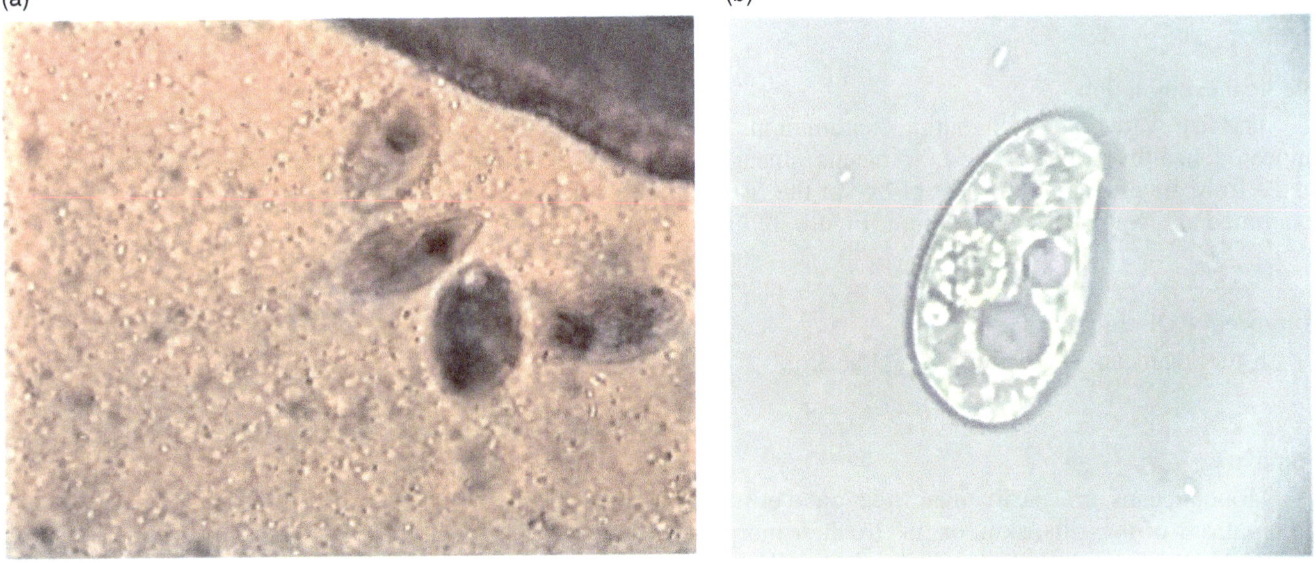

Fig. 32.6. (a), (b) View of the wet mount at 40× objective.

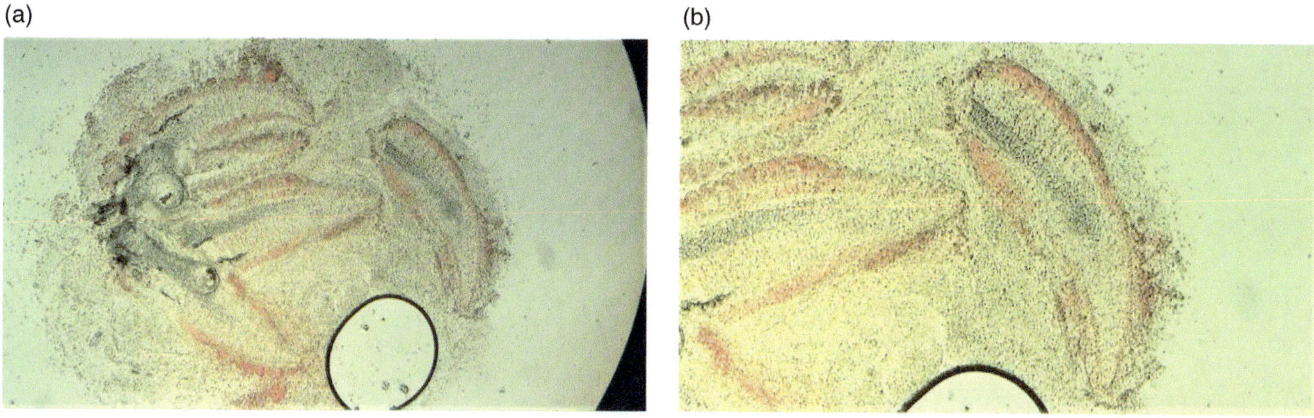

Fig. 32.7. (a) Low magnification of a gill biopsy from a pepper cory catfish. (b) Higher magnification of the same image as in Figure 32.7a.

Case 4: Catfish with Rapid Breathing and Lethargy

Signalment

Pepper cory catfish (*Corydoras paleatus*) in a freshwater aquarium

History

This fish was one of several fish in the aquarium exhibiting rapid breathing and lethargy. Fish were beginning to die. This fish died immediately after capture.

Physical Examination

The fish appeared thin and was gilling rapidly before it died. The fish appeared light in color and was covered with a thick layer of mucus.

A gill biopsy was performed and examined as a wet-mount preparation (Figures 32.7a and 32.7b).

Interpretive Discussion

The wet-mount preparation revealed secondary gill lamellae with a thick coating of hyperplastic epithelium and mucus.

Summary

Gill damage from bacteria, parasites, and poor water quality causes epithelial proliferation and thickened gill filaments. Because evidence of bacterial and parasitic involvement was not found, poor water quality was suspected. Water quality testing revealed elevated ammonia concentration in the aquarium water.

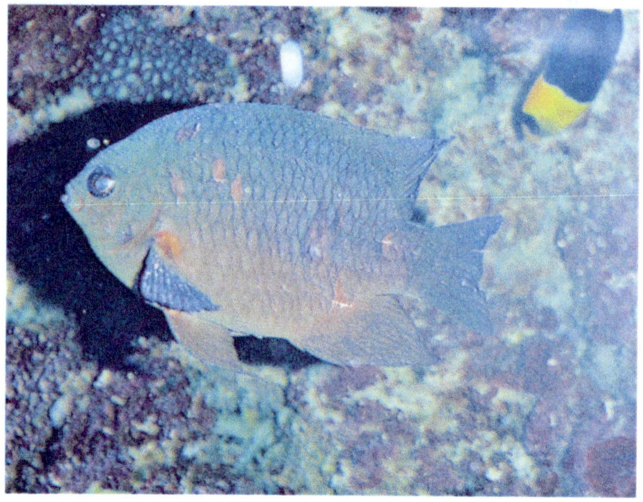

Fig. 32.8. Damselfish exhibiting skin ulcerations and slightly raised white lesions on the fins.

Case 5: Damselfish with Skin Lesions and Behavior Changes

Signalment

Damselfish (Pomacentridae) in a marine aquarium

History

This fish and a few others housed in a mixed-species marine aquarium as part of a large public aquarium were exhibiting skin and behavior changes.

Physical Examination

The fish exhibited skin ulcerations and slightly raised white spots on the fins (Figure 32.8). Some exhibited flashing behavior and rapid respiration.

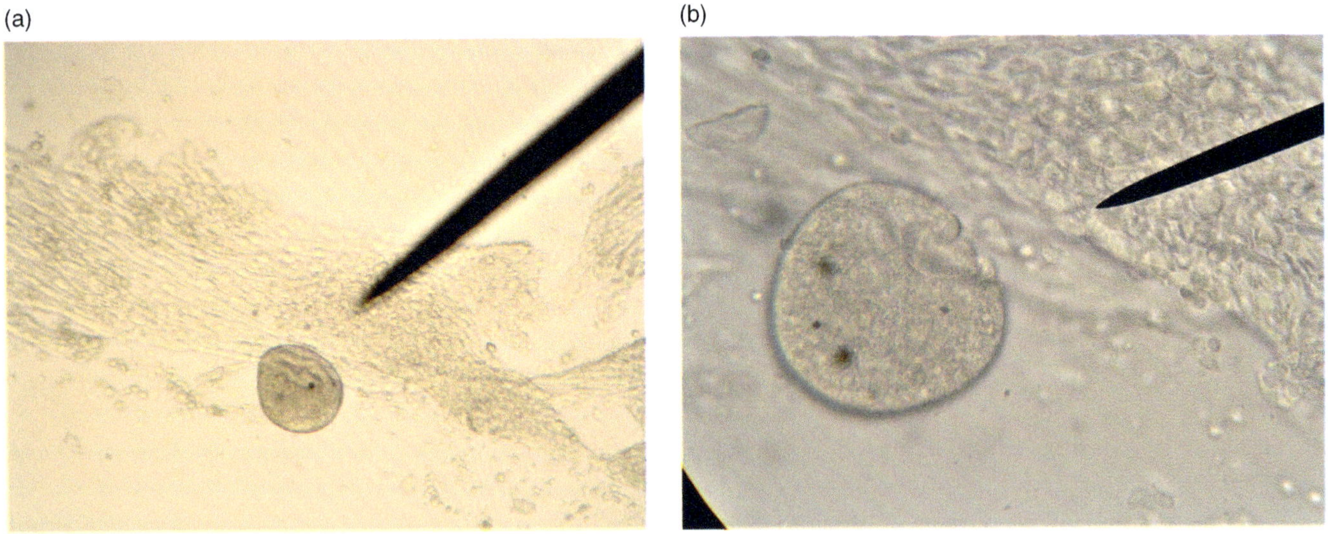

Fig. 32.9. (a) Wet mount of white spot lesions on the fins (20×). (b) Wet mount of white spot lesions on the fins (40×).

A mucus scraping over the white spots revealed numerous round protozoa moving about in a slow rolling motion across the wet-mount preparation (Figures 32.9a and 32.9b).

Interpretive Discussion

The wet-mount preparation revealed motile round, holotrich ciliate protozoan. The protozoa were identified as *Cryptocaryon irritans*, the marine counterpart of the freshwater *Ichthyophthirius multifiliis*.

Summary

Cryptocaryon irritans is a protozoan parasite that causes a disease known as marine "ich" or marine "white spot" disease in wild and cultured marine fish. Infections with this parasite cause significant disease problems for marine aquarists and commercial mariculture worldwide. The organism is known to infect many species of marine fish.

33

Piscine Cytodiagnosis

Interpretation of cytological preparations from fish is more challenging compared to that of mammals, birds, and herptiles. The basic cytological responses of fish can be classified as inflammation, tissue hyperplasia/benign neoplasia, malignant neoplasia, or normal cellularity. The inflammatory lesions can be classified as neutrophilic (heterophilic), mixed cell (pyogranulomatous), macrophagic, or rarely, eosinophilic based upon the predominant types of inflammatory cells in the sample. Fish granulomas are often characterized cytologically by the presence of lymphocytes, macrophages, neutrophils, or heterophils (eosinophilic granulocytes), and melanomacrophage aggregates (Molter et al., 2019).

In fish, macrophages accumulate melanin from phagocytosis (melanosynthesis has also been reported in visceral macrophages), where the melanin has a protective role in neutralizing free radicals during oxidative stress or producing bactericidal compounds (Matsche et al., 2021).

Melanomacrophages are unique melanin-containing cells of the mononuclear phagocyte system that have been reported in the liver, spleen, kidney, and at sites of chronic inflammation in fish (Agius and Roberts, 2003) (Figure 33.1). In agnathan and elasmobranch fish, melanomacrophages are found in isolation, whereas in osseous fish, they exist in clusters (melanomacrophage clusters) in the spleen and the posterior kidney as well as in less discrete groupings or individually in other tissues including the liver and intestine; except the salmonids, where clusters are neither dense nor well defined (Agius and Roberts, 2003; Vigliano et al., 2006; Santos et al., 2011; Gutierre et al., 2018; Matsche et al., 2021).

Goldfish melanomacrophages are distinguishable from tissue macrophages and neutrophils by being Sudan black B positive (unlike tissue macrophages) and nonspecific esterase positive (unlike neutrophils), but like tissue macrophages they are also acid phosphatase and CSF-1R positive (Diaz-Satizabal and Magor, 2015). Despite their name, the dominant pigment in these cells is lipofuscin, with melanin being the second most frequently observed pigment (Agius and Roberts, 2003).

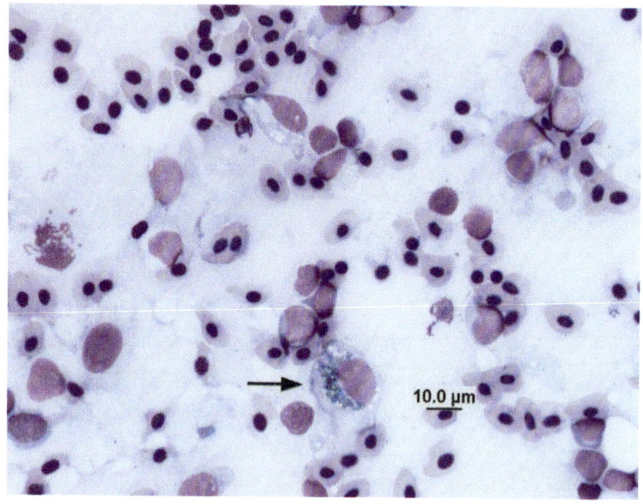

Fig. 33.1. A melanomacrophage (arrow) in an imprint of a black pigmented inflammatory skin lesion from a koi (*Cyprinus carpio*). Wright–Giemsa stain.

Skin

Ulcerative cutaneous lesions with reddened scales are common skin lesions of fish. Impression smear cytologic preparations are often helpful in identifying the causative agent. Macrophagic inflammation or mixed-cell inflammation with degenerative neutrophils (or heterophils), plasma cells, and lymphocytes are

Exotic Animal Hematology and Cytology, Fifth Edition. Terry W. Campbell and Krystan R. Grant.

Companion website: www.wiley.com/go/campbell/exotic

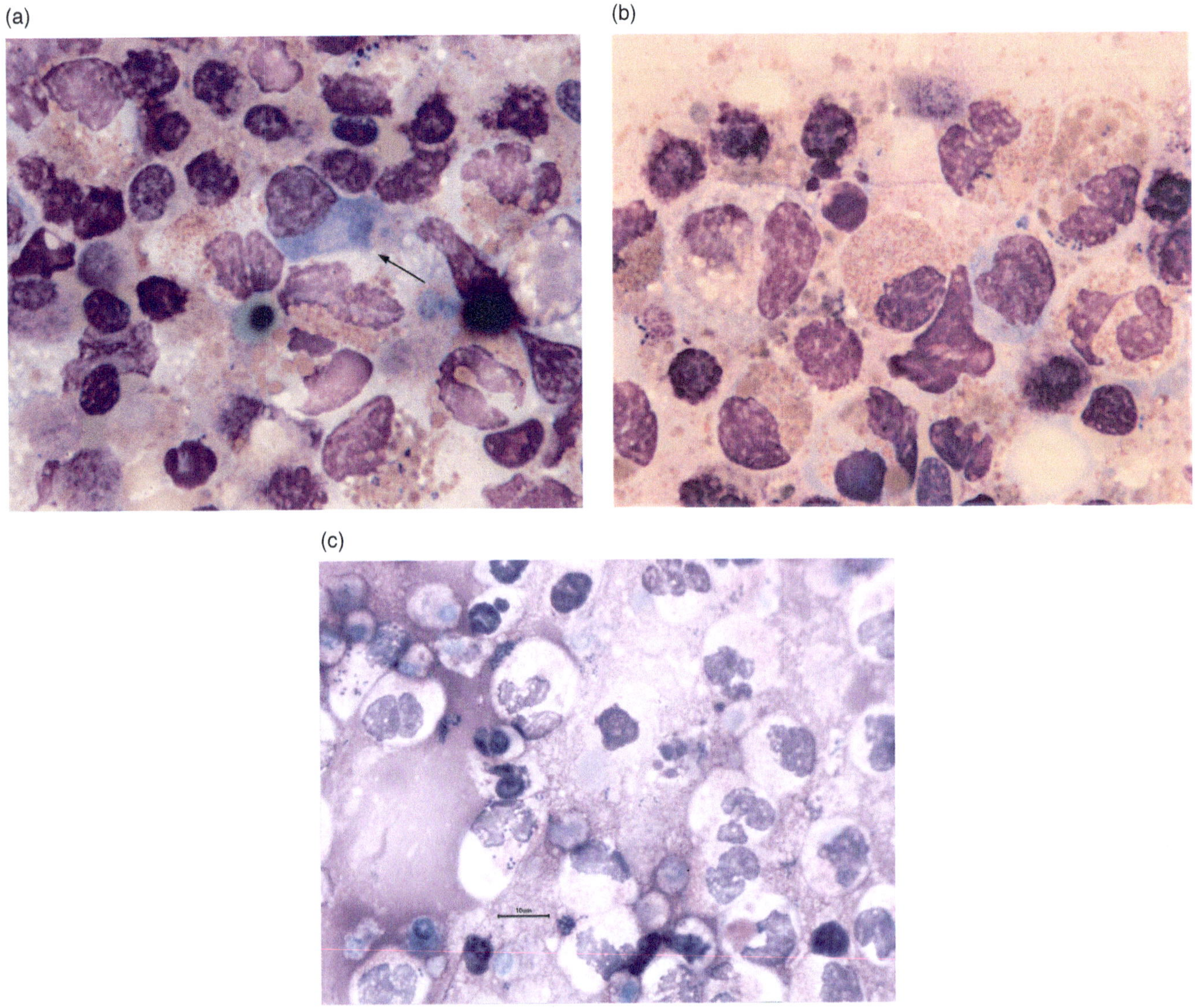

Fig. 33.2. (a) Mixed-cell inflammation in a white tip reef shark (*Triaenodon obesus*). Note the plasma cell (arrow) among the nondegenerate G_1 (heterophil) granulocytes. Wright–Giemsa stain (100× oil). (b) Mixed-cell inflammation in a white tip reef shark (*Triaenodon obesus*) showing nondegenerate G_1 (heterophil) granulocytes and macrophages. Wright–Giemsa stain (100× oil). (c) Septic inflammation in an aspirate from an abscess in the skin of a white tip reef shark (*Triaenodon obesus*) showing degenerate G_1 (heterophil) granulocytes and bacterial phagocytosis. Wright–Giemsa stain (100× oil).

common cytological responses along with lysed cells and a mixed population of extracellular bacteria in the background (Figures 33.2a–33.2c, 33.3a, 33.3b, 33.4a, 33.4b, 33.5, and 33.7). Frequently found objects in cytological preparations of the skin of fish include the following (see Chapter 31):

- Fish scales vary greatly in size, shape, structure, and coverage. They originate in the dermis, and the exposed portion is covered by a layer of epithelium that prevents direct contact with the surrounding water.
- Fish epithelial cells are small, polygonal, squamous cells lacking keratinization, with basophilic cytoplasm, and occasionally, a pyknotic central nucleus.
- *Lymphocystis* is an iridoviral disease that causes marked dermal fibroblast hypertrophy (infected cells can be up to 100 000 times their normal size), leading to wart-like tumorous skin and fin lesions.
- *Trichodina* spp. are mobile peritrich ciliates, present in both marine and freshwater environments. On cytological preparations, they are circular in shape with cilia lining the external edge (measuring 45–50 μm) with a characteristic internal denticular ring (measuring 25–30 μm) that consists of 18–22 interlinking hook-shaped structures (denticles) with a circular adhesive disk (measuring 30–40 μm) encompassing the denticles (Varvil et al., 2018).
- *Ichthyophthirius multifiliis* is a large (up to 1 mm in diameter) holotrich ciliate parasite with a large C-shaped nucleus.

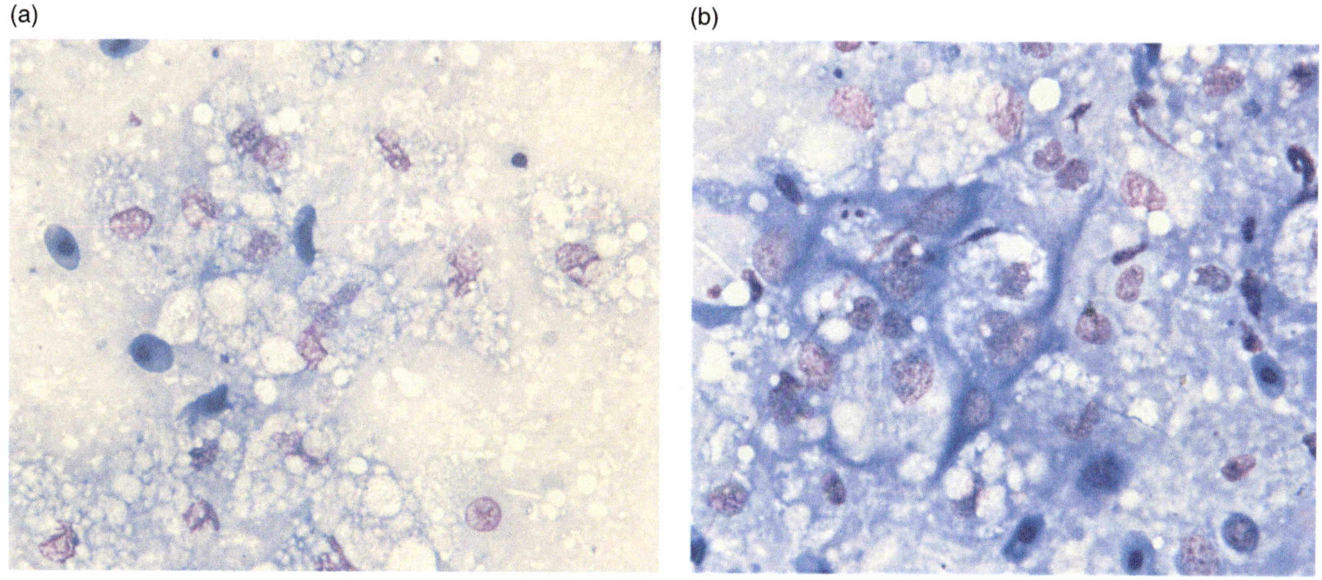

Fig. 33.3. (a) Macrophagic inflammation in a wolf eel (*Anarrhichthys ocellatus*). Wright–Giemsa stain (100× oil). (b) An imprint of a biopsy of a cutaneous mass in a wolf eel (*Anarrhichthys ocellatus*) showing numerous foamy macrophages with fat droplets in the noncellular background. A macrophagic inflammation with fat droplets is suggestive of a lipid disorder of the skin. Histology of the biopsy indicated a chronic granulomatous dermatitis possibly associated with a dyslipidosis. Wright–Giemsa stain (100× oil). Source: Image from Campbell and Grant (2010, p. 326).

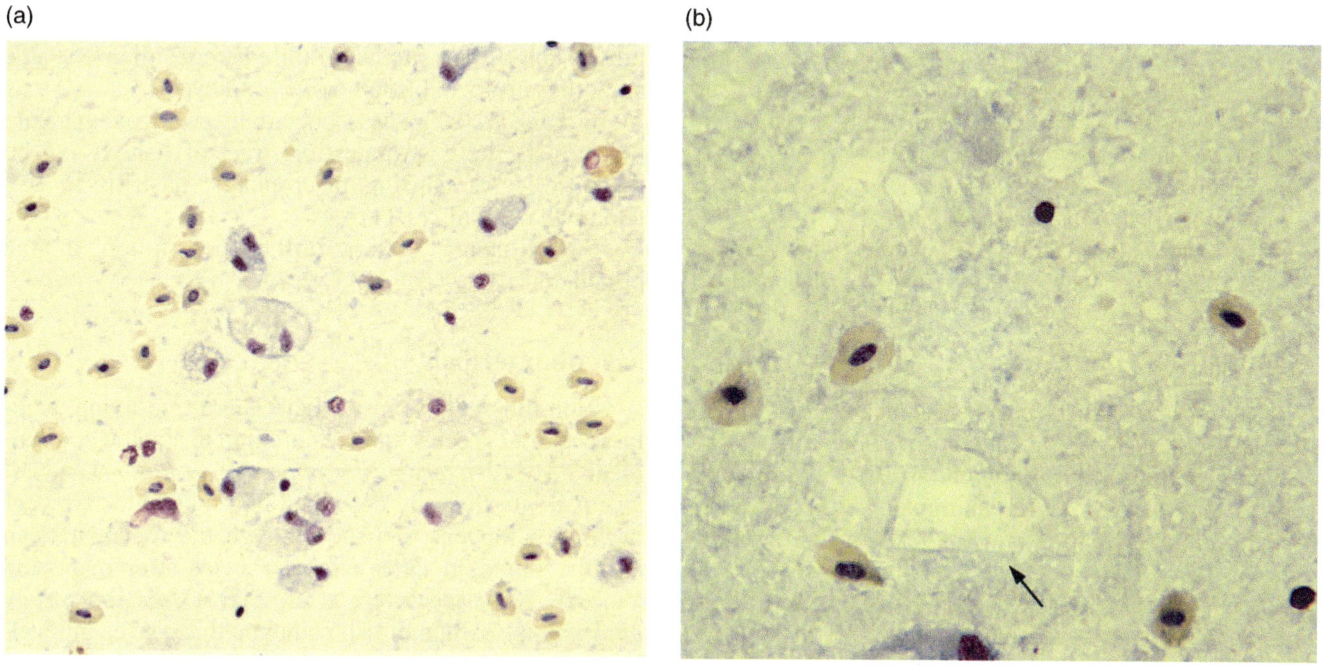

Fig. 33.4. (a) A fine-needle aspirate of a cutaneous mass reveals a highly cellular sample with a predominance of macrophages with foamy cytoplasm indicative of macrophagic inflammation in a Plecostomus (*Hypostomus plecostomus*) with a cholesterol granuloma. Wright–Giemsa stain (50×). (b) Cholesterol crystals (arrow) in a fine-needle aspiration biopsy of a cutaneous mass in a Plecostomus (*Hypostomus plecostomus*) with a cholesterol granuloma in the same sample as in Figure 33.4a. Wright–Giemsa stain (100× oil). Source: Image from Campbell and Grant (2010, p. 352).

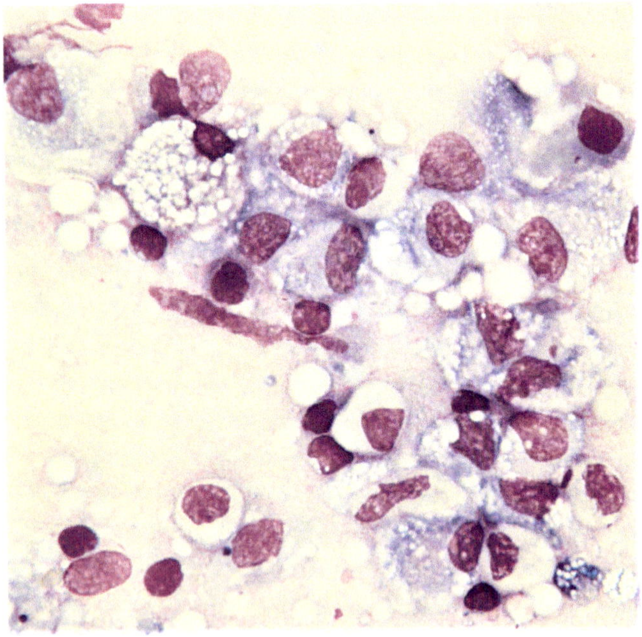

Fig. 33.5. Macrophagic inflammation in an impression of a cutaneous mass from a red-eye tetra (*Moenkhausia sanctaefilomenae*) with a *Mycobacterium* sp. infection. Wright–Giemsa stain (50×). Source: Image from Campbell and Grant (2010, p. 366).

- *Chilodonella* spp. are dorsoventrally flattened oval ciliate protozoan with cilia located in distinct bands along the body.
- *Epistylis* spp. are sessile, colonial stalked peritrich ciliate protozoa with an oral infraciliature feeding structure.
- Saprolegnia appears as branched nonseptate fungal hyphae 7–30 µm wide that are often associated with other pathogens, such as bacteria and protozoa.
- Monogeneans are parasitic flatworms with holdfast organs, such as hooks, hooklets, suckers, or clamps.

Calcinosis Circumscripta

Calcinosis circumscripta is a benign lesion presumed to be associated with mineralization of necrotic tissue secondary to trauma or inflammation. This condition has been primarily reported in mammals; however other animals, such as the southern stingray (*Hypanus americanus* formerly *Dasyatis americana*) can also develop the lesion (Campbell and Grant, 2010). Cytological features of the lesions reveal numerous refractile crystals of various shapes and sizes along with an inflammatory response that consists predominantly of macrophages and fibroblasts (Figure 33.6).

Fecal Cytology

Diatoms and algae are commonly found in fecal and other cytology specimens collected from aquatic animals, especially in herbivorous species, and can be present in variable numbers and morphologic diversity. The silica cell wall of these organisms prevents examination of internal structures on routine cytological preparations (Stacy et al., 2014). They are incidental findings and must be differentiated from more important structures, such as parasite helminth ova, coccidian oocysts, and other protozoal trophozoites and cysts.

Cryptosporidium is a coccidian protozoal parasite that affects the gastrointestinal tract of fish. It can be responsible for causing macrophagic gastritis in fish (Baragahare et al., 2011).

See Chapter 23 for further description of the organism.

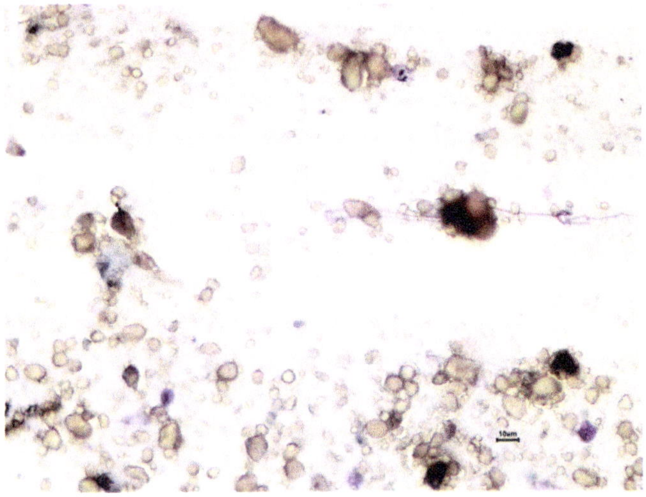

Fig. 33.6. Numerous refractile crystals of various shapes and sizes in a fine-needle aspiration biopsy from a cutaneous calcinosis circumscripta lesion in a southern stingray (*Hypanus americanus* formerly *Dasyatis americana*). Wright–Giemsa stain (400×).

Mycobacteriosis

Non-tuberculosis mycobacteria are free-living, acid-fast bacterial species that are common in aquatic environments. *Mycobacterium marinum*, *M. fortuitum*, and *M. chelonae* are the only described non-tuberculosis mycobacteria pathogens of fish, although the organisms can also be found in other animal species (Bercovier and Vincent, 2001; Decostere et al., 2004). *Mycobacterium marinum* is a common fish pathogen that causes intracellular granulomatous infections in fish and humans. *Mycobacterium fortuitum* is a ubiquitous species broadly present worldwide in various habitats such as lakes, surface water, potable water, and soil and has been frequently isolated from fish and wild animals including reptiles, amphibians, and invertebrates. *Mycobacterium chelonae* infection in fish generally progresses toward a chronic inflammatory granulomatous disease. In aquaculture, outbreaks of mycobacteriosis are associated with stressful

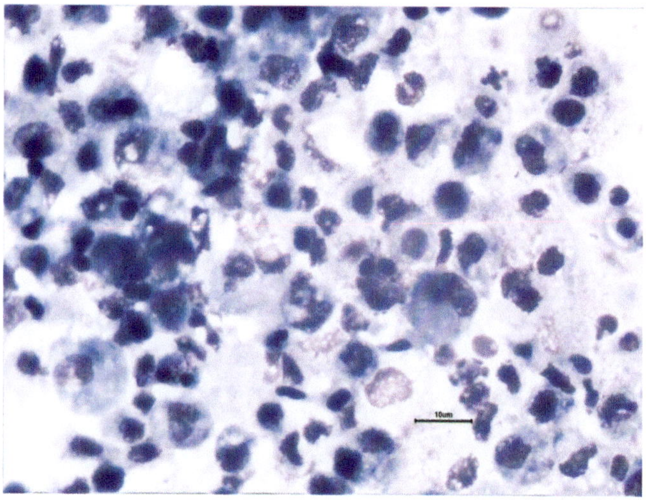

Fig. 33.7. Macrophagic inflammation in an impression smear of a cutaneous lesion from a walleye (*Sander vitreus*). Wright–Giemsa stain (100× oil).

environmental conditions and are invariably lethal (Lapointe et al., 2014). Cytological preparations reveal non-staining bacilli with Romanowsky-stains and beaded, slender, acid-fast bacilli with acid-fast stain (Clarke et al., 2013). A macrophagic inflammatory response is typical in cytological samples (Figure 33.7).

Saprolegniasis

Saprolegniasis is a catch-all term for white, fuzzy mold growth on the skin of fish. Oomycetes fungi, such as *Saprolegnia* and related genera, are common water molds that are frequently associated with skin infections on fish (Noga, 2000). Gross lesions caused by these fungi appear as white, cotton-like growths on the skin and gills. Wet-mount preparations reveal wide (7–30 µm) aseptate hyphae that are often associated with other pathogens, such as bacteria and protozoa.

Further description of *Saprolegnia* is found in Chapter 31.

Thyroid

There is a need to exercise caution in diagnosing thyroid growths as neoplastic in bony fishes, due to unique features of the normal and proliferating teleost thyroid. Whether it is ectopic or pharyngeal, follicular cell hyperplasia in fishes can be extensive (Fournie et al., 2005, Jalenques et al., 2020). Neoplastic cells should exhibit cytological features of malignant neoplasia, such as cellular pleomorphism, nuclear atypia, and/or increased mitotic figures.

Because the elasmobranch thyroid is an encapsulated organ, local invasion of the surrounding tissues is a valid criterion for malignancy from a histologic perspective; however, "invasiveness" is less meaningful in teleosts due to the diffuse distribution of their normal thyroid tissue (Crow et al., 2001). Most proliferative lesions reported from elasmobranchs are goiters, not neoplasms, and would be classified as nodular hyperplasia.

A cytological description of thyroid tissue is found in Chapter 7.

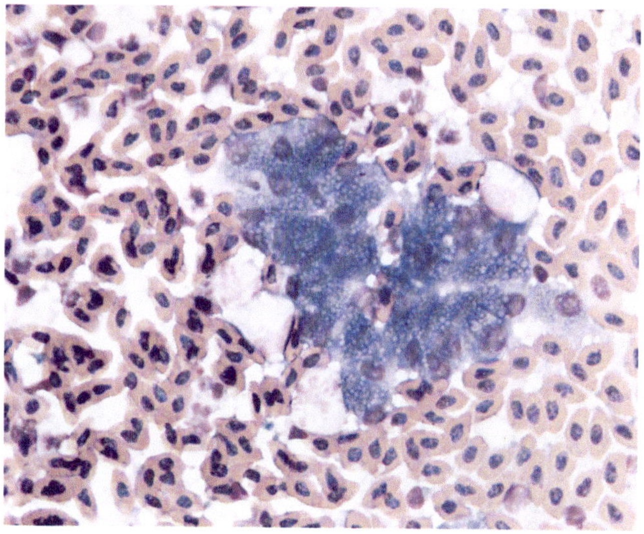

Fig. 33.8. Hepatocytes distended by small clear vacuoles (presumed to be lipid) and a background containing numerous round structures presumed to be free lipid droplets in a contact smear of a liver from a goldfish (*Carassius auratus*). Wright–Giemsa stain (100× oil).

Hepatic Lipidosis

Hepatic lipidosis (fatty liver syndrome or steatosis) is represented by the appearance of hepatocytes with many small or large clear cytoplasmic vacuoles, which represent the lipid that has dissolved during the staining process (Figure 33.8). Unstained smears made from livers with fatty change may appear "greasy" on gross inspection of the slide.

Fat storage in the liver occurs in many elasmobranchs as a source for energy between meals and to assist with buoyancy (Janse et al., 2004). Samples exhibiting lipid vacuoles collected from the liver of elasmobranchs should not be considered an abnormal finding.

Neoplasia

Neoplasms are common in fish, classified similarly to those in higher vertebrates, and described in nearly all organs and tissues (Groff, 2004). Fish, especially teleosts, primarily develop mesenchymal tumors, whereas higher vertebrates more commonly develop tumors of ectodermal or endodermal origin (Marino et al., 2006; Culp et al., 2017).

Cutaneous neoplasms represent the most frequently reported type of neoplasia in fish species, although this

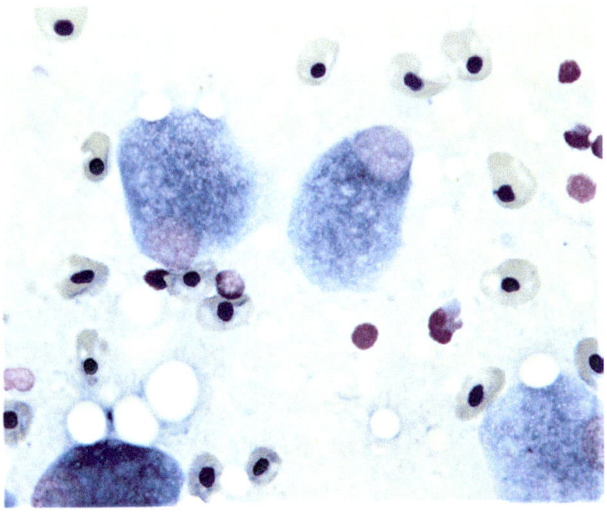

Fig. 33.9. Large mesenchymal cells with eccentric nuclei and exfoliating as single cells that exhibit features of malignancy in an imprint from a mass with a histologic diagnosis of a hemangiosarcoma removed from a red oscar (*Astronotus ocellatus*). Wright–Giemsa stain (100× oil). Source: Image from Campbell and Grant (2010, p. 334).

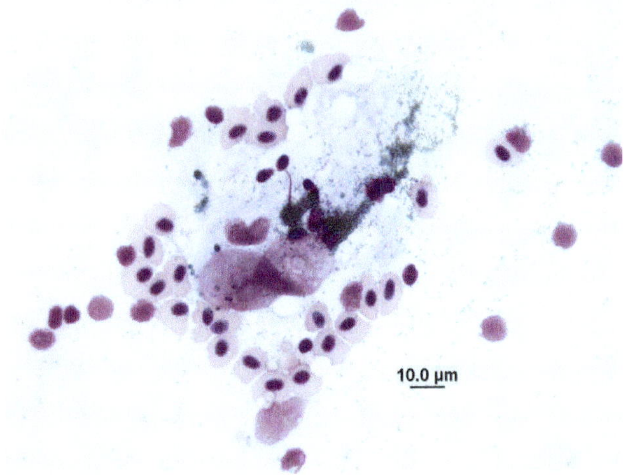

Fig. 33.10. Numerous large, spindled to round-shaped pleomorphic cells containing spherical, brown-black melanin granules such as this cell were found in an imprint from a cutaneous melanoma in a goldfish (*Carassius auratus*). Cells such as this one are difficult to differentiate from melanomacrophages based upon cytology alone. Wright–Giemsa stain.

information may be somewhat biased owing to the relative ease of detection of cutaneous masses (Groff, 2004). In teleosts, cutaneous tumors are generally classified as benign; however, recurrence is common if complete excision is not achieved. Cutaneous spindle cell neoplasms are a commonly diagnosed tumor of fish in general and are characterized by elongated to spindle-shaped cells arranged in streaming to interlacing bundles, and include tumors of mesenchymal origin such as fibromas, fibrosarcomas, myxomas, chromatophoromas, leiomyomas, and tumors of peripheral nerve origin (Reavill, 2010) (Figure 33.9). Squamous cell carcinoma is rarely reported in fish (Hanjavanit and Mulcahy, 2004; Quaglio et al., 2016; Culp et al., 2017).

Oral tumors are rare and include odontomas, ameloblastomas, papillomas, myxomas, and fibromas (Dill et al., 2017; Singaravel et al., 2017).

The cytology of ossifying fibromas reveals a uniform population of well-differentiated, spindle-shaped mesenchymal cells (fibroblasts) within a background matrix (Murphy and Imai, 2016).

Chromatophoromas (i.e., melanophoromas or melanomas, xanthophoromas, and iridophoromas) are cutaneous tumors that originate from dermal pigment cells (chromatophores) normally present in the skin of fish (Singaravel et al., 2016). Iridophores are cutaneous pigment cells responsible for the iridescent appearance of skin (Okihiro, 1988). Benign melanocytic proliferative masses are typically classified as melanocytomas or nevi, in veterinary medicine, while the term *melanoma* implies malignancy (Nau et al., 2016). Cutaneous melanomas have been reported in teleost fish, but are rare in elasmobranchs (Sakamoto and White, 2002; Waldoch et al., 2010; Nau et al., 2016) (Figure 33.10). Chromatophoromas are typically locally aggressive and can appear as unsightly masses (Yaw et al., 2016). Identifying mitotic figures, a criterion for malignancy, can be challenging in heavily pigmented cells.

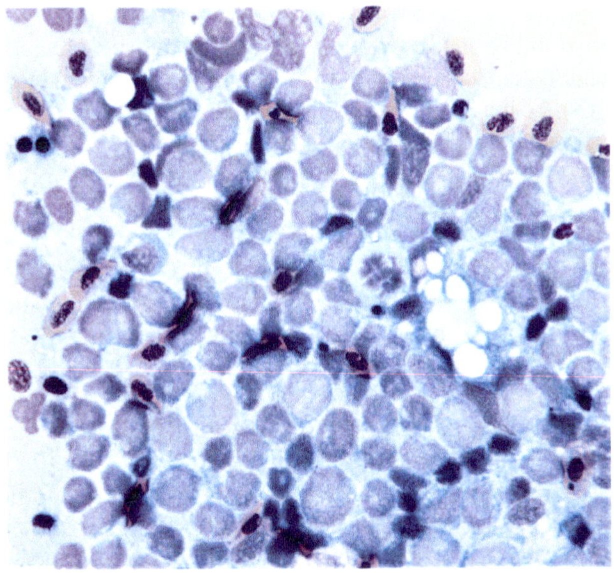

Fig. 33.11. An impression of a scraping from a lesion on the mouth of a banded rainbow fish (*Melanotaenia trifasciata*) reveals a highly cellular sample populated by round cells and erythrocytes. Most of the round cells are large lymphocytes with scant amount of blue cytoplasm and nuclei with smooth nuclear chromatin. The nuclei frequently reveal prominent nucleoli and mitotic figures. The cytology indicates lymphoid neoplasia, lymphoma. Wright–Giemsa stain (100× oil). Source: Image from Campbell and Grant (2010, p. 346).

Lipomas are rare tumors in freshwater and marine fish (Marino et al., 2006; De Stefano et al., 2012). Lipomas are indistinguishable from normal adipose tissue cytologically, histologically, and chemically (Sood et al., 2017). Lipomas have been reported in several fish orders such as Cypriniformes (bream), Perciformes (largemouth bass, black crappie, striped seabream, and European seabass), Scombriformes (southern bluefin tuna and northern bluefin tuna), Siluriformes (channel catfish), Anguilliformes (European eel), Mugiliformes (striped mullet), Pleuronectiformes (common dab), and Cyprinodontiformes (molly) (Easa et al., 1989; Marino et al., 2006; Sharon et al., 2015; Rahmati-Holasoo et al., 2016; Kehoe et al., 2020). In teleosts, lipomas typically occur as a dermal or hypodermal mass that may develop cutaneous ulceration (Harshbarger et al., 1993). Lipomas have been reported to develop internally in the hepatic parenchyma and coelomic membranes of fish (Grizzle and Goodwin, 1998; Roberts, 2012; Rahmati-Holasoo et al., 2016). Also, dermis-associated lipomas have been found to infiltrate the underlying muscle (Kehoe et al., 2020).

Hematopoietic neoplasia, such as lymphosarcoma and lymphoma, have been reported in multiple species of teleost fish (Figure 33.11). Histiocytic sarcomas (malignant tumors of histiocytes) have also been reported in fish and exhibit atypical, mononuclear, round, macrophagic cells with abundant cytoplasmic vacuolation that often exhibit bizarre nuclear pleomorphism (Kiryu et al., 2018).

Cytologic preparations of a schwannoma in fish demonstrate moderately pleomorphic medium-sized spindle cells (oval to elongated) with intermediate to high nuclear to cytoplasmic ratio occurring individually or in a storiform pattern amid a moderate amount of extracellular faintly eosinophilic matrix material (Sirri et al., 2015). The cells have scant to moderate cytoplasm that stains slightly basophilic cytoplasm (some cells having small vacuolation) with indistinct cell borders and wispy cytoplasmic extensions. The nuclei are oval to cigar-shaped with finely stippled to lacy chromatin, and 1–3 variably sized prominent nucleoli. The cells displayed moderate anisocytosis and anisokaryosis consistent with a malignant mesenchymal neoplasm.

Chordomas are neoplasms arising from notochord remnants that commonly occur in the axial skeleton. Although uncommon, spontaneous vertebral chordomas have been reported in aged zebrafish as well as spontaneous primary intestinal chordomas that have no axial or peripheral skeletal or other nonvisceral involvement (Cooper et al., 2015).

Leiomyosarcomas in fish can be associated with a viral etiology, such as a retrovirus (Bowser et al., 2012).

Osteosarcoma and chondrosarcoma are uncommon tumors of fish. Chondromas and chondrosarcomas are neoplasia of cartilage (chondrocytes and cartilaginous cells). The cytology often reveals mesenchymal cells embedded in a bright, pink, smooth to slightly granular background material (chondroid) (Figures 33.12a

(a) (b)

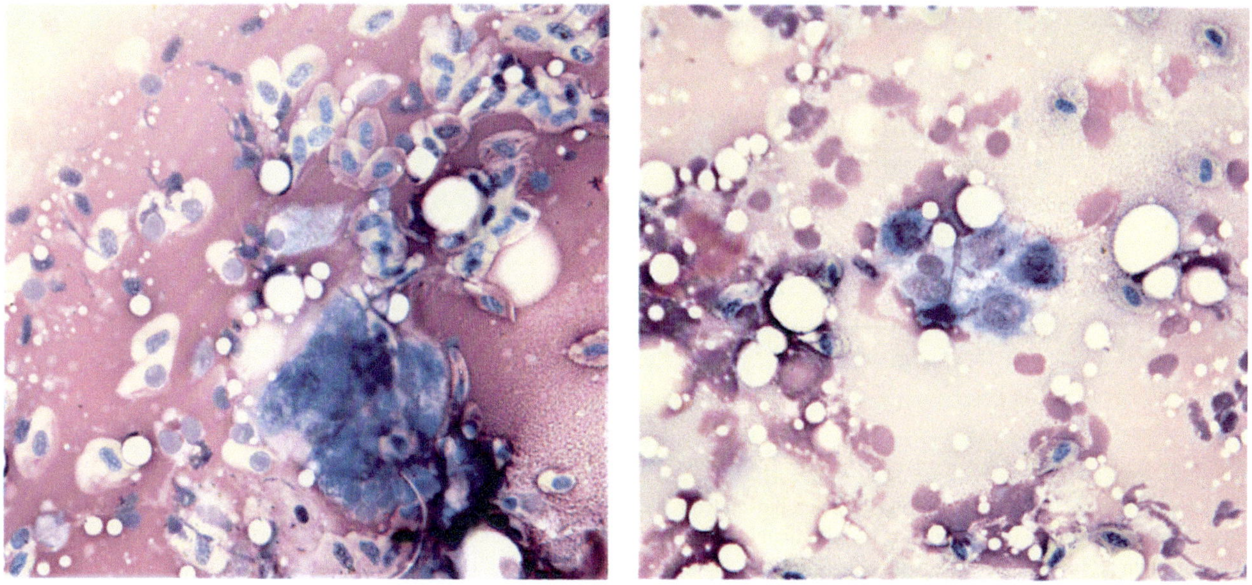

Fig. 33.12. (a) Fine-needle aspiration biopsy of a chondrosarcoma mass on operculum of a tinfoil barb (*Barbus schwanenfeldi*) reveals cells embedded in a heavy eosinophilic background substance. The pleomorphic cells tend to be elongated to spindle-shaped with a basophilic cytoplasm and an eccentrically positioned nucleus that contains coarsely granular nuclear chromatin and large, prominent nucleoli. Wright–Giemsa stain (100× oil). (b) Fine-needle aspiration biopsy of a chondrosarcoma mass on operculum of a tinfoil barb (*Barbus schwanenfeldi*) reveals cells embedded in a heavy eosinophilic background substance. The pleomorphic cells tend to be elongated to spindle-shaped with a basophilic cytoplasm and an eccentrically positioned nucleus that contains coarsely granular nuclear chromatin and large prominent nucleoli. Wright–Giemsa stain (100× oil). Source: Image from Campbell and Grant (2010, p. 362).

(a) (b) (c)

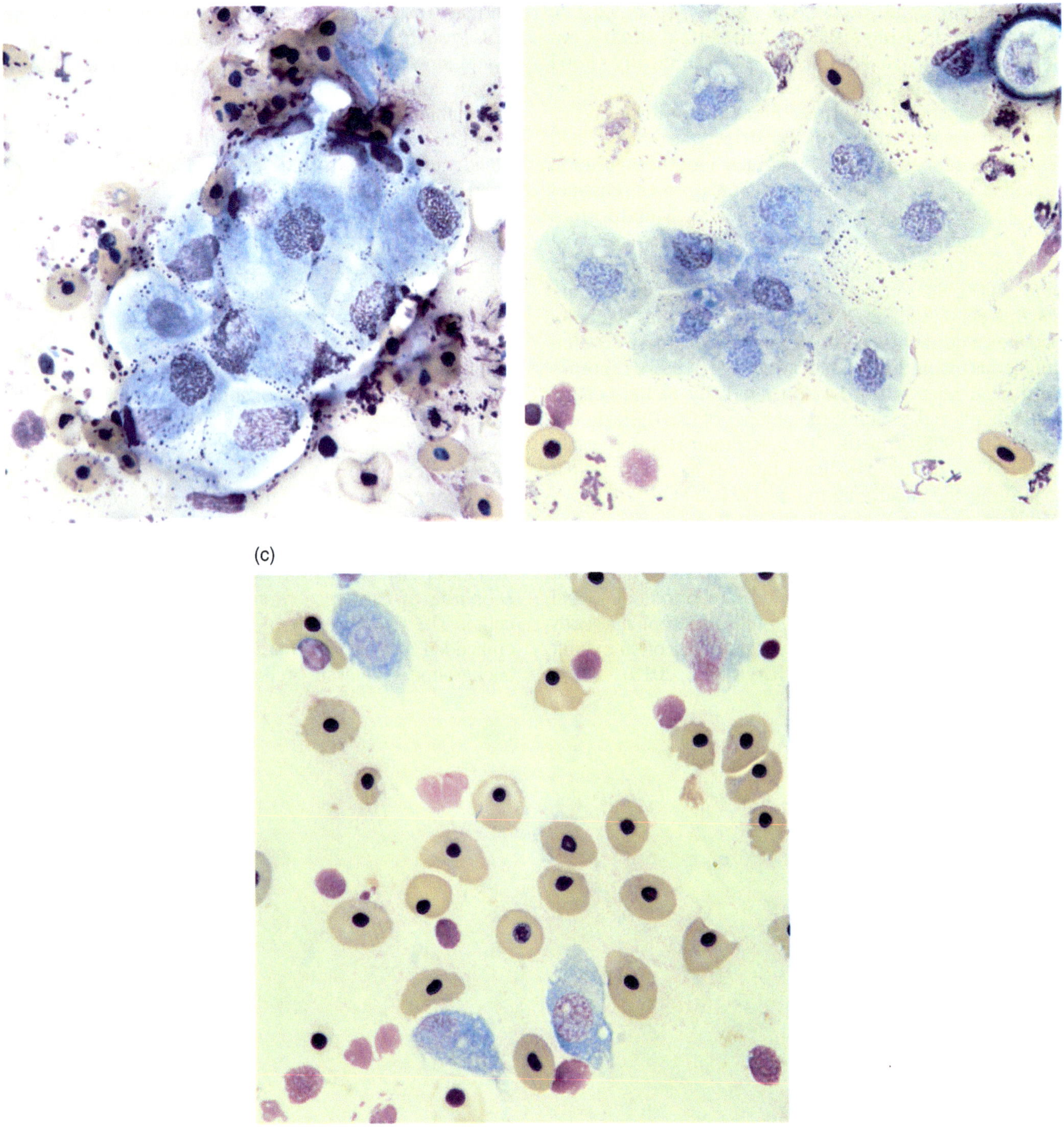

Fig. 33.13. (a) An imprint of a fibropapilloma removed from the operculum of a clown knife (*Chitala chitala*) reveals numerous erythrocytes and an aggregate of epithelial cells with abundant blue-gray cytoplasm and large nuclei with coarse nuclear chromatin. Wright–Giemsa stain (100× oil). (b) Squamous cells from the same sample as Figure 33.13a resemble those in that image, but appear more mature. Wright–Giemsa stain (100× oil). (c) Erythrocytes and three mesenchymal cells with dark blue cytoplasm and oval nuclei with coarse chromatin from the same sample as Figures 33.13a and 33.13b. There is no evidence of inflammation, and the cells do not have prominent features of malignant neoplasia; therefore, the cells in these images likely represent epithelial cell and mesenchymal cell hyperplasia as part of the fibropapilloma. Wright–Giemsa stain (100× oil). Source: Image from Campbell and Grant (2010, p. 340).

and 33.12b). The cells share an appearance to those found in osteosarcomas (primary neoplasia of bone) and can vary from round to fusiform with large nuclei and deeply basophilic cytoplasm. Like cells from osteosarcomas, chondrosarcomas can contain small intracytoplasmic vacuoles and fine eosinophilic granules.

Reports of renal tubular cell tumors in fish have been rare (Rahmati-Holasoo et al., 2017).

Cutaneous papillomas are difficult to diagnose by cytology alone because they reveal predominantly cornified squamous epithelial cells and mesenchymal cells from a connective tissue stroma on the cellular sample (Figures 33.13a–33.13c).

Effusions

Samples of fluids found in fish should be collected for cytological evaluation. Fluid samples from the coelomic cavity of fish are simply obtained by aspiration following the insertion of a needle with attached syringe through the skin and body wall along the ventral aspect of the animal. The effusions are classified as transudates, modified transudates, exudates, hemorrhagic effusions, and malignant effusions. The cytological appearances of these effusions resemble those found in other animals (Figures 33.14–33.16).

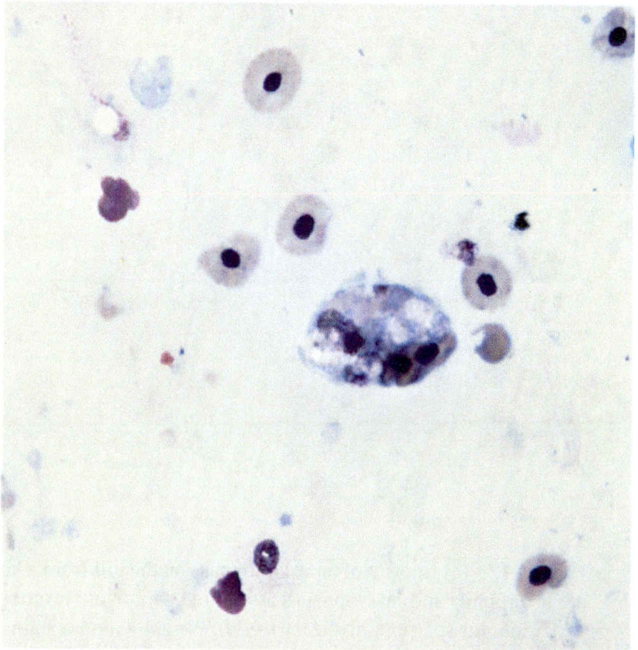

Fig. 33.15. A macrophage exhibiting erythrophagocytosis seen in the gastric fluid from a red oscar (*Astronotus ocellatus*) with hemorrhagic gastritis. Wright–Giemsa stain (100× oil). Source: Image from Campbell and Grant (2010, p. 343).

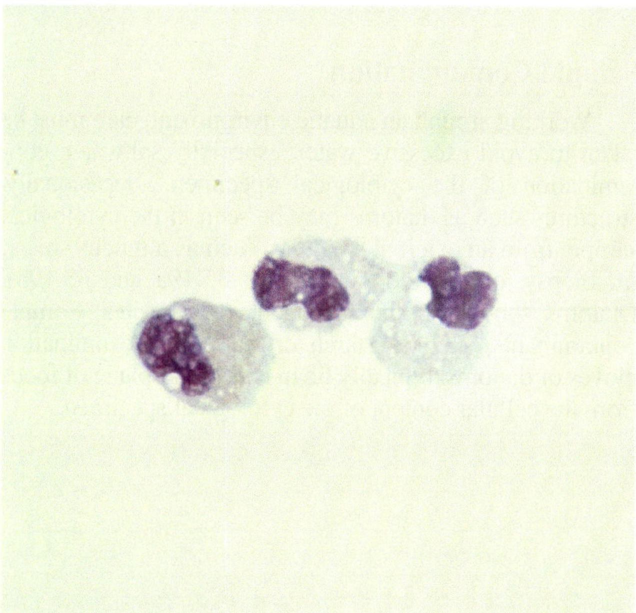

Fig. 33.14. Heterophils indicating an exudative effusion in the coelomic fluid from a goldfish (*Carassius auratus*) with generalized pyogranulomatous coelomitis. Wright–Giemsa stain (100× oil). Source: Image from Campbell and Grant (2010, p. 331).

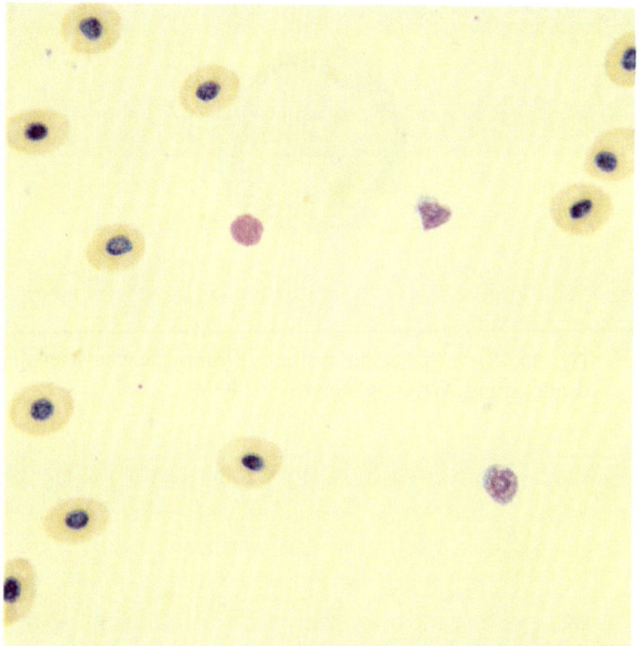

Fig. 33.16. A poorly cellular sample with a few erythrocytes and two lymphocytes in a fluid-filled subcutaneous swelling (seroma) in a red-tailed catfish (*Phractocephalus hemioliopterus*). Wright–Giemsa stain (100× oil). Source: Image from Campbell and Grant (2010, p. 350).

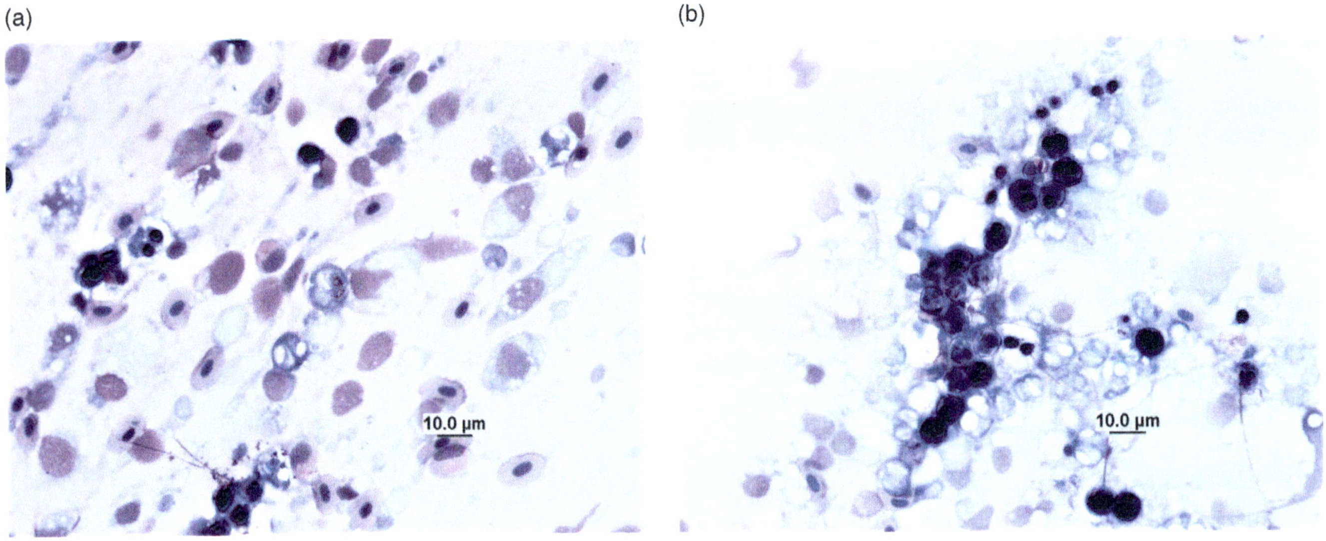

Fig. 33.17. (a) Imprint of an excised mass on the gill from a koi (*Cyprinus carpio*) with granulomatous pharyngitis showing nondegenerate heterophils and macrophages associated with ovoid protozoal spores with two polar capsules indicative of a myxozoan parasite, such as *Myxobolus* sp. (possibly *M. cyprinid*). Wright–Giemsa stain (100× oil). (b) The same imprint as Figure 33.17a showing ovoid protozoal spores with two polar capsules that stain poorly. These spores are indicative of a myxozoan parasite, such as *Myxobolus* sp. (possibly *M. cyprinid*). Wright–Giemsa stain (100× oil).

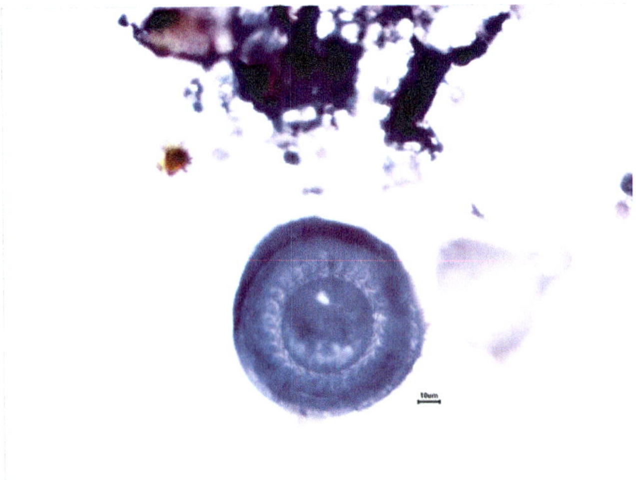

Fig. 33.18. A trichodinid parasite revealing the characteristic denticle rings. Wright–Giemsa stain (400×).

Parasites

Parasites of fish are generally identified on wet-mount preparations; however, some may be identified on air-dried stained preparations. For example, spores from myxozoan parasites and trichodinid ciliates may be seen on stained preparations (Figures 33.17a, 33.17b, and 33.18).

Sample Contamination

Working around an aquatic environment, care must be taken to avoid excessive water, especially saltwater, contamination of the cytological specimen. Occasionally, structures such as diatoms may be seen in the cytological sample from an external structure, such as a mucus smear, fin biopsy, or gill biopsy (Figures 33.19a and 33.19b). Diatoms should not be mistaken for parasites. Sample contaminants, such as starch crystals from examination gloves or diatoms, typically lie in a different plane of focus from the cellular content of the cytological specimen.

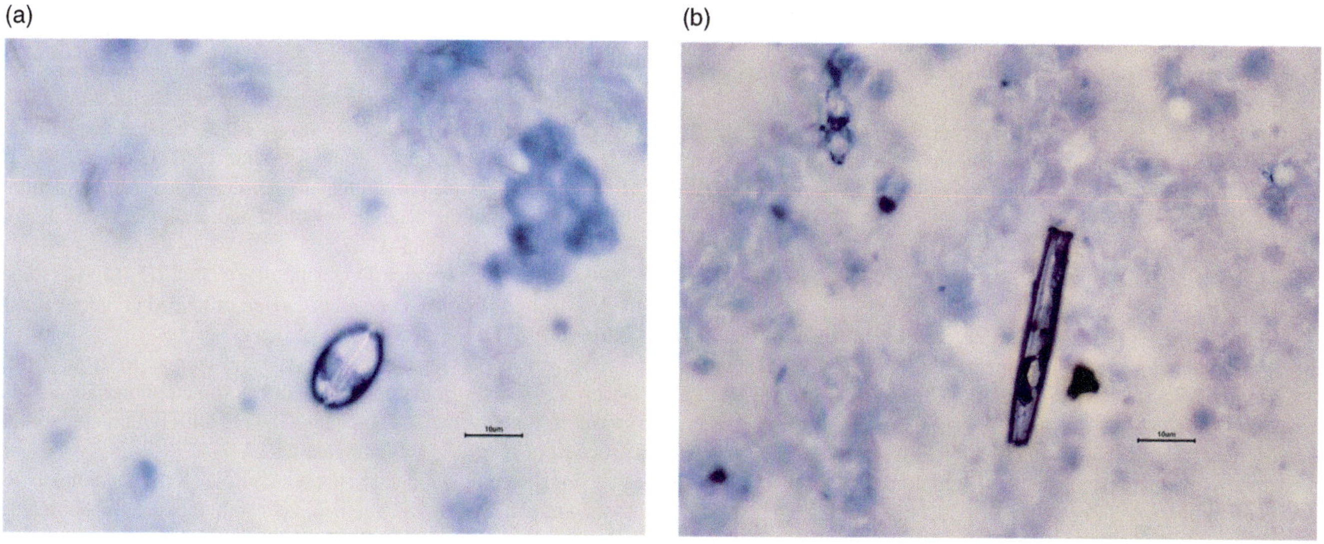

Fig. 33.19. (a) A diatom in a mucus smear from an orbicular batfish (*Platax orbicularis*). (b) A diatom in an aspirate of a cutaneous mass on the tail of a seahorse (*Hippocampus* sp.).

References

Agius C, Roberts RJ. 2003. Melanomacrophage centers and their role in fish pathology. *J Fish Dis* 26:499–509.

Baragahare R, Becker JA, Landos M, Šlapeta J, Dennis MM. 2011. Gastric cryptosporidiosis in farmed Australian murry cod, *Maccullochella peelii peelii*. *Aquac* 314(1–4):1–6.

Bercovier H, Vincent V. 2001. Mycobacterial infections in domestic and wild animals due to *Mycobacterium marinum*, M. *fortuitum*, M. *chelonae*, M. *porcinum*, M. *farcinogenes*, M. *smegmatis*, M. *scrofulaceum*, M. *xenopi*, M. *kansasii*, M. *simiae*, and M. *genavense*. *Rev Sci Tech Off Int Epiz* 20(1):265–290.

Bowser PR, Casey JW, Casey RN, et al. 2012. Swimbladder leiomyosarcoma in Atlantic salmon (*Salmo salar*) in North America. *J Wildl Dis* 48(3):795–798.

Campbell TW, Grant KR. 2010. *Clinical Cases in Avian and Exotic Animal Hematology and Cytology*. Ames: Wiley-Blackwell.

Clarke III EO, Dorn B, Boone A, Risatti G, Gilbert-Marcheterre K, et al. 2013. Mycobacteriosis, *Mycobacterium chelonae*, in captive yellow stingray (*Urobatis jamaicensis*). *J Zoo Wildl Med* 44(2):470–474.

Cooper TK, Murray KN, Spagnoli S, Spitsbergen JM. 2015. Primary intestinal and vertebral chordomas in laboratory Zebrafish (*Danio rerio*). *Vet Pathol* 52(2):388–392.

Crow GL, Luer WH, Harshbarger JC. 2001. Histological assessment of goiters in elasmobranch fishes. *J Aquat Anim Health* 13:1–7.

Culp BE, Haulena M, Britt K, Evans H, Raverty S. 2017. Squamous cell carcinoma of the rostral maxilla in an adult captive whitespotted bamboo shark (*Chiloscyllium plagiosum*). *J Zoo Wildl Med* 48(3):902–905.

Decostere A, Hermans K, Haesebrouck R. 2004. Piscine mycobacteriosis: a literature review covering the agent and the disease it causes in fish and humans. *Vet Microbiol* 99(3–4):159–166.

De Stefano C, Bonfiglio R, Montalbano G, Giorgianni P, Lanteri G. 2012. Multicentric lipoma in a molly (*Poecilia velifera*). *Bull Eur Assoc Fish Pathol* 32:220–224.

Diaz-Satizabal L, Magor BG. 2015. Isolation and cytochemical characterization of melanomacrophages and melanomacrophage clusters from goldfish (*Carassius auratus*, L.). *Dev Comp Immunol* 48:221–228.

Dill JA, Williams SM, Leary JH, Ng TFF, Camus AC. 2017. Investigation of epizootic papillomatosis in Bluegill *Lepomis macrochirus* (Rafinesque 1810) using next-generation sequencing. *J Fish Dis* 40(7):947–952.

Easa ME, Harshbarger JC, Hetrick FM. 1989. Hypodermal lipoma in a striped (grey) mullet *(Mugil cephalus)*. *Dis Aquat Organ* 6:157–160.

Fournie JW, Wolfe MJ, Wolf JC, et al. 2005. Diagnostic criteria for proliferative thyroid lesions in bony fishes. *Toxicol Pathol* 33:540–551.

Grizzle JM, Goodwin AE. 1998. Neoplasms and related lesions. In: Leatherland AF, Woo PTK, (eds), *Fish Diseases and Disorders. Vol 2: Non-Infectious Disorders*. Wallingford, England: CABI Publishing, pp. 37–104.

Groff JM. 2004. Neoplasia in fishes. *Vet Clin North Am Exot Anim Pract* 7:705–756.

Gutierre RC, Jared C, Antoniazzi MM, Coppi AA, Egami MI. 2018. Melanomacrophage functions in the liver of the caecilian *Siphonops annulatus*. *J Anat* 232:497–508.

Hanjavanit C, Mulcahy MF. 2004. Squamous cell carcinoma in Rudd *Scardinius erythrophthalmus*: histopathology, ultrastructure, and transmission. *Dis Aquat Org* 61:215–226.

Harshbarger JC, Spero PM, Wolcott NM. 1993. Neoplasms in wild fish from the marine ecosystem emphasizing environmental interactions. In: Couch JA, Fournie JW, (eds), *Pathobiology of Marine and Estuarine Organisms*. Boca Raton, Fl: CRC Press, pp. 157–176.

Jalenques M, Vergneau-Grosset C, Summa N, et al. 2020. A cluster of cases of thyroid hyperplasia in aquarium-housed tropical marine teleosts following a change of salt mix brand. *J Zoo Wildl Med* 51(3):725–728.

Janse M, Firchau B, Mohan PJ. 2004. Elasmobranch nutrition, food handling, and feeding techniques. In: Smith M, Warmolts D, Thoney D, Hueter R (eds), *Elasmobranch Husbandry Manual: Captive Care of Sharks, Rays, and their Relatives*. Columbus, OH: Ohio Biological Survey, Inc. pp. 183–200.

Kehoe SP, Divers SJ, Mayer J, et al. 2020. Computed tomographic and ultrasonographic diagnosis with successful excision of a lipoma in a shusui koi (*Cyprinus carpio*). *J Am Vet Med Assoc* 256(12):1379–1385.

Kiryu Y, Landsberg JH, Bakenhaster MD, Tyler-Jedlund AJ, Wilson PW. 2018. Putative histiocytic sarcoma in redfin needlefish *Strongylura notata* (Beloniformes: Belonidae) in Florida, USA. *Dis Aquat Org* 132:57–78.

Lapointe D, Vogelbein WK, Fabrizio MC, Gauthier DT, Brill RW. 2014. Temperature, hypoxia, and mycobacteriosis: effects on adult striped bass *Morone saxatilis* metabolic performance. *Dis Aquat Org* 108:113–127.

Marino F, Monaco S, Salvaggio A, Macri B. 2006. Lipoma in a farmed northern bluefin tuna, *Thunnus thynnus* (L.). *J Fish Dis* 29:697–699.

Matsche MA, Blazer VS, Pulster EL, Mazik PM. 2021. Biological and anthropogenic influences on macrophage aggregates in white perch *Morone americana* from Chesapeake Bay, USA. *Dis Aquat Org* 143:79–100.

Molter CM, Marrow JV, Flanagan JP, Baseler LJ. 2019. Clinical challenge: a spermatocele and sperm granulomas in a four-eyed fish (*Anableps anableps*). *J Zoo Wildl Med* 50(1):287–290.

Murphy B, Imai DM. 2016. Cutaneous ossifying fibroma in a Neon Tetra (*Paracheirodon innesi*). *J Comp Pathol* 155:272–275.

Nau MR, Gardiner DW, Nilson E, et al. 2016. Cutaneous malignant melanoma in a Haller's round ray *Urobatis helleri*. *Dis Aquat Org* 120:245–250.

Noga EJ. 2000. Fish disease: diagnosis and treatment. In Noga E (ed), *Fish Disease: Diagnosis and Treatment*. Ames, IA: Iowa State University Press, pp. 116–120.

Okihiro MS. 1988. Chromatophoromas in two species of Hawaiian butterflyfish, *Chaetodon multicinctus* and *C. miliaris*. *Vet Pathol* 25:422–431.

Quaglio F, Zappulli V, Poppi L, et al. 2016. Squamous cell carcinoma in a wild European bullhead *Cottus gobio*. *Dis Aquat Org* 122:73–76.

Rahmati-Holasoo H, Shokrpoor S, Tavakkoli A, et al. 2016. Liposarcoma or invasive lipomatosis in flower horn fish, hybrid cichlid: clinical, radiological, ultrasonographical and histopathological study. *J Fish Dis* 39:309–315.

Rahmati-Holasoo H, Shokrpoor S, Masoudifard M, et al.2017. Renal cystic adenocarcinoma in a flowerhorn cichlid with metastatic involvement of the spleen. *J Aquat Anim Health* 29:158–164.

Reavill D. 2010. Neoplasia in fish. In: Roberts HE (ed), *Fundamentals of Ornamental Fish Health*. Ames, IA: Wiley-Blackwell, pp. 204–212.

Roberts RJ. 2012. Neoplasia of teleosts. In: Roberts RJ (ed), *Fish Pathology*, 4th edn. London: WB Saunders Co, pp. 167–185.

Sakamoto K, White MR. 2002. Dermal melanoma with schwannoma-like differentiation in a brown bullhead catfish (*Ictalurus nebulosus*). *J Vet Diagn Invest* 14:247–250.

Santos AA, Gutierre RC, Antoniazzi MM, et al. 2011. Morphocytochemical, immunohistochemical and ultrastructural characterization of the head kidney of fat snook *Centropomus parallelus*. *J Fish Biol* 79:1685–1707.

Sharon G, Benharroch D, Kachko L, et al. 2015. Liposarcoma in clownfish, *Amphiprion ocellaris Cuvier*, produced in indoor aquaculture. *J Fish Dis* 38:575–580.

Singaravel V, Gopalakrishnan A, Vijayakumar R, et al. 2016. Occurrence of chromatophorma or chromatophoromatosis in *Sardinella longiceps* (Valenciennes, 1847) from Tamilnadu, southeast coast of India. *J Appl Ichthyol* 32:712–717.

Singaravel V, Gopalakrishnan A, Raja K, Vijayakumar R, Asrafuzzaman S. 2017. Oral neoplasms in pickhandle barracuda *Sphyraena jello* from India. *Dis Aquat Org* 125:115–124.

Sirri R, Diana A, Scarpa F, et al. 2015. Case report: ultrasonographic and pathologic study of schwannoma in a Goldfish (*Carassius auratus*). *Vet Clin Pathol* 44(4):586–590.

Sood N, Swaminathan TR, Yadav MK, et al. 2017. First report of cutaneous infiltrative lipoma in goldfish *Carassius auratus*. *Dis Aquat Org* 125:243–247.

Stacy N, de Wit M, Boylan S, Gulland F, Frankovich T. 2014. Diatoms in cytologic specimens of aquatic animals–Part II, dermal, respiratory, and gastric samples. *Vet Clin Pathol* 43(4):473–474.

Varvil MS, Corriveau LA, Thompson CA. 2018. What is your diagnosis? Ulcerative epidermal lesions in a koi fish. *Vet Clin Pathol* 47(4):672–673.

Vigliano FA, Bermudez R, Quiroga MI, et al. 2006. Evidence for melano-macrophage centres of teleost as evolutionary precursors of germinal centres of higher vertebrates: an immunohistochemical study. *Fish Shellfish Immunol* 21:467–471.

Waldoch JA, Burke SS, Ramer JC, Garner MM. 2010. Melanoma in the skin of a nurse shark (*Ginglymostoma cirratum*). *J Zoo Wildl Med* 41:729–731.

Yaw TJ, Michaels B, Reavill D, Zaffarano BA. 2016. Liquid nitrogen cryosurgery for a chromatophoroma in a captive Largemouth bass (*Micropterus salmoides*). *J Exotic Pet Med* 25:305–310.

34

Piscine Cytology and Clinical Chemistry: Clinical Case Presentations

Case 1: Shark with Cutaneous Nodules

Signalment

Adult sand tiger shark (*Carcharias taurus*)

History

This female shark was housed in a large public aquarium with other elasmobranchs and bony fish. She developed numerous cutaneous nodules along both sides of her body that have slowly increased in number and size (Figure 34.1). Otherwise, she appeared normal.

Physical Examination

The female sand tiger shark with the skin lesions was removed from the exhibit and examined in a holding area where she was restrained in a vinyl stretcher (Figure 34.2). Blood was drawn for a blood profile (Tables 34.1 and 34.2). Biopsy samples were obtained using a punch biopsy for histopathology. A milky fluid was discovered from the punch biopsy site and collected for microbial culture and cytology (Figures 34.3a–34.3d). She was weighed and determined to weigh 130 kg.

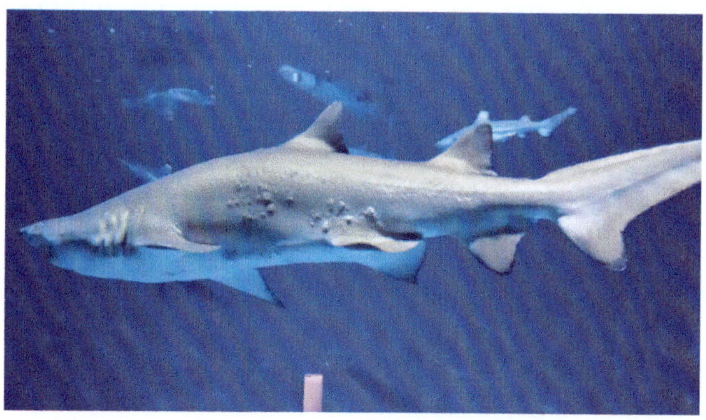

Fig. 34.1. Appearance of the female sand tiger shark with skin lesions.

Interpretive Discussion

No normal hematology and plasma biochemistry values for sand tiger sharks (*Carcharias taurus*) were available. However, compared to other species of elasmobranchs, the plasma chemistry values appeared to be within normal limits, and the hemogram indicated an

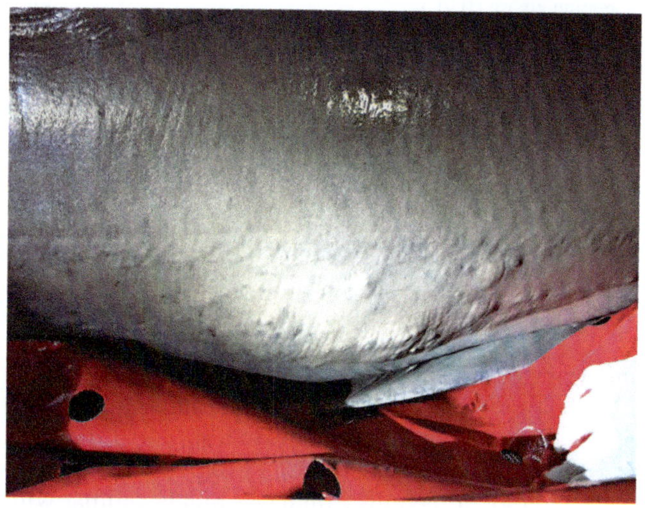

Fig. 34.2. Close-up view of the skin lesions in the female sand tiger shark during a physical examination.

Exotic Animal Hematology and Cytology, Fifth Edition. Terry W. Campbell and Krystan R. Grant.

Companion website: www.wiley.com/go/campbell/exotic

Table 34.1. Sand tiger shark hematology results (Case 1).

PCV (%)		18
Leukocytes		
WBC (×10³/μL)		21.0
Heterophils (G1) (×10³/μL)		4.0*
(%)		19
Neutrophils (G2) (×10³/μL)		5.0*
(%)		24
Lymphocytes (×10³/μL)		9.5
(%)		45
Monocytes (×10³/μL)		0
(%)		0
Eosinophils (×10³/μL)		2.5
(%)		12
Basophils (×10³/μL)		0
(%)		0
Thrombocytes		
Estimated number	Adequate	1–5/1000× field
Morphology	Normal	
Plasma protein (refractometry) (g/dL)		7.8

*Toxicity noted.

Table 34.2. Plasma biochemical results for case 1.

Glucose (mg/dL)	33
BUN (mg/dL)	878
Uric acid (mg/dL)	0.1
Total protein (biuret) (g/dL)	4.4
Albumin (g/dL)	0.6
Globulin (g/dL)	3.8
A/G ratio	0.2
Aspartate aminotransferase (IU/L)	17
Creatine kinase (IU/L)	409
Calcium (mg/dL)	14.5
Phosphorus (mg/dL)	5.0
Sodium (mEq/L)	247
Potassium (mEq/L)	3.3
Chloride (mEq/L)	249
Bicarbonate (mEq/L)	4.9
Anion gap (calculated)	−4
Cholesterol (mg/dL)	33
Calculated osmolality	781

inflammatory response based upon cell numbers and morphology (toxic heterophils and neutrophils) (Cain et al., 2004; Arnold, 2005; Dove et al., 2010; Ferreira et al., 2010; Cusack et al., 2016; Phillips et al., 2016).

Cytology of the milky fluid was highly cellular with marked numbers of heterophils with macrophages. The heterophils were degenerate, and the macrophages often revealed leukophagocytosis (not shown). No etiologic agent could be found for the marked mixed-cell inflammation. The cytodiagnosis of the fluid was indicative of an abscess that was likely associated with a bacterial infection in the skin.

Summary

Histopathology of the decalcified skin biopsy consisted of armored skin with significant crush artifact, several placoid scales, and dermis. The superficial epidermis was partially eroded, and the epidermis was infiltrated with moderate numbers of intact heterophils and clusters of stippled basophilic material. Placoid scales were mineralized and histologically normal. The dermis was normal with no inflammation detected. Additional sections of skin were stained for microorganisms (Gram), and cutaneous lesions were associated with small colonies of gram-negative coccobacilli. The histopathologic diagnosis was a subacute, moderate heterophilic epidermitis most consistent with a superficial infection with gram-negative coccobacilli.

Microbial culture was positive for coagulase-negative *Staphylococcus* sp., *Vibrio* sp., and *Photobacterium damselae*.

The shark was treated with antibiotics (florfenicol intramuscular for one dose followed by daily oral doses for 5 days and oral trimethoprim sulfa once every 48 h for 7 treatments). Following treatment, the shark's skin lesions were disappearing (Figures 34.4a and 34.4b). Also, the hemogram had improved (no toxic heterophils and neutrophils were noted along with increased number of lymphocytes). She was also gaining weight (136.8 kg).

Case 2: Trout with a Mass on Mandible

Signalment

Cutthroat trout (*Oncorhynchus clarkii*)

History

This trout was housed in a large public aquarium with many other trout. It was examined because a growth was observed on the ventral aspect of the mandible (Figure 34.5). Otherwise, the fish appeared normal.

Physical Examination

The trout was netted for examination. A small excisional biopsy of the mass was obtained for histopathology. An imprint of the biopsy sample was made for cytological examination (Figures 34.6a–34.6d).

Interpretive Discussion

Cytology of the mass revealed predominantly large spindle-shaped cells on a heavy eosinophilic noncellular background with many free degenerate nuclei. The cells exhibited significant pleomorphism. Most had abundant blue cytoplasm, and many had prominent Golgi. The nuclei were large with coarse nuclear chromatin. Nuclei with prominent and multiple nucleoli were frequently

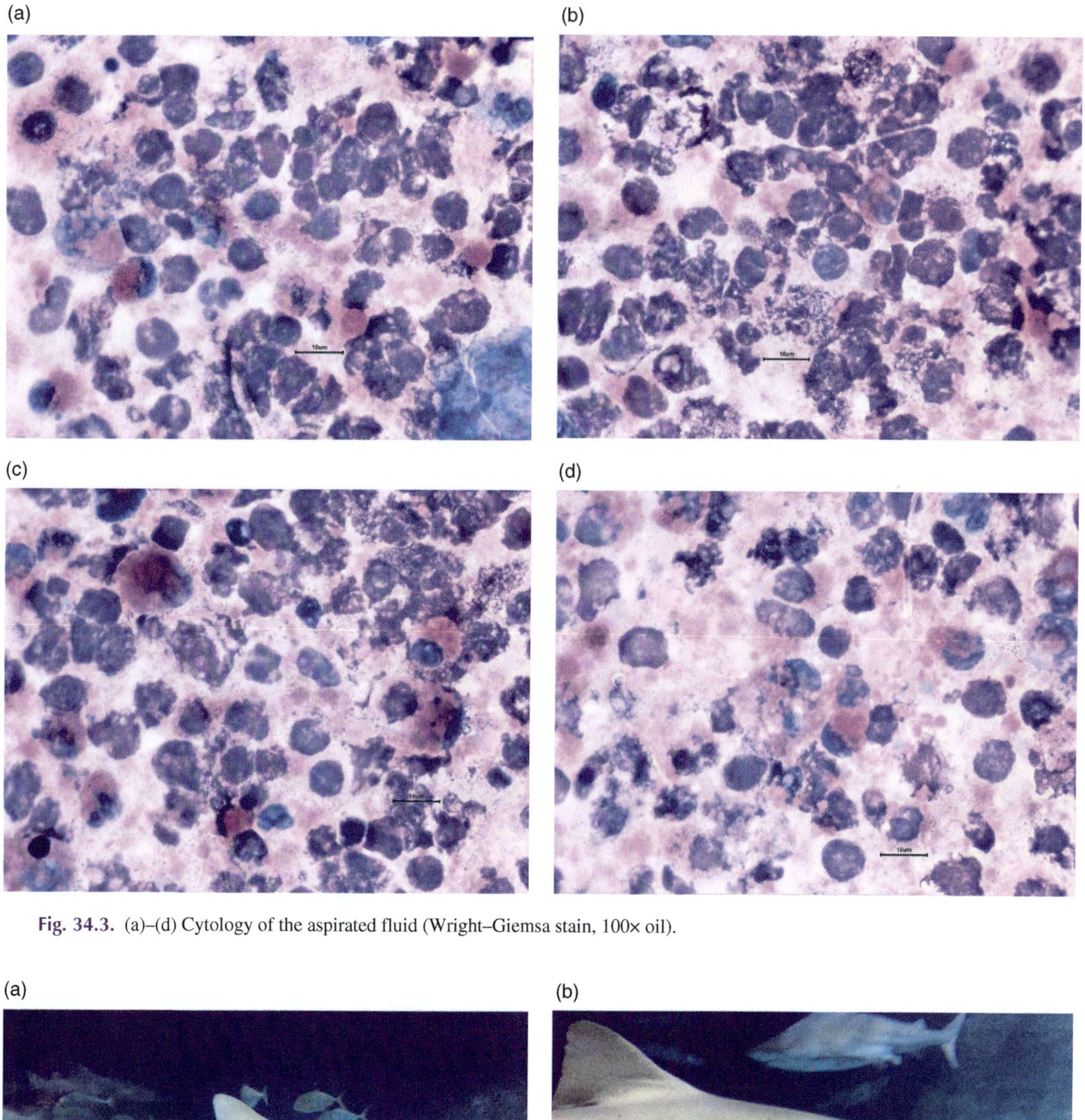

Fig. 34.3. (a)–(d) Cytology of the aspirated fluid (Wright–Giemsa stain, 100× oil).

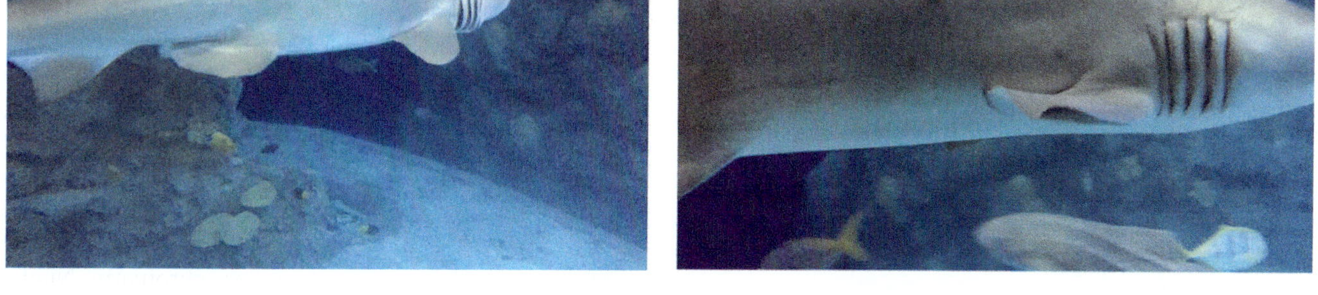

Fig. 34.4. (a), (b) Appearance of the female sand tiger shark following antibiotic treatment.

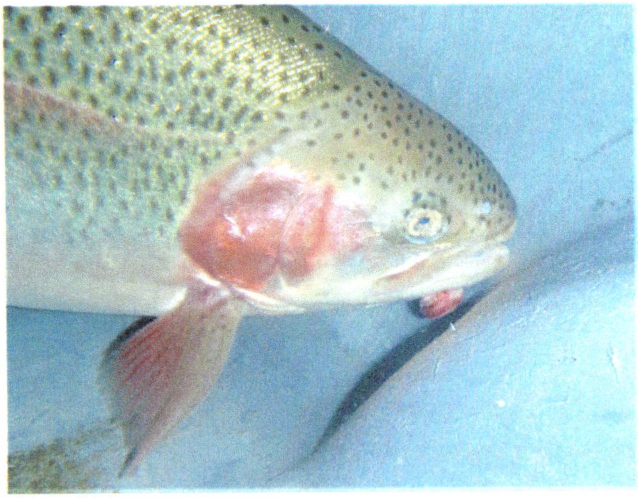

Fig. 34.5. Appearance of the mandibular mass on the trout.

observed. Binucleated cells were also found. Because the cells exhibited features of malignant neoplasia and there was no evidence of inflammation, a cytodiagnosis of mesenchymal cell neoplasia was made. The eosinophilic background was suggestive of a matrix substance as would be observed associated with osteosarcomas or chondrosarcomas. Because the cells did not resemble typical osteoblasts, a cytological diagnosis of a chondrosarcoma was considered.

Summary

Histopathology of the biopsy of the mass indicated a chondroma. The fish was placed under a general anesthetic, and the mass was surgically removed in its entirety (Figure 34.7). Skin sutures were removed six weeks later. The mass did not return.

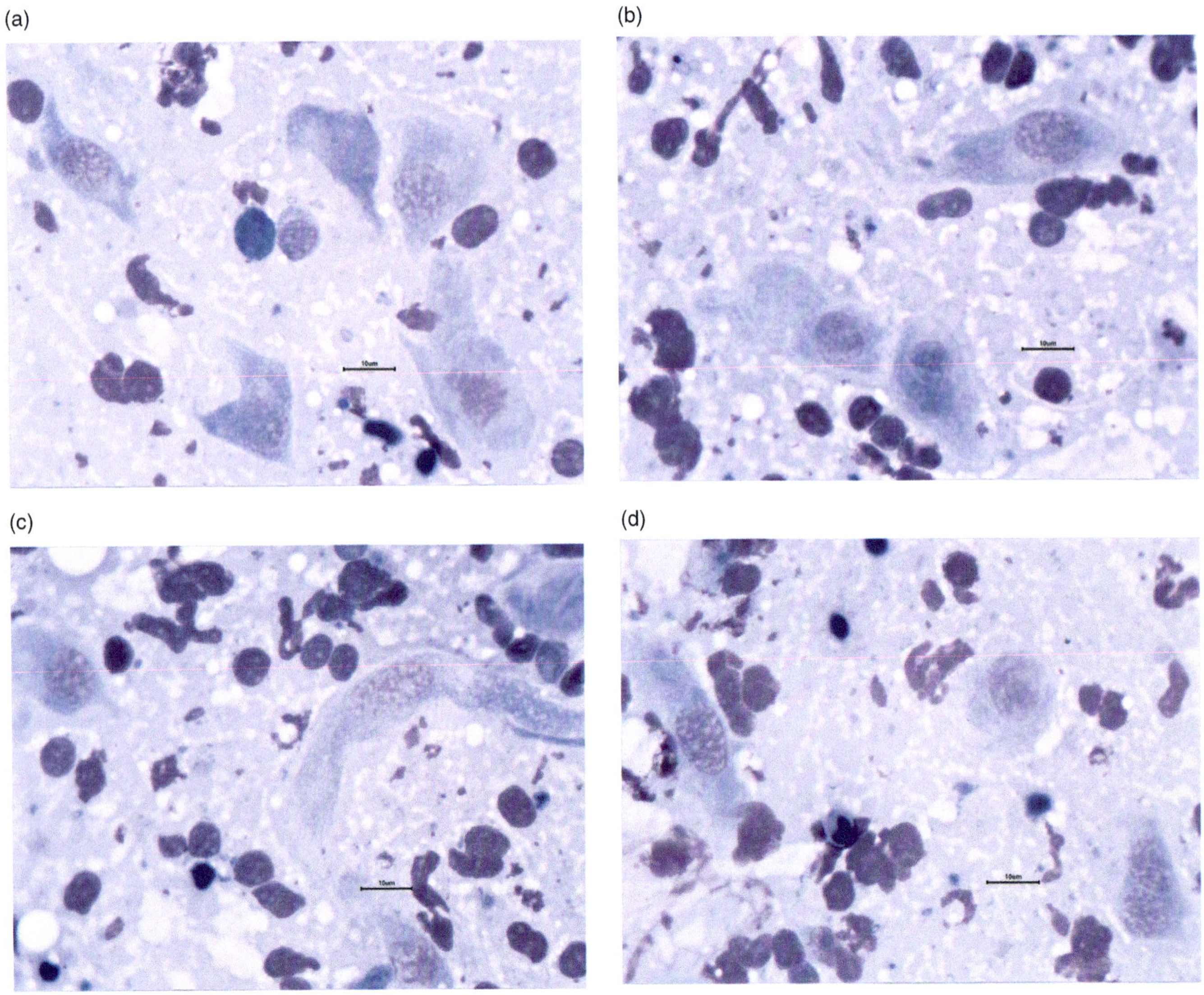

Fig. 34.6. (a)–(d) Cytology of the imprinted mass (Wright–Giemsa stain, 100× oil).

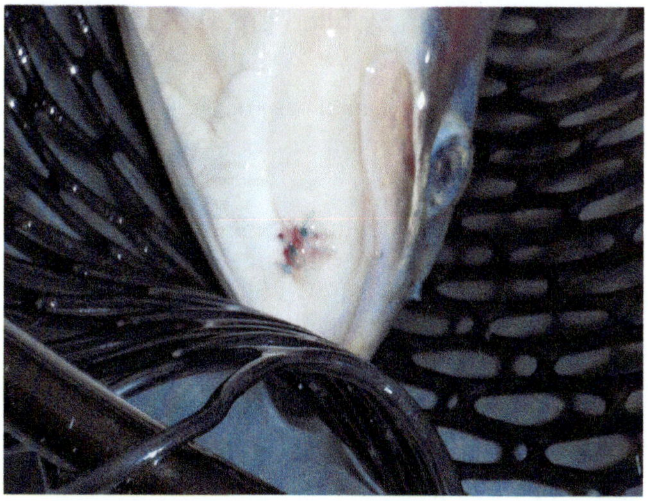

Fig. 34.7. Appearance of the surgical site on the trout following removal of the mass.

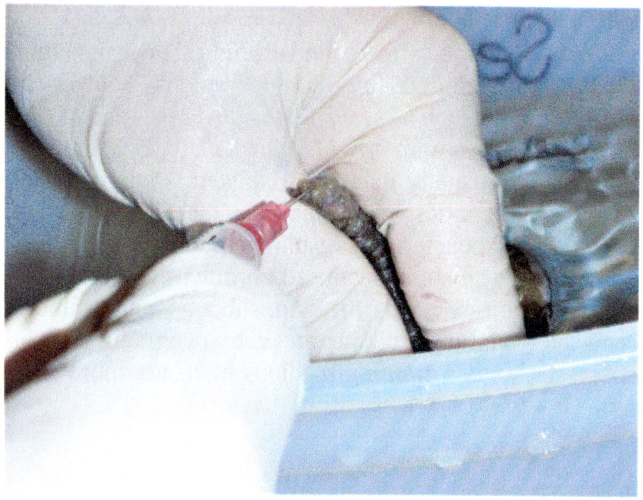

Fig. 34.8. Fine-needle aspiration biopsy of lesion on the tail of the seahorse.

(a) (b)

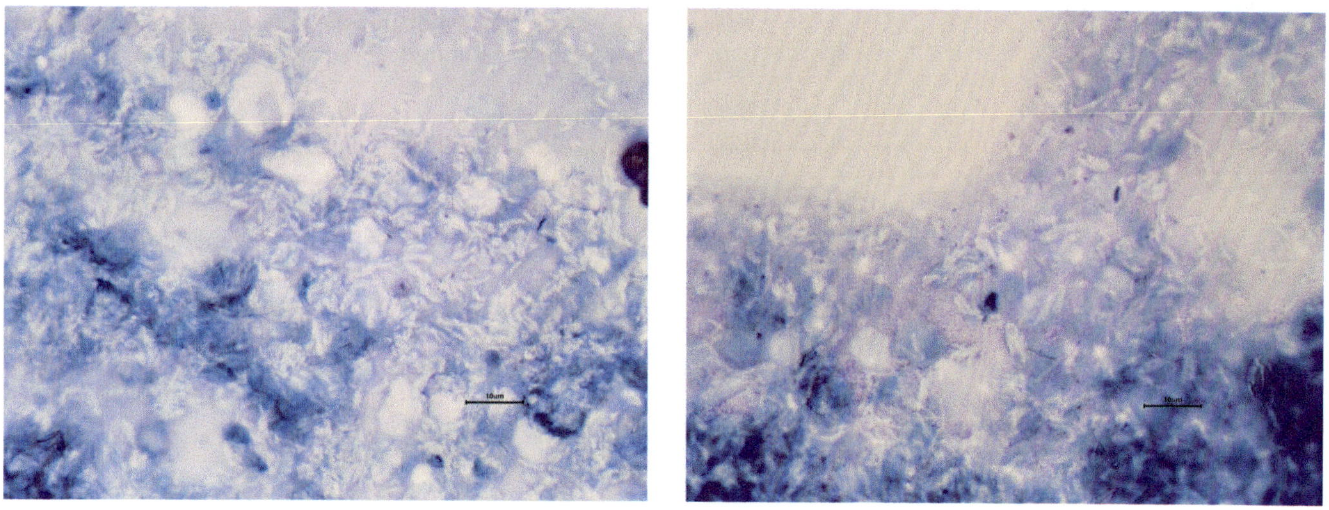

Fig. 34.9. (a), (b) Cytology of the fine-needle aspiration biopsy of the mass (Wright–Giemsa stain, 100× oil).

Case 3: Seahorse with Possible Gas Bubble Disease

Signalment

Adult seahorse (*Hippocampus* sp.)

History

This seahorse was housed alone in a tank in the quarantine area of a large public aquarium. It was removed from the exhibit where it was housed with other seahorses because of a lesion on its tail that was considered to be gas bubble disease (a condition caused by supersaturation of gases in the water leading to gas bubbles in a fish's tissues).

Physical Examination

The seahorse appeared normal except for a lesion on the tail that appeared to be a cluster of blister-like swellings in the skin. The seahorse was netted for examination. A fine-needle aspiration biopsy of the lesions was obtained for cytologic examination (Figures 34.8, 34.9a, and 34.9b).

Interpretive Discussion

Cytology of the aspirate of the tail mass revealed degenerate cells and a marked number of rod-shaped bacteria that failed to stain with the Wright–Giemsa stain. These "ghost" bacteria are suspicious for *Mycobacterium*. Confirmation was obtained when the bacteria stained positive with acid-fast stain.

Summary

Mycobacteriosis in seahorses and other syngnathids is typically caused by nontuberculous species of *Mycobacteria*, such as *M. chelonae abscessus* and *M. fortuitum* and less commonly *M. marinum*. Mycobacteriosis in these fish usually occurs as isolated, sporadic cases; however, epizootics in the tank can be seen. Although peracute mycobacteriosis resulting in sudden death can occur in these fish, subacute to chronic, pyogranulomatous infection involving the skin, subcutis, and/or underlying skeletal muscle characterized by pyogranulomatous abscesses, and/or draining fistulous tracts are more common (Berzins, 2005).

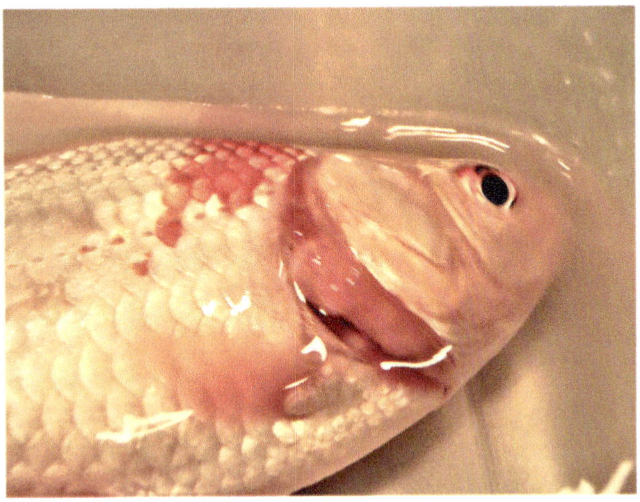

Fig. 34.10. Appearance of a mass under the right operculum.

Case 4: Carp with Swollen Operculum

Signalment

9-month-old ornamental carp (*Cyprinus carpio*)

History

The fish presented with the complaint of a swollen right operculum of two-day duration and not eating for a month's duration. The fish was housed in a large deep outdoor pond with several other ornamental carp. It was hatched in this pond. The client was concerned about pesticides sprayed in the area by a farmer on the adjacent property.

Physical Examination

A firm lobulated mass was found under the right operculum (Figure 34.10). The fish was anesthetized (MS-222), and a CO_2 laser was used to remove the mass, which consisted of three separate masses. Recovery from the procedure was uneventful. An imprint of the tissue was made for cytodiagnosis, and the tissue was submitted for histopathology (Figures 34.11a and 34.11b).

Interpretive Discussion

The imprint of an excised mass stained with Wright–Giemsa–Romanowsky stain revealed numerous inflammatory cells consisting of nondegenerate heterophils, lymphocytes, plasma cells, and macrophages. There were also numerous ovoid protozoal spores with two polar capsules. The cytology indicated a mixed-cell inflammation associated with a myxozoan parasite, such as *Myxobolus* sp. (possibly *M. cyprinid*).

(a) (b)

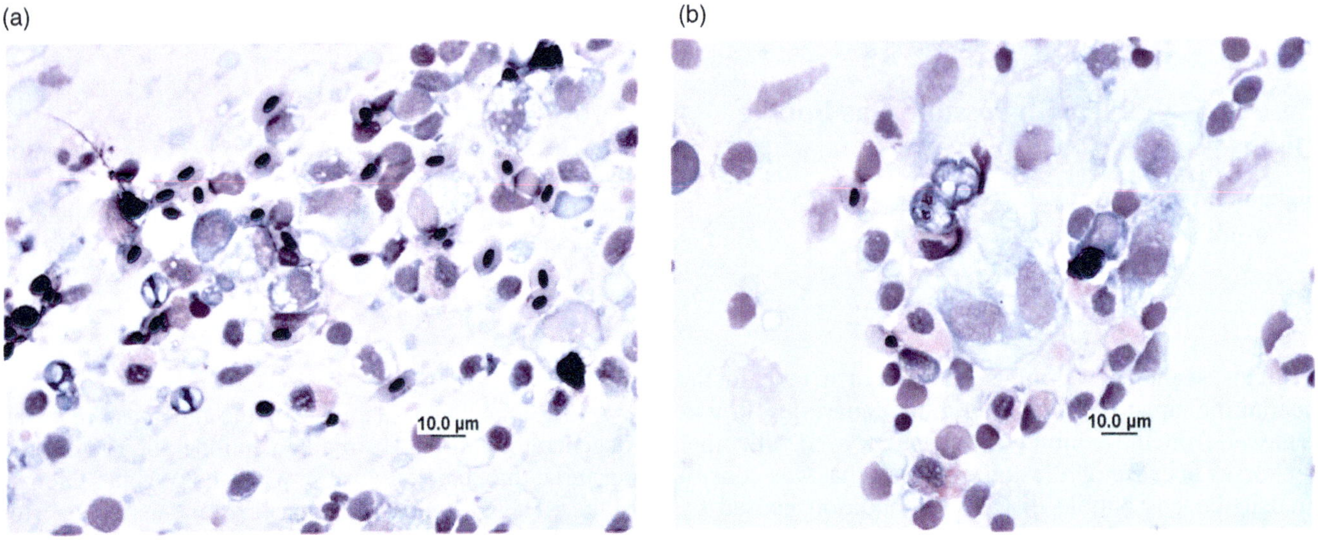

Fig. 34.11. (a), (b) Cytology of imprint of the opercular mass (Wright–Giemsa stain, 100× oil)

Summary

Due to the poor prognosis associated with a myxozoan parasite as well as the fish being a potential source of infection to other fish in the pond, the fish was euthanized and submitted for necropsy.

Gross necropsy revealed a mass expanding and effacing the left cranial gill and infiltrating and elevating the right operculum. The tan to brown mass was poorly demarcated and un-encapsulated. It was soft, heterogeneous upon cut section, and measured approximately 8×5×4 mm. Three surgically removed gill masses were submitted with the carcass that measured 7×5×3 mm, 5×4×3 mm, and 4×4×3 mm.

Histopathology of the left gill revealed multifocal to coalescing accumulations of marked numbers of large foamy macrophages that were surrounded by concentric bands of intact and degenerate heterophils, small lymphocytes, and plasma cells, all expanding and effacing the left gill. At the center of the macrophage aggregates were coalescing foci of marked numbers of round to ovoid protozoal spores ranging in size from 15–25 μm in diameter and separated by a pale, thin, 5–10 μm thick capsule. These spores were diffusely multicellular and contained 1–2 sporoblasts and 2 polar capsules. Within remnant gill structures, these spores expanded and largely replaced the primary and secondary laminae, cartilaginous matrix, and surrounding adipose tissue. Coalescing areas of granulomatous inflammation with intralesional protozoal spores extended to adjacent soft-tissue structures overlying the oropharynx. In addition, there were regionally extensive areas of cartilage necrosis that were characterized by eosinophilic chondrocytes and empty lacunae.

Histopathology of the right gill indicated that the primary and secondary laminae were diffusely expanded and effaced by marked numbers of previously described protozoal spores, as well as moderate to marked numbers of macrophages, intact and degenerate heterophils, and smaller numbers of small lymphocytes and plasma cells.

Histopathology of the oropharynx indicated the mucosa was diffusely expanded and effaced by marked numbers of previously described protozoal spores, as well as moderate to marked numbers of macrophages and intact and degenerate heterophils. The submucosa was diffusely expanded by moderate numbers of scattered small lymphocytes, plasma cells, and macrophages. Likewise, histopathology of the operculum indicated that the epithelium was diffusely expanded and effaced by marked numbers of previously described protozoal spores, as well as moderate to marked numbers of macrophages, intact and degenerate heterophils, and small lymphocytes and plasma cells.

Histopathology of the surgically removed gill masses revealed that they were composed entirely of granulomatous inflammation with intralesional protozoal cysts as previously described for the left gill. In addition, there were marked amounts of clear fluid that separated individual fibrous connective tissue fibrils (edema).

In conclusion, the gill pathology indicated a severe, chronic, diffuse, granulomatous and heterophilic, lymphoplasmacytic branchitis with intralesional protozoa consistent with Myxozoa sp. and regionally extensive chondronecrosis. In addition, there was a severe, diffuse, chronic, granulomatous and heterophilic, lymphoplasmacytic pharyngitis with intralesional protozoa, also consistent with *Myxozoa* sp. There was also a severe, diffuse, chronic hepatocellular degeneration with moderate hepatic lipidosis.

Case 5: Perch with Mass on Left Gill

Signalment

Adult black surf perch (*Embiotica jacksoni*)

History

The fish presented with the complaint of a mass associated with the left gill. The fish is housed in a large public aquarium with numerous other fish represented by a variety of species.

Physical Examination

A large soft-tissue, lobulated mass was found involving the left opercular chamber, but not involving the gills (Figures 34.12a and 34.12b). The fish was anesthetized (MS-222), and a CO_2 laser was used to biopsy the mass for histopathology. An imprint of the biopsy sample was made for cytodiagnosis (Figures 34.13a–34.13c).

Interpretive Discussion

The imprint of the biopsy stained with Wright–Giemsa–Romanowsky stain revealed numerous epithelial cells that appeared in aggregates. The cells had distinct cell margins and had squamous differentiation based upon their polygonal shape and baby blue cytoplasm indicative of keratinization. These epithelial cells demonstrated anisokaryosis, pleomorphic nuclei, and nuclear chromatin clumping and sometimes prominent large nucleoli. Mitotic figures of these cells were present. A few erythrocytes could be seen in the background. The cytology was supportive of a squamous cell carcinoma.

Summary

Histopathology of the biopsy indicated that the epithelium and submucosa of the opercular chamber were multifocally infiltrated and effaced by a densely cellular multilobulated neoplasm. The neoplasm consisted of

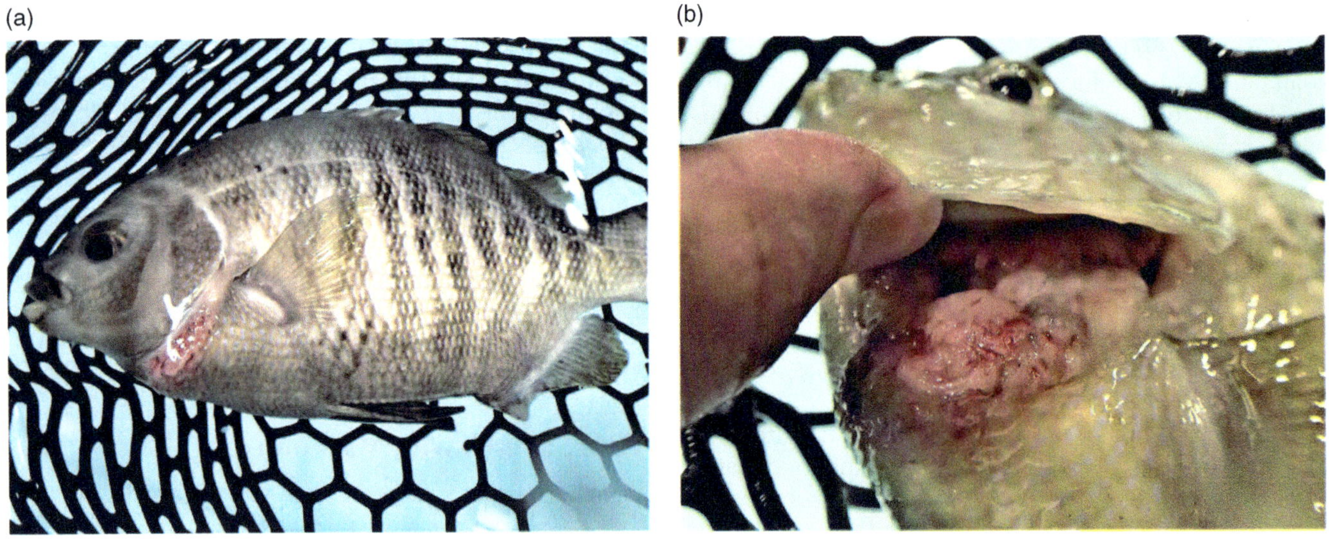

Fig. 34.12. (a), (b) Appearance of a mass in left operculum.

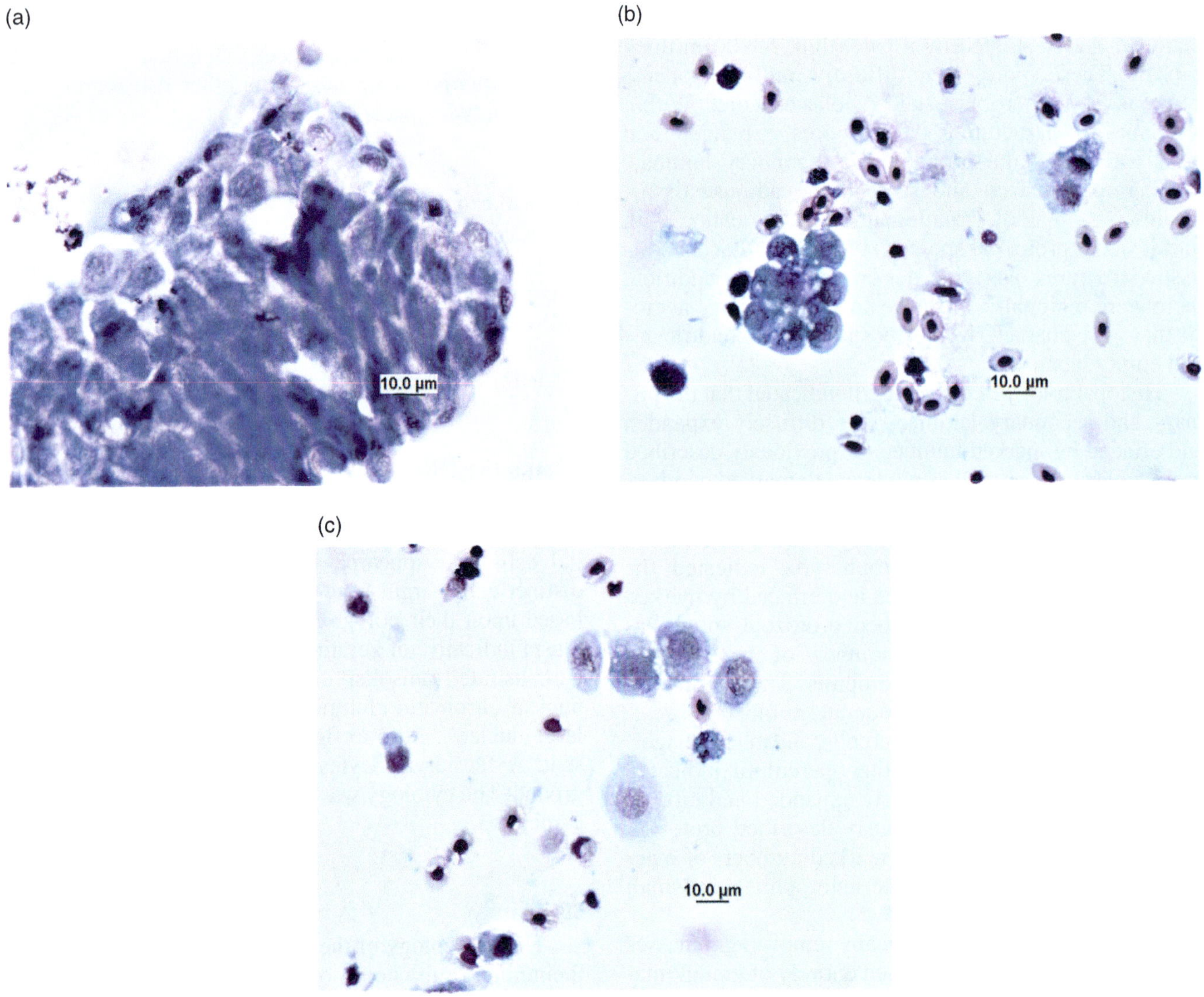

Fig. 34.13. (a)–(c) Cytology of imprint of the opercular mass (Wright–Giemsa stain, 100× oil).

polygonal squamous epithelial-like cells arranged in nests and trabeculae supported by moderate amounts of fibrovascular stroma. The cells had indistinct borders with moderate amounts of granular eosinophilic cytoplasm. The nuclei varied from medium to large and ovoid to polygonal with finely stippled chromatin and 1–2 medium nucleoli. The mitotic rate was high with 4–6 mitoses per 400× field. The neoplasm was stippled with individual apoptotic cells, and multifocal satellite masses were possibly within dilated blood vessels. Therefore, the conclusion was a squamous cell carcinoma that was highly invasive with local invasion and possible vascular metastasis.

References

Arnold JE. 2005. Hematology of the Sandbar shark, *Carcharhinus plumbeus*: standardization of complete blood count techniques for elasmobranchs. *Vet Clin Pathol* 34(2):115–123.

Berzins IK. 2005. Syngnathid health management. In: Koldewey H (ed), *Syngnathid Husbandry in Public Aquariums 2005 Manual. Zoological Society of London*. Regents Park, London, p. 32.

Cain DK, Harms CA, Segars A. 2004. Plasma biochemistry reference values of wild-caught Southern stingrays (*Dasyatis americana*). *J Zoo Wildl Med* 35(4):471–476.

Cusack L, Field CL, Hoopes L, McDermott A, Clauss T. 2016. Comparison of pre- and postquarantine blood chemistry and hematology values from wild-caught cownose rays (*Rhinoptera bonasus*). *J Zoo Wildl Med* 47(2):493–500.

Dove ADM, Arnold J, Clauss TM. 2010. Blood cells and serum chemistry in the world's largest fish: the whale shark *Rhincodon typus*. *Aquat Biol* 9:177–183.

Ferreira CM, Field CL, Tuttle AD. 2010. Hematological and plasma biochemical parameters of aquarium-maintained Cownose rays. *J Aquat Anim Health* 22:123–128.

Phillips BE, Christiansen EF, Stoskopf MK, et al. 2016. Comparison of hematology, plasma biochemistry, and blood gas variables between 2 venipuncture sites in Southern Stingrays (*Dasyatis americana*). *Vet Clin Pathol* 45(4):627–633.

APPENDIX A

Stains and Solutions Used in Hematology and Cytology

Acid-Fast Stain

Commercially prepared acid-fast stains are available and make the staining procedure relatively simple.

Staining Solution

1. Ziehl–Neelsen carbolfuchsin: Dissolve 3.0 g basic fuchsin in 100 mL 95% ethyl alcohol. Prepare a 5% phenol solution by dissolving 5.0 g phenol in 100 mL distilled water. Prepare the Ziehl–Neelsen carbolfuchsin by mixing 10 mL alcoholic basic fuchsin and 90 mL 5% phenol and allowing the mixture to stand for 24 h. Filter the solution prior to use.
2. Acid alcohol: Mix 2.0 mL concentrated hydrochloric acid and 98.0 mL 95% ethyl alcohol.
3. Methylene blue: Prepare a saturated solution of methylene blue by adding 1.5 g powdered methylene blue to 100 mL 95% ethyl alcohol. Slowly add the alcohol to dissolve the powder. Add 30 mL saturated alcoholic solution of methylene blue to 100.0 mL distilled water and 0.1 mL 10% potassium hydroxide. Filter this solution, and dilute it 1:20 with distilled water to prepare the final methylene blue counterstain.

Staining Procedure

1. Allow the film to air-dry and then gently heat-fix it (see Gram's stain procedure below).
2. Cover the slide with Ziehl–Neelsen carbolfuchsin, and steam it gently using a water bath for 3–5 min.
3. Rinse the slide with tap water.
4. Decolorize the slide with acid alcohol until little red color remains visible to the unaided eye.
5. Rinse again with tap water.
6. Counterstain the slide with aqueous methylene blue solution for 5–20 s, depending upon the thickness of the sample.
7. Rinse the slide with tap water and allow to air-dry.

Staining Results

Acid-fast positive organisms, such as *Mycobacterium* spp. and *Cryptosporidium* spp., appear distinctly red, whereas other bacteria, leukocytes, and debris appear blue.

Gram's Stain

Commercially prepared Gram's stains are available and make the staining procedure relatively simple.

Staining Solution

1. Crystal violet stain: Dissolve 2.0 g powdered crystal violet into 20 mL 95% ethyl alcohol and mix with 80 mL 1.0% aqueous ammonium oxalate. The solution is stable and can be stored for months.
2. Gram's iodine: Dissolve 1.0 g iodine (I_2) and 2.0 g potassium iodide (KI) into 300 mL distilled water. Prepare a fresh solution every 3 weeks.
3. 95% ethyl alcohol
4. Safranin stain: Dissolve 0.25 g Safranin O into 10 mL 95% ethyl alcohol. Add this solution to 100 mL distilled water.

Exotic Animal Hematology and Cytology, Fifth Edition. Terry W. Campbell and Krystan R. Grant.

Companion website: www.wiley.com/go/campbell/exotic

Staining Procedure

1. Heat-fix an air-dried slide by passing the slide (film side up) five or six times through a low flame (i.e., Bunsen burner or lighter). Allow the slide to cool.
2. Flood the heat-fixed film with crystal violet for 1 min, and gently wash the slide with water for 1–5 s.
3. Flood the slide with Gram's iodine solution for 1 min, and gently wash it with water.
4. Decolorize the film with 95% ethyl alcohol until the stain no longer elutes from the film (15–30 s). Wash the slide with water.
5. Counterstain the slide with Safranin stain solution for 1–2 min. Wash the slide with water for 1–5 s and allow to air-dry.

Staining Results

A satisfactorily stained smear should show gram-positive organisms as deep violet and gram-negative organisms as red. The Gram stain may be affected by the nature of the material on the smear. Smears often vary in thickness on the slide and excessive decolorization may occur in very thin areas, causing the gram-positive organisms to appear gram-negative. Likewise, thicker areas may be poorly decolorized, causing gram-negative organisms to appear gram-positive. Because Gram staining has a varied technique, the procedure requires practice before the cytologist gains confidence in the stain.

Macchiavello's Stain

Staining Solution

1. Basic fuchsin stain: Prepare a 0.1 M phosphate buffer (pH 7.3–7.4) by adding 80 mL 0.1 M anhydrous dibasic sodium phosphate ($Na_2 HPO_4$) to 20 mL 0.1 M monobasic sodium phosphate ($NaH_2PO_4 \cdot H_2O$). Dissolve 0.25 g basic fuchsin chloride into 100 mL 0.1 M phosphate buffer to make the stain. Prepare the 0.25% stain solution fresh each day of use, and filter the stain prior to staining the slide.
2. Citric acid solution: Dissolve 0.5 g citric acid in 100 mL distilled water. Make fresh 0.5% citric acid solution when mold growth occurs.
3. Methylene blue stain: Prepare a stock solution by adding 1.0 g methylene blue chloride to 10 mL 95% ethyl alcohol and slowly adding 100 mL distilled water and 5 mL phenol (melted crystals). Make a working solution by diluting the stock solution 1:10 with distilled water.

Staining Procedure

1. Heat-fix the air-dried film (see Gram's stain procedure).
2. Flood the slide with the basic fuchsin stain, and allow it to stain for 5 min.
3. Quickly wash the slide in tap water, and dip it one to three times in the citric acid solution (1–3 s).
4. Rinse the slide in tap water.
5. Counterstain the slide with the methylene blue stain for 20–30 s.
6. Wash the slide in tap water and allow to air-dry.

Staining Results

In satisfactorily stained smears, the elementary bodies (0.2–0.3 μm) of the *Chlamydophila* (*Chlamydia*) spp. organism stain red and the larger initial bodies (0.9–1.0 μm) stain blue. Some films contain nonchlamydophial particles that stain red, making the interpretation difficult. Heterophil and eosinophil granules frequently stain red. *Mycoplasma* colonies may resemble *Chlamydophila* (*Chlamydia*). Excessive decolorization with citric acid may decolorize the elementary bodies, making them appear blue; therefore, the citric acid decolorization step may be omitted or shortened in some films.

Modified Giménez Stain

Staining Solutions

1. Carbol basic fuchsin
   a. Stock solution: Dissolve 10 g basic fuchsin in 100 mL ethyl alcohol. Add 250 mL 4.0% phenol solution to 100 mL basic fuchsin–ethanol solution. Finally, add 650 mL distilled water and incubate the solution at 37°C for 48 h.
   b. Buffer solution: Dissolve 27.60 g $NaH_2PO_4 \cdot H_2O$ (dibasic sodium phosphate) into 100 mL distilled water. Prepare the buffer solutions by adding 3.5 mL monobasic sodium phosphate solution (0.2 M) and 15.5 mL dibasic sodium phosphate solution (0.2 M) to 10.0 mL distilled water.
   c. Working carbol basic fuchsin solution: Mix 4.0 mL carbol fuchsin stock solution with 10 mL buffer solution, and filter twice before using. Filtration is required to minimize the amount of red stain precipitate, which may interfere with the staining results.
2. Malachite green: Dissolve 0.8 g powdered malachite green into 100 mL distilled water.

Staining Procedure

1. Allow the film to air-dry, and then gently heat-fix the slide (see Gram's stain procedure above).
2. Cover the slide with a working solution of carbol fuchsin and allow to stand for 1–2 min.
3. Rinse the slide with tap water.
4. Cover the slide with malachite green solution for 6–9 s.
5. Rinse the slide in tap water, and recover the slide with malachite green solution for an additional 6–9 s.
6. Wash the slide with tap water, and allow it to air-dry.

Staining Results

Chlamydophila (*Chlamydia*) inclusions are circular and stain red against a blue-green cellular background. *Chlamydophila* (*Chlamydia*) organisms may be seen as intracellular and extracellular red organisms.

New Methylene Blue Stain

New methylene blue stain is used for reticulocyte staining and counting procedures. It can also be used to examine cytology specimens.

Staining Solution

1. Dissolve 0.5 g powdered new methylene blue into a solution containing 99.0 mL 0.85% saline and 1.0 mL 40% formalin.
2. Filter the stain solution, and store it in a brown bottle.

Staining Procedure

1. Reticulocyte stain: Mix equal parts of whole blood, and stain in a test tube and allow it to stand for 15–20 min. Prepare a standard blood film and allow it to air-dry.
2. Cytology stain: Use new methylene blue stain as a wet mount on a dried film. Apply a small drop of the stain to an air-dried film, and place a coverslip over the film for microscopic examination.

Staining Results

New methylene blue does not stain hemoglobin; therefore, erythrocytes have a colorless cytoplasm, distinct cytoplasmic borders, and, in the case of lower vertebrates, a purple nucleus. Erythrocytes of many of the lower vertebrates contain a variable amount of reticulum, which appears as blue cytoplasmic precipitate or clumps. Granulocytes have purple nuclei and pale blue cytoplasm. The cytoplasmic granules of heterophils and eosinophils do not stain with new methylene blue. New methylene blue stain provides a more distinctive chromatin and nucleolar appearance to nuclei than do alcohol-based stains, such as Wright's stain. Since new methylene blue stain is water soluble, it can be used to demonstrate fibrin, lipid droplets, and fungal hyphae, which either dissolve or do not stain well with alcohol-based stains.

Standard Natt and Herrick's Solution and Stain

Staining Solution

Add the following ingredients together, and bring them to a total volume of 1000 mL with distilled water, using a volumetric flask:

Sodium chloride	NaCl	3.88 g
Sodium sulfate	$NaSO_4$	2.50 g
Sodium phosphate	Na_2HPO_4	1.74 g
Potassium phosphate	KH_2PO_4	0.25 g
Formalin (37%)		7.50 mL
Methyl violet		0.10 g

Allow the solution to stand overnight, and filter through Whatman No. 10 medium filter paper before use.

Staining Procedure and Staining Results

Draw whole blood to the 0.5 mark of the red-blood-cell-diluting pipette, and draw Natt and Herrick's solution to the 101 mark to dilute the blood for obtaining total cell counts, using a hemacytometer.

The diluted blood is discharged onto the hemacytometer counting chamber and allowed to settle for a minimum of 5 min before counting. Nonmammalian erythrocytes have a small, dark blue nucleus surrounded by a colorless to faint pink cytoplasm with this stain. The total number of erythrocytes in the four corner and central red blood cell squares of the central large square of a Neubauer-ruled hemacytometer chamber is counted using 400× (40×, high-dry objective) magnification. Both sides of the hemacytometer are counted in order to obtain duplicate counts. The duplicate counts are averaged if they are in at least a 15% agreement between the two sides. The TRBC (total red blood cell count per microliter) is then calculated by multiplying the number of erythrocytes by 10 000.

For the total leukocyte determination, the same charged Neubauer-ruled hemacytometer used for obtaining a TRBC from blood diluted 1:200 in Natt and Herrick's diluent is used. The small, dark-blue-staining leukocytes are counted in nine large squares in the Neubauer-ruled hemacytometer chamber using 400× (40×, high-dry objective) magnification. Both sides of the hemacytometer should be counted in order to obtain duplicate counts. The duplicates are averaged if they are within at least 15% agreement between the two sides. If the two sides do not agree within 15% of each other, then the process should be repeated using a freshly charged hemacytometer. The TWBC (total white blood cell count per microliter) per microliter is then calculated using the following formula:

$$\text{TWBC}/\mu\text{L} + \left(\text{total cells in nine large squares} + 10\%\right) \times 200$$

It may be difficult to distinguish small mature lymphocytes from thrombocytes if counts are made using a 100× magnification (10× objective). In general, thrombocytes typically stain lighter than lymphocytes; however, staining the sample for 60 min in Natt and Herrick's solution may improve the differentiation between small lymphocytes and thrombocytes.

Elasmobranch-Modified Natt and Herrick's Solution and Stain

Source: Walsh CJ, Luer CA. 2004. Elasmobranch hematology: identification of cell types and practical applications. In: Smith M, Warmolts D, Thoney D, Hueter R (eds), *The Elasmobranch Husbandry Manual: Captive Care of Sharks, Rays, and Their Relatives*. Columbus, OH: Ohio Biological Survey, Inc.

Staining Solution

Add the following ingredients together, and bring them to a total volume of 100 mL with distilled water, using a volumetric flask:

NaCl	2.28 g
Na_2SO_4	0.25 g
NaH_2PO_4	0.29 g
KH_2PO_4	0.025 g
Formalin (37% formaldehyde)	750 µL
Methyl violet 2B	0.01 g

Allow the solution to stand overnight, and filter through Whatman No. 10 medium filter paper before use. Store at room temperature.

Staining Procedure and Staining Results

The procedure is the same as that described for the standard Natt and Herrick's solution. This solution protects elasmobranch cells from osmotic effects of the stain. Hemolysis of elasmobranch blood can also be decreased using a modified heparin–EDTA or citric acid (ACD) solution as an anticoagulant when collecting blood samples as follows.

Elasmobranch-Modified Heparin–EDTA

Source: Walsh CJ, Luer CA. 2004. Elasmobranch hematology: identification of cell types and practical applications. In: Smith M, Warmolts D, Thoney D, Hueter R (eds), *The Elasmobranch Husbandry Manual: Captive Care of Sharks, Rays, and Their Relatives*. Columbus, OH: Ohio Biological Survey, Inc.

1. Prepare an Elasmobranch-modified phosphate buffered saline (E-PBS) in distilled water as follows:

	g/100 mL	g/500 mL	g/1000 mL
NaCl	2.63	13.15	26.3
NaH_2PO_4	0.12	0.6	1.2

   Adjust the pH to 7.0 with 1N HCl. Filter through 0.2 µm sterile filter, and store at 4°C. The final osmolarity is approximately 920 mOsm.
2. Prepare a stock solution of the anticoagulant by adding 200 mg EDTA and 2000 units heparin in 10 mL E-PBS.
3. Filter through 0.2 µm sterile filter, and use the following volumes for specified amounts of blood: 0.5 mL for 10 mL blood; 0.25 mL for 5 mL blood; 0.15 mL for 3 mL blood. Store at 4°C; or premeasured aliquots can be frozen and thawed when needed.

Elasmobranch-Modified ACD Solution

Source: Walsh CJ, Luer CA. 2004. Elasmobranch hematology: identification of cell types and practical applications. In: Smith M, Warmolts D, Thoney D, Hueter R (eds), *The Elasmobranch Husbandry Manual: Captive Care of Sharks, Rays, and Their Relatives*. Columbus, OH: Ohio Biological Survey, Inc.

	100 mL	200 mL	500 mL
Citric acid (anhydrous)	0.73 g	1.46 g	3.65 g
Citric acid (monohydrate)	0.795 g	1.59 g	3.98 g
Sodium citrate (hydrous)	2.2 g	4.4 g	11 g
Dextrose (hydrous)	2.45 g	4.9 g	12.25 g

For 100 mL, dissolve above ingredients in approximately 67 mL E-PBS, and adjust to a final volume of 100 mL with distilled water. Filter through 0.2 µm sterile filter, and store at 4°C. Use this anticoagulant in amounts equal to the ratio of 7 mL ACD to 40 mL whole blood. For 5 mL samples, add 875 mL per tube.

Quick or Stat Stains

Staining Solutions

These commercially prepared stains are designed to provide the staining characteristics of Wright–Giemsa stains and make the staining procedure relatively simple. Examples of two commonly used quick stains are Diff–Quik (American Scientific Products, Division of American Hospital Supply Corporation, McGraw Park, IL) and Hema-Tek (Ames Division, Miles Laboratories, Inc., Elkhart, IN).

Staining Procedure

1. Dip the air-dried slide into the methanol fixative solution for five 1 s dips, and allow the excess to drain.
2. Dip the alcohol-fixed slide into Solution I (Diff–Quik's buffered Eosin Y solution) for five 1 s dips, and drain off the excess.

3. Dip the slide into Solution II (Diff–Quik's buffered solution of methylene blue and azure A dyes) for five 1 s dips, and drain off the excess.
4. Rinse the slide with distilled or deionized water for five 1 s dips, and allow it to air-dry.

Staining Results

The staining procedure can be modified according to the desired staining effects or thickness of the film. Increasing the number of dips in Solution I or II will intensify the overall staining of the film. A paler stain is obtained by fewer dips (a minimum of three dips is required). Eosinophilic staining is enhanced by increasing the number of dips in Solution I, and basophilic staining is increased by additional dips in Solution II. Overall, the staining qualities for the films are similar to those of Wright–Giemsa stain.

Sudan III and Sudan IV Stains

Staining Solutions

Because of the difficulty of preparing stain solutions, it is advisable to use commercially prepared Sudan stains.

Staining Procedure

Use Sudan stains as wet-mount stains.

Staining Results

Fat droplets or globules stain a red-orange color.

Wright's Stain

Commercially prepared Wright's stains are available and make the staining procedure relatively simple.

Staining Solution

1. Wright's stain: Dissolve 0.1 g Wright's stain into 60 mL absolute methanol. Allow the solution to stand in a tightly sealed brown bottle for 1–2 weeks. Filter the solution before using.
2. Wright's buffer: Dissolve 3.80 g Na_2HPO_4 (dibasic sodium phosphate) and 5.47 g KH_2PO_4 (monobasic potassium phosphate) into 500 mL distilled water. Bring the total volume to 1000 mL with distilled water.

Staining Procedure

1. Flood an air-dried film with Wright's stain, and allow to stand for 1–3 min.
2. Add an equal amount of Wright's buffer, and mix by gently blowing on the slide until a metallic green sheen forms on the surface. Allow it to stand for 2–6 min (the exact time must be determined for each batch of stain).
3. Gently rinse the stain from the slide using tap water or distilled water and a wash bottle or beaker.
4. Prop up the slide, and allow it to air-dry.

Staining Results

A satisfactorily stained blood film will reveal erythrocytes with a yellowish red cytoplasm. The erythrocytes of lower vertebrates and leukocytes will have dark violet nuclei. Heterophils of lower vertebrates will exhibit red-orange, rod-shaped cytoplasmic granules. Eosinophils will exhibit a pale blue cytoplasm and red-orange round granules in many species. Basophils will exhibit dark purple cytoplasmic granules. The cytoplasm of thrombocytes of lower vertebrates and the platelets of mammals will stain colorless to light blue with red granules.

Wright–Giemsa Stain

Commercially prepared Wright–Giemsa stains are available and make the staining procedure relatively simple.

Staining Solution

1. Dissolve 300 mg powdered Wright's stain and 30 g powdered Giemsa stain into 100 mL absolute methanol. Allow the solution to stand for 1–2 days in a tightly sealed brown bottle.
2. Filter the solution and use as indicated for the Wright's staining procedure.

Staining Results

The results are similar to Wright's stain alone except that the cell nuclei become reddish purple instead of violet.

APPENDIX B

Hematologic Values

Table B.1 Comparison of erythrocytes between common mammalian species.

Species	Diameter (μm)	PCV (%)	Hgb (g/dL)	MCV (fL)	MCHC (g/dL)	Reticulocytes (%)[a]
Mice[b]	5–7	35–52	10–17	45–55	30–38	–
Rats[b]	6–7	38–51	12–16	55–62	30–34	2–5
Gerbil[c]	–	44–52	14–17	46–60	31–33	3–7
Hamster[d]	5–7	44–49	13–16	59–71	26–33	–
Prairie dog[e]	–	36–54	13–20	54–71	32–39	–
Guinea pig[f]	7–8	37–50	11–17	71–96	28–39	2
Chinchilla[g]	–	38	12–14	–	–	–
Rabbit[h]	7	33–50	10–17	58–67	29–37	1–7
African hedgehog[i]	–	22–64	7–21	41–94	17–48	–
Ferret[j]	5–8	34–47	12–17	44–53	35–42	4–5

[a]With normal packed cell volume.
[b]Bolliger AP, Everds NE, Zimmerman KL, et al. 2010. Hematology of laboratory animals. In: Weiss DJ, Wardrop KJ (eds), *Schalm's Veterinary Hematology*, 6th edn. Ames, IA: Wiley-Blackwell, pp. 852–887.
[c]Mays A, Jr. 1969. Baseline hematological and blood biochemical parameters of the Mongolian gerbil (*Meriones unguiculatus*). *Lab Anim Care* 19:838–842.
[d]Reznik G. 1975. Comparative studies of blood from hibernating and nonhibernating European hamsters (*Cricetus cricetus* L). *Lab Anim Sci* 25:210–215.
[e]Funk RS. 2003. Medical management of Prairie dogs. In: Quesenberry KE, Carpenter JW (eds), *Ferrets, Rabbits, and Rodents, Clinical Medicine and Surgery*, 2nd edn. St. Louis, MO: WB Saunders, pp. 266–273.
[f]Mitruka BM, Rawnsley HM. 1981. *Clinical Biochemical and Hematological Reference Values in Normal Experimental Animal*, 2nd edn. New York: Masson.
[g]Quesenberry KE, Donnelly TM, Hillyer EV. 2003. Biology, husbandry, and clinical techniques of guinea pigs and chinchillas. In: Quesenberry KE, Carpenter JW (eds), *Ferrets, Rabbits, and Rodents, Clinical Medicine and Surgery*, 2nd edn. St. Louis, MO: WB Saunders, pp. 232–265.
[h]Zimmerman KL, Moore DM, Smith SA. 2010. Hematology of laboratory rabbits (*Oryctolagus cuniculus*). In: Weiss DJ, Wardrop KJ (eds), *Schalm's Veterinary Hematology*, 6th edn. Ames, IA: Wiley-Blackwell, pp. 862–869.
[i]Ivey E, Carpenter JW. 2003. African hedgehogs. In: Quesenberry KE, Carpenter JW (eds), *Ferrets, Rabbits, and Rodents, Clinical Medicine and Surgery*, 2nd edn. St. Louis, MO: WB Saunders, pp. 339–353.
[j]Zimmerman KL, Moore DM, Smith SA. 2010. Hematology of the guinea pig. In: Weiss DJ, Wardrop KJ (eds), *Schalm's Veterinary Hematology*, 6th edn. Ames, IA: Wiley-Blackwell, pp. 893–898.

Exotic Animal Hematology and Cytology, Fifth Edition. Terry W. Campbell and Krystan R. Grant.

Companion website: www.wiley.com/go/campbell/exotic

Table B.2 Erythrocyte parameters for laboratory animals and miscellaneous mammalian species (mean and reference range).

	PCV (%)	RBC (×10⁶/μL)	Hb (g/dL)	MCV (fL)	MCHC (g/dL)	MCH (pg)	Reticulocytes (%)
Mice[a]	40.4	8.3	13.1	49.1	32.3	15.9	4.7
	32.8–48.0	6.5–10.1	10.1–16.1	42.3–55.9	29.5–35.1	13.7–18.1	0–11.3
Rats[a]	46.1 ± 2.5	7.8	14.8	59.0 ± 6.4	32.4	18.9	2.2
	41.1–51.1	6.6–9.0	13.2–16.4	52.6–65.4	30.2–34.6	16.5–21.3	0–4.6
Guinea	42.1	5.1	12.9	83.0	30.6		2.3
pigs[a]	35.9–48.3	4.1–6.1	10.5–15.3	75.0–91.0	28.2–33.0		0–6.1
Hamsters[a]	52.5	7.5	16.8	71.2			
	47.9–57.1	2.7–12.3	13.4–19.2	64.8–77.6			
Chinchilla[a]	38.3	6.6	11.7	58.0			
	25.0–52.0	5.2–9.9	8.8–15.4				
Rabbits[a]	42.0	6.0	13.3	70.4	31.7	22.3	3.7
	36.6–47.4	5.2–6.8	11.5–15.1	64.6–76.2	29.5–33.9	21.1–24.5	1.1–6.3
Ferrets[b]	49.2	8.11	16.2	47.1	32.0	15.0	5.3
	42–55	6.8–9.8	14.8–17.4	42.6–51.0	30.3–34.9	13.7–16.0	2–14
Hedgehogs[c]	36	6	12.0	67	34	22	–
	22–64	3–16	7.0–21.1	41–94	17–48	11–31	

[a]Modified from Jain NC. 1993. *Essentials of Veterinary Hematology*. Philadelphia, PA: Lea & Febiger, pp. 54–71.
[b]Modified from Fox JG (ed). 1988. Normal clinical and biologic parameters. In: *Biology and Diseases of the Ferret*. Philadelphia, PA: Lea & Febiger, pp. 159–173.
[c]Ivey E, Carpenter JW. 2003. African hedgehogs. In: Quesenberry KE, Carpenter JW (eds), *Ferrets, Rabbits, and Rodents; Clinical Medicine and Surgery*, 2nd edn. St. Louis, MO: Saunders, p. 345.

Table B.3 Leukocyte parameters of laboratory animals and miscellaneous mammalian species (mean and reference ranges).

	WBC (×10³/μL)		Bands	Neutrophil	Lymphocytes	Monocytes	Eosinophils	Basophils	Platelets (×10³/μL)
Mice[a]	6.33	× 10³/μL	0	1.20	4.86	0.14	0.08	0	1.16
	2.61–10.05		0–0.02	0.4–2.0	1.27–8.44	0–0.29	0–0.17	0–0.02	0.78–1.54
Rats[a]	9.98	× 10³/μL	0	2.48	7.07	0.25	0.17	0	1.04
	7.30–12.66		0–0.02	1.25–3.71	5.07–9.07	0.05–0.44	0.04–0.30	0–0.03	0.84–1.24
Guinea pigs[a]	11.11	× 10³/μL	0	2.50	8.01	0.31	0.27	0	0.55
	8.22–14.0		0–0.01	1.35–3.65	5.47–10.55	0.06–0.56	0–0.69	0–0.02	0.39–0.71
Hamsters[a]	7.62	%	–	29.9 ± 8.0	73.5 ± 9.4	2.5 ± 0.8	1.1 ± 0.02	0	–
	6.32–7.92								
Chinchilla[a]	8.0	%	–	44.6	53.6	1.2	0.5	0.4	–
	2.2–45.1			10.0–78.0	19.0–98.0	0.0–5.0	0.0–9.0	0.0–11.0	
Rabbits[a]	8.18	× 10³/μL	0	2.35	5.18	0.25	0.08	0.21	0.43
	6.30–10.06			1.49–3.21	3.36–7.00	0.05–0.45	0.01–0.15	0.06–0.36	0.25–0.61
Ferrets[b]	10.5	%	–	59.5	33.4	4.4	2.6	0.2	545
	4–18			43–84	12–50	2–8	0–5	0–1	310–910
Hedgehogs[c]	11	× 10³/μL	–	5.1	4.0	0.3	1.2	0.4	229
	3–43			0.6–37.4	0.9–13.1	0.0–1.6	0.0–5.1	0.0–1.5	60–347

[a]Modified from Jain NC. 1993. *Essentials of Veterinary Hematology*. Philadelphia, PA: Lea & Febiger, pp. 54–71.
[b]Modified from Fox JG (ed). 1988. Normal clinical and biologic parameters. In: *Biology and Diseases of the Ferret*. Philadelphia, PA: Lea & Febiger, pp. 159–173.
[c]Ivey E, Carpenter JW. 2003. African hedgehogs. In: Quesenberry KE, Carpenter JW (eds), *Ferrets, Rabbits, and Rodents; Clinical Medicine and Surgery*, 2nd edn. St. Louis, MO: Saunders, p. 345.

Table B.4 Semiquantitative microscopic evaluation of avian erythrocyte morphology.[a]

	1+	2+	3+	4+
Anisocytosis	5–10	11–20	21–30	>30
Polychromasia	2–10	11–14	15–30	>30
Hypochromasia	1–2	3–5	6–10	>10
Poikilocytosis	5–10	11–20	21–50	>50
Erythroplastids	1–2	3–5	6–10	>10

[a]Based on the average number of abnormal cells per 1000 × monolayer field.

Table B.5 Erythrocyte parameters for selected birds.

	PCV (%)	RBC (× 10^6/μL)	Hb (g/dL)	MCV (fL)	MCHC (g/dL)
Psittacines					
African grey parrot[c,e]	43–55	2.4–4.5	11.0–16.0	90–180	23–33
Amazon parrots[c,d]	45–55	2.5–4.5	12.5–25	160–175	29.1–31.0
Blue-fronted Amazon[g]	44–58	2.1–3.5	16.0–18.4	163–209	31.7–37.8
Cuban Amazon[g]	44–54	3.1–3.5	15.2–17.7	142–162	31.4–37.2
Festive Amazon[g]	47–53	3.1–3.8	16.1–17.4	135–164	31.5–34.5
Orange-wing Amazon[g]	46–51	2.8–3.3	15.5–17.5	151–166	32.1–36.0
Vinaceous Amazon[g]	46–52	3.0–3.3	15.0–17.5	145–174	31.7–35.6
Yellow Amazon[g]	38–51	2.1–3.5	12.1–17.4	135–175	31.0–34.1
Budgerigar[c,e]	44–58	2.3–3.9	13–18	90–190	22–32
Cockatiel[c,e]	45–54	2.5–4.7	11–16	90–200	22–33
Cockatoos[c,e]	42–54	2–4	12–16	120–175	28–33
Black cockatoo[g]	40–46	2.4–2.7	12–17	154–184	32–37
Goffin's cockatoo[g]	37–47	2.4–3.4	12–16	119–175	33–39
Palm cockatoo[g]	36–47	2.0–3.6	13–17	131–235	31–36
White cockatoo[g]	37–48	2.8–3.2	14–18	132–171	30–39
Conures[c,e]	42–54	2.9–4.5	12–16	90–190	23–31
Golden conure[g]	50–54	3.6–4.0	17.6–20.4	126–144	33.9–40.7
Patagonian conure[g]	45–52	3.2–4.1	14.3–16.2	127–146	30.9–32.3
Eclectus parrot[c,e]	45–55	2.7–3.8	13.5–16.0	125–175	29–32
Jardine's parrot[c]	35–48	2.4–4.0	11–16	90–190	21–33
Lovebird[c,e]	44–57	3.0–5.1	13–18	90–190	22–32
Macaw[c,e]	47–55	2.7–4.5	15–17	125–170	29–35
Green-wing macaw[g]	39–54	2.7–4.1	9.6–18.7	116–177	21.9–34.9
Military macaw[g]	37–55	2.7–5.2	11.1–19.6	106–173	33.9–40.7
Scarlet macaw[g]	40–54	2.3–3.7	13.1–19.9	135–169	29.7–37.3
Pionus parrot[c]	35–54	2.4–4.0	11–16	85–210	24–31
Quaker[c,e]	30–58	2.8–3.9	11–15	90–200	22–32
Senegal parrot[c]	36–48	2.4–4.0	11–16	90–200	23–32
Others					
Canary[c,e]	37–49	2.5–3.8	12–16	90–210	22–32
Pigeon[e]	38–50	3.1–4.5	13–17.5	85–200	22–33
Chicken[c,e]	23–55	1.3–4.5	7.0–18.6	100–139	20–34
Turkey[c]	30.4–45.6	1.74–3.70	8.8–13.4	112–168	23.2–35.3
Quail[c]	30.0–45.1	4.0–5.2	10.7–14.3	60–100	28.0–38.5
Canada goose[c]	38–58	1.6–2.6	12.7–19.1	118–144	20–30
[a]Mallard duck[f]	46–51	3.05–3.65	14.8–16.4	134–162	31.4–31.8
[b]Mallard duck[f]	34–44	1.61–2.41	11–13	172–227	27–31
Peregrine falcon[c]	37–53	3–4	11.8–18.8	118–146	31.9–35.2
Red-tailed hawk[c]	31–43	2.41–3.59	10.7–16.6	150–178	29.7–34.5
Tawny owl[h]	29–47	1.5–2.4	8.0–13.3	154–221	33.1–62.1
White-back vulture[i]	35–54	21–3.0	16.32–23.0	186–208	36.2–42.3

[a]January.
[b]June.
[c]Pollack C, Carpenter JW, Antinoff N. 2005. Birds. In: Carpenter J (ed), *Exotic Animal Formulary*, 3rd edn. St. Louis, MO: Elsevier Saunders.
[d]Tell LA, Citino SB. 1992. Hematologic and serum chemistry reference intervals for Cuban mazon parrots (*Amazona leucocephala leucocephala*). *J Zoo Wildlife Med* 23:62–64
[e]Cray C. 2000. Blood and chemistry tables. In: Olsen G, Orosz S (eds), *Manual of Avian Medicine*. St. Louis, MO: Mosby.
[f]Campbell TW. 2000. Normal hematology of waterfowl. In: Feldman B, Zinkl J, Jain M (eds), *Schalm's Veterinary Hematology*, 5th edn. Philadelphia, PA: Lippincott Williams & Wilkins.
[g]Polo FJ, Peinado VI, Viscor G, Palomeque J. 1998. Hematologic and plasma chemistry values in captive psittacine birds. *Avian Dis* 42:523–535.
[h]Spagnolo V, Crippa V, Marzia A, Alberti I, Sartorelli P. 2008. Hematologic, biochemical, and protein electrophoretic values in captive tawny owls (*Strix aluco*). *Vet Clin Pathol* 37:225–228.
[i]Naidoo V, Diekmann M, Wolters K, Swan GE. 2008. Establishment of selected baseline blood chemistry and hematologic parameters in captive and wild-caught African white-backed vultures (*Gyps africanaus*). *J Wild Dis* 44:649–654.

Table B.6 Leukocyte parameters for selected birds.

	WBC (×10³/μL)	Heterophils (%)	Lymphocytes (%)	Monocytes (%)	Eosinophils (%)	Basophils (%)
Psittacines						
African grey parrot[c,e]	5–15	45–75	20–50	0–3	0–2	0–22
Grey parrot[g]	4.0–20.0	29–83	16–68	1–6	0–3	0
Amazon parrots[c,d]	6–11	30–75	20–65	0–3	0–1	0–5
Blue-fronted Amazon[g]	4.7–11.0	12–47	52–84	1–3	0–1	0–1
Cuban Amazon[g]	1.9–24.7	19–28	71–75	0–5	0–5	0–1
Festive Amazon[g]	2.2–7.0	22–32	66–76	0–4	0–2	0
Orange-wing Amazon[g]	1.2–10.1	22–41	56–73	2–5	0–5	0–2
Yellow Amazon[g]	2.2–7.2	12–52	48–80	0–8	0–1	0–1
Budgerigar[c,e]	3–8	40–65	20–45	0–1	0–1	0–1
Caique[c]	8–15	39–72	20–61	0–2	0–2	0–2
Cockatiel[c,e]	5–13	40–70	25–55	0–2	0–2	0–6
Cockatoos[c,e]	5–10	55–80	20–45	0–2	0–1	0–3
Black cockatoo[g]	3.7–22.1	7–61	33–90	3–7	0	0–2
Palm cockatoo[g]	1.4–17.6	24–75	24–69	1–7	0–1	0–1
White cockatoo[g]	1.3–18.7	18–83	15–80	0–4	0–1	0–1
Conures[c,e]	4–13	40–70	20–50	0–3	0–3	0–5
Golden conure[g]	4.2–8.0	22–49	49–69	1–3	0–2	0
Patagonian conure[g]	2.5–8.7	24–63	35–66	0–3	0–1	0
Eclectus parrot[c,e]	9–20	35–50	45–65	0–2	0–1	0–3
Grey-cheek parakeet[c]	4.5–12.0	40–75	20–60	0–3	0–1	0–5
Jardine's parrot[c]	4–10	55–75	25–45	0–2	0–1	0–1
Lory[c]	8–13	40–60	22–69	0–2	0–1	0–1
Red lory[g]	0.8–9.0	26–79	19–70	0–5	0–5	0–1
Lovebird[c,e]	3–16	40–75	20–55	0–2	0–1	0–6
Macaw[c,e]	7–22	40–60	35–60	0–3	0–1	0–1
Blue & gold macaw[g]	1.7–36.0	13–60	36–84	0–2	0–2	0–2
Green-wing macaw[g]	3.8–30.0	14–62	35–84	0–8	0–3	0–2
Hyacinthine macaw[g]	1.5–19.2	52–89	10–77	0–2	0–4	0
Military macaw[g]	13.7–18.0	12–63	43–80	0–8	0–2	0–1
Scarlet macaw[g]	4.7–22.0	26–67	36–68	0–8	0–4	0–2
Pionus parrot[c]	4.0–11.5	50–75	25–45	0–2	0–2	0–1
Quaker[c,e]	4–10	55–80	20–45	0–4	0–2	0–6
Senegal parrot[c]	4–14	55–75	25–45	0–2	0–1	0–1
Others						
Canary[c,e]	4–9	50–80	20–45	0–1	0–2	0–1
Finch[c,e]	3–8	20–65	20–65	0–1	0–1	0–5
Mynah[c]	6–11	25–65	20–60	0–3	0–3	0–7
Toucan[c]	4–10	35–65	25–50		0–4	0–5
Pigeon[c,d]	1.3–2.3	50–60	20–40	0–3	0–3	0–3
Chicken[c,e]	0.9–3.2	15–50	29–84	0–7	0–16	0–8
Ringneck pheasant[c]	1.8–3.9	12–30	63–83	2–9	0–1	0–3
Turkey[c]	1.6–2.5	29–52	35–48	3–10	0–5	0–9
Quail[c]	1.3–2.5	25–50	50–70	0–4	0–15	0–2
Canada goose[c]	1.3–1.9					
[a]Mallard duck[f]	2.3–2.5	35–40	52–56	0–6	0–1	0–4
[b]Mallard duck[f]	2.3–2.5	27–31	64–68	0–3	0–1	0–3
Golden eagle[c]	1.2–1.5	81–86	14–22	0–1	2–5	0–1
Peregrine falcon[c]	3.3–11.0	1–9	1–3	0–1	0–1	0–1
Tawny owl[h]	4.0–59.0	(1.6–9.6)×10³/μL	(2.1–7.2)×10³/μL	(0–0.5)×10³/μL	(0.2–3.0)×10³/μL	(0.1–0.4)×10³/μL
White-back vulture[i]	1.3–2.0	(1.5–25.9)×10³/μL	(0–4.8)×10³ /μL	(0–3.7)×10³/μL	(0–2.2)×10³/μL	(0–0)×10³/μL

[a]January.
[b]June.
[c]Pollack C, Carpenter JW, Antinoff N. 2005. Birds. In: Carpenter J (ed), *Exotic Animal Formulary*, 3rd edn. St. Louis, MO: Elsevier Saunders.
[d]Tell LA, Citino SB. 1992. Hematologic and serum chemistry reference intervals for Cuban mazon parrots (*Amazona leucocephala leucocephala*). *J Zoo Wildlife Med* 23:62–64.
[e]Cray C. 2000. Blood and chemistry tables. In: Olsen G, Orosz S (eds), *Manual of Avian Medicine*. St. Louis, MO: Mosby.
[f]Campbell TW. 2000. Normal hematology of waterfowl. In: Feldman B, Zinkl J, Jain M (eds), *Schalm's Veterinary Hematology*, 5th edn. Philadelphia, PA: Lippincott Williams & Wilkins.
[g]Polo FJ, Peinado VI, Viscor G, Palomeque J. 1998. Hematologic and plasma chemistry values in captive psittacine birds. *Avian Dis* 42:523–535.
[h]Spagnolo V, Crippa V, Marzia A, Alberti I, Sartorelli P. 2008. Hematologic, biochemical, and protein electrophoretic values in captive tawny owls (*Strix aluco*). *Vet Clin Pathol* 37:225–228.
[i]Naidoo V, Diekmann M, Wolters K, Swan GE. 2008. Establishment of selected baseline blood chemistry and hematologic parameters in captive and wild-caught African white-backed vultures (*Gyps africanaus*). *J Wild Dis* 44:649–654.

Table B.7 Erythrocyte parameters for selected reptiles.

	PCV (%)	RBC ($\times10^6/\mu L$)	Hb (g/dL)	MCV (fL)	MCHC (g/dL)
Lizards					
Argentine lizard[a] winter	24–28	0.8–1.1	10–14	252–300	36–48
Argentine lizard[a] summer	18–26	0.8–1.1	7–13	198–262	41–49
Adult male iguanas[b]	29–39	1.0–1.7	6.7–10.2	228–303	22.7–28.0
Adult female iguanas[b]	33–44	1.2–1.8	9.1–12.2	235–331	24.9–31.0
Juvenile iguanas[b]	30–47	1.3–1.6	9.2–10.1	–	–
Prehensile-tailed skink[c]	24–60	0.8–1.4	7.4–11.6	152–600	17–56
Adult male leopard gecko[d]	18–31	0.5–1.1	5.5–9.6	–	–
Bobtail lizard[e]	18–38	0.35–1.27	5.0–12.6	271–659	18–35
Snakes					
Boa constrictor[f,g]	24–40	1.0–2.5	3.3–15.3	159–625	21–42
Ball pythons[h]	16–21	0.3–1.3	5.5–7.9	211–540	25–40
Yellow rat snake[i]	9–46	0.2–1.6	2.8–15.2	179–961	26–54
Jungle carpet python[j]	23–37	0.5–1.3	4.0–15.5	178–414	23.5–53.2
Chelonians					
Aldabra tortoise[k]	11–34	0.13–0.77	3.8–10.5	195–742	21–42
Desert tortoise[l]	23–37	1.2–3.0	6.9–7.7	377–607	19–34

[a]Troiano JC, Gould EG, Gould I. 2008. Hematological reference intervals in argentine lizard *Tupinambis merianae* [Sauria-Teiidae]. *Comp Clin Pathol* 17:93–97.

[b]Harr KE, Alleman AR, Dennis PM, et al. 2001. Morphologic and cytochemical characteristics of blood cells and hematologic and plasma biochemical reference ranges in green iguanas. *J Am Vet Med Assoc* 218(6):915–921.

[c]Wright KM, Skeba S. 1992. Hematology and plasma chemistries of captive prehensile-tailed skinks (*Corcucia zebrata*). *J Zoo Wildl Med* 23:429–432.

[d]Knotkova Z, Morici M, Oliveri M, Knotek Z. 2019. Blood profile in captive adult male leopard geckos (*Eublepharis macularius*). *Vet Med* 64(4):172–177.

[e]Moller CA, Gaal T, Mills JN, 2016. The hematology of captive bobtail lizards (*Tiliqua rugosa*): blood counts, light microscopy, cytochemistry, and ultrastructure. *Vet Clin Pathol* 45(4):634–647.

[f]Chiodini RJ, Sundberg JP. 1982. Blood chemical values of the common boa constrictor (*Constrictor constrictor*). *Am J Vet Res* 43:1701–1702.

[g]Rosskopf WJ, Woerpel RW, Yanoff SR. 1982. Normal hemogram and blood chemistry values for boa constrictors and pythons. *Vet Med Small Anim Clin* May: 822–823.

[h]Johnson JH, Benson PA. 1996. Laboratory reference values for a group of captive ball pythons (*Python regius*). *Am J Vet Res* 57:1304–1307.

[i]Ramsey EC, Dotson TK. 1995. Tissue and serum enzyme activities in the yellow rat snake (*Elaphe obsolete quadrivitatta*). *Am J Vet Res* 56:423–428.

[j]Centini R, Klaphake E. 2002. Hematologic values and cytology in a population of captive jungle carpet pythons, *Morelia spilota cheynei*. *Proc Assoc Rept Amph Vet* 107–111.

[k]Carpenter JW. 2018. *Exotic Animal Formulary*, 5th edn. St. Louis, MO: Elsevier Saunders, p. 128.

[l]Gottdenker NL, Jacobson ER. 1995. Effect of venipuncture sites on hematologic and clinical biochemical values in desert tortoises (*Gopherus agassizii*). *Am J Vet Res* 56:19–21.

Table B.8 Summary of selected cytochemical staining reactions for normal leukocytes and thrombocytes in various reptiles.

Species/Cell	PER	SBB	CAE	AP	PAS	NSE	BG	TB	LAP
Giant Lizard[a]									
Heterophil	pos	–	neg	neg	±	pos	–	neg	–
Eosinophil	neg	–	pos	pos	neg	pos	–	pos	–
Basophil	neg	–	neg	neg	neg	pos	–	neg	–
Lymphocyte	neg	–	neg	±	neg	neg	–	neg	–
Monocyte	neg	–	neg	neg	neg	neg	–	neg	–
Azurophil	neg	–	±	pos	neg	pos	–	neg	–
Thrombocyte	–	–	–	–	–	–	–	–	–
Iguana[b]									
Heterophil	pos	pos	neg	pos	pos	pos	–	neg	neg
Eosinophil	neg	neg	neg	neg	neg	neg	–	neg	neg
Basophil	neg	neg	neg	neg	±	neg	–	neg	neg
Lymphocyte	neg	neg	neg	neg	neg	neg	–	neg	neg
Mono/Azuro	neg	neg	neg	pos	±	pos	–	neg	neg
Thrombocyte	neg	neg	neg	neg	pos	pos	–	neg	neg
Rainbow Lizard[c]									
Heterophil	±	pos	–	pos	pos	pos	–	–	pos
Eosinophil	±	neg	–	pos	pos	neg	–	–	pos
Basophil	neg	neg	–	neg	±	neg	–	–	pos
Lymphocyte	neg	neg	–	neg	neg	pos	–	–	neg
Mono/Azuro	±	±	–	pos	pos	neg	–	–	pos
Thrombocyte	pos	neg	–	neg	neg	pos	–	–	neg
Bobtail Lizard[d]									
Heterophil	pos	–	–	–	pos	–	–	neg	–
Eosinophil	neg	–	–	–	neg	–	–	neg	–
Basophil	neg	–	–	–	pos	–	–	pos	–
Lymphocyte	neg	–	–	–	neg	–	–	neg	–
Mono/Azuro	neg	–	–	–	±	–	–	pos	–
Thrombocyte	neg	–	–	–	pos	–	–	neg	–
Gila Monster[e]									
Heterophil	±	±	±	–	–	±	–	–	neg
Eosinophil	–	–	–	–	–	–	–	–	–
Basophil	neg	±	neg	–	–	neg	–	–	neg
Lymphocyte	neg	neg	±	–	–	neg	–	–	neg
Mono/Azuro	pos	pos	pos	–	–	pos	–	–	neg
Thrombocyte	neg	neg	neg	–	–	neg	–	–	neg
Asian Water Monitor[f]									
Heterophil	neg	pos	–	–	–	pos	pos	–	–
Eosinophil	–	–	–	–	–	–	–	–	–
Basophil	neg	pos	–	–	–	pos	pos	–	–
Lymphocyte	neg	neg	–	–	–	neg	neg	–	–
Monocyte	pos	neg	–	–	–	pos	neg	–	–
Azurophil	pos	neg				pos	neg		
Thrombocyte	neg	neg	–	–	–	pos	pos	–	–
King Cobra[g]									
Heterophil	–	pos	–	±	neg	pos	pos	–	–
Eosinophil	–	pos	–	–	–	–	±	–	–
Basophil	–	pos	–	neg	pos	pos	pos	–	–
Lymphocyte	–	neg	–	±	±	±	±	–	–
Mono/Azuro	–	pos	–	±	pos	pos	±	–	–
Thrombocyte	–	neg	–	±	pos	neg	±	–	–

Table B.8 (Continued)

Species/Cell	PER	SBB	CAE	AP	PAS	NSE	BG	TB	LAP
Rattle Snake[h]									
Heterophil	neg	neg	±	neg	±	±	–	neg	neg
Eosinophil	–	–	–	–	–	–	–	–	–
Basophil	neg	neg	neg	neg	pos	neg	–	neg	neg
Lymphocyte	neg	neg	neg	neg	neg	neg	–	neg	neg
Mono/Azuro	pos	pos	neg	neg	±	neg	–	neg	neg
Thrombocyte	neg	neg	neg	neg	±	±	–	neg	neg
Yellow Rat Snake[i]									
Heterophil	neg	–	–	neg	–	–	–	–	neg
Eosinophil	–	–	–	–	–	–	–	–	–
Basophil	–	–	–	–	–	–	–	–	–
Lymphocyte	–	–	–	pos	–	–	–	–	–
Mono/Azuro	pos	pos	pos	pos	pos	pos	–	–	neg
Thrombocyte	–	–	–	–	–	–	–	–	–
Green Turtle[j]									
Heterophil	neg	neg	neg	neg	pos	pos	–	neg	–
Eosinophil	neg	neg	pos	neg	±	±	–	neg	–
Basophil	neg	neg	neg	neg	neg	neg	–	pos	–
Lymphocyte	neg	neg	neg	neg	neg	neg	–	neg	–
Mono/Azuro	neg	neg	neg	pos	pos	neg	–	neg	–
Thrombocyte	neg	neg	neg	neg	pos	pos	–	neg	–
Asian Pond Turtle[k]									
Heterophil	±	–	–	–	neg	–	–	–	–
Eosinophil	pos	–	–	–	neg	–	–	–	–
Basophil	pos	–	–	–	neg	–	–	–	–
Lymphocyte	neg	–	–	–	neg	–	–	–	–
Mono/Azuro	neg	–	–	–	±	–	–	–	–
Thrombocyte	neg	–	–	–	pos	–	–	–	–
European Pond Turtle[l]									
Heterophil	neg	–	–	neg	pos	pos	–	neg	–
Eosinophil	neg	–	–	neg	neg	neg	–	neg	–
Basophil	neg	–	–	neg	neg	neg	–	pos	–
Lymphocyte	neg	–	–	neg	neg	neg	–	neg	–
Mono/Azuro	neg	–	–	±	neg	neg	–	neg	–
Thrombocyte	neg	–	–	neg	pos	neg	–	neg	–
Mediterranean Pond Turtle[l]									
Heterophil	neg	–	±	neg	pos	pos	–	neg	pos
Eosinophil	pos	–	±	neg	neg	pos	–	neg	pos
Basophil	neg	–	±	neg	neg	±	–	pos	±
Lymphocyte	neg	–	±	±	neg	neg	–	neg	neg
Mono/Azuro	neg	–	pos	pos	±	pos	–	neg	±
Thrombocyte	neg	–	neg	neg	pos	neg	–	neg	neg
Juvenile Loggerhead[m]						F/NF			
Heterophil	pos	pos	pos	pos	pos	neg/neg	–	neg	–
Eosinophil	neg	pos	pos	pos	pos	pos/neg	–	neg	–
Basophil	neg	neg	neg	neg	neg	neg/neg	–	pos	–
Lymphocyte	neg	neg	neg	neg	neg	neg/pos	–	neg	–
Mono/Azuro	neg	neg	neg	neg	neg	neg/pos	–	neg	–
Thrombocyte	neg	neg	neg	neg	pos	neg/neg	–	neg	–
Yellow-Bellied Slider[n]						F/NF			
Heterophil	pos	pos	pos	pos	pos	pos/pos	–	neg	–
Eosinophil	neg	pos	pos	pos	pos	neg/pos	–	neg	–

(Continued)

Table B.8 (Continued)

Species/Cell	PER	SBB	CAE	AP	PAS	NSE	BG	TB	LAP
Basophil	neg	neg	pos	pos	pos	pos/pos	–	pos	–
Lymphocyte	neg	neg	pos	pos	pos	pos/pos	–	neg	–
Mono/Azuro	neg	neg	pos	pos	pos	neg/pos	–	neg	–
Thrombocyte	neg	neg	neg	neg	pos	pos/pos	–	neg	–
Desert Tortoise[o]									
Heterophil	neg	neg	pos	pos	neg	pos	–	neg	±
Eosinophil	pos	neg	pos	neg	neg	neg	–	neg	neg
Basophil	neg	neg	neg	neg	neg	neg	–	pos	neg
Lymphocyte	neg	neg	neg	neg	neg	neg	–	neg	neg
Mono/Azuro	neg	neg	±	pos	neg	pos	–	neg	neg
Thrombocyte	–	–	–	–	–	–	–	–	–
American Alligator[p]									
Heterophil	neg	–	neg	pos	pos	pos	–	–	pos
Eosinophil	pos	–	neg	neg	pos	neg	–	–	pos
Basophil	neg	–	neg	pos	pos	neg	–	pos	neg
Lymphocyte	neg	–	pos	neg	pos	neg	–	–	neg
Mono/Azuro	neg	–	pos	pos	pos	pos	–	–	pos
Thrombocyte	neg	–	neg	neg	pos	neg	–	–	neg
Chinese Alligator[q]									
Heterophil	pos	pos	pos	pos	±	pos	–	–	pos
Eosinophil	pos	±	pos	pos	pos	±	–	–	pos
Basophil	pos	neg	±	pos	pos	pos	–	–	pos
Lymphocyte	neg	neg	neg	neg	±	±	–	–	neg
Mono/Azuro	neg	neg	neg	±	±	±	–	–	±
Thrombocyte	neg	neg	neg	neg	±	neg	–	–	neg

PER, peroxidase; SBB, Sudan black B; CAE, chloroacetate esterase; AP, acid phosphatase; PAS, periodic acid-Schiff; NSE, nonspecific esterase (alpha naphthyl butyrate esterase), BG, beta glucuronidase; TB, toluidine blue; LAP, leukocyte alkaline phosphatase; F/NF, with sodium fluoride/without sodium fluoride; mono/azuro, monocyte/azurophil; neg, no reaction; pos, easily detectable; ±, weak, focal, or occasional reactive; –, undetermined.

[a]Martínez-Silvestre A, Marco I, Rodriguez-Dominguez MA, Lavín S, Cuenca R. 2005. Morphology, cytochemical staining, and ultrastructural characteristics of the blood cells of the giant lizard of El Hierro (*Gallotia simonyi*), Res Vet Sci, 78(2):127–34.

[b]Harr KE, Alleman AR, Dennis PM, et al, 2001. Morphologic and cytochemical characteristics of blood cells and hematologic and plasma biochemical reference ranges in green iguanas. *J Am Vet Med Assoc* 218:915–921.

[c]Caxton-Martins AE, Nganwuchu AM. 1978. A cytochemical study of the blood of the rainbow lizard (*Agama agama*). *J Anat* 125(3):477–480.

[d]Moller CA, Gaal T, Mills JN. 2016. The hematology of captive bobtail lizards (*Tiliqua rugosa*): blood counts, light microscopy, cytochemistry, and ultrastructure. *Vet Clin Pathol* 45(4):634–647.

[e]Cooper-Bailey K, Smith SA, Zimmerman K, et al. 2011. Hematology, leukocyte cytochemical analysis, plasma biochemistry, and plasma electrophoresis of wild-caught and captive-bred Gila monsters (*Heloderma suspectum*). *Vet Clin Pathol* 40(3):316–323.

[f]Salakij C, Salakij J, Prihirunkit K, et al. 2014. Quantitative and qualitative morphologic, cytochemical, and ultrastructural characteristics of blood cells in captive Asian water monitors. *Vet Clin Pathol* 43(4):538–546.

[g]Salakij C, Salakij J, Apibal S, et al. 2002. Hematology, morphology, cytochemical staining, and ultrastructural characteristics of blood cells in king cobras (*Ophiophagus hannah*). *Vet Clin Pathol* 31:116–126.

[h]Alleman AR, Jacobson ER, Raskin RE. 1999. Morphological, cytochemical staining, and ultrastructural characteristics of blood cells from eastern diamondback rattlesnakes (*Crotalus adamaneus*). *Am J Vet Res* 60:507–514.

[i]Bounous DI, Dotson TK, Brooks RJ, et al. 1996. Cytochemical staining and ultrastructural characteristics of peripheral blood leukocytes from the yellow rat snake (*Elaphe obsoleta quadrivitatta*). *Comp Haematol Int* 6:86–91.

[j]Work TM, Raskin RE, Balazs GH, et al. 1998. Morphologic and cytochemical characteristics of blood cells from Hawaiian green turtles. *Am J Vet Res* 59:1252–1257.

[k]Chung CS, Cheng CH, Chin SC, Lee AH, Chi CH. 2009. Morphologic and cytochemical characteristics of Asian yellow pond turtle (*Ocadia sinensis*) blood cells and their hematologic and plasma biochemical reference values. *J Zoo Wildl Med* 40(1):76–85.

[l]Perpinan D, Sanchez C. 2009. Morphologic and cytochemical characteristics of blood cells from European pond turtle (Emys orbicularis) and the Mediterranean pond turtle (Mauremys leprosa). *J Herpetol Med and Surg* 19(4):119–127.

[m]Casal AB, Oros J. 2007. Morphologic and cytochemical characteristics of blood cells of juvenile loggerhead sea turtles (*Caretta caretta*). *Res Vet Sci* 82:158–165.

[n]Hernandez JD, Castro P, Saavedra P, Ramirez R, Oros J. 2017. Morphologic and cytochemic characteristics of the blood cells of the yellow-bellied slider (*Trachemys scripta scripta*), *Anat Histol Embryol* 46:446–455.

[o]Alleman AR, Jacobson ER, Raskin RE. 1992. Morphologic and cytochemical characteristics of blood cells from the desert tortoise (*Gopherus agassizii*). *Am J Vet Res* 53:1645–165.

[p]Mateo MR, Roberts ED, Enright FM. 1984. Morphologic, cytochemical, and functional studies of peripheral blood cells of young healthy American alligators (*Alligator mississippiensis*). *Am J Vet Res* 45:1046–1053.

[q]Chen X, Wei Q, Wang J, et al. 2018. Cytochemical patterns of the peripheral blood cells in Chinese alligator (*Alligator sinensis*). *Tissue and Cell* 55:71–76.

Table B.9a Leukocyte parameters for selected reptiles.

	WBC (×10³/μL)	Heterophils (×10³/μL)	Lymphocytes (×10³/μL)	Monocytes (×10³/μL)	Eosinophils (×10³/μL)	Basophils (×10³/μL)
Lizards						
Argentine lizard[a] winter	13.1–18.1	1.5–2.2	6.7–7.7	1.8–3.0	3.4–4.4	0.2–0.4
Argentine lizard[a] summer	16.0–20.8	1.9–2.9	7.8–8.5	1.6–2.6	3.8–5.0	0.3–0.5
Adult male iguanas[b]	11.1–24.6	1.0–5.4	5.0–16.5	0.2–2.7	0.0–0.3	0.1–1.0
Adult female iguanas[b]	8.2–25.2	0.6–6.4	5.2–14.4	0.4–2.3	0.0–0.4	0.2–1.2
Juvenile iguanas[b]	8.0–22.0	1.0–3.8	6.2–17.2	0.3–0.6	0.0–0.4	0.1–0.7

Table B.9b Leukocyte parameters for selected reptiles.

	WBC (×10³/μL)	Heterophils (%)	Lymphocytes (%)	Monocytes (%)	Eosinophils (%)	Basophils (%)
Lizards						
Prehensile-tailed skink[c]	3.9–22.4	16–58	2–40	0–6	0–18	4–26
Snakes						
Boa constrictor[d,e]	4–10	20–65	10–60	0–6	0–3	0–20
Ball pythons[f]	7.9–16.4	56–67	7–21	12–22	–	0–2
Yellow rat snake[g]	0.4–32.0	–	–	–	–	–
Jungle carpet python[h]						
Chelonians						
Aldabra tortoise[i]	1.0–8.3	32–79	2–40	0–8	0–7	0–4
Desert tortoise[j]	6.6–8.9	35–60	25–50	0–4	0–4	2–15

[a]Troiano JC, Gould EG, Gould I. 2008. Hematological reference intervals in argentine lizard *Tupinambis merianae* [Sauria-Teiidae]. *Comp Clin Pathol* 17:93–97.
[b]Harr KE, Alleman AR, Dennis PM, et al. 2001. Morphologic and cytochemical characteristics of blood cells and hematologic and plasma biochemical reference ranges in green iguanas. *J Am Vet Med Assoc* 218(6):915–921.
[c]Wright KM, Skeba S. 1992. Hematology and plasma chemistries of captive prehensile-tailed skinks (*Corcucia zebrata*). *J Zoo Wildl Med* 23:429–432.
[d]Chiodini RJ, Sundberg JP. 1982. Blood chemical values of the common boa constrictor (*Constrictor constrictor*). *Am J Vet Res* 43:1701–1702.
[e]Rosskopf WJ, Woerpel RW, Yanoff SR. 1982. Normal hemogram and blood chemistry values for boa constrictors and pythons. *Vet Med Small Anim Clin* May: 822–823.
[f]Johnson JH, Benson PA. 1996. Laboratory reference values for a group of captive ball pythons (*Python regius*). *Am J Vet Res* 57:1304–1307.
[g]Ramsey EC, Dotson TK. 1995. Tissue and serum enzyme activities in the yellow rat snake (*Elaphe obsolete quadrivitatta*). *Am J Vet Res* 56:423–428.
[h]Centini R, Klaphake E. 2002. Hematologic values and cytology in a population of captive jungle carpet pythons, *Morelia spilota cheynei*. *Proc Assoc Rept Amph Vet* 107–111.
[i]Carpenter JW. 2001. *Exotic Animal Formulary*, 3rd edn. St. Louis, MO: Elsevier Saunders, p. 107.
[j]Gottdenker NL, Jacobson ER. 1995. Effect of venipuncture sites on hematologic and clinical biochemical values in desert tortoises (*Gopherus agassizii*). *Am J Vet Res* 56:19–21.

Table B.10 Erythrocyte parameters for selected amphibians.

	PCV (%)	RBC (×10⁶/μL)	Hb (g/dL)	MCV (fL)	MCHC (g/dL)
American bullfrog[a,b]	39–42	0.450	9.3–9.7	–	21.1–25.9
Australian common green tree frog[c]	34–40.8	0.63–0.82	6.1–8.2	374–486	23.6–26.8
Australian white-lipped tree frog[c]	26–34	0.63–0.82	6.1–8.2	374–486	21–25
Cuban tree frog[a]	20–24	–	5.6–6.8	–	25–31
Fire-bellied toad (male)[d]	14–26	0.190–0.465	5.0–12.2	412–758	29–55
Fire-bellied toad (female)[d]	12–23	0.240–0.355	3.4–8.3	363–917	19–60
Leopard frog (male)[a]	19–52	0.227–0.767	3.8–14.6	722–916	23–27
Leopard frog (female)[a]	16–51	0.174–0.701	2.7–14.0	730–916	20–28
Mudpuppy[e]	21	0.020	4.6	10 070	22
Tiger salamander[a]	40	1.66	9.4	–	–

[a]Whitaker BR, McDermott CT. 2018. Amphibians. In: Carpenter J (ed), *Exotic Animal Formulary*, 5th edn. St. Louis, MO: Elsevier Saunders, p. 68.
[b]Cathers T, Lewbart GA, Correa M, Stevens JB. 1997. Serum chemistry and hematology values for anesthetized American bull frogs [*Rana catesbeiana*]. *J Zoo Wildl Med* 28:171–174.
[c]Young S, Warner J, Speare R, et al. 2012. Hematologic and plasma biochemical reference intervals for health monitoring of wild Australian tree frogs. *Vet Clin Pathol* 41(4):478–492.
[d]Wojtaszek J, Adamowicz A. 2003. Haematology of the fire-bellied toad, *Bombina bombina* L. *Comp Clin Pathol* 12:129–134.
[e]Wright KM. 2005. Amphibians. In: Carpenter J (ed), *Exotic Animal Formulary*, 3rd edn. St. Louis, MO: Elsevier Saunders, p. 46.

Table B.11 Erythrocyte parameters for selected teleost fish.

	PCV (%)	RBC (× 10^6/μL)	Hb (g/dL)	MCV (fL)	MCHC (g/dL)
Bass, hybrid[a]	23–47	3.66–4.96	8–12	81–106	22–30
Channel catfish[b]	40	2.44	–	–	–
Flounder[c]	17–26	1.7–2.6	4.2–6.0	90–126	–
Goldfish[d]	38–40	1.6–1.8	9.7–10.6	241–245	26
Red pacu[e]	25	1.68	–	–	–
Tilapia[f]	27–37	1.91–2.83	7.0–9.8	115–183	22–29
Trout[g]	21–44	0.77–1.67	1.5–7.7	192–420	14.4–70.0

[a]Hrubec TC, Smith SA, Robertson JL, et al. 1996. Comparison of hematologic reference intervals between cultured system and type of hybrid striped bass. *Am J Vet Res* 57:618–623.
[b]Grizzle JM, Rogers WA. 1976. *Anatomy and Histology of the Channel Catfish*. Opelika, AL: Craftmaster Printers, p. 18.
[c]Bridges DW, Cech JJ Jr, Pedro DN. 1976. Seasonal hematological changes in winter flounder. *Pseudopleuronectes americanus. Trans Am Fish Soc* 105:596–600.
[d]Burton CB, Murray SA. 1979. Effects of density on goldfish blood: I, hematology. *Comp Biochem Physiol* 62A:555–558.
[e]Tocidlowski ME, Lewbart GA, Stoskopf MK. 1997. Hematologic study of the red pacu [*Colossoma brachypornum*]. *Vet Clin Pathol* 26:119–125.
[f]Hrubec TC, Cardinale JL, Smith SA. 2000. Hematology and plasma chemistry reference intervals for cultured Tilapia [*Oreochromis hybrid*]. *Vet Clin Pathol* 29:7–12.
[g]Miller WR, Hendricks AC, Cairns J. 1983. Normal ranges for diagnostically important hematological and blood chemistry characteristics of rainbow trout [*Salmo gairdneri*]. *Can J Fish Aquat Sci* 40:420–425.

Table B.12 Leukocyte parameters for selected teleost fish.

	WBC (×10^3/μL)	Neut/Heterophils (×10^3/μL)	Lymphocytes (×10^3/μL)	Monocytes (×10^3/μL)	Eosinophils (×10^3/μL)	Basophils (×10^3/μL)
Bass, hybrid[a]	32.6–115.1	0.4–3.5	22.5–115.1	1.5–7.5	0–0.4	0
Channel catfish[b]	8.9–124.0	4.5–86.8	1.4–23.6	0.7–14.7	0	0–7.1
Flounder[c]	88.0–282.0	2.5–26.6	38.7–154.5	–	–	–
Goldfish[d]	10.1–14.7	–	9.5–13.7	–	–	–
Red pacu[e]	33.5	3.2	21.0	1.2	0.2	0
Tilapia[f]	21.6–154.7	0.6–9.9	6.8–136.4	0.4–4.3	0–1.6	0
Trout[g]	21.0	1.6	18.8	0.6	0	0

[a]Hrubec TC, Smith SA, Robertson JL, et al. 1996. Comparison of hematologic reference intervals between cultured system and type of hybrid striped bass. *Am J Vet Res* 57:618–623.
[b]Tavares-Dias M, de Moraes FR. 2007. Leukocyte and thrombocyte reference values for channel catfish [*Ictalurus punctatus* Raf], with an assessment of morphologic, cytochemical, and ultrastructural features. *Vet Clin Pathol* 36:49–54.
[c]Bridges DW, Cech JJ Jr, Pedro DN. 1976. Seasonal hematological changes in winter flounder. *Pseudopleuronectes americanus. Trans Am Fish Soc* 105:596–600.
[d]Murray SA, Burton CB. 1979. Effects of density on goldfish blood: II, cell morphology. *Comp Biochem Physiol* 62A:559–562.
[e]Tocidlowski ME, Lewbart GA, Stoskopf MK. 1997. Hematologic study of the red pacu [*Colossoma brachypornum*]. *Vet Clin Pathol* 26:119–125.
[f]Hrubec TC, Cardinale JL, Smith SA. 2000. Hematology and plasma chemistry reference intervals for cultured Tilapia [*Oreochromis hybrid*]. *Vet Clin Pathol* 29:7–12.
[g]Hunn JB, Wiedmeyer RH, Greer IE, Grady AW. 1992. Blood chemistry of laboratory-reared golden trout. *J Aquat Anim Health* 4:218–221.

Erythrocyte parameters (Table B.13) and Leukocyte parameters (Table B.14) for selected elasmobranchs can be found on the companion website.

APPENDIX C

Plate Captions

Mammal Plates

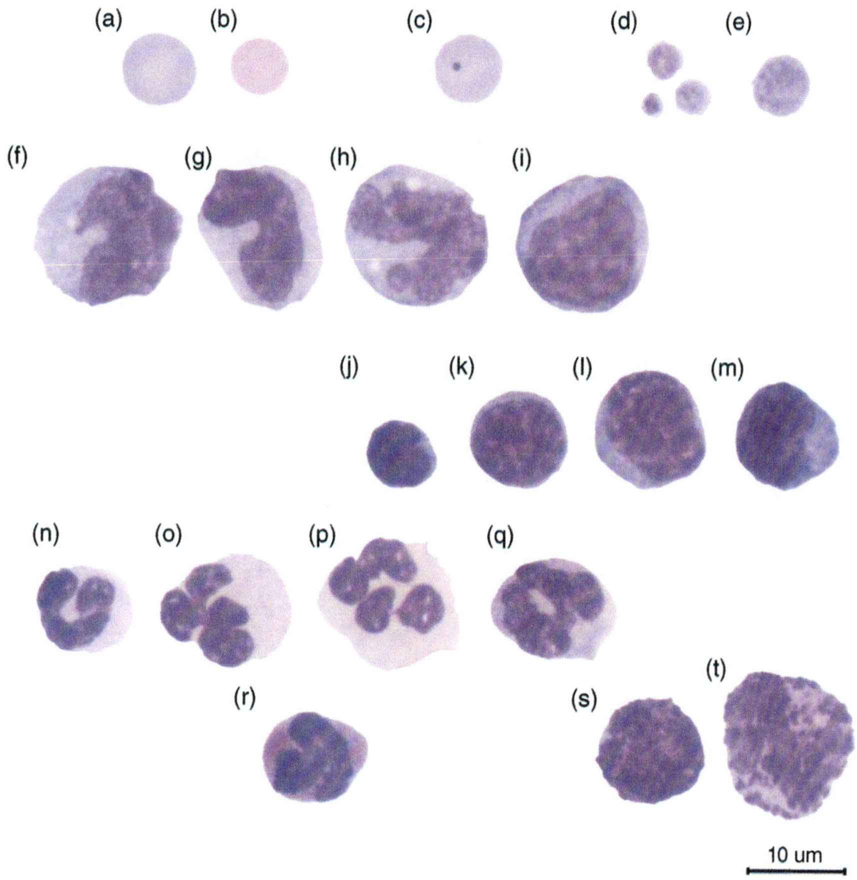

Plate. C.01. Ferret (*Mustela putorius furo*) Erythrocytes: (a) polychromatic erythrocyte, (b) mature erythrocyte, (c) erythrocyte with Howell–Jolly body Platelets: (d) platelet cluster, (e) giant platelet Mononuclear cells: (f) monocyte, (g) monocyte, (h) vacuolated (reactive) monocyte, (i) monocyte, (j) small lymphocyte, (k) medium lymphocyte, (l) large lymphocyte, (m) plasma cell Granulocytes: (n) band neutrophil, (o) neutrophil, (p) neutrophil, (q) toxic neutrophil, (r) eosinophil, (s) basophil, (t) basophil (either partially degranulated or some granules have failed to stain)

Exotic Animal Hematology and Cytology, Fifth Edition. Terry W. Campbell and Krystan R. Grant.

Companion website: www.wiley.com/go/campbell/exotic

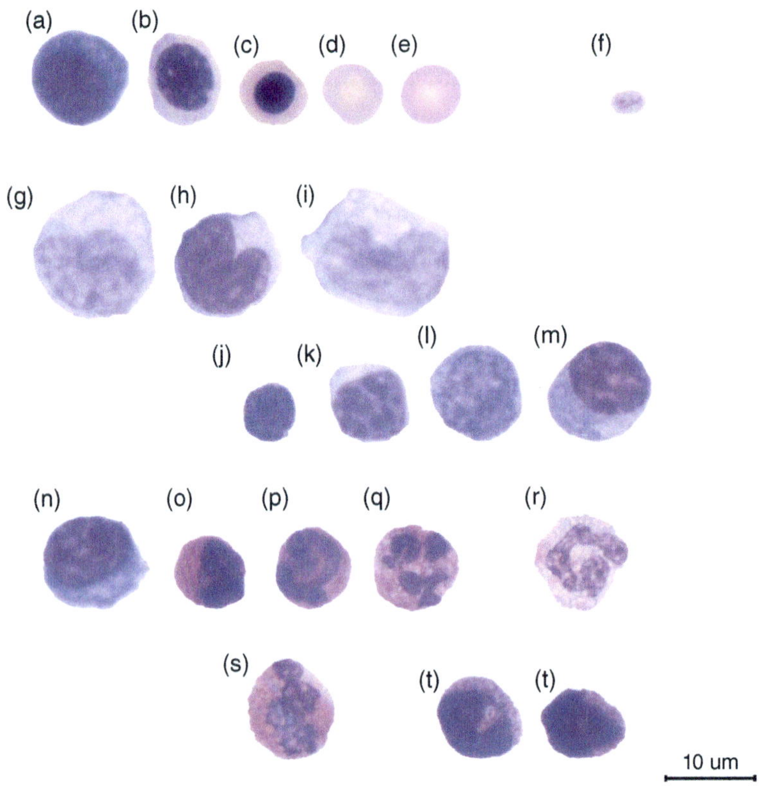

Plate. C.02. Rabbit (*Oryctolagus cuniculus*) Erythrocytes: (a) prorubricyte, (b) rubricyte, (c) metarubricyte, (d) polychromatophilic erythrocyte, (e) mature erythrocyte Platelets: (f) Platelet Mononuclear cells: (g) monocyte, (h) monocyte, (i) monocyte (reactive), (j) small lymphocyte, (k) medium lymphocyte, (l) large lymphocyte, (m) plasma cell Granulocytes: (n) myeloblast, (o) metamyelocyte, (p) band heterophil, (q) mature heterophil, (r) toxic heterophil, (s) eosinophil, (t) basophil

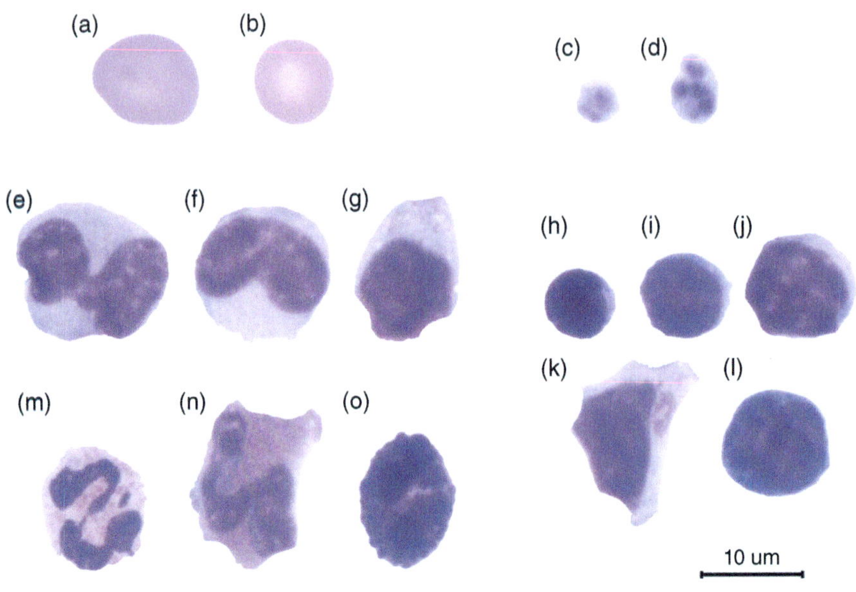

Plate. C.03. Guinea Pig (*Cavia porcellus*) Erythrocytes: (a) polychromatic erythrocyte, (b) mature erythrocyte Platelets: (c) platelet, (d) clumped platelets Mononuclear cells: (e) monocyte, (f) monocyte, (g) monocyte with azurophilic granules, (h) small lymphocyte, (i) medium lymphocyte, (j) large lymphocyte, (k) lymphocyte with Kurloff body, (l) reactive lymphocyte Granulocytes: (m) heterophil, (n) eosinophil, (o) basophil

Avian Plates

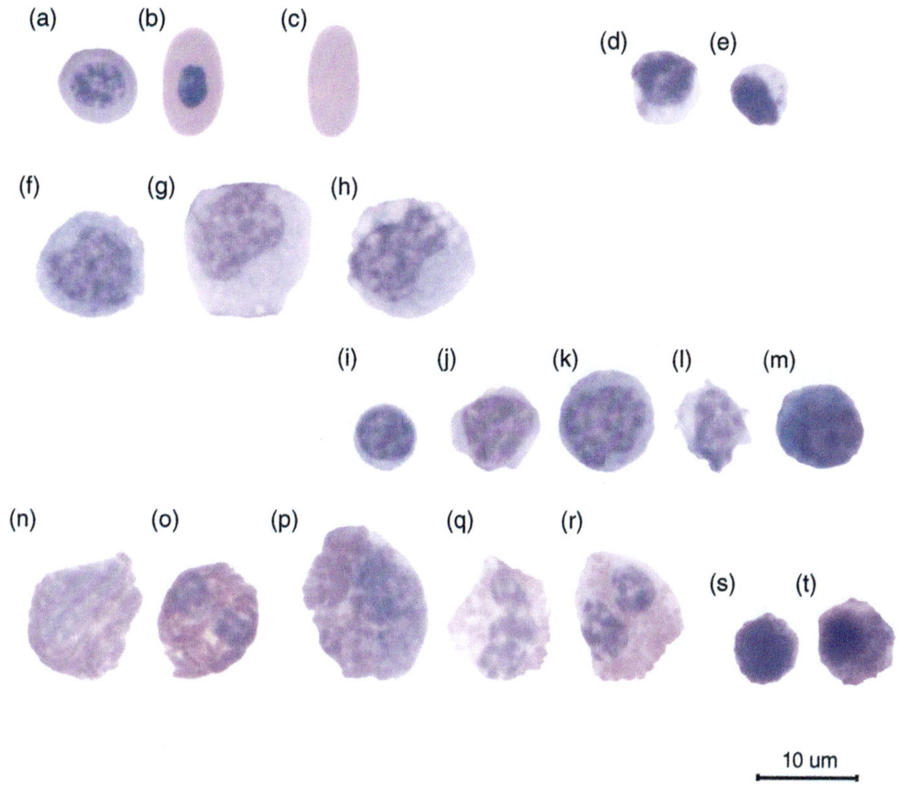

Plate. C.04. Chicken (*Gallus gallus domesticus*) Erythrocytes: (a) late polychromatic rubricyte, (b) mature erythrocyte, (c) erythroplastid Thrombocytes: (d) thrombocyte (note granule at one pole of the cell), (e) reactive thrombocyte (with fine eosinophilic granules) Mononuclear cells: (f) monocyte, (g) monocyte (with fine azurophilic granules), (h) vacuolated monocyte (reactive), (i) small lymphocyte, (j) medium lymphocyte, (k) large lymphocyte, (l) degenerating lymphocyte, (m) reactive lymphocyte Granulocytes: (n) heterophil band, (o) mature heterophil, (p) eosinophil myelocyte, (q) eosinophil band, (r) mature eosinophil, (s) basophil, (t) basophil (degranulating or partial staining)

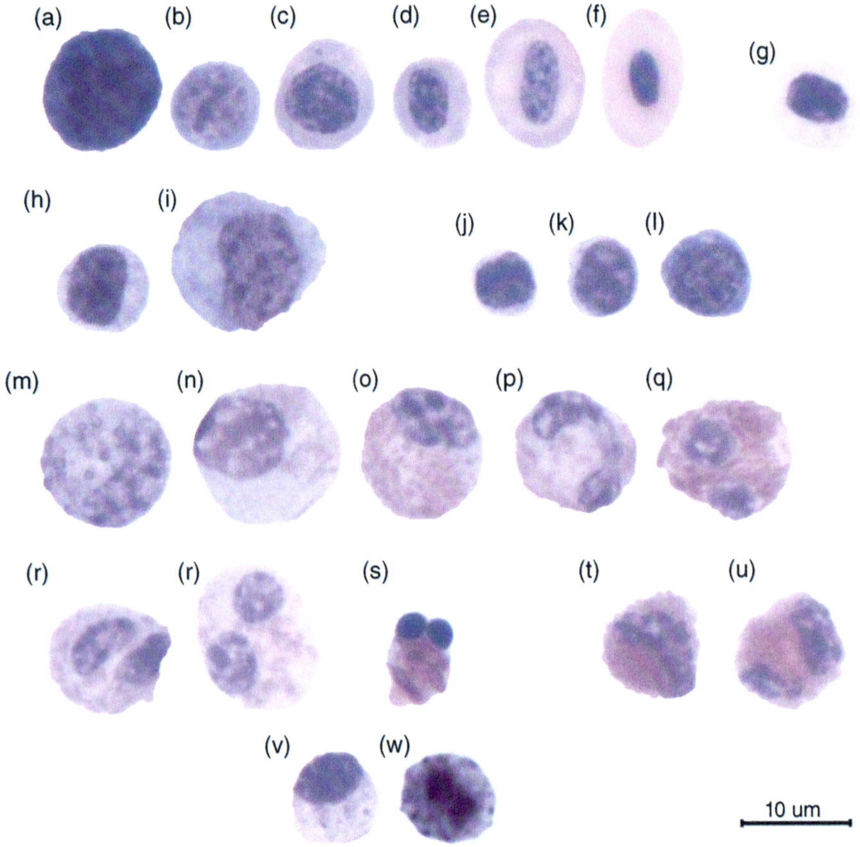

Plate. C.05. Ferruginous Hawk (*Buteo regalis*) Erythrocytes: (a) prorubricyte, (b) early polychromatic rubricyte, (c) mid polychromatic rubricyte, (d) late polychromatic rubricyte, (e) polychromatic erythrocyte, (f) mature erythrocyte Thrombocytes: (g) mature thrombocyte Mononuclear cells: (h) small monocyte, (i) large monocyte, (j) small lymphocyte, (k) medium lymphocyte, (l) reactive lymphocyte Granulocytes: (m) heterophil promyelocyte, (n) heterophil myelocyte, (o) heterophil metamyelocyte, (p) heterophil band, (q) mature segmented heterophil, (r) mild heterophil toxicity, (s) pyknotic nuclei, (t) eosinophil band, (u) mature segmented eosinophil, (v) basophil, (w) basophil (granules are poorly stained)

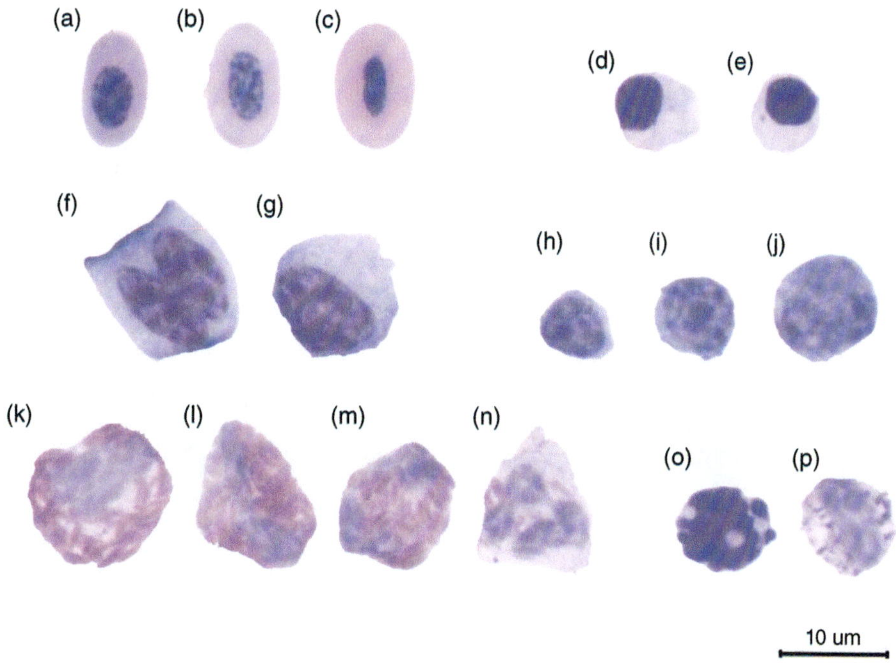

Plate. C.06. Macaw spp. (*Ara* spp.) Erythrocytes: (a) polychromatic erythrocyte, (b) polychromatic erythrocyte, (c) mature erythrocyte Thrombocytes: (d) late immature thrombocyte, (e) mature thrombocyte (note granule at one pole of the cell) Mononuclear cells: (f) monocyte, (g) monocyte (with fine azurophilic granules), (h) small lymphocyte, (i) medium lymphocyte, (j) large lymphocyte Granulocytes: (k) heterophil metamyelocyte, (l) heterophil band, (m) mature segmented heterophil, (n) toxic heterophil (degranulation, blue cytoplasm), (o) basophil, (p) basophil (degranulating or partially stained)

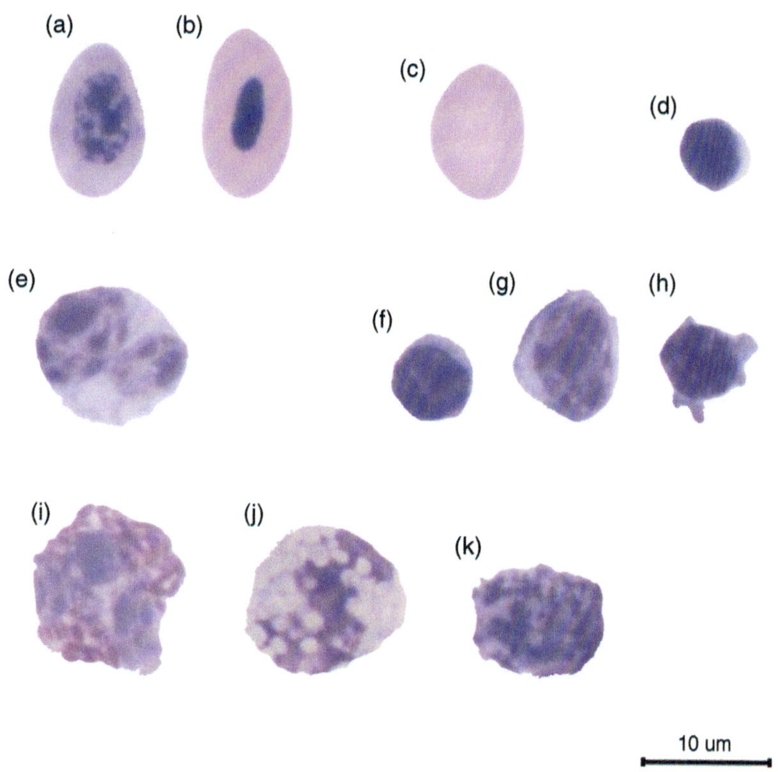

Plate. C.07. Blue-headed Pionus Parrot (*Pionus menstruus*) Erythrocytes: (a) polychromatic erythrocyte, (b) mature erythrocyte, (c) erythroplastid Thrombocytes: (d) thrombocyte Mononuclear cells: (e) monocyte, (f) small lymphocyte, (g) large lymphocyte, (h) degenerating lymphocyte Granulocytes: (i) mature segmented heterophil, (j) eosinophil, (k) basophil

Herptile Plates

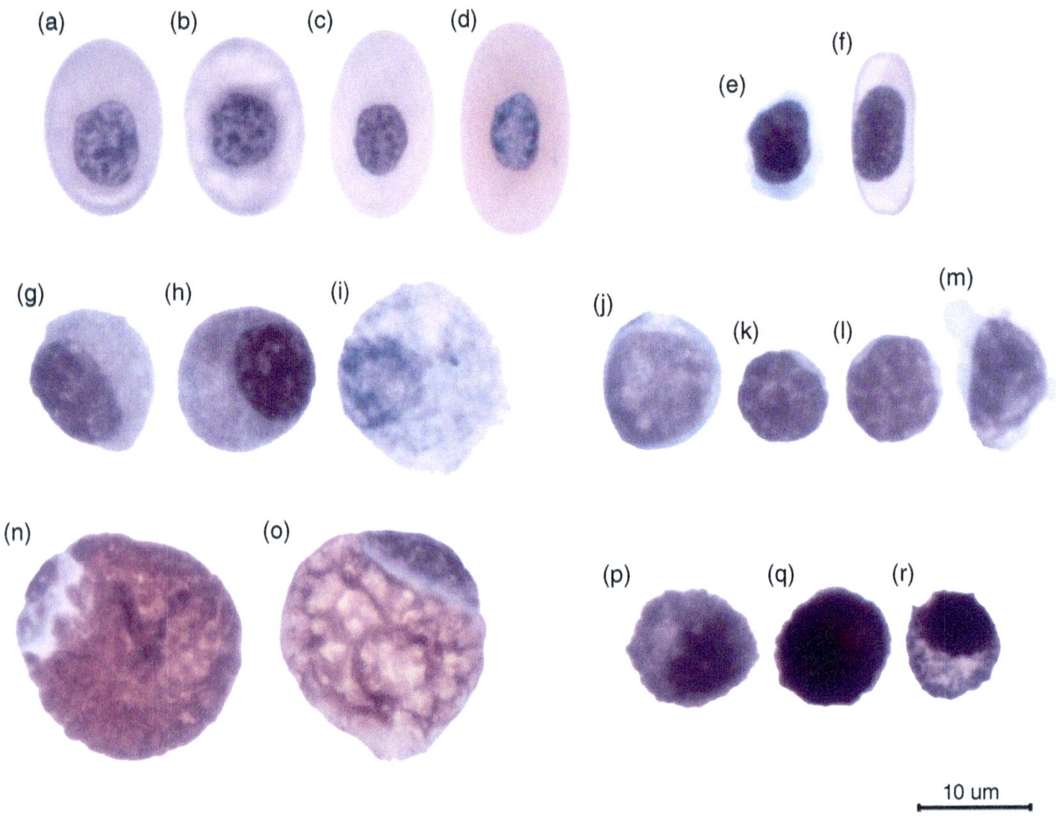

Plate. C.08. California King Snake (*Lampropeltis getula californiae*) Erythrocytes: (a) polychromatic erythrocyte, (b) polychromatic erythrocyte, (c) polychromatic erythrocyte, (d) mature erythrocyte Thrombocytes: (e) immature thrombocyte, (f) mature thrombocyte Mononuclear cells: (g) monocyte, (h) azurophilic monocyte/azurophil, (i) vacuolated monocyte (reactive), (j) lymphoblast, (k) small lymphocyte, (l) large lymphocyte, (m) degenerate lymphocyte Granulocytes: (n) heterophil, (o) heterophil with staining artifact (common presentation), (p) basophil, (q) basophil with densely packed granules, (r) basophil (degranulating or partially stained)

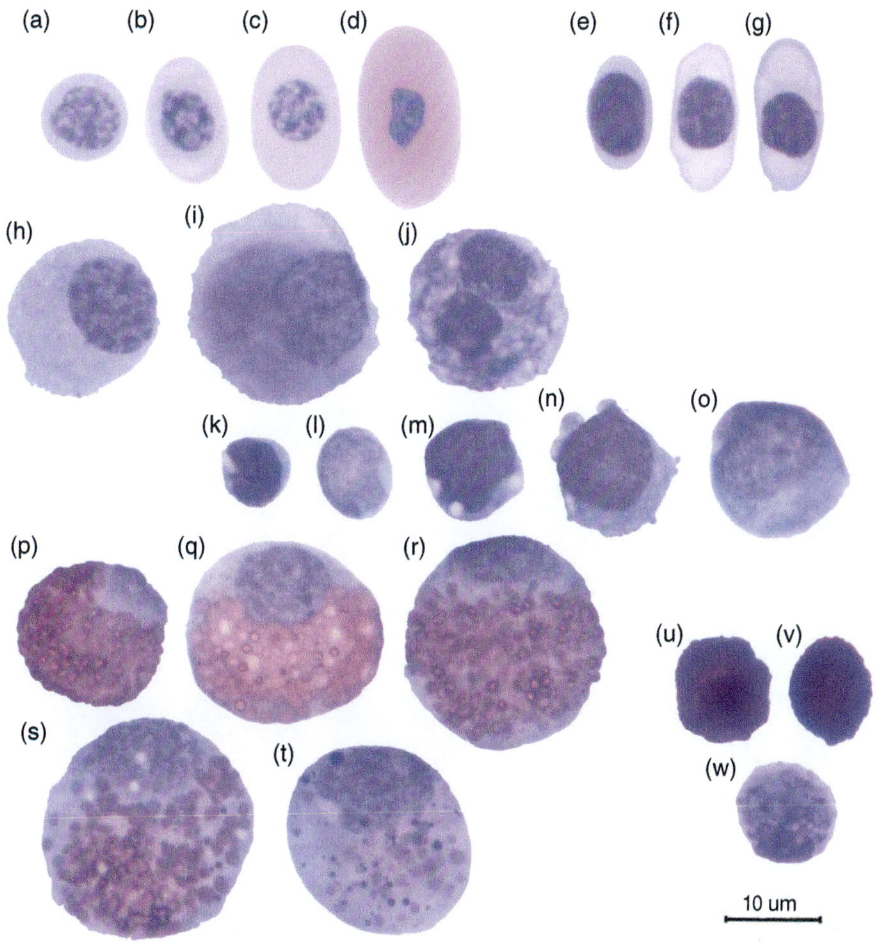

Plate. C.09. Common Boa (*Boa constrictor*) Erythrocytes: (a) mid-polychromatic rubricyte, (b) polychromatic erythrocyte, (c) polychromatic erythrocyte, (d) mature erythrocyte Thrombocytes: (e) immature thrombocyte, (f) mature thrombocyte, (g) mature thrombocyte (reticulated cytoplasm suggestive of becoming reactive) Mononuclear cells: (h) mature monocyte, (i) vacuolated azurophilic monocyte/ azurophil, (j) vacuolated azurophilic monocyte/azurophil (reactive), (k) small lymphocyte, (l) medium lymphocyte, (m) large lymphocyte (Mott cell variant), (n) degenerate lymphocyte, (o) plasma cell Granulocytes: (p) heterophil, (q) heterophil with mild toxic changes (1+; partial degranulation, and basophilic cytoplasm), (r) heterophil with moderate toxic changes (2+; partial degranulation, basophilic cytoplasm, and a few primary granules), (s) heterophil with moderate toxic change (3+; degranulation, basophilic cytoplasm, and presence of primary granules), (t) heterophil with marked toxic change (4+; moderate degranulation, and presence of primary granules), (u) basophil, (v) basophil with densely packed granules, (w) basophil (degranulating or partial stained granules)

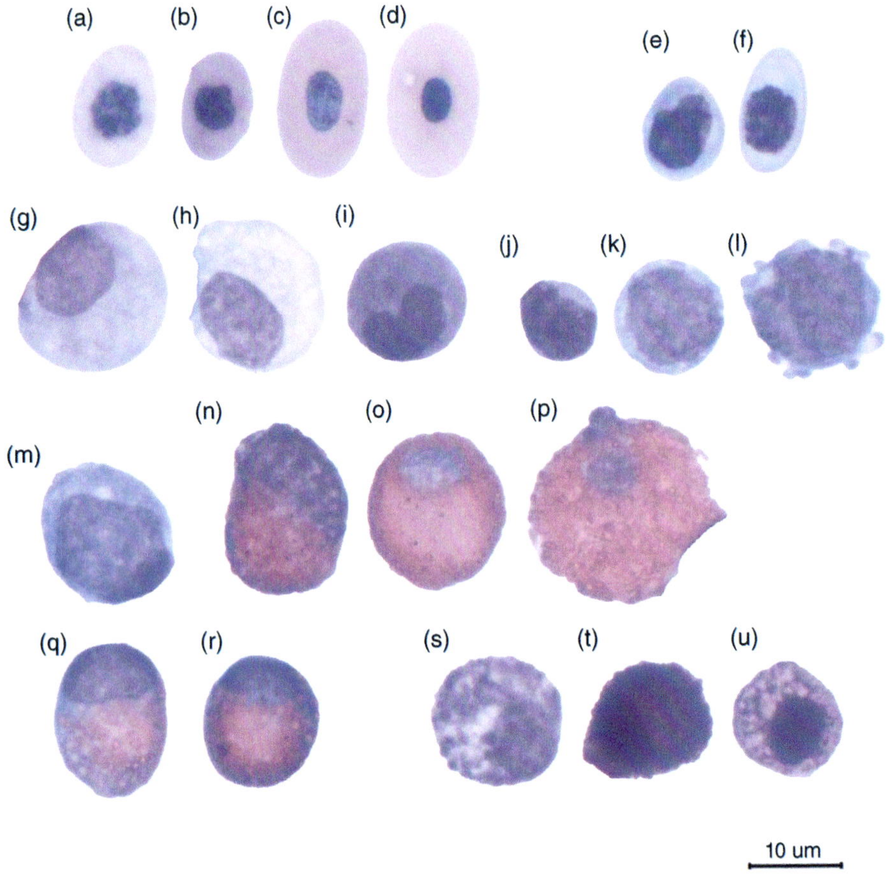

Plate. C.10. Jungle Carpet Python (*Morelia spilota cheynei*) Erythrocytes: (a) polychromatic erythrocyte, (b) mature erythrocyte, (c) mature erythrocyte, (d) mature erythrocyte (with cytoplasmic artifact and not an inclusion body) Thrombocytes: (e) immature thrombocyte, (f) mature thrombocyte Mononuclear cells: (g) monocyte, (h) vacuolated monocyte, (i) azurophilic monocyte/azurophil, (j) small lymphocyte, (k) large lymphocyte, (l) degenerate lymphocyte Granulocytes: (m) myeloblast, (n) heterophil myelocyte, (o) mature heterophil, (p) mature heterophil, (q) eosinophil, (r) eosinophil, (s) basophil, (t) basophil, (u) basophil (degranulating or partial stained granules)

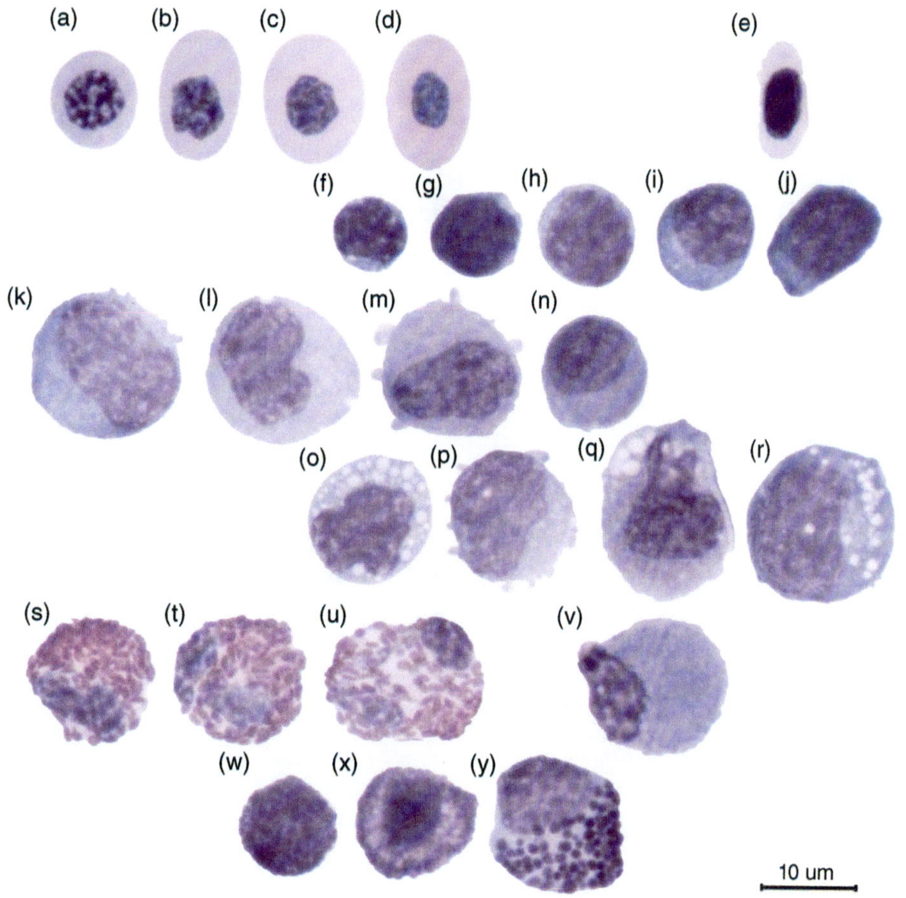

Plate. C.11. Green Iguana (*Iguana iguana*) Erythrocytes: (a) mid-polychromatic rubricyte, (b) polychromatic erythrocyte, (c) mature erythrocyte, (d) mature erythrocyte Thrombocytes: (e) mature thrombocyte Mononuclear cells: (f) small lymphocyte, (g) medium lymphocyte, (h) large lymphocyte, (i) plasma cell, (j) reactive lymphocyte, (k) monocyte with round to oval nucleus, (l) monocyte with indented nucleus, (m) monocyte with cytoplasmic pseudopodia, (n) azurophilic monocyte, (o) reactive monocyte (vacuoles), (p) monocyte with vacuolization and pseudopodia, (q) azurophilic monocyte with vacuolization (reactive), (r) monocyte with vacuolization (reactive) Granulocytes: (s) heterophil with nonlobed nucleus, (t) mature heterophil with lobed/segmented nucleus, (u) heterophil with dispersed granules, (v) eosinophil with round to oval nucleus and blue cytoplasmic granules, (w) mature basophil with densely packed granules, (x) basophil with dispersed granules, (y) basophil (degranulating or partial stained granules)

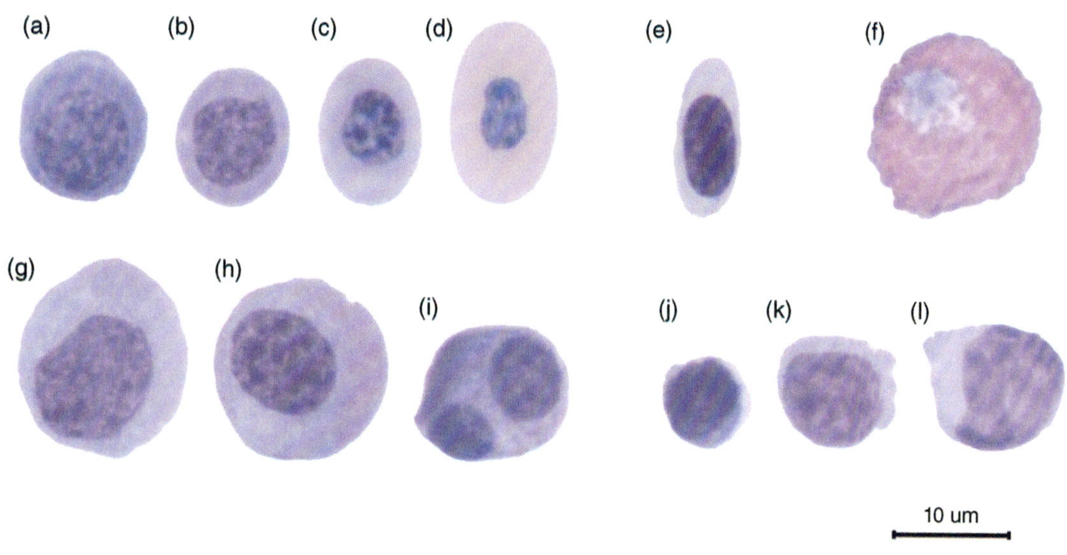

Plate. C.12. Savannah Monitor (*Varanus exanthematicus*) Erythrocytes: (a) basophilic polychromatic rubricyte, (b) mid-polychromatic rubricyte, (c) polychromatic erythrocyte, (d) mature erythrocyte Thrombocytes: (e) mature thrombocyte Granulocytes: (f) mature heterophil Mononuclear cells: (g) monocyte, (h) azurophilic monocyte/azurophil, (i) azurophilic monocyte/azurophil with bilobed nucleus, (j) small lymphocyte, (k) medium lymphocyte, (l) large lymphocyte

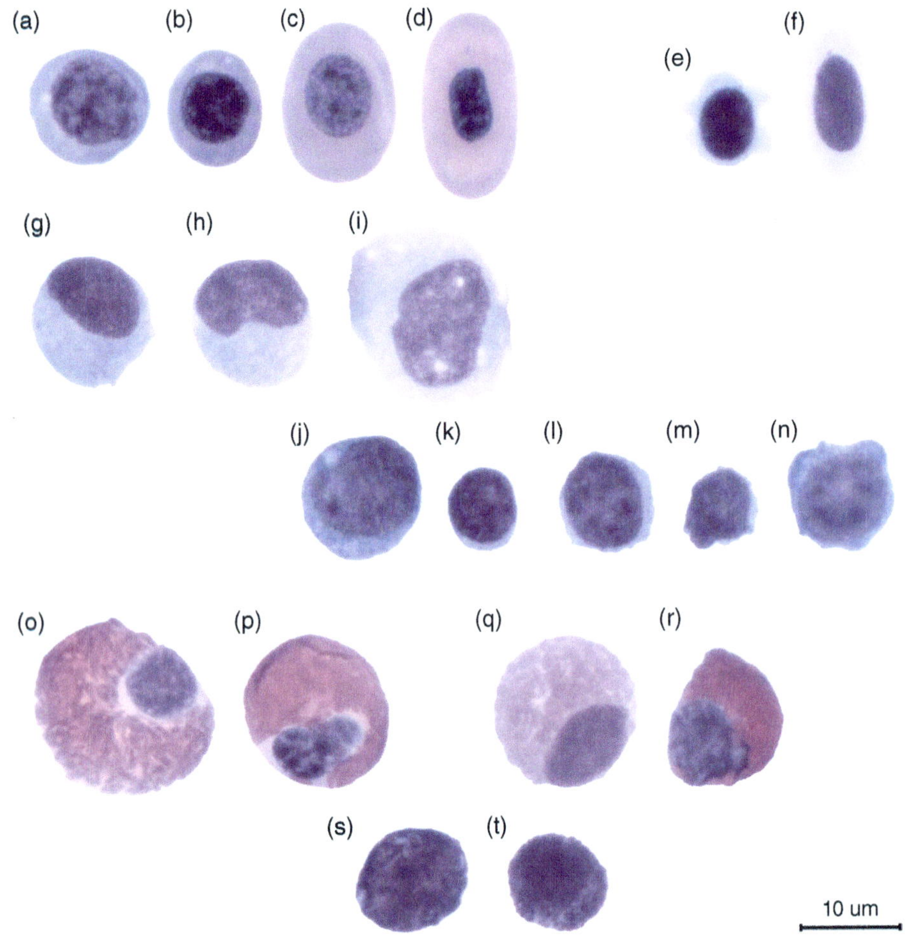

Plate. C.13. Russian Tortoise (*Testudo horsfieldii*) Erythrocytes: (a) early/basophilic polychromatic rubricyte, (b) mid-polychromatic rubricyte, (c) late polychromatic rubricyte, (d) mature erythrocyte Thrombocytes: (e) immature thrombocyte, (f) mature thrombocyte Mononuclear cells: (g) monocyte, (h) azurophilic monocyte, (i) vacuolated azurophilic monocyte (reactive), (j) lymphoblast, (k) small lymphocyte, (l) large lymphocyte, (m) small degenerate lymphocyte, (n) reactive lymphocyte Granulocytes: (o) heterophil, (p) heterophil with staining artifact (cytoplasmic folding is a common presentation), (q) eosinophil, (r) eosinophil, (s) basophil with densely packed granules, (t) basophil with dispersed granules

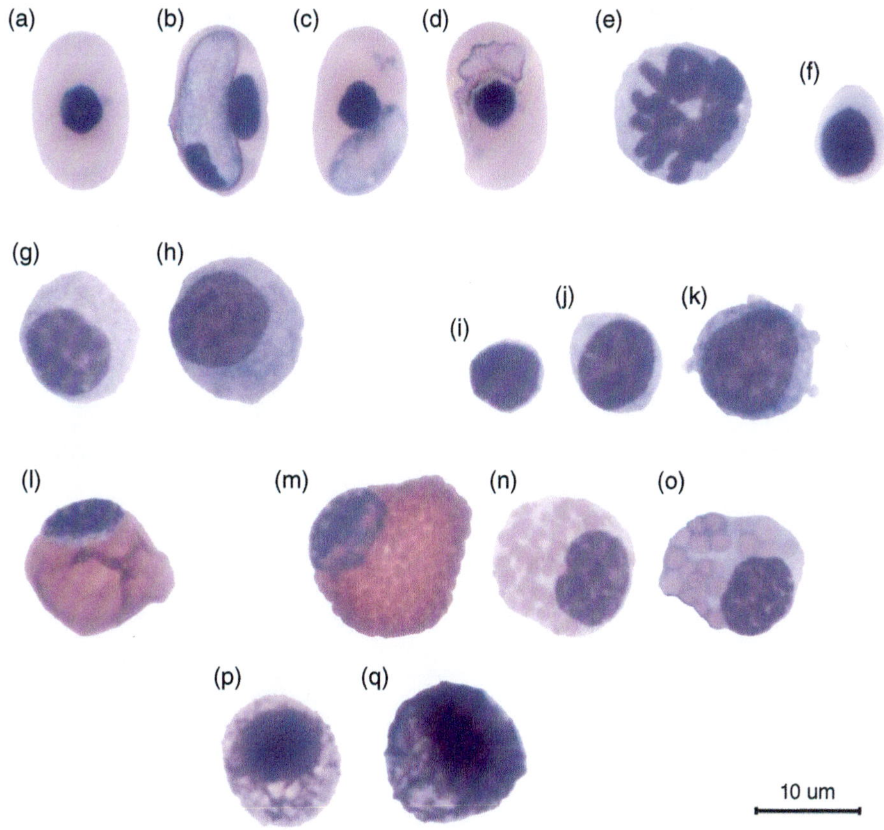

Plate. C.14. Red-Eared Slider (*Trachemys scripta elegans*) Erythrocytes: (a) mature erythrocyte, (b) mature erythrocyte with a hemogregarine, (c) mature erythrocyte with a developing hemogregarine, (d) mature erythrocyte with a cytoplasmic staining artifact (should not be confused with a parasitic inclusion), (e) mitotic figure (unknown cell type) Thrombocytes: (f) mature thrombocyte Mononuclear cells: (g) monocyte, (h) monocyte, (i) small lymphocyte (j) medium lymphocyte, (k) large lymphocyte Granulocytes: (l) heterophil, (m) large eosinophil, (n) small eosinophil, (o) small eosinophil, (p) basophil, (q) basophil

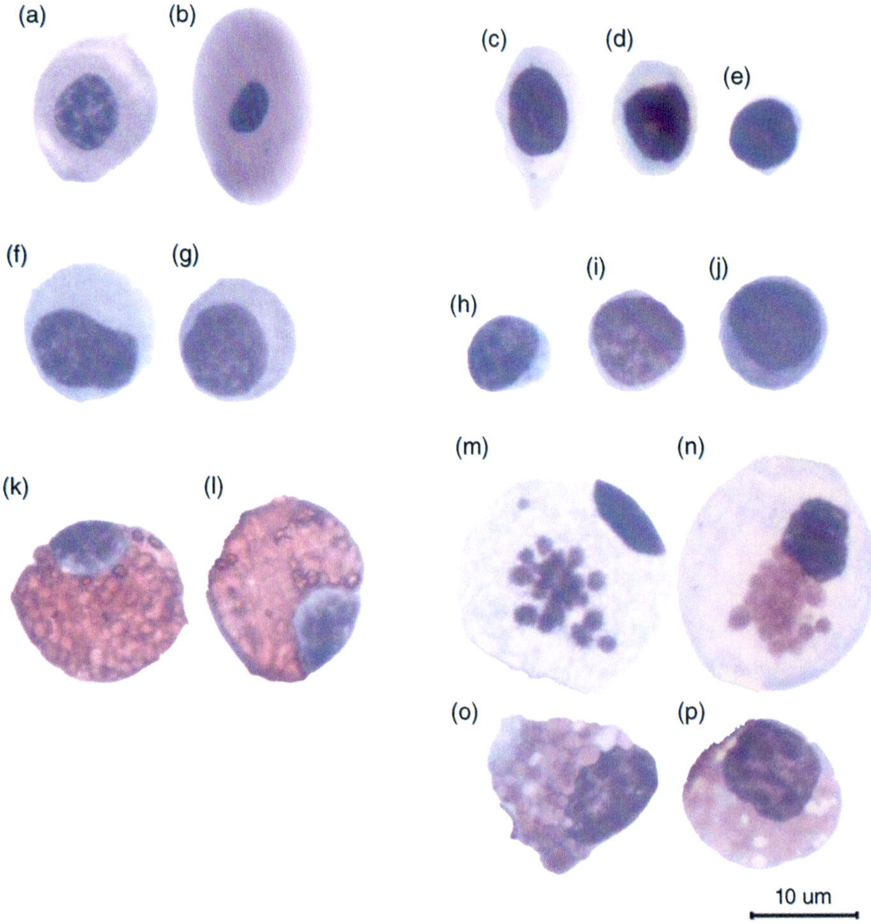

Plate. C.15. Green Sea Turtle (*Chelonia mydas*) Erythrocytes: (a) polychromatic erythrocyte, (b) mature erythrocyte Thrombocytes: (c) thrombocyte, (d) thrombocyte, (e) thrombocyte Mononuclear cells: (f) monocyte, (g) monocyte, (h) small lymphocyte, (i) medium lymphocyte, (j) large reactive lymphocyte Granulocytes: (k) heterophil, (l) heterophil, (m) large eosinophil showing region of concentrated stained granules in the cytoplasm, (n) large eosinophil showing region of concentrated stained granules in the cytoplasm, (o) small eosinophil, (p) small eosinophil

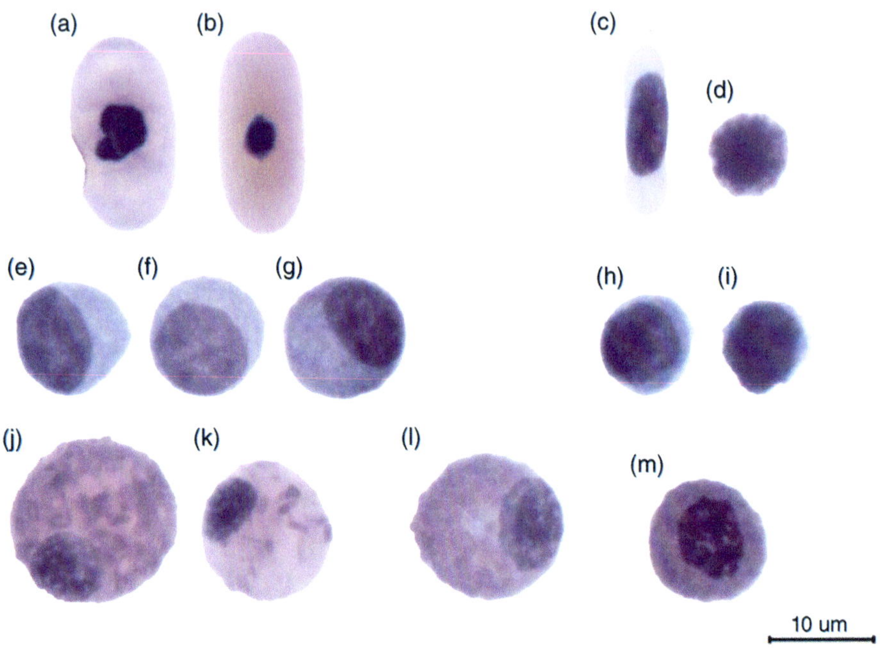

Plate. C.16. Dwarf Caiman (*Paleosuchus palpebrosus*) Erythrocytes: (a) polychromatic erythrocyte, (b) mature erythrocyte Thrombocytes: (c) mature thrombocyte, (d) thrombocyte (reactive with eosinophilic cytoplasmic granules) Mononuclear cells: (e) monocyte, (f) monocyte with mild azurophilic granulation, (g) azurophilic monocyte, (h) lymphocyte, (i) lymphocyte Granulocytes: (j) heterophil, (k) heterophil with sparsely stained granules, (l) eosinophil, (m) basophil

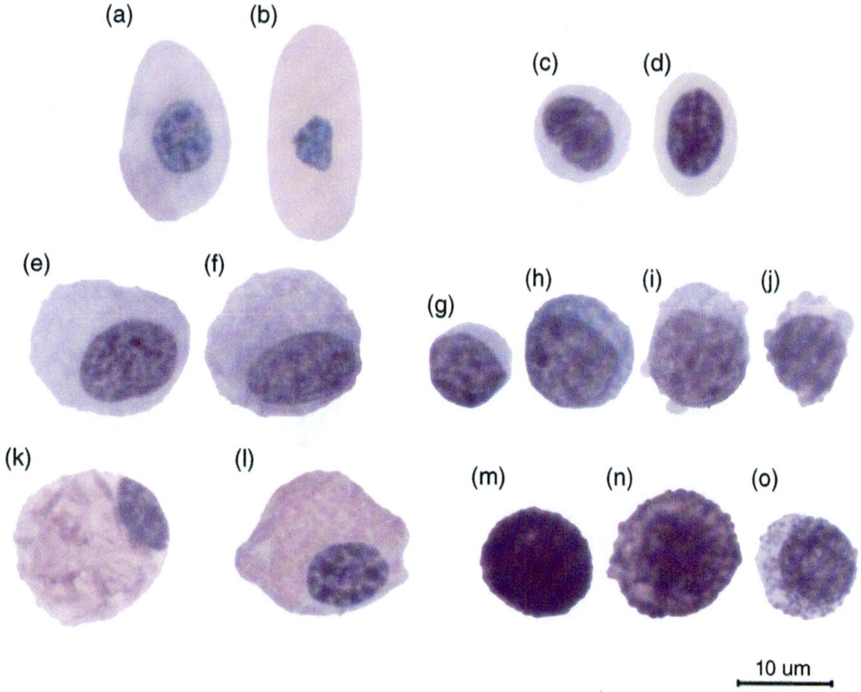

Plate. C.17. American Alligator (*Alligator mississippiensis*) Erythrocytes: (a) polychromatic erythrocyte, (b) mature erythrocyte Thrombocytes: (c) immature thrombocyte, (d) mature thrombocyte Mononuclear cells: (e) monocyte, (f) azurophilic monocyte, (g) small lymphocyte, (h) large lymphocyte, (i) large lymphocyte (degenerate), (j) small lymphocyte (degenerate) Granulocytes: (k) heterophil with unstained/sparsely stained granules, (l) eosinophil, (m) basophil with densely packed granules, (n) basophil with dispersed granules, (o) basophil (degranulating or partial stained granules)

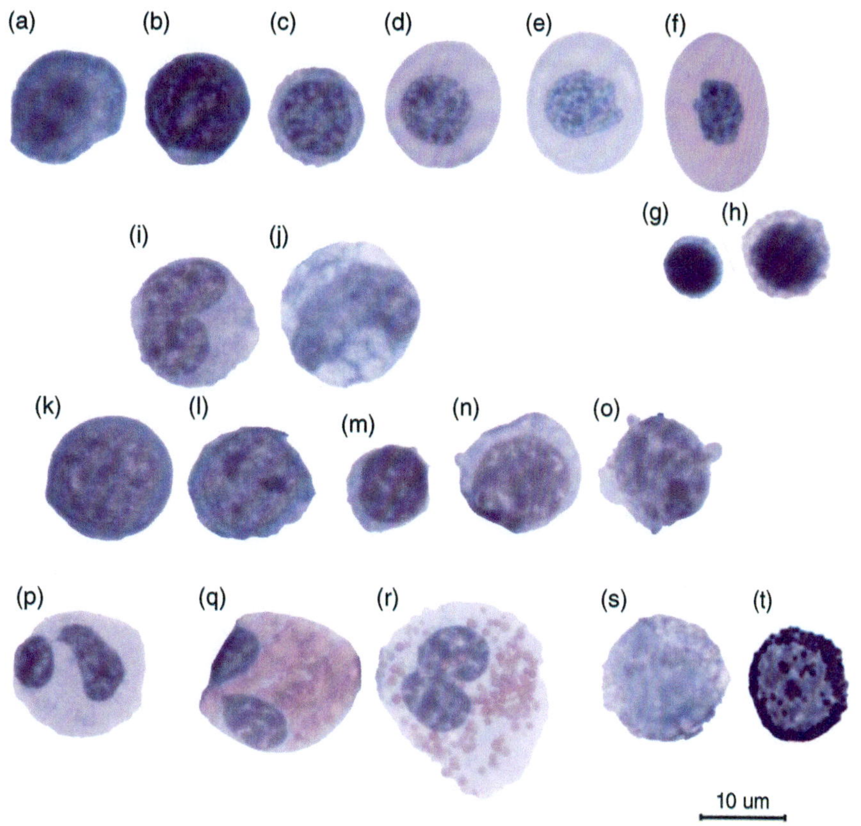

Plate. C.18. Colorado River Toad (*Incilius alvarius*) Erythrocytes: (a) rubriblast, (b) prorubricyte, (c) basophilic/early polychromatic rubricyte, (d) late polychromatic rubricyte, (e) polychromatic erythrocyte, (f) mature erythrocyte Thrombocytes: (g) thrombocyte, (h) thrombocyte (reactive) Mononuclear cells: (i) monocyte, (j) vacuolated monocyte (reactive), (k) lymphoblast, (l) prolymphocyte, (m) small lymphocyte, (n) large lymphocyte, (o) lymphocyte (degenerate) Granulocytes: (p) neutrophil, (q) eosinophil, (r) eosinophil, (s) basophil, (t) basophil (degranulating or partial stained granules)

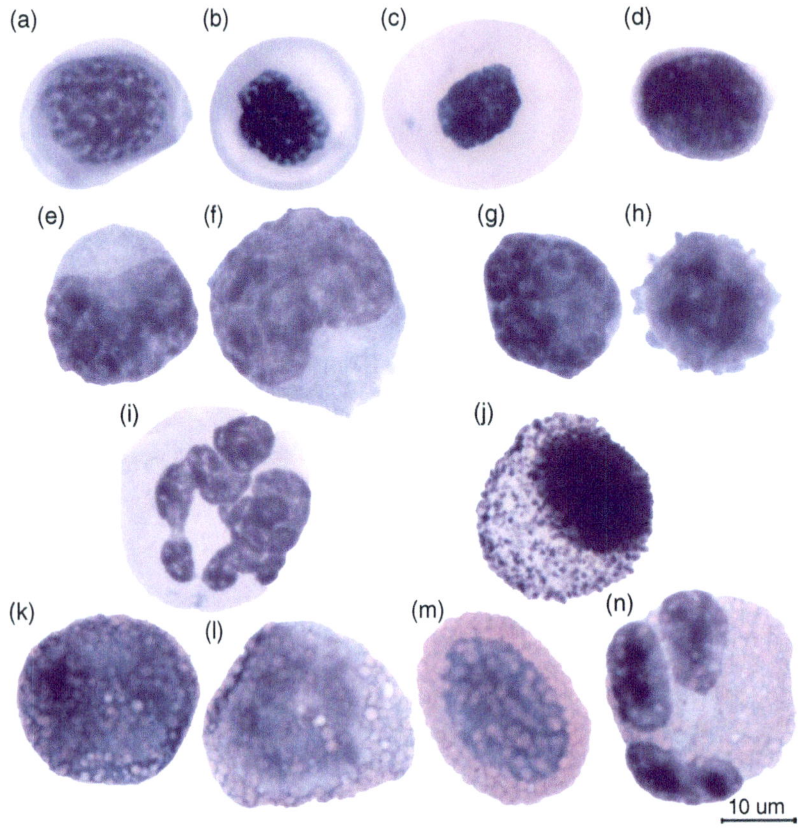

Plate. C.19. Tiger Salamander (*Ambystoma tigrinum*) Erythrocytes: (a) mid-to-late polychromatic rubricyte, (b) polychromatic erythrocyte, (c) mature erythrocyte Thrombocytes: (d) thrombocyte (reactive) Mononuclear cells: (e) monocyte, (f) monocyte, (g) lymphocyte, (h) lymphocyte (degenerate) Granulocytes: (i) neutrophil, (j) basophil, (k) eosinophil myelocyte, (l) eosinophil metamyelocyte, (m) eosinophil (nonsegmented nucleus), (n) mature eosinophil (segmented nucleus)

Piscine Plates

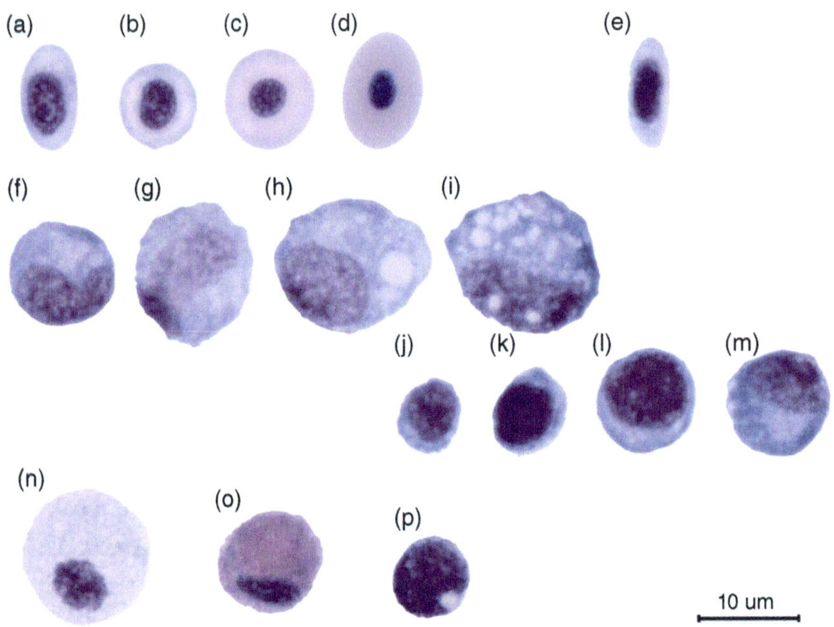

Plate. C.20. Iridescent Catfish (*Pangasianodon hypophthalmus*) Erythrocytes: (a) polychromatic erythrocyte, (b) polychromatic erythrocyte, (c) mature erythrocyte, (d) mature erythrocyte (senescent with pyknotic nucleus) Thrombocytes: (e) thrombocyte Mononuclear cells: (f) monocyte, (g) monocyte, (h) vacuolated monocyte (reactive), (i) vacuolated monocyte (reactive), (j) small lymphocyte, (k) medium lymphocyte, (l) large lymphocyte, (m) plasma cell Granulocytes: (n) neutrophil, (o) eosinophil, (p) basophil

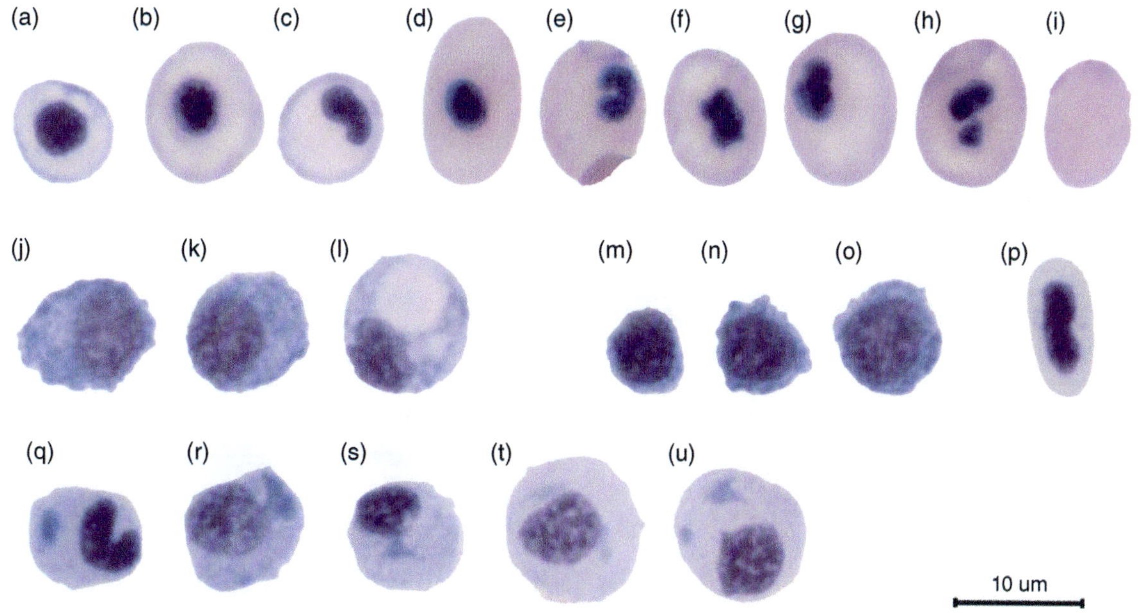

Plate. C.21. Largemouth Bass (*Micropterus salmoides*) Erythrocytes: (a) late polychromatic rubricyte, (b) polychromatic erythrocyte, (c) polychromatic erythrocyte with eccentric, indented nucleus, (d)–(h) mature erythrocytes with varying nuclear size and shape, (i) erythroplastid Mononuclear cells: (j) monocyte, (k) monocyte, (l) vacuolated monocyte, (m) small lymphocyte, (n) medium lymphocyte, (o) large lymphocyte Thrombocytes: (p) thrombocyte Granulocytes: (q) neutrophil (band), (r)–(u) neutrophil (most contain Döhle bodies in the cytoplasm)

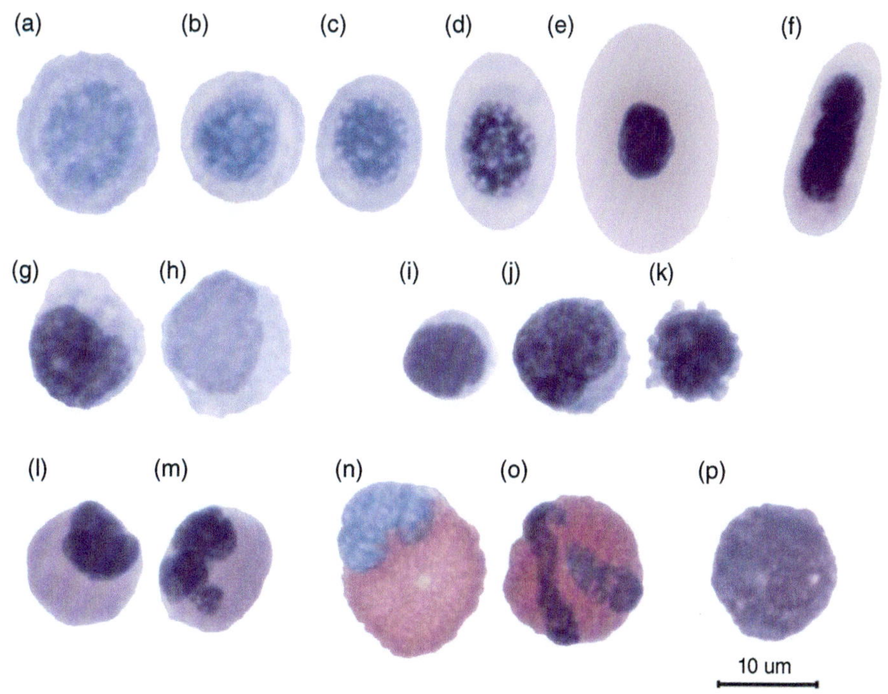

Plate. C.22. Leopoldi Stingray (*Potamotrygon leopoldi*) Erythrocytes: (a) early polychromatic rubricyte, (b) mid-to-late polychromatic rubricyte, (c) mid-to-late polychromatic rubricyte, (d) polychromatic erythrocyte, (e) mature erythrocyte Thrombocytes: (f) mature thrombocyte Mononuclear cells: (g) monocyte, (h) monocyte, (i) small lymphocyte, (j) large lymphocyte, (k) lymphocyte (degenerate) Granulocytes: (l) G_1/fine eosinophilic granulocyte (nonsegmented nucleus), (m) G_1/fine eosinophilic granulocyte (segmented nucleus), (n) G_3/coarse eosinophilic granulocyte (nonsegmented nucleus), (o) G_3/coarse eosinophilic granulocyte (segmented nucleus), (p) basophil

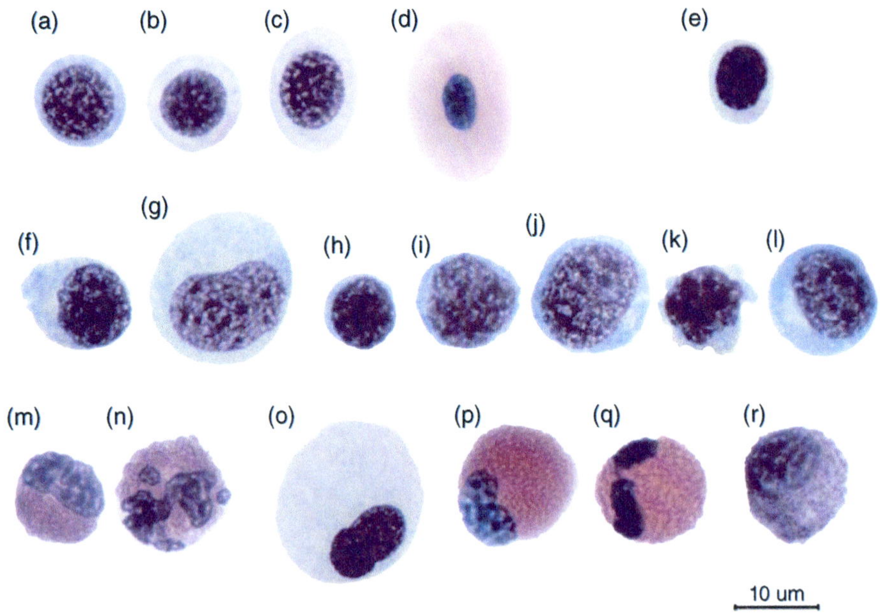

Plate. C.23. Cownose Ray (*Rhinoptera bonasus*) Erythrocytes: (a) mid-polychromatic rubricyte, (b) late polychromatic rubricyte, (c) polychromatic erythrocyte, (d) mature erythrocyte Thrombocytes: (e) Thrombocyte Mononuclear cells: (f) monocyte, (g) monocyte, (h) small lymphocyte, (i) medium lymphocyte, (j) large lymphocyte, (k) lymphocyte (degenerate), (l) plasma cell Granulocytes: (m) G_1/fine eosinophilic granulocyte (nonsegmented nucleus), (n) G_1/fine eosinophilic granulocyte (segmented nucleus), (o) G_2/neutrophil, (p) G_3/ coarse eosinophilic granulocyte (nonsegmented nucleus), (q) G_3/coarse eosinophilic granulocyte (segmented nucleus), (r) basophil

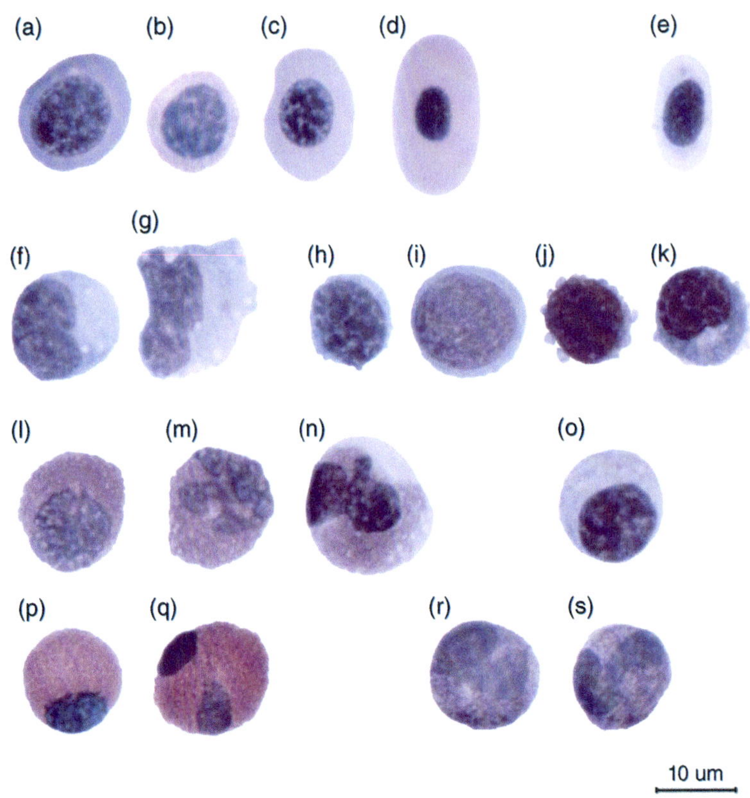

Plate. C.24. Southern Stingray (*Hypanus americanus*) Erythrocytes: (a) early to mid-polychromatic rubricyte, (b) late polychromatic rubricyte, (c) polychromatic erythrocyte, (d) mature erythrocyte Thrombocytes: (e) thrombocyte Mononuclear cells: (f) monocyte, (g) monocyte with vacuoles (reactive), (h) small lymphocyte, (i) large lymphocyte, (j) lymphocyte (degenerate), (k) plasma cell granulocytes: (l) g_1/fine eosinophilic granulocyte (nonsegmented nucleus), (m) g_1/fine eosinophilic granulocyte (segmented nucleus), (n) toxic g_1/fine eosinophilic granulocyte, (o) g_2/neutrophil, (p) G_3/coarse eosinophilic granulocyte (nonsegmented nucleus), (q) G_3/coarse eosinophilic granulocyte (segmented nucleus), (r) basophil, (s) basophil with band nucleus

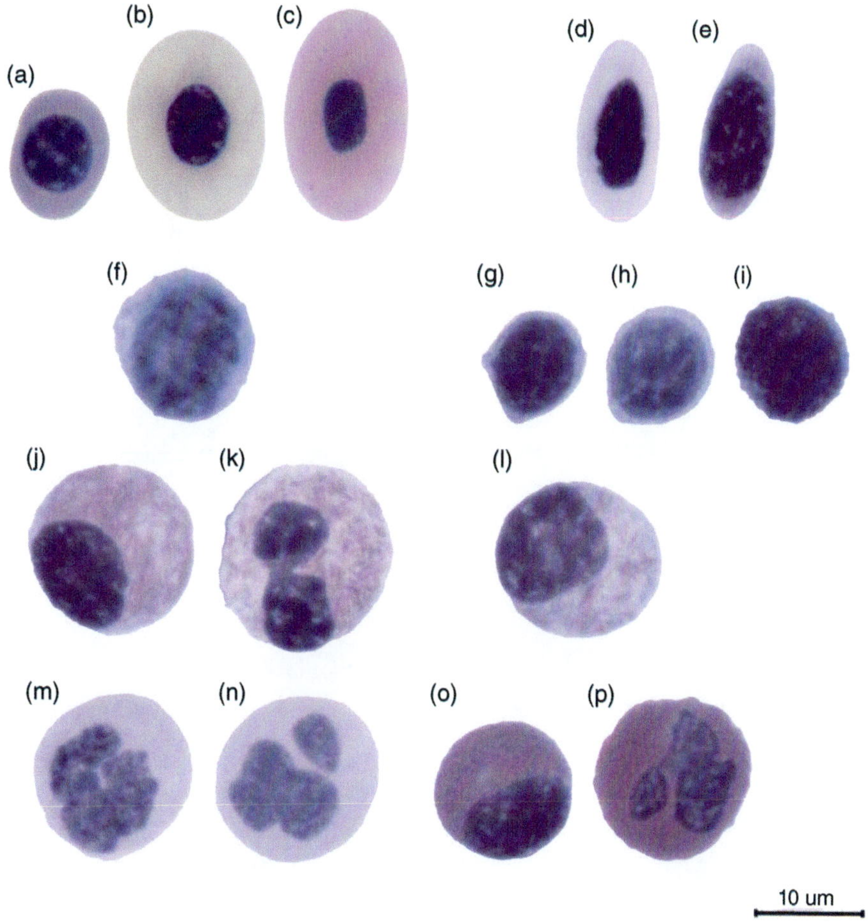

Plate. C.25. White Spotted Bamboo Shark (*Chiloscyllium plagiosum*) Erythrocytes: (a) polychromatic erythrocyte, (b) mature erythrocyte, (c) mature erythrocyte Thrombocytes: (d) thrombocyte, (e) reactive thrombocyte (with cytoplasmic granules) Mononuclear cells: (f) monocyte, (g) small lymphocyte, (h) medium lymphocyte, (i) reactive lymphocyte Granulocytes: (j) G_1/fine eosinophilic granulocyte (nonsegmented nucleus), (k) G_1/fine eosinophilic granulocyte (segmented nucleus), (l) toxic G_1 (degranulation, basophilic cytoplasm), (m) G_2/neutrophil, (n) G_2/neutrophil, (o) G_3/coarse eosinophilic granulocyte (nonsegmented nucleus), (p) G_3/coarse eosinophilic granulocyte (segmented nucleus)

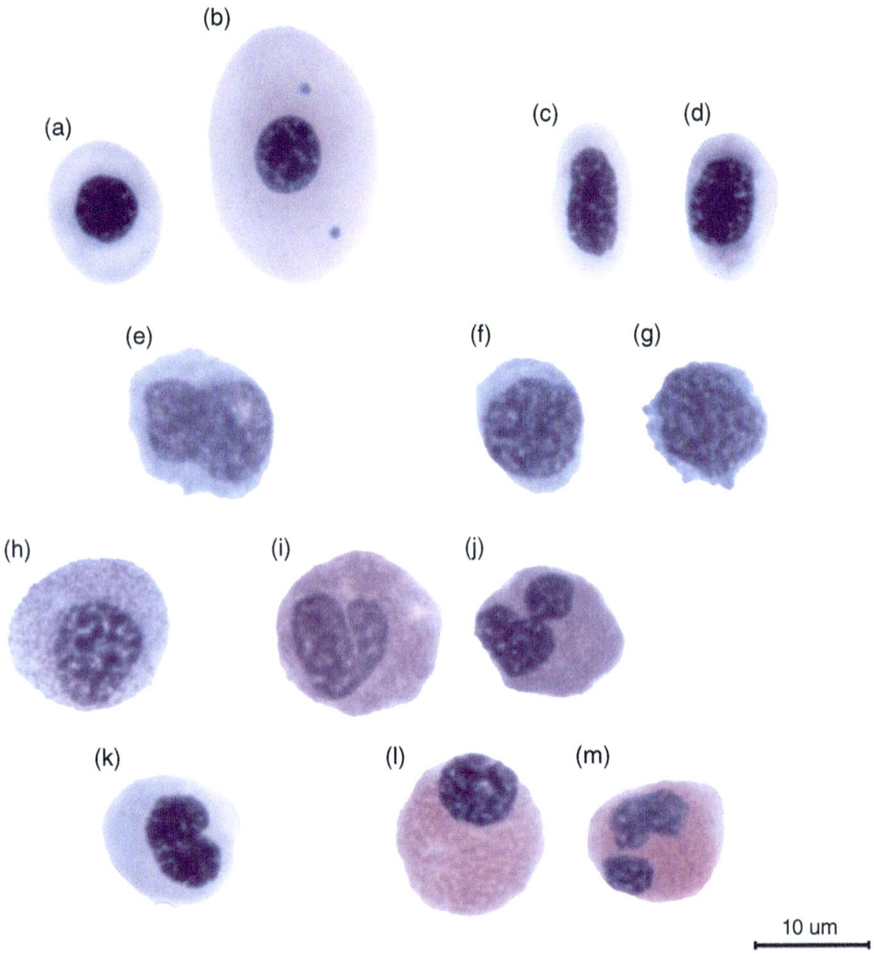

Plate. C.26. Nurse Shark (*Ginglymostoma cirratum*) Erythrocytes: (a) polychromatic erythrocyte, (b) mature erythrocyte Thrombocytes: (c) mature thrombocyte, (d) reactive thrombocyte (with cytoplasmic granules) Mononuclear cells: (e) monocyte, (f) lymphocyte, (g) lymphocyte (degenerative) Granulocytes: (h) immature granulocyte (progranulocyte, blue cytoplasm with primary granules), (i) G_1/fine eosinophilic granulocyte (nonsegmented nucleus), (j) G_1/fine eosinophilic granulocyte (segmented nucleus), (k) G_2/neutrophil, (l) G_3/ coarse eosinophilic granulocyte (nonsegmented nucleus), (m) G_3/coarse eosinophilic granulocyte (segmented nucleus)

APPENDIX D

Common Artifacts Found in Blood Film and Cytologic Samples

Artifacts in cytologic samples and blood films can occur as contaminants of the specimen or because of poor sample preparation. One must be familiar with the common artifacts that can occur so as not to confuse them with infectious agents, abnormal cells, or important cytologic findings to prevent a false-positive cytodiagnosis.

Artifacts Associated with Contamination of the Sample

Contaminants of specimens are not associated with cellular responses; therefore, they can be present in normal cytologic preparations. Sample contaminants, such as talc or starch crystals originating from examination gloves, pollen, feather or hair fragments, ultrasound gel, and stain precipitate, can mimic abnormal cells or infectious agents. Talc or starch crystals can be confused with neoplastic cells, parasites, or yeast (e.g., *Cryptococcus*). These crystals are refractile and are not in the same plane of focus as the cellular elements on the blood film or cytologic slide. Instead, they appear to lie on top of the cellular plane (Figures D.1a and D.1b).

Pollen is often mistaken for infectious agents (e.g., parasites and fungal elements). Pollen granules are rigid structures with a capsule, uniformly staining cytoplasm, and swollen polar structures (often seen in elongated

(a) (b)

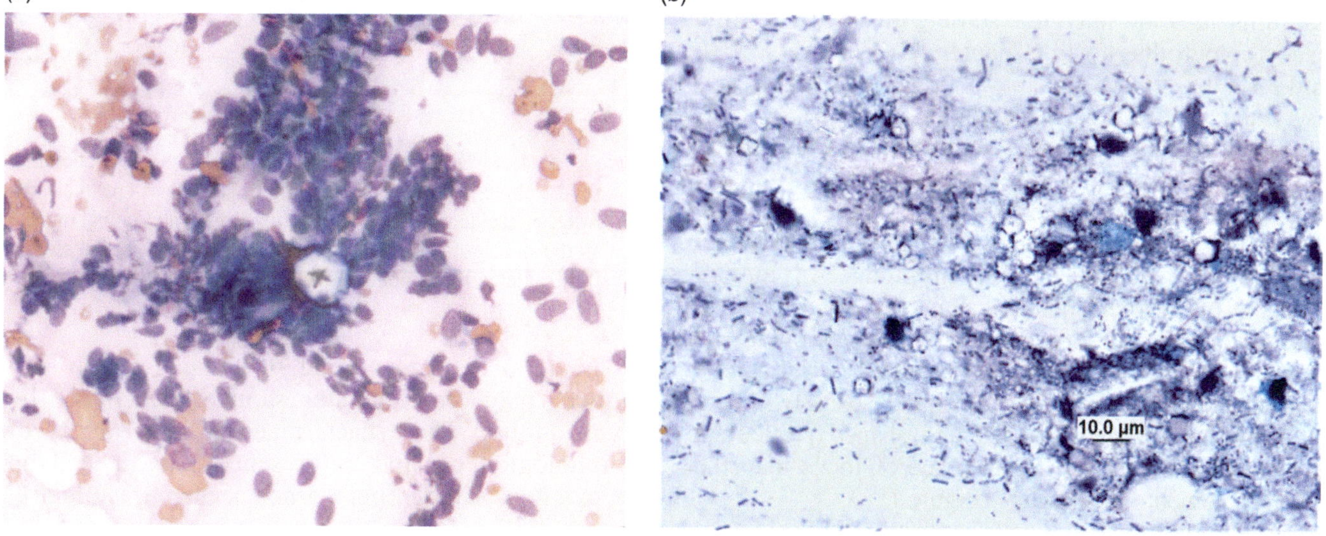

Fig. D.1. (a) A polygonal granule with a central X-shaped fissure that is refractile when the focus of the image is changed. The granule is out of focus when the cells are in focus. Wright–Giemsa stain (100× oil). (b) Numerous starch granules in a fecal smear. Wright–Giemsa stain.

Exotic Animal Hematology and Cytology, Fifth Edition. Terry W. Campbell and Krystan R. Grant.

Companion website: www.wiley.com/go/campbell/exotic

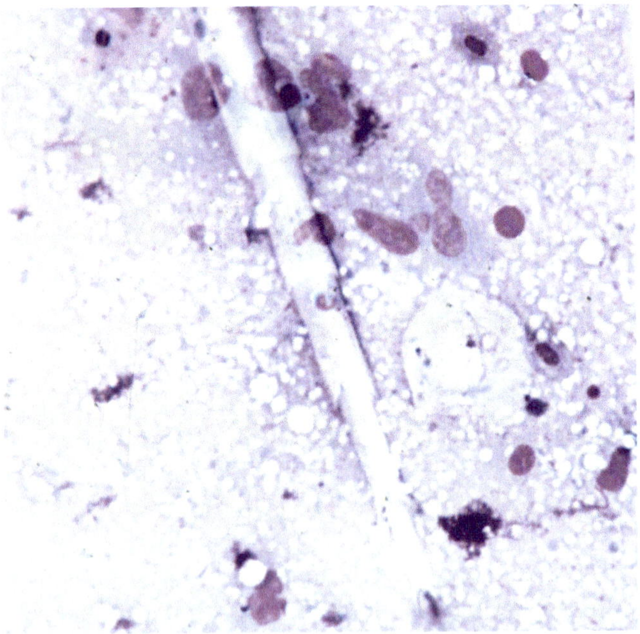

Fig. D.2. A feather fragment in a contact smear from a cutaneous lesion from a bird. Artifacts such as this in cytologic specimens could also result from contamination of the staining solutions. Diff–Quik stain (100× oil).

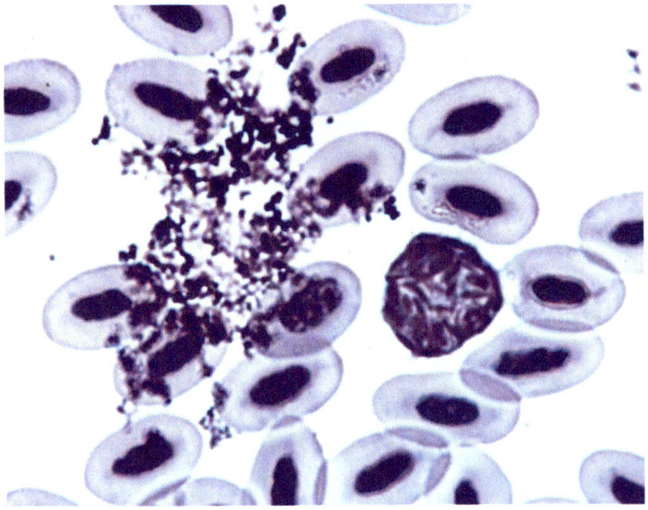

Fig. D.3. The dark purple material that appears to be on top of the cells in this image is the result of stain precipitate, a common artifact found on cytologic specimens. This material should not be confused with bacteria or other pathogens. Wright–Giemsa stain (100× oil).

forms) that are variable in appearance depending on their source.

Diatoms may be contaminants of cytologic specimens from aquatic animals. Diatoms are single cell algae encased in a transparent exoskeleton (frustule) made of hydrated silica consisting of two halves. Diatoms may or may not stain with routine stains used for cytodiagnosis (Chapter 33, Figures 33.19a and 33.19b).

Hair and feather fragments are occasionally confused with fungal elements; however, they are much larger and more rigid in appearance (Figure D.2).

The use of ultrasound to assist in the collection of cytologic samples may result in ultrasound gel contamination of the specimen. This produces a granular magenta background material that may suggest secretory products or necrotic material. Stain precipitate is a frequent finding in many cytologic samples and can be confused with bacteria. The precipitate usually occurs in refractile, irregularly sized and shaped particulate clumps that are in a different plane of focus than the cellular elements on the slide (Figure D.3).

Squamous epithelial cells or stratified muscle cells may appear in some cytology samples because of traumatic exfoliation of skin or muscle during fine-needle aspiration biopsy procedures (Chapter 7, Figures 7.4 and 7.5, and Figure D.4). When these cells occur in sheets or clusters, they may be mistaken for metastatic disease.

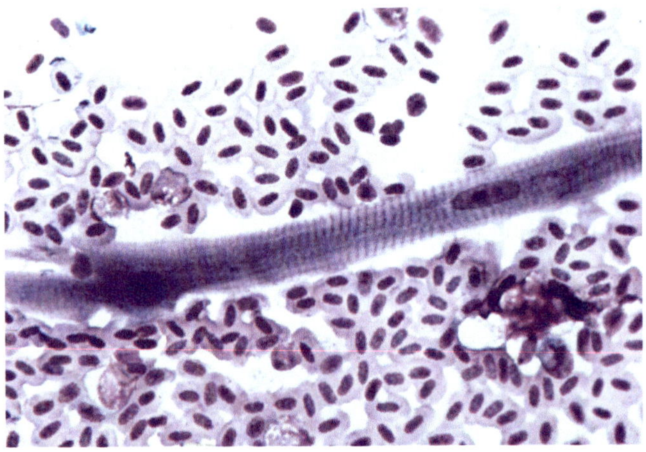

Fig. D.4. Striated muscle fibers that are found in a coelomic fluid sample from a bird following celiocentesis are likely the result of accidental fine-needle biopsy of the abdominal muscle as the needle passed through the body wall during coelomic fluid collection, Wright–Giemsa stain (100× oil).

Bacteria that are normal inhabitants of the skin surface may contaminate samples obtained by needle biopsy. These bacteria occur in a variety of morphologic types and are present among the cells in the cytology sample, but do not occur intracellularly (Figure 7.7).

Peripheral blood samples are sometimes contaminated by bacteria, which then multiply during shipment of the sample to the laboratory or prolonged storage of the sample (Figure D.5). Films produced from such samples reveal a marked number of extracellular bacteria (usually of one morphologic type).

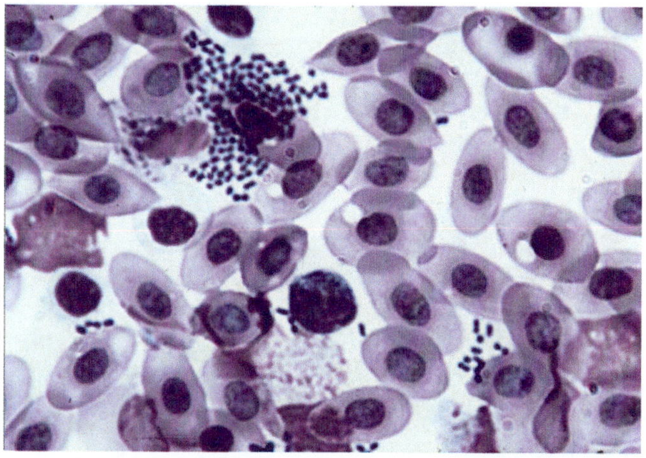

Fig. D.5. An avian blood film that was prepared from a blood sample shipped two days prior to preparation of the specimen reveals bacterial contamination of the sample. The result is a uniform population of extracellular bacteria resulting from the growth of the bacteria in the sample during shipment. Wright–Giemsa stain (100× oil).

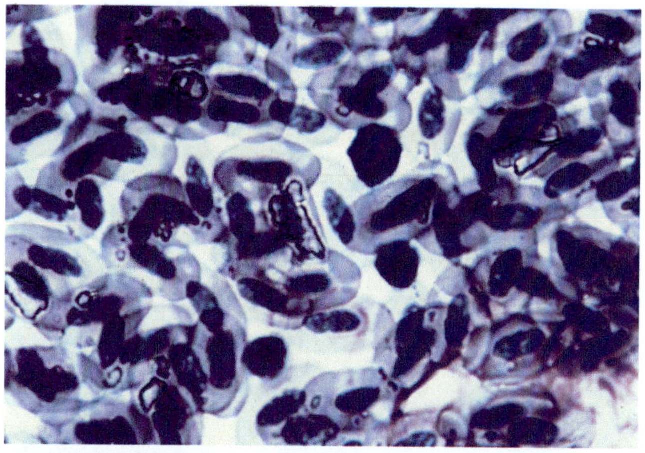

Fig. D.6. This image of a blood film from a bird is in an area of the smear that is too thick for proper evaluation. Areas that are too thick do not allow the cells to spread out to reveal their cytologic features. As a result, many of the cells in such areas appear as lymphocytes. Wright–Giemsa stain (100× oil).

Bacterial phagocytosis is rarely found and the erythrocytes and leukocytes in these samples often appear degenerate. Preparation and submission of a fresh blood film made immediately following blood sample collection helps to eliminate the need to differentiate bacterial contamination of the blood sample from a true bacteremia.

Contamination of staining solutions can also create artifacts. Bacteria or yeast can grow in certain staining solutions and will appear on cytology slides during staining. Bacteria, yeast, fat, oil, and cells (especially sperm cells) from previously stained cytology slides can contaminate the staining solution and appear on subsequent slides as well. Frequent replacement with fresh stains will eliminate this type of contamination.

Artifacts Associated with Poor Sample Preparation

Blood films that are too thick do not allow cells to spread properly on the surface of the slide. Cells in thick films are often misidentified because their cellular features cannot be properly evaluated (Figure D.6). For example, many leukocytes in thick films resemble lymphocytes, and the interpretation of the cellular response is often misleading. Ideally, properly prepared blood films for cytologic examination contain many monocellular areas for evaluation.

Preparing blood films and other cytologic samples by applying too much pressure on the spreader slide can rupture cells, resulting in the presence of nuclear protein strands. These strands of nuclear material streak across the slide and are often misidentified as chains of bacteria or fungal elements because they appear as purple linear structures (Figures D.7a and D.7b). Often, these strands can be traced back to the ruptured nucleus where they originated.

Rough handling of blood and cytologic samples can also result in large numbers of free erythrocyte nuclei and smudge cells in samples from lower vertebrates. The free erythrocyte nuclei are condensed, dark-staining, oval structures that should not be confused with yeast or other infectious agents. Smudge cells are ruptured cells that have a varied appearance on the slide depending upon the degree of rupture.

Staining artifacts and improper staining techniques can result in samples that are confusing and difficult to evaluate. One type of erythrocyte artifact occurs frequently in peripheral blood films of lower vertebrates allowed to dry too slowly before staining. The affected erythrocytes undergo a form of erythrocyte crenation and have clear, refractile spaces in the cytoplasm (Figure D.8). Such artifacts resemble blood parasites, such as gametocytes of *Hemoproteus* and *Plasmodium*. However, they differ from blood parasites because they are refractile, transparent, demonstrate marked pleomorphism, and disappear with proper sample preparation.

Exposure of the cytologic sample to chemical vapors, such as formaldehyde, can cause staining artifacts. Formaldehyde in an aqueous solution of 10% or greater readily vaporizes when exposed to air, and cytology specimens exposed to these vapors stain poorly. The effects of exposure to formaldehyde vapors result in erythrocytes that appear blue-green and are surrounded by a halo formed due to shrinkage of the cell from the

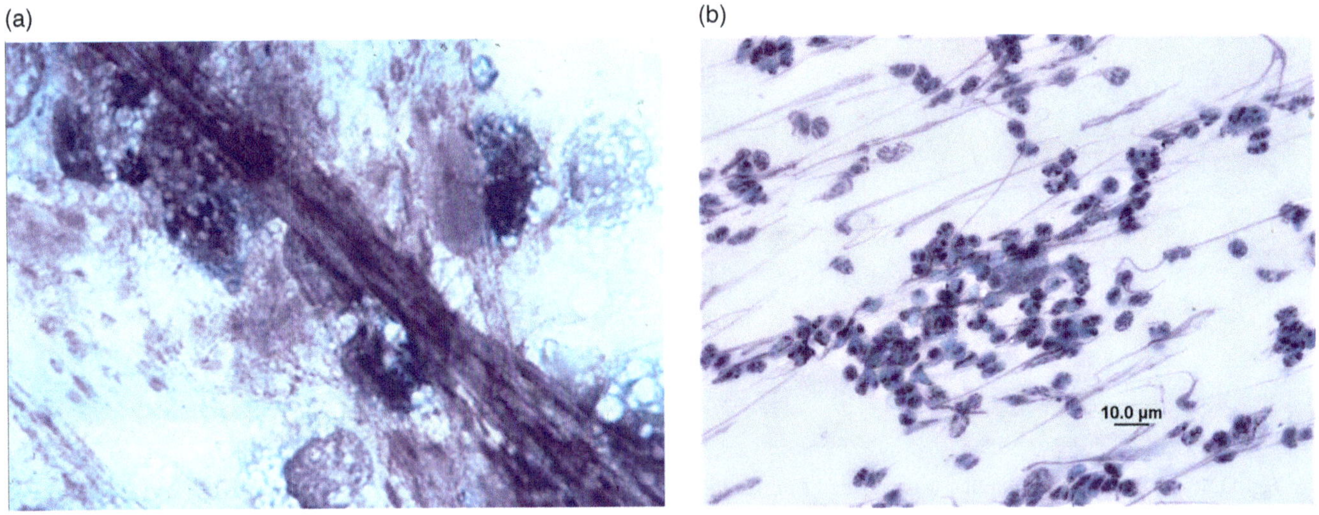

Fig. D.7. (a) Nucleoprotein strands from ruptured cell nuclei. These streaks of nuclear material are an artifact of slide preparation and should not be confused with fungal elements or other pathogens. Diff–Quik stain (100× oil). (b) Nucleoprotein strands from ruptured cell nuclei in the cytology of a joint aspirate from a cockatiel. Wright–Giemsa stain (100× oil).

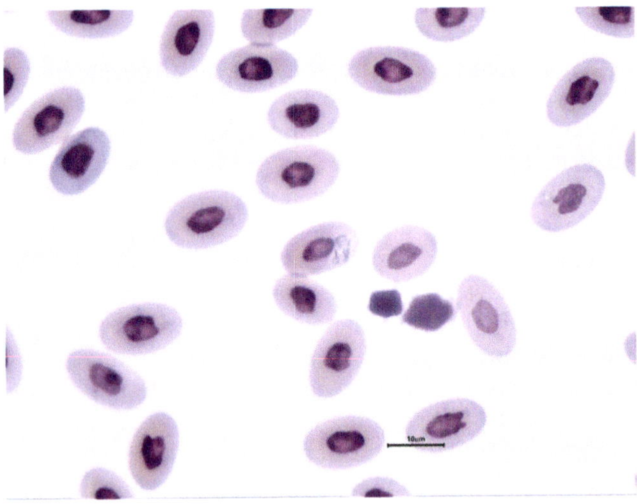

Fig. D.8. The transparent refractile artifact in the cytoplasm of the reptilian erythrocyte resembles a blood parasite, such as the gametocytes of *Hemoproteus* and *Plasmodium*; however, artifacts such as this one are variable in appearance and often appear in a different plane of focus from the cells in the cytologic specimen. Diff–Quik stain (100× oil).

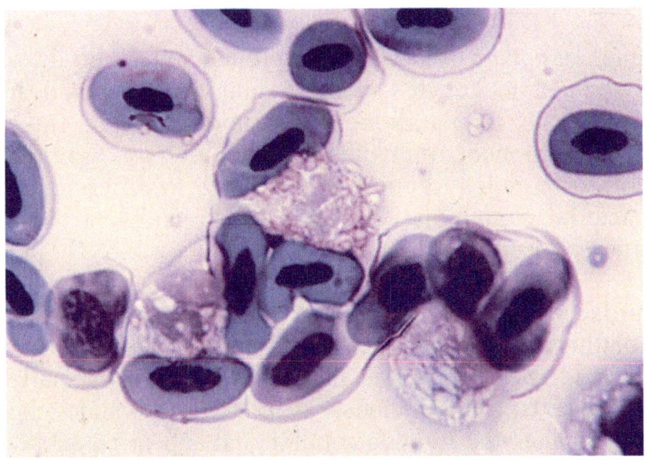

Fig. D.9. The effects of formaldehyde vapors on cytologic specimens reveal cell shrinkage that leaves a halo around the cells. The fumes also interfere with proper staining and generally gives a blue-green appearance to erythrocytes, and heterophil granules fail to stain. Wright–Giemsa stain (100× oil).

background material when stained with Wright's stain (Figure D.9). Heterophil granules do not stain after exposure to formaldehyde vapors and appear as rod-shaped ghost images within the cell (Figure D.9). Bacteria do not stain well when exposed to formaldehyde fumes and often appear as ghost images (Figure D.10). These non-staining bacteria should not be confused with bacteria that normally do not stain with Romanowsky stains (i.e. *Mycobacterium*). Properly stained slides that have not been exposed to chemical vapor should show normal staining heterophil granules. If the bacteria in these films do not stain, then an acid-fast stain should be applied to confirm the presence of organisms such as *Mycobacterium*. Formaldehyde shrinks other cells as well, making cytologic specimens difficult to evaluate.

Aging of the sample can affect the staining quality and appearance of cells. For example, peripheral blood films made from blood that contains EDTA and is stored at room temperature (27°C) for 48 h show cellular

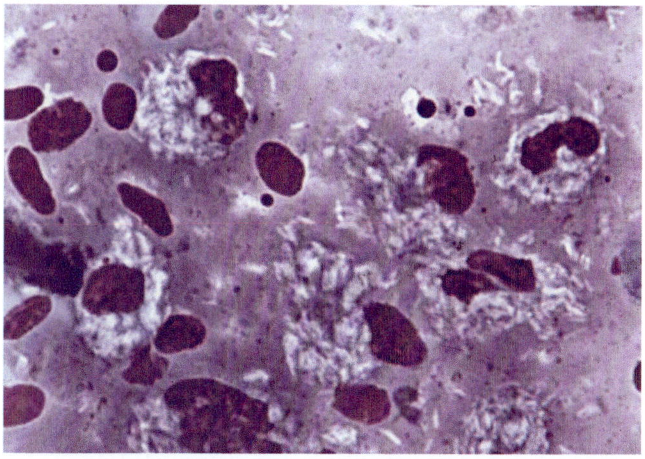

Fig. D.10. The effects of formaldehyde vapors on the appearance of heterophils in this lung imprint from a bird. Note that the cytoplasmic granules of the heterophils do not stain. This may be confused with *Mycobacterium* organisms that normally do not stain with Romanowsky stains. Diff–Quik stain (100× oil).

changes that differ from films made from the same blood sample prepared immediately following blood collection. The erythrocytes from the aged sample are pale staining, have pyknotic nuclei (in the case of lower vertebrates), and show less polychromasia when compared to erythrocytes from the freshly prepared sample. Heterophils and neutrophils with aging effects show increased cytoplasmic basophilia that resembles toxic changes, swollen and sometimes fused cytoplasmic granules, and nuclear pyknosis. Monocytes demonstrate increased cytoplasmic basophilia and vacuolation with large vacuoles. Thrombocytes of lower vertebrates show increased nuclear pyknosis and cellular pleomorphism with aging effects. An increased number of smudge cells is expected in aged samples.

INDEX

Exotic Animal Hematology and Cytology, Fifth Edition. Terry W. Campbell and Krystan R. Grant.

Companion website: www.wiley.com/go/campbell/exotic